Energy Efficiency, Environment and Health—Volume I

Energy Efficiency, Environment and Health—Volume I

Editors

Roberto Alonso González Lezcano
Francesco Nocera
Rosa Giuseppina Caponetto

MDPI • Basel • Beijing • Wuhan • Barcelona • Belgrade • Manchester • Tokyo • Cluj • Tianjin

Editors
Roberto Alonso González Lezcano
Departamento de Arquitectura y Diseño, Escuela Politécnica Superior, Universidad CEU San Pablo, Madrid, Spain

Francesco Nocera
Department of Civil Engineering and Architecture, University of Catania, Catania, Italy

Rosa Giuseppina Caponetto
Department of Civil Engineering and Architecture, University of Catania, Catania, Italy

Editorial Office
MDPI
St. Alban-Anlage 66
4052 Basel, Switzerland

This is a reprint of articles from the Topic published online in the open access journals *Energies* (ISSN 1996-1073), *International Journal of Environmental Research and Public Health* (ISSN 1660-4601), *Processes* (ISSN 2227-9717), *Buildings* (ISSN 2075-5309), and *Atmosphere* (ISSN 2073-4433) (available at: https://www.mdpi.com/topics/energy_health).

For citation purposes, cite each article independently as indicated on the article page online and as indicated below:

LastName, A.A.; LastName, B.B.; LastName, C.C. Article Title. *Journal Name* **Year**, *Volume Number*, Page Range.

Volume I
ISBN 978-3-0365-8222-1 (Hbk)
ISBN 978-3-0365-8223-8 (PDF)

Volume I-III
ISBN 978-3-0365-8220-7 (Hbk)
ISBN 978-3-0365-8221-4 (PDF)

Contents

About the Editors

Roberto Alonso González Lezcano

Accredited as full professor by AQU Catalunya (March 2023). Extraordinary Doctorate Award. San Pablo CEU University Tenured Professor at the Department of Architecture and Design, the area of Building Systems, within the Institute of Technology of Universidad CEU San Pablo. Coordinator of the Mechanical Systems area. Professor Accredited by ANECA in the position of Tenured Professor. Two six-year research periods at CNEAI (last period 2016–2021). Coordinator of the post-graduate degree of Energy Efficiency and Mechanical Systems in Buildings and Coordinator of the Laboratory of Building Systems within Universidad CEU San Pablo. Member of the PhD Program in "Health Science and Technology" and the PhD Program "Composition, History and Techniques pertaining to Architecture and Urbanism", where he is the Coordinator of the Construction, Innovation and Technology line and Coordinator of the complementary training program "Methodology of technical and statistical experimentation". Ángel Herrera Award for the best research work in the areas of Architecture and Engineering for the year 2020/2021 in the XXV Edition of the Ángel Herrera Awards of the CEU San Pablo University. Coordinator of the Wind Energy Section within the master's course in Renewable Energy of the Institute of Technology (Universidad CEU San Pablo).

Architecture and Solidarity Award (2019) of the 1st Housing Excellence Awards of the newspaper La Razón for the VEM Project financed by Airbus Defense and Space and developed at the CEU San Pablo University. Award won due to the VEM project developed with the AIRBUS company, 2015. Member of the Team Crew and Advisor of the Universidad Autónoma de Occidente and Universidad de San Buenaventura in the MIHOUSE Project team in the Solar Decathlon Latin American and Caribbean 2015.

Francesco Nocera

Qualified as a Full Professor through the Italian National Scientific Qualification, sector 09/C2—Building Physics and Energy Systems in the year 2020. He is the author of more 200 research papers dealing with several research topics experimentally as well as numerically and analytically, including basic thermodynamics, thermo-fluid dynamics, heat transmission, lighting, acoustics, the rational use of energy, the use of renewable energy sources, buildings energy analysis, IEQ, UHI, and HAVC systems.

He was a postdoctoral researcher in Fluid Dynamics Modeling of Aeraulic Ducts, University of Catania (01-10-2007–31-10-2007) and gained a Ph.D. in Applied Environmental Physics, University di Palermo (01-10-2003–10-02-2006).

Scientist responsible for the Computer Laboratory at Special Didactic Structures of Architecture Siracusa (2010–) and responsible for the Energetic Sustainability and Environmental Control (SECA) Laboratory at Special Didactic Structures Architecture (2020–). Rector's Delegate for the UN Sustainable Development Solutions Network (SDSN) (17-05-2018; 02-07-2019). Member of the Quality Management Board of the Architecture Degree Course, University of Catania (2018–2019) Member of the Joint Committee of the DICAR Department, the University of Catania (2020–). Secretary of Special Didactic Structure of Architecture, University of Catania (2020–2021). Visiting Professor at the University of Valladolid (2020) Scientific Responsible of Memorandum of understanding, cooperation agreement of general interest: CEU Cardenal Herrera University (Spain), Faculty of Urban Construction and Environmental Engineering of Chongqing University (China), Applied Science and Arts of Southern Switzerland University (SUPSI), Lega Ambiente, EURAC center.

Member of International Building Physics Association—IABP (2018). Member of the International Commission on Illumination (CIE)—UNI/CT 023/GL 02 Lighting of Work Places and Schools.

Rosa Giuseppina Caponetto

Qualified as a Full Professor through the Italian National Scientific Qualification, sector 08/C1—Design and Technological Architecture Design, in the year 2022. Her main research topics are: materials and technologies for sustainable construction; the durability of building materials and components; the experimental assessment of building materials' performance; self-build; knowledge of local building tradition and innovative scenarios; the assessment of buildings' sustainability; and energy and seismic upgrading of existing buildings.

She is the scientific director of the LaTPrE laboratory, Laboratory of Building Production Technologies (University of Catania). She is a member of the "Smart Cities & Communities" National Laboratory by CINI (focus group: "ICT for Smart Energy & Smart Buildings"). She is the head of operations management and a member of the scientific committee of "MuRa", Museum of Representation (University of Catania), as well as a member of the "Technical College for Building Consultancy" (University of Catania).

She is the co-inventor of the patent idea entitled "Anti-seismic construction system: technology and production process". She has developed several research works in collaboration with national research institutes (e.g., CNR) and/or with some municipalities (cooperative agreements).

She has been involved in the following projects: the VVITA project "Modernizing Learning and Teaching for Architecture through Smart and Long-lasting Partnerships leading to sustainable and inclusive development strategies to Vitalize Heritage Villages through Innovative Technologies", ERASMUS + KA2 program funded by the European Community (2016–2019), U.O Scientific Responsible; the EWAS project "An Early Warning System for cultural-heritage", funded by the PNR program (2017–2022).

International Journal of
Environmental Research and Public Health

MDPI

Article

Knowledge, Attitudes and Practices of Eye Health among Public Sector Eye Health Workers in South Africa

Zamadonda Xulu-Kasaba [1,*], Khathutshelo Mashige [1] and Kovin Naidoo [1,2]

[1] Discipline of Optometry, School of Health Sciences, University of KwaZulu-Natal, Durban 4000, South Africa; mashigek@ukzn.ac.za (K.M.); NaidooK6@ukzn.ac.za (K.N.)
[2] Department of Optometry, University of New South Wales, Sydney, NSW 2052, Australia
* Correspondence: XuluKasabaZ@ukzn.ac.za

Abstract: In South Africa, primary eye care is largely challenged in its organisational structure, availability of human and other resources, and clinical competency. These do meet the standard required by the National Department of Health. This study seeks to assess the levels of knowledge, attitudes, and practices on eye health amongst Human Resources for eye health (HReH) and their managers, as no study has assessed this previously. A cross-sectional study was conducted in 11 districts of a South African province. A total of 101 participants completed self-administered, close-ended, Likert-scaled questionnaires anonymously. Binary logistic regression analysis was conducted, and values of $p < 0.05$ were considered statistically significant. Most participants had adequate knowledge (81.6%), positive attitudes (69%), and satisfactory practices (73%) in eye health. HReH showed better knowledge than their managers ($p < 0.01$). Participants with a university degree, those aged 30–44 years, and those employed for <5 years showed a good attitude ($p < 0.05$) towards their work. Managers, who supervise and plan for eye health, were 99% less likely to practice adequately in eye health when compared with HReH (aOR = 0.012; $p < 0.01$). Practices in eye health were best amongst participants with an undergraduate degree, those aged 30–44 years (aOR = 2.603; $p < 0.05$), and participants with <5 years of employment (aOR = 26.600; $p < 0.01$). Knowledge, attitudes, and practices were found to be significantly moderately correlated with each other ($p < 0.05$). Eye health managers have poorer knowledge and practices of eye health than the HReH. A lack of direction is presented by the lack of adequately trained directorates for eye health. It is therefore recommended that policymakers review appointment requirements to ensure that adequately trained and qualified directorates be appointed to manage eye health in each district.

Keywords: visual impairment; human resources for eye health; avoidable blindness; eye health; public health; eye health directorate

Citation: Xulu-Kasaba, Z.; Mashige, K.; Naidoo, K. Knowledge, Attitudes and Practices of Eye Health among Public Sector Eye Health Workers in South Africa. *Int. J. Environ. Res. Public Health* **2021**, *18*, 12513. https://doi.org/10.3390/ijerph182312513

Academic Editors: Roberto Alonso González Lezcano, Francesco Nocera and Rosa Giuseppina Caponetto

Received: 5 November 2021
Accepted: 22 November 2021
Published: 27 November 2021

1. Introduction

Visual impairment is a serious public health problem globally. It is estimated that 253 million people worldwide are affected by visual impairment. In Sub-Saharan Africa (SSA), 22 million people are blind or visually impaired mainly from avoidable causes such as cataracts and uncorrected refractive errors [1]. Over 100 million adults in SSA are estimated to have near visual impairment [1]. Blindness from avoidable causes is said to have increased in all four regions of SSA in the past decade [2]. The age-standardised prevalence of blindness (>50 years) was found to be 5.1% in western and 4.3% in eastern SSA [1]. The disproportionate burden of visual impairment in low-and-middle-income countries (LMIC) compared to high-income countries was observed to be a direct cause of socioeconomic factors, poor health systems and concomitant human immunodeficiency virus (HIV), and tuberculosis epidemics [3–7]. The World Health Organization's 2014–2019 global action plan (GAP) for universal eye health aimed to reduce avoidable vision loss, thereby curbing the quality-of-life limitations and economic demands associated with visual disabilities [8–10].

The World Health Organisation (WHO) has recommended that primary eye care (PEC) be included in primary healthcare (PHC) as a strategy to increase sustainability and access to ocular health services [11,12]. To effectively control visual impairment, the WHO highlighted the importance of accessible eye care services and called on member states to secure the inclusion of PEC within PHC, as previously recommended by the International centre for eye health [8,13]. Many challenges such as lack of agreement on the scope of PEC and lack of clear guidelines on the technical eye-related skills required by PHC workers were reported as challenges for the effective implementation of PEC in SSA. These affect the extent of training, supervision, and the type of equipment and consumables required [14].

In South Africa, PEC is mainly provided at the PHC level, but if need arises, patients are referred to higher-level institutions. The country does not have a dedicated directorate for eye health, nor does it have an integrated eye health promotional policy [15]. This results in inadequate eye care services, similar to other African countries [16,17]. Challenges in the South African eye care programme include insufficient human resources, unaffordable or unavailable medication, unsatisfactory programme evaluation and inadequate service coverage for Vitamin A supplementation, vision assessments, spectacle provision, cataract surgery, and screening for eye complications in patients with diabetes [18–23]. In addition, coordination between the different levels of the eye health system is lacking, with poor communication, a complex referral system and problems transporting patients to specialised services [19].

Studies from South Africa have reported on the prevalence of visual loss/visual impairment in different districts/provinces [24–27]. Another study performed an evaluation of primary eye care services in three districts of South Africa to assess whether an ophthalmic health system strengthening (HSS) package could improve these services [28]. The study concluded that primary eye care in South Africa faces multiple challenges with regard to the organisation of care, and clinical competency [28]. Training of all cadres of eye health was said to be crucial if the goals of VISION 2020 were to be attained, and universal access to ocular health achieved [29]. Very little is known about the knowledge, attitudes, and practices of eye health care workers and their supervisors towards eye health. Therefore, this study aimed to establish the level of knowledge, attitudes, and practices of eye health amongst HReH and their supervisors/managers. In this study, participants were tasked with responding to questions on the definitions of the different HReH, their roles in their work, resources needed in eye health, and challenges that exist in eye health daily. Policies guiding HReH work were also included in the questions.

Based on the responses, study findings will assist in clarifying the levels to which management and HReH each understand staffing roles and needs within the province, leading to possible interventions needed for optimal service provision. This study will also inform policymakers, healthcare administrators, and eye care professionals on areas that need attention in public health policies, further promoting efficient and equitable allocation of resources to alleviate the burden of vision loss in South Africa.

2. Methods

A cross-sectional study was conducted in the 56 eye clinics and 11 district offices in the province of KwaZulu-Natal, South Africa. The population for the study comprised two levels of managers, district office-based NCD coordinators and medical managers, who manage HReH within the various HCFs. Included HReH were Optometrists, Ophthalmologists, Ophthalmic Medical Officers (OMOs), and Ophthalmic Nurses, as well as an administrator, working in the various eye clinics.

Purposive sampling was used to identify 196 role-players within eye health in KwaZulu-Natal, a total population of 174 HReH and 22 Managers. Due to this sample size being relatively small, a sample size calculation was deemed to be irrelevant. In an attempt to obtain a saturated sample, the PI contacted all the eye clinics and made arrangements to personally visit each institution so as to ensure a saturated sample. Of the 196 eye health workers, 91 were either on leave, ill, occupied by other work, or unavailable for other reasons. The remaining 105 employees who were available all accepted the invitation to take part in the study. Ultimately, 101 eye health workers returned the self-administered, completed questionnaire after the allocated 20 min time frame, yielding a response rate of 96.2%.

The questionnaire comprised four sections. The first section of the questionnaire contained demographic information such as age, race, district, role in eye health, period of service, and highest level of qualification. The second, third, and fourth sections of the questionnaire comprised ten statements for each section to determine participants' knowledge, attitudes, and practices on eye health. All the statements were 5-point Likert type with the categories ranging from "Strongly Disagree" to "Strongly Agree".

The questionnaire was pretested among 10 HReH members who had resigned from the public sector eye clinics within two years prior to the commencement of this study. They responded to the questions and gave comments on the questionnaire. Amendments were made wherever needed, and the tool was modified and validated for this study. The Cronbach alpha scores were 0.72 for knowledge, 0.85 for attitude, and 0.84 for practices (Table S1).

Ethical clearance for the study was granted by the University of KwaZulu-Natal (BE155/19) and the Department of Health Research Ethics Committee. Anonymity and confidentiality were maintained at all times. Participation in the study was voluntary.

Data were cleaned, coded, captured, and analysed using SPSS version 25. The Likert scale responses were condensed to elicit binary responses. Where the correct response was an agreement, "Strongly agree and Agree" were accepted as favourable responses while "Neutral, Disagree and Strongly disagree" were considered to be unfavourable. Similarly, where the correct response was a disagreement, "Strongly Disagree" and "Disagree" were accepted as favourable responses while "neutral", "I don't know", "Agree" and "Strongly Agree" were rejected as unfavourable responses. Participants who correctly answered a minimum of 75% of the questions were considered to have adequate knowledge, a positive attitude, and satisfactory practicing skills.

3. Results

Most of the study participants were Africans (91%). About half (44.6%) were aged between 30 and 44 years, and HReH contributed 76.2% of the responses (Table 1). The highest qualification levels amongst the participants were a university degree (48.5%), a post-basic diploma in ophthalmic nursing (20.8%), a postgraduate degree (17.8%), a diploma (6.9%), and those with a grade 12 or a certificate for a short course were 6% were 6% of the study population.

Table 1. Distribution of managers and HReH.

Managers	**24**	**23.76%**	**HReH**	**77**	**76.24%**
District Director of NCD (trained as Ophthalmic Nurses)	1	0.99	Ophthalmologists	3	2.97
District Director of NCD (not trained as Ophthalmic Nurses)	4	3.96	OMO	2	1.98
Hospitals CEOs	5	4.95	Optometrists	38	37.62
Medical Managers	13	12.87	Ophthalmic Nurses	24	23.76
Medical Managers/OMO	1	0.99	Nurses	9	8.91
			Eye Clinic clerk	1	0.99

3.1. Analysis of Knowledge

Table 2 shows a summary of the responses related to knowledge regarding eye health. Results show that the majority of the participants answered correctly to most of the statements. It was found that almost all the participants (95%) knew which eye health services were provided in their hospitals. An overwhelming majority of the participants agreed that an Ophthalmic Nurse provides the role of performing eye screening and assisting in theatre (83%), and an Optometrist is central in performing refraction and low vision services (87%), respectively. About two-thirds (65%) of the participants disagreed that an Optometrist is the HReH performs general primary eye health. Overall, 82% of the participants had good knowledge regarding eye health.

Table 2. Frequency distribution of responses related to knowledge regarding eye health.

Statements	D	N	A
An optician is mainly trained to measure and cut lenses.	13.9	7.9	78.2
An Ophthalmic Nurse provides the role of performing eye screening and assisting in theatre.	11.9	5.0	83.2
An Optometrist is central in performing refraction and low vision services.	11.9	1.0	87.1
An Optometrist is an eye health professional trained through a 4-year university degree.	17.8	5.9	76.2
An Optician is an eye health professional trained through a university of technology diploma.	35.6	17.8	46.5
An Ophthalmologist is an eye health professional trained with a basic medical degree and further training after that.	19.8	73.3	6.9
An Optometrist is the HReH performs general primary eye health.	65.3	3.0	31.7
An Ophthalmologist works in theatre performing eye surgery.	14.9	11.9	73.3
I know which eye health services we provide in my hospital/district/province.	1.0	4.0	95.0
I am fully aware of the programmes that we have in place as a hospital/district/province, in order to assist with prevention of blindness in this region.	5.0	12.9	82.2
In Our district/province we have not yet met the HReH targets in line with the Global Action Plan.	7.9	55.4	36.6
Eye health has not been specified amongst the priority programmes of the NHI.	5.0	41.6	53.5

D = Disagree, N = Neutral, A = Agree.

Table 3 shows the results from binary logistic regression analysis to determine the significant factors for having good knowledge. According to binary logistic regression analysis, HReH were 14 times more likely to have better knowledge (aOR = 14.21; $p < 0.01$) than their managers. Participants having a certificate qualification were 98% less likely to have good knowledge (aOR = 0.02; $p < 0.05$) compared to those with a higher level of education (a university degree and a postgraduate qualification). Respondents in the middle-aged (30–44) group were 12 times more likely to have better knowledge (aOR = 12.02; $p < 0.01$) than those in the oldest age group (>44 years).

Table 3. Logistic regression output for having good knowledge.

Variables	Adjusted Odds Radio (aOR)	95%CI		*p*-Value
		Lower	Upper	
Role in Department of Health				
HReH	14.21	1.99	101.28	0.008
Management	1			
Highest Qualification				
Certificate	0.02	0.01	0.38	0.010
Post-basic Diploma	0.09	0.01	1.04	0.054
Postgraduate Qualification	0.07	0.00	1.32	0.076
Undergraduate Diploma	0.35	0.05	2.71	0.315
University Degree	1			

Table 3. *Cont.*

Variables	Adjusted Odds Radio (aOR)	95%CI		*p*-Value
		Lower	Upper	
Age				
<30 years	2.36	0.10	58.42	0.599
30–44 years	12.02	2.00	72.09	0.007
>44 years	1			
Period of service				
<5 years	0.21	0.01	5.27	0.344
5–10 years	0.35	0.04	2.85	0.326
11–15 years	0.68	0.08	5.92	0.725
16–20 years	0.80	0.09	7.39	0.846
21–25 years	3.13	0.22	44.47	0.400
>25 years	1			

Figure 1 reports the frequency distribution of the statements regarding attitudes towards eye health. It was found that most of the participants showed positive attitudes towards eye health. For example, 90% of the participants thought that Glaucoma, Diabetic Retinopathy, and Uncorrected Refractive Error should be treated as priority areas of care, and eye health is not about cataract surgery, which should be known to the directorate. Just over half of the participants agreed that the prevention of blindness should be prioritised, as most blinding conditions are preventable. Overall, 69% of the participants showed positive attitudes towards eye health.

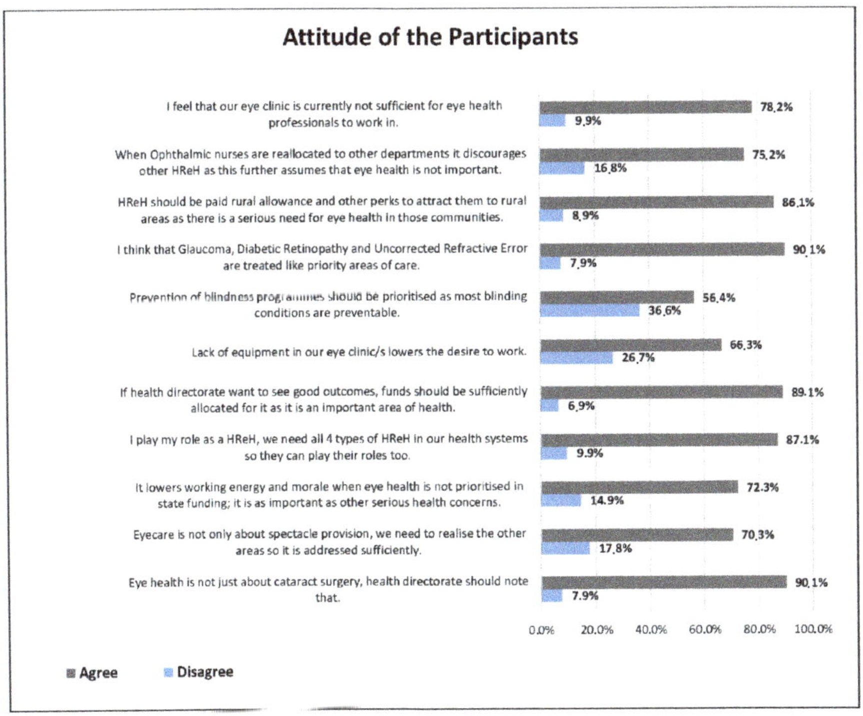

Figure 1. Summary of responses related to attitude towards eye health.

Binary logistic regression analysis (Table 4) showed that participants who were <30 years old were 94% less likely to have positive attitudes when compared with participants >44 years (aOR = 0.06; $p < 0.05$). It was found that participants working <5 years and between 5 and 10 years were 30 times and 17 times more likely to have positive attitudes towards eye health when compared with participants having >25 years of experience. No other variables were found to be significantly associated with positive attitudes regarding eye health ($p > 0.05$).

Table 4. Association between attitude and demographic variables.

Variables	aOR	95%CI		*p*-Value
		Lower	Upper	
Role in Department of Health				
HReH	2.08	0.43	10.03	0.362
Management (ref)	1			
Highest Qualification				
Certificate	0.79	0.08	8.16	0.840
Post-basic Diploma	0.72	0.14	3.63	0.689
Postgraduate Qualification	2.49	0.36	17.44	0.357
Undergraduate Diploma	0.51	0.07	3.65	0.502
University Degree	1			
Age				
<30 years	0.06	0.01	0.98	**0.0411**
30–44 years	0.25	0.04	1.68	0.152
>44 years	1			
Period of service				
<5 years	30.28	1.52	603.24	**0.025**
5–10 years	17.17	2.28	33.94	**0.009**
11–15 years	3.96	0.42	36.87	0.227
16–20 years	4.48	0.48	41.65	0.187
>25 years	1			

3.2. Analysis of Practices

Table 5 shows the frequency distribution of practice-related statements. It was found that almost all the participants (95%) prioritise prevention of blindness programmes. More than two-thirds (71%) reported that their spectacle service has a satisfactory turnaround time. Another 70% disagreed that their administration (drug stock/frame stock/IOL stock) is efficiently managed by our ward clerk/s, and 67% indicated that they do not perform noncontact tonometry on all patients. Overall, about three-quarters (73.27%) of the participants were well acquainted with practices on eye health.

Using binary logistic regression, there were statistically significant associations in every category assessed (Table 6). Management were 99% less likely to practice properly towards eye health when compared with RHeH (aOR = 0.012; $p < 0.01$). The Participants Qualified with Certificates and Grade 12 were 92% less likely and participants with postgraduate qualifications were 89% (aOR = 0.106; $p < 0.01$) less likely to know practices related to eye health when compared with participants having a university degree. With regards to age, the middle age group (30–44 years) were about three times more likely to have the best information on practices within the eye clinics (aOR = 2.603; $p < 0.05$) when compared with the >44 years age group. Having <5 years of experience were 27 times more likely to practice properly than those having more than 27 years of experience (aOR = 26.600; $p < 0.01$).

Table 5. Practices towards eye health by eye health workers (%).

Statements	D	N	A
Optometrists are restricted to refraction in our hospital/district/province	79 4	7.5	44.6
We perform non—contact tonometry on all patients	67.3	28.7	4.0
We perform a DFE on all chronic patients seen in our clinics	65.3	14.9	19.8
We have equipment that is useable and modern	62.4	22.8	14.9
Our spectacle service has a satisfactory turnaround time	71.3	9.9	18.8
We/our staff have the resources to perform basic slitlamp techniques on all our diabetic patients	62.4	33.7	4.0
We are unable to practice fully in our scopes as we do not have basic equipment for that.	13.9	119	74.3
Our referrals to Ophthalmologists have a turnaround time of up to three weeks	87.1	2.0	10.9
We are aware of prevention of blindness programmes, and we prioritise them in our eye clinic/hospital/district/province.	1.0	4.0	95.0
Our administration (drug stock/frame stock/IOL stock) is efficiently managed by our ward clerk/s	70.3	14.9	14.9
I am satisfied with the district/provincial directorate, as they understand eye health and provide sufficient budgets for it	63.4	15.8	20.8

Table 6. Association between practices and demographic variables.

Variables	aOR	95%CI		*p*-Value
		Lower	Upper	
Role within Department of Health				
Management	**0.012**	**0.003**	**0.052**	**<0.01**
HReH	1			
Highest Qualification				
Certificate and grade 12	**0.083**	**0.013**	**0.544**	**0.009**
Post-basic Diploma	0.708	0.183	2.736	0.617
Postgraduate Qualification	1.000	0.104	9.614	1.000
Undergraduate Diploma	**0.106**	**0.031**	**0.367**	**0.000**
University Degree	1			
Age				
30–44 years	**2.603**	**1.006**	**6.737**	**0.034**
>44 years	1			
Period of service				
<5 years	**26.600**	**2.626**	**269.409**	**0.005**
5–10 years	**7.560**	**1.700**	**33.629**	**0.008**
11–15 years	2.600	0.598	11.310	0.203
16–20 years	2.100	0.381	11.589	0.395
21–25 years	1.867	0.283	12.310	0.517
>25 years	1			

Spearman's correlation (Table 7) test found significant moderate positive correlation exists between knowledge, attitudes, and practices among the participants.

Table 7. Spearman's correlation test output.

			Practice	Knowledge	Attitude
Spearman's rho	Practice	Correlation Coefficient	1.000	**0.499**	0.114
		Sig. (2-tailed)		0.000	0.251
		N	101	101	101
	Knowledge	Correlation Coefficient	**0.499**	1.000	**0.421**
		Sig. (2-tailed)	0.000		0.000
		N	101	101	101
	Attitude	Correlation Coefficient	0.114	**0.421**	1.000
		Sig. (2-tailed)	0.251	0.000	0.000
		N	101	101	101

Correlation is significant at the 0.01 level (2-tailed).

4. Discussion

The study aimed to determine the levels of knowledge, attitudes, and practices of eye health care workers and their supervisors towards eye health. Knowledge, attitude, and practice (KAP) surveys are useful in public health planning, as they collect focused, essential information that is useful in guiding public health programmes [30].

4.1. Knowledge on Eye Health

Good knowledge of health is always associated with satisfactory health behaviours and outcome [30]. Therefore, understanding the correlates of good eye health through knowledge leads to improved eye care in a society [31]. The present study found a good level of knowledge among the participants. The study also found that eye health managers had poorer knowledge than the HReH that they supervise. Similarly, other studies conducted in South Africa and Swaziland reported poor knowledge of eye health management, factors attributed to the absence of policies and guidelines on eye health [32,33]. Authors reported a lack of eye health knowledge amongst general practitioners and attributed this to their short training period in this area of healthcare [34]. Other studies that reported reasons for poor knowledge in eye health said that it was due to the fact that it was not a critical "life or death" issue, a lack of adequately trained personnel, a shortage of refresher courses, and that focusing on it would unnecessarily add to their already high workload [35,36]. A recent Ethiopian study found poor knowledge among paediatricians of eye diseases [37].

In this study, education levels were significantly associated with knowledge levels. This finding is similar to that of other studies conducted elsewhere [33,38,39]. These studies showed a correlation between eye health knowledge, age, and the respondents' education level [31,38]. On the contrary, another study showed no correlation between knowledge of eye health and education level or age [40]. As a result, regardless of how qualified another physician was in another area of health such as orthopaedics, paediatrics, or even general health practice, their knowledge was still poor when it came to eye health. Considering that medical officers and specialists initially qualify as medical doctors, their reported minimal exposure to ocular health in their training is a possible reason for their poor knowledge. As they also spend a few weeks in their ophthalmology block, they do not learn much in this area of health care and as such have poor knowledge in it [39–41].

4.2. Attitudes towards Eye Health

Health workers who have positive attitudes are more likely to follow standard procedures and apply themselves to their duties, whereas those with negative attitudes would not do the same [42]. In this study, the majority of the participants had positive attitudes regarding eye health. It was also found that the youngest participants had the most negative attitudes. The possible explanation for this is that the youngest participants generally came from the safe and sheltered environment of an academic institution, where there were systems and clear protocols. They had since entered a system that does not have clear processes and guidelines, no dedicated directorate, and no easily available supervision. In addition to the working environment, they generally did not have the basic equipment that they required to perform their basic tasks [24,43]. In realising this, they did not have an understanding supervisor who would realise that urgent procurement of basic equipment was a critical enabler for them to perform their duties. As a result, they found themselves lost. The reality of their internal managers not being trained in eye health, and being incapable of providing clinical guidance and support, might be part of the reason for their negative attitude towards it. In another study, HReH attitudes were far more favourable amongst themselves when they were discussing task sharing as opposed to when they were discussing it with management [44]. A recent study conducted among paediatricians in Jordan reported satisfactory attitudes regarding eye health and disorders [45].

Those who had recently started working in eye health had the most positive attitude compared to those who had been working for more than 15 years. Evidence has shown that even though financial remuneration drives employees, it does not compare to the attainment of certain personal goals, either by progression or vertical promotion [46,47]. Intrinsic drivers include promotion and more responsibility within the employment context, driving better performance, self-actualisation, and job satisfaction in an employee [47,48]. The fulfilment that comes with greater responsibility and decision making often drives millennials (those up to age 40) to work hard as they value climbing the corporate ladder [46,47]. As this is lacking in some areas of HReH employment within DoH, it lowers the employee drive and nurtures a negative attitude towards work. Further to this, the lack of professional support and understanding is a challenge within these eye clinics. Most respondents in this study (78.2%) did not feel that their working space was sufficient for eye health professionals to work in. This is further supported by the majority (89.1%) of respondents who agreed that if directorates want to see positive outputs, they need to provide resources in the eye clinics. Sithole conducted a study among the Directorate Managers and found that there were no guidelines on eye screening, eye protection, and basic eye care [32]. Since the management group generally had a slightly older population, with a long service period, their negative attitude was largely due to a lack of ocular guidelines. They further did not have any ocular directorate at a senior level to look to for guidance, possibly resulting in a negative attitude, and shifted their focus more to their familiar health areas such as geriatrics and NCD [32].

4.3. Practices towards Eye Health

Overall, participants were practicing satisfactorily towards eye health. Almost all the participants confirmed that their eye clinics/districts prioritised blindness prevention in their daily practice. This shows that in light of their working circumstances, these eye health workers still aim to practice the highest level of clinical care in their workplaces. Two-thirds (67%) of the participants indicated that eye clinics did not perform tonometry or fundus examinations due to a lack of equipment, showing that the lack of understanding and prioritising of eye health has severe consequences. Another South African study reported that the conventional practice in hospitals is for trainees to perform cataract surgery under the supervision of consultants, and evaluation of the progress in ophthalmic surgical training was essentially an apprenticeship model [47]. To improve cataract surgical outcomes in Africa, "improved training of surgeons" was ranked as the top priority [49,50].

Both managers and HReH were clear about the severe shortage of basic equipment in the eye clinics, as well as the inefficient spectacle supply chain. Furthermore, the replacement of dysfunctional and old equipment is not honoured or prioritised by managers. Another study reported similar findings indicating that South Africa's primary eye health services lack the organisation and resources to address the leading causes of visual impairment, namely uncorrected refractive error and cataract [23,51,52]. Resource constraints, both human and equipment, are common inhibitors to the delivery of ocular services in African countries [17,52,53]. The shortage of these resources impedes basic practices aimed to ensure the prevention of blindness and PEC. The WHO states that an efficient supply chain and the availability of medicines, and medical devices, are crucial contents in their framework of health systems, to ensure health systems strengthening [8]. This will continue to be unsuccessful if these issues persist as they impede the practices of HReH.

Future studies should seek to include financiers and supply chain managers in public health services, in an effort to understand the details involved in the financing of eye health overall. This will add valuable information and provide further context on the issues raised in this study.

5. Conclusions

The overall knowledge, attitudes and practices on eye health were satisfactory among the participants but differed significantly between managers and HReH. It is evident that an appropriate eye health professional should be appointed as part of management at both operational and directorate levels. Resources, both human and equipment, would need to be better allocated by knowledgeable professionals for improvement of clinical practice and eye health services overall. There is a need to review the current management structure, as HReH currently work under difficult conditions.

Despite adding new information to the body of existing knowledge, the limitation of this study was the exclusion of supply chain and finance personnel, who could have given context to the issues that were raised by respondents.

The appointment of a sufficiently trained directorate to manage eye health in each district would be beneficial to eye health and prevention of blindness strategies. This will further ensure that an efficient eye health workforce is placed and managed through optimal governance, resulting in improved eye health outcomes and better service delivery to the communities within the province.

Supplementary Materials: The following are available online at https://www.mdpi.com/1660-4601/18/23/12513/s1, Table S1: Validation of questionnaire.

Author Contributions: Z.X.-K. conceptualised the study and prepared the manuscript, K.M. and K.N. supervised the study and reviewed the manuscript. All authors have read and agreed to the published version of the manuscript.

Funding: The authors thank the UKZN University Capacity Development Programme for funding the study.

Institutional Review Board Statement: The study was conducted according to the guidelines of the Declaration of Helsinki and approved by the Biomedical Review Ethics Committee of the University of KwaZulu-Natal (BE155/19 on 19 May 2019).

Informed Consent Statement: Informed consent was obtained from all participants involved in the study.

Data Availability Statement: Data are included in the manuscript.

Acknowledgments: The authors thank the HReH in the KZN eye clinics and their managers both in the hospitals and at the various district offices for their participation in this study.

Conflicts of Interest: The authors declare that they have no competing interest or financial relationships that could have influenced the writing of this manuscript.

References

1. Bourne, R.R.A.; Flaxman, S.R.; Braithwaite, T.; Cicinelli, M.V.; Das, A.; Jonas, J.B.; Keeffe, J.; Kempen, J.H.; Leasher, J.; Limburg, H.; et al. Magnitude, temporal trends, and projections of the global prevalence of blindness and distance and near vision impairment: A systematic review and meta-analysis. *Lancet Glob. Health* **2017**, 5, e888–e897. [CrossRef]
2. Xulu-Kasaba, Z.; Kalinda, C. Prevalence of Blindness and its major causes in Sub-Saharan African in 2020: A systematic review and meta-analysis. *Br. J. Vis. Impair.* **2021**. accepted for publication.

3. Ramke, J.; Zwi, A.B.; Palagyi, A.; Blignault, I.; Gilbert, C.E. Equity and blindness: Closing evidence gaps to support universal eye health. *Ophthalmic Epidemiol.* **2015**, *22*, 297–307. [CrossRef]
4. Freeman, E.E.; Roy-Gagnon, M.-H.; Samson, S.; Haddad, S.; Aubin, M.-J.; Vela, C.; Zunzunegui, M.V. The global burden of visual difficulty in low, middle, and high income countries. *PLoS ONE* **2013**, *8*, e63315. [CrossRef] [PubMed]
5. Cockburn, N.; Steven, D.; Lecuona, K.; Joubert, F.; Rogers, G.; Cook, C.; Polack, S. Prevalence, causes and socioeconomic determinants of vision loss in Cape Town, South Africa. *PLoS ONE* **2012**, *7*, e30718. [CrossRef]
6. Kestelyn, P.G.; Cunningham, E.T.J. HIV/AIDS and blindness. *Bull. World Health Organ.* **2001**, *79*, 208–213. [PubMed]
7. Smit, D.P.; Esterhuizen, T.M.; Meyer, D. The prevalence of intraocular tuberculosis in HIV-positive and HIV negative patients in South Africa using a revised classification system. *Ocul. Immunol. Inflamm.* **2016**, *26*, 830–837. [CrossRef]
8. World Health Organization. Universal Eye Health: A Global Action Plan 2014–2019. 2013. Available online: https://www.who.int/blindness/AP2014_19_English.pdf (accessed on 28 March 2021).
9. Koberlein, J.; Beifus, K.; Schaffert, C.; Fingerm, R.P. The economic burden of visual impairment and blindness: A systematic review. *BMJ Open* **2013**, *3*, e003471. [CrossRef]
10. Langelaan, M.; de Boer, M.R.; van Nispen, R.M.; Woutersm, B.; Moll, A.C.; van Rens, G.H. Impact of visual impairment on quality of life: A comparison with quality of life in the general population and with other chronic conditions. *Ophthalmic Epidemiol.* **2007**, *14*, 119–126. [CrossRef] [PubMed]
11. Andriamanjato, H.; Mathenge, W.; Kalua, K.; Courtright, P.; Lewallen, S. Task shifting in primary eye care: How sensitive and specific are common signs and symptoms to predict conditions requiring referral to specialist eye personnel? *Hum. Resour. Health* **2014**, *12*, S3. [CrossRef]
12. Graham, R. Facing the crisis in human resources for eye health in sub-Saharan Africa. *Community Eye Health* **2017**, *30*, 85. [PubMed]
13. Gilbert, C. The importance of primary eye care. *Community eye Health.* **1998**, *11*, 1719.
14. Courtright, P.; Seneadza, A.; Mathenge, W.; Eliah, E.; Lewallen, S. Primary eye care in sub-Saharan African: Do we have the evidence needed to scale up training and service delivery? *Ann. Trop. Med. Parasitol.* **2010**, *104*, 361–367. [CrossRef]
15. Sithole, H.L. A situational analysis of ocular health promotion in the South African primary health-care system. *Clin. Exp. Optom.* **2017**, *100*, 167–173. [CrossRef] [PubMed]
16. Naidoo, K. Poverty and blindness in Africa. *Clin. Exp. Optom.* **2007**, *90*, 415–421. [CrossRef]
17. Sukati, V.N.; Moodley, V.R.; Mashige, K.P. A situational analysis of eye care services in Swaziland. *J. Public Health Afr.* **2018**, *9*, 892. [CrossRef]
18. Lecuona, K.; Cook, C. South Africa's cataract surgery rates: Why are we not meeting our targets? *S. Afr. Med. J.* **2011**, *101*, 510–512.
19. De Wet, M.; Ackermann, L. Improving eye care in the primary health care setting. *Curationis* **2000**, *23*, 36–42. [CrossRef]
20. Hendricks, M.; Beardsley, J.; Bourne, L.; Mzamo, B.; Golden, B. Are opportunities for vitamin A supplementation being utilised at primary health-care clinics in the Western Cape Province of South Africa? *Public Health Nutr.* **2007**, *10*, 1082–1088. [CrossRef] [PubMed]
21. Webb, E.M.; Rheeder, P.; Van Zyl, D.G. Diabetes care and complications in primary care in the Tshwane district of South Africa. *Prim. Care Diabetes* **2015**, *9*, 147–154. [CrossRef]
22. Mathee, A.; de la Rey, A.; Swart, A.; Plagerson, S.; Naicker, N. 'Urban insight': A high level of undiagnosed need reflects limited access to and availability of eye-care services in South Africa. *S. Afr. Med. J.* **2014**, *104*, 407–408. [CrossRef] [PubMed]
23. Xulu Kasaba, Z.N.; Mashige, K.P.; Naidoo, K.S. An assessment of human resource distribution for public eye health services in KwaZulu-Natal, South Africa. *Afr. Vis. Eye Heath* **2021**, *80*, 8. [CrossRef]
24. South African Department of Health. *National Guideline—Prevention of Blindness in South Africa*; South African Department of Health: Pretoria, South Africa, 2002.
25. Naidoo, K.S.; Sweeney, D.; Jaggernath, J.; Holden, B. A population-based study of visual impairment in the lower Tugela health district in KwaZulu Natal, South Africa. *Afr. Vis. Eye Health* **2013**, *72*, 110–118. [CrossRef]
26. Xulu-Kasaba, Z.; Mashige, K.; Naidoo, K.; Kalinda, C. Prevalence of visual impairment and blindness in South African in the period 2010–2020: A systematic scoping review and meta-analysis. Unpublished work. 2021.
27. Magakwe, T.; Xulu-Kasaba, Z.; Hansraj, R. Prevalence and distribution of visual impairment and refractive error amongst school-going children aged 6–18 years in Sekhukhune District (Limpopo, South Africa). *Afr. Vis. Eye Health* **2020**, *79*, 8. [CrossRef]
28. Lilian, R.R.; Railton, J.; Schaftenaar, E.; Mabitsi, M.; Grobbelaar, C.J.; Khosa, N.S.; Maluleke, B.H.; Struthers, H.E.; McIntyre, J.A.; Peters, R.P.H. Strengthening primary eye care in South Africa: An assessment of services and prospective evaluation of a health systems support package. *PLoS ONE* **2018**, *13*, e0197432. [CrossRef]
29. Courtright, P.; Mathenge, W.; Kello, A.B.; Cook, C.; Kalua, K.; Lewallen, S. Setting targets for human resources for eye health in sub-Saharan Africa: What evidence should be used? *Hum. Resour. Health* **2016**, *14*, 11. [CrossRef]
30. Chandler, C.I.R. Knowledge, Attitudes, and Practice Surveys. The International Encyclopedia of Anthropology. 2020. Available online: https://www.spring-nutrition.org/sites/default/files/publications/tools/spring_context_assessment_tools_all.pdf (accessed on 22 May 2021).
31. McClure, L.A.; Tannenbaum, S.L.; Zheng, D.D.; Joslin, C.E.; Perera, M.J.; Gellman, M.D.; Arheart, K.L.; Lam, B.L.; Lee, D.J. Eye Health Knowledge and Eye Health Information Exposure Among Hispanic/Latino Individuals: Results from the Hispanic Community Health Study/Study of Latinos. *JAMA Ophthalmol.* **2017**, *135*, 878–882. [CrossRef]

32. Sithole, L. Perceptions of Health Directorates Managers on Eye Health Promotion in South Africa. *Eur. J. Public Health* **2017**, *27* (Suppl. 3), ckx186.066. [CrossRef]
33. Sukati, V.; Moodley, V.R.; Mashige, K.P. Knowledge and practices of eye health professionals about the availability and accessibility of child eye care services in the public sector in Swaziland. *Afr. Vis. Eye Heal.* **2019**, *78*, a471. [CrossRef]
34. Fatima, I.; Ahmad, I. Knowledge, Attitude, Practice (KAP) study regarding optometric services among general practitioners in Lahore. *Ophthalmol. Pak.* **2018**, *8*, 14–17.
35. Fashafsheh, I.H.D.; Morsy, W.Y.M.; Ismaeel, M.S.; Alkaiasi, A.A.E. Impact of a designed eye care protocol on nurses knowledge, practices and on eye health status of unconscious mechanically ventilated patients at North Palestine hospitals. *J. Educ. Pract.* **2013**, *4*, 107–120.
36. Kandel, H.; Murthy, G.V.; Bascaran, C. Human resources for refraction services in Central Nepal. *Clin. Exp. Optom.* **2015**, *98*, 335–341. [CrossRef] [PubMed]
37. Regassa, T.T.; Daba, K.T.; Fabian, I.D.; Mengasha, A.A. Knowledge, attitude and practice of Ethiopian pediatricians concerning childhood eye diseases. *BMC Ophthalmol.* **2021**, *21*, 91. [CrossRef] [PubMed]
38. Katibeh, M.; Ziaei, H.; Panah, E.; Moein, H.-R.; Hosseini, S.; Kalantarion, M.; Eskandari, A.; Yaseri, M. Knowledge and awareness of age related eye diseases: A population-based survey. *J. Ophthalmic Vis. Res.* **2014**, *9*, 223. [PubMed]
39. Achigbu, E.O.; Chuka-Okosa, C.M. The knowledge and attitude of non-ophthalmic medical doctors towards glaucoma in two tertiary institutions in south eastern Nigeria. *Niger. Postgrad. Med. J.* **2014**, *21*, 144–149.
40. Razak, A.; Sarpan, S.; Ramlan, R. Influence of Promotion and Job Satisfaction on Employee Performance. *J. Account. Bus. Financ. Res.* **2018**, *3*, 18–27. [CrossRef]
41. Altangerel, U.; Nallamshetty, H.S.; Uhler, T.; Fontanarosa, J.; Steinmann, W.C.; Almodin, J.M.; Chen, B.H.; Henderer, J.D. Knowledge about glaucoma and barriers to follow-up care in a community glaucoma screening program. *Can. J. Ophthalmol.* **2009**, *44*, 66–69. [CrossRef]
42. Permana, M.A.B.; Hidayah, N. The Influence of Health Workers' Knowledge, Attitudes and Compliance on Implementation of Standard Precautions in Hospital-Acquired Infections Prevention at X Hospital Bantul. *Arch. Bus. Res.* **2018**, *6*. [CrossRef]
43. Aboobaker, S.; Courtright, P. Barriers to cataract surgery in Africa: A systematic review. *Middle East Afr. J. Ophthalmol.* **2016**, *23*, 145–149. [CrossRef]
44. Shah, M.; Noor, A.; Ormsby, G.M.; Chakrabarti, R.; Harper, C.A.; Islam, F.A.; Keeffe, J. Attitudes and perceptions of eye care workers and health administrators regarding task sharing in screening and detection for management of diabetic retinopathy in Pakistan. *Ophthalmic Epidemiol.* **2018**, *25*, 169–175. [CrossRef]
45. Ababneh, L.T.; Khriesat, W.; Abu Dalu, S.; Hanania, R.J.; Ababneh, B.F.; Amer, N.A.B.; Jahmani, T. Knowledge of and attitude to eye disorders among pediatricians in North Jordan. *Ann. Med. Surg.* **2021**, *67*, 102430. [CrossRef]
46. Franco, L.M.; Bennett, S.; Kanfer, R. Health sector reform and public sector health worker motivation: A conceptual framework. *Soc. Sci. Med.* **2002**, *54*, 1255–1266. [CrossRef]
47. PWC. Millennials at Work—Reshaping the Workplace 2012. Available online: https://www.pwc.com/co/es/publicaciones/assets/millennials-at-work.pdf (accessed on 21 October 2020).
48. Van Zyl, L.; Fernandes, N.; Rogers, G.; Du Toit, N. Primary health eye care knowledge among general practitioners working in the Cape Town metropole. *South Afr. Fam. Pract.* **2011**, *53*, 52–55. [CrossRef]
49. Haastrup, O.O.O.; Buchan, J.C.; Cassels-Brown, A.; Cook, C. Are we monitoring the quality of cataract surgery services? A qualitative situation analysis of attitudes and practices in a large city in South Africa. *Middle East Afr. J. Ophthalmol.* **2015**, *22*, 220–225. [CrossRef] [PubMed]
50. Buchan, J.C.; Dean, W.H.; Foster, A.; Burton, M.J. What are the priorities for improving cataract surgical outcomes in Africa? Results of a Delphi exercise. *Int. Ophthalmol.* **2018**, *38*, 1409–1414. [CrossRef] [PubMed]
51. Flaxman, S.R.; Bourne, R.R.A.; Resnikoff, S.; Ackland, P.; Braithwaite, T.; Cicinelli, M.V.; Das, A.; Jonas, J.B.; Keeffe, J.; Kempen, J.H.; et al. Global causes of blindness and distance vision impairment 1990-2020: A systematic review and meta-analysis. *Lancet Glob. Health* **2017**, *5*, e1221–e1234. [CrossRef]
52. Onakpoya, O.H.; O Adeoye, A.; O Adegbehingbe, B.; Akinsola, F.B. Assessment of human and material resources available for primary eye-care delivery in rural communities of southwestern Nigeria. *West Indian Med. J.* **2009**, *58*, 472–475.
53. Bozzani, F.M.; Griffiths, U.K.; Blanchet, K.; Schmidt, E. Health systems analysis of eye care services in Zambia: Evaluating progress towards VISION 2020 goals. *BMC Health Serv. Res.* **2014**, *14*, 94. [CrossRef]

International Journal of
Environmental Research and Public Health

MDPI

Article

Feasible Distributed Energy Supply Options for Household Energy Use in China from a Carbon Neutral Perspective

Yingxin Zhang [1,*], Sainan Wang [1], Wei Shao [2] and Junhong Hao [3]

1 School of Economy, Beijing Technology and Business University, Beijing 100048, China; wangsainan@btbu.edu.cn
2 Institute of Thermal Science and Technology, Shandong University, Jinan 250061, China; shao@sdu.edu.cn
3 School of Energy Power and Mechanical Engineering, North China Electric Power University, Beijing 102206, China; hjh@ncepu.edu.cn
* Correspondence: yingxin.z@btbu.edu.cn

Abstract: This contribution firstly proposed the concept of annual average power generation hours and analyzed per capita energy consumption, carbon emission, and the human development index from a macro perspective. On this basis, we compared the average household electrical energy consumption of urban and rural residents based on the data from CGSS-2015 from a micro perspective. The results show the positive correlation between carbon emissions per capita and the human development index and China's regional imbalance characteristics between household electricity consumption and renewable energy distribution. Therefore, the distributed energy supply system is proposed as an effective complement to centralized power generation systems and is the key to synergizing human development and carbon emissions in China. Moreover, we analyzed the characteristics of distributed energy supply systems in the context of existing energy supply systems, pointing out the need to fully use solar energy and natural gas. Finally, two types of typical distributed energy supply systems are proposed for satisfying the household energy requirements in remote or rural areas of western and the eastern or coastal areas of China, respectively. Two typical distributed energy systems integrate high-efficiency energy conversion, storage, and transfer devices such as electric heat pumps, photovoltaic thermal, heat and electricity storage, and fuel cells.

Keywords: household energy consumption; carbon neutrality; distributed energy system; high-efficiency; human development index

Citation: Zhang, Y.; Wang, S.; Shao, W.; Hao, J. Feasible Distributed Energy Supply Options for Household Energy Use in China from a Carbon Neutral Perspective. *Int. J. Environ. Res. Public Health* **2021**, *18*, 12992. https://doi.org/10.3390/ijerph182412992

Academic Editors: Roberto Alonso González Lezcano, Francesco Nocera and Rosa Giuseppina Caponetto

Received: 15 November 2021
Accepted: 7 December 2021
Published: 9 December 2021

1. Introduction

1.1. Background and Status

To fight against climate warming and environmental pollution, carbon peaking and carbon neutrality have become the main energy development strategies worldwide. At present, in China, various industries such as electric power, transportation, construction, steel, etc., have proposed different routes for achieving carbon peaking and carbon neutrality [1]. The carbon emission of electricity generation based on fossil fuel provides a larger proportion [2]. That is, reducing carbon emissions from electricity production processes is vital to achieving carbon neutrality for China. Recently, the primary solution is the improvement of energy utilization efficiency and increase of renewable energy generation. The rapid development of renewable energy, such as wind power and photovoltaic, has formed an integrated energy system with traditional coal-fired power generation and hydroelectric power generation, turning into China's main centralized energy supply [3].

For the development of the integrated energy system, many studies have explored carbon peaking and carbon-neutral pathways in energy use from technical, economic, and social perspectives [4–7]. For example, Liu et al. [8] proposed a differentiated model for evaluating the impact of the emissions trading scheme (ETS) on the development of non-fossil energy sources, and it is concluded that the ETS significantly promotes the development of non-fossil energy sources in China, and the higher the carbon price, the stronger the effect of ETS on promoting the development of non-fossil energy sources. Li et al. [9] developed a collaborative hierarchical framework to coordinate electricity and heat interactions and analyzed the impact of carbon tax, electricity and heat demand responses on the outcome of multi-stakeholder interaction problems. The results show a win-win situation for all participants, with significant reductions in total costs and CO_2 emissions. Zhao et al. [10] investigated the technical and economic feasibility of New York State's energy transition goals. They developed an energy conversion optimization framework, pointed out that air-source heat pumps and geothermal technologies will provide 47% and 41% of heat demand, respectively, by 2050. Bao et al. [11] proposed a classification method for renewable energy-led distributed energy supply models. They provided an integrated economic and environmental evaluation model and concluded that the biomass waste-based supply model could achieve "zero" carbon emissions and "zero" energy consumption. In addition, it is advisable to promote waste-based energy utilization and wind and solar energy-based supply modes in new rural and remote areas with abundant resources.

Meanwhile, the distributed energy system has become an attractive alternative technology that has received much attention. Especially on the customer side, distributed energy supply systems can be used to increase the flexibility of the customer side and further improve the consumption and utilization of renewable energy [12–16]. For example, Huo et al. [17] innovatively developed an integrated dynamic simulation model and explored possible emission peaks and peak times by scenario analysis and Monte Carlo simulation methods. The dynamic sensitivity analysis shows that GDP per capita, carbon emission factor, and urban residential floor area play an essential role in driving carbon emissions' peak and peaking times. Zhang et al. [18] reviewed the distributed generation PV policy changes since 2013. They examined their impact on China's domestic distributed generation PV market, presented a cost and time breakdown for installing distributed generation PV projects in China, and identified the major barriers to distributed generation PV installation. Zhao et al. [19] calculated the internal rate of return (IRR) and static payback period for some distributed PV systems in five cities with different resource zones in China. The effects of relevant policy variables such as subsidies, benchmark prices, tariffs, and taxes on the economic performance of distributed power systems were discussed. Duan et al. [20] analyzed the influence of solar energy substitution for coal-fired power generation on future greenhouse gas emission trajectories and peak arrival times based on the full-spectrum and life-cycle perspective based on an integrated energy–economic–environment model and a simple climate response model. Moreover, from the application and evaluation perspective of the distributed energy system, Zeng et al. [21] described the current situation of distributed energy development in China. Sameti et al. [22] established the optimal design emissions of the district energy system based on a trade-off between annualized total cost and annual CO_2 and showed that a district energy system with energy storage provides the best solution to environmental and economic problems. Ren et al. [23] studied the feasibility of distributed energy systems for three typical building clusters in one major city in each of China's five climate zones. Huang et al. [24] constructed a practical evaluation index system that integrates soft and hard competitiveness and classified distributed energy supply system scenarios according to development characteristics. Yoon et al. [25] artificially assessed the possibility of introducing cogeneration distributed energy systems in existing multi-family dwellings. The annual energy consumption of a typical urban multifamily dwelling was estimated based on primary energy consumption reduction, CO_2 emission reduction, simple payback period, and recurring cost values.

The above existing research on distributed energy supply systems has been carried out from various aspects such as system energy source, process construction, operation strategy, economic evaluation, and application scenarios. Combined with carbon emission requirements, different distributed energy supply schemes are given from cities, industrial estates, buildings, etc. [26–28]. These studies provide the necessary basis for the development of distributed energy supply systems. Besides, household energy consumption playing a vital role as main energy consumption on the user side is also significant for carbon peaking and carbon neutrality [29–32]. For example, Wu et al. [33] provided a systematical overview of rural household energy consumption in China from 1985 to 2013 and illustrated the pattern of rural household energy consumption using a comprehensive household survey, the Chinese Residential Energy Consumption Survey (CRECS, 2013). Zou et al. [34] presented a detailed analysis of rural household energy consumption characteristics based on the data of 1472 rural households from the Chinese General Social Survey of 2015 (CGSS2015). Ren et al. [35] predicted energy consumption and carbon emissions using both the carbon emissions coefficient and the sector energy consumption method and concluded that urbanization positively affects energy consumption and carbon emissions in China. Chen et al. [36] proposed a spatial downscaling framework to identify different provinces and sectors' roles in promoting carbon emission peaks. Zhang et al. [37] developed a questionnaire survey to investigate and evaluate the carbon emissions of household energy consumption and analyzed the influence factors, including residential consumption, housing conditions, daily travel distance, etc.

1.2. Research Gap

Currently, many studies have been conducted on various aspects of planning, modeling, operation, and evaluation of integrated energy system, local energy system, and community energy system by combining with the renewable energy. Meanwhile, some studies have focused more on household energy consumption in rural or urban areas of a particular Chinese province. These researches provide some feasible and significant technological guides for the future energy supply systems from the city-level, community-level, and household-level. However, due to the considerable difference in household energy consumption in each province of China, more research about the choice of household energy supply pathway is desirable and should be developed by simultaneously considering the energy resource distribution and social development characteristics in the context of carbon neutrality. That is, the synergy between household energy consumption and renewable energy distribution in different regions of China is crucial for the current development of distributed energy supply systems and the choice of household energy supply pathways under the carbon neutrality target.

1.3. Resrarch Content and Novelty

This contribution analyzes the energy consumption, power generation, carbon emission, and human development index of China near 40 years. It presents the average household electrical energy consumption of urban and rural residents in 28 provinces based on the data from the Chinese General Social Survey 2015 (CGSS-2015). Based on the above macro and micro statistical analysis, we analyze the characteristic of the distributed energy system and present the future energy system that should be the solar energy-based energy supply system. Moreover, two types of typical distributed energy supply systems are proposed by integrating high-efficiency energy conversion, storage, and exchange devices that are feasible pathways for the choice of household energy supply in China from a carbon neutral perspective. The following provides the novelty of the work,

(1) The research proposes a new concept of annual average power generation hours to analyze the development of the energy generation, analyzes the relationship between carbon emission and the human development index in China.
(2) The research first presents the household electricity consumption distribution of urban and rural areas in each province of China based on the CGSS-2015, and obtain the imbalance characteristic between the renewable energy distribution and the household electricity consumption.
(3) The research concludes the characteristics of solar energy-based distributed energy supply system based on the macro and micro analysis, and proposes two types of distributed energy system by integrating clean, high-efficiency, and low/zero carbon technologies for eastern and western areas in China under the carbon neutral perspective.

2. Energy Consumption and Carbon Emission in China

2.1. Energy Generation and Consumption in China

In China, thermal power (TP), hydropower (HP), nuclear power (NP), wind power (WP), and photovoltaic (PV) have been the primary generation. Figure 1 shows the variation in the installed capacity share of different power generation methods. The installed capacity of thermal power generation occupies the largest share and has decreased from 73.8% to 56.4% in the last 30 years. The total installed capacity of wind power and PV has increased rapidly in the last decade and has already surpassed the installed capacity of hydropower, reaching 43.2% of the total installed capacity of thermal power in 2020. Currently, coal-fired power generation is still the primary method of electricity production in China. However, last year, for the first time, the installed capacity of renewable energy surpassed that of coal-fired units. Besides, the continuous increase of installed capacity of wind power and PV will become an important step to achieving the carbon peak and carbon neutral strategy in the future.

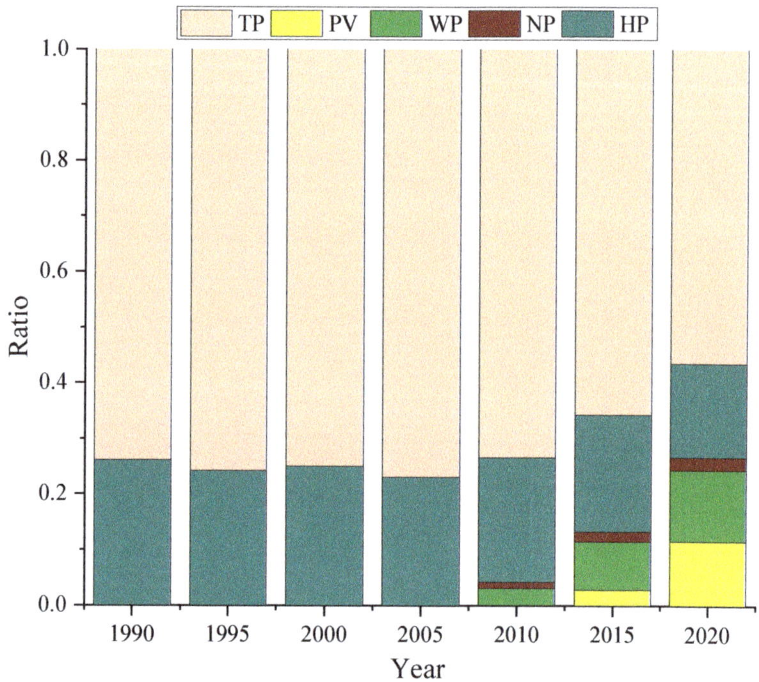

Figure 1. The power generation installed capacity ratio (1990–2020) in China.

Changes in the structure of the installed power capacity of energy will cause changes in the production and consumption of electricity. Figure 2 presents the annual average power generation hours, including all-power generation ways as thermal power, wind power, hydropower, nuclear, and PV shown in Figure 1, and meanwhile shows the annual per capita power production from 1980 to 2020 in China. Figure 3 shows the power generation utilization hours of different power generation ways in China. The annual average power generation hours are a new concept proposed in this paper and equals the total power generation ratio to the total installed capacity. Although the installed capacity of power generation continuously increases, the power generation hours reached up to the maximum 4964.7 h in 2004 and the minimum 3463.6 h in 2020.

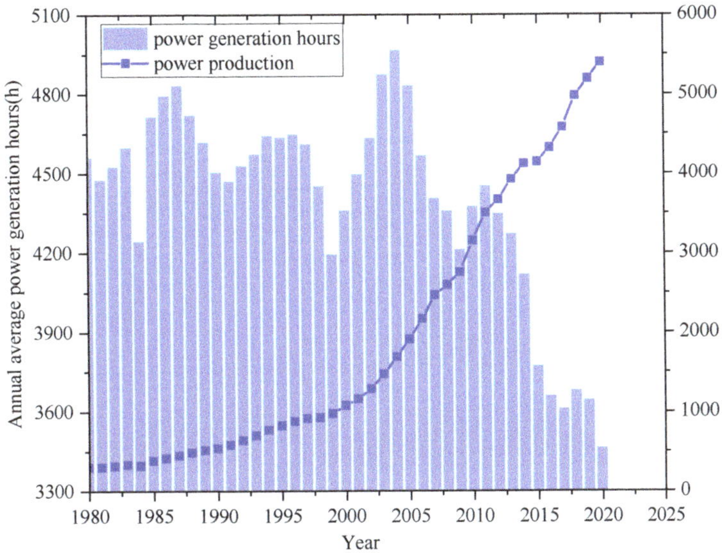

Figure 2. Annual average power generation hours and power production (1980–2020) in China.

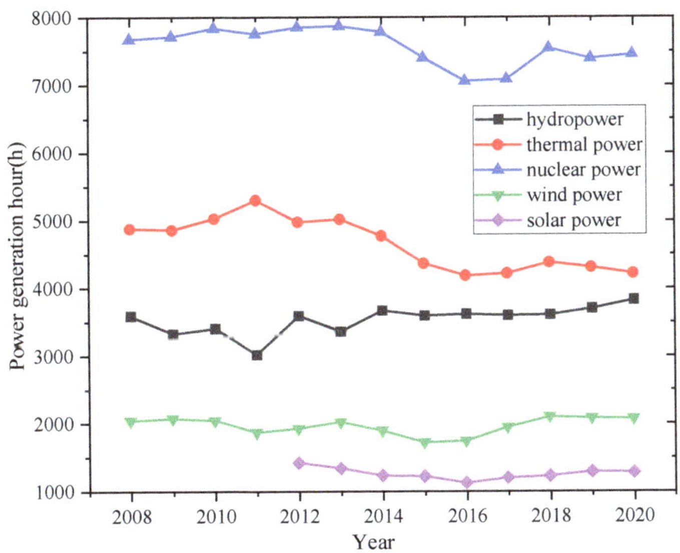

Figure 3. Power generation utilization hours of different power generation ways in China (2008–2020).

On the one hand, the wind power and PV generation installation ratios increase with lower generation hours due to their essential characteristics. On the other hand, the ratio of thermal power generation and the generating equipment availability hour decrease. On the other hand, since 2010, the average annual number of hours of electricity generated has decreased to 91 h per year. The thermal plant has the same trend shown in Figure 3. Especially in 2020, the annual average power generation hours will reduce 180.8 h due to the impact of the COVID-19 pandemic. Besides, the annual per capita power production has continued to grow, increasing nearly 18-fold in 40 years. In particular, it has increased from 3153 kW to 5397 kW in the last decade, almost 71.2%.

2.2. Carbon Emission and Human Development Index

In the past four decades, the rapid development of energy and electricity in China has dramatically improved people's social quality of life, bringing about serious environmental problems. Meanwhile, HDI is an indicator of economic and social development and is a comprehensive evaluation containing the financial standard, education measure, and life expectation [38]. Therefore, Figure 4a presents the annual per capita carbon emission of China from 1980 to 2020 and the human development index (HDI) of China from 1990 to 2020 and their relationship. Over the past four decades, the annual per capita carbon emissions have increased from 1.467 tons to 7.008 tons, an average increase of 0.138 t per year. Besides, the HDI increases from 0.499 to 0.761 from 1990 to 2020 in China. Figure 4b also shows that the HDI is positively correlated with carbon emissions per capita. In other words, to a certain extent, the increase in carbon emissions per capita contributes to the improvement of HDI.

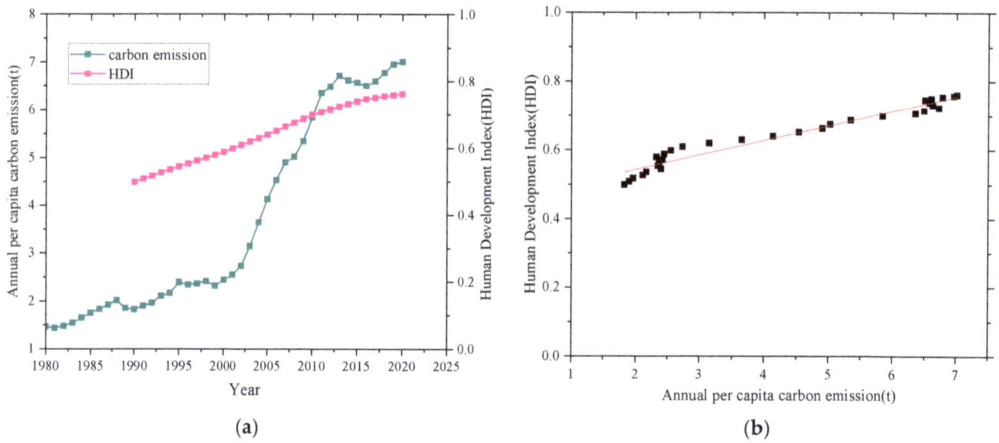

Figure 4. (**a**) Annual per capita carbon emission and HDI of China, (**b**) HDI varies with the annual per capita carbon emission.

3. Household Electricity Consumption Distribution

3.1. Household Electricity Consumption in Urban and Rural Areas

The above analysis provides a macroscopic view of China's energy production and social development from different data such as installed capacity, per capita electricity generation, per capita carbon emissions and human development index. Besides, from the microscopic view, household electricity consumption also greatly influences the total energy consumption in China, in particular, electric power consumption. This article analyzes the corresponding electricity power consumption data based on the 2015 Chinese General Social Survey (CGSS-2015). Figure 5 presents the average household electricity consumption of urban and rural residents in 28 provinces of China, respectively. We can find that the urban electricity consumption is almost more than the rural electricity consumption. According to the statistical data, the average annual electricity consumption per household of urban residents in Fujian Province is the highest. The average annual electricity consumption per household of urban residents in Gansu, Inner Mongolia, Shaanxi, and Sichuan is the lowest in addition to the national position. Geographically, it can be seen that the average annual electricity consumption per household of urban residents in the northern region is slightly lower than that in the south, and the trend of electricity consumption increases gradually from the northwest to the southeast. In addition, the average annual electricity consumption per household of urban residents has a regional concentration distribution pattern, with high electricity consumption areas concentrated in the capital, east China, south China, and southeast coastal areas, which is closely related to the high level of political and economic development in these areas. Meanwhile, considering that the overall development level of the central and northern regions still has more room for improvement, the lower overall electricity consumption in this region also supports this status quo.

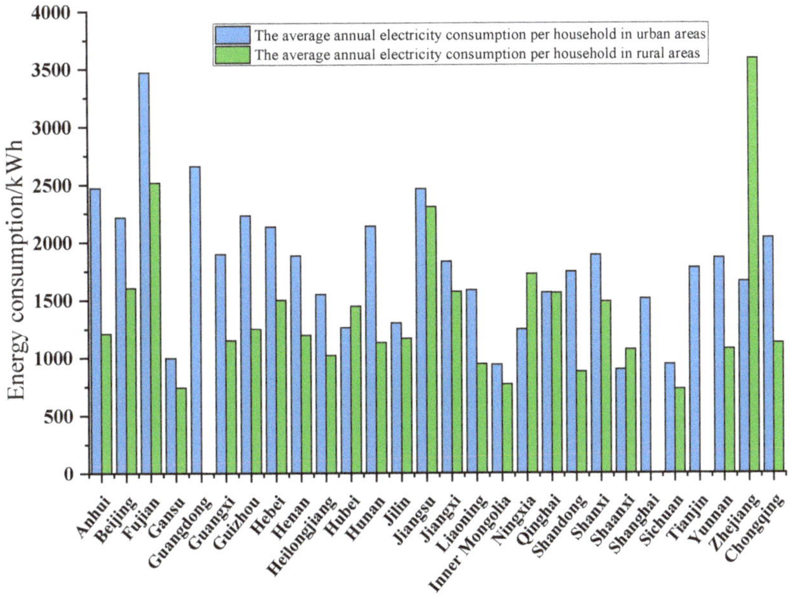

Figure 5. The average annual electricity consumption per household in urban and rural residents in 28 provinces of China, 2014.

Moreover, Figure 6 presents the average household electricity consumption of urban residents in 28 provinces of China, 2014. For urban residents, the average annual electricity consumption per household in Fujian Province, Guangdong Province, and Anhui Province resides in the top three statistical provinces in order. The average annual electricity consumption per household is concentrated in the range of 1500 2000 kWh in more provinces, with 12, which better reflects the average level of urban residents nationwide. For the electricity consumption of rural residents, there are missing data for Guangdong Province, Tianjin, and Shanghai. The average annual electricity consumption per household in Zhejiang, Fujian, and Jiangsu provinces is in the top three statistical provinces in order of residence. Comparing the average annual electricity consumption per household in different regions, we can see that the overall electricity consumption of urban residents is higher than that of rural residents. The average annual electricity consumption per household of urban residents in Shandong Province, Guizhou Province, Hunan Province, and Chongqing City is already about twice that of rural residents, indicating a large imbalance between urban and rural development in the regions as mentioned above. In comparison, the average annual electricity consumption per household of rural residents in Zhejiang Province, Ningxia Province, Hubei Province, and Shaanxi Province is higher than rural residents. The average annual electricity consumption per household in Zhejiang Province, Ningxia Province, Hubei Province, and Shaanxi Province is higher than that of urban residents, which indicates to a certain extent that the development level of local villages and cities is more average and the electricity consumption is comparable. In particular, the average annual electricity consumption per household in Zhejiang Province is more than twice that of urban residents, which laterally indicates that the development level of local rural areas is higher.

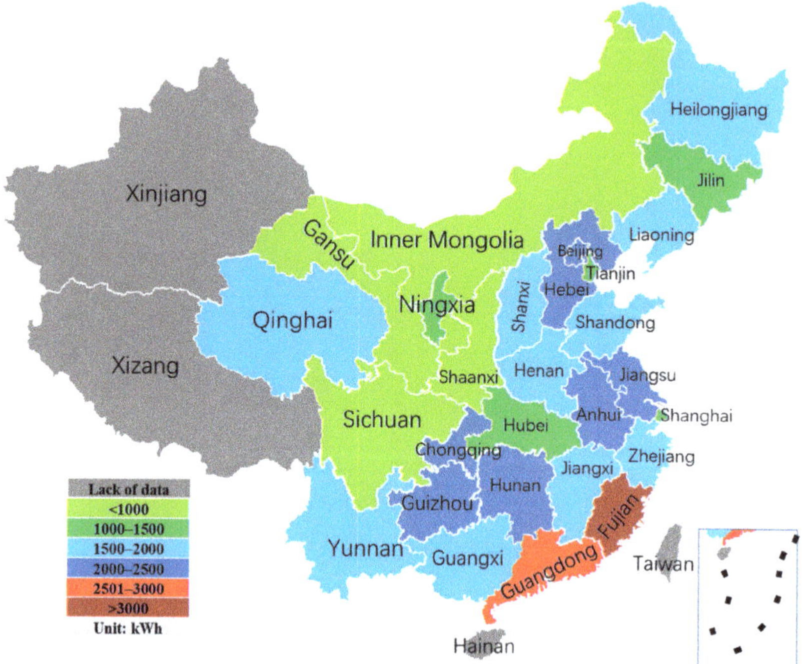

Figure 6. The average household electricity consumption of urban residents in 28 provinces of China, 2014.

3.2. Wind and Solar Distribution in China

Finally, the more economically developed coastal areas, such as Beijing, Shanghai, Jiangsu, Zhejiang, and Guangdong, have greater household electrical energy consumption on average than the lower Midwest regions in China. Figures 7 and 8 show wind power and solar energy installed capacity until 2020 in China. In addition, more renewable energy sources such as wind energy and solar energy are located in the Midwest of China, such as Xinjiang, Qinghai, Gansu, Inner Mongolia, etc. Therefore, the non-balance between energy generation and energy consumption generates some obstacles for achieving the carbon peak and carbon neutral strategies of China. Therefore, developing an extra-high voltage power grid is an effective solution for improving renewable energy utilization and reducing carbon emissions. Besides, in these energy consumption regions such as Beijing, Shanghai, and Guangdong, distributed energy systems have also become a feasible solution for ensuring energy demands with low or zero carbon emissions.

In summary, from a macro perspective, the installed capacity of power generation based on fossil fuels and renewable energy sources has both continued to increase in the last decade. Although the average annual power generation utilization hours decrease year by year, it is conducive to improving China's human development index. However, a continuous increase in carbon emissions per capita comes with this. Meanwhile, from a micro perspective, the statistical and comparative analysis of the average household electricity consumption and wind power generation in each province in China shows regional and urban–rural development imbalances in China. There is also a large regional inconsistency between energy production and consumption. Therefore, under the carbon neutral perspective, the selection of future household energy supply paths should fully consider the characteristics of household electricity consumption in different regions, the characteristics of renewable energy distribution, and China's HDI targets.

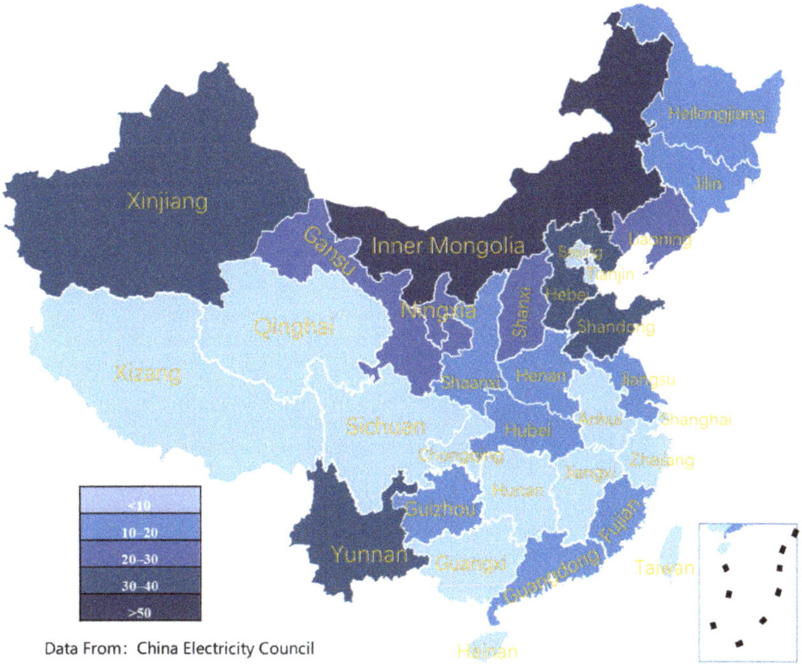

Figure 7. Superior wind power plant distribution in China until 2020.

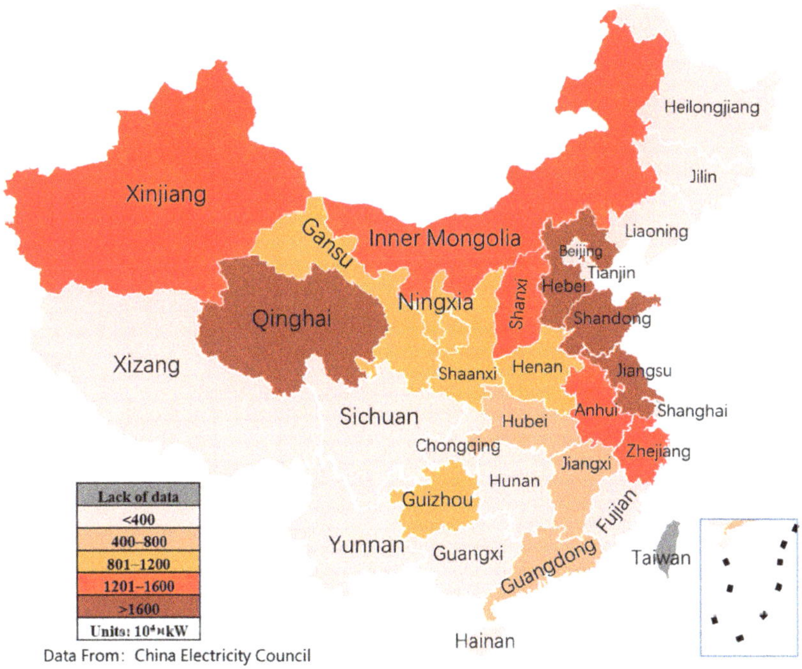

Figure 8. PV installed capacity distribution in China until 2020.

4. Characteristics of the Distributed Energy Supply System

4.1. An Alternative Future Energy System

According to the above macro and micro energy consumption and carbon emission analysis, it can be seen that carbon emission, electricity consumption, and human development index are positively correlated, while there are regional imbalance characteristics of energy consumption and production. Therefore, the development and selection of future energy systems must simultaneously consider human development, regional energy resources distribution, users' energy demand, etc. The improvement of the contradiction between carbon emission and human development is more significant for China.

Recently, the energy demands of the industry, commerce, and residential life have focused more on electricity and heat/cool. Various energy generation units provide electricity, heat, and cool. Based on the current feature of China's energy structure and future development plan, this research provides an alternative sketch of the future integrated energy system under the carbon neutral perspective shown in Figure 9. On the energy generation side, various thermal power, combined heat, and power (CHP), wind power, hydroelectric power, nuclear power, photovoltaic (PV), and solar thermal power are the main power generation ways in China, which can meet large amounts of electricity demand. There are power grid, gas network, and heat network in the energy transport processes. There are electricity, heat, and cool demands on the energy consumption side. Meanwhile, various energy storage units (such as electrochemical energy storage, mechanical energy storage, thermal energy storage, etc.), power to gas units, and electricity to heat conversion units (such as heat pump, electrical heating) are in the integrated energy system. Besides, the power generation units such as wind power and PV are also arranged on the customer side. There are two main types of energy production: centralized and distributed in the future integrated energy system. Meanwhile, the future integrated energy system can achieve efficient, flexible, safe, and stable operation by coordinating source, network, load, and storage.

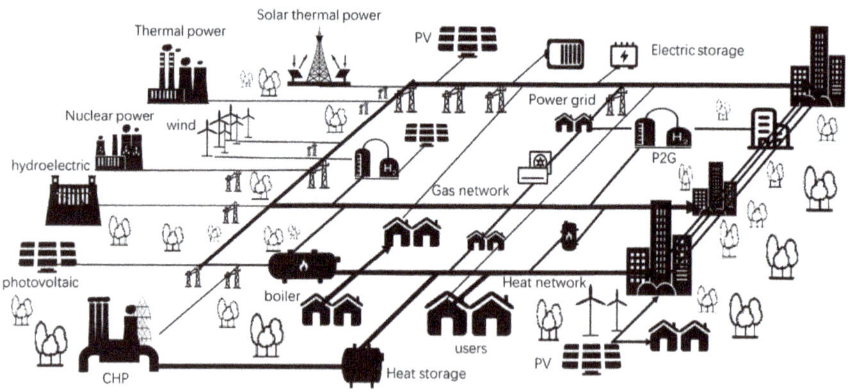

Figure 9. The sketch of the future integrated energy system.

Based on the data shown in Figure 4, China's human development needs to be further enhanced, yet the traditional centralized, fossil fuel-based approach to energy utilization needs to change under the strategy of carbon peaking and carbon neutrality in China. In the context of synergistic consideration of China's social development and carbon neutrality, an energy supply system based on renewable energy is necessary and significant. However, the imbalance characteristic between the renewable energy source and the user demands becomes the main obstacle of renewable energy utilization. Therefore, as a complement to the traditional centralized energy production methods, the development of distributed energy systems is essential to balance the regional contradictions in energy production and consumption and increase the efficient utilization of renewable energy [21,39].

Typically, distributed energy systems are placed on the customer side, and there are various types [40–44]. Therefore, the choice and construct of the distributed energy system are significant and necessary for the household energy consumption in a carbon neutral perspective for different regions in China.

4.2. Solar Energy-Based Energy Supply System

It is well known that solar energy is the most widely distributed energy. Therefore, the solar energy-based distributed energy supply system is desirable and will be a significant viable energy supply option for future household energy demand. However, due to its intermittent nature and unavailability at night, the comprehensive utilization of solar energy is provided and required to satisfy the electricity, heat/cool, and gas requirements of users. This utilization can achieve high efficiency, flexibility, low carbon, and security of the distributed energy system.

Figure 10 shows the comprehensive utilization ways of solar energy. All energy comes from the sun, and solar energy is capable of producing heat and electricity through photovoltaics (PV) and photovoltaic thermal (PVT), and fuels, such as hydrogen and methanol, through photochemistry (PC) and other technologies. In order to solve the problem of indirectness and uncertainty of solar energy, energy storage can be used through electricity storage (ES), heat storage (HS), power to gas (P2G), and other energy storage methods. Finally, it further meets the different needs of users for electricity, heat, cold, and gas through high-efficient energy conversions such as fuel cells (FC), heat pumps (HP), and air conditioners (AC). As the research from Frankea et al. [45], the interdependencies of renewable energy and flexibility options such as hydrogen and batteries may be the most cost-effective solutions for the future Chinese energy system under different scenarios. China's carbon-neutral energy system is mainly based on solar power plants that use batteries and hydrogen reconversion to meet nighttime demand.

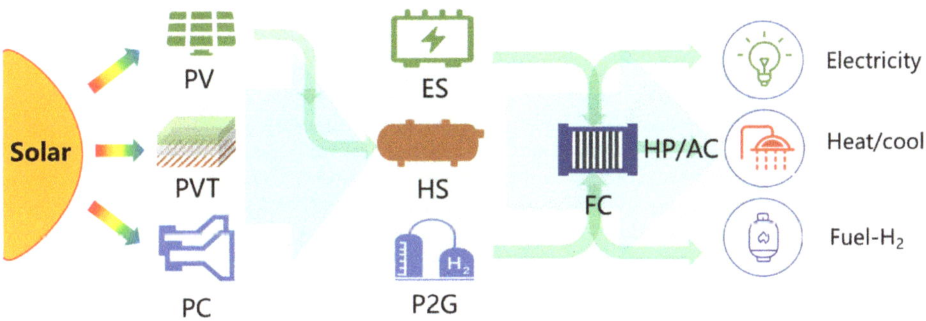

Figure 10. Comprehensive utilization ways of solar energy.

5. Two Types of Distributed Energy Systems

According to the above-mentioned distributed energy system based on solar energy utilization, photovoltaic and photovoltaic thermal utilization can generate different grades of energy such as electricity and heat to meet various needs of users. Whether in urban or rural areas, in western or eastern China regions, solar energy through building walls, house roofs, etc., is a viable way to produce energy. Therefore, the following will propose two types of typical distributed energy supply systems based on wind, photovoltaic and photovoltaic thermal utilization.

5.1. Heat Pump and PVT Integration Solutions

In remote or rural areas of western China, good wind and solar resources are shown in Figures 7 and 8. Meanwhile, the energy and electricity consumption are relatively decentralized, and the demand for electricity and heat from retail households is prominent.

Therefore, to satisfy the electricity and heat demands of households, wind turbines, PV and PVT can be integrated to form a distributed energy system with the complementary scenery. As shown in Figure 11, this distributed integrated energy system includes wind turbine power generation, photovoltaic power generation, a high-efficiency electric heating device composed of PVT and heat pump, and energy storage devices such as batteries and heat storage, which together meet the electricity and heat needs of users. For the PVT-heat pump subsystem, the working medium flows through the photovoltaic panels, which on the one hand, reduces the temperature of the photovoltaic back and improves the efficiency of photovoltaic power generation. On the other hand, the heated air goes into the evaporator of the heat pump to further enhance the electric–heat conversion coefficient of the heat pump.

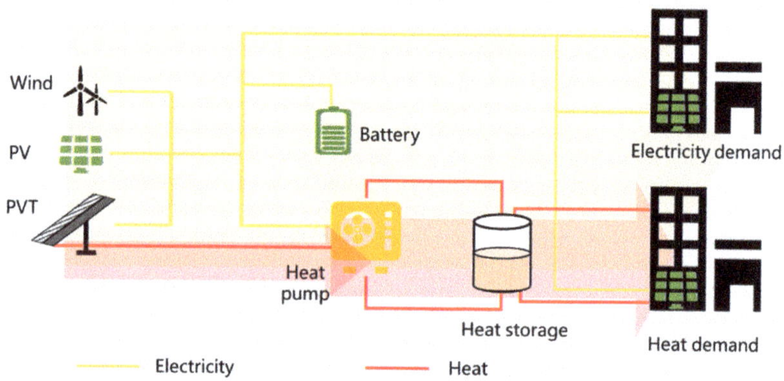

Figure 11. The integration of heat pump, wind, PV, PVT, and energy storage units.

Meanwhile, energy storage is significant for this distributed energy system, including electricity and heat storage devices. The electricity storage equipment can be electrochemical batteries to improve user-side wind power and photovoltaic power generation. In addition, the thermal storage equipment can be water storage or ice storage to meet the different thermal needs of users. That is, this electricity and heat storage device ensures the stable electricity and heat output of this distributed energy system and guarantees the energy demand of customers without carbon emissions.

5.2. Fuel Cells and PVT Integration Solutions

Unlike the western areas in China, wind power resources are relatively scarce in the eastern or coastal areas, as shown in Figure 7. Therefore, solar energy should be better utilized in household energy consumption. Due to the intermittent nature of solar energy utilization, a certain amount of energy storage technology is required to guarantee the stability and reliability of energy consumption by users. In addition, solar energy should be stored directly as electricity or converted into fuels, such as hydrogen and methane.

Therefore, this research proposes an alternative distributed energy system containing PV, PVT, and fuel cells shown in Figure 12. The fuel cell is a high-efficiency combined heat and power generation technology [46,47]. Among them, building PV and PVT can be used to generate electricity. Using natural gas and solar fuel, etc., the combined heat and power supply is carried out by means of fuel cells. For example, fuel cells can use solar fuel (natural gas or hydrogen) to directly convert the chemical energy of the fuel into electricity without producing mission pollutants and can provide both electricity and heat with an efficiency of over 80%. The combination of PVT and heat pump can improve the coefficient of performance of the heat pump that produces the heat for users. Besides, batteries and heat storage are introduced to overcome the temporal mismatches between the solar energy distribution and the electricity and heat needs of the users.

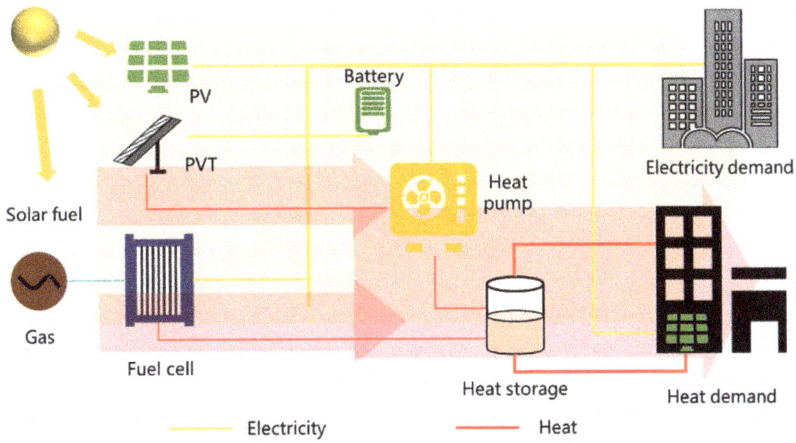

Figure 12. The integration of PV, PVT, FC, and energy storage units.

Figures 11 and 12 propose two types of distributed energy supply systems based on wind power and solar power, so they do not have carbon emissions. Meanwhile, these two types of distributed energy supply systems are two possible conceptual solutions based on the basic situation of renewable energy distribution and household energy consumption in China and are not real systems. However, they provide a feasible reference for the design of real systems in the future. In the future, we still need to plan and design, working conditions optimization and operational control from the technical and economic point of view for the actual user needs and the geographical characteristics of the location.

6. Conclusions

In the context of carbon neutrality, making full use of renewable energy is key to further improving China's human development index. To improve China's HDI under the carbon neutrality constraint, effectively reducing household energy consumption and selecting appropriate household energy supply options are significant. Therefore, this research obtained some conclusions

(1) This contribution analyzed the proportion of installed capacity of thermal, hydropower, nuclear, wind, and photovoltaic power, and firstly proposed and calculated the annual average power generation utilization, annual per capita power generation, carbon emission, and human development index in China in the past four decades, and concluded the positive correlation between energy consumption, carbon emission and social development from a macro perspective.

(2) Based on the 2015 Chinese General Social Survey (CGSS-2015) data, we analyzed the average electrical energy consumption of urban and rural households in 28 provinces across China from a micro perspective. The results show regional imbalance characteristics between household electricity consumption and renewable energy distribution characteristics in China.

(3) In order to better consume renewable energy and promote the carbon neutral strategy, this paper proposes that distributed energy supply system is a feasible option as an effective complement to the centralized power generation system based on the distribution of household energy consumption and scenic resources in the mid-western and eastern regions.

(4) Two types of typical distributed energy supply systems can be provided by integrating efficient energy conversion, storage, and exchange devices, such as electric heat pumps, PV, PVT, heat storage, electricity storage, and fuel cells, all of which are clean, efficient, low-carbon, and safe. In conclusion, the proposed two distributed energy systems can achieve carbon neutrality while meeting the energy needs of households.

Author Contributions: Conceptualization, Y.Z.; Data curation, S.W.; Formal analysis, Y.Z.; Funding acquisition, Y.Z.; Methodology, Y.Z.; Writing—original draft, Y.Z.; Writing—review & editing, W.S.; visualization, J.H. All authors have read and agreed to the published version of the manuscript.

Funding: The research is support by Capacity Building of Science and Technology Innovation Services Basic Research Operation Fund (PXM2020_014213_000017) and Research Foundation for Youth Scholars of Beijing Technology and Business University (QNJJ2020-150).

Institutional Review Board Statement: Not applicable.

Informed Consent Statement: Not applicable.

Data Availability Statement: Restrictions apply to the availability of these data. Data was obtained from Chinese General Social Survey and are available at http://cgss.ruc.edu.cn/ with the permission of Chinese General Social Survey.

Conflicts of Interest: The authors declare no conflict of interest.

References

1. Xie, Y.; Liu, X.; Chen, Q.; Zhang, S. An integrated assessment for achieving the 2 C target pathway in China by 2030. *J. Clean. Prod.* **2020**, *268*, 122238. [CrossRef]
2. Wang, Q.; Su, M.; Li, R. Toward to economic growth without emission growth: The role of urbanization and industrialization in China and India. *J. Clean. Prod.* **2018**, *205*, 499–511. [CrossRef]
3. Tahir, M.F.; Haoyong, C.; Mehmood, K.; Ali, N.; Bhutto, J.A. Integrated energy system modeling of China for 2020 by incorporating demand response, heat pump and thermal storage. *IEEE Access* **2019**, *7*, 40095–40108. [CrossRef]
4. Pehl, M.; Arvesen, A.; Humpenöder, F.; Popp, A.; Hertwich, E.G.; Luderer, G. Understanding future emissions from low-carbon power systems by integration of life-cycle assessment and integrated energy modelling. *Nat. Energy* **2017**, *2*, 939–945. [CrossRef]
5. Liu, L.; Zhou, C.; Huang, J.; Hao, Y. The impact of financial development on energy demand: Evidence from China. *Emerg. Mark. Financ. Trade* **2018**, *54*, 269–287. [CrossRef]
6. Li, L.; Mu, H.; Li, N.; Li, M. Economic and environmental optimization for distributed energy resource systems coupled with district energy networks. *Energy* **2016**, *109*, 947–960. [CrossRef]
7. Huang, J.; Shen, J.; Miao, L. Carbon emissions trading and sustainable development in China: Empirical analysis based on the coupling coordination degree model. *Int. J. Environ. Res. Public Health* **2021**, *18*, 89. [CrossRef]
8. Jing-Yue, L.; Yue-Jun, Z. Has carbon emissions trading system promoted non-fossil energy development in China? *Appl. Energy* **2021**, *302*, 117613. [CrossRef]
9. Li, L.; Yu, S. Optimal management of multi-stakeholder distributed energy systems in low-carbon communities considering demand response resources and carbon tax. *Sustain. Cities Soc.* **2020**, *61*, 102230. [CrossRef]
10. Zhao, N.; You, F. Can renewable generation, energy storage and energy efficient technologies enable carbon neutral energy transition? *Appl. Energy* **2020**, *279*, 115889. [CrossRef]
11. Hong, B.; Li, Q.; Chen, W.; Huang, B.; Yan, H.; Feng, K. Supply modes for renewable-based distributed energy systems and their applications: Case studies in China. *Glob. Energy Interconnect.* **2020**, *3*, 259–271. [CrossRef]
12. Sun, L.; Hu, J.; Jin, H. Research and Application of Distributed Energy Integration Optimization for Sino-German Building in the Cold Area of China. *IFAC-Pap.* **2018**, *51*, 90–95. [CrossRef]
13. Jia, X.; Du, H.; Zou, H.; He, G. Assessing the effectiveness of China's net-metering subsidies for household distributed photovoltaic systems. *J. Clean. Prod.* **2020**, *262*, 121161. [CrossRef]
14. Yang, Y.; Campana, P.E.; Yan, J. Potential of unsubsidized distributed solar PV to replace coal-fired power plants, and profits classification in Chinese cities. *Renew. Sustain. Energy Rev.* **2020**, *131*, 109967. [CrossRef]
15. Wang, Y.; He, J.; Chen, W. Distributed solar photovoltaic development potential and a roadmap at the city level in China. *Renew. Sustain. Energy Rev.* **2021**, *141*, 110772. [CrossRef]
16. Krarti, M.; Aldubyan, M. Role of energy efficiency and distributed renewable energy in designing carbon neutral residential buildings and communities: Case study of Saudi Arabia. *Energy Build.* **2021**, *250*, 111309. [CrossRef]
17. Huo, T.; Xu, L.; Feng, W.; Cai, W.; Liu, B. Dynamic scenario simulations of carbon emission peak in China's city-scale urban residential building sector through 2050. *Energy Policy* **2021**, *159*, 112612. [CrossRef]

18. Zhang, F.; Deng, H.; Margolis, R.; Su, J. Analysis of distributed-generation photovoltaic deployment, installation time and cost, market barriers, and policies in China. *Energy Policy* **2015**, *81*, 43–55. [CrossRef]
19. Zhao, X.; Zeng, Y.; Zhao, D. Distributed solar photovoltaics in China: Policies and economic performance. *Energy* **2015**, *88*, 572–583. [CrossRef]
20. Duan, H.-B.; Zhang, G.-P.; Zhu, L.; Fan, Y.; Wang, S.-Y. How will diffusion of PV solar contribute to China's emissions-peaking and climate responses? *Renew. Sustain. Energy Rev.* **2016**, *53*, 1076–1085. [CrossRef]
21. Ming, Z.; Shaojie, O.; Hui, S.; Yujian, G.; Qiqi, Q. Overall review of distributed energy development in China: Status quo, barriers and solutions. *Renew. Sustain. Energy Rev.* **2015**, *50*, 1226–1238. [CrossRef]
22. Sameti, M.; Haghighat, F. Integration of distributed energy storage into net-zero energy district systems: Optimum design and operation. *Energy* **2018**, *153*, 575–591. [CrossRef]
23. Ren, H.; Zhou, W.; Gao, W. Optimal option of distributed energy systems for building complexes in different climate zones in China. *Appl. Energy* **2012**, *91*, 156–165. [CrossRef]
24. Huang, X.; Ouyang, S.; Ma, S. A Practical Classification Evaluation Approach for Comprehensive Competitiveness of Distributed Energy Supply Systems. *IOP Conf. Ser. Earth Environ. Sci.* **2018**, *168*, 012041. [CrossRef]
25. Yoon, G.; Naruse, K. Evaluation of the feasibility of distributed energy supply system for existing multi-family housing in Nagoya City. *IOP Conf. Ser. Earth Environ. Sci.* **2019**, *238*, 012058. [CrossRef]
26. Zhu, X.; Yang, J.; Pan, X.; Li, G.; Rao, Y. Regional integrated energy system energy management in an industrial park considering energy stepped utilization. *Energy* **2020**, *201*, 117589. [CrossRef]
27. Zhang, Y.; Hao, J.; Ge, Z.; Zhang, F.; Du, X. Optimal clean heating mode of the integrated electricity and heat energy system considering the comprehensive energy-carbon price. *Energy* **2021**, *231*, 120919. [CrossRef]
28. Luo, X.; Liu, Y.; Liu, J.; Liu, X. Energy scheduling for a three-level integrated energy system based on energy hub models: A hierarchical Stackelberg game approach. *Sustain. Cities Soc.* **2020**, *52*, 101814. [CrossRef]
29. Hu, Z.; Wang, M.; Cheng, Z.; Yang, Z. Impact of marginal and intergenerational effects on carbon emissions from household energy consumption in China. *J. Clean. Prod.* **2020**, *273*, 123022. [CrossRef]
30. Wang, Q.; Jiang, R. Is carbon emission growth decoupled from economic growth in emerging countries? New insights from labor and investment effects. *J. Clean. Prod.* **2020**, *248*, 119188. [CrossRef]
31. Zhang, J.; Teng, F.; Zhou, S. The structural changes and determinants of household energy choices and energy consumption in urban China: Addressing the role of building type. *Energy Policy* **2020**, *139*, 111314. [CrossRef]
32. Han, X.; Wei, C. Household energy consumption: State of the art, research gaps, and future prospects. *Environ. Dev. Sustain.* **2021**, *23*, 12479–12504. [CrossRef]
33. Wu, S.; Zheng, X.; You, C.; Wei, C. Household energy consumption in rural China: Historical development, present pattern and policy implication. *J. Clean. Prod.* **2019**, *211*, 981–991. [CrossRef]
34. Zou, B.; Luo, B. Rural household energy consumption characteristics and determinants in China. *Energy* **2019**, *182*, 814–823. [CrossRef]
35. Ren, L.; Wang, W.; Wang, J.; Liu, R. Analysis of energy consumption and carbon emission during the urbanization of Shandong Province, China. *J. Clean. Prod.* **2015**, *103*, 534–541. [CrossRef]
36. Chen, H.; Yang, L.; Chen, W. Modelling national, provincial and city-level low-carbon energy transformation pathways. *Energy Policy* **2020**, *137*, 111096. [CrossRef]
37. Zhang, J.; Li, F.; Sun, M.; Sun, S.; Wang, H.; Zheng, P.; Wang, R. Household consumption characteristics and energy-related carbon emissions estimation at the community scale: A study of Zengcheng, China. *Clean. Responsible Consum.* **2021**, *2*, 100016. [CrossRef]
38. Hossain, M.A.; Chen, S. Nexus between Human Development Index (HDI) and CO_2 emissions in a developing country: Decoupling study evidence from Bangladesh. *Environ. Sci. Pollut. Res.* **2021**, *28*, 58742–58754. [CrossRef]
39. Wen, Q.; Liu, G.; Rao, Z.; Liao, S. Applications, evaluations and supportive strategies of distributed energy systems: A review. *Energy Build.* **2020**, *225*, 110314. [CrossRef]
40. Liu, Z.; Fan, G.; Sun, D.; Wu, D.; Guo, J.; Zhang, S.; Yang, X.; Lin, X.; Ai, L. A novel distributed energy system combining hybrid energy storage and a multi-objective optimization method for nearly zero-energy communities and buildings. *Energy* **2021**, 122577. [CrossRef]
41. Sun, X.; Zhong, X.; Wang, C.; Zhou, T. Simulation research on distributed energy system based on coupling of PV/T unit and wind-to-heat unit. *Sol. Energy* **2021**, *230*, 843–858. [CrossRef]
42. Hao, J.; Chen, Q.; He, K.; Chen, L.; Dai, Y.; Xu, F.; Min, Y. A heat current model for heat transfer/storage systems and its application in integrated analysis and optimization with power systems. *IEEE Trans. Sustain. Energy* **2020**, *11*, 175–184. [CrossRef]
43. Wang, Y.; Zhang, Y.; Hao, J.; Pan, H.; Ni, Y.; Di, J.; Ge, Z.; Chen, Q.; Guo, M. Modeling and operation optimization of an integrated ground source heat pump and solar PVT system based on heat current method. *Sol. Energy* **2021**, *218*, 492–502. [CrossRef]
44. Zhang, Y.; Xiong, N.; Ge, Z.; Zhang, Y.; Hao, J.; Yang, Z. A novel cascade heating system for waste heat recovery in the combined heat and power plant integrating with the steam jet pump. *Appl. Energy* **2020**, *278*, 115690. [CrossRef]
45. Franke, K.; Sensfuß, F.; Bernath, C.; Lux, B. Carbon-neutral energy systems and the importance of flexibility options: A case study in China. *Comput. Ind. Eng.* **2021**, *162*, 107712. [CrossRef]

46. Olabi, A.; Wilberforce, T.; Abdelkareem, M.A. Fuel cell application in the automotive industry and future perspective. *Energy* **2021**, *214*, 118955. [CrossRef]
47. Manoharan, Y.; Hosseini, S.E.; Butler, B.; Alzhahrani, H.; Senior, B.T.F.; Ashuri, T.; Krohn, J. Hydrogen fuel cell vehicles; current status and future prospect. *Appl. Sci.* **2019**, *9*, 2296. [CrossRef]

International Journal of
Environmental Research and Public Health

MDPI

Article

Effects of Elevation and Distance from Highway on the Abundance and Community Structure of Bacteria in Soil along Qinghai-Tibet Highway

Zhuocheng Liu [1,2], Yangang Yang [2], Shuangxuan Ji [1,2], Di Dong [1], Yinruizhi Li [1], Mengdi Wang [1], Liebao Han [1,*] and Xueping Chen [2,*]

1 School of Grassland Science, Beijing Forestry University, Beijing 100083, China; liuzhuocheng@bjfu.edu.cn (Z.L.); jsx11223345@163.com (S.J.); didoscori@163.com (D.D.); liyinruizhi@163.com (Y.L.); mengdi0627@163.com (M.W.)
2 Environmental Protection and Soil and Water Conservation Research Center, China Academy of Transportation Sciences, Beijing 100029, China; Ecologyoung@126.com
* Correspondence: hanliebao@163.com (L.H.); chenxueping@vip.sina.com (X.C.)

Abstract: In recent years, highway construction in the Qinghai-Tibet Plateau (QTP) has developed rapidly. When the highway passes through grassland, the soil, vegetation, and ecological environment along the line are disturbed. However, the impact on soil bacteria is still unclear. Soil bacteria play an important role in the ecological environment. The Qinghai-Tibet Highway (QTH) was selected as the research object to explore the changes in bacterial community structure, vegetation, soil, and other indicators. The results showed that the highway-related activities increased the degradation of vegetation along the road, significantly changed the physical and chemical properties of soil, and caused heavy metal pollution. These environmental factors affected the diversity and community structure of soil bacteria. This kind of disturbance shows a trend of gradually increasing from near to far from the highway. *Gemmatimonas*, *Terrimonas*, *Nitrospira* and *Bacillus* are more tolerant to environmental changes along the highway, while *Barnesiella*, and *Blastococcus* are more sensitive. The content of nitrate decreased and the content of ammonium nitrogen increased in the disturbed area, increasing the abundance of nitrifying bacteria. Therefore, the main factor of the disturbance of the QTH on the grassland is the decline of soil nutrient content, and the supplement of soil nutrients such as carbon and nitrogen should be taken into account in the process of ecological restoration of grassland along the line.

Keywords: Qinghai-Tibet Plateau; plant community structure; bacterial community structure; heavy metals; Tibet Highway

Citation: Liu, Z.; Yang, Y.; Ji, S.; Dong, D.; Li, Y.; Wang, M.; Han, L.; Chen, X. Effects of Elevation and Distance from Highway on the Abundance and Community Structure of Bacteria in Soil along Qinghai-Tibet Highway. *Int. J. Environ. Res. Public Health* **2021**, *18*, 13137. https://doi.org/10.3390/ijerph182413137

Academic Editors: Roberto Alonso González Lezcano, Francesco Nocera and Rosa Giuseppina Caponetto

Received: 5 November 2021
Accepted: 4 December 2021
Published: 13 December 2021

1. Introduction

As the highest geographical unit in the world, the Qinghai-Tibet Plateau (QTP) has a particular and representative ecological environment. The QTP is of great significance to global climate change, carbon cycle, and biological germplasm resources [1–4]. As a fragile ecosystem, the QTP ecosystem is particularly vulnerable to human activities [5,6]. In recent years, with the rapid economic development of the Qinghai-Tibet region, road transportation has also continued to develop [7,8]. The total length of highways in the Tibet Autonomous Region increased from 15,852 km in 1978 to 117,000 km in 2021 [9]. Highway traffic inevitably disturbs natural grasslands and has a series of negative influences on the ecosystem, including soil erosion, vegetation destruction, and water quality deterioration [10–13]. The sharp increase in negative impacts has resulted in imbalances in the self-regulation of the grassland ecosystem, and varying degrees of degradation of grasslands along highways [14].

As an important part of the ecosystem, soil microorganisms participate in the degradation of organic matter, biogeochemical cycles, and the maintenance of soil structure and are closely related to the degradation of grassland ecosystems [15]. In natural grassland, vegetation growth, soil nutrients, moisture, pH value, etc. determine the community composition and structure of soil microorganisms [16,17]. In addition, it changes with depth due to factors such as redox conditions and soil nutrients. In the QTP, soil microorganisms are mainly distributed in the topsoil (0–20 cm) [18]. Many scholars point out that soil bacterial communities are extremely sensitive to human activities [19]. However, the response of soil bacterial communities to environmental changes resulting from road traffic is currently unclear.

Road traffic and construction will produce different types of heavy metal pollutants [20,21]. The components, fuels, and lubricants of vehicles and paving materials may contain heavy metals such as copper, copper, lead, zinc, and cadmium [22]. The burning of liquid fuels, the use of lubricating oil, the wear of vehicles and the loss of pavement will bring in heavy metal ion particles. These particles enter the ecosystem on both sides of the road, possibly through sedimentation pavement runoff and splashing [23]. Studies have shown that the concentrations of heavy metals in soil were significantly affected by road construction and traffic. The degree of impact is inversely proportional to the distance from the road [24,25]. Many studies have shown that the deposition of heavy metal pollutants in soil will affect the composition and structure of soil bacterial communities [26,27]. Additionally, soil nutrient content is another important factor affecting soil bacterial communities. Road construction and traffic drainage will cause varying degrees of soil erosion, topsoil stripping, and other changes. Many studies have shown that soil erosion can change physical and chemical properties such as soil density, soil moisture, and pH, leading to soil nutrient loss [28,29]. As the mediator of more than 90% of the energy and material exchange in the soil ecosystem, the bacterial community structure is bound to be affected to varying degrees [30].

In general, exploration of the influences of soil nutrient changes and heavy metal on the structure of soil bacteria communities can provide data support for grassland ecological restoration along the highway, and can also provide a decision for road construction in the QTP. The Qinghai-Tibet Highway (QTH) provides favorable conditions for exploring the relationship between the highway and soil microorganisms [25]. The grassland ecosystems in most areas along the route are well preserved, are very sensitive to external influences, and have poor natural recovery capabilities [21]. As an uninhabited area and nature reserve, there is almost no human disturbance in this area except for traffic [31,32]. The Golmud-Lhasa section of the QTH passes through areas of different altitudes, climates, soil types, and vegetation types. We assume that the QTH has an impact on the structure of the grassland soil bacterial community by changing soil and heavy metals factors. In this study, treatments at different distances from the highway and altitude were selected, and the bacterial communities along the QTH were determined by high-throughput sequencing technology. The results showed that: (1) The soil bacterial community structure changes with the distance from the QTH; (2) In high altitude areas, the soil bacterial community is more susceptible to highway impacts; (3) Soil nutrients are the main driving factor of soil bacterial community structure change; (4) Within a certain distance from the QTH, the heavy metal content was correlated with soil bacterial community diversity.

2. Materials and Methods

2.1. Study Area and Sampling Lines

This study selects the QTH (G109 National Highway) Golmud to Lhasa section as the research object. The region where the QTH passes through has a temperate/sub-frigid continental climate, with long and cold winters, strong winds, little rain in summer, and short spring and autumn. This section of the highway crosses two major soil types: alpine prairie soils (Cryuborolls) and alpine meadow soils (Cryaquet) and a small portion of gray-brown desert soils (Gypsic Haplosalid). In this area, the highway passes through the Hoh Xil National Nature Reserve and the Sanjiangyuan Nature Reserve. There is no large-scale agriculture, animal husbandry, and manufacturing industries, and the natural grassland is less affected except for the highway. The effect of traffic activity on the deposition of soil pollutants was stronger closer to the road and weakened with the increase of distance from the road [25,32]. Therefore, a plot 400 m from the highway was collected as a control in each area that may not be affected by traffic activity.

More than 91% of the studied sections have an altitude of >4000 m, and the highest altitude is 5231 m, which is located at Tanggula Mountain Pass. In this study, 3 sampling zones at 4000 m, 4600 m, and 5231 m were selected, and one sampling zone was set in an area within 400 m of each altitude where there were no other human influence factors except roads (sampling zone 35°47′ N, 94°20′ E; sampling line 2 at 34°27′ N, 92°44′ E; sampling zone 3 at 32°53′ N, 91°55′ E). The sampling lines were perpendicular to the highway and is 400 m long and 10 m wide (Figure 1). The altitude drop in the sampling zone is less than 30 m. For each sampling zone, 4 plots were set at a distance of 5 m, 20 m, 50 m, and 100 m away from the highway shoulder, and 1 plot was set at a distance of 400 m from the shoulder, which was used as a control plot. Four samples of 1 m × 1 m are randomly set for each plot.

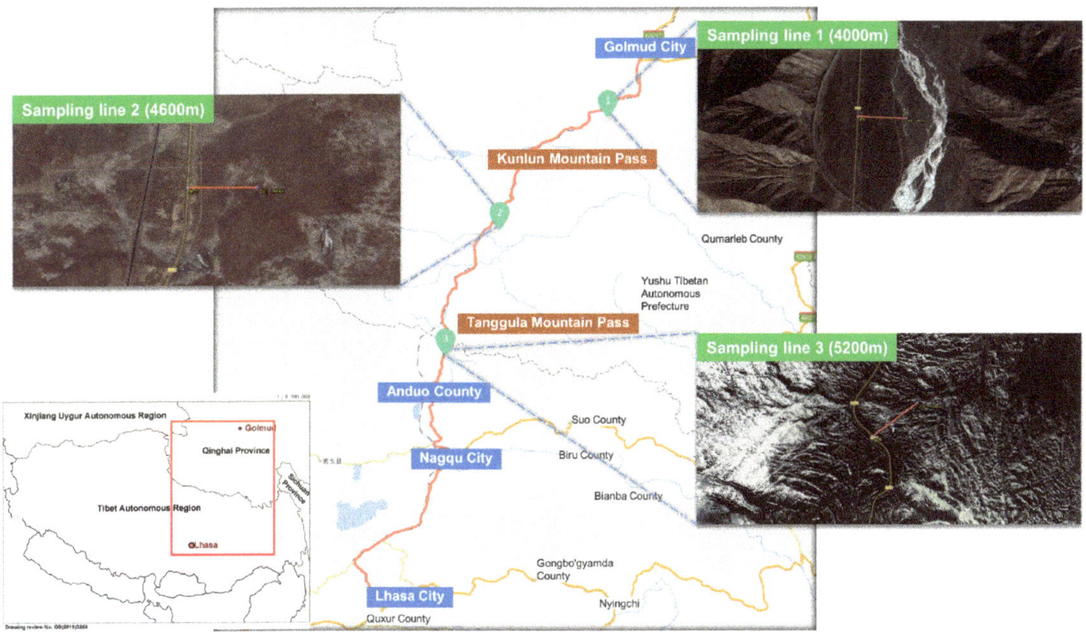

Figure 1. Sampling sites along the Qinghai–Tibet highway, China.

2.2. Vegetation Samples

In each plot, we investigated plant species, abundance, height, coverage and other indicators, and calculate important values. Species diversity is measured by species richness index and Shannon diversity index. All the above-ground parts of the sample were collected to determine the above-ground biomass.

2.3. Soil Sampling

July is the growing season for plateau vegetation. The middle of July 2019 was selected as the time of soil sample collection. Use a thermometer to measure the soil temperature before sampling. The soil density was determined by a soil compaction meter (TJSD-7500II). Soil samples were collected using a soil auger with a diameter of 5 cm and a sampling depth of 0–20 cm. Ten soil cores were evenly distributed in each quadrat. Five plots were set for each site. Four quadrats were set for each plot for repetition, and 5 times of sampling were set in each quadrat for mixing. Thus, a total of 15 treatments were set and 60 soil samples were collected.

After removing the rocks and grass roots, the sample is thoroughly mixed and passed through a 2 mm sieve. Approximately 5 g of samples were immediately put in a 2 mL centrifuge tube and brought back at low temperature, and kept in a refrigerator at −80 °C for DNA analysis. About 300 g samples were sealed and brought back into the refrigerator at 4 °C for soil physical and chemical analysis. About 1000 g of Soil samples are dried for soil nutrient and heavy metal analysis. During the entire collection and processing of soil samples, bacteria and heavy metal contamination should be avoided.

2.4. Soil Laboratory Analysis

Chemical Analysis

Soil pH was determined by mixing the soil sample and water in a ratio of 1:5 using a pH meter. Soil organic C content was determined by a potassium dichromate external heating method [33]. Soil total N was determined by Kjeldahl digestion and automatic azotometer [34]. Soil alkali-hydrolytic nitrogen, total nitrogen, available P, and available K were determined by the method of previous studies [35,36].

The contents of Cu and Zn in the soil were determined by flame atomic absorption spectrophotometry. The main instrument is a TAS-990F atomic absorption spectrophotometer. Soil Pb and Cd contents were determined by graphite furnace atomic absorption spectrophotometry using a 240ZAA atomic absorption spectrophotometer [37].

2.5. DNA Extraction, PCR Amplification

According to the manufacturer's instructions, use the Fast DNA SPIN Kit for Soil (DNeasy PowerSoil Kit, QIAGEN, Hilden, Germany) to extract total soil DNA. Finally, the DNA was eluted with 100 μL DNA eluent in the kit. Dilute the successfully extracted DNA to a concentration of 1 ng/μL and store at −20 °C until further processing.

The barcoded primers and Takara Ex Taq (Takara) were used to amplify the *16S rRNA* genes of bacteria using the diluted DNA as a template, and V3-V4 variable regions of *16S rRNA* genes were amplified with universal primers 343F and 798R for bacterial diversity analysis [38]. To verify the size and quality of the PCR products, all of them were electrophoresed in 1.5% (wt/vol) agarose [39,40].

2.6. Cloning, Sequencing and Phylogenetic Analysis

The quality of the amplicons was visualized using gel electrophoresis, purified with AMPure XP beads (Agencourt), and subjected to another round of PCR amplification. After purification again using AM-Pure XP magnetic beads, the final amplicons were quantified using the Qubit dsDNA Detection Kit. Equal amounts of purified amplicons were pooled for subsequent sequencing [41,42].

The raw sequencing data were in FASTQ format [43]. Pre-processing of double-ended reads, including detection and cleavage of ambiguous bases (N), was performed using Trimmomatic software (Bolger AM: Golm, Brandenburg, Germany) [44]. Low-quality sequences with an average quality score below 20 were cut off using the sliding window pruning method [40]. Parameters of assembly were: 10 bp of minimal overlapping, 200 bp of maximum overlapping, and 20% of maximum mismatch rate. Assembly parameters were: minimum overlap of 10 bp, maximum overlap of 200 bp, and maximum mismatch of 20%. Reads with 75% of bases above Q20 were retained. Reads with chimeras were then detected and deleted. QIIME software (version 1.8.0, Caporaso JG: Boulder, CO, USA) was used to implement the above two steps [45].

Using the Vsearch software (Edgar RC: Cambridge, MD, USA) with 97% similarity threshold, the clean readings were generated by primer sequencing and clustering to generate surgical taxons (OTUs) [46]. We used the QIIME package to choose a representative reading for each OTU; the RDP classifier (confidence threshold 70%) to annotate all representative readings and annotate the Silva database version 123 (*16s rDNA*) [42]; and the blast to annotate all representative reads and blast the Unite database (ITSs rDNA) [43].

2.7. Statistical Analyses

Statistical analysis software such as Excel 2010 (Microsoft: Seattle, WA, USA) and SPSS 22 (International Business Machines Corporation: Armonk, NY, USA) were used to arrange and plot the measured data. The data were analyzed by Microsoft Excel 2010, and the differences of vegetation data, soil physical, and chemical properties and soil bacterial diversity index were analyzed by One-way ANOVA in SPSS 22. R 3.5.2 was used to perform analyses of species composition and diversity, non-metric multidimensional scaling (NMDS), Adonis and Mantel tests. The OmicShare tool was used to perform the FAPROTAX analysis (https://www.omicshare.com/tools, accessed on 10 September 2021).

3. Results

3.1. Environmental Factors

The coverage in the area within 100 m from the highway reduced more significantly than the control (400 m) at three sites (Figure 2B). The coverage at 20 m decreased by 64.44% (0.20), 67.24% (0.24) and 64.86% (0.33) in 4000 m, 4600 m and 5200 m sites, respectively. The aboveground biomass was negatively correlated with distance in three sites. The aboveground biomass decreased significantly within 100 m, 50 m, and 100 m from the road, respectively (Figure 2A). The plant Shannon index decreased significantly in 4000 m and 5200 m sites within 20 m from the highway and decreased significantly at the 4600 m site within 50 m from the highway. For the plots 20 m away from the highway, the values decreased by 28.14% (1.62), 14.05% (1.56), and 28.80% (1.21) compared with the control (400 m) in 4000 m, 4600 m, and 5200 m sites, respectively (Figure 2C). The Simpson index (Figure 2D) of plants also shows similar changes in the areas close to the road (50 m, 20 m, and 5 m plots). Compared with the control (400 m), the plants' heights were significantly higher. The increase ranges were 561.17% (35.59 cm), 250.46% (16.15 cm) and 59.38% (8.54 cm).

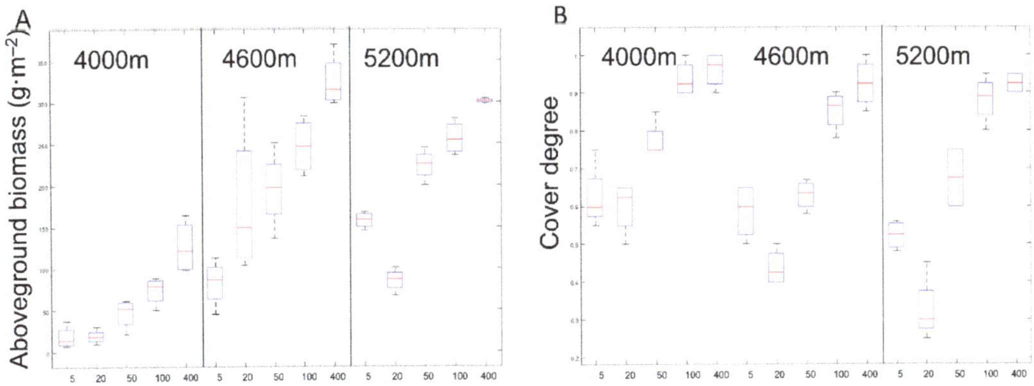

Figure 2. *Cont.*

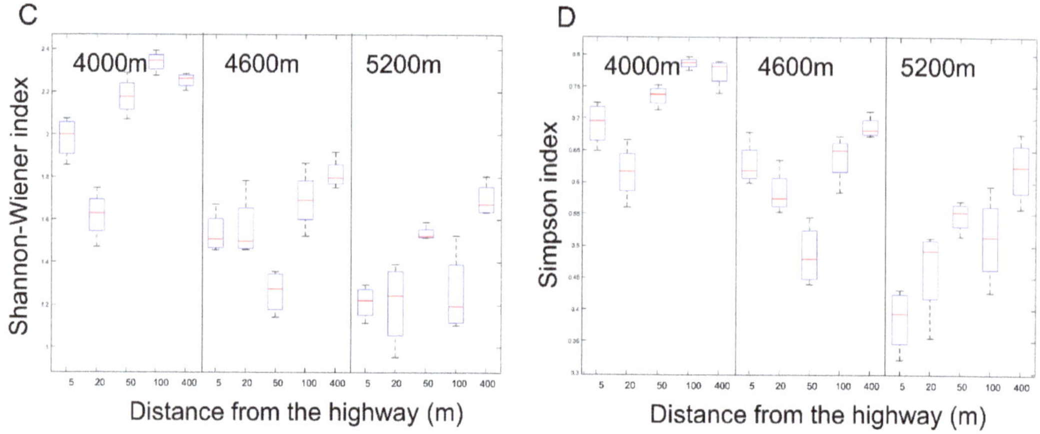

Figure 2. Comparison of (**A**) above-ground biomass, (**B**) plant cover degree, (**C**) plant simpson and (**D**) above-ground biomass between treatments at 5, 20, 50, 100 and 400 m from the curb G109 highways at altitudes of 4000 m (L), 4600 m (M) and 5200 m (H).

The soil moisture (SM) was significantly reduced by 58.63%, 38.45%, and 73.04% within 100 m along the highway at 20 m plots from the highway in 4000 m, 4600 m, and 5200 m sites, respectively (Figure 3A). In the 5200 m site, soil pH significantly decreased by 6.26%, 6.07%, 3.47%, and 2.11% at 5 m, 20 m, 50 m, and 100 m from the road, respectively (Figure 3B). At the same time, smaller changes occurred at 4000 m and 4600 m, with only significant decreases of 2.75% and 1.29% at 5 m from the road, respectively. The soil temperature in the areas 100 m and 50 m away from the highway decreased significantly compared with the control, 4000 m site and 5200 m site, respectively (Figure 3C). Soil compaction only changed significantly at 5200 m and decreased by 9. 14% (1715.75 Pa) and 5.69% (1780.75 Pa) at 5 m and 20 m away from the road, respectively (Figure 3D).

SOC is negatively related to the distance from the road. This trend is most obvious at 5200 m (Figure 4A). Roads significantly reduced soil organic carbon by 33.85% (.84 $g \cdot kg^{-1}$), 36.43% (8.49 $g \cdot kg^{-1}$), and 32.72% (8.99 $g \cdot kg^{-1}$) at plots 5 m, 50 m, and 100 m away from the road, respectively. Soil organic carbon content decreased by 70.19% (8.35 $g \cdot kg^{-1}$) and 66.01% (9.52 $g \cdot kg^{-1}$) at 5 m and 20 m plots from the road, respectively, compared with the control (400 m) at 5200 m. Soil total nitrogen content decreased by 67. 48%, 60.98%, 19.86% and 21.12% at 5 m, 20 m, 50 m, and 100 m away from the highway, respectively (Figure 4B). In the 4600 m site, soil total nitrogen content significantly decreased by 27.17% at 20 m from the road. At the same time, the change of soil total nitrogen content was not significant at the 4000 m site. The change trend of alkali-hydrolyzable nitrogen (AN) was the same as TN in the 5200 m site (Figure 4C). The difference is that angle in which the content of soil AN decreased significantly became within 50 m from the road. On the contrary, at the site of 4600 m, the content of soil AN at 5 m plot away from the road was significantly increased by 16.36% (67.02 $mg \cdot kg^{-1}$) compared with the control (400 m). At the same time, at the site of 4000 m, the content of soil AP (Figure 4D) at the plot of 20 m from the road was significantly increased by 30.34% (80.00 $mg \cdot kg^{-1}$) compared with the control (400 m). In 5200 m site, the content of soil available phosphorus increased by 119.04% (4.80 $mg \cdot kg^{-1}$) and 198.97% (6.56 $mg \cdot kg^{-1}$) at 5 m and 20 m distance respectively. The content of soil available phosphorus increased at the distance of 50 m (56.15%) and 20 m (169.42%) from the highway, and at the distance of 4000 m and 4600 m, respectively. The change of soil AK with distance was not significant (Figure 4E).

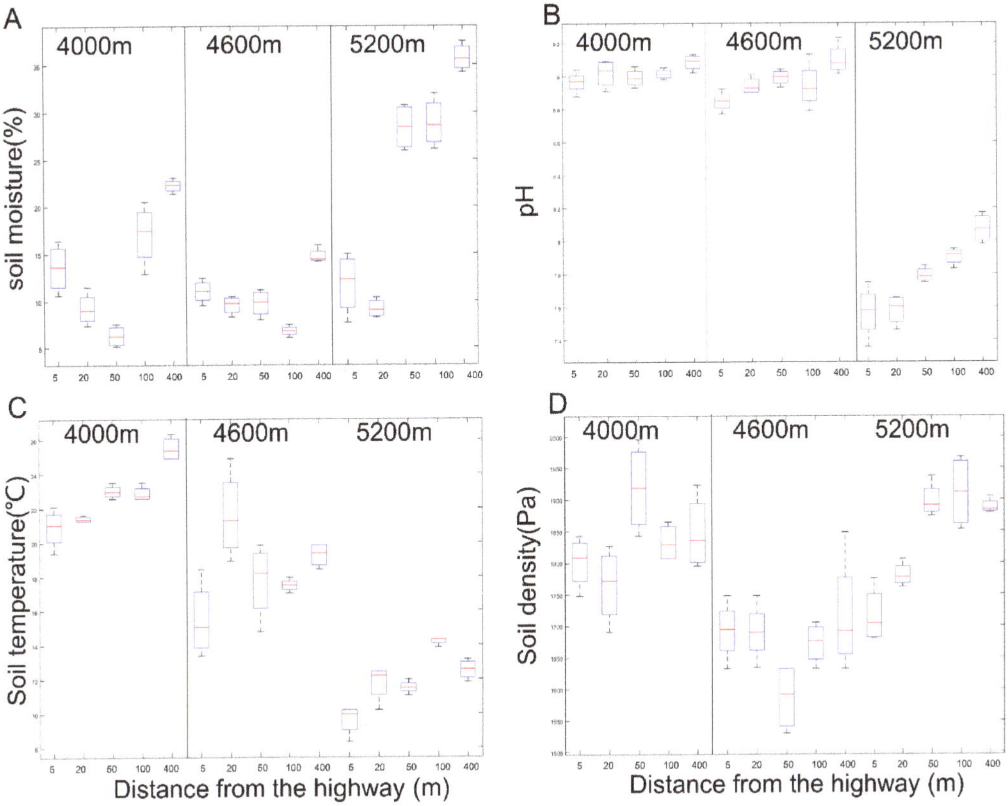

Figure 3. Comparison of soil: (**A**) soil moisture content, (**B**) pH, (**C**) soil temperature and (**D**) soil density between treatments at 5, 20, 50, 100, and 400 m from the curb G109 highways at altitudes of 4000 m (L), 4600 m (M), and 5200 m (H).

The Contents of Cu, Zn, and Cd increased significantly in the 4000 m site, and the increasing areas were mainly concentrated in the area 20 m away from the road (Figure 5). The three heavy metals contents increased by 17.18%, 14.73%, and 31.58% at 20 m from the road, compared with the control(400 m in 4000 m sites).The total lead content in the soil increased by 41.92% and 63.57% at 5 m and 20 m, respectively, in the 4600 m sites.

3.2. Bacterial α-Diversity

Alpha Diversity Index is used to reflect species diversity. Observed Species and Chao1 are used to indicate the actual number of OTUs in the community. The larger the Shannon Wiener and Simpson values are, the higher the community diversity is and the more uniform the individual distribution is. The Good's Coverage index reflects the sequencing depth, and the closer the index is to 1, it indicates that the sequencing depth has covered all species in the sample. The larger the value of the Phylogenetic Diversity index, indicates that the species that make up the biome are further apart in evolution. Specaccum accumulation curves determine whether the amount of sequenced data completely covers the species on the total sample. After pruning and quality filtering, 98,532 high-quality readings were obtained from a total of 60 samples from three altitudes, and the amount of clean tags data after quality control ranged from 4802 to 52,373. The data size of the valid tags (used for analysis) ranged from 11,648 to 42,192, with an average length of 426.58 to 432.68 bp.

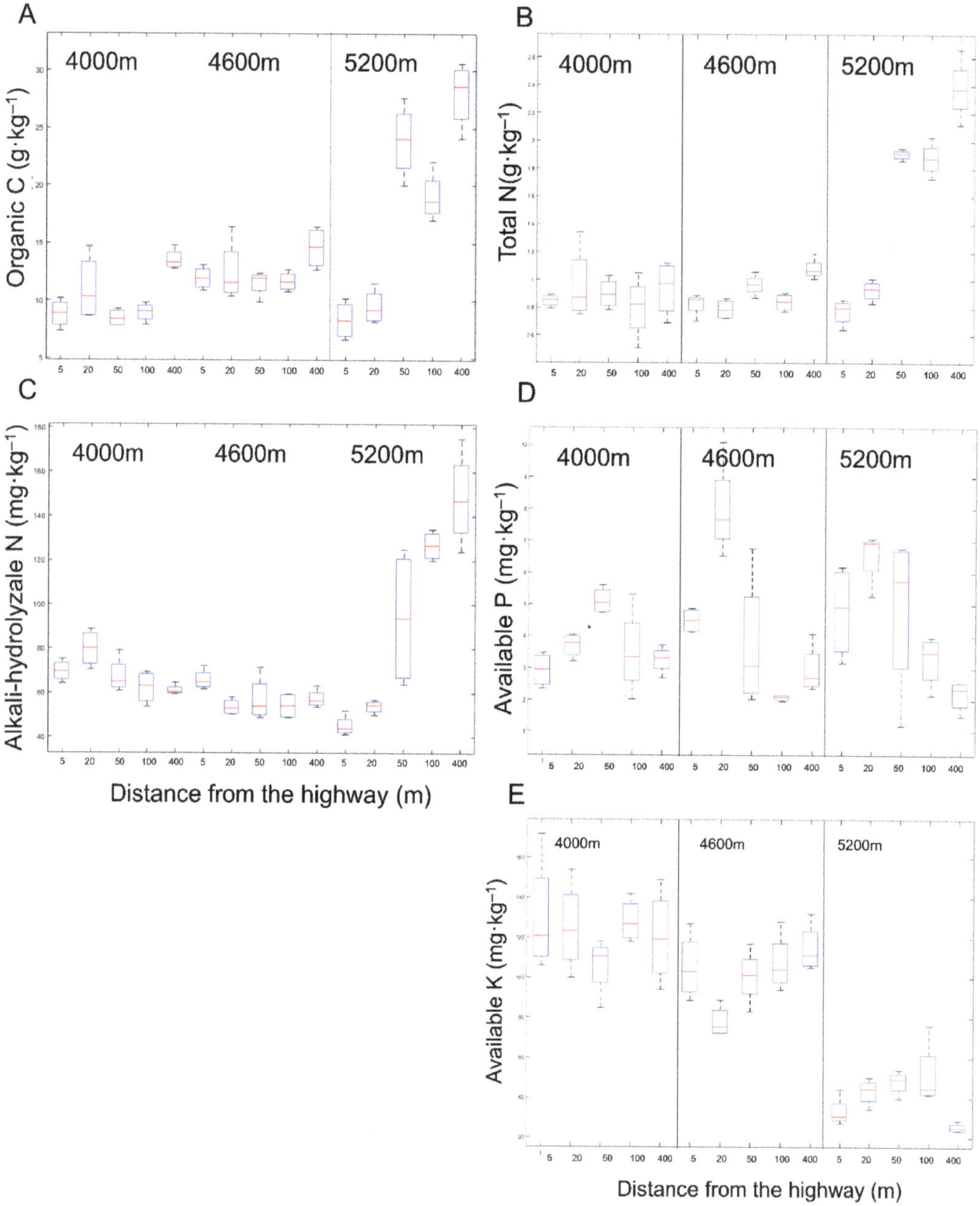

Figure 4. Comparison of soil: (**A**) organic carbon (SOC), (**B**) total nitrogen (TN), (**C**) alkali-hydrolyzable nitrogen (AN), (**D**) available phosphorus (AP), and (**E**) available potassium (AK) between treatments at 5, 20, 50, 100, and 400 m from the curb G109 highways at altitudes of 4000 m (L), 4600 m (M), and 5200 m (H).

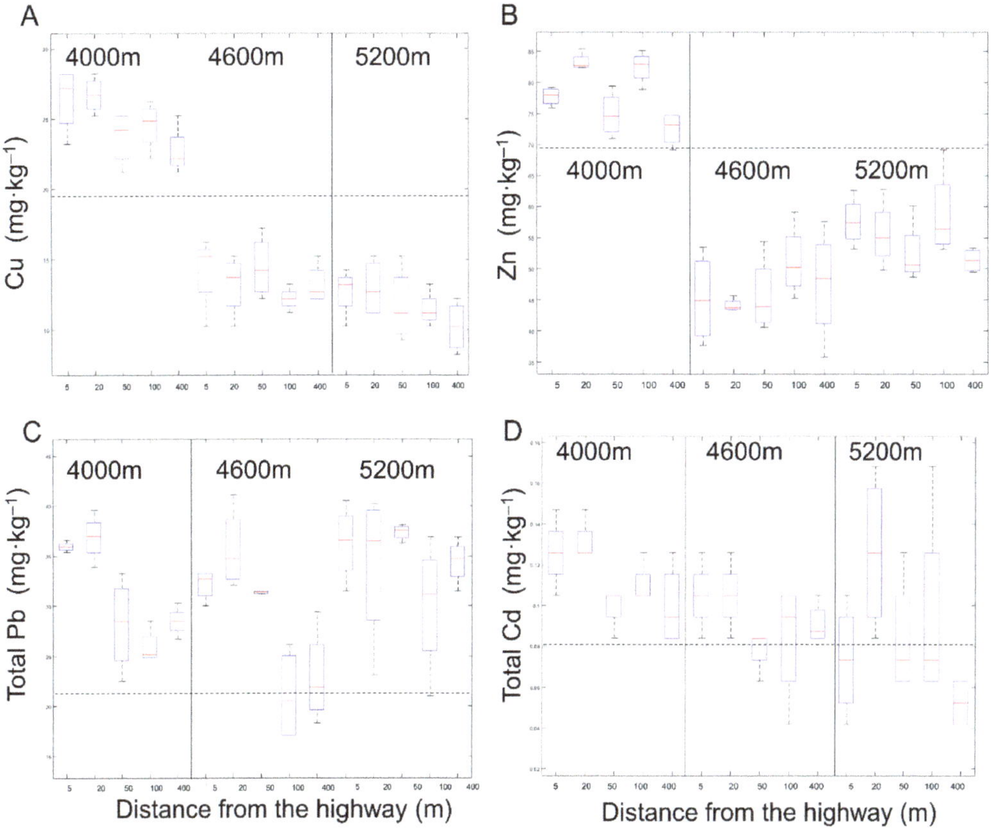

Figure 5. Concentrations of Cu (**A**), Zn (**B**), Pb (**C**), and Cd (**D**) in the 0–20 cm soil in sites 5, 20, 50, 100, and 400 m away from the G109 highway at altitudes of 4000 m (L), 4600 m (M), and 5200 m (H). The dotted line in the figure represents the background value of heavy metals in the Qinghai-Tibet Plateau.

The number of OTUs obtained from all treated soil samples ranged from 786 to 1987, and the species coverage (Good's Coverage index) was more than 90%. Based on a genetic distance of 3%, the sparse curve tends to saturate the plateau, indicating that the sequencing depth is sufficient (Figure 6D). The species accumulation curve showed that the sample size was sufficient for subsequent data analysis (Figure 6E).

The impact of highway traffic on bacterial α-diversity was mainly reflected in the 5200 m site, and the OTUs of soil bacteria significantly increased by 12.78% (1713) and 11.67% (1696) in the 5 m and 20 m plots in the 5200 m sites, respectively. Consistently, the bacterial Shannon index also increased significantly by 4.40% (9.40) and 3.86% (9.35) at 5 m and 20 m from the road, respectively, at 5200 m. In the 4600 m site, the bacterial CHAO1 index significantly increased by 8.93% (2901.93) at the 5 m site. On the contrary, the number of bacterial OTUs and Shannon index decreased significantly by 13.35% (1544.7) and 7.61% (8.56), respectively at 50 m from the road in 4000 m site (Figure 6).

Pearson correlation analysis showed that the environmental factors, especially altitude, SOC, AK, TN, AN, SM, pH, Density, Cu, and Simpson were significantly correlated with the bacterial α diversity index. OUT number and CHAO were negatively correlated with the PD whole tree index. In addition, there was a significant positive correlation between altitude and bacterial Simpson index. Cu content was significantly negatively correlated with Simpson index and Good's Coverage index. The Simpson index of plants was negatively correlated with that of bacteria (Figure 6D).

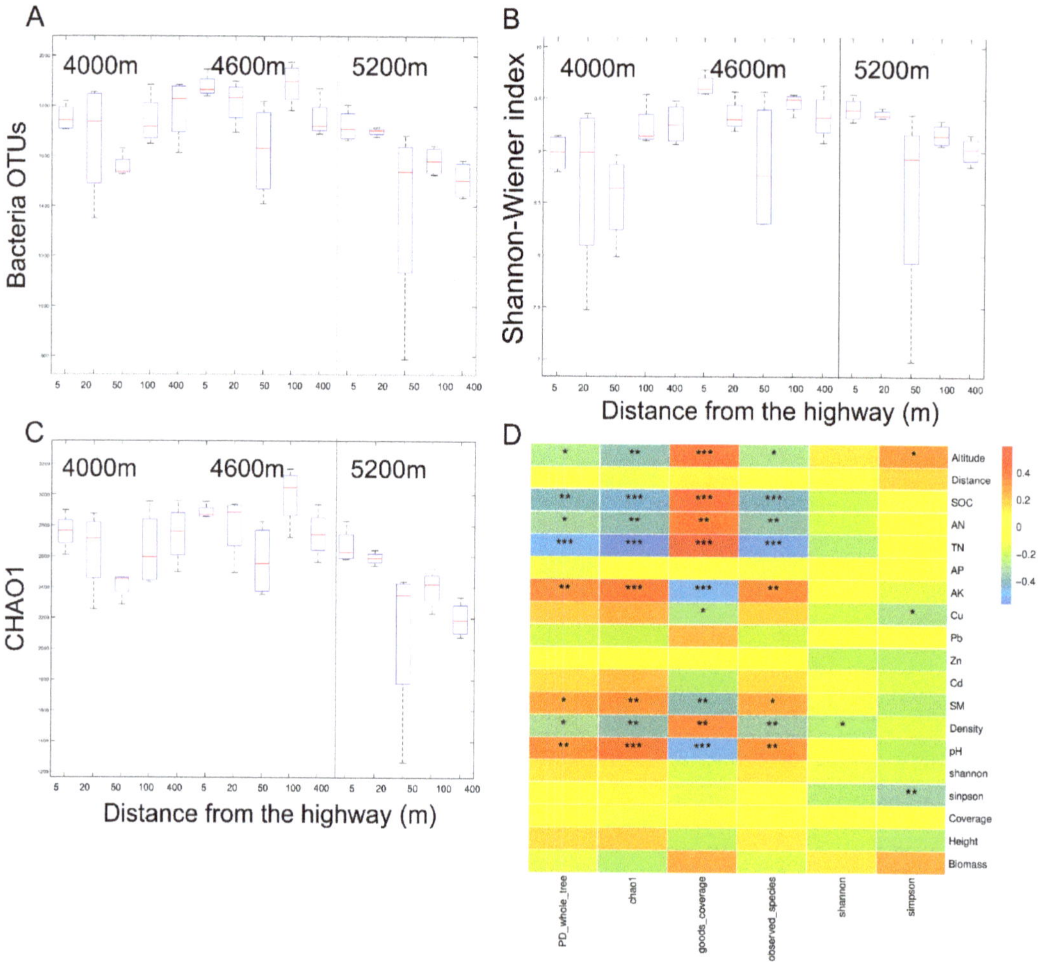

Figure 6. Box Diagram of (**A**) bacterial operational taxonomic unit (OTU), (**B**) bacterial Shannon and (**C**) bacterial CHAO1 in the 0–20 cm soil depths at 5, 20, 50, 100, and 400 m from G109 highway at altitudes of 4000 m (L), 4600 m, (M) and 5200 m (H). Pearson correlation heatmaps are based on bacterial alpha diversity estimators and environmental factors (**D**). * Means $p < 0.05$ for significance test; ** means $p < 0.01$ for significance test; *** means $p < 0.001$ for significance test.

3.3. Bacterial Community Structure

The relative abundance of phylum-level bacterial communities is shown in Figure 7. The major phyla in all samples were *Proteobacteria* (20.83–40.02%), *Actinobacteria* (15.28–31.09%), *Bacteroidetes* (13.16–27.99%), *Firmicutes* (9.72–27.99%), *Gemmatimonadetes* (1.61–8.10%), *Acidobacteria* (1.39–5.06%), *Nitrospirae* (0.15–1.13%), *Chloroflexi* (0.13–0.86%), *Cyanobacteria* (0.15–1.08%) and *Chlorobi* (0.13–0.47%), with a total of more than 98% in each sample (Table S1).

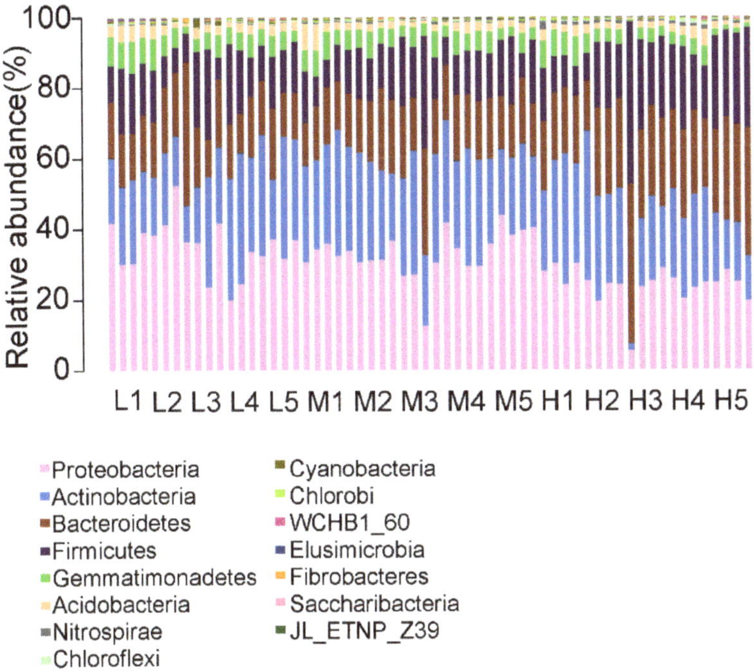

Figure 7. Chart of the relative abundance of the different levels of bacteria at the phylum level in the 0–20 cm depths soil at 5, 20, 50, 100, and 400 m from the curb G109 highways at altitudes of 4000 m, 4600 m, and 5200 m.

The *Proteobacteria* abundance decreased by 30.65% (28.03%) at the 50 m site than the control (400 m). The *Actinomycetes* abundance significantly decreased by 47.07% (20 m plot, 15.28%) in the 4000 m and 4600 m sites than the control. Conversely, the abundance of *Actinomycetes* significantly increased by 87.71% (29.03%) and 98.43% (28.03%) at 5 m and 20 m, respectively. *Bacteroides* abundance in the 20 m plot significantly increased by 75.92% (23.15%) in the 4000 m site compared with the control, while in the 5 m plot it significantly decreased by 34.82% (19.08%) in the 5200 m site compared with the control. The same results occurred with acid bacilli. At the 4000 m and 4600 m sites in the highway disturbance area, the abundance of acid bacilli at the 20 m and 50 m plots showed a significant decrease than control. However, the abundance of *Acidobacteria* significantly increased by 88.16% (2.61%) and 138.27% (3.31%) in the 5 m and 100 m sites, respectively. In addition, *Firmicutes* abundance in the 5 m and 20 m plots decreased significantly by 59.50% (10.61%) and 42.23% (15.13%) compared with the control in the 5200 m site. The abundance of *Nitrospirillum*, *Chlorospirillum*, *Cyanobacteria* and *Chlorobacteria* increased significantly in different degrees in the highway disturbance area.

In the genus level, the abundance of bacteria was analyzed by LEfSe in each site at each elevation, and the results are shown in Figure 8. Road traffic significantly increased the number of 4, 8, and 14 taxa of soil bacterial communities within 100 m (4000 m, 4600 m, and 5200 m), and significantly decreased the number of 5, 2, and 4 taxa of soil bacterial communities. *Flavisolibacter*, *Gemmatimonas*, *Microvirga*, *Nocardioides*, and *Rubrobacter* are enriched at sites of 4600 m and 5200 m in the disturbed area of the highway. *Crossiella* and *Gaiella* are enriched in the disturbed area at 4000 m and 5200 m sites respectively. At the same time, *Barnesiella* and *Blastococcus* were the main bacterial genera enriched in the unaffected area. *Flavisolibacter* abundance increased significantly at 5 m and 20 m sites at 4600 m and 5200 m sites, respectively. In addition, *Flavisolibacter* is also the genus with the highest importance index in 5200 m site in the random forest analysis. *Alistipes* and

Barnesiella increased in abundance in the undisturbed area at the 5200 m site. In the 4600 m site, *Gemmatimonas*, *Rubrobacter*, and *Microvirga* all increased in abundance close to the road, consistent with the 5200 m site. *Pseudomonas* was the most important genus in random forest analysis at the 4000 m site, and its abundance increased significantly at the 20 m site, and the content of soil alkali-hydrolysable nitrogen also increased significantly at the 20 m site. *Marmoricola* abundance was lower in the highway disturbance area compared to the control in the 4000 m site. *Nocardioides* were enriched at 5 m in 4600 m and 5200 m sites, in contrast to 4000 m in the control (400 m) group. In random forest analysis, the top 10 genera were *Skermanella, Prevotella* 9, *Rubrobacter, Gaiella, Blastococcus, Crossiella, Flavisolibacter, Faecalibacterium, Pseudomonas,* and *Microvirga* (Figure 8A).

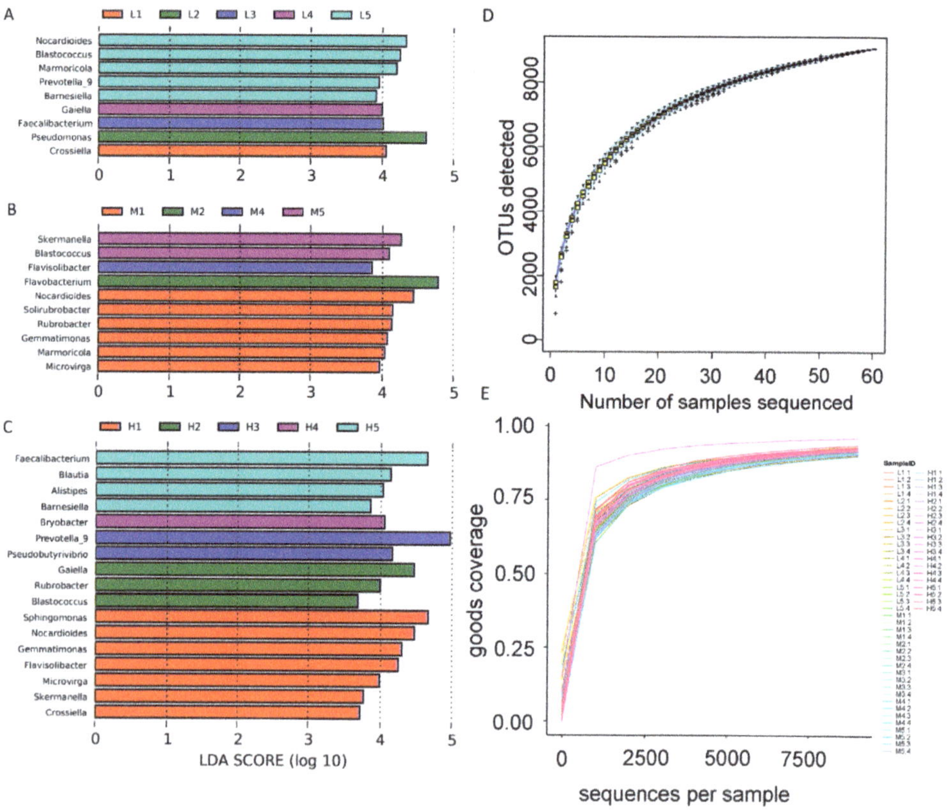

Figure 8. Linear discriminant analysis (LDA) of soil bacterial community in 3 sites of (**A**) 4000 m, (**B**) 4600 m, and (**C**) 5200 m. Rarefaction curve (**D**) and species accumulation curves (**E**) of the 60 soil samples.

3.4. Bacterial *β*-Diversity

ADONIS analysis showed significant differences in vegetation and bacterial community structure between distances at the same elevation, as well as between elevations (Table S2). From the results of NMDS analysis(Figure 9), it can be seen that there are significant differences in the structure of soil bacterial community among the samples at different altitudes (Stress value is 0.084), and the effect of altitude on bacterial community structure was more significant than that of distance. In different regions, significant differences in soil bacterial community structure were revealed among different distances (Stress values were 0. 058, 0.045, and 0. 043), which indicated that the soil bacterial community structure in the highway disturbed zone had changed significantly.

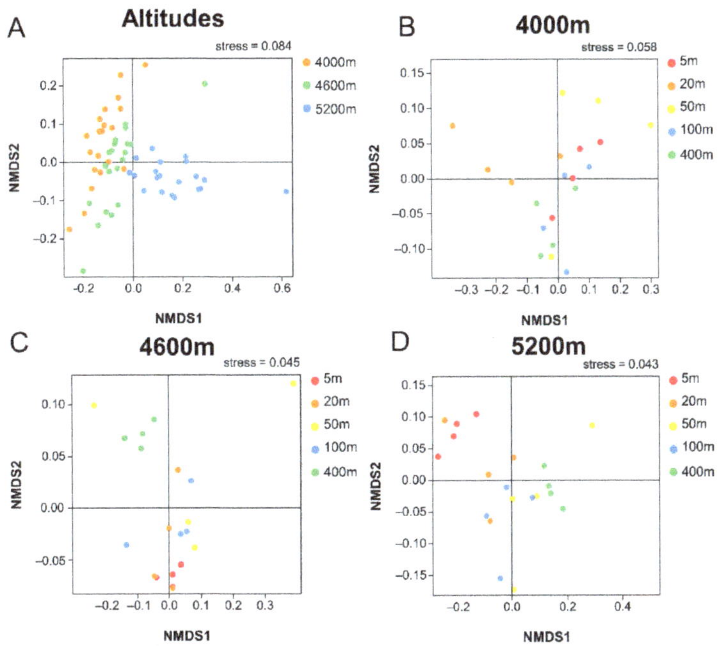

Figure 9. Non-metric multidimensional scaling (NMDS) analysis of (**A**) overall bacterial in 3 altitudes and bacterial in 3 sites of (**B**) 4000 m, (**C**) 4600 m, and (**D**) 5200 m.

According to the RDA results, soil bacterial community structures in three sites could be distinguished by plant and soil factors (Figure 10). In the site of 4000 m, AN had the greatest impact on the bacterial community. The first and second axes explained 54.70% and 18.53% of the variation, respectively. AK, SOC, and Zn are the main correlation factors of axis 1. Associated with axis 2 are mainly AN and AK (Figure 10A). In the 4600 m site, the most important factor is distance, followed by TN and coverage (Figure 10B). The first axis (mainly related to distance and TN) and the second axis (mainly related to SM and AP) described 35.70% and 33.37% of the variation, respectively. In the 5200 m site, SOC and pH had the greatest impact on the bacterial community, followed by distance (Figure 10C). The first axis, mainly related to SOC, pH, and AN explained 60.96% of the variation. At that same time, the second axis was mainly related to Cd and AN explained 9.95% of the variation.

3.5. Relative Effects of Environmental Factors on Bacterial Communities

Pearson correlation coefficient analysis results between bacterial abundance and environmental factors are shown in Figure 11. At the phylum level, the abundance of *Proteobacteria* and *Fibrobacteres* was positively correlated with AK, SM, pH, and Cu ($p < 0.01$), and negatively correlated with SOC and TN ($p < 0.05$). *Actinobacteria* abundance was positively correlated with AK, SM, Zn, and Cu ($p < 0.05$). *Bacteroidetes* were negatively correlated with AK, SM, pH, Zn, and Cu ($p < 0.05$) and positively correlated with SOC, TN, and AN ($p < 0.01$). At the genus level, the abundance of *Lactobacillus* and *Enterococcus* was positively correlated with Cu, Zn, pH, and SM ($p < 0.01$), and negatively correlated with SOC ($p < 0.05$). The abundance of *Sphingomonas* and *Rubrobacter* was positively correlated with AK, Cu, pH, and SM ($p < 0.001$), and negatively correlated with SOC, TN, Density, and AN ($p < 0.01$). *Faecalibacterium*, *Prevotella* 9, and *Blautia* were negatively correlated with AK, SM, pH, and Cu ($p < 0.01$), and positively correlated with SOC and TN ($p < 0.001$). The abundance of *Bacteroides* was negatively correlated with AK, Zn, pH, and SM ($p < 0.05$). In addition, *Gemmatimonas* was positively correlated with Zn ($p < 0.05$) and negatively correlated with SOC ($p < 0.01$). These results show that soil properties, especially SOC, TN, AN, AK, SM, pH, Cu, and Zn have significant effects on soil bacterial communities.

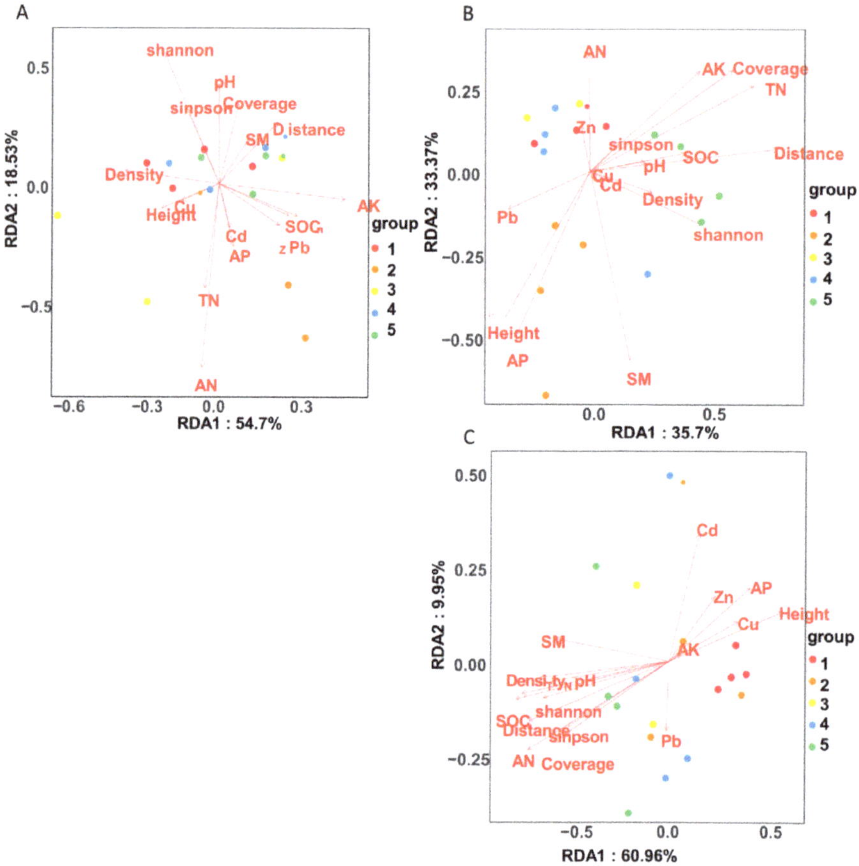

Figure 10. Ordination biplots of redundancy analysis (RDA) analysis of bacteria community structure, physical and chemical properties of soil and plant between treatments at 5, 20, 50, 100, and 400 m from the curb G109 highways at altitudes of (**A**) 4000 m, (**B**) 4600 m, and (**C**) 5200 m.

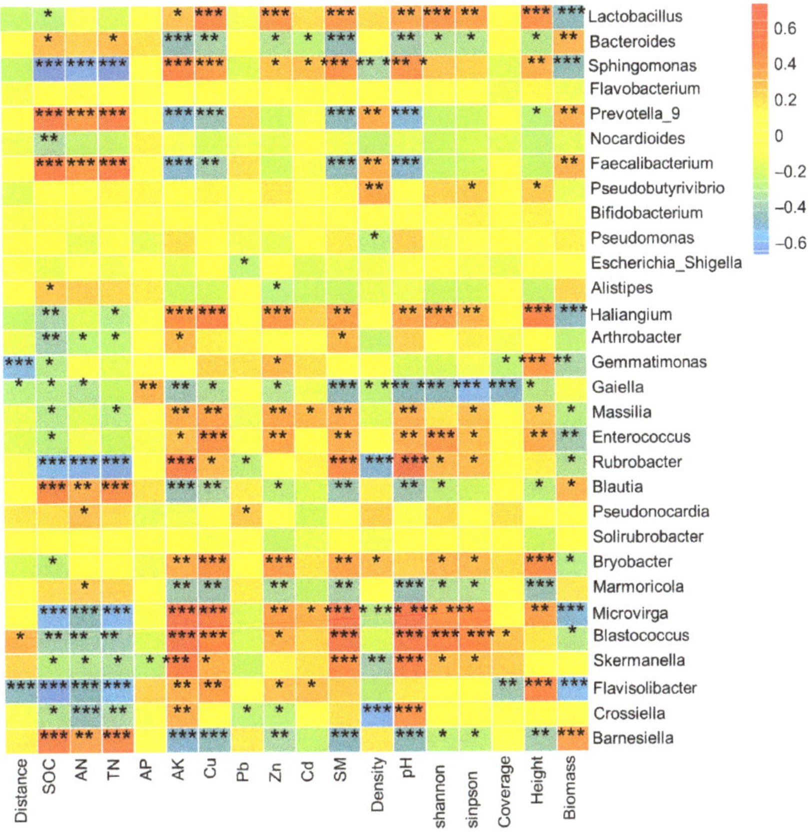

Figure 11. Pearson correlation heat map with correlation coefficient and significance levels based on the relative abundance of bacteria at the genus level and environmental factors. * Means $p < 0.05$ for significance test; ** means $p < 0.01$ for significance test; *** means $p < 0.001$ for significance test.

3.6. Bacterial Functional Community

Effect of road traffic on soil bacterial function FAPROTAX function prediction results (Figure 12) showed that chemoheterotrophy, fermentation, animal parasites or symbionts, and nitrate reduction are the main functional groups along the highway. Among the top 30 functional predicted relative abundances, 25 species showed significant differences ($p < 0.05$): chemoheterotrophy, human pathogens, predatory or exoparasitic, aerobic ammonia oxidation, ureolysis, cellulolysis. The functional groups of ligninolysis, sulfate respiration and aromatic compound degradation increased in the disturbed area. The functional groups showing a downward trend in the highway disturbance area included fermentation, animal symbionts, photoheterotrophy, chlorate reducers and other functional groups. In addition, soil nitrifying bacteria such as ammonia oxidation, nitrite oxidation and nitrification showed an increasing trend in the disturbed area from the road compared with the control. Nitrate reduction and nitrogen fixation related to soil denitrification were significantly decreased in the sites within 100 m from the road.

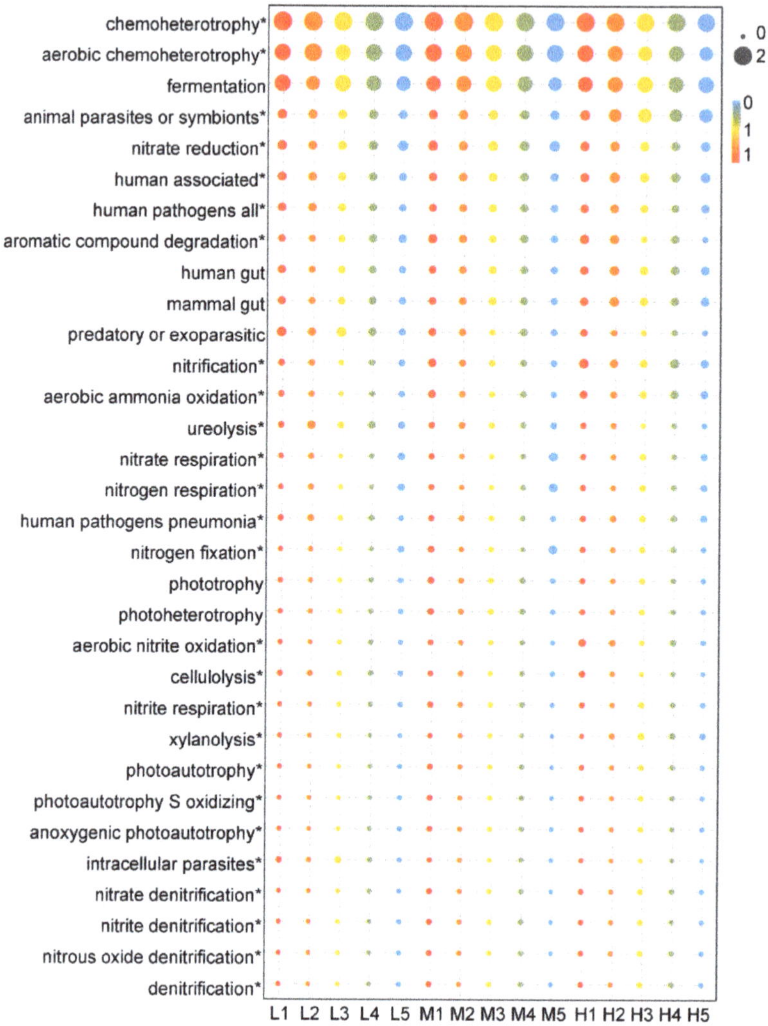

Figure 12. Ecological functional diversity of soil bacterial community in different altitudes and distances. * $p < 0.05$.

3.7. Variation Partitioning

The results of variation partitioning analysis (VPA) showed that environmental factors such as altitude, vegetation, soil, and heavy metals could explain 32.71% of the variation in soil bacterial community structure, and the unexplained rate was 67.29%, of which the interaction of soil, vegetation, and heavy metals could explain 12.42% (Figure 13A). Environmental factors such as altitude, vegetation, soil, and heavy metals accounted for 34.89% and 65.11% of the changes in the ecological functional structure of soil bacteria FAPROTAX, of which the soil factor alone accounted for 8.02% and the interaction of soil, vegetation, and heavy metals accounted for 14.76% (Figure 13B). Compared to the soil bacterial community structure, the coupling effect of soil and vegetation had a greater impact on the functional structure of bacteria.

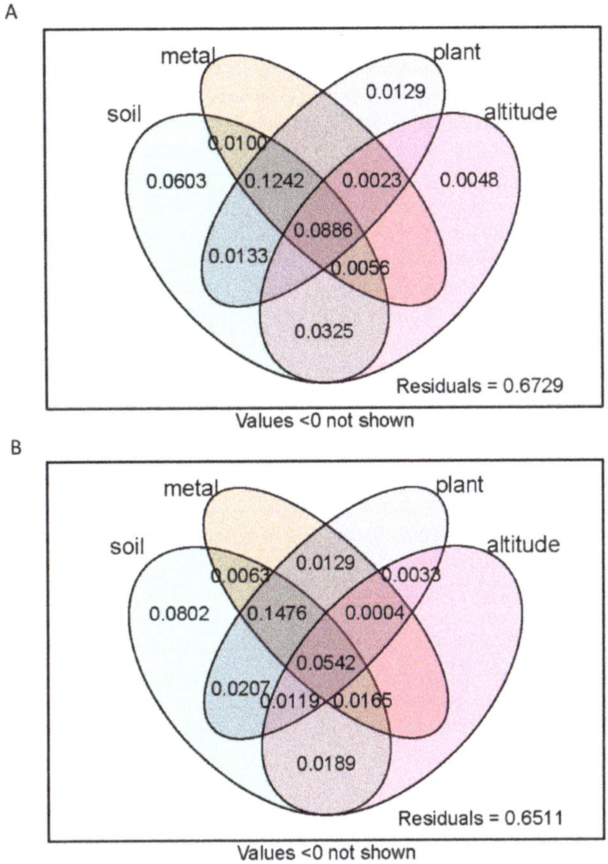

Figure 13. Variation partitioning analysis (VPA) which showed the relative proportions of total (**A**) bacterial and (**B**) functional diversity composition variations that can be explained by different types of environmental factors. The circles show the variation explained by each group of environmental factors alone.

4. Discussion

4.1. Impact of Highway on Plant and Soil Physical and Chemical Properties

During the highway construction and operation, different degrees of impact were inevitable on the grassland soil environment and vegetation along the highway. As we can predict, the grassland vegetation in the areas close to the highway has been degraded to varying degrees. In general, results showed the closer to the highway, the lower the coverage and diversity and biomass of grassland vegetation were. This is consistent with many previous research results [47]. This damage includes the direct excavation and rolling of grassland vegetation by construction and access vehicles [11]. It may also be indirectly caused by soil erosion caused by the change of terrain on both sides of the highway [12,48]. In this study, the vegetation height was higher in areas closer to the road. In the field investigation, we found that this was because some invasive plants such as *Stipa purpurea* appeared after the original low grassland of the QTP was disturbed and degraded [49]. At the same time, heavy metal pollution caused by road traffic has further aggravated the degradation of grassland vegetation [50]. In different altitude environments, the degradation of grassland vegetation is also different, of which 4600 m is similar to 5200 m, and the degradation is most obvious in the 4000 m environment. There may be two reasons, one is that the 4000 m section is closer to the city (Golmud), and the traffic flow is larger. On the other hand, because the vegetation type of the 4000 m site is desert grassland, the vegetation diversity is low, and the ecological environment is fragile. It is more vulnerable to the interference of environmental factors.

Consistent with previous studies, our results indicate that highway slopes affect soil nutrient content, resulting in lower pH. Our results show that the soil moisture decreased significantly in the highway disturbed area. Engineering disturbance may cause soil compaction or decomposition by destroying original vegetation, altering soil porosity, and disrupting soil aggregates [51–53]. At the same time, the destruction of vegetation in the disturbed area of the highway leads to the decrease of the fixation ability of roots to soil, and the process of soil erosion may cause the loosening of soil structure. Our results show that soil pH is sensitive to engineering disturbance, which may be related to soil parent material [54,55]. Road disturbance affects soil pH by destroying native vegetation and affecting soil pH and nitrogen levels in plant material [56]. In addition, increased soil acidification may lead to increased leaching of cationic nutrients from the soil, thereby exacerbating the deficiency of certain nutrients essential for plant growth and ultimately leading to reduced plant productivity [57]. Because of the decrease of plant litter, the activity of soil denitrifying bacteria was promoted, and the mineralized nitrogen tended to nitrify, which led to the decrease of soil pH [56]. The decrease of soil moisture content (SM) in the highway disturbance area is related to the coverage of vegetation [53,58]. A reduction in the capacity of the soil to retain water due to degradation of vegetation. The change of soil temperature is contrary to the results of previous studies, which may be related to the weather at the time of sampling, or because the change of vegetation cover affects the thermal insulation performance. This requires further study.

Our results show that the soil SOC, TN, and AK in the disturbed areas of the highway do not change significantly compared to the control areas at 4000 m and 4600 m sites. The research of Pan and Jiang on highway slopes also shows the same situation [53,59]. All study areas are located below 4000 m and include the Tibetan Plateau region. In contrast, at the 5200 m site, the SOC, TN, and AK of highway disturbed area decreased significantly in our study, suggesting that SOC, TN, and AK may be more sensitive to the impact of the highway at higher altitudes. He et al.'s study showed that SOC and TN of highway disturbed areas significantly reduced compared with control [14]. The results of this study are consistent with this. However, there are few studies on the soil SOC and N contents in the highway disturbed area at an altitude of more than 5000 m. Therefore, we analyzed the differences of soil nitrate and ammonium nitrogen contents and related bacterial abundances among the three altitudes in this study. Our study revealed that due to the low oxygen content in high altitude areas, a low-oxygen environment is more conducive to denitrification, resulting in significantly higher soil ammonium nitrogen content and significantly lower nitrate content at other altitudes (Figure 14A,B). At the same time, the contents of TN and MBN and the abundance of Nitrospirillum in the soil at the altitude of 5200 m were significantly higher than those at other altitudes (Figure 14C,D), possibly due to the differences in biomass and coverage of grasslands and human disturbance. This also led to a significantly higher abundance of bacteria associated with the soil nitrogen cycle, including nitrifying and denitrifying bacteria. This indicates that the soil nitrogen content is higher and the activity of related bacteria is more vigorous at the altitude of 5200 m, which may cause the soil N indicators more sensitive to the impact of the highway at high altitudes. The abundance of nitrifying bacteria is proportional to that of denitrifying bacteria. This result is in accordance with the law expounded by the predecessors [60].

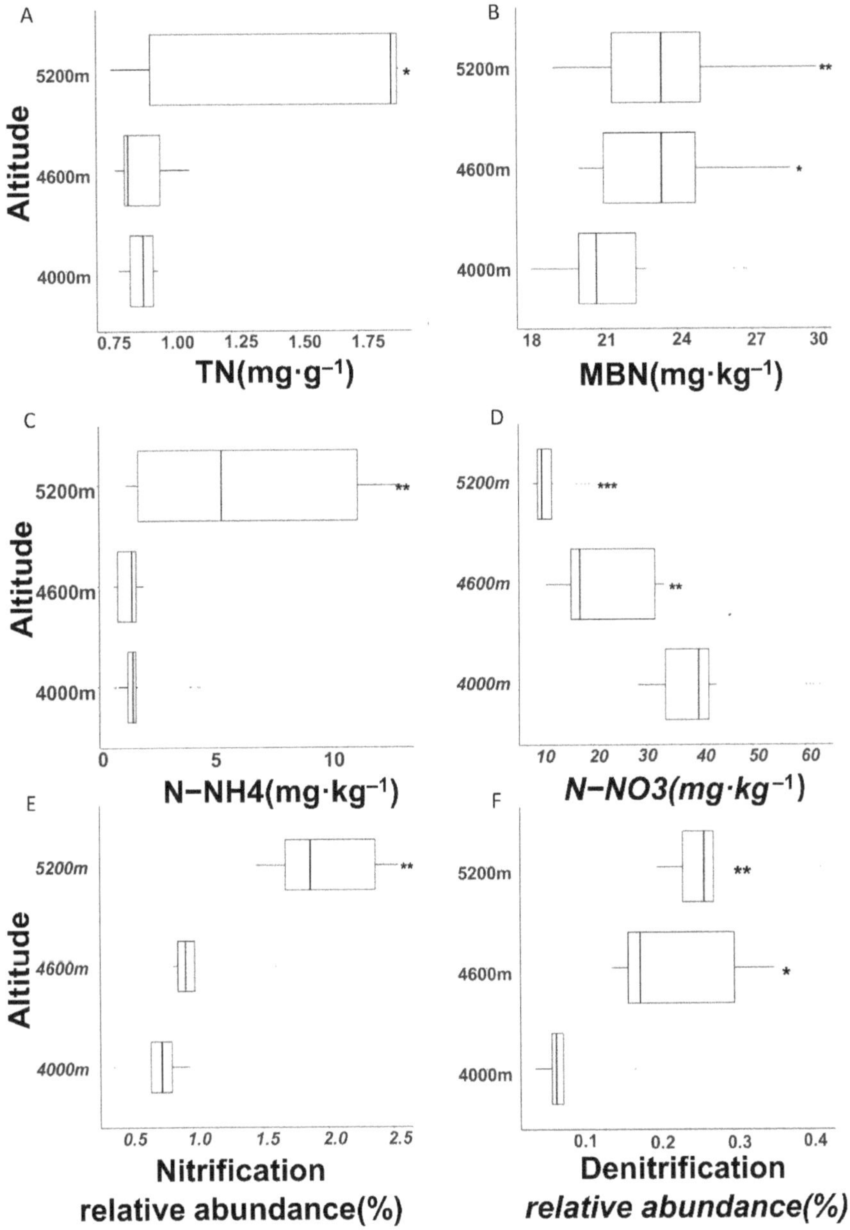

Figure 14. N cycle related indicators: (**A**) total soil nitrogen content, (**B**) soil microbial nitrogen content, (**C**) soil ammonia nitrogen N-NH_4, (**D**) soil nitrate N-NO_3, (**E**) nitrification bacteria relative content, (**F**) the relative content of denitrification bacteria at 4000 m (L), 4600 m (M), and 5200 m (H). * Means $p < 0.05$ for significance test; ** means $p < 0.01$ for significance test; *** means $p < 0.001$ for significance test.

The increase of soil available phosphorus may be affected by many factors. In alkaline soils, the content of calcium ions is usually high in alkaline or calcareous soils, and phosphate ions are easy to form calcium phosphate precipitation with calcium ions, thus reducing the content of available phosphorus. In this study, the pH value of the road disturbance area decreased, which promoted the dissolution of the P element in alkaline soil into AP and increased soil AP. Simultaneously, the abundance of some bacteria (such as *Bradyrhizobium* and *Mycobacterium*) related to phosphorus dissolution increased in the disturbed area of the highway, which may also be the reason for the significant increase of available phosphorus content. Ma et al. (2013) recorded relatively rich AP levels on the slopes of the Beijing-Chengde Phase III Expressway [61], consistent with the findings of this research. The ratio of carbon to nitrogen increased significantly in the disturbed zone.

Many heavy metals have been proved by previous researches to enter the soil on both sides of the highway from vehicle mechanical wear and fuel consumption [11,62]. Our findings are consistent with their results. The Zn content in the study area did not increase significantly and was generally lower than the background value of Tibet in China [23]. Parts of the vehicle that are galvanized or contain zinc, such as fuel tanks and tires, may be a source of zinc contamination [63]. This may be due to the fact that there is little human activity other than the normal driving of vehicles in the study section, and there is little exposure and wear of galvanized parts. The research shows that the enrichment of heavy metals in the 4000 m area is more obvious in the highway disturbance area, and the overall content is higher, which may be related to the differences in traffic flow and vegetation types. Heavy metals might be transferred to the soil along the highway through airflow or pavement runoff [64,65]. In this study, the range of significant increase of heavy metal content along the highway was mainly limited to 25–50 m from the highway, which may be related to the location of the transect in this study. This study area is selected in the no man's land and nature reserve without other human activities except roads, with few people and no grazing except for normal vehicle driving and road maintenance. Wildlife activity is also relatively low, which may lead to weak diffusion of heavy metal particles.

4.2. Effects of Environmental Factors on Soil Bacterial Community Structure at Different Altitudes

Therefore, the construction and traffic of the highway will significantly change the vegetation growth, soil physical, and chemical properties and content in grassland soil of heavy metal along the highway, thus affecting the diversity and structure of soil microbial communities. For example, Li et al. reported that the species composition of soil bacteria changed significantly during the degradation of vegetation [66]. Kang et al. studied the microbial community in an alpine wetland ecosystem and showed that human-induced pH changed microbial diversity and community structure in the upper soil layer as the main driving factors [67]. Underground coal mining has been reported to cause changes in soil conductivity and water content in sandy areas of western China, which can change the structure and diversity of soil microbial communities [68]. Research on the stressed soil near the QTH and Qinghai-Tibet Railway (QTR) proved heavy metals were important factors in the formation of bacterial community diversity [26]. In the Changbai mountain area, the disturbance of the highway was studied alongside the microbial diversity and communities in turf marsh soils, with the result that the microbial composition of turf marsh soils were mainly changed by road runoff and heavy metals emission [14]. In this study, the sequence data obtained indicate that the microbial communities differ significantly at the genus level.

In this study, the main dominant species at the phylum level are consistent with many previous studies (Figure 15A) [14,69,70]. In general, in disturbed or stressed soils, the abundance of *Proteobacteria* significantly decreased, while *Acidobacteria* abundance significantly increased compared with the undisturbed grassland [14,71]. In this study, this change was only consistent and significant in some areas, which may be related to the different degrees of environmental factors in different areas (Figure 15B). The ratio of *Proteobacteria* to *Acidobacteria* has been proved to be an indicator of changes in soil environmental conditions by several scholars [18]. This ratio between the road disturbed area and the control area was significantly different at three sites, with a significant increase at the 4000 m site and a significant decrease at the 5200 m site, indicating that the soil environmental conditions in the road-disturbed area have indeed changed in this study. He et al.'s research shows that the significant decrease of this ratio in the grassland affected by the highway is related to the fact that the altitude of the study area is much lower than 4000 m. This can be explained by geographical location and soil properties. *Alistipes* and *Barnesiella* are derived from faeces and are more abundant in unaffected areas. *Barnesiella* is in a similar situation.

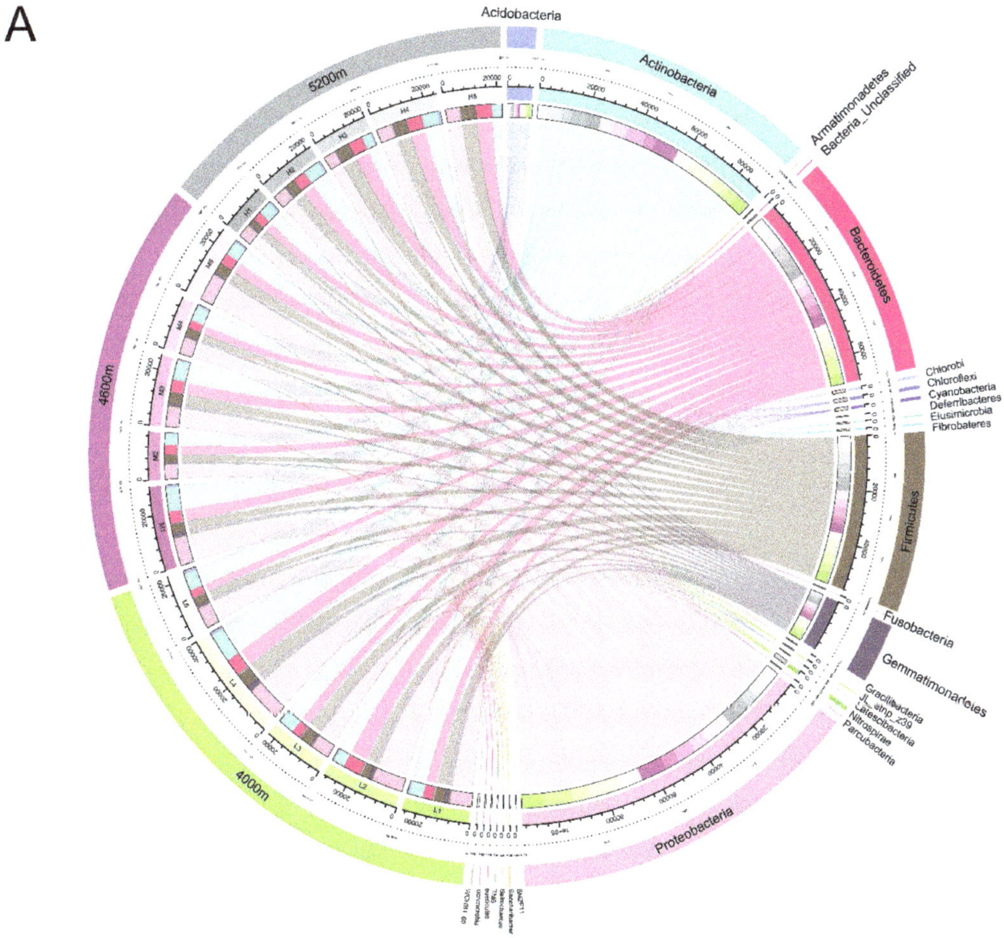

Figure 15. *Cont.*

B

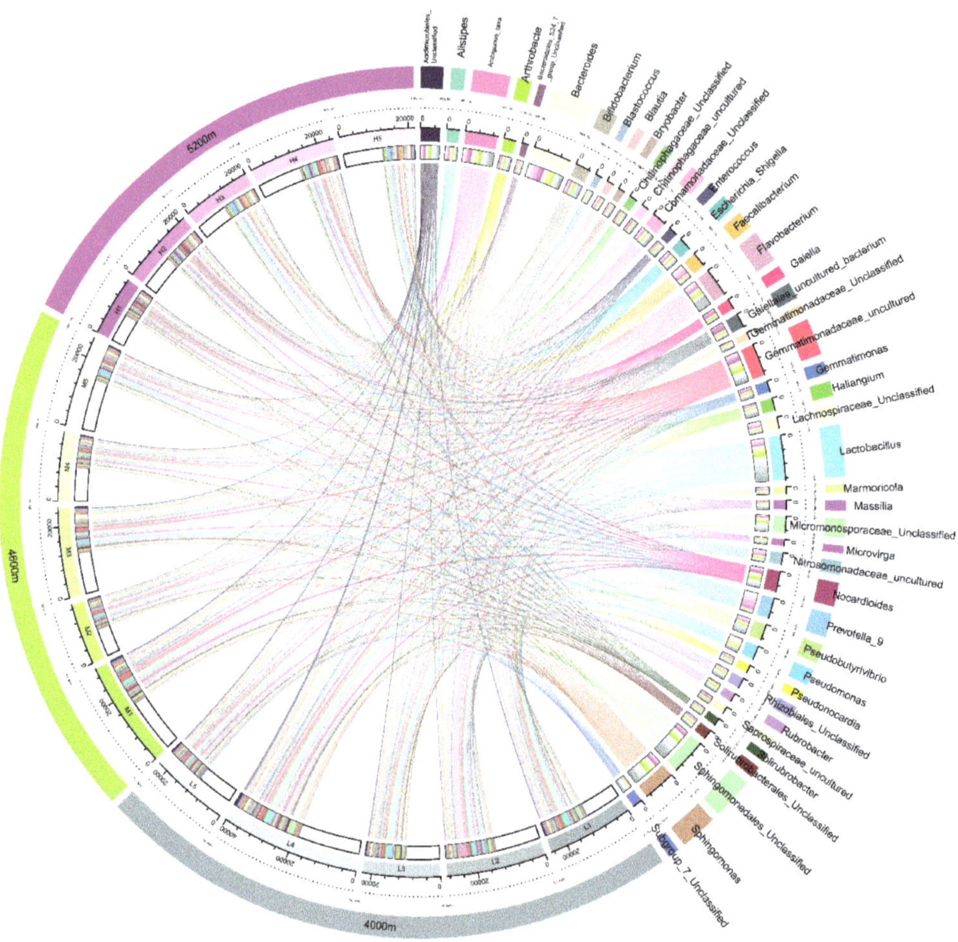

Figure 15. Circos circular plot of the bacterial community (**A**) at the phylum level and (**B**) at the genus level.

At the genus level, the changes of different bacteria in this study showed a variety of patterns, which may be related to their characteristics. For example, *Flavisolibacter* was isolated from automotive air conditioners in previous studies [70]. Its significant enrichment occurred within 20 m from the road, which may be due to the movement of the vehicle. The *Blautia* abundance significantly increased in the control which was isolated from animals and humans [69,72]. This could be due to the fact that the vegetation in the unaffected area remained in the original state, the quality of grassland was high, and there were more wildlife activities. It could be seen that due to the impact of highway construction and operation, the activities of wildlife were reduced in the area near the highway, as were *Alistipes* and *Barnesiella*, which may also come from animal dung [73–75]. This was also confirmed by the increase in abundance in the unaffected areas. Abundance of *Microvirga*, *Skermanella* and *Crossiella* correlates with pH [76]. Due to the optimum pH (7.0) for growth, the abundance of those was negatively related to pH in the alkaline environment of the study area, which was also confirmed by the results of this research. Consistently in this study, a significant positive correlation was found between *Pseudomonas* abundance and N content [77]. Another study proved [78] that *Pseudomonas* abundance in the soil samples of the non-plant area was significantly enriched compared with the composite rhizosphere soil samples. Consistent with previous studies, the vegetation coverage of the 20 m treatment declined significantly, while *Pseudomonas* abundance significantly increased. Liu et al. reported that the *Pseudomonas* can promote the degradation of weathered diesel-oil pollutants to some extent. The increased abundance of *Pseudomonas* in the area near the highway in this study may be related to its adaptability to diesel pollutants caused by the highway. Consistent with previous studies, *Marmoricola* abundance correlated with soil carbon content positively [8]. There was a reported significant positive correlation between *Nocardioides* abundance and soil phosphorus content [79], which is consistent with the enrichment of soil-available phosphorus in this study. At 5200 m and 4600 m, soil-available phosphorus increased significantly near the highway. In addition, different bacteria responded differently to heavy metals, and those sensitive to toxicity decreased, while resistant bacteria could adapt to environmental changes and their relative abundance increased. For example, the relative abundance of *Flavobacterium, Gemmatimonas, Terrimonas, Nitrospira,* and *Bacillus* had increased, while *Barnesiella* and *Blastococcus'* relative abundance decreased in metal-enriched soil [14,80,81]. Our results are consistent with these observations. *Flavobacterium* and *Pseudomonas* were more significantly enriched in the disturbed area at the height of 4000 m. Accordingly, the content of heavy metals at 4000 m is relatively high. This indicated that heavy metals had an impact on the soil bacterial community structure. *Prevotella* 9, *Blautia, Marmoricola,* and *Barnesiella* were significantly enriched in the control group and negatively correlated with the concentration of heavy metals, which were sensitive to heavy metals. Consistent with the results of this study, *Marmoricola* abundance was shown to be significantly negatively correlated with soil heavy metal content [82]. *Gemmatimonas, Microvirga, Massilia, Sphingomonas,* and *Blastococcus* were significantly enriched in the highway disturbed area, and were positively correlated with heavy metals, indicating that they were heavy metal tolerant bacterium [83–85].

4.3. Changes in Soil Bacterial Functional Groups under the Influence of Highway

FAPROTAX analysis showed that the functional groups with significant changes in different sites were mainly concentrated in bacteria related to soil nitrogen cycling. Ammonia oxidation, nitrite oxidation, nitrification and other soil nitrifying bacteria in the disturbed area from the road showed an upward trend compared with the control. Ammonia oxidation by ammonia-oxidizing bacteria is the first step in nitrification and the rate limiting step [60]. The conversion of ecosystem types may have important potential impacts on soil microorganisms involved in ammonia oxidation, and there is a significantly positively correlation between the number of soil ammonia-oxidizing bacteria and soil NH_4^+-N content [86]. NH_4^+-N significantly affected the population composition of soil ammonia-oxidizing bacteria in previous studies [80]. The results showed that the content of soil ammonium nitrogen increased significantly after the moderate degradation stage of alpine meadow, and the soil ammonium accumulation was obvious in the later stage of grassland degradation. Consistent with previous studies, the number of aerobic nitrite oxidation bacterial at 5 m significantly increased compared with the control in the 4600 m site, which was similar to the change trend of soil ammonium nitrogen. The increase of soil ammonium nitrogen was the main reason for the enrichment of ammonia-oxidizing functional genes. Nitrite oxidation is the second step of nitrification. At the 5200 m and 4600 m sites, the number of nitrite-oxidizing bacteria increased significantly at 5 m sites compared with the control, which may be due to the accumulation of ammonium nitrogen in the degraded grassland affected by the highway, which promoted ammonia oxidation, thus providing a material basis for the nitrite oxidation process. However, the content of nitrite in the soil was not measured in this study, so the specific reasons for this process need further study.

In the process of soil denitrification, the bacterial communities related to nitrate reduction decreased significantly in the sites within 100 m from the road, which was opposite to the change of nitrification. Nitrate reduction and nitrite ammonification are two important processes of soil denitrification. Nitrate reduction is the first step of denitrification.

Nitrate-reducing bacteria decreased significantly in the disturbed area of the highway, and their abundance was positively correlated with distance. There is a positive correlation between distance and nitrate bacteria. In the road disturbed area, the content of soil nitrate decreased, the material base of nitrate-reducing bacteria decreased, and the substrate of nitrate reduction reaction decreased, so the abundance of nitrate-reducing bacteria decreased. Nitrate bacteria relative abundance significantly correlated with altitude, and the same correlation occurs between nitrate-reducing bacteria and altitude. The reason is that with the increase of altitude, the oxygen content and the relative abundance of anaerobic nitrate-reducing bacteria increase, and the nitrate reduction reaction becomes more intense, consuming nitrate, therefore the content of nitrate decreases.

In the disturbed areas of 4600 m and 5200 m, the content of nitrate decreased and the content of ammonium nitrogen increased, indicating that soil denitrification was dominant. These might be due to the deterioration of soil aeration caused by the slight degradation of grassland, the decrease of vegetation coverage, the increase of soil compaction and the compression of soil pore structure [81], and then the promotion of the growth of anaerobic denitrifying bacteria. Firstly, because of the decrease of nitrate content, nitrate-reducing bacteria, and the reaction product nitrite and the nitrogen-fixing bacteria, nitrous oxide denitrifying bacteria increases, and part of nitrogen in soil enters the air in the form of nitrous oxide and nitrogen. This also confirms the results of the decrease of total soil nitrogen and AN content. Nitrogen-fixing bacteria decreased, but the content of ammonium nitrogen increased, indicating that the way of denitrification to produce ammonium nitrogen may be mainly through nitrite ammonification [87]. The decrease of SM proved it could significantly increase nitrite-oxidizing bacteria abundance, which also confirmed the significant increase of nitrite-ammonifying bacteria in this study. This may also be due to the deterioration of soil aeration, which reduces the performance of soil respiration, weakens nitrogen fixation, and promotes the production of anaerobic bacteria in the soil. According to Yu et al., in farmland soil, the abundance of denitrifying bacteria and nitrogen-fixing bacteria decreased significantly due to the decrease of nitrogen content after long-term nitrogen application [88]. It was further confirmed that the growth of denitrifying bacteria was limited by the decrease of soil nitrogen content. On the contrary, the nitrate and ammonium nitrogen decreased significantly at 4000 m, which may be due to the more serious grassland degradation and the overall decrease of nitrate and ammonium nitrogen. At the same time, denitrification-related bacteria also decreased in the disturbed area and significantly reduced. Combined with the results of vegetation index, it can be seen that the degradation degree of grassland in the highway disturbance area of the 4000 m site is higher, referring to the classification standards commonly used by predecessors [86], to the extent of moderate or severe degradation. Studies have shown that the soils C and N in severely degraded grassland are significantly reduced. The abundance of bacteria related to the nitrogen cycle showed a downward trend because of the lack of material basis for growth.

In addition, the chemoheterotrophic bacterial community showed a significant upward trend within 50 m from the road, and showed a consistent rule in the three areas, as the similar trend of previous studies. Sulfide respiration bacteria in the road disturbance area showed a downward trend compared with the control, and the lowest value (50 m) was found in the moderately degraded grassland soil, which was consistent with previous studies.

4.4. Relative Contribution of Vegetation, Soil, and Spatial Factors to Bacterial Community Structure in Different Altitudes

Mantel test results showed that biomass significantly affected the soil bacterial community structure (R = 0.241, $p = 0.001$). Among the soil factors, SOC, TN, AN, and NH4 were the main driving factors for the difference of soil bacterial community structure. AK and SM were the main driving factors for the difference of soil bacterial functional groups. This study found that soil nutrients are the most critical. As the most important nutrients for organisms, SOC and TN have been proved by many studies to be significantly related to soil microorganisms in different ecosystems [89,90]. Due to the anoxic soil conditions in the QTP, the decomposition of organic matter is slow. The lack of available nutrients, especially in areas disturbed by roads, limits the growth of bacteria. According to the traditional niche theory, the niches of many organisms may be related to available nitrogen, which causes impact on their coexistence in the ecosystem and changes the community structure [91]. Changes in TN, AN, and NH_4 can lead to changes in niche size, which can alter bacterial diversity [92].

According to the results of redundancy analysis (RDA), altitude played an important role in affecting the soil bacterial community structure. The responses of soil bacterial communities to environmental factors at different altitudes were further discussed, and the main driving factors of soil bacterial communities varied with different altitudes. For example, in the 4000 m site, the content of Zn and Pb were important factors driving the change of the soil bacterial community. Consistently, the soil heavy metal content was higher at 4000 m. This shows that the heavy metal pollution is more serious in the 4000 m environment of the disturbed area. The toxicity of heavy metals leads to the change of the soil bacterial community structure. The results of the RDA analysis at different altitudes also proved that the distance from the road greatly affected the structure of soil bacterial communities. The community structure and functional groups of soil bacteria were significantly changed by the changes of grassland vegetation and soil in the disturbed area of the highway.

In general, the effects of the highway on soil bacterial community structure and functional groups in the disturbed area are multifaceted, which is the result of the joint action of vegetation and soil. The effects of soil-vegetation coupling on the bacterial community structure and function were greater than the effects of soil-vegetation coupling alone. This phenomenon has also been reflected in previous studies. This shows that the influence of the environment on the growth of soil bacteria is a very complex process. Road traffic has a significant impact on all aspects of environmental factors, and the resulting changes in soil bacterial communities need to be explained in many ways. Therefore, further research is of great need in this area.

4.5. Uncertainty and Perspectives

Our study describes above-ground vegetation, soil chemistry, and bacterial communities at different elevations along the QTH. In addition, the driving mechanism of microbial community diversity and community structure changes in the highway-disturbed area of the QTP explored.

Several shortcomings of this study need to be considered. First, there is no repetition in the same altitude environment; however, the results of the study at different altitudes are generally consistent and can be verified by each other, which does not affect the reliability of our conclusions. Secondly, due to legal and policy requirements, we have no way to obtain specific traffic flow of data in the sampling zone. This might also play an important role in the change of grassland vegetation and soil bacteria. By further measuring more comprehensive indicators related to the soil nitrogen cycle (such as nitrate, nitrite, etc.), the response mechanism of bacterial functional groups related to the soil nitrogen cycle can be more clearly expounded. These problems deserve further study.

The impact of highway construction and transportation on soil microbial diversity of the ecosystem along the highway has attracted more and more attention [93–95]. A recent study found that soil nitrogen was a key factor driving changes in soil microbial biomass and enzyme activity in cutting slopes [96]. Interactions between potentially toxic substances from vehicle emissions, roadside soils, and associated biota have also recently been reviewed [97]. Soil nutrients such as TOC and TN were found to be the most important variables affecting soil bacterial diversity and community structure along the QTH in our research which was significant for the research of the ecological restoration process along the plateau highway in the future.

5. Conclusions

Based on high-throughput sequencing, physical and chemical parameters, and statistical analysis, this study explored the effects of traffic and construction of the Qinghai-Tibet Highway on soil bacterial communities and diversity along the highway. The results showed that the road-related activities led to vegetation degradation, significantly changed the physical and chemical properties of soil, and caused heavy metal pollution. These environmental factors significantly affected the soil bacteria diversity and community structure. Soil organic carbon (SOC) and total nitrogen (TN) were the main factors driving the difference of the soil bacterial community structure in the disturbed area. The main factor of grassland disturbance along the Qinghai-Tibet Highway is caused by the decrease of soil-nutrient content. This disturbance shows a trend of increasing gradually from closer to farther distances. Therefore, in the restoration stage of the highway slope, it is very important to maintain the balance of soil nutrient supply for the restoration of the underground ecosystem function. The bacteria that showed heavy metal tolerance in the study may be explored for potential use in soil bioremediation in future studies. These results may provide guidance for the grassland ecosystem restoration along the highway and the selection of highway construction schemes in the Qinghai-Tibet region.

Supplementary Materials: The following are available online at https://www.mdpi.com/1660-4601/18/24/13137/s1, Table S1: The relative abundance of the top 10 dominant bacteria in the phylum level abundance at different altitudes and distances; Table S2: Adonis analysis in 5 m, 20 m, 50 m, 100 m and 400 m from the highway for plant and soil bacterial respectively in 3 sites and adonis analysis in altitudes of 4000 m, 4600 m and 5200 m for plant and soil bacterial.

Author Contributions: Conceptualization, L.H. and X.C.; methodology, Z.L.; validation, Z.L. and Y.Y.; formal analysis, Z.L.; investigation, Z.L., Y.Y., S.J., Y.L. and X.C.; resources, Z.L., S.J., D.D. and M.W.; data curation, Z.L.; writing—original draft preparation, Z.L.; writing—review and editing, L.H. and X.C.; visualization, Z.L.; supervision, L.H.; funding acquisition, X.C. All authors have read and agreed to the published version of the manuscript.

Funding: This research was funded by [the Second Tibetan Plateau Scientific Exploration] grant number [2021QZKK0203], [Science and Technology Project of Tibet Department of Transportation] grant number [XZJTKJ[2019]01] and [National Natural Science Foundation of China] grant number [31971770].

Institutional Review Board Statement: Not applicable.

Informed Consent Statement: Not applicable.

Conflicts of Interest: The authors declare no conflict of interest.

References

1. Qiu, J. The third pole. *Nature* **2008**, *454*, 393–396. [CrossRef]
2. Su, F.; Duan, X.; Zhang, L.; Hao, Z.; Cuo, L. *21 Century Climatic Change Impacts on the Hydrology of Major Rivers in the Tibetan Plateau*; American Geophysical Union: Washington, DC, USA, 2011.
3. Cui, X.; Graf, H.-F. Recent land cover changes on the Tibetan Plateau: A review. *Clim. Chang.* **2009**, *94*, 47–61. [CrossRef]
4. Miehe, G.; Miehe, S.; Bach, K.; Nölling, J.; Hanspach, J.; Reudenbach, C.; Kaiser, K.; Wesche, K.; Mosbrugger, V.; Yang, Y.P.; et al. Plant communities of central Tibetan pastures in the Alpine Steppe/Kobresia pygmaea ecotone. *J. Arid Environ.* **2011**, *75*, 711–723. [CrossRef]
5. Yu, B.H.; Lü, C.H. Assessment of ecological vulnerability on the Tibetan Plateau. *Geogr. Res.* **2011**, *30*, 2289–2295.
6. Klein, J.A.; Harte, J.; Zhao, X.Q. Experimental warming causes large and rapid species loss, dampened by simulated grazing, on the Tibetan Plateau. *Ecol. Lett.* **2004**, *7*, 1170–1179. [CrossRef]
7. Fu, D.; Yang, H.; Wang, L.; Yang, S.; Li, R.; Zhang, W.; Ai, X.; Ai, Y. Vegetation and soil nutrient restoration of cut slopes using outside soil spray seeding in the plateau region of southwestern China. *J. Environ. Manag.* **2018**, *228*, 47–54. [CrossRef]
8. Liu, H.; Chen, L.-P.; Ai, Y.-W.; Yang, X.; Yu, Y.-H.; Zuo, Y.-B.; Fu, G.-Y. Heavy metal contamination in soil alongside mountain railway in Sichuan, China. *Environ. Monit. Assess.* **2008**, *152*, 25–33. [CrossRef] [PubMed]
9. Wang, X. Tibet has 117,000 kilometers of highways open to traffic. *People's Daily Online*. Available online: http://xz.people.com.cn/n2/2021/0208/c138901-34571170.html (accessed on 8 February 2021).

10. Bocking, E.; Cooper, D.J.; Price, J. Using tree ring analysis to determine impacts of a road on a boreal peatland. *For. Ecol. Manag.* **2017**, *404*, 24–30. [CrossRef]
11. Wang, H.; Nie, L.; Xu, Y.; Lv, Y. The Effect of Highway on Heavy Metal Accumulation in Soil in Turfy Swamps, Northeastern China. *Water Air Soil Pollut.* **2017**, *228*, 292. [CrossRef]
12. Bohemen, H.; Laak, W. The Influence of Road Infrastructure and Traffic on Soil, Water, and Air Quality. *Environ. Manag.* **2003**, *31*, 50–68. [CrossRef]
13. Chen, Z.; Ai, Y.; Fang, C.; Wang, K.; Li, W.; Liu, S.; Li, C.; Xiao, J.; Huang, Z. Distribution and phytoavailability of heavy metal chemical fractions in artificial soil on rock cut slopes alongside railways. *J. Hazard. Mater.* **2014**, *273*, 165–173. [CrossRef]
14. He, Y.; Xu, Y.; Lv, Y.; Nie, L.; Wang, H. Soil Bacterial Community Structure in Turfy Swamp and Its Response to Highway Disturbance. *Int. J. Environ. Res. Public Health* **2020**, *17*, 7822. [CrossRef] [PubMed]
15. Schmidt, M.; Torn, M.S.; Abiven, S.; Dittmar, T.; Guggenberger, G.; Janssens, I.A.; Kleber, M.; KGel-Knabner, I.; Lehmann, J.; Manning, D. Persistence of soil organic matter as an ecosystem property. *Nature* **2011**, *478*, 49–56. [CrossRef]
16. Jaatinen, K.; Fritze, H.; Laine, J.; Laiho, R. Effects of short- and long-term water-level drawdown on the populations and activity of aerobic decomposers in a boreal peatland. *Glob. Chang. Biol.* **2010**, *13*, 491–510. [CrossRef]
17. Fisk, M.C.; Ruether, K.F.; Yavitt, J.B. Microbial activity and functional composition among northern peatland ecosystems. *Soil Biol. Biochem.* **2003**, *35*, 591–602. [CrossRef]
18. Thormann, M.N.; Currah, R.S.; Bayley, S.E. Patterns of distribution of microfungi in decomposing bog and fen plants. *Can. J. Bot.* **2004**, *82*, 710–720. [CrossRef]
19. Muneer, M.A.; Wang, P.; Zhang, J.; Li, Y.; Ji, B. Formation of Common Mycorrhizal Networks Significantly Affects Plant Biomass and Soil Properties of the Neighboring Plants under Various Nitrogen Levels. *Microorganisms* **2020**, *8*, 230. [CrossRef] [PubMed]
20. Wiseman, C.; Zereini, F.; Püttmann, W. Metal translocation patterns in Solanum melongena grown in close proximity to traffic. *Environ. Sci. Pollut. Res.* **2014**, *21*, 1572–1581. [CrossRef] [PubMed]
21. Hua, Z.; Zhang, Y.; Wang, Z.; Ding, M.; Jiang, Y.; Xie, Z. Traffic-related metal(loid) status and uptake by dominant plants growing naturally in roadside soils in the Tibetan plateau, China. *Sci. Total Environ.* **2016**, *573*, 915–923.
22. Al-Awadhi, J.M.; Aldhafiri, B.T. Heavy metal concentrations in roadside-deposited sediments in Kuwait city. *Arab. J. Geoences* **2016**, *9*, 1–14. [CrossRef]
23. Werkenthin, M.; Kluge, B.; Wessolek, G. Metals in European roadside soils and soil solution—A review. *Environ. Pollut.* **2014**, *189*, 98–110. [CrossRef]
24. Silva, S.D.; Ball, A.S.; Huynh, T.; Reichman, S.M. Metal accumulation in roadside soil in Melbourne, Australia: Effect of road age, traffic density and vehicular speed. *Environ. Pollut.* **2015**, *208*, 102–109. [CrossRef]
25. Zhang, H.; Wang, Z.; Zhang, Y.; Ding, M.; Li, L. Identification of traffic-related metals and the effects of different environments on their enrichment in roadside soils along the Qinghai-Tibet highway. *Sci. Total Environ.* **2015**, *521–522*, 160–172. [CrossRef]
26. Zhao, X. Influence of proximity to the Qinghai-Tibet highway and railway on variations of soil heavy metal concentrations and bacterial community diversity on the Tibetan Plateau. *Sci. Cold Arid. Reg.* **2019**, *11*, 407–418.
27. Belyaeva, O.N.; Haynes, R.J.; Birukova, O.A. Barley yield and soil microbial and enzyme activities as affected by contamination of two soils with lead, zinc or copper. *Biol. Fertil. Soils* **2005**, *41*, 85–94. [CrossRef]
28. Forman, R.T.; Alexander, L.E. Roads and Their Major Ecological Effects. *Annu. Rev. Ecol. Syst.* **1998**, *29*, 207–231. [CrossRef]
29. Assaeed, A.M.; Al-Rowaily, S.L.; El-Bana, M.I.; Abood, A.; Dar, B.; Hegazy, A.K. Impact of Off-Road Vehicles on Soil and Vegetation in a Desert Rangeland in Saudi Arabia. *Saudi J. Biol. Sci.* **2018**, *26*, 1187–1193. [CrossRef] [PubMed]
30. Benbi, D.K., Nieder, R. *Handbook of Processes and Modelling in Soil-Plant System*; CRC Press: Boca Raton, FL, USA, 2003.
31. Guan, Z.H.; Li, X.G.; Wang, L. Heavy metal enrichment in roadside soils in the eastern Tibetan Plateau. *Environ. Sci. Pollut. Res.* **2017**, *25*, 7625–7637. [CrossRef] [PubMed]
32. Yan, X.; Gao, D.; Zhang, F.; Zeng, C.; Xiang, W.; Zhang, M. Relationships between Heavy Metal Concentrations in Roadside Topsoil and Distance to Road Edge Based on Field Observations in the Qinghai-Tibet Plateau, China. *Int. J. Environ. Res. Public Health* **2013**, *10*, 762–775. [CrossRef] [PubMed]
33. Sparks, D.L.; Page, A.; Helmke, P.; Loeppert, R.H. *Methods of Soil Analysis, Part 3: Chemical Methods*; John Wiley & Sons: Hoboken, NJ, USA, 2020; Volume 14.
34. Bremner, J.M.; Mulvaney, C.S. Total nitrogen. In *Methods of Soil Analysis*; Page, A.L., Miller, R.H., Keeny, D.R., Eds.; 1965; Available online: https://acsess.onlinelibrary.wiley.com/doi/abs/10.2136/sssabookser5.3.c37 (accessed on 8 February 2021).
35. Wen, Y.; You, J.; Zhu, J.; Hu, H.; Gao, J.; Huang, J. Long-term green manure application improves soil K availability in red paddy soil of subtropical China. *J. Soils Sediments* **2020**, *21*, 63–72. [CrossRef]
36. Zi, H.I.; Hu, L.; Ade, L.; Wang, C. Distribution Patterns of Ratio of Root to Soil and Soil Physical Chemical Characteristics at the Different Degraded Successional Stages in an Alpine Meadow. *Acta Agrestia Sin.* **2015**, *23*, 1151–1160. [CrossRef]
37. Hua, Z.; Wang, Z.; Zhang, Y.; Hu, Z. The effects of the Qinghai–Tibet railway on heavy metals enrichment in soils. *Sci. Total Environ.* **2012**, *439*, 240–248. [CrossRef]
38. Nossa, C.W.; Oberdorf, W.E.; Yang, L.; Aas, J.A.; Paster, B.J., DeSantis, T.Z.; Brodie, E.L.; Malamud, D.; Poles, M.A.; Pei, Z. Design of 16S rRNA gene primers for 454 pyrosequencing of the human foregut microbiome. *World J. Gastroenterol.* **2010**, *16*, 4135–4144. [CrossRef]

39. Magoč, T.; Steven, S.L. FLASH: Fast length adjustment of short reads to improve genome assemblies. *Bioinformatics* **2011**, *27*, 2957–2963. [CrossRef] [PubMed]
40. Reyon, D.; Tsai, S.Q.; Khayter, C.; Foden, J.A.; Sander, J.D.; Joung, J.K. FLASH assembly of TALENs for high-throughput genome editing. *Nat. Biotechnol.* **2012**, *30*, 460–465. [CrossRef] [PubMed]
41. Rognes, T.; Flouri, T.; Nichols, B.; Quince, C.; Mahé, F. VSEARCH: A versatile open source tool for metagenomics. *PeerJ* **2016**, *4*, e2584. [CrossRef] [PubMed]
42. Wang, Q. Naive Bayesian classifier for rapid assignment of rRNA sequences into the new bacterial taxonomy. *Appl. Environ. Microbiol.* **2007**, *73*, 5261–5267. [CrossRef] [PubMed]
43. Altschul, S.F. Basic local alignment search tool (BLAST). *J. Mol. Biol.* **2012**, *215*, 403–410. [CrossRef]
44. Bolger, A.M.; Marc, L.; Bjoern, U. Trimmomatic: A flexible trimmer for Illumina sequence data. *Bioinformatics* **2014**, *30*, 2114–2120. [CrossRef]
45. Caporaso, J.G.; Kuczynski, J.; Stombaugh, J.; Bittinger, K.; Bushman, F.D.; Costello, E.K.; Fierer, N.; Pena, A.G.; Goodrich, J.K.; Gordon, J.I. QIIME allows analysis of high-throughput community sequencing data. *Nat. Methods* **2010**, *7*, 335–336. [CrossRef]
46. Edgar, R.C.; Haas, B.J.; Clemente, J.C.; Quince, C.; Knight, R. UCHIME improves sensitivity and speed of chimera detection. *Bioinformatics* **2011**, *27*, 2194–2200. [CrossRef] [PubMed]
47. Dörfer, C.; Kühn, P.; Baumann, F.; He, J.S.; Scholten, T. Soil Organic Carbon Pools and Stocks in Permafrost-Affected Soils on the Tibetan Plateau. *PLoS ONE* **2013**, *8*, e57024.
48. Buckeridge, K.M.; Jefferies, R.L. Vegetation loss alters soil nitrogen dynamics in an Arctic salt marsh. *J. Ecol.* **2007**, *95*, 283–293. [CrossRef]
49. Chen, Y.; Li, Y.; Zhao, X.; Awada, T.; Wen, S. Effects of Grazing Exclusion on Soil Properties and on Ecosystem Carbon and Nitrogen Storage in a Sandy Rangeland of Inner Mongolia, Northern China. *Environ. Manag.* **2012**, *50*, 622–632. [CrossRef]
50. Pagotto, C.; Rémy, N.; Cloirec, M.L.; Le, P. Heavy Metal Pollution of Road Dust and Roadside Soil near a Major Rural Highway. *Environ. Technol.* **2001**, *22*, 307–319. [CrossRef] [PubMed]
51. Chen, S.; Ai, X.; Dong, T.; Li, B.; Luo, R.; Ai, Y.; Chen, Z.; Li, C. The physico-chemical properties and structural characteristics of artificial soil for cut slope restoration in Southwestern China. *Sci. Rep.* **2016**, *6*, 20565. [CrossRef]
52. Huang, Z.; Jiao, C.; Ai, X.; Li, R.; Ai, Y.; Wei, L. The texture, structure and nutrient availability of artificial soil on cut slopes restored with OSSS—Influence of restoration time. *J. Environ. Manag.* **2017**, *200*, 502. [CrossRef] [PubMed]
53. Jiang, X.; Ai, S.; Yang, S.; Zhu, M.; Huang, C. Effects of Different Highway Slope Disturbance on Soil Bulk Density, pH, and Soil Nutrients. *Environ. Eng. Sci.* **2020**, *38*, 256–265. [CrossRef]
54. Arbestain, M.C.; Mourenza, C.; Álvarez, E.; Macıas, F. Influence of parent material and soil type on the root chemistry of forest species grown on acid soils. *For. Ecol. Manag.* **2004**, *193*, 307–320. [CrossRef]
55. Tan, M.Z.; Zhan, Q.H.; Chen, J. Spatial Similarity Analysis of Soil pHS Influence Factor Based on Information Entropy Theory. *Soils* **2007**, *39*, 953–957.
56. Hong, S.; Piao, S.; Chen, A.; Liu, Y.; Liu, L.; Peng, S.; Sardans, J.; Sun, Y.; Peñuelas, J.; Zeng, H. Afforestation neutralizes soil pH. *Nat. Commun.* **2018**, *9*, 520. [CrossRef] [PubMed]
57. Bowman, W.D.; Cleveland, C.C.; Halada, U.; Hreko, J.; Baron, J.S. Negative impact of nitrogen deposition on soil buffering capacity. *Nat. Geosci.* **2008**, *1*, 767–770. [CrossRef]
58. Jia, X.; Wang, D.; Liu, F.; Dai, Q.M. Evaluation of highway construction impact on ecological environment of Qinghai-Tibet plateau. *Environ. Eng. Manag. J.* **2020**, *19*, 1157–1166.
59. Pan, S.L.; Zhou, S.T.; Bin, G.U. Effect of Slope Degree and Slope Position on Soil Nutrient Variability in the Early Succession of Rocky Slope Revegetation. *Res. Soil Water Conserv.* **2012**, *19*, 289–292.
60. Nelson, M.B.; Martiny, A.C.; Martiny, J. Global biogeography of microbial nitrogen-cycling traits in soil. *Proc. Natl. Acad. Sci. USA* **2016**, *113*, 8033–8040. [CrossRef]
61. Ma, S.-S.; Wang, Y.Y.; Song, G.L.; Xu, H.-Y.; Wang, F.; Liu, X.H. Soil Nutrient Characteristics and Their Influence Factors in Vegetation Restoration on Rocky Slope. *Bull. Soil Water Conserv.* **2013**, *194*, 24–28.
62. Yan, X.; Zhang, F.; Zeng, C.; Zhang, M.; Devkota, L.P.; Yao, T. Relationship between Heavy Metal Concentrations in Soils and Grasses of Roadside Farmland in Nepal. *Int. J. Environ. Res. Public Health* **2012**, *9*, 3209–3226. [CrossRef]
63. Falahi-Ardakani, A. Contamination of environment with heavy metals emitted from automotives. *Ecotoxicol. Environ. Saf.* **1984**, *8*, 152–161. [CrossRef]
64. Nabulo, G.; Oryem-Origa, H.; Diamond, M. Assessment of lead, cadmium, and zinc contamination of roadside soils, surface films, and vegetables in Kampala City, Uganda. *Environ. Res.* **2006**, *101*, 42–52. [CrossRef] [PubMed]
65. Viard, B.; Pihan, F.; Promeyrat, S.; Pihan, J.C. Integrated assessment of heavy metal (Pb, Zn, Cd) highway pollution: Bioaccumulation in soil, Graminaceae and land snails. *Chemosphere* **2004**, *55*, 1349–1359. [CrossRef] [PubMed]
66. Zhang, W.; Bahadur, A.; Sajjad, W.; Zhang, G.; Chen, T. Bacterial Diversity and Community Composition Distribution in Cold-Desert Habitats of Qinghai—Tibet Plateau, China. *Microorganisms* **2021**, *9*, 262. [CrossRef]
67. Kang, E.; Li, Y.; Zhang, X.; Yan, Z.; Wu, H.; Li, M.; Yan, L.; Zhang, K.; Wang, J.; Kang, X. Soil pH and nutrients shape the vertical distribution of microbial communities in an alpine wetland. *Sci. Total Environ.* **2021**, *774*, 145780. [CrossRef]
68. Shi, P.; Zhang, Y.; Hu, Z.; Ma, K.; Wang, H.; Chai, T. The response of soil bacterial communities to mining subsidence in the west China aeolian sand area. *Appl. Soil Ecol.* **2017**, *121*, 1–10. [CrossRef]

69. Ghimire, S.; Wongkuna, S.; Kumar, R.; Nelson, E.; Scaria, J. Genome sequence and description of Blautia brookingsii SG772 sp. nov., a novel bacterial species isolated from the human feces. *New Microbes New Infect.* **2020**, *34*, 100648. [CrossRef] [PubMed]
70. Kim, D.U.; Lee, H.; Lee, S.; Kim, S.G.; Ka, J.O. Flavisolibacter metallilatus sp. nov., isolated from an automotive air conditioning system and emended description of the genus Flavisolibacter. *Int. J. Syst. Evol. Microbiol.* **2018**, *68*, 917. [CrossRef]
71. Hui, S.; Terhonen, E.; Koskinen, K.; Paulin, L.; Asiegbu, F.O. Bacterial diversity and community structure along different peat soils in boreal forest. *Appl. Soil Ecol.* **2014**, *74*, 37–45.
72. Lawson, P.A.; Finegold, S.M. Reclassification of Ruminococcus obeum as Blautiaobeum comb. nov. *Int. J. Syst. Evol. Microbiol.* **2015**, *65*, 789–793. [CrossRef] [PubMed]
73. Ormerod, K.L.; Wood, D.; Lachner, N.; Gellatly, S.L.; Daly, J.N.; Parsons, J.D.; Dal'Molin, C.; Palfreyman, R.W.; Nielsen, L.K.; Cooper, M.A. Genomic characterization of the uncultured Bacteroidales family S24-7 inhabiting the guts of homeothermic animals. *Microbiome* **2016**, *4*, 36. [CrossRef]
74. Song, Y. Alistipes onderdonkii sp. nov. and Alistipes shahii sp. nov., of human origin. *Int. J. Syst. Evol. Microbiol.* **2006**, *56*, 1985. [CrossRef]
75. Sakamoto, M.; Ikeyama, N.; Ogata, Y.; Suda, W.; Iino, T.; Hattori, M.; Ohkuma, M. Alistipes communis sp. nov., Alistipes dispar sp. nov. and Alistipes onderdonkii subsp. vulgaris subsp. nov., isolated from human faeces, and creation of Alistipes onderdonkii subsp. onderdonkii subsp. nov. *Int. J. Syst. Evol. Microbiol.* **2020**, *70*, 473–480. [CrossRef]
76. Rodríguez-Berbel, N.; Ortega, R.; Lucas-Borja, M.E.; Benet, A.S.; Miralles, I. Long-term effects of two organic amendments on bacterial communities of calcareous Mediterranean soils degraded by mining. *J. Environ. Manag.* **2020**, in press. [CrossRef] [PubMed]
77. Chen, S.; Li, Y.; Fan, Z.; Liu, F.; Liu, H.; Wang, L.; Wu, H. Soil bacterial community dynamics following bioaugmentation with Paenarthrobacter sp. W11 in atrazine-contaminated soil. *Chemosphere* **2021**, *282*, 130976. [CrossRef] [PubMed]
78. Kaur, I.; Gaur, V.K.; Regar, R.K.; Roy, A.; Srivastava, P.K.; Gaur, R.; Manickam, N.; Barik, S.K. Plants exert beneficial influence on soil microbiome in a HCH contaminated soil revealing advantage of microbe-assisted plant-based HCH remediation of a dumpsite. *Chemosphere* **2021**, *280*, 130690. [CrossRef] [PubMed]
79. Wang, Y.; Huang, Q.; Gao, H.; Zhang, R.; Yang, L.; Guo, Y.; Li, H.; Awasthi, M.K.; Li, G. Long-term cover crops improved soil phosphorus availability in a rain-fed apple orchard. *Chemosphere* **2021**, *275*, 130093. [CrossRef]
80. Dong, S.K.; Wen, L.; Li, Y.Y.; Wang, X.X.; Li, X.Y. Soil-Quality Effects of Grassland Degradation and Restoration on the Qinghai-Tibetan Plateau. *Soil Sci. Soc. Am. J.* **2012**, *76*, 2256–2264. [CrossRef]
81. Sorensen, L.H.; Mikola, J.; Olofsson, M. Trampling and Spatial Heterogeneity Explain Decomposer Abundances in a Sub-Arctic Grassland Subjected to Simulated Reindeer Grazing. *Ecosystems* **2009**, *12*, 830–842. [CrossRef]
82. Li, S.; Wu, J.; Huo, Y.; Zhao, X.; Xue, L. Profiling multiple heavy metal contamination and bacterial communities surrounding an iron tailing pond in Northwest China. *Sci. Total Environ.* **2021**, *752*, 141827. [CrossRef]
83. An, M.; Chang, D.; Hong, D.; Fan, H.; Wang, K. Metabolic regulation in soil microbial succession and niche differentiation by the polymer amendment under cadmium stress. *J. Hazard. Mater.* **2021**, *416*, 126094. [CrossRef]
84. Wang, M.; Chen, S.; Chen, L.; Wang, D. Responses of soil microbial communities and their network interactions to saline-alkaline stress in Cd-contaminated soils. *Environ. Pollut.* **2019**, *252*, 1609–1621. [CrossRef]
85. Yang, J.; Wang, Y.; Cui, X.; Xue, K.; Zhang, Y.; Yu, Z. Habitat filtering shapes the differential structure of microbial communities in the Xilingol grassland. *Sci. Rep.* **2019**, *9*, 19326. [CrossRef]
86. Shen, J.P.; Zhang, L.M.; Di, H.J.; He, J.Z. A review of ammonia-oxidizing bacteria and archaea in Chinese soils. *Front. Microbiol.* **2012**, *3*, 296. [CrossRef]
87. Yan, G.; Xing, Y.; Han, S.; Zhang, J.; Changcheng, M.U. Long-time precipitation reduction and nitrogen deposition increase alter soil nitrogen dynamic by influencing soil bacterial communities and functional groups. *Pedosphere* **2020**, *30*, 363–377. [CrossRef]
88. Yu, L.; Luo, S.; Gou, Y.; Xu, X.; Wang, J. Structure of rhizospheric microbial community and N cycling functional gene shifts with reduced N input in sugarcane-soybean intercropping in South China. *Agric. Ecosyst. Environ.* **2021**, *314*, 107413. [CrossRef]
89. Peng, D.; Yang, G.; Liu, J.; Yu, S.; Zhong, Z. Effects of thinning intensity on understory vegetation and soil microbial communities of a mature Chinese pine plantation in the Loess Plateau. *Sci. Total Environ.* **2018**, *630*, 171–180.
90. Liu, J.; Dang, P.; Gao, Y.; Zhu, H.; Zhu, H.; Zhao, F.; Zhao, Z. Effects of tree species and soil properties on the composition and diversity of the soil bacterial community following afforestation. *For. Ecol. Manag.* **2018**, *427*, 342–349. [CrossRef]
91. Harpole, W.S.; Tilman, D. Grassland species loss resulting from reduced niche dimension. *Nature* **2007**, *446*, 791–793. [CrossRef] [PubMed]
92. Zhang, X.; Han, X. Nitrogen deposition alters soil chemical properties and bacterial communities in the Inner Mongolia grassland. *J. Environ. Sci.* **2012**, *24*, 1483–1491. [CrossRef]
93. Diana, N.; Petra, T.; Petr, K.; Pavel, D.; Karel, F.; Milan, C.; Petr, B. Diversity of fungi and bacteria in species-rich grasslands increases with plant diversity in shoots but not in roots and soil. *FEMS Microbiol. Ecol.* **2018**, *95*, fiy208. [CrossRef]
94. Schmid, M.W.; Hahl, T.; Moorsel, S.J.V.; Wagg, C.; Deyn, G.B.D.; Schmid, B. Feedbacks of plant identity and diversity on the diversity and community composition of rhizosphere microbiomes from a long-term biodiversity experiment. *Mol. Ecol.* **2019**, *28*, 863–878. [CrossRef]
95. Nobuhiko, S.; Kiyoshi, U.; Toshihide, H. Plant functional diversity and soil properties control elevational diversity gradients of soil bacteria. *FEMS Microbiol. Ecol.* **2019**, *4*, fiz025.

96. Liao, H.; Sheng, M.; Liu, J.; Ai, X.; Li, C.; Ai, S.; Ai, Y. Soil N availability drives the shifts of enzyme activity and microbial phosphorus limitation in the artificial soil on cut slope in southwestern China. *Environ. Sci. Pollut. Res. Int.* **2021**, *28*, 33307–33319. [CrossRef] [PubMed]
97. De Silva, S.; Ball, A.S.; Indrapala, D.V.; Reichman, S.M. Review of the interactions between vehicular emitted potentially toxic elements, roadside soils, and associated biota. *Chemosphere* **2021**, *263*, 128135. [CrossRef] [PubMed]

International Journal of
Environmental Research and Public Health

MDPI

Article

Impact of DST (Daylight Saving Time) on Major Trauma: A European Cohort Study

André Nohl [1,2,3,4,*], Christine Seelmann [5], Robert Roenick [6], Tobias Ohmann [5], Rolf Lefering [7], Bastian Brune [3,8], Veronika Weichert [4,9], Marcel Dudda [3,4,8,9] and The TraumaRegister DGU [10,†]

1 Department of Emergency Medicine, BG Klinikum Duisburg, 47249 Duisburg, Germany
2 Emergency Medical Services, Fire Brigade Oberhausen, 46047 Oberhausen, Germany
3 Department of Trauma, Hand and Reconstructive Surgery, University Hospital Essen, 45147 Essen, Germany; bastian.brune@uk-essen.de (B.B.); marcel.dudda@uk-essen.de (M.D.)
4 Helicopter Emergency Medical Service (HEMS), 47249 Duisburg, Germany; veronika.weichert@bg-klinikum-duisburg.de
5 Research Department, BG Klinikum Duisburg, 47249 Duisburg, Germany; christine.seelmann@bg-klinikum-duisburg.de (C.S.); tobias.ohmann@bg-klinikum-duisburg.de (T.O.)
6 Clinic for Arthroscopic Surgery, Sports Traumatology and Sports Medicine, BG Klinikum, 47249 Duisburg, Germany; robert.roenick@bg-klinikum-duisburg.de
7 Institute for Research in Operative Medicine (IFOM), University of Witten/Herdecke, 51109 Cologne, Germany; rolf.lefering@uni-wh.de
8 Emergency Medical Services, Fire Brigade Essen, 45139 Essen, Germany
9 Department of Trauma Surgery, BG Klinikum Duisburg, 47249 Duisburg, Germany
10 Committee on Emergency Medicine, Intensive Care and Trauma Management (Sektion NIS) of the German Trauma Society (DGU), 10623 Berlin, Germany
* Correspondence: andre.nohl@uk-essen.de or andre.nohl@bg-klinikum-duisburg.de
† A.N. and R.L. are members of the Committee on Emergency Medicine, Intensive Care and Trauma Management (Sektion NIS) of the German Trauma Society (DGU).

Citation: Nohl, A.; Seelmann, C.; Roenick, R.; Ohmann, T.; Lefering, R.; Brune, B.; Weichert, V.; Dudda, M.; The TraumaRegister DGU. Impact of DST (Daylight Saving Time) on Major Trauma: A European Cohort Study. *Int. J. Environ. Res. Public Health* **2021**, *18*, 13322. https://doi.org/10.3390/ijerph182413322

Academic Editors: Roberto Alonso González Lezcano, Francesco Nocera and Rosa Giuseppina Caponetto

Received: 20 November 2021
Accepted: 15 December 2021
Published: 17 December 2021

Abstract: (1) Background: Approximately 73 countries worldwide implemented a daylight saving time (DST) policy: setting their clocks forward in spring and back in fall. The main purpose of this practice is to save electricity. The aim of the present study was to find out how DST affects the incidence and impact of seriously injured patients. (2) Methods: In a retrospective, multi-center study, we used the data recorded in the TraumaRegister DGU® (TR-DGU) between 2003 and 2017 from Germany, Switzerland, and Austria. We compared the included cases 1 week before and after DST. (3) Results: After DST from standard time to summertime, we found an increased incidence of accidents of motorcyclists up to 51.58%. The result is consistent with other studies. (4) Conclusion: However, our results should be interpreted as a tendency. Other influencing factors, such as time of day and weather conditions, were not considered.

Keywords: DST; daylight saving time; major trauma

1. Introduction

In 2021, 73 nations worldwide conducted DST transitions in a biannual manner, adjusting the clock in order to establish a scenario in which the daylight is maximal utilized for waking activity.

In 2019, the EU Parliament accepted the EU Commission's proposal to abolish the time change in 2021. However, nothing has happened since then. The changeover is now to remain until at least 2026. The basis for the abolition of the clock changeover was a survey of people living in the EU.

In this (non-representative) online survey, 84 percent voted in favor of ending the switch between summer and winter time. A total of 4.6 million people took part, two-thirds of them from Germany [1].

The first transition takes place in spring, when the clock is set one hour forwards, and the second in autumn, when the clock is set one hour back again. The main arguments for this adjustment were economic reasons (energy saving) and changing illumination conditions for peak traffic density to likely avoid accidents due to bad light conditions in the evening, when the number of traffic accidents are elevated due to driver fatigue. The rationale of this approach is to shift one extra hour of daylight to the evening hours to compensate for the driver's lack in concentration.

There is evidence that especially the DST transition might have a negative impact on people's health, leading to sleep deprivation and circadian misalignment [2–7]. A study by Kantermann et al. suggests that the human circadian system does not adapt to daylight saving time and that its seasonal adaptation to changing photoperiods is disrupted by the introduction of daylight saving time. This disruption could also affect other aspects of human seasonal biology [3]. Jin et al. used an empirical approach to exploit the end of daylight saving time in a quasi-experimental setting on a daily basis. Due to the time reset in the fall, sleep time was extended by one hour. The study group found significant health benefits as hospital admissions decreased. For example, hospital admissions for cardiovascular disease decreased by 10 per day per million population. Using an event study approach, they found that the effect continued for four days after the time change. Admissions for heart attacks and injuries also showed the same characteristic four-day decline [8]. Toro et al. analyzed the effects of acute light sleep deprivation and circadian rhythm disturbances due to daylight saving time on the incidence of acute myocardial infarction using daily data for Brazil. They found robust evidence of a significant increase (7.4–8.5%) in the number of acute myocardial infarctions in Brazilian states with a time change to summer time but no statistical relationship between states without a time change [9].

A possible connection between DST transition and fatal traffic accidents is controversially discussed in literature. Fritz et al. (2020), for example, found acute consequences of the DST transition in spring on traffic accidents in a chronobiologic context [10]. Here, the spring DST transition increased fatal motor vehicle accidents by 6% in the DST week, whereas the fallback transition in autumn to Standard Time had no effects. Lahti et al. 2011 found that the sleep deprivation after DST transition is not harmful enough to have an influence on the incidence of occupational accident rates [11]. In a recent systematic review, Carey and Sarma addressed the topic about the impact of DST on road traffic collision risk [12]. A total of 24 studies were included in this overview. The complex picture emerging from this review showed day- and time-dependent potentially positive or negative short-term effects of DST and a possible positive long-term effect.

Because of inconsistent findings and conclusions across the mostly heterogeneous studies, no conclusion about a positive or negative overall impact of DST on traffic accidents could be drawn.

Traffic accidents represent only a part of all trauma patients. As a whole, trauma accounts for 10% of deaths worldwide and is the leading cause of death in people younger than 40 years [13]. Therefore, advancements in the prevention of accidents are inevitable. However, external factors such as time of the day, day of the week, and seasons are thought to affect trauma events [14]. Here, it seems obvious that the incidence of traumata might be affected by DST transition markedly.

Previous studies concentrated on the analysis of the impact of DST on traffic accidents, but none investigated the incidence of trauma that occurred from other reasons.

In this present study, our approach was to analyze the very extensive database of the TraumaRegisters DGU®, which has not been used for this purpose thus far and provides an excellent data collection to address the question if DST has an impact on the incidence and impact on major trauma.

2. Materials and Methods

2.1. Data Set

The TraumaRegister DGU® (TR-DGU, AUC - Akademie der Unfallchirurgie GmbH, Munich, Germany) of the German Trauma Society was founded in 1993 to create a multicenter database for pseudonymized and standardized documentation of severely injured patients for quality assurance and research [15].

Participating hospitals are predominantly located in Germany (90%), but an increasing number of hospitals from other countries have also started to contribute their data (e.g., Austria, Belgium, Finland). Currently, approximately 30,000 cases from more than 650 hospitals are entered into the database annually. Participation in TR-DGU is voluntary; however, hospitals associated with TraumaNetzwerk DGU® are required to enter at least a basic dataset for reasons of quality assurance.

Documentation in the TR-DGU includes detailed information on:

- Demographics;
- Injury patterns;
- Comorbidities;
- Prehospital data;
- Course of hospital treatment, including intensive care unit, relevant laboratory findings, transfusions, and interventions;
- Outcome.

Inclusion criteria for the TR-DGU are admission to hospital via the emergency department followed by intensive care or admission to hospital with vital signs and death before admission to the intensive care unit (ICU).

The infrastructure for documentation and data management is provided by the AUC - Academy of Trauma Surgery, a society affiliated with the German Trauma Society. Scientific management is provided by the Committee on Emergency Medicine, Intensive Care and Trauma Management (Sektion NIS) of the German Trauma Society. The scientific evaluation of the data is performed according to a peer-review process defined in the publication guideline of the TR-DGU [15]. The present study complies with the publication guideline of the TR-DGU and is registered under the TR-DGU project ID 2018-047. The inclusion criteria of our study are shown in Figure 1.

Permission by the ethics committee (Ärztekammer Nordrhein/Medical Association North Rhine; no. 310/2018).

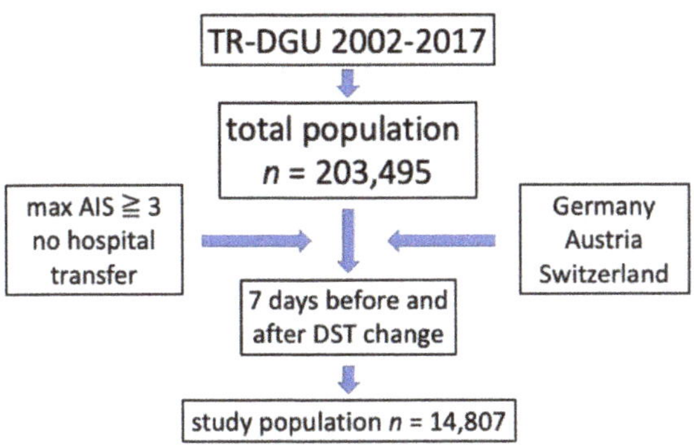

Figure 1. Inclusion criteria; max = maximum; AIS = abbreviated injury score; DST daylight saving time.

2.2. Statistics

The day of DST change was excluded (usually a Sunday), and a time period of 7 days before and after DST change in spring and autumn was selected for comparison (the comparison of 7 days was chosen because the direct comparison of individual days showed a low number of cases; in the studies cited, the procedure was comparable). Both pre- and post-change phases thus contained each weekday once. Data are presented as number of cases with percentage for counts, and as mean with standard deviation (SD) for metric data. In seriously skewed data, median and inter-quartile range were given instead. Observed differences were evaluated with the chi-squared test or the Mann–Whitney *U*-test.

Statistical analysis was performed using SPSS Statistical software (Version 27.0, IBM Inc., Armonk, NY, USA). The level of statistical significance was set at $p < 0.05$.

The RISC II score was developed and validated using TR-DGU data and represents a summary of the 13 variables, including pattern and severity of injuries, age, sex, prior diseases, and initial physiology [16].

3. Results

A total of 14,807 trauma patients were included in the study. The mean age was 51 (±22) years. The majority were males (71%). In Table 1, the mechanism of accident 1 week before and 1 week after the time change are listed. More traffic accidents occurred after the time change (n = 3459 vs. 3582), but it was not statistically significant (p = 0.131). The mean ISS was higher after the time change. Although, this difference did not reach the significance level, we observed a strong tendency (p = 0.052). There was a noticeable increase in the number of motorcycle and bicycle accidents during the time change from spring to summer (motorcycle n = 349 vs. 529, increase of 51.58%; bicycle n = 245 vs. 280, increase of 14.29%). After the time change in autumn, these incidents decreased in number compared to the previous week.

Table 1. Impact of daylight saving time change in patients with major trauma.

Accident History, *n* = 14,488				
		Pre-Week	**Post-Week**	**Total**
DST standard to summer time	car/lorry, *n* (%)	758 (21.9)	778 (20.8)	1534 (21.3)
	motorcycle, *n* (%)	349 (10.1)	529 (14.1)	878 (12.2)
	bicycle, *n* (%)	245 (7.1)	280 (7.5)	525 (7.3)
	pedestrians, *n* (%)	218 (6.3)	209 (5.6)	427 (5.9)
	high fall > 3 m, *n* (%)	589 (17.0)	610 (16.3)	1199 (16.6)
	low fall < 3 m, *n* (%)	869 (25.1)	870 (23.2)	1739 (24.1)
	others, *n* (%)	430 (12.4)	472 (12.6)	902 (12.5)
	total, *n*	3456	3748	7204
DST summer to standard time	car/lorry, *n* (%)	863 (23.0)	830 (23.5)	1693 (23.2)
	motorcycle, *n* (%)	412 (11.0)	319 (9.0)	731 (10.0)
	bicycle, *n* (%)	288 (7.7)	244 (6.9)	532 (7.3)
	pedestrians, *n* (%)	243 (6.5)	303 (8.6)	546 (7.5)
	high fall > 3 m, *n* (%)	653 (17.4)	638 (18.1)	1291 (17.7)
	low fall < 3 m, *n* (%)	866 (23.1)	803 (22.8)	1669 (22.9)
	others, *n* (%)	430 (11.5)	392 (11.1)	822 (11.3)
	total, *n*	3755	3529	7284
Total	car/lorry, *n* (%)	1619 (22.5)	1608 (22.1)	3227 (22.3)
	motorcycle, *n* (%)	761 (10.6)	848 (11.7)	1609 (11.1)
	bicycle, *n* (%)	533 (7.4)	524 (7.2)	1057 (7.3)
	pedestrians, *n* (%)	461 (6.4)	512 (7.0)	973 (6.7)
	fall > 3 m, *n* (%)	1242 (17.2)	1248 (17.1)	2490 (17.2)
	fall < 3 m, *n* (%)	1735 (24.1)	1673 (23.1)	3408 (23.5)
	others, *n* (%)	860 (11.9)	864 (11.9)	1724 (11.9)
	total, *n* (%)	7211	7277	14,488

DST = daylight saving time.

Table 2 shows demographics and the distribution of different injury regions before and after the time change. Increased deaths after time change *n* (%) = 900 (12.2) vs. 950 (12.8). The age, injury severity, expected mortality (RISC II), ICU, and hospitalization days are shown in Table 3.

Table 2. Cross tabulation.

Impact of DST in Major Trauma				
		Pre-DST	**Post-DST**	***p*-Value**
Traffic accident, *n* (%)	no	3752 (52.0)	3695 (50.8)	$p = 0.131$
	yes	3459 (48.0)	3582 (49.2)	
Blunt/penetrating trauma, *n* (%)	blunt	6749 (95.8)	6808 (95.6)	$p = 0.595$
	penetrating	295 (4.2)	311 (4.4)	
Sex, *n* (%)	female	2172 (29.6)	2066 (27.8)	$p = 0.017$
	male	5175 (70.4)	5367 (72.2)	
Age 70+ years, *n* (%)	<70	5459 (74.4)	5502 (74.2)	$p = 0.778$
	>70	1877 (25.6)	1912 (25.8)	
Died, *n* (%)	no	6482 (87.8)	6495 (87.2)	$p = 0.325$
	yes	900 (12.2)	950 (12.8)	
AIS head ≥ 3, *n* (%)	<3	3968 (58.9)	3993 (53.6)	$p = 0.746$
	≥3	3394 (46.1)	3452 (46.4)	
AIS thorax ≥ 3, *n* (%)	<3	3898 (52.9)	3942 (52.9)	$p = 0.999$
	≥3	3464 (47.1)	3503 (47.1)	
AIS abdomen ≥ 3, *n* (%)	<3	6384 (86.7)	6473 (86.9)	$p = 0.681$
	≥3	978 (13.3)	972 (13.1)	
AIS extremities ≥ 3, *n* (%)	< 3	5166 (70.2)	5106 (68.6)	$p = 0.036$
	≥3	2196 (29.8)	2339 (31.4)	

AIS = abbreviated injury scale, *DST* = daylight saving time.

Table 3. Impact of DST in major trauma—spring and autumn.

	Pre-DST	**Post-DST**	***p*-Value**
Age, mean (SD)	51 (22)	51 (22)	0.501
ISS, mean (SD)	21.8 (11.7)	22.3 (12.1)	0.052
Prognosis based on RISC II, mean %	13.2	13.4	0.439
ICU days, median (IQR)	2 (1–8)	3 (1–8)	0.035
Hospital days, median (IQR)	13 (5–23)	13 (6–23)	0.457

DST = daylight saving time, ICU = intensive care unit, ISS = Injury Severity Score, IQR = interquartile range, RISC II = Revised Injury Severity Classification II, SD = standard deviation.

4. Discussion

The results of this study showed an increased incidence of traffic accidents (bicycle and motorcycle) after the spring DST. Motorcycle accidents showed an increase of 51.58%, whereas accidents involving motorcyclists slightly decreased again after the time change in autumn. However, it is worth mentioning that many motorcyclists have summer license plates from March to October. Central European Summer Time begins on the last Sunday in March at 2:00 CET. Therefore, there is an interval of over 4 weeks from the seasonal registration of the motorcycles to the change of time.

However, a possible cause could also be the general trend that motorcycle and bicycle accidents occur more frequently in the summertime and decrease again in the winter. External influences, such as time of day, lighting conditions, days of the week, weather conditions, and temperatures were not considered in our study.

The number of registered motorcycles in Germany has risen steadily, reaching 4.31 million in 2017. We detected 10 of the busiest highways in the most populous state of North Rhine-Westphalia and compared 10 automatic counting stations for traffic measurement between March 2017 and April 2017. The 10 automatic counting stations counted 5848 motorcycles in March 2017 and 6362 motorcycles in April 2017. Thus, there is an increase of 8.79% in the number of motorcycles counted on the 10 busiest highways in North Rhine-Westphalia from March to April. The increase of 8.79% more motorcycles counted from March to April contrasts with the 51.58% increase in motorcyclists seriously injured after the time change in spring. Although only 10 measuring points were evaluated, the sample of a total of 12,210 was representative. However, a sample of a German state is compared here with a European cohort in our study [17].

A comparable study by Pape-Köhler et al. (2014) showed that the time of day shows a high variation in the incidence of trauma. In particular, the frequency of accidents increased during rush hour [14]. However, these external factors could also have an influence on accident frequency. In addition, our data do not show whether the motorcyclists caused the traffic accidents themselves or were harmed by other road users.

Importantly one should take into account that due to our inclusion criteria, only accidents with serious injuries were considered. Thus, no conclusion can be drawn about the general frequency of accidents.

Fritz et al. (2020) showed similar results in their study. The study group was able to show that the incidence of serious car accidents increased by 6% after the time change in spring. They attributed the result to sleep deprivation due to the one-hour time shift. Here, the frequency of accidents was increased, especially in the early morning hours. The research team concluded that leaving out the time change could prevent up to 27 serious traffic accidents annually [10].

Besides the disturbance of the circadian rhythm, another reason could be the fact that due to the time shift by one hour later, it is correspondingly darker in the early morning and thus an increased accident frequency could be explained.

In a study by Robb et al. (2018), an increased accident frequency was proven in the first 2 days after the time change in New Zealand [18].

Another study from Spain showed that the time change is associated with fatal accidents of 1.5 people per year in 52 Spanish capital cities [19].

What is slightly noticeable in our study is the increased accident frequency explicitly among motorcyclists. There are a number of confounding factors that influence the frequency of motorcycle accidents. The biggest disruptive factors are certainly the winter break and a colder season at the beginning of the motorcycle season. It has been proven that the frequency of accidents increases with age (young, inexperienced riders, as well as seniors), general riding experience and frequency, weight of the motorcycle, male gender, weather conditions, etc. [20].

However, here, the period of 1 week before and 1 week after the time change was quite short to conclude.

Thus, according to our results, if the time change were eliminated, up to 12 serious motorcycle accidents could be prevented each year if these accidents were indeed related to DST.

However, we cannot confirm this statement with a probability bordering on certainty. Nevertheless, due to the external influences not taken into account and the lack of statistical significance, it should rather be seen as a tendency. Our result is certainly not conclusive enough for a clear recommendation.

Strengths and Limitations

Due to the high number of cases and the study period of almost two decades, our study has a high level of representativeness.

This study has several limitations. It is a retrospective analysis.

Patients who died in the prehospital setting are not included in the TraumaRegister DGU®. Data from patients who were admitted to the hospital without activation of the trauma team are not captured by the TraumaRegister DGU®. Another limitation of this study is that treatment restrictions, for example due to a living will, were not recorded. The participation of hospitals in the TraumaRegister DGU® is voluntary [15].

5. Conclusions

There is a noticeable increase in the number of motorcycle and bicycle accidents during the DST from standard to summer time. Our results should be understood as a tendency, since various influencing factors, such as times of day and weather, were not taken into account.

Author Contributions: Conceptualization, A.N., R.R., R.L.; methodology, A.N., R.R., R.L.; software, R.L.; validation, A.N., R.R., R.L.; formal analysis, A.N., R.R., R.L.; investigation, A.N., R.R., R.L.; resources, A.N., R.R., R.L.; data curation, R.L.; writing—original draft preparation, A.N., C.S.; writing—review and editing, A.N., C.S., R.L., M.D., T.O., B.B., V.W.; visualization, A.N.; supervision, M.D.; project administration, A.N., R.R., C.S., T.O.; funding acquisition, A.N., M.D. All authors have read and agreed to the published version of the manuscript.

Funding: The APC was funded by the Open Access Publication Fund of the University of Duisburg-Essen. A grant no. is not applicable.

Institutional Review Board Statement: The study was conducted according to the guidelines of the Declaration of Helsinki and is approved by the Ärztekammer Nordrhein (no. 310/2018). The present study complies with the publication guideline of the TR-DGU and is registered under the TR-DGU project ID 2018-047.

Informed Consent Statement: Not applicable.

Data Availability Statement: Data are available from andre.nohl@bg-klinikum-duisburg.de.

Conflicts of Interest: The authors declare no conflict of interest The funders had no role in the design of the study; in the collection, analyses, or interpretation of data; in the writing of the manuscript; or in the decision to publish the results.

Abbreviations

Abbreviations

AIS	abbreviated injury scale
DST	daylight saving time
ICU	intensive care unit
ISS	Injury Severity Score
IQR	interquartile range
RISC II	Revised Injury Severity Classification II

References

1. Summertime Consultation: 84% Want Europe to Stop Changing the Clock. Available online: https://ec.europa.eu/commission/presscorner/detail/en/IP_18_5302 (accessed on 8 December 2021).
2. Varughese, J.; Allen, R.P. Fatal Accidents Following Changes in Daylight Savings Time: The American Experience. *Sleep Med.* **2001**, *2*, 31–36. [CrossRef]
3. Kantermann, T.; Juda, M.; Merrow, M.; Roenneberg, T. The Human Circadian Clock's Seasonal Adjustment Is Disrupted by Daylight Saving Time. *Curr. Biol. CB* **2007**, *17*, 1996–2000. [CrossRef] [PubMed]
4. Janszky, I.; Ljung, R. Shifts to and from Daylight Saving Time and Incidence of Myocardial Infarction. *N. Engl. J. Med.* **2008**, *359*, 1966–1968. [CrossRef] [PubMed]

5. MONK, T.H.; APLIN, L.C. Spring and Autumn Daylight Saving Time Changes: Studies of Adjustment in Sleep Timings, Mood, and Efficiency. *Ergonomics* **1980**, *23*, 167–178. [CrossRef] [PubMed]
6. Smith, A.C. Spring Forward at Your Own Risk: Daylight Saving Time and Fatal Vehicle Crashes. *Am. Econ. J. Appl. Econ.* **2016**, *8*, 65–91. [CrossRef]
7. Czeisler, C.A.; Wickwire, E.M.; Barger, L.K.; Dement, W.C.; Gamble, K.; Hartenbaum, N.; Ohayon, M.M.; Pelayo, R.; Phillips, B.; Strohl, K.; et al. Sleep-Deprived Motor Vehicle Operators Are Unfit to Drive: A Multidisciplinary Expert Consensus Statement on Drowsy Driving. *Sleep Health* **2016**, *2*, 94–99. [CrossRef] [PubMed]
8. Jin, L.; Ziebarth, N.R. Sleep, Health, and Human Capital: Evidence from Daylight Saving Time. *J. Econ. Behav. Organ.* **2020**, *170*, 174–192. [CrossRef]
9. Toro, W.; Tigre, R.; Sampaio, B. Daylight Saving Time and Incidence of Myocardial Infarction: Evidence from a Regression Discontinuity Design. *Econ. Lett.* **2015**, *136*, 1–4. [CrossRef]
10. Fritz, J.; VoPham, T.; Wright, K.P.; Vetter, C. A Chronobiological Evaluation of the Acute Effects of Daylight Saving Time on Traffic Accident Risk. *Curr. Biol.* **2020**, *30*, 729–735.e2. [CrossRef] [PubMed]
11. Lahti, T.; Sysi-Aho, J.; Haukka, J.; Partonen, T. Work-Related Accidents and Daylight Saving Time in Finland. *Occup. Med.* **2011**, *61*, 26–28. [CrossRef] [PubMed]
12. Carey, R.N.; Sarma, K.M. Impact of Daylight Saving Time on Road Traffic Collision Risk: A Systematic Review. *BMJ Open* **2017**, *7*, e014319. [CrossRef] [PubMed]
13. MacKenzie, E.J. Epidemiology of Injuries: Current Trends and Future Challenges. *Epidemiol. Rev.* **2000**, *22*, 112–119. [CrossRef] [PubMed]
14. Pape-Köhler, C.I.A.; Simanski, C.; Nienaber, U.; Lefering, R. External Factors and the Incidence of Severe Trauma: Time, Date, Season and Moon. *Injury* **2014**, *45*, S93–S99. [CrossRef] [PubMed]
15. AUC: TraumaRegister. Available online: https://www.traumaregister-dgu.de/ (accessed on 12 May 2021).
16. Lefering, R.; Huber-Wagner, S.; Nienaber, U.; Maegele, M.; Bouillon, B. Update of the Trauma Risk Adjustment Model of the TraumaRegister DGU^{TM}: The Revised Injury Severity Classification, Version II. *Crit. Care* **2014**, *18*, 476. [CrossRef] [PubMed]
17. Dauerzählstellen | Straßen.NRW. Available online: https://www.strassen.nrw.de/de/wir-bauen-fuer-sie/verkehr/verkehrsbelastung/dauerzaehlstellen.html (accessed on 8 December 2021).
18. Robb, D.; Barnes, T. Accident Rates and the Impact of Daylight Saving Time Transitions. *Accid. Anal. Prev.* **2018**, *111*, 193–201. [CrossRef] [PubMed]
19. Prats-Uribe, A.; Tobías, A.; Prieto-Alhambra, D. Excess Risk of Fatal Road Traffic Accidents on the Day of Daylight Saving Time Change. *Epidemiology* **2018**, *29*, e44. [CrossRef] [PubMed]
20. Bäumer, M.; Hautzinger, H.; Pfeiffer, M. Motorräder: Mobilitätsstrukturen und Expositionsgrößen = Motorcycles: Mobility structure and exposition data. 2020. Available online: https://bast.opus.hbz-nrw.de/opus45-bast/frontdoor/deliver/index/docId/2457/file/M301_barrfreiPDF.pdf; (accessed on 8 December 2021).

energies

MDPI

Article

Determination of the Model Basis for Assessing the Vehicle Energy Efficiency in Urban Traffic

Miroslaw Śmieszek [1,*], Nataliia Kostian [2], Vasyl Mateichyk [1], Jakub Mościszewski [1] and Liudmyla Tarandushka [2]

1 Department of Technical Systems Engineering, Rzeszow University of Technology, al. Powstancow Warszawy 10, 35-959 Rzeszow, Poland; vmate@prz.edu.pl (V.M.); j.mosciszews@prz.edu.pl (J.M.)
2 Department of Automobiles and Technologies for their Operating, Cherkasy State Technological University, 333 Shevchenko, 18006 Cherkasy, Ukraine; 438knl@gmail.com (N.K.); tarandushkal@ukr.net (L.T.)
* Correspondence: msmieszk@prz.edu.pl

Abstract: The paper studies the problem of assessing the vehicle energy efficiency on the streets of urban road network. As a result of morphological analysis of the system "Vehicle—Traffic flow—Road—Traffic Environment" 18 significant morphological attributes of its functional elements, that affect the energy efficiency of vehicles, were identified. Each attribute is characterized by 3–6 implementation variants, which are evaluated by the relevant quantitative or qualitative parameters. The energy efficiency of vehicles is determined by the criteria of their energy consumption considering the vehicle category, type of energy unit, mode of vehicle movement and adjustment factors—road, climatic and others. The input parameters values of the system in the process of traffic flow on the linear fragments of streets and road networks of the cities of Ukraine and Poland were measured. The set of independent system parameters is determined by applying the Farrar-Glober method based on statistical estimates. The specified set is the basis of the studied system and is formed of 10 independent input parameters. The presence in the basis of parameters that correspond to the morphological features of all four functional elements, confirmed the importance of these elements of the system. The mathematical dependence of the impact of vehicle characteristics, traffic flow, road and environment on vehicle energy efficiency is built. The standard deviation of the model values from the tabular ones equals $\acute{\sigma} = 0.0091$. Relative standard deviation equals $\acute{S}_r = 1.5\%$. The results of the study could be used in the development of new and optimization of existing intelligent traffic control systems of urban transport.

Keywords: energy efficiency; urban traffic; traffic flow; level of vehicle energy efficiency; morphological matrix; multiple linear regression

Citation: Śmieszek, M.; Kostian, N.; Mateichyk, V.; Mościszewski, J.; Tarandushka, L. Determination of the Model Basis for Assessing the Vehicle Energy Efficiency in Urban Traffic. *Energies* **2021**, *14*, 8538. https://doi.org/10.3390/en14248538

Academic Editors: Roberto Alonso González-Lezcano, Francesco Nocera and Rosa Giuseppina Caponetto

Received: 25 November 2021
Accepted: 14 December 2021
Published: 17 December 2021

1. Introduction

The development of the world economy and population growth inevitably led to an increase in freight and passenger traffic. The needs for population mobility are growing every year. Around 70% of the European Union population lives in urban areas (cities, towns and suburbs) and generate around 85% of European Union's GDP [1]. At the same time, the level of motorization of large cities is growing rapidly. Urbanization coupled with motorization directly causes several issues, such as environmental pollution by harmful emissions and noise, congestion, and accidents. Urban transport is still mainly based on conventional private passenger vehicles equipped with internal combustion engines, which are the main sources of greenhouse gas emissions. Around 40% of all CO_2 emissions from transport and up to 70% of other pollutants generated by transport are emitted by urban traffic [2]. Inefficient traffic control and poorly designed urban road network causes unnecessary energy consumption while the vehicle is driving in heavy traffic or idling in traffic jams. Idling refers to engine working while vehicle is not moving. Idling fuel consumption of conventional vehicles can be as high as 15 mL per minute [3]. Conventional vehicles are still emitting exhaust gases while idling, hence they are polluting air under idling conditions. Reduction of emissions can be achieved by redesigning of intersections. Authors of [4] found that change of one specific roundabout layout can reduce up to 30% of emissions from this intersection.

City's inhabitants should be encouraged to use public transport, as fuel consumption per passenger of city bus can be much lower than of private passenger vehicles what confirms high energy efficiency of public transport [5]. City's authorities might take measures to encourage its inhabitants to use public transport instead of private vehicles, i.e., creation of proper urban infrastructure (bus lanes and parking lots), replacement of public transport fleet, development of Integrated Traffic and Public Transportation Management System [6]. Authors of [7] found that urban mobility planning can affect number of passengers of urban public transport.

The intensity of traffic has a great influence on the level of roadside pollution. Authors of [8] calculated that during pandemic, decrease of daily traffic intensity by 66% accounted for decrease of total daily emissions of: CO by factor of 2.25, CnHm by factor of 3.55, PM concentration by factor of 1.39–3.42, NOx, by factor of 2.64 and PM by factor of 1.96. In addition, there is a global trend of rising energy prices. These factors require the optimization of traffic management systems in large cities and identification of energy reserves during vehicle operation to ensure sufficient air quality in cities, as most of the cities in European Union do not meet the air quality requirements [9].

In developed countries, the transition of transport to alternative fuels and the creation of appropriate infrastructure is carried out, which requires significant financial investment. Therefore, it is important to identify and implement alternative ways to reduce energy consumption by ensuring energy-efficient traffic in urban mobility to reduce cost of urban transportation. One way of reducing energy consumption is to provide guidance of eco-driving to drivers [10,11].

Energy consumption and the harmful effects of the vehicle movement on the environment can be determined by real-time measurements while the vehicle is in motion or by computer simulation. In the case of measurements of harmful substances emitted into the atmosphere by vehicles, the applied test method requires appropriate equipment and is most often used to assess pollution in a limited area [8]. In the case of measurements performed over a large area, it is required to have an extensive measuring and monitoring system. A method that requires the use of a much smaller amount of specialized measuring equipment is the use of a computer simulation based on a mathematical model of fuel consumption, emissions or energy efficiency. The available literature describes 2 simulation methods. The first one consists in determining the quantities values, such as fuel consumption, energy efficiency and emissions, separately for each vehicle [12–14]. The input data for the simulation process may be the measured traffic profiles [15–17] or driving cycles characteristic for a given section of the route [18–21]. A driving cycle is defined as the speed over time profile of a representative vehicle that can be obtained by combining a series of micro journeys. A micro journey is defined as the journey between the starts of two periods of idling. Driving cycles may be divided into 2 types: standard and real-world. Usually, standard driving cycles are used to ensure emission norms and real-world driving cycles are used to test and evaluate field performance [22]. Authors of [23] developed a model to estimate diesel bus fuel consumption. Authors of [24] developed a model to estimate influence of changing traffic conditions on fuel consumption of public urban bus. The process of simulating selected quantities separately for each vehicle requires additional knowledge of the Brake-Specific Fuel Consumption (BSFC) characteristics [25,26]. But these characteristics are not always available.

One of those methods, that do not require such knowledge, is estimation based on VSP (Vehicle Specific Power) model [24,27,28]. VSP is defined as the required engine power to offset vehicle acceleration, wind, rolling and road slope resistances. VSP model is a function of a vehicle velocity, acceleration, deceleration and road slope. VSP model connects instantaneous driving state, required engine power and fuel consumption. VSP model could be used for comparisons of fuel consumption characteristics between different vehicles [29].

The second method does not consider individual vehicles but takes a comprehensive approach to the entire traffic flow in the entire area. In this method, vehicles are divided into categories [30] and for each category, assuming specific traffic conditions, fuel consumption, emission and energy efficiency are determined. With a comprehensive approach to the issue, the most advanced is the method of morphological analysis. Morphological analysis is defined as a method for structuring and evaluation of the total set of relationships contained in complex, multidimensional, non-quantifiable problem [31]. The morphological analysis begins by identifying and defining dimensions of the investigated complex problem, that are the most important for this problem. Then, each of these dimensions is given a range values or conditions, that are relevant. These together make up the structure of variables or parameters of the problem. Then, a morphological field is created by making the table of the parameters placed in parallel columns, representing an n-dimensional configuration space. The last step is to examine each configuration (created by selecting a single value from each of the variables) or to reduce number of configurations by a process of cross-consistency assessment before examination (by applying logical, empirical and normative constrains) [32].

To assess the efficiency of vehicle motion on the urban road network in the paper [33] a morphological analysis of the system "Vehicle-Traffic flow-Road-Means of traffic flow control" was performed. For each functional element the variants of realization of its morphological attributes and ranges of their values are given. However, the methods of calculating the values of individual parameters are not described in detail and the criteria for assessing the energy efficiency of vehicles moving on the urban road network are not defined. The authors of [34] provide regression equations describing the dependence of energy consumption of vehicles on their speed. When choosing the parameters values of these equations, the category, energy unit type and operation mode of the vehicle are considered significant. For hybrid and electric vehicles, these mathematical dependencies are not defined. The parameters of the road and the flow of traffic, in which the vehicle is moving, are not considered. In the article [35], in assessment of the vehicle's energy efficiency, the following functional elements of the transport system are considered: the driver, the vehicle, the environment. The functional element "Driver" is characterized by the following functional characteristics: aggressiveness of driving, psychological and behavioral traits. The parameters of the element "Vehicle" are determined by the type of engine and type of gearbox (for vehicles with internal combustion engine), battery efficiency and regenerative braking (for hybrid and electric vehicles), vehicle body type, geometric parameters, weight and age of the vehicle, tire pressure. Environmental factors include traffic (e.g., heaviness, time of day, day of the year, exceptional situations), type of roads (small public or private roads with city's traffic, city's highways and highways), weather conditions. The total energy consumption of a vehicle is defined as the sum of the energy consumption of the vehicle and the standby energy consumption. In [36] the comparative analysis of dependencies of energy efficiency of vehicles on their technical parameters for vehicles with internal combustion engines and with electric energy units is carried out. It is determined that for vehicles with an internal combustion engine, fuel consumption depends significantly on the rated engine power. In electric vehicles, increasing the battery capacity by 10 kWh increases energy consumption by 0.7–1.0 kWh/100 km. Modern mass-produced electric passenger vehicles are 2.1 $\pm$ 0.8 kWh/100 km more efficient than first-generation cars. Vehicles with gas-balloon energy units are not considered. The authors [37] study the energy consumption of vehicles with a hybrid engine. The value of the total energy consumption depends on the energy consumption of the internal combustion engine (1.25–2.95 (J/(kg·m)) and the electric drive (0.27–1.1 (J/(kg·m)). The power consumption of an internal combustion engine is 3.4 times higher than the power consumption of an electric drive. Ref. [38] proposes a methodology for estimating the energy consumption of vehicles for different traffic models, what takes into account the parameters that characterize the vehicle, the environment and the driver's behavior when moving along a given route. It was found that among the considered parameters the greatest influence on energy consumption has the speed and acceleration of the vehicle. Regeneration of energy from braking gave significant energy savings and weakened the correlation between most of the source and the resulting parameters. The authors [39] consider that movement energy consumption is largely determined by driving behavior, terrain information and the situation on the road, which is difficult to predict. The paper develops a model for estimating the energy consumption of electric vehicles. The number of passengers, weather conditions, road category, parameters that characterize the traffic flow, driver and route were determined as the significant parameters. Two algorithms for estimating energy consumption are presented: under the condition of maximum speed and to achieve maximum efficiency.

Despite the large number of scientific studies on the energy efficiency of vehicles, the development of a mathematical apparatus for comprehensive assessment and forecasting of energy consumption of a wider range of vehicles, considering the characteristics of all functional elements of the transport system remains relevant.

The object of research is the system "Vehicle—Traffic flow—Road—Traffic Environment" (the TrEECS system).

The purpose of the article is to determine the character of influence exerted independent parameters of the TrEECS system on the energy efficiency of vehicles.

To achieve this goal the following tasks were solved:

- to identify significant morphological attributes of the TrEECS system;
- to investigate the state of functional elements of TrEECS in the traffic process on linear sections of street and urban road networks and to form an array of initial data;
- on the basis of statistical estimates to determine the basic parameters corresponding to the morphological attributes of the TrEECS system;
- build the analytical dependence of energy efficiency on system parameters and evaluate its accuracy.
- In order to achieve the assumed goals, the article includes the following sections:
- Section 1 introduces the subject of the article and provides an overview of the literature;
- Section 2 presents a description of the used methodology and includes a description of the model;
- Section 3 presents the input data and an example of the model application for the analysis of energy efficiency on a linear road section. In this section, the Farrar-Glober method was used to evaluate the significance of the model parameters;
- Section 4 summarizes the work and contains conclusions concerning further research directions.

2. Materials and Methods

The movement of traffic flows on the urban road network forms a complex system (hereinafter the TrEECS system), the internal processes of which occur according to certain laws, the mathematical representation of which is necessary to assess both individual processes and the efficiency of the system. This system is represented by four functional elements: "Vehicle" (V), "Traffic flow" (TF), "Road" (R) and "Traffic environment" (Env). Morphological analysis of the TrEECS system [33] allowed to determine 18 morphological attributes of its functional elements that are significant in terms of assessing the energy efficiency of a vehicle in urban traffic, namely: X_1—vehicle category, X_2—vehicle energy unit type, X_3—vehicle age, X_4—degree of use of load capacity and/or passenger capacity of the vehicle, X_5—vehicle motion mode, X_6—vehicle autonomy level, X_7—traffic intensity, X_8—traffic density, X_9—traffic flow complexity level, X_{10}—traffic flow phase, X_{11}—number of lanes on the road in both directions, X_{12}—road resistance degree, X_{13}—carriageway curvature degree, X_{14}—group of localities determined by the city population, X_{15}—population density, X_{16}—level of motorization, X_{17}—time interval, X_{18}—complexity of weather conditions. The results of morphological analysis of the TrEECS system presented in the form of a morphological matrix of the system (Tables 1 and 2).

Table 1. Results of the analysis of the functional elements "Vehicle" and "Traffic flow".

Vehicle						Traffic Flow			
1. Category	**2. Energy Unit Type**	**3. Vehicle age**	**4. The Degree of Use of Load Capacity and/or Passenger Capacity**	**5. Movement Mode**	**6. Autonomy Level**	**7. Traffic Intensity, Reduced Units/Hour**	**8. Traffic Density, Reduced Units/km**	**9. Traffic Flow Complexity Level**	**10. Traffic Flow Phase**
1.1. M1 1	2.1. Petrol 1	3.1. Up to 5 years 1	4.1. Low 0–0.4	5.1. Acceleration dV/dt > 0 1	6.1. Null 1	7.1. Very small 0–200	8.1. Small 0–12	9.1. Very low 0–0.25	10.1. Free 1
1.2. M2 2	2.2. Diesel 2	3.2. 5–10 years 2	4.2. Medium 0.41–0.5		6.2. First 2	7.2. Small 200–400	8.2. Medium 12–36	9.2. Low 0.25–0.5	10.2. Stable 2
1.3. M3 3	2.3. Gas 3	3.3. 10–15 years 3	4.3. High 0.051–0.7	5.2. Movement at a constant speed V = const 2	6.3. Second 3	7.3. Medium 400–600	8.3. Large 36–60	9.3. Medium 0.5–0.75	10.3. Unstable 3
1.4. N1 4		3.4. 15–20 years 4				7.4. Large 600–800			
1.5. N2 5	2.4. Hybrid and electric 4	3.5. More than 20 years 5	4.4. Very high 0.71–1	5.3. Idle mode V = 0 3	6.4. Third 4	7.5. Very large >800	8.4. The largest >60	9.4. High 0.75–1	10.4. Intense 4
1.6. N3 6									

Table 2. Results of the analysis of the functional elements "Road" and "Traffic environment".

Road			Traffic Environment				
11. Number of Lanes on the Road in Both Directions	**12. Road Resistance Degree, *f* + *i***	**13. Carriageway Curvature Degree**	**14. Group of Localities Determined by the City Population, Thousand People**	**15. Population Density, People/km^2**	**16. Level of Motorization, Cars/1000 Inhabitants**	**17. Time Interval**	**18. Complexity of Weather Conditions**
11.1 2	12.1. Low 0.007–0.05	13.1. Low 2maxR/3-maxR 1	14.1. Small <50 1	15.1. Low <500 1	16.1. Low <200 1	17.1. Night hours 1	18.1. Low 0–0.2
11.2 3			14.2. Medium 50–250 2	15.2. Medium 500–1000 2		17.2. Hours of decreasing traffic intensity 2	18.2. Medium 0.21–0.4
11.3 4	12.2. Medium 0.05–0.1	13.2. Medium maxR/3-2maxR/3 2	14.3. Large 250–500 3	15.3. High 1000–4000 3	16.2. Medium 200–300 2	17.3. Hours of steady intensity during the day 3	18.3. High 0.41–0.7
11.4 6							
11.5 8	12.3. High 0.1–0.15	13.3. High 0-maxR/3 3	14.4. Significant 500–1000 4	15.4. Very high >4000 4	16.3. High >300 3	17.4. Hours of increasing traffic intensity 4	18.4. Very high 0.71–1
			14.5. Most important >1000 5			17.5. Rush hours 5	

The choice of morphological features is based on the results of a survey conducted within the studied transport networks with the involvement of experts—employees in the field of organization and provision of road safety, including specialists of the civil service "Ukrtransbezpeka". For the functional elements, the features that, according to experts, have an impact on the energy efficiency of vehicles, and the value of which can be determined based on current statistical information within the information space, are selected. When choosing features that are quantitative in nature, the possibility of studying their structure and obtaining calculation algorithms is considered. The characteristics of the element "Traffic environment" are unmanageable within transport systems but must be taken into account in the process of finding strategies to improve the vehicle energy efficiency.

Each morphological attribute is characterized by 3 to 6 implementation variants. A numeric value or range of values is defined for each implementation (Tables 1 and 2). The combination of specific values of all implementation variants forms a certain structure of the system, which determines the degree of energy consumption of the vehicle under given conditions. To choose the rational structure of the system it is necessary to comprehensively assess the impact of morphological attributes of its functional elements on the energy consumption of vehicles based on developed mathematical models.

Morphological attributes of the TrEECS system are estimated by quantitative or qualitative parameters of the corresponding model. The parameters x_4, x_7–x_9, x_{11}–x_{12}, x_{18} are quantitative. The degree of use of the load capacity and/or passenger capacity of the vehicle x_4 is the ratio of the actual weight of cargo and passengers carried to the nominal load capacity of the vehicle. By analogy with the distribution of the values of the coefficient of utilization of load capacity by load classes for trucks in this study, we take the following ranges of values x_4:

- low—from 0 to 0.4;
- middle—from 0.41 to 0.5;
- high—from 0.51 to 0.7;
- very high—from 0.71 to 1.

Parameters x_7 and x_8 are standard traffic flow meters. The traffic flow complexity level x_9 is defined as the share of freight and public vehicles in the flow. Parameter x_{12}—road resistance degree $\psi = f + i$, where f is the coefficient of rolling resistance; i—the slope of the road.

The complexity of weather conditions x_{18} is an integral indicator, calculated as the sum of the evaluations of the four components:

- strong wind—from 0 to 0.2;
- ice—from 0 to 0.3;
- atmospheric precipitation—from 0 to 0.2;
- fog—from 0 to 0.3.

Qualitative parameters x_1–x_3, x_5–x_6, x_{10}, x_{13}–x_{17} are described in detail in the paper [33].

The ranges of values of the parameters x_1–x_3 and x_5 correspond to the ranges of values of the corresponding morphological features, which are exhaustively presented in Table 1.

The area of definition of the parameter x_6 is a set containing four options for implementing the levels of autonomy of the car:

1. zero level—lack of automation of operational tasks;
2. the first level—automation of only certain functions, but acceleration, braking and monitoring of the situation around the car is not automated;
3. second level—partial automation of control functions;
4. third level—an autonomous system can monitor the situation on the road with the help of leaders, under safe conditions to perform braking functions.

Four phases of the transport flow x_{10} are selected in accordance with the values of the congestion coefficient K: free flow, stable, unstable and tense. The congestion coefficient is determined by expression (1) [40]:

$$K = \frac{H_x - H_{opt}}{H_{max} - H_{opt}} \quad (1)$$

where H_x, H_{opt}, H_{max}—the density of the transport flow to its stop at point x and the optimal and maximum density of the transport flow, vehicle/km. H_{opt} is achieved provided that the maximum intensity is reached at the optimal speed of the traffic flow.

Carriageway curvature degree x_{13} has the following implementations:

- low—from 2maxR/3 to maxR (maxR is maximum radius of the road on fragments of the studied system);
- medium—from maxR/3 to 2maxR/3;
- high—from 0 to maxR/3.

The larger the turning radius of the road, the lower the level of curvature of the carriageway x_{13}.

The ranges of values of the variants of the implementation of the features corresponding to the parameters x_{14}–x_{16} are given in the corresponding cells of Table 2.

The same implementations of the parameter x_{17} may have different ranges of values depending on the settlement. In the process of further modeling, the reduced value of this qualitative parameter to the number of the variant of realization of the corresponding feature is used.

When reduced to quantitative values, these parameters are equated to the number of the implementation variant of the corresponding morphological attribute. Quantitative values (ranges of values) of system parameters are given in the corresponding cells Tables 1 and 2.

The resulting parameter of the system is the level of energy efficiency of vehicle LEE in the process of traffic on the road network of the city, which is calculated as follows:

$$\text{LEE} = \frac{E_{\text{reason}}}{E_{\text{fact}}} \quad (2)$$

where E_{reason}—energy needed for a movement at a given mode of movement of the vehicle on a horizontal road in moderate weather conditions, MJ;

E_{fact}—energy in fact consumed by the engine, MJ.

For example, for cars and buses with internal combustion engines at steady motion and in acceleration mode, the energy in fact consumed by the engine, E_{fact}, is equal to the quantity of heat released by fuel combustion, and is calculated by the Formula (3):

$$E_{\text{fact}} = \text{LHV} \cdot m = \text{LHV} \cdot 0.001 \cdot H_S \cdot S \cdot (1 + 0.01 \cdot K_e) \quad (3)$$

where LHV—lower heating value of combustion of fuel, MJ/kg;

m—fuel consumption for cars and buses, kg;

H_S—the basic rate of fuel consumption, g/km, the regression equation for the calculation of which and the values of the corresponding regression coefficients are given in [22];

S—distance travelled by the car, km;

K_e—total adjustment coefficient, %.

$$K_e = \sum_{i=1}^{n} K_i - \sum_{j=n+1}^{n+m} K_j \quad (4)$$

where K_i, K_j—the i-th increasing and j-th lowering coefficients to fuel consumption rates [41], respectively, %;

n, m—the number of increasing and decreasing coefficients accordingly.

Correction coefficients that are significant in accordance with the purpose of the study are systematized and presented in Table 3. The parameter H_S takes into account the category, type of energy unit, the mode of movement and speed of the vehicle. If the necessary information is available, this parameter can be replaced by a basic linear fuel consumption.

Table 3. List of significant adjustment coefficients to fuel consumption rates.

Marking	Title	Maximum Value, %	Condition of Application
K_1	increase depending on the ambient temperature	2	$T \in [-5, 0]$
		4	$T \in [-10, -5)$
		6	$T \in [-15, -10)$
		8	$T \in [-20, -15)$
		10	$T \in [-25, -20)$
		12	$T < -25$
K_2	increase depending on movement up the slope or alternating climbing/descent	5	$i \in [0.04,\ 0.08)$
		10	$i \geq 0.08$
K_3	increase depending on a movement of vehicles on roads with a complex plan	10	the average presence of more than 5 curves with a radius of less than 40 m per 1 km of road
K_4	increase within the city	5	at $k < 250$ in the presence of adjustable controlled intersections
		10	$k \in [250,\ 500)$
		15	$k \geq 500$
K_5	increase in heavy road conditions of cities	10	at frequent traffic stops (in particular, in the central parts of cities)
K_6	increase in satisfactory road conditions of cities	10	when driving in traffic jams, including during peak hours, $V < 20$ km/h.
K_7	increase for new cars	10	in the case of the first thousand kilometers
K_8	increase depending on the age and mileage of the vehicle	3	age $\in (5,\ 8]$, $L \in (100, 150]$
		5	age $\in (8,\ 11]$, $L \in (150, 250]$
		7	age $\in (11, 14]$, $L \in (250, 400]$
		9	age > 14, $L > 400$
K_9	increase for cooling the interior of the vehicle	5	$T \in [+20, +25]$
		7	$T \in (+25, +30]$
		10	$T > +30$
K_{10}	increase depending on increased aerodynamic resistance	5	for vans, trucks during the transportation of bulky goods
K_{11}	reduction for city buses not on regular routes	5–10	including in the mode "on demand"

For the above vehicles when running at idle energy consumed by the engine E_{fact} is determined by expression (5):

$$E_{\text{fact}} = \text{LHV} \cdot m = \text{LHV} \cdot 0.001 \cdot H_i \cdot t \cdot (1 + 0.01 \cdot K_e) \quad (5)$$

where H_i—the basic rate of fuel consumption at idle running, g/s; tabular values are presented in [34];

t—time interval, seconds.

In the Table 3 the following notation is adopted: T—ambient air temperature, °C; i—the slope of the road; k—population, thousand people; V—vehicle speed, km/h; age—vehicle age, years; L—mileage of the vehicle, thousand km, $\in$—"is element of".

3. Results

Energy efficiency assessment was implemented on the example of vehicles of categories M1–M3, N1–N3 with energy units of different types (petrol, diesel, gas, hybrid and electric) with the air conditioning turned off, constant speed and idling. Measurements of TrEECS system parameters were performed for road networks of cities: Boryspil, Zolotonosha, Kaniv, Kyiv, Lviv, Odesa, Smila, Cherkasy (Ukraine) and Rzeszow (Poland).

Numerical values of road parameters x_{11}, x_{12} and x_{13} are obtained using the Internet service Google Earth Pro version 7.3.

The results of measuring parameters of linear fragments of road networks considering Tables 1 and 2 are given in Tables 4 and 5.

Table 4. Observation results for the functional elements "Vehicle" and "Traffic flow".

Observation Number	Vehicle						Traffic Flow			
	Category	Energy Unit Type	Vehicle Age	The Degree of Use of Load Capacity and/or Passenger Capacity	The Movement Mode	The Autonomy Level	Traffic Intensity, Reduced Units/Hour	Traffic Density, Reduced Units/km	The Traffic Flow Complexity Level	The Traffic Flow Phase
	x_1	x_2	x_3	x_4	x_5	x_6	x_7	x_8	x_9	x_{10}
1	1	1	3	0.75	1	4	655	22	0.03	2
2	1	3	5	0.49	1	1	655	20	0.03	2
3	5	2	2	0.64	2	1	770	31	0.24	3
4	3	2	4	0.72	2	1	770	33	0.24	3
5	1	1	4	0.57	1	1	710	42	0.52	4
6	3	4	2	0.8	3	3	864	216	0.04	4
7	1	3	5	0.3	2	1	828	207	0.06	4
8	1	1	1	0.36	2	4	577	46.27	0.35	3
9	1	1	3	0.13	1	2	10	2	0	1
10	2	2	3	0.77	3	1	550	11	0.06	1
11	6	2	3	0.71	2	2	710	27	0.22	4
12	4	2	4	0.69	3	1	376	125	0.31	4
13	4	2	2	0.86	2	1	534	13	0.25	2
14	3	2	5	0.5	1	1	279	5.58	0.17	2
15	5	2	4	0.91	2	1	592	22	0.33	2
16	1	3	5	0.2	1	1	417	18	0.21	2
17	1	2	5	0.15	2	1	535	12	0.49	2
18	1	1	3	0.42	2	2	133	5	0.21	1
19	4	3	5	0.37	1	1	26	1	0.038	1
20	4	2	4	0.73	2	1	875	25	0.58	3
21	3	2	3	0.82	2	2	775	31	0.76	4
22	1	1	3	0.27	1	3	956	90	0.01	4
23	1	1	1	0.31	2	4	1130	113	0.015	4
24	4	2	2	0.65	1	1	120	16	0.19	1
25	2	2	2	0.53	1	1	400	40	0.05	2

Table 5. Observation results for the functional elements "Road" and "Traffic environment".

Observation Number	Road				Traffic environment			
	Number of Lanes in Both Directions	Road Resistance Degree, $f + i$	Carriageway Curvature Degree	Group of Localities, Thousand People	Population Density, People/km^2	Level of Motorization, Cars/1000 Inhabitants	Time Interval	Complexity of Weather Conditions
	x_{11}	x_{12}	x_{13}	x_{14}	x_{15}	x_{16}	x_{17}	x_{18}
1	2	0.09	2	3	4	2	2	0.4
2	2	0.068	2	3	4	2	2	0.2
3	4	0.023	1	3	4	2	3	0
4	4	0.023	1	3	4	2	3	0
5	4	0.023	1	3	4	2	4	0.5
6	8	0.015	1	5	3	3	5	0.2
7	8	0.017	1	5	3	3	4	0.2
8	4	0.065	1	4	4	1	3	0.1
9	4	0.02	2	3	4	2	1	0.7
10	4	0.02	2	3	4	2	3	0.2
11	4	0.023	1	3	4	2	4	0.5
12	4	0.018	1	2	3	1	5	0
13	4	0.03	1	1	3	1	5	0.4
14	4	0.03	1	1	3	1	2	0.4
15	2	0.077	1	2	3	1	3	0.2
16	2	0.077	1	2	3	1	2	0.2
17	2	0.049	1	3	4	2	5	0
18	2	0.049	1	3	4	2	2	0
19	2	0.049	1	3	4	2	1	0.1
20	6	0.025	1	3	4	2	3	0.2
21	6	0.025	1	3	4	2	4	0.1
22	2	0.029	3	3	4	2	3	0
23	2	0.037	1	5	4	3	5	0.2
24	2	0.13	3	1	3	2	3	0.7
25	2	0.08	3	1	3	2	4	0.3

The development of regression models of the system requires the independence of all input parameters. Estimation of the degree and elimination of multicollinearity in the array of data was performed by the Farrar-Glober method [42,43]. This algorithm is based on the consistent application of Pearson criterion χ^2—to test for multicollinearity in the array, Fisher's F—criterion to evaluate each TrEECS parameter by the degree of multicollinearity to others and Student's t—criterion to assess the dependence of each variant for its implementation to others. At each stage of the algorithm, the input parameters, which are more correlated with others, are removed from further consideration. Generalized block diagram of algorithm for eliminating multicollinearity of input parameters of the TrEECS model based on the Farrar-Glober method is shown in Figure 1.

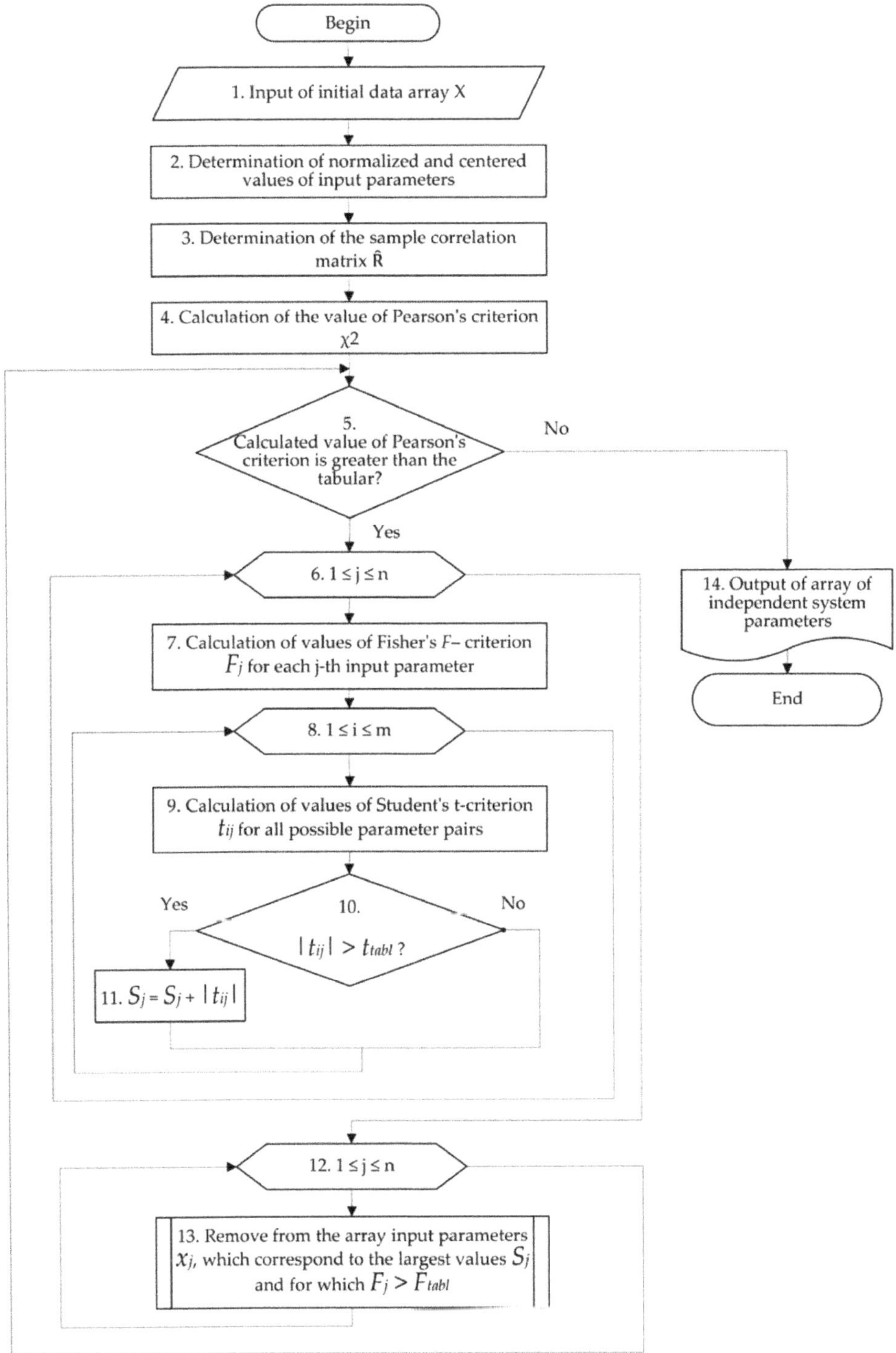

Figure 1. Algorithm for eliminating multicollinearity of input parameters of the TrEECS model based on the Farrar-Glober method.

In block 1, a two-dimensional array of initial data $X = \{x_{ij}\}$ is formed, x_{ij} is the initial value of the j-th parameter of the i-th observation.

In block 2, a matrix X^N of normalized and centered values of input parameters is formed. The elements of the matrix X^N are calculated by the formula:

$$x_{ij}^N = \frac{x_{ij} - \acute{x}_j}{\delta_j}, 1 \le i \le 25,\ 1 \le j \le n, \tag{6}$$

where: x_{ij}^N is the normalized value of the j-th parameter of the i-th observation, $\acute{x}_j$ is the average value of the j-th parameter, δ_j is the j-th parameter variance, n is the number of input parameters in this iteration.

In block 3, a sampling correlation matrix is formed:

$$\hat{R} = \frac{1}{m}\left(X^N\right)^T X^N, \tag{7}$$

where: m is the number of observations, $m = 25$.

In blocks 4, 7, 9, relevant statistical criteria are calculated.

In blocks condition check units 5, 10 and in block of call subprogram 13 Pearson criterion χ^2, Fisher's F—criterion F_j, Student's t–criterion t_{ij} $(1 \le i \le 25, 1 \le j \le n)$ are compared with their tabular values χ^2_{tabl}, F_{tabl} and t_{tabl}, respectively. The significance level $\alpha = 0.05$.

At each iteration of the algorithm, the dependent parameters of the system are deleted from the data array in accordance with the procedure of block 13. The algorithm terminates if condition 5 is not met.

In total, 4 iterations of the algorithm were performed. Intermediate results obtained at each iteration are given in Table 6.

Table 6. The results of the step-by-step execution of the Farrar-Glober method.

Iteration No	Number of Parameters, n	Value of the Pearson Criterion, χ^2		Presence of Multicollinearity in the Data Array	Parameters Deleted
		Calculated	Tabular		
I	18	326.707	182.865	yes	x_8, x_{14}, x_{15}
II	15	175.505	129.918	yes	x_5, x_{11}
III	13	120.091	99.617	yes	x_6, x_7, x_{10}
IV	10	56.774	61.656	no	–

Based on the results of the evaluation of the states of the TrEECS system (Table 6), for its further modeling an input data array containing the values of the 10 remaining independent parameters is formed. Then the influence of the characteristics of the functional elements on the level of energy efficiency of the vehicle in general can be written by the following mathematical dependence:

$$\text{LEE} = f(x_1, x_2, x_3, x_4, x_9, x_{12}, x_{13}, x_{16}, x_{17}, x_{18}) \tag{8}$$

where: x_1–x_4—basic parameters that correspond to the attributes of the functional element "Vehicle", x_9—basic parameter of the functional element "Transport flow", x_{12}–x_{13}—basic parameters that specify the state of the functional element "Road", x_{16}–x_{18}—basic parameters that characterize the functional element "Traffic environment":

- x_1—vehicle category;
- x_2—vehicle energy unit type;
- x_3—vehicle age;
- x_4—the degree of use of load capacity and/or passenger capacity;

- x_9—the traffic flow complexity level;
- x_{12}—road resistance degree;
- x_{13}—the carriageway curvature degree;
- x_{16}—level of motorization;
- x_{17}—time interval;
- x_{18}—complexity of weather conditions.

Thus, within this study, all functional elements of the TrEECS system are essential.

Table 7 shows the input and output data arrays used for further modeling of the dependence of the energy efficiency of the vehicle on the TrEECS parameters. The elements of the source array were obtained using (2) based on observations of the state of the system under different initial conditions.

Table 7. Values of basic and resulting parameters of the TrEECS system.

Observation Number	x_1	x_2	x_3	x_4	x_9	x_{12}	x_{13}	x_{16}	x_{17}	x_{18}	LEE	Sampling Variance, D_i
1	1	1	3	0.75	0.03	0.09	2	2	2	0.4	0.669	0.59478
2	1	3	5	0.49	0.03	0.068	2	2	2	0.2	0.746	0.90731
3	5	2	2	0.64	0.24	0.023	1	2	3	0	0.712	0.91001
4	3	2	4	0.72	0.24	0.023	1	2	3	0	0.784	0.11239
5	1	1	4	0.57	0.52	0.023	1	2	4	0.5	0.592	0.51240
6	3	4	2	0.8	0.04	0.015	1	3	5	0.2	0.676	1.19375
7	1	3	5	0.3	0.06	0.017	1	3	4	0.2	0.641	0.92145
8	1	1	1	0.36	0.35	0.065	1	1	3	0.1	0.813	1.07520
9	1	1	3	0.13	0	0.02	2	2	1	0.7	0.658	1.01842
10	2	2	3	0.77	0.06	0.02	2	2	3	0.2	0.803	0.09806
11	6	2	3	0.71	0.22	0.023	1	2	4	0.5	0.525	1.45173
12	4	2	4	0.69	0.31	0.018	1	1	5	0	0.707	0.75227
13	4	2	2	0.86	0.25	0.03	1	1	5	0.4	0.719	0.89939
14	3	2	5	0.5	0.17	0.03	1	1	2	0.4	0.806	0.61767
15	5	2	4	0.91	0.33	0.077	1	1	3	0.2	0.719	0.86156
16	1	3	5	0.2	0.21	0.077	1	1	2	0.2	0.840	0.97870
17	1	2	5	0.15	0.49	0.049	1	2	5	0	0.746	0.96579
18	1	1	3	0.42	0.21	0.049	1	2	2	0	0.787	0.56846
19	4	3	5	0.37	0.038	0.049	1	2	1	0.1	0.775	1.26295
20	4	2	4	0.73	0.58	0.025	1	2	3	0.2	0.760	0.33934
21	3	2	3	0.82	0.76	0.025	1	2	4	0.1	0.787	0.16389
22	1	1	3	0.27	0.01	0.029	3	2	3	0	0.730	0.68212
23	1	1	1	0.31	0.015	0.037	1	3	5	0.2	0.667	1.46929
24	4	2	2	0.65	0.19	0.13	3	2	3	0.7	0.548	0.75604
25	2	2	2	0.53	0.05	0.08	3	2	4	0.3	0.671	0.57780
$\acute{x}_j$	2.52	1.96	3.32	0.546	0.2161	0.0437	1.4	1.88	3.24	0.232		

To build an adequate mathematical model, the input data set is divided into training and control samples. For this purpose, an algorithm based on the calculation of the values of the sampling variance Di [43] was used, calculated by the formulas:

$$D_i = \frac{1}{n-1}\sum_{j=1}^{n}\left(x_{ij} - \acute{x}_j\right)^2 = \frac{1}{9}\sum_{j=1}^{10}\left(x_{ij} - \acute{x}_j\right)^2,\ i = \overline{1,25}, \tag{9}$$

$$\acute{x}_j = \frac{1}{25}\sum_{i=1}^{25} x_{ij}, j = \overline{1,10}, \tag{10}$$

where: n—number of independent system parameters.

The obtained values of the sampling variance for each observation and the average values of the basic parameters are presented in the Table 7.

The control sample included five arrays (20% of the initial sample), which have the lowest values of the sampling variance and correspond to the following numbers of observations: 4, 5, 10, 20, 21.

A mathematical model in the form of multiple linear regression is built on the educational sample. The coefficients of the regression equation a_j are determined by the Formula (11) [43]:

$$\left(a_0,\ a_1, a_2, a_3,\ a_4, a_9, a_{12},\ a_{13}, a_{16}, a_{17},\ a_{18}\right)^T = \left(X^T \times X\right)^{-1} \times X^T \times \left(\overline{LEE}\right)^T, \tag{11}$$

where: X—the matrix of dimension 20 × 11, the columns of which contain the values of the basic parameters at different states of the system (column x_0 contains units), ($L\acute{E}E$)—vector of statistical values of the resulting parameter.

Thus, the following analytical dependence is obtained, which reflects the influence of TrEECS parameters on the level of the vehicle energy efficiency:

$$\begin{gathered} LEE = 1.06414 - 0.02128{\cdot}x_1 + 0.02675{\cdot}x_2 - 0.01139{\cdot}x_3 - \\ -0.02787{\cdot}x_4 - 0.07902{\cdot}x_9 - 0.0187{\cdot}x_{12} - 0.02774{\cdot}x_{13} - \\ -0.082{\cdot}x_{16} - 0.01742{\cdot}x_{17} - 0.18435{\cdot}x_{18}. \end{gathered} \tag{12}$$

Mathematical modeling is an alternative to field experiment. The advantages of the model approach are determined by economic considerations. Experimental determination of the energy in fact consumed by the engine of vehicles, and accordingly the level of energy efficiency according to Formula (2), in some cases causes difficulties. Determining the input parameters of the model (12) is less complicated, and the calculation of the resulting parameter using the application software does not require much time. Therefore, model (12) is more productive than calculating the level of energy efficiency according to Formula (2).

Figures 2 and 3 present a graphical representation of the simulation results of the states of the studied TrEECS system.

The largest error in the calculation of the resulting parameter is observed in the study of the movement of buses and trucks of category N1 aged more than 10 years with a high and very high degree of use of passenger capacity/load capacity.

The accuracy of the obtained model was evaluated for five TrEECS states of the control sample. The standard deviation of the model values from the tabular ones equals $\acute{\sigma} = 0.0091$. Relative standard deviation equals $\acute{S}_r = 1.5\%$.

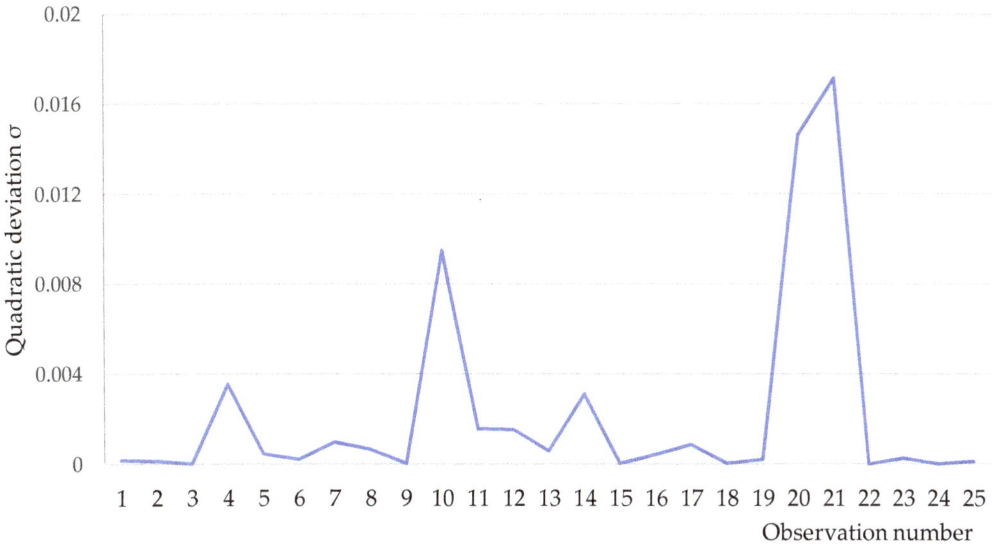

Figure 2. The error of the regression model.

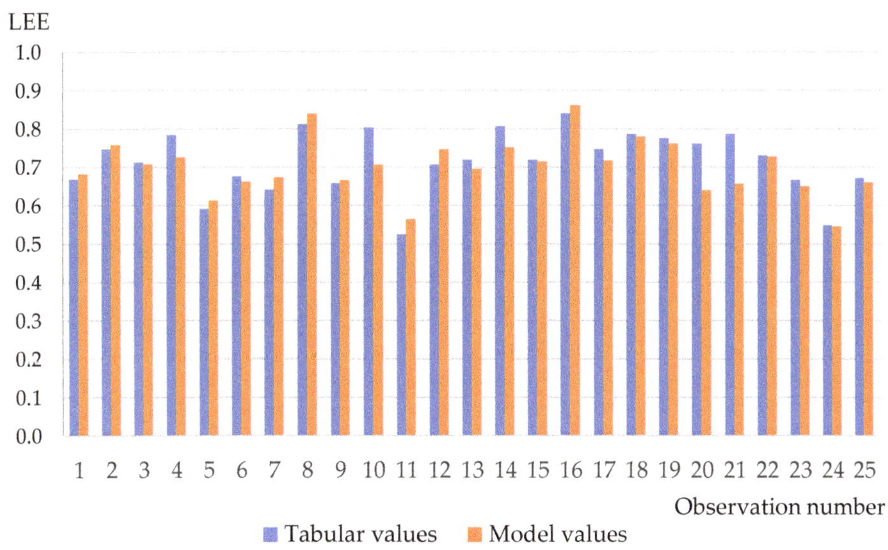

Figure 3. The results of comparison of statistical and model values of the level of the vehicles energy efficiency in the training sample.

4. Discussion

Based on the performed morphological analysis of the TrEECS system, 18 significant morphological attributes of its main functional elements have been identified. The input parameters of the corresponding system model take values from a set of implementation variants of each attribute. Each set has 3–6 variants. The degree of energy efficiency of the vehicle at a certain state of the system is chosen as the resulting parameter. A survey of the state of the system on the linear fragments of the road network of nine typical cities of Ukraine and Poland was performed. The basis of the system includes parameters that correspond to the following morphological attributes of its functional elements: vehicle category, vehicle energy unit type, vehicle age, the degree of use of load capacity and/or passenger capacity, traffic flow complexity level, road resistance degree, the carriageway curvature degree, level of motorization, time interval, complexity of weather conditions. It can be argued that all four functional elements are essential for this study and the basic parameters determine the most important attributes of these functional elements. Usage of the obtained model is more productive in terms of time and level of complexity than the calculation of the level of energy efficiency according to the statistical values of the energy in fact consumed by the vehicle engine. This mathematical model shows high accuracy of the resulting parameter and allows to quantify the impact of each of the basic parameters on the level of energy efficiency of vehicles. The developed mathematical model makes requirements for constructive properties of vehicles, their operating conditions, road infrastructure and can be used in the process of developing design solutions for planning and modernization of roads and buildings, taking into account the efficiency of transport and its impact on the environment. In addition, the results of the study can be applied in mathematical models of intelligent traffic control systems for urban traffic flows. This study is an intermediate stage in the development of a generalized methodology for improving the vehicle energy efficiency in terms of urban mobility. The integrated energy efficiency indicator is determined based on partial indicators for individual fragments of the road network. At this stage, an analytical dependence has been developed to calculate the level of the vehicle energy efficiency when driving on linear sections of the network. In the future it is planned to conduct a similar study for other structural elements of the network. In addition, further research will be aimed at solving problems of identification of nonlinear models of the system and determining the degree of impact of each morphological attribute on the vehicle energy efficiency.

Author Contributions: Conceptualization, L.T. and N.K.; methodology, L.T. and N.K.; software, L.T. and N.K.; validation, L.T., N.K. and V.M.; formal analysis, L.T. and N.K.; investigation, L.T. and N.K.; resources, J.M.; data curation, L.T. and N.K.; writing—original draft preparation, L.T., N.K., V.M. and M.Ś.; writing—review and editing, J.M.; visualization, V.M. and J.M.; supervision, M.Ś. and V.M.; project administration, V.M. and M.Ś. All authors have read and agreed to the published version of the manuscript.

Funding: This research received no external funding.

Institutional Review Board Statement: Not applicable.

Informed Consent Statement: Not applicable.

Data Availability Statement: Not applicable.

Conflicts of Interest: The authors declare no conflict of interest.

References

1. Lozzi, G.; Rodrigues, M.; Marcucci, E.; Gatta, V.; Teoh, T.; Ramos, C.; Jonkers, E. *Research for TRAN Committee—Sustainable and Smart Urban. Transport*; European Parliament, Policy Department for Structural and Cohesion Policies: Brussels, Belgium, 2020.
2. Nanaki, E.; Koroneos, C.; Roset, J.; Susca, T.; Christensen, T.; Hurtado, S.D.G.; Rybka, A.; Kopitovic, J.; Heidrich, O.; López-Jiménez, P.A. Environmental assessment of 9 European public bus transportation systems. *Sustain. Cities Soc.* **2017**, *28*, 42–52. [CrossRef]
3. Kumar, P.; Anil, S.; Niraj, S.; Chalumuri, R.S. Evaluation of Idling Fuel Consumption of Vehicles across Different Cities. In Proceedings of the Recent Advances in Traffic Engineering, Surat, India, 21–22 December 2015.
4. Mądziel, M.; Campisi, T.; Jaworski, A.; Kuszewski, H.; Woś, P. Assessing Vehicle Emissions from a Multi-Lane to Turbo Roundabout Conversion Using a Microsimulation Tool. *Energies* **2021**, *14*, 4399. [CrossRef]
5. Chen, X.; Shan, X.; Ye, J.; Yi, F.; Wang, Y. Evaluating the Effects of Traffic Congestion and Passenger Load on Feeder Bus Fuel and Emissions Compared with Passenger Car. *Transp. Res. Procedia* **2017**, *25*, 616–626. [CrossRef]
6. Smieszek, M.; Dobrzanska, M.; Dobrzanski, P. Rzeszow as a City Taking Steps towards Developing Sustainable Public Transport. *Sustainability* **2019**, *11*, 402. [CrossRef]
7. Rabay, L.; Meira, L.H.; Andrade, M.O.D.; Oliveira, L.K.D. A portrait of the crisis in the Brazilian urban bus system: An analysis of factors influencing the reduction in usage. *Case Stud. Transp. Policy* **2021**, *9*, 1879–1887. [CrossRef]

8. Smieszek, M.; Mateichyk, V.; Dobrzanska, M.; Dobrzanski, P.; Weigang, G. The Impact of the Pandemic on Vehicle Traffic and Roadside Environmental Pollution: Rzeszow City as a Case Study. *Energies* **2021**, *14*, 4299. [CrossRef]
9. Eißel, D.; Chu, C. The future of sustainable transport system for Europe. *AI Soc.* **2014**, *29*, 387–402. [CrossRef]
10. Chen, Y.; Zhu, L.; Gonder, J.; Young, S.; Walkowicz, K. Data-driven fuel consumption estimation: A multivariate adaptive regression spline approach. *Transp. Res. Part. C Emerg. Technol.* **2017**, *83*, 134–145. [CrossRef]
11. Wang, Y.; Boggio-Marzet, A. Evaluation of Eco-Driving Training for Fuel Efficiency and Emissions Reduction According to Road Type. *Sustainability* **2018**, *10*, 3891. [CrossRef]
12. Duarte, G.O.; Gonçalves, G.A.; Farias, T.L. A Methodology to Estimate Real-world Vehicle Fuel Use and Emissions based on Certification Cycle Data. *Procedia-Soc. Behav. Sci.* **2014**, *111*, 702–710. [CrossRef]
13. Oprešnik, S.R.; Seljak, T.; Vihar, R.; Gerbec, M.; Katrašnik, T. Real-World Fuel Consumption, Fuel Cost and Exhaust Emissions of Different Bus Powertrain Technologies. *Energies* **2018**, *11*, 2160. [CrossRef]
14. Soylu, S. The effects of urban driving conditions on the operating characteristics of conventional and hybrid electric city buses. *Appl. Energy* **2014**, *135*, 472–482. [CrossRef]
15. Oh, Y.; Park, J.; Lee, J.; Eom, M.D.; Park, S. Modeling effects of vehicle specifications on fuel economy based on engine fuel consumption map and vehicle dynamics. *Transp. Res. Part. D Transp. Environ.* **2014**, *32*, 287–302. [CrossRef]
16. Pathak, S.K.; Sood, V.; Singh, Y.; Channiwala, S. Real world vehicle emissions: Their correlation with driving parameters. *Transp. Res. Part. D Transp. Environ.* **2016**, *44*, 157–176. [CrossRef]
17. Grote, M.; Williams, I.; Preston, J.; Kemp, S. A practical model for predicting road traffic carbon dioxide emissions using Inductive Loop Detector data. *Transp. Res. Part. D Transp. Environ.* **2018**, *63*, 809–825. [CrossRef]
18. Huzayyin, O.A.; Salem, H.; Hassan, M.A. A representative urban driving cycle for passenger vehicles to estimate fuel consumption and emission rates under real-world driving conditions. *Urban. Clim.* **2021**, *36*, 100810. [CrossRef]
19. Qi, X.; Wu, G.; Boriboonsomsin, K.; Barth, M.J. Data-driven decomposition analysis and estimation of link-level electric vehicle energy consumption under real-world traffic conditions. *Transp. Res. Part. D Transp. Environ.* **2018**, *64*, 36–52. [CrossRef]
20. Gallet, M.; Massier, T.; Hamacher, T. Estimation of the energy demand of electric buses based on real-world data for large-scale public transport networks. *Appl. Energy* **2018**, *230*, 344–356. [CrossRef]
21. Łebkowski, A. Studies of Energy Consumption by a City Bus Powered by a Hybrid Energy Storage System in Variable Road Conditions. *Energies* **2019**, *12*, 951. [CrossRef]
22. Kancharla, S.R.; Ramadurai, G. Incorporating driving cycle based fuel consumption estimation in green vehicle routing problems. *Sustain. Cities Soc.* **2018**, *40*, 214–221. [CrossRef]
23. Wang, J.; Rakha, H.A. Fuel consumption model for conventional diesel buses. *Appl. Energy* **2016**, *170*, 394–402. [CrossRef]
24. Śmieszek, M.; Mateichyk, V. Determining the fuel consumption of a public city bus in urban traffic. In Proceedings of the 2021 IOP Conference Series: Materials Science and Engineering, Bardejovské Kúpele, Slovak Republic, 13–15 September 2021; Volume 1199, p. 012080.
25. Macor, A.; Rossetti, A. Fuel consumption reduction in urban buses by using power split transmissions. *Energy Convers. Manag.* **2013**, *71*, 159–171. [CrossRef]
26. He, H.; Tang, H.; Wang, X. Global Optimal Energy Management Strategy Research for a Plug-In Series-Parallel Hybrid Electric Bus by Using Dynamic Programming. *Math. Probl. Eng.* **2013**, *2013*, 708261. [CrossRef]
27. Guo, J.; Ge, Y.; Hao, L.; Tan, J.; Peng, Z.; Zhang, C. Comparison of real-world fuel economy and emissions from parallel hybrid and conventional diesel buses fitted with selective catalytic reduction systems. *Appl. Energy* **2015**, *159*, 433–441. [CrossRef]
28. Yu, H.; Liu, Y.; Li, J.; Liu, H.; Ma, K. Real-Road Driving and Fuel Consumption Characteristics of Public Buses in Southern China. *Int. J. Automot. Technol.* **2020**, *21*, 33–40. [CrossRef]
29. Frey, H.C.; Rouphail, N.; Zhai, H.; Farias, T.; Gonçalves, G.A. Comparing real-world fuel consumption for diesel- and hydrogen-fueled transit buses and implication for emissions. *Transp. Res. Part. D Transp. Environ.* **2007**, *12*, 281–291. [CrossRef]
30. Grote, M.; Williams, I.; Preston, J.; Kemp, S. Including congestion effects in urban road traffic CO2 emissions modelling: Do Local Government Authorities have the right options? *Transp. Res. Part. D Transp. Environ.* **2016**, *43*, 95–106. [CrossRef]
31. Ritchey, T. General Morphological Analysis (GMA). In *Wicked Problems—Social Messes*; Risk, Governance and Society; Springer: Berlin/Heidelberg, Germany, 2011; Volume 17, pp. 7–18. [CrossRef]
32. Ritchey, T. General Morphological Analysis—A General Method for Non-Quantified Modelling privately published. Fritz Zwicky, Morphologie and Policy Analysis. In Proceedings of the 16th EURO Conference on Operational Analysis, Brussels, Belgium, 12–15 July 1998.
33. Kostian, N.L.; Smieszek, M. Do Vyznachennia Produktyvnosti ta Enerhoefektyvnosti Transportnykh Zasobiv v Umovakh Miskoi Mobilnosti [To Determining the Performance and Energy Efficiency of Vehicles in the Context of Urban Mobility]. Visnyk Natsionalnoho Transportnoho Universytetu [Bulletin of the National Transport University]. *Bull. Natl. Transp. Univ.* **2021**, *3*, 113–122. (In Ukrainian)
34. Dmytriiev, M.M. *M 218-02070915-694:2011 Metodika Otsenki Ingredientnogo i Parametricheskogo Zagryazneniya Pridorozhnogo Sredyi Sistemoy Transportnyiy Potok—Doroga [Methods for Assessing the Ingredient and Parametric Pollution of the Roadside Environment by the System Traffic Flow—Road]*; National Transport University: Kyiv, Ukraine, 2011; p. 28.
35. Tseng, C.-M.; Chau, C.-K. Personalized Prediction of Vehicle Energy Consumption Based on Participatory Sensing. *IEEE Trans. Intell. Transp. Syst.* **2017**, *18*, 3103–3113. [CrossRef]

36. Weiss, M.; Cloos, K.C.; Helmers, E. Energy efficiency trade-offs in small to large electric vehicles. *Environ. Sci. Eur.* **2020**, *32*, 1–17. [CrossRef]
37. Mamala, J.; Śmieja, M.; Prażnowski, K. Analysis of the Total Unit Energy Consumption of a Car with a Hybrid Drive System in Real Operating Conditions. *Energies* **2021**, *14*, 3966. [CrossRef]
38. Wang, J.; Besselink, I.; Nijmeijer, H. Electric Vehicle Energy Consumption Modelling and Prediction Based on Road Information. *World Electr. Veh. J.* **2015**, *7*, 447–458. [CrossRef]
39. Braun, A.; Rid, W. The influence of driving patterns on energy consumption in electric car driving and the role of regenerative braking. In Proceedings of the 19th EURO Working Group on Transportation Meeting, EWGT2016, Istanbul, Turkey, 5–7 September 2016; pp. 174–182.
40. Polishchuk, V.P.; Dziuba, O.P. *Teoriia Transportnoho Potoku: Metody ta Modeli Orhanizatsii Dorozhnoho Rukhu: Navchalnyi Posibnyk [Theory of Traffic Flow: Methods and Models of Traffic Organization]*; Znannia Ukrainy—Knowledge of Ukraine: Kyiv, Ukraine, 2008; p. 175.
41. *Pro Zatverdzhennia Zmin do Norm Vytrat Palyva ta Mastylnykh Materialiv na Avtomobilnomu Transporti: Nakaz Ministerstva Infrastruktury Ukrainy [About the Statement of Changes to Standards of Expenses of Fuel and Lubricants on Motor Transport: Order of the Ministry of Infrastructure of Ukraine]. (24.01.2012 No. 36)*; Ministry of Infrastructure of Ukraine: Kyiv, Ukraine, 2012. Available online: https://zakon.rada.gov.ua/rada/show/v0036733-12#Text (accessed on 5 December 2021).
42. Tarandushka, L.; Mateichyk, V.; Kostian, N.; Tarandushka, I.; Rud, M. Assessing the quality level of technological processes at car service enterprises. *East.-Eur. J. Enterp. Technol.* **2020**, *2*, 58–75.
43. Snytiuk, V.Y. *Prohnozuvannia. Modeli. Metody. Alhorytmy [Prognostication. Models. Methods. Algorithms]*; Maklaut: Kyiv, Ukraine, 2008; p. 364.

International Journal of
Environmental Research and Public Health

Article

Quantification of Sound Exposure from Wind Turbines in France

David Ecotière [1], Patrick Demizieux [1], Gwenaël Guillaume [1], Lise Giorgis-Allemand [2] and Anne-Sophie Evrard [2,*]

1 UMRAE, Cerema, Univ Gustave Eiffel, IFSTTAR, F-67035 Strasbourg, France; david.ecotiere@cerema.fr (D.E.); patrick.demizieux@laposte.net (P.D.); gwenael.guillaume@cerema.fr (G.G.)
2 Umrestte UMR T9405, Univ Lyon, Univ Gustave Eiffel, IFSTTAR, Univ Lyon 1, F-69675 Bron, France; lise.giorgis-allemand@univ-eiffel.fr
* Correspondence: anne-sophie.evrard@univ-eiffel.fr

Abstract: The WHO guidelines on environmental noise highlight that evidence on the health effects of wind turbine sound levels is either non-existent or of poor quality. In this context, a feasibility study was conducted in France in 2017. The objective was to suggest a methodology for calculating wind turbine sound levels in order to quantify the number of windfarms' residents exposed to this sound. Based on a literature review, the Harmonoise model was selected for sound exposure calculation. It was validated by quantifying its uncertainties, and finally used to estimate the population exposed to wind turbine sound in metropolitan France. Compared to other environmental noise sources (e.g., transportation), sound exposure is very moderate, with more than 80% of the exposed people exposed to sound levels below 40 dBA. The total number of people exposed to more than 30 dBA is about 686,000 and 722,000 people for typical daytime and night-time meteorological conditions respectively, i.e., about 1% of the French population in 2017. These results represent the first ever assessment of sound exposure from wind turbines at the scale of the entire metropolitan France.

Keywords: wind turbine; sound exposure; environmental noise; public health

Citation: Ecotière, D.; Demizieux, P.; Guillaume, G.; Giorgis-Allemand, L.; Evrard, A.-S. Quantification of Sound Exposure from Wind Turbines in France. *Int. J. Environ. Res. Public Health* **2022**, *19*, 23. https://doi.org/10.3390/ijerph19010023

Academic Editors: Roberto Alonso González Lezcano, Francesco Nocera and Rosa Giuseppina Caponetto

Received: 9 November 2021
Accepted: 17 December 2021
Published: 21 December 2021

Publisher's Note: MDPI stays neutral with regard to jurisdictional claims in published maps and institutional affiliations.

1. Introduction

Wind energy is expanding rapidly in France, as it is everywhere else in the world. Specific rules govern the design and implementation of wind farms in order to limit the noise they produce when in operation. However, the population living near these installations is often concerned about the health impacts of sound levels emitted by wind turbines (WT) and there is a lack of available scientific data on this topic.

Most studies have found a significant positive association between WT sound levels and the percentage of highly annoyed people [1,2]. Very few studies have investigated the effects of WT sound on sleep disturbance, cardiovascular disease, effects on metabolic or endocrine systems, or on cognition or mental health. Therefore, the WHO guidelines on environmental noise published in October 2018 pointed out that the evidence on the health effects of wind turbines noise is either non-existent or of low quality [3]. The WHO and Anses (French Agency for Food, Environmental and Occupational Health & Safety) in France therefore recommended implementing epidemiological studies [3–5]. However, a number of issues remained to be overcome before such a study can be carried out in France.

The first issue concerned the estimation of exposure to WT sound. Indeed, the quality of epidemiological studies evaluating the risks related to environmental exposures depends in part on the quality of the estimation or measurement of the participants' exposure. However, there was no real consensus on a WT sound prediction model and it was necessary to provide validation criteria to identify the most relevant model.

The second issue concerned the count of the number of people exposed to WT sound. Unlike other sources of noise pollution (e.g., transportation noise), wind farms are generally built in sparsely populated areas, and consequently the number of people potentially exposed to WT sound seemed a priori to be much smaller than the number of residents exposed to other sources of anthropogenic noise, such as transportation noise, for example. In order to conduct an epidemiological study, it would be necessary to recruit a sufficient number of individuals exposed to different and relatively contrasting WT sound levels. Thus, it was necessary to be able to estimate the population exposed to various WT sound levels at the scale of an entire country. This had never been done before in France.

In this context, a feasibility study for an epidemiological study called Cibélius (Knowing the impact of wind turbine noise on health) was conducted in France between 2017 and 2019. The objective was to propose a methodology for calculating WT sound levels and to identify the number of French residents exposed to different sound levels of wind turbine.

The aim of the research presented in this paper was to quantify the number of wind-farms' residents in France exposed to audible WT sound. For this purpose, a WT sound prediction model was selected and validated for the calculation of sound exposure. Then a methodology was suggested for estimating the number of people exposed to WT sound at the scale of all metropolitan France. A brief comparison with transportation noise exposure was also investigated.

2. Material and Methods

2.1. Overview of the Methodology

As it would not be feasible to make sound levels measurements in all the dwellings of people exposed to WT sound at the scale of the whole French national territory, it was necessary to estimate sound exposure by using an appropriate numerical modeling of WT sound emission and propagation. We first presented the numerical model used, and its performances for WT sound prediction by quantifying its uncertainties. Then, we detailed the method of calculation of sound exposure at the scale of the metropolitan French territory. Finally, the method for evaluating the count of people exposed to WT sound was shown.

2.2. Selection and Validation of a Numerical Wind Turbine Sound Model

The sound levels prediction model was selected from a literature review based on the following essential criteria in the context of WT sound: ability to account for a high noise source (hub height above 60 m), topography properties, meteorological (vertical profiles of wind speed, wind direction and temperature) and ground effects on sound propagation. The model must also be able to parameterize the sound power of the source as a function of wind speed. Although some research propagation models could meet these criteria for WT sound [6–9], they were not suitable for sound levels modeling on a scale as large as a country's territory, because of their high computational time.

Although it was less frequently used [10,11] than other engineering models that can handle a large-scale territory (e.g., ISO 9613-2 [12], NMPB-2008 [13] or CNOSSOS-EU [14]), the Harmonoise model [15] was preferred here for WT sound prediction because it takes into account ground effects more accurately, and because it is able to model the effects of different wind speeds and directions, and different classes of atmospheric stability on sound propagation. These properties are essential for the modeling of WT sound propagation, and several authors have mentioned the capabilities of this model for WT sound predictions [16–18].

The uncertainties of the Harmonoise model were estimated by comparison between numerical modeling and in situ measurements. For this purpose, an experimental campaign was carried out near a wind farm whose characteristics were representative of the vast majority of French wind farms: flat site (terrain slope lower than 2% over 2000 m), quiet environment, good diversity of wind speeds and directions. The wind farm consisted of five wind turbines with a rated electrical power of 2 MW each. Each WT had a hub located at 100 m high, and three 46 m long blades. During the eight days of the measurement period, the wind farm operated in 1-h /1-h on/off cycles, in order to select only measurements with a satisfactory signal to noise ratio between WT sound and background noise of the site, and thus not to retain sound samples containing extraneous noise.

LAeq (10 min) sound levels were recorded using 15 sound level meters located on the two dominant wind directions of the site, and at distances from the wind farm ranging from 0 to 1500 m (Figure 1). This arrangement enabled sound levels to be measured for downwind and upwind situations, for which sound propagation differs [19]. The sound level meters (B&K 2250, ACOEM Solo and Cube, Rion NL62) were placed at a height of 1.5 ± 0.1 m above the ground and measured in the frequency bands [12.5 Hz; 20 kHz] or [1 Hz; 20 kHz] depending on the point. In addition to these sound level measurements, the sound level power of the wind turbines was derived according to the protocol described in the standard IEC 61400-11 [20], based on sound levels measurements made with a flush-mounted microphone on a circular reflective plate of 1 m diameter, placed on the ground 143 m from a wind turbine (Figure 1).

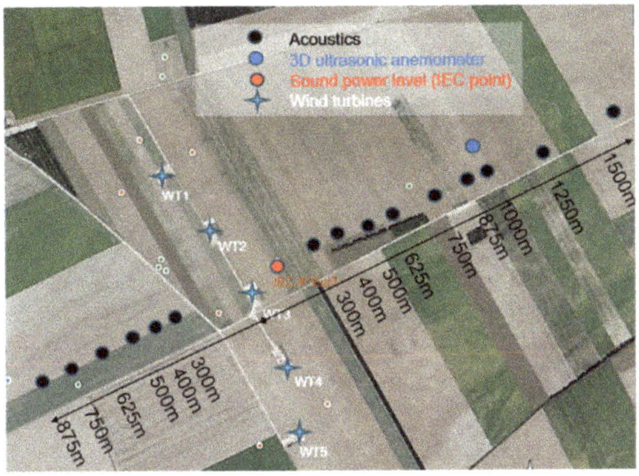

Figure 1. General overview of the experimental set-up for the validation of the numerical model. Location of sound level measurements (black points), wind measurements (blue points), wind turbine sound power level measurements (red points), wind turbines (blue crosses).

Meteorological measurements were made in order to obtain the influence of wind speed and direction on both emission and propagation of WT sound. Wind speed and direction measured from a 3D ultrasonic anemometer (Campbell CSAT3) located at 3 m high were used to classify sound propagation conditions as required by the Harmonoise modeling [10]. Wind speed at hub height and wind turbine operation data (speed rotation of the rotor, electrical production) were obtained from the wind farm's Supervisory Control And Data Acquisition system (SCADA). The accuracy of the anemometers (of the Campbell device or the WT hub) was typically 0.1 m/s, which was satisfactory for not inducing a significant uncertainty in the wind speed classification required for the analysis.

The WT emission was modeled using the manufacturer's WT technical specifications, which give the sound power level as a function of wind speed. An additional 2.2 dBA was added to these values to match the actual sound power level measured at the IEC point. The uncertainties of the sound levels prediction model were estimated by calculating the distribution of the deviation between the predicted and measured sound levels. The bias was estimated with the mean of this distribution, and the standard uncertainty with its standard deviation [21]. The hypothesis adopted for the calculation process of WT sound assumed WT operating at full power (see Section 2.3.2). To be in line with this hypothesis, only periods when wind speed was above 6 m/s at 10 m high were kept for the calculation of the bias and the standard uncertainty. Similarly, in order to be consistent with French regulations that do not allow wind farms to be installed less than 500 m from local residents, only measurements for which the distance to the wind farm was greater than 500 m were kept. Bias was used to correct the sound levels predicted by the Harmonoise model, while the standard uncertainty was used to bound the estimate of the population exposed to WT sound and to account for the uncertainty in the Harmonoise model's estimate of sound levels on the count of the exposed population. Indeed, the population count was performed by considering three scenarii of sound exposure: the first one (average scenario) used the sound levels predicted by the Harmonoise model, only corrected by the estimated bias, and the other two scenarii (upper and lower scenarii) used the sound levels predicted by the model, corrected by the bias, and increased or decreased respectively by a standard uncertainty in the sound level estimate. It should be noted that the range given by the uncertainty estimates based on the lower and upper scenarii did not correspond to confidence intervals associated with a level of reliability. They did, however, provide information on the best and worst-case values.

As meteorological conditions (wind and temperature vertical profiles) could have significant effects on long-range propagation of outdoor sound, resulting in decreased or increased noise levels at dwellings, it was essential to separate daytime and night-time periods where the meteorological influence on propagation often differs [19]. The uncertainties were thus calculated for two propagation conditions representative of daytime and night-time meteorological conditions.

2.3. Estimation of Sound Exposure from Wind Turbines

The selected sound levels prediction model was used to produce a noise map of all the wind farms on the metropolitan French territory. This mapping was built following the three steps detailed below.

2.3.1. Constitution of a Database with the Characteristics Required for the Prediction of Sound Levels from Wind Farms in Metropolitan FRANCE

The location of the wind farms (Figure 2), the hub height and the rated electrical power of the wind turbines were obtained from a 2017 database provided by www.thewindpower.net (accessed on 1 December 2021), which was the most complete database publicly available at the beginning of this research. This database listed existing wind farms as of 30 August 2017, of which only wind farms in operation in metropolitan France were considered here. The absolute position of each WT within each wind farm was obtained from the BDTOPO® topographic database [22] from the National Institute of Geographic and Forestry Information (IGN).

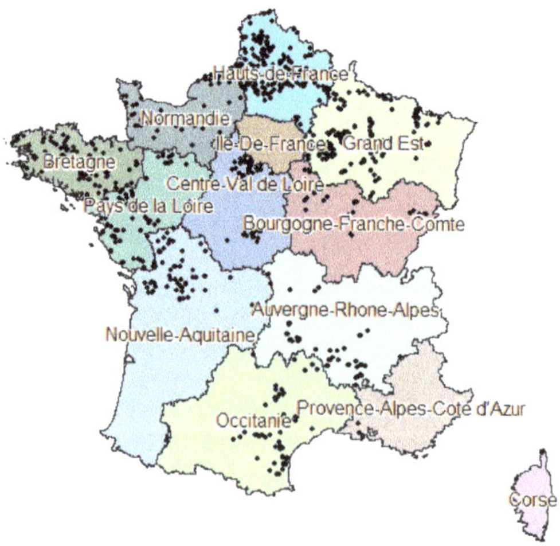

Figure 2. Localisation of metropolitan French wind farms (2017, www.thewindpower.net, accessed on 1 December 2021).

2.3.2. Calculation of Sound Contributions of Wind Turbines near the Dwellings of Wind Farm Residents

Sound levels calculations with the Harmonoise model presented earlier were performed with the environmental noise prediction software CadnaA from DataKustik [23]. In this software, each wind turbine was modeled as a point source located at the height of the wind turbine hub. Following the results of Botha et al. [24], Møller et al. [25] and Tachibana et al. [26], the sound emission of each wind turbine was estimated considering a linear sound emission spectrum (−4 dB/octave), whose overall sound power level was estimated from its rated electrical power [25], considering a wind speed of 7 m/s at 10 m height (nominal operation of the wind turbines in full operation).

The topographic data used in the propagation model came from the BDTOPO® database [22]. Sound levels were predicted for standard environmental conditions (temperature 10 °C, humidity 70%, partially sound absorbing ground) and for eight wind directions (from 0° to 315°, in 45° steps). The sound level assigned to each building corresponds to the sound level in front of the most exposed façade, and to the maximum of the sound levels predicted for the eight wind directions. Two propagation conditions typical of the daytime and night-time periods were also considered. These conditions could be parametrized in the Harmonoise model by choosing classes of meteorological stability adapted to these periods (three classes for day, and two classes for night). For each time period, the class that favored sound propagation was chosen (classes S3 for daytime and S5 for night-time [27]). It is important to note that the assessment of daytime and night-time exposures was not related to the sound a resident would be exposed to during an entire daytime or night-time period (as an equivalent sound level indicator would quantify), but they were related to two different meteorological scenarii that influence the sound propagation differently during these two periods. Sound levels exposures below 30 dBA were excluded as too low to be significant. Finally, the calculations provided the sound level exposure at each building façade in BDTOPO database around all the wind farms. Figure 3 shows an example of the sound radiated from a wind farm (Figure 3a) and the exposure of nearby buildings (Figure 3b) estimated with these calculations.

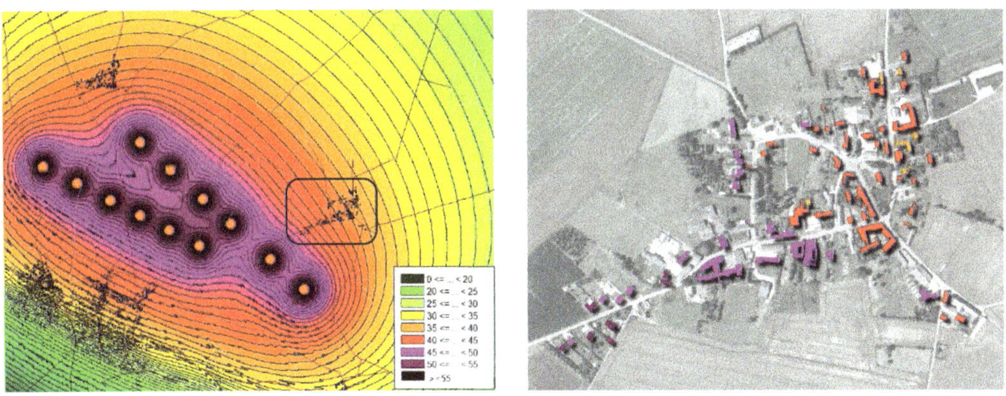

(**a**) (**b**)

Figure 3. Example of the result of the calculation of the radiated sound from a wind farm (**a**), and of the exposure of the buildings in the nearby village enclosed by the black block in (**a**,**b**).

2.4. Count of the Number of People Exposed to WT Sound

Building exposures were cross-referenced using a GIS software (QGIS [28]) with the populations provided by the national database of land use files MAJIC updated in 2016 [29]. Only residential buildings were included in the counting.

Finally, the number of people exposed to WT sound for day- and night-time propagation conditions was determined at the scale of the whole metropolitan France, as well as of the 13 administrative regions in metropolitan France.

2.5. Comparison of WT Sound Exposure with Other Environmental Noise Sources

A comparison of WT sound exposure with transportation noise exposure was conducted. Transportation noise exposure data were derived from calculations performed in 2017 [30] as part of the European directive related to the assessment and management of environmental noise [31].

3. Results

3.1. Evaluation of the Wind Turbine Sound Prediction Model

The distribution of differences between the predicted and measured sound levels was obtained from 77 and 79 measurements where the wind speed was greater than 6 m/s and the distance from the wind turbine ranged from 500 m to 1500 m, for daytime and night-time propagation conditions respectively. The bias was −4.4 dBA and −0.2 dBA, and the standard uncertainty was 3.9 dBA and 4.7 dBA, for daytime and night-time propagation conditions, respectively (Figure 4).

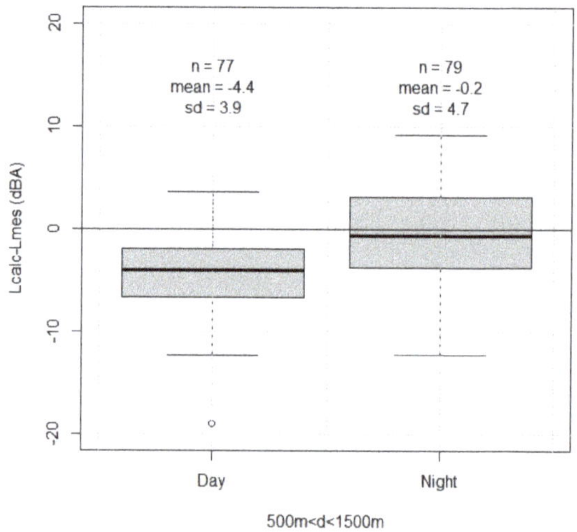

Figure 4. Boxplot of the difference between predicted and measured sound levels, for two typical meteorological conditions during the day and night. The wind speed was above 6 m/s and the distance from the wind turbine ranged from 500 m to 1500 m. Number of samples (n), bias (mean), standard uncertainty (sd).

3.2. Wind Turbine Sound Exposure in Metropolitan France

The total number of people in metropolitan France exposed to WT sound levels above 30 dBA was 685,770 people for daytime propagation conditions and 721,559 people for night-time conditions (Table 1). Taking into account the standard uncertainty from the model validation resulted in a range of this estimate of [430,036; 905,967] people for daytime meteorological conditions and [303,976; 1,029,390] for night-time. These results corresponded to 1.0% [0.6%; 1.3%] of people living in France in 2017 for daytime, and 1.0% [0.4%; 1.5%] for night-time. It should be noted that the range of these estimates did not correspond to confidence intervals, but to estimates based on the lower and upper scenarii.

Table 1. Number of people in metropolitan France exposed to WT sound levels above 30 dBA for daytime and night-time propagation conditions. The lower/upper scenarii correspond to +/−1 standard deviation on the Harmonoise sound level estimate.

Sound Levels Scenario	Daytime	Night-Time
Average scenario	685,770	721,559
Lower scenario	430,036	303,976
Upper scenario	905,967	1,029,390

Finally, 48% and 61% of the people exposed to sound levels above 30 dBA were exposed to sound levels below 35 dBA for daytime and night-time propagation conditions respectively, and 82% and 93% of the people exposed to sound levels between 30 dBA and 40 dBA for both daytime and night-time propagation conditions respectively (Figure 5).

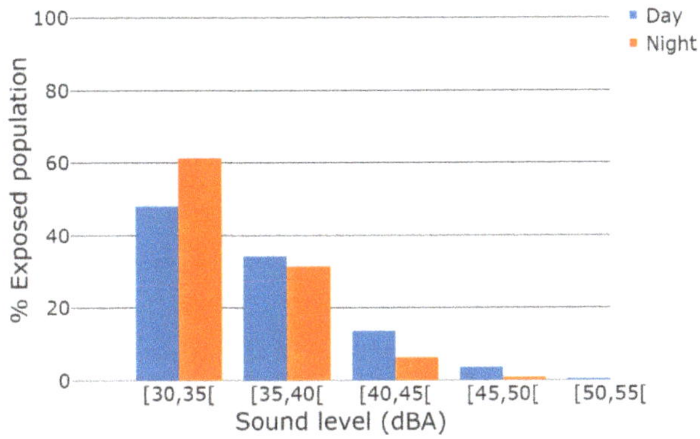

Figure 5. Number of people in metropolitan France exposed to WT sound as a function of WT sound level for daytime and night-time meteorological conditions, normalized by the total number of people exposed to WT sound level above 30 dBA.

3.3. Wind Turbine Sound Exposure by Region

Most of the population exposed to WT sound levels above 30 dBA was located in the Hauts-de-France region (daytime: 265,227 people, night-time: 275,846 people). Bretagne, Grand-Est and Normandie regions accounted for 62,728 to 86,770 people for daytime, and for 65,285 to 94,742 people for night-time (Figure 6).

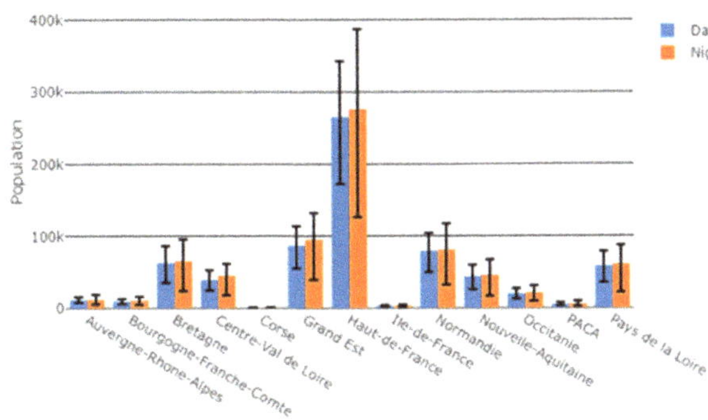

Figure 6. Number of people exposed to WT sound level above 30 dBA, by region. Error bars account for the uncertainty of +/−1 standard deviation on the Harmonoise sound level estimate.

For daytime, 39% of the French population exposed to WT sound levels above 30 dBA lived in Hauts-de-France (38% for night-time) (Figure 7). Bretagne, Grand-Est and Normandie represented 9% to 13% (daytime) and 9% to 13% (night-time) of the population exposed to WT sound levels above 30 dBA.

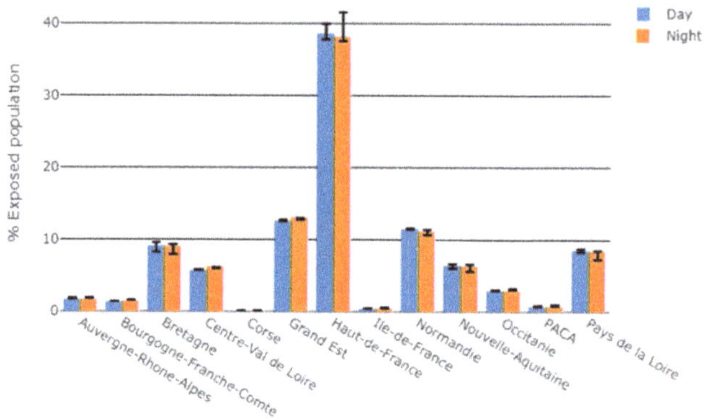

Figure 7. Number of people exposed to WT sound levels above 30 dBA for daytime and night-time meteorological conditions, by region, normalized by the total number of exposed people in metropolitan France. Error bars account for the uncertainty of +/−1 standard deviation on the Harmonoise sound level estimate.

Considering the exposed population in relation to the total population of each region, two northern regions had a higher percentage of people exposed to WT sound: Hauts-de-France and Normandie accounted for 4% and 6% for daytime, and 5% and 6% for night-time, respectively, (Figure 8) of the total population of each region.

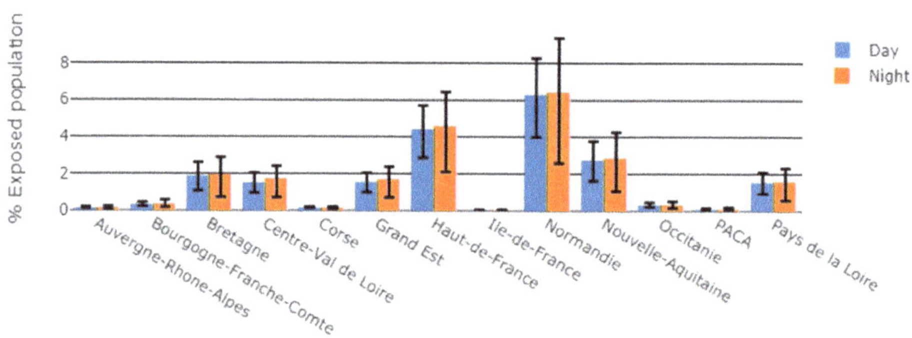

Figure 8. Number of people exposed to WT sound level above 30 dBA for daytime and night-time meteorological conditions, by region, normalized by the total population of each region. Error bars account for the uncertainty of +/−1 standard deviation on the Harmonoise sound level estimate.

Figure 9 shows a comparison of the WT sound level distributions of the exposed populations between all regions of France, for both daytime and night-time meteorological conditions. Except for Corse and Provence-Alpes-Côte d'Azur (PACA) regions, for all other regions, the majority of exposed people are exposed to WT sound levels below 35 dBA.

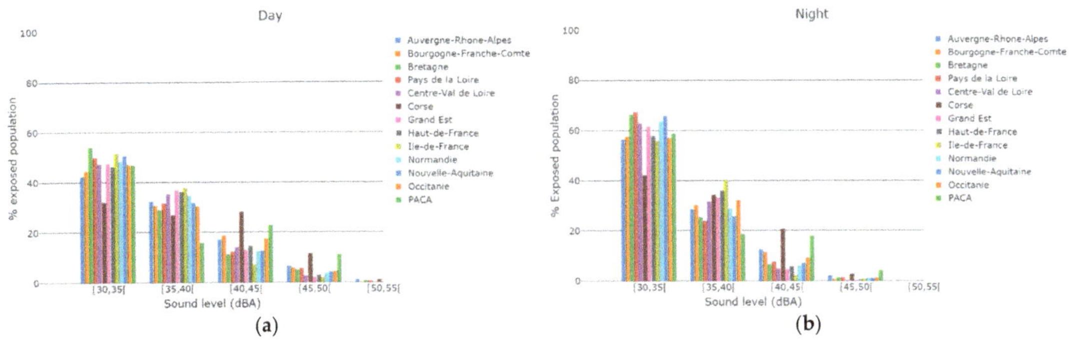

Figure 9. Number of people exposed to WT sound as a function of WT sound levels, normalized by the total number of people exposed to WT sound levels above 30 dBA: daytime (**a**) and night-time (**b**) meteorological conditions.

3.4. Comparison of WT Sound Exposure with Transportation Noise Exposure

Figure 10 shows a comparison of the proportion of people exposed to transportation sound levels above 40 dBA during the night (L_{night}) [30] with the population exposed to WT sound levels above 40 dBA for night-time propagation conditions. The French population in 2017 exposed to night-time noise was 10,394,293 for road traffic noise, 5,113,159 for railway noise and 463,611 for aircraft noise, which can be compared to 53,752 people for night-time WT sound exposure; i.e., 15.0%, 7.0%, 0.7% and 0.08% of the 2017 French population, respectively.

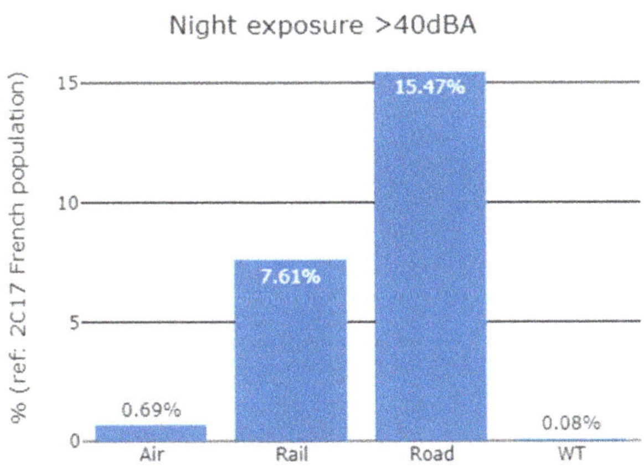

Figure 10. Proportion (%) of the 2017 French population exposed to sound levels above 40 dBA during the night, for four noise sources: aircraft noise (Air), railway noise (Rail), road traffic noise (Road) and wind turbine noise (WT).

4. Discussion

The aim of the research presented in this paper was to quantify the number of wind-farms' residents in France exposed to wind turbine sound. The first objective was to validate a sound level prediction model for the calculation of WT sound levels. The performance of the Harmonoise model was evaluated through the quantification of its uncertainties on the WT sound levels predictions. For both daytime and night-time propagation conditions, the bias between predicted and measured WT sound levels was regarded as sufficiently small (bias between −4.4 dBA and −0.2 dBA) to allow a correction of predicted sound levels. The value of the standard uncertainty was considered sufficiently low to validate the use of Harmonoise model for the prediction of WT sound levels in this research. It is consistent with what is encountered for engineering models of outdoor noise prediction, for which the standard uncertainty can typically range from 2 to 4 dBA, depending on the model [12,32–34].

The second objective was to count the number of people in metropolitan France exposed to WT sound levels. The proportion of those exposed to WT sound levels above 30 dBA represented a small proportion of the total population in France (1% for both daytime and night-time propagation conditions). The WT sound exposure of these people was very moderate: the majority of people were exposed to sound levels below 35 dBA, and more than 80% were exposed to sound levels below 40 dBA, for both daytime and night-time propagation conditions. Most of the exposed population was located in the Hauts-de-France region (about 40%). A very large majority of the exposed population was located in the North of France: Bretagne, Grand-Est, Normandie and Hauts-de-France represented more than 75% of the people exposed to WT sound.

Compared to other regions, the two northern regions, Hauts-de-France and Normandie have more people exposed to WT sound compared to the total population of each region. Nevertheless, this difference was rather small (less than 5%) and could be partly explained by the combination of several regional factors: the number of wind farms, the number of people living in rural areas, where wind farms were generally installed, and the spatial distribution of people within each region.

The distributions of sound levels between regions were compared in order to investigate regional specificities in the WT sound exposure. This could happen, for example, if WT would be noisier or closer to residents' dwellings in some regions. Except for Corse and PACA regions, the distributions of sound levels of exposed populations seemed very similar across regions, for both daytime and night-time meteorological conditions. In metropolitan France, people exposed to WT sound were exposed in a similar manner, with no regional specificity. In addition, for almost all regions, the sound exposure of the majority of exposed people was between 30 dBA and 35 dBA. The cases of Corse and PACA were marginal given the small number of exposed people for those regions.

If any significant health effects from WT sound were to be demonstrated in the future, it would be useful to assess this potential public health issue in comparison to other exposures to common noise source for which health effects have already been demonstrated [3]. The comparison of the proportion of the French population in 2017 exposed to sound levels above 40 dBA during the night for transportation noise and for WT sound showed that far few people were exposed to WT sound than to transportation noise (0.08% for WT sound, compared to 15.0%, 7.0%, 0.7% for road traffic noise, aircraft noise and railway noise respectively). This is especially true as the sound levels of the population exposed to transportation noise were underestimated. Indeed, only major transportation infrastructures, and cities with more than 100,000 inhabitants were considered (see [31] for more details). Conversely, WT sound exposure was probably overestimated here (see below). The fact that the proportion of people exposed to WT sound was much lower than that exposed to transportation noise could be explained by the much smaller number of wind farms on the metropolitan territory, compared to transportation infrastructures, by the installation of wind farms in rural areas where the population density is lower, by sound levels at dwellings that are lower for WT, and finally by distances between dwellings and noise sources that are greater for WT due to French legislation about wind farms implantation.

The methodology for assessing the population exposed to WT sound had some limitations. The first limitation, as briefly mentioned above, was that the count of exposed people was likely to be overestimated because the WT sound levels were estimated by considering (i) a constant wind speed corresponding to the nominal operation of the wind turbines, as if WT were constantly in operation throughout the day or night, (ii) the sound exposure based on the maximum sound level among all the sound levels predicted for the different wind directions, (iii) the sound level of the most exposed façade of each dwelling and (iv) the meteorological conditions corresponding to favorable conditions for sound propagation.

The initial objective of the paper was to investigate the worst-case scenario that maximized noise exposure levels. Therefore, only one wind speed value was considered (7 m/s at 10 m height). This corresponded to the maximum sound emission of the wind turbine and to the nominal WT operation. It should be noted that the sound emission is constant for wind speeds above 7 m/s. Three scenarii were then considered: the best, the worst and the average scenario, named in the paper lower, upper and average scenario in order to bound the estimates of population counts. The range of estimates could sometimes be wide, but this was not a major problem, the most important being the orders of magnitude of the population counts, and also the values corresponding to the lower scenario, which indicated whether there are enough people exposed to different and relatively contrasting WT sound levels to conduct an epidemiological study and to demonstrate, in a statistically rigorous way, an association between a health condition and the level of wind turbine noise, if such an association exists. In the on-going RIBeolH project [35], information from regional wind statistics will be used to take into account the regional influence of wind direction and speed on exposure. Considering that all inhabitants of a house were assigned to the most exposed façade could also lead to an overestimation of the number of people exposed to the WT sound. This overestimation was not a major concern in this research since one of its original aims was to obtain an upper limit of WT sound exposure. Conversely, if the www.thewindpower.net (accessed on 1 December 2021) database (was the most complete publicly available database of WT in France in 2017, pending the exhaustive database that the French Ministry of the Environment is building and which should be accessible in 2022, its completeness was not perfect and the missing wind farms could be a cause of underestimating the number of residents exposed to WT sound in this study. A comparison of national wind capacity from the database with other data sources [36,37] showed that the underestimation could nevertheless be limited because the database contains 94% of the installed capacity as of mid-2017.

A second limitation was that the predicted sound exposure did not correspond to an actual exposure over a day or night period, as would for example an equivalent noise level, but took into account typical propagation conditions of daytime and night-time periods. However, they could possibly be interpreted as an equivalent sound level exposure if it was assumed that the meteorological conditions and wind speed were the same during all the periods. While this was not the most realistic situation, it nevertheless did provide useful information on the upper limit of the number of people exposed to WT sound.

Another limitation of this research concerned the estimation of uncertainties. Estimating the uncertainties in the population counts (associated with the level of reliability and the percentage of error) was rather difficult because there was no simple relationship between sound exposure and population count: this relationship differed strongly from one wind farm to another due to the propagation influence (e.g., the presence or absence of obstacles), and the spatial distribution of the population around each wind farm. Some procedures based on Monte Carlo or bootstrapping techniques could have been considered, but they were deemed too time-consuming in relation to the time available for this research. They will nevertheless be explored for the update of this research in the framework of the RIBEolH project. Thus, in order to give a range of estimates of the population counts, three noise exposure scenarii (upper scenario, average scenario and upper scenario) were preferred for estimating these uncertainties.

The aim of this study was to deal only with audible noise, which is a first step before going further. It was out of the scope to deal with all phenomena involved in WTN, in particular:

- Tonalities: audible tonalities phenomena than can occur in WT is very often due to a malfunction of the WT (e.g., in the hub machinery). In this study, we have assumed that wind turbines were operating normally.
- Amplitude modulation: nowadays, no available engineering model can model amplitude modulation, and amplitude modulation modeling is still a research challenge (see for example the PIBE project [38], http://www.anr-pibe.fr, (accessed on 1 December

2021). Moreover, the few available research models on amplitude modulation cannot be applied at the scale of a national territory because of their complexity and because they require input information that is not available at this large geographical scale.

The methodology proposed in this paper could be improved: the introduction of annual wind speed and direction statistics for each region in the calculation process could provide a more realistic sound exposure for daytime or night-time periods. An investigation of the low frequency noise exposure could also be done. An update of this work is in progress as part of the preparation of the epidemiological study planned in the RIBEolH project [35], to adapt to the rapid growth in the number of wind farm installations in France and the evolution of the French population, but also to improve the calculation process and to extent the assessment to low frequency noise exposure.

The results presented above, being the first assessment of exposure to wind turbine noise in France, may lead to a relevant epidemiological study in the RIBEolH project. Indeed, in order to conduct an epidemiological study and to demonstrate, in a statistically rigorous way, an association between a health condition and the level of wind turbine noise, if such an association exists, it would first be necessary to recruit a sufficient number of individuals exposed to different and relatively contrasting WT sound levels. It will be possible to reach this first step thanks to the count of the number of people exposed to contrasted levels of WT sound for all wind farms of the whole metropolitan France. Then, the quality of epidemiological studies assessing the risks associated with environmental exposures depends in part on the quality of the estimation or measurement of participants' exposure. However, in a large-scale epidemiological study, noise measurements in a large number of residents will not be feasible because of the cost and it will be necessary to use noise prediction models. The use of Harmonoise prediction model proposed and validated in this paper will thus make it possible to estimate the exposure to wind noise at the home of each participant who will be included in the epidemiological study of the RIBEolH project.

5. Conclusions

The objective of the Cibelius feasibility study was to propose a methodology for calculating WT sound exposure at a national geographical scale and to identify the number of people exposed to WT sound in metropolitan France.

The total number of people exposed to WT sound was approximately 686,000 during the day and 722,000 during the night, thus about 0.1% of the 2017 French population. More than 80% of the population exposed to WT sound levels above 30 dBA was exposed to levels below 40 dBA. It is important to note that, due to some assumptions (wind speed corresponding to WT nominal operation, wind turbines constantly in operation throughout the day), the sound exposure, and therefore the number of people exposed to WT sound, was probably overestimated.

These results constitute the first assessment of WT sound exposure at a national geographical scale, and more specifically for metropolitan France. The results and methodology proposed in this paper were the first step in preparing an epidemiological study in France in the few next years. This study will be conducted in the RIBEolH project, which is investigating the impact of WT sound on human health and annoyance. The results of this study will provide useful information for public authorities to assess whether or not regulations concerning WT should be adapted.

Author Contributions: Conceptualization, D.E.; Formal analysis, D.E.; Funding acquisition, D.E. and A.-S.E.; Investigation, D.E.; Methodology, D.E.; Project administration, A.-S.E.; Software, D.E., P.D. and G.G.; Supervision, A.-S.E.; Validation, D.E. and P.D.; Writing—original draft, D.E., L.G.-A. and A.-S.E.; Writing—review & editing, D.E., L.G.-A. and A.-S.E. All authors have read and agreed to the published version of the manuscript.

Funding: This research was funded by Ifsttar (now Gustave Eiffel University), Cerema and by a grant provided by the Environment-Health-Work Program of Anses (French Agency for Food, Environmental and Occupational Health & Safety) with the support of the ministries in charge of ecology (EST-2016/1/007).

Institutional Review Board Statement: Not applicable.

Informed Consent Statement: Not applicable.

Data Availability Statement: The data for each wind farm is publicly available at www.thewindpower.net, but the complete database was purchased from that site by the authors for this project under a research agreement. The topography and building databases are freely available online (see ref. [22]).

Acknowledgments: The authors thank the French Agency for Food, Environmental and Occupational Health & Safety (Anses) who funded this study.

Conflicts of Interest: The authors declare no conflict of interest.

References

1. Van Kamp, I.; van den Berg, F. Health effects related to wind turbine sound, including low-frequency sound and infrasound. *Acoust. Aust.* **2018**, *46*, 31–57. [CrossRef]
2. Van Kamp, I.; van den Berg, F. Health effects related to wind turbine sound: An update. *Int. J. Environ. Res. Public Health* **2021**, *18*, 9133. [CrossRef]
3. WHO. *Environmental Noise Guidelines for the European Region*; World Health Organisation: Copenhague, Denmark, 2018.
4. ANSES. *Évaluation des Effets Sanitaires des Basses Fréquences Sonores et Infrasons dus Aux Parcs Eoliens, Saisine 2013-SA-0115: Avis de l'ANSES*; Collective Expertise Report; French Agency for Food, Environmental and Occupational Health & Safety: Paris, France, 2017.
5. Lepoutre, P.; Avan, P.; Cadene, A.; Ecotière, D.; Evrard, A.S.; Moati, F.; Topilla, E. Health effects of low frequency noise and infrasound from wind farms: Results from an independent collective expertise in France. In Proceedings of the 12th ICBEN Congress on Noise as a Public Health Problem, Zurich, Switzerland, 18–22 June 2017.
6. Kayser, B.; Cotté, B.; Ecotière, D.; Gauvreau, B. Environmental parameters sensitivity analysis for the modelling of wind turbine noise in downwind conditions. *J. Acoust. Soc. Am.* **2020**, *148*, 3623–3632. [CrossRef] [PubMed]
7. Heimann, D.; Englberger, A.; Schady, A. Sound propagation through the wake flow of a hilltop wind turbine—A numerical study. *Wind Energy* **2018**, *21*, 650–662. [CrossRef]
8. Barlas, E.; Zhu, W.J.; Shen, W.Z.; Dag, K.O.; Moriarty, P. Consistent modelling of wind turbine noise propagation from source to receiver. *J. Acoust. Soc. Am.* **2017**, *142*, 3297–3310. [CrossRef] [PubMed]
9. Cotté, B. Extended source models for wind turbine noise propagation. *J. Acoust. Soc. Am.* **2019**, *145*, 1363–1371. [CrossRef] [PubMed]
10. Keith, S.E.; Feder, K.; Voicescu, S.A.; Soukhovtsev, V.; Denning, A.; Tsang, J.; Broner, N.; Leroux, T.; Richarz, W.; van den Berg, F. Wind turbine sound pressure level calculations at dwellings. *J. Acoust. Soc. Am.* **2016**, *139*, 1436–1442. [CrossRef] [PubMed]
11. Verheijen, E.; Jabben, J.; Schreurs, E.; Smith, K.B. Impact of wind turbine noise in The Netherlands. *Noise Health* **2011**, *13*, 459–463. [PubMed]
12. Standard ISO 9613-2:1996*Acoustics—Attenuation of Sound during Propagation Outdoors—Part 2: General Method of Calculation*, International Organization for Standardization: Geneva, Switzerland, 1996.
13. Dutilleux, G.; Defrance, J.; Ecotière, D.; Gauvreau, B.; Bérengier, M.; Besnard, F.; Duc, E.L. NMPB-routes-2008: The revision of the french method for road traffic noise prediction. *Acta Acust. United Acust.* **2010**, *96*, 452–462. [CrossRef]
14. Kephalopoulos, S.; Paviotti, M.; Anfosso-Lédée, F. *Common Noise Assessment Methods in Europe (CNOSSOS-EU), EUR 25379 EN*; Publications Office of the European Union: Luxembourg; European Commission Joint Research Centre, Institute for Health and Consumer Protection: Ispra, Italy, 2012; 180p.
15. Salomons, E.; van Maercke, D.; Defrance, J.; de Roo, F. The Harmonoise Sound Propagation Model. *Acta Acust. United Acust.* **2011**, *97*, 62–74. [CrossRef]
16. Forssén, J.; Schiff, M.T.; Pedersen, E.; Persson Waye, K. Wind Turbine Noise Propagation over Flat Ground: Measurements and Predictions. *Acta Acust. United Acust.* **2010**, *96*, 753–760. [CrossRef]
17. Bowdler, D.; Leventhall, G. (Eds.) *Wind Turbine Noise*; Multi-Science Publishing Co Ltd.: London, UK, 2011; 215p.
18. Méthode D'évaluation du Bruit des Eoliennes—Comparaison Entre Modélisation et Mesurage, Rapport Final, Office Fédéral de L'énergie OFEN, Confédération Suisse. 2016. Available online: https://www.aramis.admin.ch/Texte/?ProjectID=36116 (accessed on 1 December 2021).
19. Attenborough, K.; Li, K.; Horoshenkov, K. *Predicting Outdoor Sound*; Taylor & Francis: London, UK, 2007.
20. Standard IEC 61400-11:2012*Wind Turbine—Part 11: Acoustic Noise Measurement Techniques*, International Electrotechnical Commission: Geneva, Switzerland, 2012.

21. Standard ISO/IEC Guide 98-3:2008*Uncertainty of Measurement—Part 3: Guide to the Expression of Uncertainty in Measurement (GUM:1995)*, International Organization for Standardization: Geneva, Switzerland, 2008.
22. National Institute of Geographic and Forestry Information. Available online: https://geoservices.ign.fr/documentation/diffusion/telechargement-donnees-libres.html#bd-topo (accessed on 1 December 2021).
23. Available online: https://www.datakustik.com/products/cadnaa/ (accessed on 1 December 2021).
24. Paul, B. Ground Vibration, Infrasound and Low Frequency Noise Measurements from a Modern Wind Turbine. *Acta Acust. United Acust.* **2013**, *99*, 537–544.
25. HMøller, H.; Pedersen, C.S. Low-frequency noise from large wind turbines. *J. Acoust. Soc. Am.* **2011**, *129*, 3727–3744. [CrossRef] [PubMed]
26. Tachibana, H.; Yano, H.; Fukushima, A.; Sueoka, S. Nationwide field measurements of wind turbine noise in Japan. *Noise Control Eng. J.* **2014**, *62*, 90–101. [CrossRef]
27. Heimann, D.; Bakermans, M.; Defrance, J.; Kühner, D. Vertical Sound Speed Profiles Determined from Meteorological Measurements Near the Ground. *Acta Acust. United Acust.* **2007**, *93*, 228–240.
28. QGIS Geographic Information System. QGIS Association. Available online: http://www.qgis.org (accessed on 1 December 2021).
29. Létinois, L. *Méthodologie de Répartition Spatiale de la Population*; Laboratoire Central de Surveillance de la Qualité de l'Air: Verneuil-en-Halatte, France, 2014.
30. Reported Data on Noise Exposure Covered by Directive 2002/49/EC, European Environment Agency (EEA). Available online: https://www.eea.europa.eu/data-and-maps/data/data-on-noise-exposure-7 (accessed on 1 December 2021).
31. Directive 2002/49/EC of the European Parliament and of the Council of 25 June 2002 Relating to the Assessment and Management of Environmental Noise. Available online: https://eur-lex.europa.eu/legal-content/EN/TXT/?uri=celex%3A32002L0049 (accessed on 1 December 2021).
32. Peters, R. (Ed.) *Uncertainty in Acoustics Measurement, Prediction and Assessment*; CRC Press: Boca Raton, FL, USA, 2020; 464p, ISBN 9781498769150.
33. Ecotière, D.; Foy, C.; Dutilleux, G. Comparison of engineering models of outdoor sound propagation: NMPB2008 and Harmonoise-Imagine. In Proceedings of the Acoustics 2012 Conference, Nantes, France, 23–27 April 2012.
34. Jónsson, G.B.; Jacobsen, F.; A Comparison of Two Numerical Models for Outdoor Sound Propagation Harmonoise and Nord 2000. Proceedings of the Joint Baltic-Nordic Acoustics Meeting 2008, Reykjavik, Iceland, 17–19 August 2008; Available online: https://is.gd/K6Ogmb (accessed on 1 December 2021).
35. Evrard, A.S.; Avan, P.; Champelovier, P.; Cotté, B.; Écotière, D.; Gauvreau, B.; Giorgis-Allemand, L.; Marquis-Favre, C.; Meunier, S. Research on the impacts of wind turbine noise on humans: Sound, perception, health (RIBEolH). In Proceedings of the 13th ICBEN International Congress on Noise as a Public Health Problem, Stockholm, Sweden, 14–17 June 2021.
36. Panorama de L'électricité Renouvelable au 30 Septembre 2017. RTE, SER, Enedis, ADEeF. 2017. Available online: https://assets.rte-france.com/prod/public/2020-06/Panorama%20de%20l%27%C3%A9lectricit%C3%A9%20renouvelable%20au%2030%20septembre%202017.pdf (accessed on 1 December 2021).
37. STAT INFO Energie—Tableau de bord: Éolien—Troisième Trimestre 2017, Ministry of the Ecological Transition. Available online: https://www.statistiques.developpement-durable.gouv.fr/publicationweb/60 (accessed on 1 December 2021).
38. Ecotière, D.; Gauvreau, B.; Cotté, B.; Roger, M.; Schmich, I.; Nessi, M.-C. PIBE: A new French project for predicting the impact of wind turbine noise. In Proceedings of the 8th International Conference on Wind Turbine Noise, Lisbon, Portugal, 12–14 June 2019.

buildings

MDPI

Article

Effect of Road and Railway Sound on Psychological and Physiological Responses in an Office Environment

Boya Yu *, Linjie Wen, Jie Bai and Yuying Chai

School of Architecture and Design, Beijing Jiaotong University, Beijing 100044, China; 18311054@bjtu.edu.cn (L.W.); 18311002@bjtu.edu.cn (J.B.); 21126381@bjtu.edu.cn (Y.C.)
* Correspondence: boyayu@bjtu.edu.cn

Abstract: The present study aims to explore the psychophysiological impact of different traffic sounds in office spaces. In this experiment, 30 subjects were recruited and exposed to different traffic sounds in a virtual reality (VR) office scene. The road traffic sound and three railway sounds (conventional train, high-speed train, and tram) with three sound levels (45, 55, and 65 dB) were used as the acoustic stimuli. Physiological responses, electrodermal activity (EDA) and heart rate (HR) were monitored throughout the experiment. Psychological evaluations under each acoustic stimulus were also measured using scales within the VR system. The results showed that both the psychological and the physiological responses were significantly affected by the traffic sounds. As for psychological responses, considerable adverse effects of traffic sounds were observed, which constantly increased with the increase in the sound level. The peak sound level was found to have a better performance than the equivalent sound level in the assessment of the psychological impact of traffic sounds. As for the physiological responses, significant effects of both the acoustic factors (sound type and sound level) and the non-acoustic factors (gender and exposure time) were observed. The relationship between sound level and physiological parameters varied among different sound groups. The variation in sound level hardly affected the participants' HR and EDA when exposed to the conventional train and tram sounds. In contrast, HR and EDA were significantly affected by the levels of road traffic sound and high-speed train sound. Through a correlation analysis, a relatively weak correlation between the psychological evaluations and HR was found.

Keywords: road traffic sound; conventional train sound; high-speed train sound; tram sound; electrodermal activity; heart rate; acoustic comfort; noise annoyance

Citation: Yu, B.; Wen, L.; Bai, J.; Chai, Y. Effect of Road and Railway Sound on Psychological and Physiological Responses in an Office Environment. *Buildings* **2022**, *12*, 6. https://doi.org/10.3390/buildings12010006

Academic Editors: Roberto Alonso González Lezcano, Francesco Nocera and Rosa Giuseppina Caponetto

Received: 17 November 2021
Accepted: 17 December 2021
Published: 22 December 2021

1. Introduction

Recent surveys suggest that office employees are the most dissatisfied with the acoustic environment when various factors of the physical indoor environment are enquired [1]. Noise was found to be influential not only on the perception of the overall environment, but also on the working performance in offices [2,3]. Landström revealed the relationship between low-frequency noises and fatigue in the working environment [4]. Focusing on the open-planned offices, the most annoying sounds were found to be noises from outside, ventilation systems, office equipment, and keyboard typing [5]. As for the home working space, the sounds from other people at home, neighbors, construction, and traffic were reported as the most negatively evaluated sounds [6]. As reported, traffic sound is a major source of environmental sound pollution [7], and 81% of the workers around major streets are annoyed by traffic sounds [8]. With rapid urban growth all over the world [9,10] and increasing demand for better transportation systems, a simultaneous increase in traffic sound exposure and the associated impact on residents can be anticipated. Therefore, it is important to perform a comprehensive investigation on the adverse effect of traffic sounds on the agenda of sound policies and urban development.

Exposure to traffic sounds has been proven to be associated with an increased risk of negative health outcomes both physiologically and psychologically [11–13]. Psychological attributes, such as noise annoyance, are the most widely used measures for evaluating the impact of traffic sounds [14–17]. It was found that traffic-related noise annoyance had a considerable impact on health-related quality of life [18]. With the increase in the sound level, exponential growth in the percentage of highly annoyed people was found by large-scale surveys, namely, the dose–response curve [17]. In the past several decades, the dose–response curve has been used as direct scientific evidence for most sound policies and regulations. In addition to noise annoyance, traffic sounds were found to have a significant influence on how people perceive the overall urban soundscape [19,20]. Considering the diversity of the urban context, it has been suggested that the perception of the acoustic environment was multidimensional [21,22]. A two-dimensional scale is widely used for evaluating the psychological response to the acoustic environment, including the eventfulness (arousal) and pleasantness (pleasant) [23–25]. In addition, acoustic comfort is also widely used as a measure of the quality of the overall sound environment [26–28]. Focusing on the indoor acoustic environment, another two-dimensional scale (comfort–content) was suggested to evaluate the soundscape quality [29]. Through a virtual reality experiment, this model was proved to be efficient for evaluating the work-related quality in open-plan offices [2]. In almost all relevant studies, the traffic sounds were found to have an adverse effect on the perception of the acoustic environment, which increased with the sound level [30].

In addition to psychological responses, the physiological responses to traffic sounds were also investigated to reveal the potential effect on health [31–33]. Significant impacts of traffic sound on physiological responses have been reported in the literature. In laboratory experiments, Vera et al. found that the exposure to high-intensity traffic sound with negative self-statements produced a significant electromyography (EMG) increase [32]. Significant increases in electroencephalographic (EEG) indices and HR with the increase in sound level were reported by Basner et al. [34]. Similar results were also reported by Raggam et al. [35]; the presence of traffic sounds led to an increase in heart rate (HR), although the respiratory rate (RR) was unaffected. In a recent field study, strong associations between blood pressure and traffic sounds were found [36]. Laboratory experiments are more commonly used for investigating the physiological effect of traffic sounds and to control non-experimental factors. Under audio–video stimuli [37], higher HR, heart rate variability (HRV), RR, amplitude of the R wave, and SCL were found when close to the traffic sound source. A higher skin conductance level (SCL) was observed when the traffic sound was mixed with the natural sound [38]. In the field of soundscape research, similar results could be found when the traffic sounds were compared with other urban sounds [25,39–41]. The relationship between physiological responses and exposure time has revealed that the introduction of sound stimuli led to an immediate change in physiological parameters in the first 30 to 60 s, including EDA and HR. With the increase in exposure time, participants gradually adapted to the sound stimuli and the physiological parameters gradually returned to the baseline levels [38,41,42]. In most previous studies, it was found that the baseline level of physiological parameters was highly dependent on personal characteristics [38,41]. Therefore, the change in physiological parameters is commonly used to reveal the effect of sound stimuli on people.

There are only very few studies that have investigated the effect of traffic sounds in office spaces, and which have mainly focused on the psychological attributes. Through a questionnaire survey, traffic sound was identified as the cause of annoyance, activity disturbance, and headaches [43]. A positive correlation between the sound level and the percentage of annoyed people was identified [8]. In addition, annoyance caused by the traffic sound was found to be influential on the psychological state, including anxiety [44], fatigue, and tension [45]. As for the overall acoustic environment, the traffic sound was also found to harm the overall acoustic comfort in office buildings [46]. However, to the best of the authors' knowledge, research on the physiological responses to traffic sounds in office spaces is not detailed.

Meanwhile, most of the existing literature has mainly focused on the effect of sound level variation of road traffic sound [37], whereas very few studies have compared the responses to different traffic sounds. However, there are considerable differences between different traffic sounds on not only the physical characteristics, but also on the impact on people [30,47]. In very few studies which examined the psychophysiological responses under different sound sources [36,48], simultaneous consideration of the sound type and the sound level was not detailed, to the authors' knowledge. However, for effective sound control treatment, it is important to determine the interaction effect of the sound type and the sound level on people.

Our analysis indicated that the following questions on the topic of psychophysiological responses under the impact of traffic noises in office spaces still need to be addressed:

(a) What are the psychophysiological effects of different traffic sounds in office spaces?;
(b) Do the increases in sound levels interfere with the psychophysiological responses to traffic sounds?;
(c) Do the other factors (gender and exposure time) interfere with the psychophysiological responses to traffic sounds?;
(d) Are there correlations between psychological responses and physiological responses under the impact of traffic sounds?

Therefore, in the present study, we conducted laboratory experiments to measure the psychophysiological responses of 30 respondents under different traffic sound configurations. The interaction effects of sound type and sound level on the psychological and physiological responses were examined. This paper was organized as follows. The experiment implementations are shown in Section 2. Section 3 shows the results that reveal the influential factors of psychophysiological parameters when exposed to traffic sounds. In addition, the correlations between psychological responses and physiological responses are shown in Section 3. Sections 4 and 5 summarize the discussion on related issues and the main findings of this study.

2. Methodology

2.1. Participants

There were 30 subjects ranging in age from 19 to 26 years participating in the experiment (15 male and 15 female). All of the participants reported having normal hearing and corrected vision. None of them was taking prescription medication. All of the participants were informed about the aim and protocol of the experiment, and they voluntarily participated in the study.

2.2. Experiment Stimuli

The experiment was conducted in an office-like experimental chamber, where the physical environment was controlled (temperature = 21~23 °C; background sound level < 25 dBA). To provide a complete and realistic presentation of an office and avoid other distractions in the lab, immersive virtual reality (VR) technology was employed in this study. An omnidirectional picture of an actual open-planned office was taken and played in the VR head-mounted display (HTC VIVE Pro EYE; Resolution: 2880 × 1600; Refresh rate: 90 Hz) during the experiments, as shown in Figure 1.

In this study, four traffic sounds (including road traffic, conventional train, high-speed train, and tram sounds) were used to generate the sound stimuli. The four traffic sounds were selected for the following reasons: (1) they are very common traffic sounds in urban areas and are frequently considered in relevant studies [49–52]; and (2) they are reported to have different influences on subjective evaluation and could have potential differences on psychophysiological effects [36]. All the sound stimuli were extracted from field recordings collected in Beijing, China. The sound recordings were all collected in quiet areas to avoid accidental sounds. A sound meter (6228+, Aihua, Hangzhou, China) was used to conduct sound recordings and measurements under the same format (48 kHz, single-channel, 16 bits). Then, 2 min clips were extracted from the field recordings as the experimental stimuli. Specifically, the road traffic sound was recorded near a city highway. A continuous 2 min clip was then extracted. However, the railway sounds were discontinuous, with the duration time varying from 15 s to 45 s, as shown in Figure 2. Moreover, the time period between two trains was not the same. For standardization, a 1 min clip with one train passing by was extracted and then repeated to produce a 2 min experimental stimulus. Therefore, in each railway sound stimulus, there were two trains passing by. The spectrograms of four traffic sound stimuli are shown in Figure 2. It could be found that there were both spectral and temporal differences between different traffic sounds. In general, the spectral characteristics of all traffic sounds were similar, whereas the railway sounds contained more high-frequency components. Moreover, the temporal differences were much more significant between road traffic sounds and railway sounds. The road traffic sound was mainly continuous and steady, whereas the railway sounds were intermittent and fluctuating. Due to the differences in speed and train length, the tram sounds exhibit a minimum duration of approximately 15 s, whereas the duration of the conventional train sound was approximately 45 s.

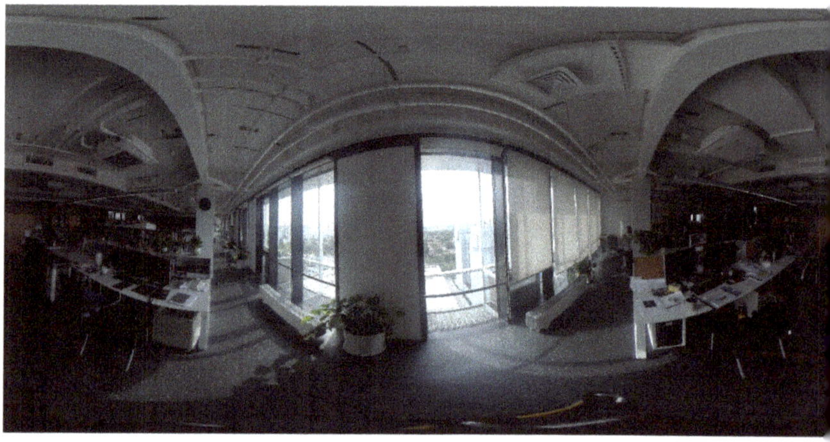

Figure 1. The panoramic view of an open-plan office.

The sound level was another considered experimental factor in the experiment. According to sound regulations and the existing literature [11,36], the sounds (A-weighted equivalent sound level) were set at 3 levels in this study: 45, 55, and 65 dBA. The sound stimuli were replayed through reference class Sennheiser 650 HD headphones to ensure the spectral accuracy of the emitted signal with respect to the real sound. The equivalent sound level of the single-channel signal was measured by a class 1 sound level meter (6228+, Aihua, Hangzhou, China) placed 1 cm away from the headphones. Then, the sound levels of the stimuli were calibrated to the standard sound levels (45, 55, and 65 dB) in Cooledit software. Finally, the single-channel signals were copied to produce the dual-channel stimuli.

In addition, silence was used as the control stimulus to conduct baseline measurements. The duration of silence was also set as 2 min. Altogether, 13 acoustic stimuli were used in the study. During the experiment, sound signals of the acoustic stimuli were delivered by a computer through the headphones.

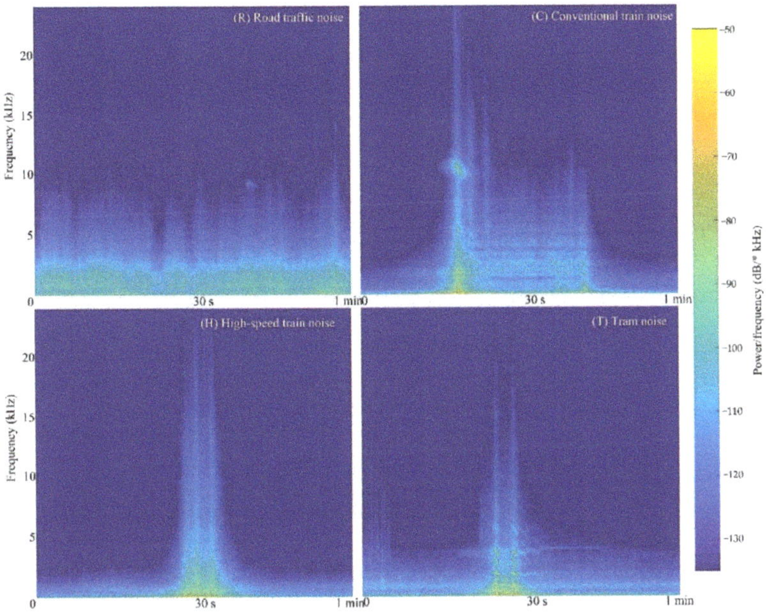

Figure 2. Spectrogram of the experiment stimuli, including road traffic sound (R), conventional train sound (C), high-speed train sound (H), and tram sound (T).

2.3. Measures

To measure the physiological responses to traffic sounds, two simple measures were applied: electrodermal activity (EDA) and heart rate (HR). These two indices are widely used to assess the physiological response to sound stimuli and are suggested as sensitive indicators for evaluating the impact of sounds [39,41,42,53]. The EDA was measured using two electrodes (HKR-11, range: 100 to 2500 kΩ; accuracy: 2.5 kΩ; sample frequency: 50 Hz) attached to the subject's index and middle fingers of the non-dominant hand. The HR was measured by a photoplethysmography (PPG) sensor (HKG-07, range: 30 to 250 bpm; accuracy: 1 bpm; sample frequency: 16 Hz) attached to the ring finger [53]. The study protocol enabled us to record EDA and ECG simultaneously while the participants were exposed to the experimental stimuli.

As for the psychological attributes, a questionnaire with four aspects was used to assess the psychological effect of traffic sounds in this study. The questionnaire was implemented in the VR system, which appeared after each sound stimulus to avoid influences caused by removing VR equipment. The first used attribute was noise annoyance (AN), which is widely used to evaluate the impact of traffic sounds. A five-point verbal ICBEN (International Commission on Biological Effects of Noise) scale was used with the verbal marks: (1) "not annoyed at all"; (2) "slightly annoyed"; (3) "moderately annoyed"; (4) "very annoyed"; and (5) "extremely annoyed" [54]. The Self-Assessment Manikin (SAM) was used to measure the evoking state associated with experiencing sound stimuli [55,56]. The SAM is commonly applied using graphic scales and cartoon characters to explain the meanings of the scales [41,56]. A modified nine-point numerical scale has been proposed to rate the psychological state when exposed to sound stimuli [25]. Due to size limitations of the questionnaire, nine-point numerical scales were used in this study for the evaluation of arousal and pleasantness evoked by the acoustic stimuli with descriptions: (1) no arousal at all/completely unpleasant; (9) complete arousal/completely pleasant) [25]. In addition, acoustic comfort (AC) was used as an assessment of the overall acoustic environment. Similar to the annoyance evaluation, a five-point verbal scale suggested by Yang and Kang was used with the verbal marks: (1) "very uncomfortable"; (2) "uncomfortable"; (3) "neither comfortable nor comfortable"; (4) "comfortable"; and (5) "very comfortable" [26]. During the experiment, the experimental operator also verbally instructed the participants before the measurements. Instructions used for evaluating acoustic quality in the laboratory study were adopted and used [57]:

"Begin by listening through the 12 traffic sounds presented in the headphone, and build your opinion about their character. Thereafter you measure the traffic sounds with the aid of four attribute scales that appears in front of you. The traffic sounds must be measured one at a time on all the attribute scales and in the order presented from up to down.

Your task is to judge to what extent the attributes listed in the protocol are applicable to the traffic sounds in the current office environment."

2.4. Experimental Procedure

The experiment was generally divided into two sessions: (1) preparation and adaptation; (2) formal experiment. The participants came into the laboratory and were seated in a comfortable chair 15 min before the formal experiment to avoid the impact of physical movement. In the first 10 min, the informed consent was read and signed, basic personal information was collected and the sensors for physiological measurements were attached. After putting on the VR equipment, the participants were asked to adapt to the scene for 4 min to reduce the personal differences caused by the VR environment. The scale for psychological attributes was presented inside the VR environment; therefore, practice was necessary to avoid misunderstandings. After the adaptation session, the participants were asked to rest for 1 min with their eyes closed to remove the impact caused by the practice session. As for the formal experiment, a baseline level was measured as the reference psychophysiological response to a quiet office environment. Then, the psychophysiological responses of the participants were measured when exposed to twelve traffic sound stimuli. For each experimental stimulus, there were three periods: (1) a 2 min period of sound exposure with the continuous measurement of EDA and HR; (2) a 30 s psychological response measurement in which the participants were asked to evaluate the acoustic comfort (AC), noise annoyance (AN), arousal (AR), and pleasantness (PL) with the scales displayed in the VR scene; and (3) a 1 min rest to reduce the effect of the previous stimuli and measurement process. The order of acoustic stimuli presentation was randomized and counterbalanced. A random order of experimental stimuli was generated for each participant. The average order of each stimulus was then calculated. If the average order of any stimulus was smaller than five or larger than eight (order unbalanced), the random order generation process was repeated to maintain the balance among the experimental stimuli. The experiment process is schematically shown in Figure 3. The total time for the formal experiment was approximately 45 min.

2.5. Data Analysis

In this study, all statistical analysis was performed within SPSS 20.0 software (IBM Corp., New York, NY, USA). For the psychological attributes, the measured data were directly used in the statistical analysis, where evaluation of the silent condition was used as the reference. However, it is suggested that non-acoustical characteristics, including gender and exposure time, have a considerable effect on the physiological data [41,42]. Therefore, the 2 min measured data were divided into 20 s segments to reveal the temporal variations of the physiological index. Then, the mean changes in physiological data (EDA and HR) were calculated by comparing with the baseline measurement [41,42]:

$$Index_{change} = \frac{Index_{i,j} - Index_{baseline}}{Index_{baseline}}, \tag{1}$$

where i and j indicate the number of traffic sound type and the time serial for each acoustic stimulus, respectively.

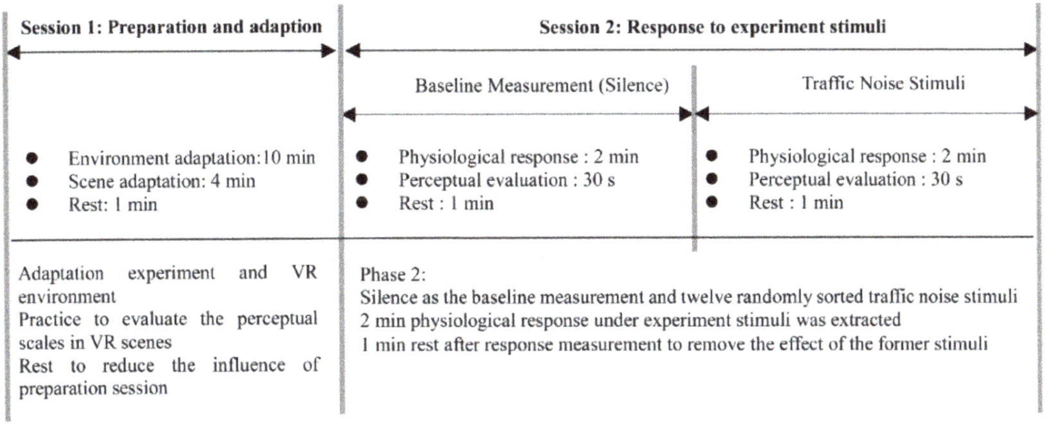

Figure 3. Schematic diagram of the experiment process.

As for the statistical method, the multivariate analysis of variance (MANOVA) was first used to reveal the effect of experimental variables on the psychophysiological response under the impact of different traffic sounds. Before the MANOVA, the normality assumptions of the measured responses for each level of independent variables were examined with the Kolmogorov–Smirnov test. Only one dataset violated the normality assumption (EDA under 55 dB tram sound: $p = 0.028$). In addition, it was suggested that ANOVA could still yield robust and valid results with non-normally distributed data [58]. The homogeneity of variance was verified with the Levene's test (acoustic comfort: $p = 0.493$; annoyance: $p = 0.608$; arousal: $p = 0.993$; pleasantness: $p = 0.791$; EDA: $p = 0.643$; HR: $p = 0.779$). Four experimental variables were considered in the MANOVA: sound level, sound type, gender, and exposure time. As for the psychological responses, the exposure time was not included because the evaluations were performed based on the overall 2 min sound stimuli. The main effects of experimental variables on psychophysiological responses were investigated. As indicated in the previous studies, the relationship between experimental variables and psychophysiological responses might depend on the sound source. Therefore, the interaction effects of sound type and other experimental factors were also included in the MANOVA, as shown in Figure 4. The pairwise comparison was then applied to further show where the differences lay. For the main effects of independent variables, the least significant difference (LSD) was used to conduct the pairwise comparison. For the significant interaction effects found in MANOVA, a nonparametric Mann–Whitney U test was used to conduct the pairwise comparison. For example, if the interaction of sound type and sound level was found to have a significant effect on EDA, pairwise comparisons were conducted between any two sound levels in each sound group to reveal how EDA varied with the sound level. In addition, a correlation analysis was applied to investigate the relationship between physiological response and psychological attributes. In all analyses, a p-value less than 0.05 was used as the criterion to determine significant differences.

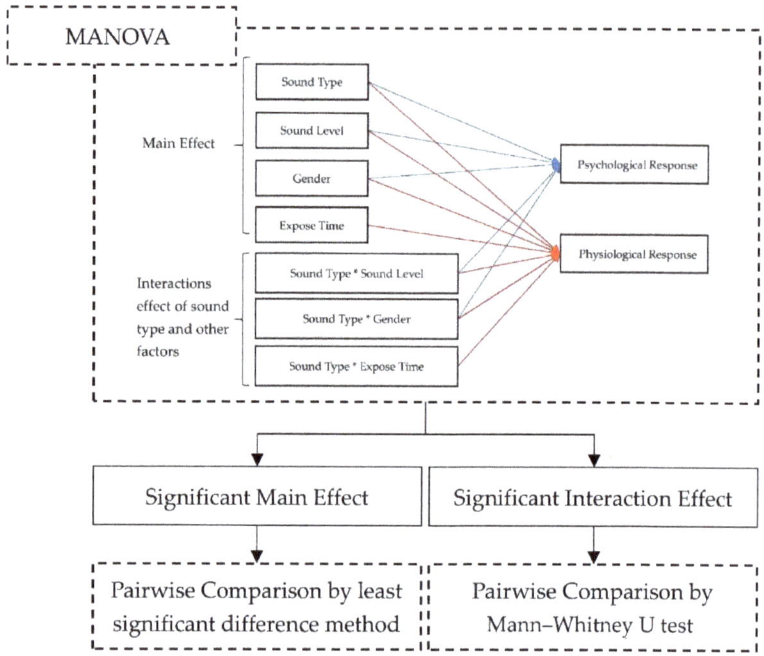

Figure 4. A flowchart of statistical analysis used in this study.

3. Results

3.1. Effect of Traffic Sounds on Psychological Responses

Four psychological dimensions were measured in this study, with greater values indicating higher perceived acoustic comfort (AC), annoyance (AN), arousal (AR), and pleasure (PL). As shown in Figure 5, a strong adverse effect of traffic sounds on psychological responses was found, which led to lower comfort, higher annoyance, higher arousal, and lower pleasure compared with the silence group. A MANOVA was conducted to investigate the effect of traffic sounds on the psychological responses, as shown in Table 1. The main effects of acoustic variables, including sound type and the sound level were found to be statistically significant (Sig. < 0.05) with no interactions. Moreover, no significant difference was found between different gender groups.

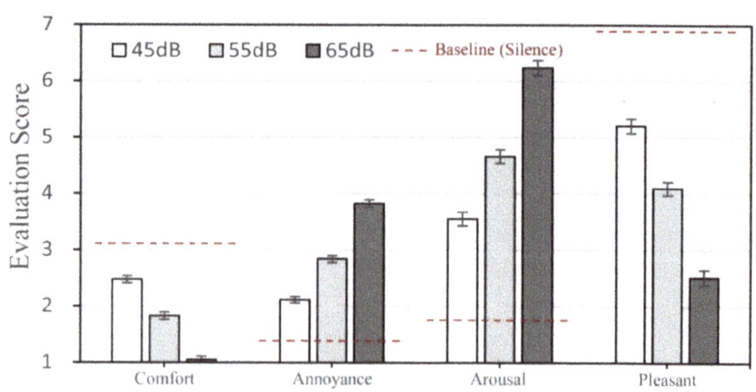

Figure 5. Effect of sound level on psychological responses. The vertical bar represents 95% confidence interval.

Table 1. Results of multivariate tests of psychological evaluations to traffic sounds. AC, AN, AR, and PL represent the evaluation of acoustic comfort, annoyance, arousal, and pleasantness, respectively. * and ** represent significant difference at 0.05 and 0.01 level, respectively.

Variables	Psychological Response	F	Sig.	η_p^2
Sound Type	AC	2.93	0.03 *	0.02
	AN	4.58	0.00 **	0.04
	AR	1.40	0.24	0.01
	PL	2.19	0.09	0.02
SPL (L_{Aeq})	AC	80.86	0.00 **	0.32
	AN	98.56	0.00 **	0.36
	AR	75.45	0.00 **	0.30
	PL	74.41	0.00 **	0.30
Gender	AC	0.65	0.42	0.00
	AN	0.66	0.42	0.00
	AR	0.00	0.96	0.00
	PL	0.00	0.96	0.00
Sound Type * SPL	AC	0.38	0.89	0.01
	AN	0.46	0.84	0.01
	AR	0.29	0.94	0.00
	PL	0.17	0.98	0.00

As for the sound level, significant differences were observed in all four psychological responses. The effect size factor (η_p^2) indicated that the sound level was the most dominant factor for all four psychological attributes. As shown in Figure 5, the decrease in the sound level led to significant improvements in psychological responses (more comfort, less annoyance, less arousing, and more pleasant). Further pairwise comparison (LSD) showed that differences between any sound levels were significant (Sig. < 0.05) for all psychological attributes. Considering that there were no interactions between the sound type and sound level, this tendency was agreed upon in all traffic sound groups.

Although less influential than the sound level, the sound type factor showed significant impacts on acoustic comfort (F = 2.93, Sig. = 0.03 < 0.05) and noise annoyance (F = 4.58, Sig. = 0.00 < 0.05). However, no significant effects of the sound type on arousal and pleasantness were found. By further pairwise comparison (Figure 6), it was found that the impact of tram sound on acoustic comfort (AC), arousal (AR), and pleasure (PL) was higher than that of road traffic sound (Sig. = 0.004 < 0.05). Meanwhile, for noise annoyance, the impact of tram sound was significantly higher than those of the other three traffic sounds ($p_{R,T} = 0.001$; $p_{C,T} = 0.004$; $p_{H,T} = 0.015$). This result showed that the tram sound had a greater impact on how people perceive the acoustic environment at the same sound level. As shown in Figure 2, the tram sound occurred for the shortest duration in this experiment. Moreover, a negative correlation between the psychological impact of traffic sounds (T > H > C > R) and the duration of the sound (T < H < C < R) can be observed in Figure 6. As discussed in Section 2, the 2 min A-weighted equivalent sound level was used to normalize the acoustic stimuli in this study. Therefore, the shortest sound duration time (tram sound) led to the highest peak sound level. The results in Figure 6 indicate that the effect of traffic sound type on psychological responses might be caused by the peak sound level. Another MANOVA was carried out by replacing the equivalent sound level (LAeq) with the peak sound level (LAFmax) to investigate the influence of the sound level parameters. It was found that the peak sound level (LAFmax) was the only influential factor for all four psychological attributes in this analysis. This result indicated that the impact of traffic sound on the perceived acoustic environment was mainly determined by the peak sound level when the traffic sounds showed significant temporal variations. In terms of sound level index for evaluating the perceptual impact, LAFmax showed better performance than LAeq when both the road traffic sound and the railway sound were considered.

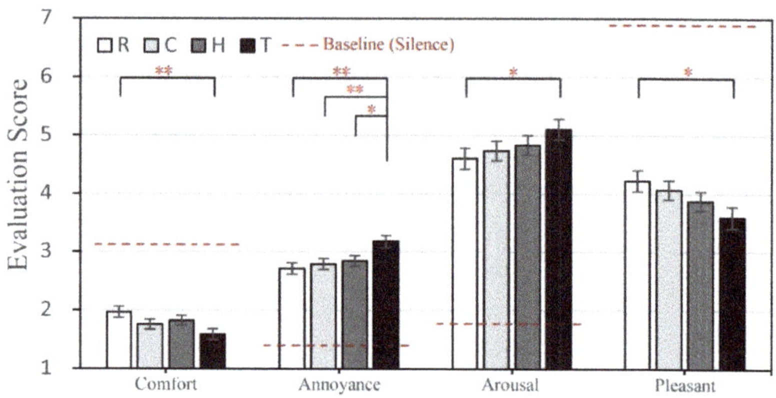

Figure 6. Effect of sound type on psychological attributes. R, C, H, and T represent the road traffic, conventional train, high-speed train, and tram, respectively. The vertical bar represents 95% confidence interval. * and ** represent significant differences in pair-wise comparison (LSD) at a 0.05 level and 0.01 level, respectively.

3.2. *Effect of Traffic Sounds on Physiological Responses*

Table 2 shows the MANOVA results between experiment variables and physiological responses (mean change in EDA and HR). It was found that the physiological responses were significantly affected by both the acoustic factors and the non-acoustic factors, including sound level, gender, and exposure time. Meanwhile, the interactions between factors, including sound type by sound level and sound type by gender, were also observed to be influential on the change in physiological parameters.

Table 2. MANOVA results of physiological evaluations to traffic sounds. * and ** represent significant difference at 0.05 and 0.01 levels, respectively.

Variables	HR			EDA		
	F	Sig.	η_p^2	F	Sig.	η_p^2
Gender	60.389	0.000 **	0.03	57.247	0.000 **	0.03
Time	2.699	0.019 *	0.01	0.113	0.989	0.00
Sound Type	0.456	0.713	0.00	2.293	0.076	0.00
SPL	6.033	0.002 **	0.01	3.615	0.027 *	0.00
Sound Type * SPL	2.365	0.028 *	0.01	2.835	0.009 **	0.01
Sound Type * Gender	0.261	0.853	0.00	6.079	0.000 **	0.01
Sound Type * Time	0.102	1.000	0.00	0.006	1.000	0.00

In terms of acoustic factors, the sound level showed significant influences on both EDA (F = 3.615, Sig. = 0.027) and HR (F = 6.033, Sig. = 0.002). The main effect of the sound type was found to not be significant on neither EDA (F = 2.293, Sig. = 0.076) nor HR (F = 0.456, Sig. = 0.713). Instead, significant interaction effects of sound type and sound level were observed on EDA (F = 2.835, Sig. = 0.009) and HR (F = 2.365, Sig. = 0.028). In general, this result indicated that the sound level played a more important role in the physiological impact of traffic sounds than the sound type. However, the tendencies between sound level and physiological indicators might be different for different traffic sounds. Therefore, a pairwise comparison by nonparametric Mann–Whitney U test was applied.

Figure 7 shows the relationship between the sound level and physiological indicators in different sound groups. From the pairwise comparison in the Mann–Whitney U test, significant differences were identified in each traffic sound group with the variation in the sound level. All the significant differences were found within the road traffic sound group (R) and high-speed train group (H). As for EDA, two significant differences were observed: (1) road traffic sound: a significant decrease with SPL increased from 55 dB to 65 dB ($\chi^2(1) = 2.227$, $p = 0.026$); (2) high-speed train sound: a significant increase with SPL increased from 45 dB to 65 dB ($\chi^2(1) = 2.320$, $p = 0.020$). As for HR, three significant differences were observed: (1) road traffic sound: a significant increase with SPL increased from 45 dB to 65 dB ($\chi^2(1) = 3.605$, $p = 0.002$); (2) road traffic sound: a significant increase with SPL increased from 55 dB to 65 dB ($\chi^2(1) = 2.807$, $p = 0.005$); (3) high speed train sound: a significant increase with SPL increased from 45 dB to 65 dB ($\chi^2(1) = 2.662$, $p = 0.008$).

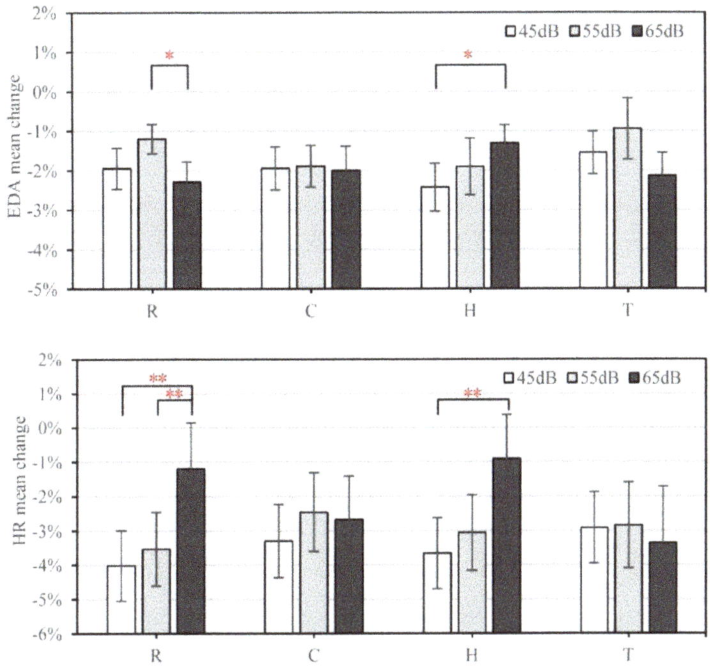

Figure 7. Interaction effect of sound level and sound type on EDA and HR. The vertical bar represents 95% confidence interval. * and ** represent significant differences in the Mann–Whitney U test at a 0.05 level and 0.01 level, respectively.

This result showed that the influence of the sound level on physiological responses depended on the sound type. In general, the relationship between the sound level and physiological parameters could be divided into two categories: (1) sound-level-sensitive group: road traffic sound (R) and high-speed train (H); (2) sound-level-insensitive group: conventional train (C) and tram (T). For the conventional train (C) and tram (T), the variation in sound level from 45 dB to 65 dB hardly affected the change in participant's physiological indicators. In contrast, considerable impacts on physiological responses were observed by the increase in sound level of road traffic sound (R) and high-speed train sound (H). This phenomenon was the same in both EDA and HR. As for HR, the tendency was agreed in the road traffic group (R) and tram group (T) that HR increased with the increase in sound level. However, the increase in sound level led to the increase in EDA under high-speed train sound (H) and the decrease in EDA under road traffic sound (R). It was also found that all the significant differences were caused by increasing the sound level to 65 dB, although the influence of the change between 45 dB and 55 dB was minimal. This result indicated that the subjects were more physiologically sensitive to the sound level when expose to high-level traffic sounds.

As for non-acoustic factors, the main effect of gender and exposure time was found to be influential on the participant's physiological responses. Regarding the effect size, gender was found to be the most influential factor for both EDA and HR ($\eta_p^2 = 0.03$). As shown in Figure 8, the changes in HR and EDA of male subjects were lower and higher than those of female subjects, respectively. Significant effects of exposure time on HR (F = 2.699, Sig. = 0.019) are exhibited in Figure 8, where no effect on EDA (F = 0.113, Sig. = 0.989) was found. With the increase in exposure time, HR significantly decreased by approximately 3% in the first 60 s, and gradually steadied after 80 s.

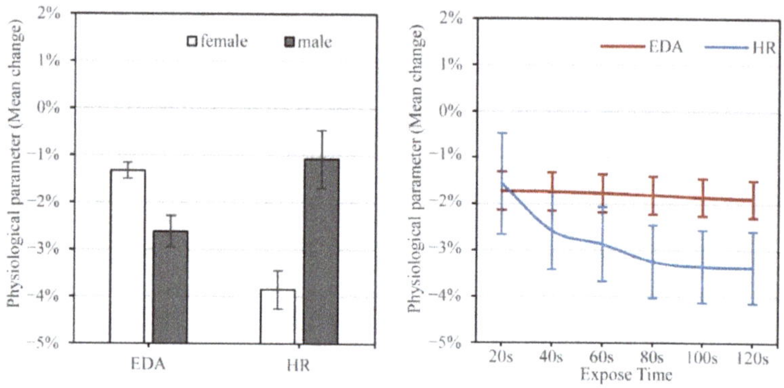

Figure 8. Effect of gender and exposure time on physiological responses to traffic sounds. The vertical bars represents 95% confidence intervals.

In addition, an interaction effect of gender and sound type was observed on EDA, as shown in Figure 9. In pairwise comparison by the Mann–Whitney U test within each gender group, three significant differences were observed: (1) the EDA of males under high-speed train sound was significantly lower than that under the tram sound ($\chi^2(1) = 2.323$, p = 0.020); (2) the EDA of female participants under high-speed train sound was significantly higher than that under the conventional train sound ($\chi^2(1) = 2.267$, $p = 0.023$); and (3) the EDA of female participants under high-speed train sound was significantly higher than that under the road traffic sound ($\chi^2(1) = 2.142$, $p = 0.032$). In general, exposure to high-speed train sound led to lower and higher EDA for male and female subjects, respectively. This result indicated that the impact of the high-speed train sound on EDA response was different from those of other sounds, which also agreed with the results in Figure 7.

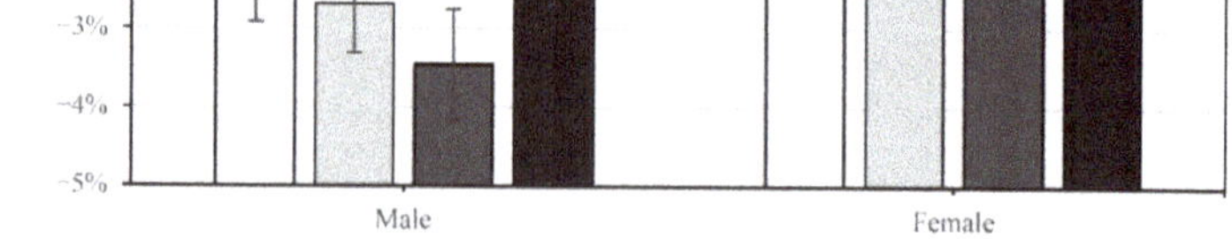

Figure 9. Interaction effect of gender and sound type on EDA. R, C, H, and T represent the road traffic, conventional train, high-speed train, and tram, respectively. The vertical bar represents 95% confidence interval. * represents significant difference in the Mann−Whitney U test at a 0.05 level.

3.3. Relationship between Psychological and Physiological Responses

A correlation analysis was applied to reveal the relationship between the psychological responses and physiological responses for the 12 experiment stimuli. As shown in Table 3, all four psychological responses were highly correlated with each other (r = 0.986~0.998, $p < 0.01$), which indicated that the psychological evaluations of the traffic sounds (AN, AR, and PL) had considerable influences on the evaluation of the overall acoustic environment (AC). It was also found that the HR was significantly correlated with all four psychological dimensions (r = 0.624~0.691, $p < 0.05$). A lower perceptual impact of sound (more comfort, less annoying, less arousal, and more pleasant) led to lower HR, as shown in Figure 10. However, the EDA was found to be independent of the psychological responses and the HR.

Table 3. Correlation analysis between psychological and physiological responses. * and ** represent significant correlations at 0.05 and 0.01 levels, respectively.

Pearson Correlation		Psychological				Physiological	
		AC	AN	AR	PL	EDA	HR
Psychological	AC	1.000					
	AN	−0.986 **	1.000				
	AR	−0.993 **	0.986 **	1.000			
	PL	0.992 **	−0.987 **	−0.998 **	1.000		
Physiological	EDA	−0.092	0.131	0.064	−0.062	1.000	
	HR	−0.689 *	0.624 *	0.691 *	−0.687 *	0.124	1.000

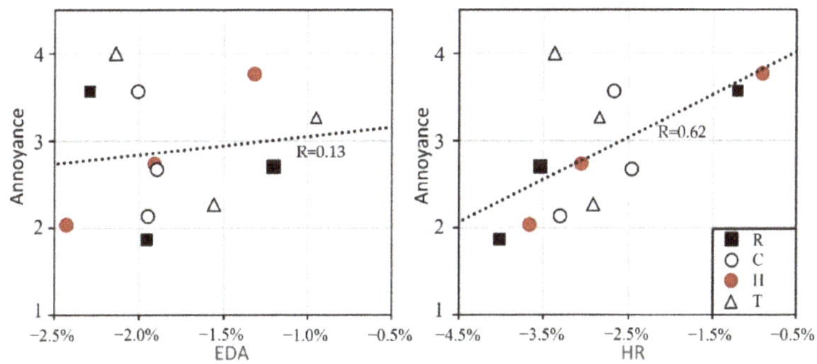

Figure 10. Relationship between psychological response (annoyance) and physiological responses. R, C, H, and T represent the road traffic, conventional train, high-speed train, and tram, respectively.

This result was based on the analysis of all four considered traffic sounds, which could be different in different traffic sound groups, as shown in Figure 10. Strong positive correlations between annoyance and physiological responses were observed in the high-speed train group (H). However, for the tram (T) and the conventional train group (C), the noise annoyance was independent of both the EDA and the HR. As for the road traffic sound (R), the noise annoyance was highly correlated with the HR, as shown in Figure 10. As discussed in Sections 3.1 and 3.2, the psychological responses were dominated by the sound level. Meanwhile, the physiological responses were also significantly affected by the interaction of the sound type and the sound level. Therefore, only weak correlations were found between the psychological responses and the physiological responses which varied in different sound groups.

4. Discussion

As for psychological evaluations, it was found that the traffic sounds brought considerable impacts on the acoustic environment in office space, which constantly increased with the increase in sound level. This result indicated that the control of traffic sound level was efficient for reducing the psychological impact at any sound level, which agreed with the dose–response curve established by the long-term field survey [59,60]. In addition, significant effects of the sound type on acoustic comfort and noise annoyance were also found, which were further revealed to be caused by the peak sound level. In this study, both the continuous sound (road traffic sound) and the intermittent sound (railway sound) were considered in the short-term sound exposure experiment. Under this condition, the peak sound level was more appropriate for evaluating the perceptual impact of sounds. This result agreed with the result in the literature in other indoor spaces [61]. However, if the analysis was conducted focusing on one single traffic sound source, for instance, the high-speed train sound, the equivalent sound level representing the average energy of the sound might be more appropriate because the temporal structures of sounds were similar. The results in this study indicated that for evaluating the perceptual impact of short-term traffic sound exposure, the peak sound level could be used as a common index for different traffic sounds, instead of setting an adjusting factor according to the sound type.

As for physiological responses, a complex interaction effect of acoustic factors and non-acoustic factors on physiological indices was found. In general, the sound level showed significant influences on both the EDA and HR. Regarding the road traffic sound, the increase in sound level led to higher HR and EDA levels, which agreed with most results in the existing literature [35,37,40].

However, different from the existing literature, the physiological impacts of three railway sounds were also examined and compared with road traffic sound in this study. The results showed that the influence of the sound level on physiological responses depended on the sound type. As for the conventional train and tram, the influence caused by sound level variation from 45 to 65 dB hardly affected the participant's HR and EDA. In contrast, the sound level was found to be influential in the road traffic group and the high-speed train group on HR and EDA. The results in this study revealed the importance of sound source recognition for evaluating the physiological impact of traffic sounds. It was also reported in the literature that the effect of other sound, for example, sound in hospitals [62], environmental sounds [23], and floor impact sounds [63], could be very different from continuous sounds. In the field of soundscape research, when multiple sound sources are considered, including artificial sounds, natural sounds, and music, it was suggested that the sound source was a dominant factor to determine the physiological effect of the acoustic environment [41,53,64]. Some other long-term exposure studies also found a difference between road traffic and railway sound, in which the road traffic sound and railway sound showed different impacts on other physiological parameters (blood pressure) [65].

Relative weak correlations between the psychological responses and physiological responses under the impact of traffic sounds were found in this study, which were also affected by the sound type. The HR was found to be significantly correlated with psychological evaluations of the sound, whereas lower HR was found under the exposure to less annoying, less arousing, and less unpleasant sounds. Similar results were also reported in relevant soundscape studies, in which pleasantness and eventfulness were found to be correlated with the HR and EDA [25,66]. Although significant associations were found, the results in this study showed that the physiological responses, which indicated the potential long-term health effect, could not be fully predicted by the self-reported psychological responses. Therefore, to comprehensively investigate the traffic sound impact, the collection of physiological responses might be necessary.

In general, the results in this study showed that the psychophysiological effects of traffic sounds on people were different. One main reason for this phenomenon is the difference in temporal characteristics. As the spectrogram shows in Figure 2, the major difference between road traffic sound and railway sounds was the duration time. The results in Section 3 further proved that the differences in duration time led to differences in psychological responses. As for the physiological responses, results in this study also found that there were significant differences between the continuous traffic sound (road traffic) and the intermittent sounds (railway sounds). However, it should be noted that some of the results could not be fully explained by the temporal characteristics. In Section 3, the high-speed train sound was found to have different physiological effects on people when compared with other railway sounds. However, the duration of high-speed train sound was similar to that of the tram sound. In addition to temporal differences, the spectral differences between different traffic sounds were also observed in this study. As shown in Figure 2, there were more high-frequency components in high-speed train sounds than in other railway sounds. Moreover, there were significant concentrations of magnitudes in the beginning and the end of the stimuli in the conventional train and tram sounds. The combination of spectral and temporal characteristics made the participants be able to recognize the traffic sound type, which could not be simply described by the sound level and duration time.

Regarding the sound control treatments, the results in this study revealed that the decrease in the sound level did not necessarily lead to the reduction in the impact from traffic sounds, because the physiological responses for some traffic sounds (conventional train and tram) were not sensitive to the sound level. Therefore, different strategies should be especially designed according to the sound type. As for the road traffic sound and the high-speed train sound, the sound control treatments, for instance, sound barrier, could be efficient both psychologically and physiologically. However, for conventional train and tram, such treatments hardly reduced the sound impact on the residents' physiological state. It has been found that the presence of natural sounds, including bird singing and water sound, could improve perceptual evaluations of the acoustic environment. Moreover, it was suggested that in the mixed soundscape, the physiological responses were correlated with the pleasantness of the overall acoustic environment [25]. A positive physiological effect of birdsong mixed with road traffic sound was reported in [38]. Therefore, introducing pleasant natural sound elements might be a potential solution for masking the physiological impacts of conventional train and tram sound.

This study also has some limitations. First, silence was chosen as the baseline condition to investigate the fundamental effect of traffic sounds on people in offices. Therefore, the scenario considered in this study was more related to offices in which traffic sounds are the dominant sound sources, including offices very close to traffic lines and quiet single working spaces (for instance, home working spaces). However, there are inevitable other sound sources in office spaces, which also have significant impacts on people [6]. As for open-plan offices, conversation sounds were reported to be the most influential sound source on the perception of acoustic quality and work-related quality [2]. Therefore, in offices with multiple sound sources, the effect of traffic sounds might be different. Future studies need to be conducted to investigate the effect of combined sounds on people in such office spaces. Second, the experimental stimuli in this study were collected adjacent to the traffic lines to avoid accidental environmental sounds. However, there were inevitable differences between the recorded traffic sounds and the sounds received inside the offices because the reflections and absorptions were not considered. In future studies, the interaction effect of traffic sound characteristics and indoor acoustic quality could be further investigated. Third, the sound level equalization of experimental stimuli was carried out without using a head and torso simulator, which could lead to errors in the traffic sound levels.

5. Conclusions

A laboratory experiment on the psychophysiological responses to traffic sounds was conducted in this study. MANOVA was applied to identify the influential factor that had significant effects on the psychophysiological responses. The following results were obtained:

(1) The traffic sounds brought considerable impacts on the psychophysiological responses of the acoustic environment in office space, which depended on the sound type. Without considering the interaction with other indoor noises, all traffic sounds were found to have adverse psychological effects on the overall acoustic environment. As

for the physiological responses, the effect of sound type was found to interact with the sound level and non-acoustic factors (gender);

(2) The sound level was found to be the most influential factor on the psychophysiological responses. The negative effects of traffic sounds on psychological responses were found to constantly increase with the increase in the sound level. The peak sound level showed better performance than the equivalent sound level in evaluating the perceptual impact of short-term sound exposure. The relationship between sound level and physiological parameters varied among different sound groups. The variation in sound level hardly affected the participants' HR and EDA when exposed to the conventional train and tram sound. In contrast, HR and EDA were significantly affected by the levels of road traffic sounds and high-speed train sounds;

(3) Non-acoustic factors were found to be influential on the physiological responses. The HR was found to decrease with the increase in exposure time. Gender was found to be an important factor of the physiological parameters, which also had an interaction effect with the noise level;

(4) Relatively weak correlations between the psychological evaluations and HR were found, whereas the relationship between the psychological attributes and EDA was found to be significantly affected by the sound type.

Although the current study was based on a laboratory experiment, the results presented in this study may serve as a supplementary tool for architects, planners, and city managers to estimate not only the impact of traffic sounds on the urban environment, but also the effectiveness of noise treatments. Future research will focus on how to reduce the impact of traffic sounds, including (a) the effect of sound barriers on the psychophysiological responses when exposed to traffic sounds; (b) effectiveness of soundscape treatments on masking traffic sounds, for example, introducing natural sounds to reduce the impact brought by traffic sounds.

Author Contributions: Conceptualization, B.Y.; methodology, B.Y., J.B. and L.W.; formal analysis, B.Y. and Y.C.; investigation, J.B., and L.W.; data curation, B.Y.; writing—original draft preparation, B.Y.; writing—review and editing, B.Y.; supervision, B.Y.; project administration, B.Y.; funding acquisition, B.Y. All authors have read and agreed to the published version of the manuscript.

Funding: This research was funded by the National Natural Science Foundation of China (Project No. 51808030).

Institutional Review Board Statement: The study was conducted according to the guidelines of the Declaration of Helsinki, and approved by the Institutional Review Board of Beijing Jiaotong University, School of architecture and design.

Informed Consent Statement: Informed consent was obtained from all subjects involved in the study.

Acknowledgments: The authors wish to thank Wu Wei and Li Junjie, for their help with the VR software.

Conflicts of Interest: The authors declare no conflict of interest.

References

1. Yang, W.; Krishnan, S. Combining temporal features by local binary pattern for acoustic scene classification. *IEEE/ACM Trans. Audio Speech Lang. Process.* **2017**, *25*, 1315–1321. [CrossRef]
2. Jo, H.I.; Jeon, J.Y. Influence of indoor soundscape perception based on audiovisual contents on work-related quality with preference and perceived productivity in open-plan offices. *Build. Environ.* 2021; 108598, *in press*. [CrossRef]
3. Meng, Q.; An, Y.; Yang, D. Effects of acoustic environment on design work performance based on multitask visual cognitive performance in office space. *Build. Environ.* **2021**, *205*, 108296. [CrossRef]
4. Landström, U. Noise and fatigue in working environments. *Environ. Int.* **1990**, *16*, 471–476. [CrossRef]
5. Zhang, M.; Kang, J.; Jiao, F. A social survey on the noise impact in open-plan working environments in China. *Sci. Total Environ.* **2012**, *438*, 517–526. [CrossRef] [PubMed]
6. Torresin, S.; Albatici, R.; Aletta, F.; Babich, F.; Oberman, T.; Stawinoga, A.E.; Kang, J. Indoor soundscapes at home during the COVID-19 lockdown in London—Part II: A structural equation model for comfort, content, and well-being. *Appl. Acoust.* **2022**, *185*, 108379. [CrossRef]

7. Saadu, A.A.; Onyeonwu, R.O.; Ayorinde, E.O.; Ogisi, F.O. Road traffic noise survey and analysis of some major urban centers in Nigeria. *Noise Control Eng. J.* **1998**, *46*, 146–158. [CrossRef]
8. Abo-Qudais, S.; Abu-Qdais, H. Perceptions and attitudes of individuals exposed to traffic noise in working places. *Build. Environ.* **2005**, *40*, 778–787. [CrossRef]
9. Kotzeva, M.M.; Brandmüller, T. *Urban Europe: Statistics on Cities, Towns and Suburbs*; 2016 edition; Publications office of the European Union: Luxembourg, 2017; ISBN 9279601407.
10. Chen, J. Rapid urbanization in China: A real challenge to soil protection and food security. *Catena* **2007**, *69*, 1–15. [CrossRef]
11. Jarosińska, D.; Héroux, M.È.; Wilkhu, P.; Creswick, J.; Verbeek, J.; Wothge, J.; Paunović, E. Development of the WHO environmental noise guidelines for the european region: An introduction. *Int. J. Environ. Res. Public Health* **2018**, *15*, 813. [CrossRef]
12. Muzet, A. Environmental noise, sleep and health. *Sleep Med. Rev.* **2007**, *11*, 135–142. [CrossRef]
13. Ndrepepa, A.; Twardella, D. Relationship between noise annoyance from road traffic noise and cardiovascular diseases: A meta-analysis. *Noise Health* **2011**, *13*, 251. [PubMed]
14. Griffiths, I.D.; Langdon, F.J. Subjective response to road traffic noise. *J. Sound Vib.* **1968**, *8*, 16–32. [CrossRef]
15. Fields, J.M.; Walker, J.G. Comparing the relationships between noise level and annoyance in different surveys: A railway noise vs. aircraft and road traffic comparison. *J. Sound Vib.* **1982**, *81*, 51–80. [CrossRef]
16. Guski, R.; Schreckenberg, D.; Schuemer, R. WHO environmental noise guidelines for the European region: A systematic review on environmental noise and annoyance. *Int. J. Environ. Res. Public Health* **2017**, *14*, 1539. [CrossRef]
17. Ouis, D. Annoyance from road traffic noise: A review. *J. Environ. Psychol.* **2001**, *21*, 101–120. [CrossRef]
18. Dratva, J.; Zemp, E.; Dietrich, D.F.; Bridevaux, P.O.; Rochat, T.; Schindler, C.; Gerbase, M.W. Impact of road traffic noise annoyance on health-related quality of life: Results from a population-based study. *Qual. Life Res.* **2010**, *19*, 37–46. [CrossRef] [PubMed]
19. Puyana Romero, V.; Maffei, L.; Brambilla, G.; Ciaburro, G. Acoustic, visual and spatial indicators for the description of the soundscape of water front areas with and without road traffic flow. *Int. J. Environ. Res. Public Health* **2016**, *13*, 934. [CrossRef]
20. Puyana Romero, V.; Maffei, L.; Brambilla, G.; Ciaburro, G. Modelling the soundscape quality of urban waterfronts by artificial neural networks. *Appl. Acoust.* **2016**, *111*, 121–128. [CrossRef]
21. Kang, J.; Zhang, M. Semantic differential analysis of the soundscape in urban open public spaces. *Build. Environ.* **2010**, *45*, 150–157. [CrossRef]
22. Yu, B.; Kang, J.; Ma, H. Development of indicators for the soundscape in urban shopping streets. *Acta Acust. United Acust.* **2016**, *102*, 462–473. [CrossRef]
23. Gomez, P.; Danuser, B. Affective and physiological responses to environmental noises and music. *Int. J. Psychophysiol.* **2004**, *53*, 91–103. [CrossRef]
24. Hall, D.A.; Irwin, A.; Edmondson-Jones, M.; Phillips, S.; Poxon, J.E.W. An exploratory evaluation of perceptual, psychoacoustic and acoustical properties of urban soundscapes. *Appl. Acoust.* **2013**, *74*, 248–254. [CrossRef]
25. Hume, K.; Ahtamad, M. Physiological responses to and subjective estimates of soundscape elements. *Appl. Acoust.* **2013**, *74*, 275–281. [CrossRef]
26. Yang, W.; Kang, J. Acoustic comfort evaluation in urban open public spaces. *Appl. Acoust.* **2005**, *66*, 211–229. [CrossRef]
27. Kang, J.; Meng, Q.; Jin, H. Effects of individual sound sources on the subjective loudness and acoustic comfort in underground shopping streets. *Sci. Total Environ.* **2012**, *435–436*, 80–89. [CrossRef] [PubMed]
28. Rey Gozalo, G.; Trujillo Carmona, J.; Barrigón Morillas, J.M.; Vílchez-Gómez, R.; Gómez Escobar, V. Relationship between objective acoustic indices and subjective assessments for the quality of soundscapes. *Appl. Acoust.* **2015**, *97*, 1–10. [CrossRef]
29. Torresin, S.; Albatici, R.; Aletta, F.; Babich, F.; Oberman, T.; Siboni, S.; Kang, J. Indoor soundscape assessment: A principal components model of acoustic perception in residential buildings. *Build. Environ.* **2020**, *182*, 107152. [CrossRef]
30. Brown, A.L.; van Kamp, I. WHO environmental noise guidelines for the European region: A systematic review of transport noise interventions and their impacts on health. *Int. J. Environ. Res. Public Health* **2017**, *14*, 873. [CrossRef]
31. Bhatia, P.; Muhar, I. Noise sensitivity and mental efficiency. *Psychol. Int. J. Psychol. Orient* **1988**, *31*, 163–169.
32. Vera, M.N.; Vila, J.; Godoy, J.F. Physiological and subjective effects of traffic noise: The role of negative self-statements. *Int. J. Psychophysiol.* **1992**, *12*, 267–279. [CrossRef]
33. Clark, C.R.; Turpin, G.; Jenkins, L.M.; Tarnopolsky, A. Sensitivity to noise on a community sample: II. Measurement of psychophysiological indices. *Psychol. Med.* **1985**, *15*, 255–263. [CrossRef]
34. Basner, M.; Samel, A.; Elmenhorst, E.M.; Maab, H.; Müller, U.; Quehl, J.; Vejvoda, M. Single and combined effects of air, road and rail traffic noise on sleep. In Proceedings of the Institute of Noise Control Engineering of the USA—35th International Congress and Exposition on Noise Control Engineering (INTER-NOISE), Honolulu, Hawaii, 3–6 December 2006; Volume 7, pp. 4629–4637.
35. Raggam, R.B.; Cik, M.; Höldrich, R.R.; Fallast, K.; Gallasch, E.; Fend, M.; Lackner, A.; Marth, E. Personal noise ranking of road traffic: Subjective estimation versus physiological parameters under laboratory conditions. *Int. J. Hyg. Environ. Health* **2007**, *210*, 97–105. [CrossRef] [PubMed]
36. Lee, P.J.; Park, S.H.; Jeong, J.H.; Choung, T.; Kim, K.Y. Association between transportation noise and blood pressure in adults living in multi-storey residential buildings. *Environ. Int.* **2019**, *132*, 105101. [CrossRef]
37. Li, Z.; Kang, J.; Ba, M. Influence of distance from traffic sounds on physiological indicators and subjective evaluation. *Transp. Res. Part D Transp. Environ.* **2020**, *87*, 102538. [CrossRef]

38. Suko, Y.; Saito, K.; Takayama, N.; Sakuma, T.; Warisawa, S. Effect of faint road traffic noise mixed in birdsong on the perceived restorativeness and listeners' physiological response: An exploratory study. *Int. J. Environ. Res. Public Health* **2019**, *16*, 4985. [CrossRef]
39. Erfanian, M.; Mitchell, A.J.; Kang, J.; Aletta, F. The psychophysiological implications of soundscape: A systematic review of empirical literature and a research agenda. *Int. J. Environ. Res. Public Health* **2019**, *16*, 3533. [CrossRef] [PubMed]
40. Li, Z.; Ba, M.; Kang, J. Physiological indicators and subjective restorativeness with audio-visual interactions in urban soundscapes. *Sustain. Cities Soc.* **2021**, *75*, 103360. [CrossRef]
41. Shu, S.; Ma, H. Restorative effects of urban park soundscapes on children's psychophysiological stress. *Appl. Acoust.* **2020**, *164*, 107293. [CrossRef]
42. Park, S.H.; Lee, P.J.; Jeong, J.H. Effects of noise sensitivity on psychophysiological responses to building noise. *Build. Environ.* **2018**, *136*, 302–311. [CrossRef]
43. Pathak, V.; Tripathi, B.D.; Mishra, V. kumar Evaluation of traffic noise pollution and attitudes of exposed individuals in working place. *Atmos. Environ.* **2008**, *42*, 3892–3898. [CrossRef]
44. Alimohammadi, I.; Nassiri, P.; Azkhosh, M.; Hoseini, M. Factors affecting road traffic noise annoyance among white-collar employees working in Tehran. *Iran. J. Environ. Heal. Sci. Eng.* **2010**, *7*, 25–34.
45. Ma, H.; Shu, S. An experimental study: The restorative effect of soundscape elements in a simulated open-plan office. *Acta Acust. United Acust.* **2018**, *104*, 106–115. [CrossRef]
46. Bourikas, L.; Gauthier, S.; En, N.K.S.; Xiong, P. Effect of thermal, acoustic and air quality perception interactions on the comfort and satisfaction of people in office buildings. *Energies* **2021**, *14*, 333. [CrossRef]
47. Hygge, S. Classroom experiments on the effects of different noise sources and sound levels on long-term recall and recognition in children. *Appl. Cogn. Psychol.* **2003**, *17*, 895–914. [CrossRef]
48. Cik, M.; Lienhart, M.; Fallast, K.; Marth, E.; Freidl, W.; Niederl, F. Psychoacoustic indicators of road and rail traffic noise, subjective perception and psychological and physiological parameters. In Proceedings of the INTER-NOISE 2016—45th International Congress and Exposition on Noise Control Engineering: Towards a Quieter Future, Hamburg, Germany, 21–24 August 2016; pp. 1967–1976.
49. Yano, T.; Sato, T.; Björkman, M.; Rylander, R. Comparison of community response to road traffic noise in Japan and Sweden—Part II: Path analysis. *J. Sound Vib.* **2002**, *250*, 169–174. [CrossRef]
50. Tetsuya, H.; Yano, T.; Murakami, Y. Annoyance due to railway noise before and after the opening of the Kyushu Shinkansen Line. *Appl. Acoust.* **2017**, *115*, 173–180. [CrossRef]
51. Kuwano, S.; Namba, S.; Okamoto, T. Psychological evaluation of sound environment in a compartment of a high-speed train. *J. Sound Vib.* **2004**, *277*, 491–500. [CrossRef]
52. Trollé, A.; Marquis-Favre, C.; Klein, A. Short-term annoyance due to tramway noise: Determination of an acoustical indicator of annoyance via multilevel regression analysis. *Acta Acust. United Acust.* **2014**, *100*, 34–45. [CrossRef]
53. Lee, Y.; Nelson, E.C.; Flynn, M.J.; Jackman, J.S. Exploring soundscaping options for the cognitive environment in an open-plan office. *Build. Acoust.* **2020**, *27*, 185–202. [CrossRef]
54. Brink, M.; Schreckenberg, D.; Vienneau, D.; Cajochen, C.; Wunderli, J.M.; Probst-Hensch, N.; Röösli, M. Effects of scale, question location, order of response alternatives, and season on self-reported noise annoyance using icben scales: A field experiment. *Int. J. Environ. Res. Public Health* **2016**, *13*, 1163. [CrossRef] [PubMed]
55. McManis, M.H.; Bradley, M.M.; Berg, W.K.; Cuthbert, B.N.; Lang, P.J. Emotional reactions in children: Verbal, physiological, and behavioral responses to affective pictures. *Psychophysiology* **2001**, *38*, 222–231. [CrossRef] [PubMed]
56. Bradley, M.M.; Lang, P.J. Measuring emotion: The self-assessment manikin and the semantic differential. *J. Behav. Ther. Exp. Psychiatry* **1994**, *25*, 49–59. [CrossRef]
57. Axelsson, Ö.; Nilsson, M.E.; Berglund, B. A principal components model of soundscape perception. *J. Acoust. Soc. Am.* **2010**, *128*, 2836–2846. [CrossRef] [PubMed]
58. Schmider, E.; Ziegler, M.; Danay, E.; Beyer, L.; Bühner, M. Is It Really Robust?: Reinvestigating the robustness of ANOVA against violations of the normal distribution assumption. *Methodology* **2010**, *6*, 147–151. [CrossRef]
59. Morihara, T.; Sato, T.; Yano, T. Comparison of dose-response relationships between railway and road traffic noises: The moderating effect of distance. *J. Sound Vib.* **2004**, *277*, 559–565. [CrossRef]
60. Fidell, S.; Mestre, V.; Schomer, P.; Berry, B.; Gjestland, T.; Vallet, M.; Reid, T. A first-principles model for estimating the prevalence of annoyance with aircraft noise exposure. *J. Acoust. Soc. Am.* **2011**, *130*, 791–806. [CrossRef] [PubMed]
61. Di, G.Q.; Lin, Q.L.; Li, Z.G.; Kang, J. Annoyance and activity disturbance induced by high-speed railway and conventional railway noise: A contrastive case study. *Environ. Health* **2014**, *13*, 12. [CrossRef]
62. Hsu, S.M.; Ko, W.J.; Liao, W.C.; Huang, S.J.; Chen, R.J.; Li, C.Y.; Hwang, S.L. Associations of exposure to noise with physiological and psychological outcomes among post-cardiac surgery patients in ICUs. *Clinics* **2010**, *65*, 985–989. [CrossRef]
63. Park, S.H.; Lee, P.J. Effects of floor impact noise on psychophysiological responses. *Build. Environ.* **2017**, *116*, 173–181. [CrossRef]
64. Lee, S.; Hwang, S. Physiological response by construction noise according to temporal characteristics. In Proceedings of the 26th International Congress on Sound and Vibration (ICSV26), Montreal, QC, Canada, 7–11 July 2019.

65. Sørensen, M.; Hvidberg, M.; Hoffmann, B.; Andersen, Z.J.; Nordsborg, R.B.; Lillelund, K.G.; Jakobsen, J.; Tjønneland, A.; Overvad, K.; Raaschou-Nielsen, O. Exposure to road traffic and railway noise and associations with blood pressure and self-reported hypertension: A cohort study. *Environ. Health* **2011**, *10*, 92. [CrossRef]
66. Medvedev, O.; Shepherd, D.; Hautus, M.J. The restorative potential of soundscapes: A physiological investigation. *Appl. Acoust.* **2015**, *96*, 20–26. [CrossRef]

International Journal of
Environmental Research and Public Health

MDPI

Article

Does Environmental Regulation Promote Environmental Innovation? An Empirical Study of Cities in China

Dezhong Duan * and Qifan Xia

Institute for Global Innovation and Development, East China Normal University, Shanghai 200062, China; 51183902025@stu.ecnu.edu.cn
* Correspondence: dzduan@geo.ecnu.edu.cn

Abstract: Promoting environmental innovation through environmental regulation is a key measure for cities to reduce environmental pressure; however, the role of environmental regulation in environmental innovation is controversial. This study used the number of environmental patent applications to measure urban environmental innovation and analyzed the role of urban environmental regulation on urban environmental innovation with the help of the spatial Durbin model (SDM). The results showed that: (1) From 2007 to 2017, the number of environmental patent applications in China has grown rapidly, and technologies related to buildings dominated the development of China's environmental innovation. (2) Although the number of cities participating in environmental innovation was increasing, China's environmental innovation activities were highly concentrated in a few cities (Beijing, Shenzhen, and Shanghai), showing significant spatial correlation and spatial agglomeration characteristics. (3) Urban environmental regulation had a positive U-shaped relationship with urban environmental innovation capability, which was consistent with what the Porter hypothesis advocates.

Keywords: environmental regulation; environmental innovation; environmental patent; spatial Durbin model; China cities

Citation: Duan, D.; Xia, Q. Does Environmental Regulation Promote Environmental Innovation? An Empirical Study of Cities in China. *Int. J. Environ. Res. Public Health* **2022**, *19*, 139. https://doi.org/10.3390/ijerph19010139

Academic Editors: Roberto Alonso González Lezcano, Francesco Nocera and Rosa Giuseppina Caponetto

Received: 12 November 2021
Accepted: 21 December 2021
Published: 23 December 2021

1. Introduction

The urban environment is a major contributor to climate change, mainly due to its high dependence on natural resources [1]; therefore, cities can be key players in combating climate change by addressing environmental sustainability actions (e.g., formulating pollution discharge standards, collecting pollution taxes, granting emission reduction subsidies, issuing pollution permits, etc.) to encourage enterprises to carry out environmental innovation in order to reduce emissions [2]. China has ushered in rapid urbanization for nearly 40 years under the "competition for growth" economic development mode since reform and opening-up; however, it is also facing increasingly severe urban environment pressures [3]. It is undeniable that the Chinese government attaches increasing importance to environmental protection, and increasingly strict environmental regulations are constantly being implemented in China [4].

The realization of strong decoupling between urban economic growth and environmental degradation crucially depends on technological improvements, which is environmental innovation. Environmental innovation is a core topic in research fields, such as environmental economics, innovation economics, and innovation management, emphasizing innovative behavior based on environmental protection or reducing environmental damage. The academic community has carried out a great deal of research on environmental innovation, including the assessment of environmental innovation ability, the determinants of environmental innovation, the economic and environmental effects of environmental innovation, environmental innovation policy design, etc. Since environmental innovation puts more emphasis on production and output [5,6], research on environmental innovation at the enterprise level has become the mainstream [7]. Similarly, environmental innovation is generally considered to be a response of enterprises to government environmental regulations. However, the academic circle has not yet formed a conclusion regarding the relationship between environmental regulation and environmental innovation, and rather has formed a binary opposition between two theories, namely the "Porter hypothesis" [8] and the "repression hypothesis" [9]. In addition, many scholars hold a wait-and-see attitude, indicating that the relationship between the two needs more verification [10].

Recently, with the promotion of regional innovation system theory [11], the relationship between environmental regulation and environmental innovation (green innovation efficiency, green development efficiency) has become a hot topic in environmental economic geography, regional economics, urban economics, innovation geography, and other fields [12,13]. Due to the large regional differences and the local competition brought by decentralization, China is the best-case field for this hot research topic. Many studies have revealed the positive correlation between environmental regulations and environmental innovation at the regional level in China [14]; however, there are some studies that have found a non-linear relationship between China's urban environmental regulation and urban environmental innovation, showing a U-shaped pattern. That is, the effect of environmental regulation on environmental innovation shows the characteristics of restraint in the short term and promotion in the long term [13]. In addition, some scholars believe that the impact of China's environmental regulation on environmental innovations presents significant spatial heterogeneity; that is, the relationship between the two in eastern China is significantly positive, while the relationship between the two in the central and western regions needs more discussion [15].

Looking at the existing regional or city-level related research, it is not difficult to find that the relationship between environmental regulation and environmental innovation still needs to be tested with more empirical research. One of the main reasons for the differences in existing research results is that scholars have used different research methods in measuring regional or urban environmental innovation capabilities. Some use the input–output analysis method to measure the efficiency of regional environmental innovation [14], some use the number of environmental patent applications (not completely covering all patent categories) to measure the environmental innovation capability [15], and others use alternative indicators to measure regional environmental innovation capability [16].

The purpose of this paper is to explore the relations between environmental regulation and environmental innovation in China from a city-level perspective. The main contributions are twofold. First, this paper has enriched the literature that uses patent data to measure urban environmental innovation. Based on the contribution of Haščič and Migotto [17], we analyzed the developments of urban environmental innovation in China from 2007 to 2017 by identifying the environment-related patents. Second, this paper has also enriched the literature on the relationships between environmental regulation and environmental innovation. Based on the spatial econometric model, we explored the relationship between urban environmental regulation and environmental innovation in China.

The remainder of the article is organized as follows. Section 2 provides a short literature review of the current research on the relationship between environmental regulations and environmental innovation. Section 3 introduces the data and methodology used in this paper. Section 4 presents the empirical results, and Section 5 discusses our findings and concludes this paper.

2. Theoretical Background

Exploring the relations between environmental regulation and environmental innovation is the core issue of environmental economics and other related disciplines. Environmental economics regards environmental regulation as a policy tool for internalizing the external costs of enterprises, focusing on the impact of environmental regulation on enterprises and the impact of different policy tools on enterprise innovation behavior. However, what kind of impact will environmental regulation have on environmental innovation? This has always been a controversial and interesting topic. The mainstream view agrees that environmental regulation can induce innovation and bring about innovation compensation and competitive advantage; this is the "Porter Hypothesis" [9], which states that market-oriented policy instruments (such as pollution taxes, emission reduction subsidies, and pollution permits) can stimulate enterprises to carry out environmental innovation more than command-and-control regulations (such as pollution standards, emission quotas, etc.) [18].

However, there are also views that strict environmental regulations may have a negative impact on enterprises, and will not only increase the production cost of the enterprise and the survival risk of the enterprise, but also bring about the transfer of pollutants. For example, some companies experienced a severe decline in financial performance after implementing environmental innovation and did not achieve Porter's "win-win" situation [19]. Some studies also found that environmental regulation can lead to the decline of enterprise productivity, even producing negative spillover effects on the national economy. Barbera and McConnell [20] found that the main reason for the decline in the performance of steel, nonferrous metals, paper, chemical, and non-metallic mineral products industries in the United States was the increase in pollution control investment caused by environmental regulation. Moreover, environmental regulations will have different effects on enterprises of different sizes and types. Numerous studies have shown that environmental innovation practices vary greatly between companies. Large companies, especially multinational companies, are pioneers and leaders in environmental innovation, while Small and Medium Enterprises (SMEs) have shown more uncertainty in environmental innovation [21,22]. In addition, according to the research of Ouyang et al. (2020) concerning China, environmental supervision is not conducive to technological innovation of state-owned enterprises due to the high cost of energy conservation and emission reduction, and industries with higher market competition and human capital investment tend to have stronger environmental innovation capabilities. It was also found that the scale of the regional economy also has a significant impact on the regional environmental innovation capacity [3,23,24].

Contrary to the above two opposing views, some scholars hold that the impact of environmental regulation on green technology innovation is uncertain. For example, Mody [25] found that there was no obvious correlation between the increased emission reduction expenditure of environmental regulation and environmental innovation. Jaffe and Palmer's research [26] on US manufacturing showed that the impact of environmental regulation on environmental innovation is not significant. In summary, the relations between environmental regulation and environmental innovation have aroused controversy in academia. Research conclusions are often different due to differences in research cases (industry differences, scale differences, type differences, etc.) and measurement methods (measures of environmental regulation and measures of environmental innovation). Environmental innovation is widely believed to be the strategic adjustment of enterprise development in response to environmental regulation to gain competitive advantages; thus, the relations between environmental regulation and environmental innovation at the enterprise level have always been the focus of attention [27], while research on the relationship between environmental regulation and environmental innovation at the city level is still rare.

Based on the perspective of urban space in China, this study first measured the intensity of urban environmental regulation and urban environmental innovation capability in China, and then used a spatial econometric model to explore the relationship between environmental regulation and urban environmental innovation ability, to make up for the spatial factors that have not been fully considered in previous studies.

3. Data and Methods

3.1. Measuring Environmental Regulation

Measuring the intensity of environmental regulation is the first step to test the relationship between environmental regulation and environmental innovation. Existing literature has launched an active attempt to quantify environmental regulations, which can be roughly divided into four categories.

The first is to use environmental governance expenditures to measure the intensity of environmental regulations. Related indicators include the government investment in pollution control and other incentive policies [28], pollutant emission reduction expenditure, and other regulatory measures [29]. The second is measurement of the emission level of pollutants or treatment level, such as the scale of pollutant emissions, pollutant treatment rate, domestic sewage treatment rate, etc. The third measurement method is based on the input–output analysis framework to build an environmental regulation intensity evaluation system. For example, Sauter [30] believed that environmental regulation is an input–output process, and the measurement of environmental regulation should include three dimensions: input, process, and result. The last method is to use alternative indicators to measure environmental regulation [31]. To avoid the complexity of the measurement of environmental regulation indicators, some studies have used alternative indicators to express the degree of environmental regulation, such as the lead content in gasoline [32] and the income level of residents [33].

Comparing the four methods mentioned above, it seems that the comprehensive construction of an environmental regulation evaluation system is a very reasonable description method; however, due to the limitations of data availability and index screening, it is difficult to apply to city-level research. Moreover, it is controversial to use alternative indicators to measure environmental regulation. For example, the income of residents in developed countries may reflect the high requirements for environmental protection, while in many developing countries, due to the limitation of the development stage, most areas may be at the left end of the environmental Kuznets curve; that is, a higher per capita GDP may correspond to a lower intensity of environmental regulation. Placing the research in the context of China, when the lower limit of the research scale is cities rather than provinces, the data for pollutant emission reduction expenditure investment is almost impossible to obtain; however, the pollutant emission level has official statistics.

According to past experiences [4], this paper constructed a comprehensive index of environmental regulation intensity in China city systems based on three indicators: the comprehensive utilization rate of industrial solid waste, domestic sewage treatment rate, and domestic waste harmless treatment rate. The relevant data are from the China City Statistical Yearbook and the specific methods are as follows: firstly, the extreme value method was used to standardize the treatment rate of the three pollutants (Equation (1)); second, considering the differences in the discharge of pollutants in each city, if a city had a large discharge of pollutants, the same treatment rate for such pollutants may mean stricter environmental regulations, so a greater weight was assigned; third, the weighted average of the treatment rates of three pollutants in a city was taken as the intensity of the city's environmental regulations (Equation (2)).

$$S\_Pr^{g}_{i,t} = \left[Pr^{g}_{i,t} - \min\left(Pr^{g}_{t}\right)\right] / \left[\max\left(Pr^{g}_{t}\right) - \min\left(Pr^{g}_{t}\right)\right] \tag{1}$$

In the above formula, $S\_Pr^{g}_{i,t}$ and $Pr^{g}_{i,t}$ are the standard and original value of the treatment rate of pollutant g in city i at time t, respectively. $\max\left(Pr^{g}_{t}\right)$ and $\min\left(Pr^{g}_{t}\right)$ are the maximum value and minimum value, respectively, of the original values of the treatment rates of pollutant g in China as a whole.

$$Environ\_Regu_{i,t} = \left[\sum_{g=1}^{3}\left(\frac{P^{g}_{i,t}}{P^{g}_{t}}\right) * S\_Pr^{g}_{i,t}\right] / 3 \tag{2}$$

In Equation (2), $Environ\_Regu_{i,t}$ is the comprehensive index of environmental regulation intensity in city i at time t. Pr^{g}_{t} is the emission of pollutant g in China as a whole.

3.2. Measuring Environmental Innovation

Given its multi and transdisciplinary features, there are many concepts related to environmental innovation, such as green innovation, eco innovation, and sustainable innovation [34]. Due to this unclear definition, these concepts are usually interchangeable [35]. However, in terms of measurement, studies to date have employed different perspectives and methods. Existing environmental innovation measurements also can be classified into four categories.

The first is the overall measurement of environmental innovation by constructing an evaluation system covering as many indicators as possible [36,37]. The second is to focus on environmental innovation input, usually measured by environmental R&D investment [38]. The third is to focus on environmental innovation output, usually measured by environmental patents [17,39]. Due to their quantifiable and available features, patents, especially those related to the environment, are widely used to measure environmental innovation [40,41]. The fourth is to focus on the process of environmental innovation, usually using environmental innovation efficiency as a proxy for environmental innovation [42–44]. Existing research has completed the measurement of the environmental innovation efficiency of some enterprises (large enterprises, SMEs, or specific enterprises), cities, regions, and countries [42].

Certainly, there are other methods for measuring environmental innovation; however, they are relatively rare and impractical. For example, determining green products based on industry and commodity classification would first require identification of the industry or commodity classes that represent environmental. In this paper, we used environmental patents to measure China's environmental innovation at the city level due to their higher availability and wider coverage when compared to environmental R&D investment, green products, and other indicators.

Through referencing the identification strategies of environment-related technologies (patents) proposed by Haščič and Migotto [17], this study obtained environmental patent application data from the China Wanfang patent database (http://g.wanfangdata.com.cn/index.html, accessed on 1 December 2021). The environment-related technologies (see Table A1 in Appendix A) in this paper include energy technology (climate change mitigation technologies, related energy generation, transmission of distribution etc.), greenhouse gas treatment technology (capture, storage, sequestration, or disposal of greenhouse gases), transportation technology (climate change mitigation technologies related to transportation), building technology (climate change mitigation technologies related to buildings), environmental management technology (technologies of air pollution abatement, water pollution abatement, waste management, soil remediation, and environmental monitoring), and water-related adaptation technology (technologies of water conservation and availability). We assigned these environmental patents to cities in China based on the address of the patent applicant, including municipalities directly under the central government (e.g., Beijing, Shanghai, Tianjin, and Chongqing), prefecture level cities (e.g., Hangzhou, Suzhou, Guangzhou, Shenzhen, Nanjing, etc.), autonomous prefectures (e.g., Dali Bai Autonomous Prefecture, Enshi Tujia and Miao Autonomous Prefecture, Chuxiong Yi Autonomous Prefecture, etc.), prefecture regions (e.g., Altay, Ali, Aksu, etc.), leagues (e.g., Xilingol League, Alashan League, and Xingan League) and counties directly under the jurisdiction of provinces (e.g., Xiantao, Qianjiang, Tianmen, etc.).

Table 1 shows the development trend of environmental innovation in China in the past decade. From 2007 to 2017, environment-related patent applications increased from 87,691 to 307,929, with an average annual growth rate of 13.4%. In addition to being slightly lower than the field of energy in 2010, technologies related to buildings have always ranked first, increasing from 35,850 in 2007 to 105,681 in 2017.

Table 2 shows the proportion of environmental patents in Chinese patent applications. Although the number of environmental patent applications has increased rapidly, its proportion in all patent applications has shown a significant decline. At the urban scale, the proportion of environmental patent applications in each city was also much lower than that of non-environmental patents. This seems to indicate that environmental innovation has a higher production cost and a higher production threshold.

Table 1. Number of environment-related patent applications in different technical fields from 2007 to 2017 in China.

Year	Envir_M.	Energy	Green_G.	Building	Water_A.	Transp.	Total
2007	6210	32,352	843	35,850	3096	9340	87,691
2008	13,792	28,279	6885	48,444	3772	9874	111,046
2009	5895	7608	4813	33,850	3647	1099	56,912
2010	17,089	57,814	12,124	56,861	3337	22,740	169,965
2011	18,540	19,153	10,646	39,759	6301	3393	97,792
2012	25,173	34,480	13,809	62,043	5279	5221	146,005
2013	35,994	46,295	20,848	61,992	9009	11,048	185,186
2014	31,122	45,123	19,122	55,958	7088	9666	168,079
2015	41,904	93,398	28,818	128,166	9834	50,700	352,820
2016	62,345	85,142	15,247	115,247	12,471	32,415	322,867
2017	83,090	79,562	10,081	105,681	13,440	16,075	307,929

Notes: Envir_M.: environmental management technology; Green_G.: greenhouse gas treatment technology; Water_A.: water-related adaptation technology; Transp.: transportation technology.

Table 2. Proportion of environmental patents in overall patents from 2007 to 2017 in China.

Year	Number of Environmental Patents	Total Number of Patent Applications	Proportion of Environmental Patents
2007	87,691	407,090	21.5%
2008	111,046	469,670	23.6%
2009	56,912	575,504	9.9%
2010	169,965	711,457	23.9%
2011	97,792	957,267	10.2%
2012	146,005	1,224,727	11.9%
2013	185,186	1,382,867	13.4%
2014	168,079	1,536,629	10.9%
2015	352,820	1,910,833	18.5%
2016	322,867	2,224,683	14.5%
2017	307,929	2,696,311	11.4%

3.3. Research Methodology

3.3.1. Variables

The interpreted variable in our study was urban environmental innovation capability (EIC). Urban EIC was measured by the environmental patent applications.

The core explanatory variable was urban environmental regulation (ER). Referring to the comprehensive index construction methods of Peng [4], this study selected three indicators, namely the comprehensive utilization rate of industrial solid waste, domestic sewage treatment rate, and domestic waste harmless treatment rate.

Innovation economics believes that, as an innovative activity that emphasizes environmental protection or reduces environmental damage [34,35], the market drivers of general innovation behavior (population, foreign direct investment (FDI), economic development level, urban construction scale, etc.) and technology drivers (investment, human capital, etc.) are also applicable and effective for explaining the determinants of environmental innovation [16,40,45]. For example, the relationship between FDI and environmental innovation has been widely explored in the fields of innovation economics and innovation management [46–48]. With the in-depth exploration of evolutionary economic and grounded theory, scholars have found that innovation willingness and innovation attitude have an important role in promoting environmental innovation, and environmental innovation is highly dependent on its own development mode, growth path, and industry environment. Meanwhile, environmental innovation is a means for enterprises (especially manufacturing) to respond to environmental regulations and participate in market competition. If a city's industrial structure is dominated by industrial manufacturing, it would bear more responsibility for environmental protection and pollution reduction, and the city will also introduce more environmental policies to stimulate enterprises to carry out environmental innovation [3,13]. Besides, in China, different cities have different administrative levels. Cities with different administrative levels have certain differences in the level of educational resources, investment in innovation resources, and convenience of patent application or transfer.

Therefore, based on the existing innovation and environmental innovation literature, we added eight control variables: urban size (U-S), urban FDI (U-FDI), urban economic development level (U-EDL), urban technological innovation capability (U-TIC), urban construction scale (U-CS), urban initial environmental innovation capacity (U-IEIC), urban industrial structure (U-IS), and urban administrative level (U-AL). In terms of the measurement of these indicators, this study used the urban population to characterize the U-S, used the amount of foreign capital used in that year to characterize the U-FDI, used the urban per capita GDP to measure the U-EDL, used the proportion of secondary industry to measure the U-IS, and used the number of environmental patents of the city in 1990 to characterize U-IEIC (the China National Intellectual Property Administration (CNIPA) began collecting patent data in 1985, and considering the incompleteness of the data in the first few years, the data of 1990 was adopted). Regarding U-AL, we constructed a dummy variable, which was 1 if the city is a provincial capital, and 0 otherwise. Unless otherwise noted, data on control variables were obtained from China City Statistical Yearbook.

As discussed above, Table 3 lists and describes the interpreted, core explanatory, and other control variables.

Table 3. Description of variables.

Variable Name	Description	Measurement
	Interpreted variable	
EIC	Urban environmental innovation capability	The number of environment-related patent applications.
	Core explanatory variable	
ER	Urban environmental regulation	The weighted average value of the treatment rates of three pollutants.
	Other control variables	
U-S	Urban size	Urban registered residence population at the end of the year.
U-EDL	Urban economic development level	Urban per capita GDP.
U-TIC	Urban technological innovation capability	Urban R&D investment.
U-FDI	Urban FDI	The amount of foreign capital actually used in that year.
U-IEIC	Urban initial environmental innovation capacity	The number of environmental patents of the city in 1990.
U-CS	Urban construction	Urban fixed asset investment.
U-IS	Urban industrial structure	The proportion of secondary industry.
U-AL	Urban administrative level	1 if the city is a provincial capital, and 0 otherwise.

3.3.2. Spatial Correlation Analysis

To explore the spatial correlation of environmental innovation in China, this study used the global Moran's I index to conduct a spatial statistical analysis of environmental innovation in China city systems [12]. The definition of the global Moran's I index is:

$$\text{Moran's I} = \frac{n\sum_{i=1}^{n}\sum_{j=1,i\neq j}^{n} W_{ij}(X_i-\overline{X})(X_j-\overline{X})}{\sigma^2\sum_{i=1}^{n}\sum_{j=1,i\neq j}^{n} W_{ij}},\ \overline{X}=\frac{1}{n}\sum_{i=1}^{n}X_i,\ \sigma^2=\frac{1}{n}\sum_{i=1}^{n}(X_i-\overline{X})^2,\ W_{ij}=1/d_{ij} \quad (3)$$

where X_i and X_j represent the *EIC* in city *i* and city *j*, respectively. W_{ij} is the spatial weighted matrix, n is the number of cities, and d_{ij} is the distance between city *i* and city *j*. The range of values of the global Moran's I index is $[-1, 1]$.

Table 4 shows the global Moran's I index results. The index of urban *EIC* in each period was positive at the 1% level, and the Moran's I of the six types of environment-related technologies all showed a rising trend that was statistically significant at $p < 0.01$, indicating a significantly positive spatial autocorrelation in the urban *EIC* of the 349 cities in China from 2007 to 2017.

Table 4. Global Moran's I index of urban EIC (2007, 2012, and 2017).

Year	Urban *EIC*	Different Types of Environment-Related Technologies					
		Envir_M.	**Energy**	**Green_G.**	**Building**	**Water_A.**	**Transp.**
2007	0.182 ***	0.193 ***	0.107 ***	0.117 ***	0.257 ***	0.111 ***	0.176 ***
2012	0.252 ***	0.201 ***	0.185 ***	0.156 ***	0.326 ***	0.178 ***	0.267 ***
2017	0.324 ***	0.330 ***	0.202 ***	0.266 ***	0.353 ***	0.267 ***	0.273 ***

Note: ***, $p < 0.01$.

3.3.3. Random Effects Model

For the coldiag2 test, the condition number using scaled variables was 13.02; thus, the variables passed the collinearity test [49]. To ensure the accuracy and credibility of the estimated results of the F test, the fixed-effect model is considered to be significantly better than mixed regression. Further, considering the addition of dummy variables and according to the least squares dummy variables (LSDV) method, a Hausman test was used to determine the use of random effects model.

3.3.4. Spatial Regression Model

Due to the significant spatial correlation of environmental innovation with cities in China, a spatial panel regression model was considered for the detection of the determinants. By comparing the spatial lag model (SLM), the spatial error model (SEM), and the spatial Durbin model (SDM) based on Stata 12.0 analysis, it was found that the goodness of fit and credibility of the SDM ($R^2 = 0.863$) was the highest among the three models, and the Hausman test results showed that the SDM random effects passed the robustness test. Therefore, this paper selected the SDM with random effects to analyze the determinants of environmental innovation of cities in China:

$$\begin{aligned} \mathrm{Ln}EIC_{i,t} = \alpha_i + \; & \beta_1 \mathrm{Ln}ER_{i,t} + \beta_2 \mathrm{Ln}U - S_{i,t} + \beta_3 \mathrm{Ln}U_{FDI i,t} + \beta_4 \mathrm{Ln}U - TIC_{i,t} + \beta_5 \mathrm{Ln}U - IEIC_{i,t} + \beta_6 \mathrm{Ln}U - CS_{i,t} \\ & + \beta_7 \mathrm{Ln}U - EDL_{i,t} + \beta_8 \mathrm{Ln}U - IS_{i,t} + \beta_9 \mathrm{Ln}U - AL_{i,t} + \lambda \sum_{k=1}^{11} w_{ij} \mathrm{Ln}EIC_{j,t} + \theta_1 \sum_{j=1}^{11} w_{ij} \mathrm{Ln}ER_{j,t} \\ & + \theta_2 \sum_{j=1}^{11} w_{ij} \mathrm{Ln}U - S_{j,t} + \theta_3 \sum_{j=1}^{11} w_{ij} \mathrm{Ln}U - FDI_{j,t} + \theta_4 \sum_{j=1}^{11} w_{ij} \mathrm{Ln}U - TIOC_{j,t} \\ & + \theta_5 \sum_{j=1}^{11} w_{ij} \mathrm{Ln}U - IEIC_{j,t} + \theta_6 \sum_{j=1}^{11} w_{ij} \mathrm{Ln}U - CS_{j,t} + \theta_7 \sum_{j=1}^{11} w_{ij} \mathrm{Ln}U - EDL_{j,t} \\ & + \theta_8 \sum_{j=1}^{11} w_{ij} \mathrm{Ln}U - IS_{j,t} + \theta_9 \sum_{j=1}^{11} w_{ij} \mathrm{Ln}U - AL_{j,t} \end{aligned} \tag{4}$$

where i indexes the city, and t indexes time.

4. Empirical Results

4.1. Environmental Innovation of Cities in China

From 2007 to 2017, the number of cities participating in environmental innovation in China increased from 330 in 2007 to 338 in 2017, among which the number of cities engaging in innovation around building technology was always the largest, while the number of cities engaging in innovation around greenhouse gas technology was always the smallest. Spatially, China's environmental innovation activities showed significant spatial heterogeneity, highly concentrated in a few cities (Table 5).

Specifically, in 2007, the top 10 cities in environmental innovation accounted for 48.1% of the environment-related patent applications in China. There were four cities with more than 5000 environment-related patents, namely Shanghai (9003), Beijing (8073), Guangzhou (6689), and Shenzhen (6174). Shanghai also ranked first in patent applications in the field of greenhouse gases, building, water adaptation, and transportation technology, while Beijing ranked first in the field of environmental management and energy technology. In different technical fields, most of the cities with outstanding performance were in eastern China. Cities in central and western China were generally backward in environmental innovation. In 2012, the proportion of the top 10 cities in environmental patents fell to 43.3%. Beijing not only surpassed Shanghai in terms of total volume, but also ranked first in all six technical fields. Chengdu and Xi-An in the central and western regions ranked sixth and seventh with 3852 and 3822 patent applications, respectively. Similarly, in different technical fields, cities with outstanding performance were mostly located in east China. Environmental innovation in central and western China was still generally backward. By 2017, Beijing continued to rank first with 26,224 patent applications and Shenzhen ranked second with 18,997 patents. Shanghai, Guangzhou, and Suzhou ranked third, fourth, and fifth with 14,801, 11,800, and 10,659 patent applications, respectively. Foshan ranked tenth with 7059 environmental patent applications. Its environmental patent applications mainly came from the field of water-related adaptation, accounting for 57.7% of the total. This is mainly because the Midea Group, which is headquartered in Foshan, applied for more than 2000 patents in the field of water-related adaptation technology in 2017. In the six categories of environment-related technologies, Beijing still ranked first in environmental management, energy, greenhouse gases, and transportation technologies, while Shenzhen ranked first in the technologies of building and water-related adaptation.

Table 5. Top 10 cities with the most environment-related technologies (2007, 2012, and 2017).

			Year = 2007				
City	**Envir_M.**	**Energy**	**Green_G.**	**Building**	**Water_A.**	**Transp.**	**Total**
Shanghai	510	3408	131	3453	356	1145	9003
Beijing	520	3589	96	3044	261	563	8073
Guangzhou	452	2758	19	2453	136	871	6689
Shenzhen	184	2489	9	2583	47	862	6174
Tianjin	248	1148	19	797	104	172	2488
Dongguan	121	745	11	894	18	405	2194
Hangzhou	152	922	32	782	110	139	2137
Ji-Nan	130	667	20	925	73	93	1908
Suzhou	120	549	36	809	47	306	1867
Ningbo	84	608	6	620	39	290	1647
			Year = 2012				
City	**Envir_M.**	**Energy**	**Green_G.**	**Building**	**Water_A.**	**Transp.**	**Total**
Beijing	2669	7286	1728	4481	471	431	17,066
Shanghai	1362	2351	720	3234	414	368	8449
Guangzhou	679	2776	420	3846	172	128	8021
Suzhou	1009	1126	558	2857	207	166	5923
Hangzhou	1088	1077	922	2044	174	186	5491
Chengdu	653	824	402	1718	107	148	3852
Xi An	423	777	292	2127	111	92	3822
Tianjin	882	667	530	1246	253	125	3703
Nanjing	746	942	649	1133	134	95	3699
Ningbo	411	495	156	1962	130	65	3219
			Year = 2017				
City	**Envir_M.**	**Energy**	**Green_G.**	**Building**	**Water_A.**	**Transp.**	**Total**
Beijing	785	5020	10,731	1136	7755	797	26,224
Shenzhen	358	2479	6116	1835	8055	154	18,997
Shanghai	608	3169	4266	947	5350	461	14,801
Guangzhou	471	2640	3430	528	4414	317	11,800
Suzhou	404	3110	2399	540	3789	417	10,659
Chengdu	376	2583	2428	466	3216	302	9371
Nanjing	319	2287	2837	358	2789	303	8893
Hangzhou	337	1953	2163	334	2460	384	7631
Tianjin	344	2463	1814	314	2153	291	7379
Foshan	245	1476	920	174	4070	174	7059

Note: The underlined numbers indicate that the corresponding city ranked first in patent applications for this type of technology.

4.2. Regression Results

Our initial data covered all cities at the prefecture level and above in China; however, due to the limitation of variable data, we finally selected 274 cities to enter the regression model. Table 6 shows the variable descriptive statistics, interpreted variables including urban EIC (total number of environmental patents), and the innovation ability of the cities in six types of environmental technology (the number of patent applications in each technology). Table 7 shows the descriptive statistics of the variables in three major regions of China. There were 114 cities in the eastern region, 108 in the central region, and 52 in the western region.

Table 6. Descriptive statistics of China city panel data and six types of environment-related technologies.

Variables	Obs	Mean	Std. Dev.	Min	Max
EIC	3014	662.066	2118.858	0	38,943
Envir_M.	3014	111.654	313.556	0	5020
Energy	3014	175.033	726.617	0	14,715
Green_G.	3014	48.516	161.997	0	2803
Building	3014	245.385	749.394	0	12,790
Water_A.	3014	25.036	65.447	0	973
Transp.	3014	56.993	230.217	0	5137
ER	3014	0.06	0.069	0	0.817
Ln *U-S*	3014	441.49	309.441	17.22	3375.2
Ln *U-EDL*	3014	10.19	0.736	7.782	13.056
Ln *U-TIC*	3014	9.302	1.696	−2.04	14.873
U-FDI	3014	69,407.898	167,333.8	0	2,113,444
U-IEIC	3014	22.984	58.506	0	718.5
Ln U-CS	3014	15.512	1.047	12.594	18.691
U-IS	3014	49.615	10.804	0	90.97
U-AL	3014	0.124	0.33	0	1

Table 7. Descriptive statistics for panel data of cities in three major regions of China.

		East China			
Variables	**Obs**	**Mean**	**Std. Dev.**	**Min**	**Max**
EIC	1254	1182.068	3050.199	0	38,943
ER	1254	0.072	0.077	0	0.752
Ln *U-S*	1254	473.962	267.289	51.19	1442.97
Ln *U-EDL*	1254	10.426	0.701	8.476	13.056
Ln *U-TIC*	1254	9.825	1.781	4.078	14.873
U-FDI	1254	114,108.5	225,575.12	10	2,113,444
U-IEIC	1254	40.243	84.366	0	718.5
Ln U-CS	1254	15.834	0.999	12.971	18.571
U-IS	1254	49.438	8.712	0	82.28
U-AL	1254	0.149	0.356	0	1
		Central China			
Variables	**Obs**	**Mean**	**Std. Dev.**	**Min**	**Max**
EIC	1188	261.213	642.137	0	6880
ER	1188	0.053	0.05	0.001	0.41
Ln *U-S*	1188	421.282	254.29	43.11	1244.35
Ln *U-EDL*	1188	10.079	0.677	8.232	12.456
Ln *U-TIC*	1188	9.038	1.503	4.344	13.433
U-FDI	1188	39,974.045	68,656.763	0	734,303
U-IEIC	1188	10.407	20.419	0	163.25
Ln U-CS	1188	15.373	0.967	12.594	18.059
U-IS	1188	49.416	11.651	15.17	85.92

Table 7. *Cont.*

U-AL	1188	0.083	0.277	0	1
		West China			
Variables	**Obs**	**Mean**	**Std. Dev.**	**Min**	**Max**
EIC	572	354.6	1180.692	0	11,445
ER	572	0.05	0.081	0	0.817
Ln *U-S*	572	412.271	458.309	17.22	3375.2
Ln *U-EDL*	572	9.903	0.77	7.782	12.322
Ln *U-TIC*	572	8.705	1.553	−2.04	13.124
U-FDI	572	32,542.272	136,893.7	0	1,121,599
U-IEIC	572	11.264	21.334	0	98
Ln U-CS	572	15.099	1.101	12.686	18.691
U-IS	572	50.415	12.9	9	90.97
U-AL	572	0.154	0.361	0	1

Table 8 shows the regression results of the random effects model. The quadratic coefficients of environmental regulation were greater than 0, and the coefficients of the primary term were less than 0, which indicated that the impact of environmental regulation on the urban environmental innovation capability was a positive U-shaped curve that first declined and then rose. In other words, our research showed that urban environmental regulation had a restraining effect on urban environmental innovation in the short term [8]; however, they presented a positive correlation in the long term [12]. To avoid the interference of regional differences and improve the robustness and accuracy of the findings, we performed the same analysis on the sample data from three regions in China. Table 9 shows the regression results of different regions of China. We obtained the same results from the analysis, which showed that at the city level, the U-shaped relationship between China's environmental regulation and environmental innovation has a certain degree of stability.

Furthermore, we continued to investigate whether the negative effect of environmental regulation on environmental innovation had spatial spillover effects or not. Table 10 reports the results of the SDM. Since the SDM contains the spatial lag terms of both the explanatory variables and the explained variables, the partial differential method was adopted to decompose the spillover effects of the SDM into direct effect, indirect effect, and total effect. Among them, the direct effect reflects the impact on the city's environmental innovation, that is, the local effect. The indirect effect reflects the impact on the environmental innovation of the surrounding cities, that is, the spillover effect. The total effect is equal to the sum of the direct effect and the indirect effect. The R^2 was 0.852 and the spatial rho was significant at a significance level of 1%, with a coefficient of 0.213, indicating that environmental innovation in China city systems has a significant positive spatial spillover effect. Regarding the relationship between environmental regulation and environmental innovation, the regression results of the SDM were consistent with the results of the random effects model. That is, the effect of environmental regulation on environmental innovation was first to inhibit and then to promote.

Through the above regression results, we verified some existing findings. Firstly, there was a significant positive correlation between urban size and urban environmental innovation capability, which is consistent with the existing studies on the relationship between enterprise environmental innovation and enterprise size [21,22], and the relationship between regional environmental innovation and regional size [3,23,24]. Secondly, the higher the level of urban economic development was, the stronger the capability of urban environmental innovation was. This is also consistent with the existing research results of environmental economics and innovation economics. Thirdly, urban FDI was not only positively correlated with the urban environmental innovation capability, but also showed positive local effects and local spillover effects. This is consistent with existing research results [38,45,47,48]. A large amount of foreign capital investment promotes the improvement of local environmental innovation ability, and also forms a strong trickle-down effect to the surrounding areas, promoting the environmental innovation of surrounding cities. Fourthly, the urban initial environmental innovation capability was obviously conducive to the urban environmental innovation capability. The direct effect of the urban initial environmental innovation capability was 18.288, and the indirect effect was −22.658, both of which were significant at the 1% significance level, indicating that urban environmental innovation had strong path dependence characteristics, while it also reflected that the cities with good performance in environmental innovation in the early stage would form a siphon effect, thus restraining the environmental innovation of surrounding cities.

Table 8. Regression results of the random effects model.

Variables	EIC	Envir_M.	Energy	Green_G.	Building	Water_A.	Transp.
ER^2	896.321 ***	145.235 ***	324.754 ***	56.231 ***	101.632 ***	10.245 ***	63.247 ***
ER	−1816.837 ***	−348.393 ***	−797.105 ***	−238.132 ***	−248.698 *	−42.23 ***	−148.083 **
Ln *U-S*	0.482 ***	0.089 ***	0.108 *	0.021	0.148 **	0.029 ***	0.079 ***
Ln *U-EDL*	538.145 ***	75.462 ***	151.808 ***	9.333	200.017 ***	15.178 ***	74.9 ***
Ln *U-TIC*	14.046	19.014 ***	−5.373	7.775 ***	−1.607	2.769 ***	−5.824
U-FDI	0.005 ***	0.001 ***	0.001 ***	0.0004 ***	0.002 ***	0.0009 ***	0.001 ***
U-IEIC	18.151 ***	1.691 ***	7.765 ***	1.522 ***	5.784 ***	0.45 ***	1.022 ***
Ln U-CS	−187.683 ***	−28.383 ***	−59.192 ***	−1.943	−65.131 ***	−6.545 ***	−24.405 ***
U-IS	−22.907 ***	−4.189 ***	−6.86 ***	−0.72 ***	−7.784 ***	−0.735 ***	−1.975 ***
U-AL	−180.225	−48.567 ***	−117.343 **	−23.03 **	−3.391	3.827	13.869
Ln *U-S*	−1754.264 ***	−304.289 ***	−314.708	−100.657 **	−689.436 ***	−50.508 ***	−263.437 ***

Note: *** $p < 0.01$, ** $p < 0.05$, * $p < 0.1$.

Table 9. Regression results from different regions of China.

Variables	China	East China	Central China	West China
ER^2	896.321 ***	103.547 ***	315.631 ***	89.243 ***
ER	−1816.837 ***	−348.393 ***	−797.105 ***	−238.132 ***
Ln *U-S*	0.482 ***	0.089 ***	0.108 *	0.021
Ln *U-EDL*	538.145 ***	75.462 ***	151.808 ***	9.333
Ln *U-TIC*	14.046	19.014 ***	−5.373	7.775 ***
U-FDI	0.005 ***	0.001 ***	0.001 ***	0.0008 ***
U-IEIC	18.151 ***	1.691 ***	7.765 ***	1.522 ***
Ln U-CS	−187.683 ***	−28.383 ***	−59.192 ***	−1.943
U-IS	−22.907 ***	−4.189 ***	−6.86 ***	−0.72 ***
U-AL	−180.225	−48.567 ***	−117.343 **	−23.03 **
Ln *U-S*	−1754.264 ***	−5115.433 ***	443.483	−1128.648 **

Note: *** $p < 0.01$, ** $p < 0.05$, * $p < 0.1$.

In addition, we also found some very interesting conclusions about the control variables. Firstly, the industrial structure dominated by the secondary industry not only did not promote urban environmental innovation, but also played an obvious inhibitory effect. This finding is clearly different from the existing related research [3,12]. To verify the correctness of this result, we replaced this variable with the proportion of tertiary industry and performed a regression analysis again and found that the industrial structure dominated by the tertiary industry had a significant role in promoting the environmental innovation of the city itself and its surrounding cities. The reason for this result may be that the traditional manufacturing industry is still the pillar industry in China's cities dominated by secondary industry, and patent applications are mostly completed by the tertiary industry, represented by the information and communication industry, real estate industry, and scientific research. Secondly, the scale of urban construction measured by the scale of urban fixed asset investment had a significant negative effect on urban environmental innovation capability. As an important driving force of economic growth, China's urban fixed asset investment is growing rapidly. However, while stimulating economic growth, it has also increased energy consumption and environmental pollution. Many studies have found that there is a significant positive correlation between urban fixed asset investment and urban environmental pollution emissions in China [50]. Thirdly, there was a negative correlation between the urban administrative level and urban environmental innovation capability. The reason for this may be that some non-capital cities have performed very well in environmental innovation, such as Suzhou, Ningbo, Shenzhen, and Foshan. However, this negative correlation did not pass the significance test, which also showed that the relationship between the two needs more verification.

Table 10. Results of the spatial Durbin model (SDM).

Variables	Factors		Elimination Effect Decomposition		
	Main	W(X)	Direct Effect	Indirect Effect	Total Effect
ER^2	864.576 ***	1124.653	1024.561 ***	554.714	746.894 ***
ER	−1717.110 ***	1242.10	−1734.926 ***	660.385	−1074.54 ***
Ln *U-S*	0.475 ***	0.00	0.483 ***	0.672	1.155
Ln *U-EDL*	437.675 ***	−51.39	448.137 ***	489.962 *	938.098 **
Ln *U-TIC*	4.26	−36.73	−5.871	−92.338	−98.21
U-FDI	0.005 ***	0.002 ***	0.005 ***	0.011 ***	0.016 ***
U-IEIC	18.288 ***	−20.246 ***	18.268 ***	−22.658 ***	−4.39
Ln U-CS	−229.288 ***	97.08	−232.795 ***	−84.863	−317.658 *
U-IS	−16.178 ***	−4.67	−16.468 ***	−34.963 ***	−51.43 ***
U-AL	−26.30	−2036.330 **	−23.97	−1675.709	−1699.679
_cons			−692.31		
Spatial rho			0.587 ***		
R^2			0.7186		
Log-likelihood			−9628.413		

Note: ***, $p < 0.01$; **, $p < 0.05$; *, $p < 0.1$.

5. Conclusions

Exploring the relationship between environmental regulation and environmental innovation is the core topic of environmental economics, innovation economics, and other research fields, and it is also one of the emerging topics in the field of environmental economic geography in recent years. This study used the number of environmental patent applications to measure urban environmental innovation, and analyzed the role of urban environmental regulation on urban environmental innovation, from which we summarize the following key findings.

Firstly, the number of environmental patents in China has grown rapidly, from 87,691 in 2007 to 307,929 in 2017. From a technical perspective, technologies related to buildings have always dominated the development of environmental innovation of cities in China, while technologies in the field of greenhouse gases and water adaptation were quite unpopular throughout China. China's urban environmental innovation showed a significant spatial correlation. The Moran's I index of both the whole (urban EIC) and the six technical fields were significant at the 1% level and greater than 0. Additionally, in the time sequence, the values of Moran's index were increasing, which indicated that the spatial correlation was strengthened with the passage of time.

Secondly, the number of cities participating in environmental innovation in China increased from 330 in 2007 to 338 in 2017, among which the number of cities engaging in innovation around building technology was always the largest, while the number of cities engaging in innovation around the greenhouse gas technology was always the smallest. Spatially, China's environmental innovation activities showed significant spatial heterogeneity, highly concentrated in a few cities [43]. From 2007 to 2017, Beijing not only surpassed Shanghai in the total number of environmental patent applications, but also ranked first in the fields of environmental management, energy, greenhouse gas treatment, and transportation technology. Shenzhen also surpassed Shanghai in the total number of environmental patent applications, ranking second in China. At the same time, Shenzhen had the largest number of environmental patent applications in the field of building and water-related adaptation in China.

Thirdly, both the random effects model and the SDM model showed that there was a U-shaped relationship between China's urban environmental regulation and urban environmental innovation, which was not only consistent with what the Porter hypothesis advocates [9,12], but is also consistent with existing research on the relationship between green innovation and urban green development [51]. Moreover, the regression results of different technical fields and different regions verified this result. These results showed that environmental regulations will first restrict environmental innovation due to increased production costs. After a period of adaptation, environmental regulations will induce environmental innovation. We also found some interesting results in the control variables. Urban size, urban economic development level, and urban FDI all played positive roles in promoting urban environmental innovation, while the urban fixed asset investment scale and industrial structure dominated by the secondary industry significantly inhibited urban environmental innovation. In addition, we also found that urban environmental innovation had significant path dependence characteristics.

6. Discussion

The discussion of the relationship between environmental regulation and environmental innovation in this article gives us many policy implications. Firstly, local governments should adhere to the innovation-driven development strategy, increasing R&D investment to promote the continuous growth of urban technological innovation capability. Secondly, local governments should continue to promote the transformation and upgrading of the urban industrial structure, especially increasing the supports for the producer service industry. Thirdly, local governments should increase the introduction of foreign capital to promote the upgrading of local production and management methods. Fourthly, local governments should conduct environmental assessments on the increasing urban fixed asset investment under the background of rapid urbanization. In addition, increasing investment in fixed assets will also reduce other financial expenditures. Fifthly, in view of the U-shaped relationship between environmental regulation and environmental innovation, local governments should adopt strategies that adapt to time and local conditions in environmental regulation.

We noticed that enterprises are becoming increasingly important as the largest actors in China's environmental innovation. Based on applicant information for environmental patents, we identified environmental innovation actors in four categories, namely universities and scientific research institutions, enterprises, individuals, and others. We found that the proportion of enterprises increased rapidly from 39.7% in 2007 to 70.2% in 2017. This showed that the difference in the spatial distribution of China's environmental innovation was seriously affected by the distribution of enterprises engaged in environmental innovation. Therefore, future research on China's environmental innovation must fully consider the impact of the spatial distribution characteristics of different types of enterprises.

There are also some limitations that may exist in our study. First, we limited our data to the patent applications from the Wanfang Patent Database, which cannot avoid criticism about neglecting other data sources. Second, using only one indicator (environmental patent applications) to measure the capacity of a city's environmental innovation is relatively weak, and building a richer evaluation system for city environmental innovation is a direction we will explore in the future. Third, although six types of environmental technologies were identified based on the work of the Organization for Economic Co-operation and Development (OECD), there are still some environmental technologies that we have not considered, such as adsorption cooling technology [52,53], advanced combustion technology, and emission reduction technology [54,55]. A broader environmental technology identification system should be constructed. Fourth, we considered the spatial relevance of urban environmental innovation but ignored the spatial diffusion of environmental innovation. In the era of innovation networking, cities participate in environmental innovation activities not only relying on their own development, but also relying on networks to obtain innovation resources. Therefore, future environmental innovation research must fully consider the externality effect brought by the innovation network.

Author Contributions: Conceptualization, D.D.; methodology, D.D. and Q.X.; software, Q.X.; validation, D.D.; formal analysis, D.D. and Q.X.; investigation, D.D.; resources, D.D.; data curation, D.D. and Q.X.; writing—original draft preparation, D.D..; writing—review and editing, D.D.; supervision, Q.X.; project administration, D.D.; funding acquisition, D.D. All authors have read and agreed to the published version of the manuscript.

Funding: This research was funded by the National Natural Science Foundation of China grant number 41901139.

Institutional Review Board Statement: Not applicable.

Informed Consent Statement: Not applicable.

Data Availability Statement: Not applicable.

Conflicts of Interest: The authors declare no conflict of interest.

Appendix A

Table A1. Search strategies for the identification of environment-related technologies.

Environment-Related Technology	Description	IPC Class
Energy	Climate change mitigation technologies related to energy generation, transmission, or distribution.	F24J2, F03D9, H01L31, F03D11, H02J3, B03B13, F03D7, F03D3, F03B13, H01L51, H02N6, F03G6, F02J7, C10L5, B01J2, B09B3, F23L15, F23J15, F23L7, C10J3, F23D14, F27D17, G21C15, G21D3, G21C13, G21D1, G22C16, G06Q10, H02J13, H01B12, G06Q50, H01M2, H01M8, H01M10, H01M4, H02J7, F28D20, C25B1, G06F17, H02J15, B01D53, B01J20, C01B31
Greenhouse gases	Capture, storage, sequestration, or disposal of greenhouse gases.	B01D53, B01J20, C01B31
Transportation	Climate change mitigation technologies related to transportation.	B60L8, F02M25, B60L15, F02M21, F01N3, B60W20, F02B29, B60W10, F01N5, F01N11, F01N9, F02M27, B61D27, B61D17, B61C3, F01D5, B64D27, B64C1, B64C23, B64D11, B64C25, B63B1, B63H19, B63H13, B63H21, B60L11, H02J7, H01M8, H02J17, B60L3, B60K1
Building	Climate change mitigation technologies related to buildings.	F03D9, F24D17, H01L31, E04H1, F21S9, H05B33, F21S8, F21S2, F21V29, H05B41, F21V23, F24F5, F24H8, F24F11, F25B15, F25B29, F24F6, F24F1, F24D3, F24F12, F24H4, F24J2, F24C3, F24B1, B66B25, B66B9, B66B1, B66B11, B66B23, G08C17, G05B19, H04W52, G06F1, H04L29, F24D19, H02M3, H02M1, H02J3, H02M7, H05B37, E04B1, A01G9, E06B3, E04D13, E04D11, H02J13, H01M8, H02J9, G01D4, H02J7
		B01D53, F23J15, F27B1, C21B7, C21C5, F23B80, F23C9, F23C10, F02M3, B01J23, F01M13, F02D21, G01M15, F02B47, F02D41, F02D43, F02D45, F02M23, F02M25, 02M27, F02M31, F02M39, F02P5, B01D46, B01D47, B01D49, B01D50, B01D51, B03C3, F01N3, F01N5, F01N7, F01N13, F01N9, C10L10, B63J4, C02F, E03C1,

Table A1. *Cont.*

Environment-Related Technology	Description	IPC Class
Environmental management	Technologies of air pollution abatement, water pollution abatement, waste management, soil remediation, and environmental monitoring.	E03F, E02B15, B63B35, C09K3, E01H15, B65F, A23K1, A43B1, A43B21, B03B9, B22F8, B29B7, B29B17, B30B9, B62D67, B65H73, B65D65, C03B1, C03C6, C04B7, C04B11, C04B18, C04B33, C08J11,C09K11, C10M175, C22B7, C22B19, C22B25, D01G11, D21B1, D21C5, D21H17, H01B15, H01J9, H01M6, H01M10, C05F1, C05F5, C05F7, C05F9, C05F17, C10L5, F23G5, F23G7, B09B, C10G1, A61L11, B09C, F01N11, G08B21
Water adaptation	Technologies of water conservation and availability.	F16K21, F16L55, E03C1, E03D3, E03D1, A47K11, E03D13, E03D5, E03B1, Y02B40, A01G25, C12N15, F01K23, F01D11, F17D5, G01M3, E03B5, E03B3, E03B9, E03B11

References

1. Aelenei, L.; Aelenei, D.; Gongalves, H.; Lollini, R.; Musall, E.; Scognamiglio, A.; Cubio, E.; Noguchi, M. Design issues for net zero-energy buildings. *Open House Int.* **2013**, *38*, 7. [CrossRef]
2. Baglivo, C.; Congedo, P.M. Implementation hypothesis of the Apulia ITACA Protocol at district level-part I: The model. *Sust. Cities Soc.* **2021**, *70*, 102931.
3. Ouyang, X.; Li, Q.; Du, K. How does environmental regulation promote technological innovations in the industrial sector? Evidence from Chinese provincial panel data. *Energy Policy* **2020**, *139*, 111310. [CrossRef]
4. Peng, X. Strategic interaction of environmental regulation and green productivity growth in China: Green innovation or pollution refuge? *Sci. Total Environ.* **2020**, *732*, 139200. [CrossRef] [PubMed]
5. Khan, Z.; Ali, S.; Umar, M.; Kirikkaleli, D.; Jiao, Z. Consumption-based carbon emissions and international trade in G7 countries: The role of environmental innovation and renewable energy. *Sci. Total Environ.* **2020**, *730*, 138945. [CrossRef]
6. Wang, Q.; Qu, J.; Wang, B.; Wang, P.; Yang, T. Green technology innovation development in China in 1990–2015. *Sci. Total Environ.* **2019**, *96*, 134008. [CrossRef]
7. Jiao, J.; Wang, C.; Yang, R. Exploring the driving orientations and driving mechanisms of environmental innovation: The case study of the China Gezhouba. *J. Clean Prod.* **2020**, *260*, 121016. [CrossRef]
8. Forsman, D.H. Environmental innovations as a source of competitive advantage or vice versa? *Bus. Strateg. Environ.* **2013**, *22*, 306–320. [CrossRef]
9. Porter, M.E.; Linde, C.V.D. Green and competitive: An underlying logic links the environment, resource productivity, innovation, and competitiveness. *Harv. Bus. Rev.* **1995**, *73*, 120–129.
10. Baker, E.; Clarke, L.; Shittu, E. Technical change and the marginal cost of abatement. *Energy Econ.* **2008**, *30*, 2799–2816. [CrossRef]
11. Asheim, B.; Coenen, L. Knowledge bases and regional innovation systems: Comparing nordic clusters. *Res. Policy* **2005**, *34*, 1173–1190. [CrossRef]
12. Fan, F.; Lian, H.; Liu, X.; Wang, X. Can environmental regulation promote urban green innovation Efficiency? An empirical study based on Chinese cities. *J. Clean Prod.* **2021**, *287*, 125060. [CrossRef]
13. Long, X.; Sun, C.; Wu, C.; Chen, B.; Boateng, K.A. Green innovation efficiency across China's 30 provinces: Estimate, comparison, and convergence. *Mitig. Adapt. Strateg. Glob. Change* **2020**, *25*, 1243–1260. [CrossRef]
14. Song, W.; Yu, H. Green innovation strategy and green innovation: The roles of green creativity and green organizational identity. *Corp. Soc. Responsib. Environ. Manag.* **2018**, *25*, 135–150. [CrossRef]
15. Li, W.; Gu, Y.; Liu, F.; Li, C. The effect of command-and-control regulation on environmental technological innovation in China: A spatial econometric approach. *Environ. Sci. Pollut. Res.* **2019**, *26*, 34789–34800. [CrossRef]
16. Ardito, L.; Petruzzelli, A.M.; Pascucci, F.; Peruffo, E. Inter-firm R&D collaborations and green innovation value: The role of family firms' involvement and the moderating effects of proximity dimensions. *Bus. Strateg. Environ.* **2019**, *28*, 185–197.
17. Haščič, I.; Migotto, M. *Measuring Environmental Innovation Using Patent Data*; OECD Environment Working Papers 2005, No. 89; OECD Publishing: Paris, France, 2005.
18. Tang, K.; Qiu, Y.; Zhou, D. Does command-and-control regulation promote green innovation performance? Evidence from China's industrial enterprises. *Sci. Total Environ.* **2020**, *712*, 136362. [CrossRef]
19. Liao, Z. Corporate culture, environmental innovation and financial performance. *Bus. Strateg. Environ.* **2018**, *27*, 1368–1375. [CrossRef]
20. Barbera, A.J.; Mcconnell, V.D. The impact of environmental regulations on industry productivity: Direct and indirect effects. *J. Environ. Econ. Manag.* **1990**, *18*, 50–65. [CrossRef]

21. Triguero, A.; Moreno-Mondéjar, L.; Davia, M.A. Leaders and laggards in environmental innovation: An empirical analysis of SMEs in Europe. *Bus. Strateg. Environ.* **2016**, *25*, 28–39. [CrossRef]
22. Marin, G.; Zanfei, A. Does host market regulation induce cross-border environmental innovation? *World Econ.* **2019**, *42*, 2089–2119. [CrossRef]
23. Yuan, B.; Ren, S.; Chen, X. Can environmental regulation promote the coordinated development of economy and environment in China's manufacturing industry? a panel data analysis of 28 sub-sectors. *J. Clean Prod.* **2017**, *149*, 11–24. [CrossRef]
24. Wang, G.; Liu, S. Is technological innovation the effective way to achieve the "double dividend" of environmental protection and industrial upgrading? *Environ. Sci. Pollut. Res.* **2020**, *27*, 18541–18556. [CrossRef] [PubMed]
25. Mody, L.A. Innovation and the international diffusion of environmentally responsive technology. *Res. Policy* **1996**, *25*, 549–571.
26. Jaffe, A.B.; Palmer, K. Environmental regulation and innovation: A panel data study. *Rev. Econ. Stat.* **1997**, *79*, 610–619. [CrossRef]
27. Huang, Y.C.; Tu, J.C.; Lin, T.W. Key success factors of green innovation for transforming traditional industries. In *Sustainability Through Innovation in Product Life Cycle Design*; Matsumoto, M., Masui, K., Fukushige, S., Kondoh, S., Eds.; EcoProduction (Environmental Issues in Logistics and Manufacturing); Springer: Singapore, 2017.
28. Pearce, D.; Palmer, C. Public and private spending for environmental protection: A cross-country policy analysis. *Fisc. Stud.* **2010**, *22*, 403–456. [CrossRef]
29. Cole, M.A.; Elliott, R.J. Do environmental regulations cost jobs? An industry-level analysis of the UK. *B E J. Econ. Anal. Policy* **2007**, *7*, 1–25. [CrossRef]
30. Sauter, C. How Should We Measure Environmental Policy Stringency? In *A New Approach*; IRENE Working Papers; IRENE Institute of Economic Research: Neuchatel, Switzerland, 2014; pp. 14–101.
31. Henderson, D.J.; Millimet, D.L. Pollution abatement costs and foreign direct investment inflows to U.S. states: A nonparametric reassessment. *Rev. Econ. Stat.* **2007**, *89*, 178–183. [CrossRef]
32. Damania, R.; Fredriksson, P.G.; List, J.A. Trade liberalization, corruption, and environmental policy formation: Theory and evidence. *J. Environ. Econ. Manag.* **2003**, *46*, 490–512. [CrossRef]
33. Antweiler, W.; Copeland, B.R.; Taylor, M.S. Is free trade good for the environment? *Am. Econ. Rev.* **2001**, *91*, 877–908. [CrossRef]
34. Zhang, D.; Rong, Z.; Ji, Q. Green innovation and firm performance: Evidence from listed companies in China. *Resour. Conserv. Recycl.* **2019**, *144*, 48–55. [CrossRef]
35. Bossle, M.B.; De Barcellos, M.D.; Vieira, L.M.; Sauvée, L. The drivers for adoption of eco-innovation. *J. Clean Prod.* **2016**, *113*, 861–872. [CrossRef]
36. Pan, X.; Han, C.; Lu, X.; Jiao, Z.; Ming, Y. Green innovation ability evaluation of manufacturing enterprises based on AHP–OVP model. *Ann. Oper. Res.* **2020**, *290*, 409–419. [CrossRef]
37. Wang, C. An environmental perspective extends market orientation: Green innovation sustainability. *Bus. Strateg. Environ.* **2020**, *29*, 3123–3134. [CrossRef]
38. Tumelero, C.; Sbragia, R.; Evans, S. Cooperation in R&D and eco-innovations: The role in companies' socioeconomic performance. *J. Clean Prod.* **2019**, *207*, 1138–1149.
39. Duan, D.; Xia, Q.; Zhang, Y.; Gao, X. Evolution pattern and impact factors of environmental innovation in the Yangtze River Economic Belt. *Sci. Geogr. Sin.* **2021**, *41*, 1158–1167. [CrossRef]
40. Leyva-de la Hiz, D.I. Environmental innovations and policy network styles: The influence of pluralism and corporativism. *J. Clean Prod.* **2019**, *232*, 839–847. [CrossRef]
41. Shen, C.; Li, S.; Wang, X.; Liao, Z. The effect of environmental policy tools on regional green innovation: Evidence from China. *J. Clean Prod.* **2020**, *254*, 120122. [CrossRef]
42. Liu, C.; Gao, X.; Ma, W.; Chen, X. Research on regional differences and influencing factors of green technology innovation efficiency of China's high-tech industry. *J. Comput. Appl. Math.* **2020**, *369*, 112597. [CrossRef]
43. Singh, S.K.; Giudice, M.D.; Chierici, R.; Graziano, D. Green innovation and environmental performance: The role of green transformational leadership and green human resource management. *Technol. Forecast. Soc. Chang.* **2020**, *150*, 119762. [CrossRef]
44. Zhang, J.; Kang, L.; Li, H.; Ballesteros-Pérez, P.; Skitmore, M.; Zuo, J. The impact of environmental regulations on urban green innovation efficiency: The case of Xi'an. *Sust. Cities Soc.* **2020**, *57*, 102123. [CrossRef]
45. Huang, Z.; Liao, G.; Li, Z. Loaning scale and government subsidy for promoting green innovation. *Technol. Forecast. Soc. Chang.* **2019**, *144*, 148–156. [CrossRef]
46. Liu, Q.; Wang, S.; Zhang, W.; Zhan, D.; Li, J. Does foreign direct investment affect environmental pollution in China's cities? A spatial econometric perspective. *Sci. Total Environ.* **2018**, *613*, 521–529. [CrossRef]
47. Tang, D.; Xu, H.; Yang, Y. Mutual influence of energy consumption and foreign direct investment on haze pollution in China: A spatial econometric approach. *Pol. J. Environ. Stud.* **2018**, *27*, 1743–1752. [CrossRef]
48. Hao, Y.; Wu, Y.; Wu, H.; Ren, S. How do FDI and technical innovation affect environmental quality? Evidence from China. *Environ. Sci. Pollut. Res.* **2020**, *27*, 7835–7850. [CrossRef]
49. Yang, H.; Lin, Z.; Peng, M. Behind acquisitions of alliance partners: Exploratory learning and network embeddedness. *Acad. Manag. J.* **2011**, *54*, 1097. [CrossRef]
50. Li, L.; Qi, P. The impact of China's investment increase in fixed assets on ecological environment: An empirical analysis. *Energy Procedia* **2011**, *5*, 501–507. [CrossRef]

51. Hu, S.; Zeng, G.; Cao, X.; Yuan, H.; Chen, B. Does technological innovation promote green development? A case study of the Yangtze River Economic Belt in China. *Int. J. Environ. Res. Public Health* **2021**, *18*, 6111. [CrossRef] [PubMed]
52. Krzywanski, J.; Grabowska, K.; Sosnowski, M.; Zylka, A.; Nowak, W. An adaptive neuro-fuzzy model of a re-heat two-stage adsorption chiller. *Therm. Sci.* **2019**, *23*, 1053–1063. [CrossRef]
53. Hinze, M.; Ranft, F.; Drummer, D.; Schwieger, W. Reduction of the heat capacity in low-temperature adsorption chillers using thermally conductive polymers as heat exchangers material. *Energy Conv. Manag.* **2017**, *145*, 378–385. [CrossRef]
54. Idziak, K.; Czakiert, T.; Krzywanski, J.; Zylka, A.; Kozlowska, M.; Nowak, W. Safety and environmental reasons for the use of Ni-, Co-, Cu-, Mn- and Fe-based oxygen carriers in CLC/CLOU applications. *Fuel* **2020**, *268*, 117245. [CrossRef]
55. Krzywanski, J.; Czakiert, T.; Shimizu, T.; Majchrzak-Kuceba, I.; Shimazaki, Y.; Zylka, A.; Grabowska, K.; Sosnowski, M. NOx Emissions from Regenerator of Calcium Looping Process. *Energy Fuels* **2018**, *32*, 6355–6362. [CrossRef]

International Journal of
Environmental Research and Public Health

MDPI

Article

Spatial-Temporal Responses of Ecosystem Services to Land Use Transformation Driven by Rapid Urbanization: A Case Study of Hubei Province, China

Xufeng Cui, Cuicui Liu, Ling Shan, Jiaqi Lin, Jing Zhang, Yuehua Jiang * and Guanghong Zhang *

School of Business Administration, Zhongnan University of Economics and Law, Wuhan 430073, China; cxf@zuel.edu.cn (X.C.); lcc@stu.zuel.edu.cn (C.L.); shanling@stu.zuel.edu.cn (L.S.); linjiaqi@stu.zuel.edu.cn (J.L.); zjing@stu.zuel.edu.cn (J.Z.)
* Correspondence: jyh@stu.zuel.edu.cn (Y.J.); z0001297@zuel.edu.cn (G.Z.)

Abstract: Exploring the changes of ecosystem services value caused by land use transformation driven by urbanization is crucial for ensuring the safety of the regional ecological environment and for enhancing the value of ecosystem services. Based on the land use remote sensing data during the rapid urbanization development period of Hubei Province from 1995 to 2015, this study analyzed the characteristics of land use/land cover change and land use transformation. The spatial–temporal response characteristics and evolution of ecosystem services value (ESV) to land use transformation driven by urbanization were measured by equivalent factor method, spatial autocorrelation analysis, hot spot analysis and gravity model. We found that: (1) Driven by urbanization, the most significant feature of land use transformation in Hubei Province was the expansion of the built-up land and the significant reduction of cropland and forest, among which 90% of the new built-up land was converted from cropland and forest. (2) This land use transformation became the main source of ESV losses. Especially, the sharp increase of the built-up land from 2010 to 2015, occupying cropland and forest, resulted in ESV losses of nearly USD 320 million. The service capacity of climate regulation, soil conservation, gas regulation and food production undertaken by cropland and forest decreased. (3) The ecosystem services value in the study area showed spatial distribution characteristics of high in the west and low in the middle and east regions. The center of gravity of ESV shifted from northwest to southeast. Due to the sharp increase of the built-up land from 2010 to 2015, the center of gravity shift rebounded. This study can help policymakers better understand the trade−offs between land use transformation and ecosystem services driven by urbanization.

Keywords: urbanization; land use transformation; ecosystem services value; spatial autocorrelation; hot spot analysis; Hubei province; gravity model

Citation: Cui, X.; Liu, C.; Shan, L.; Lin, J.; Zhang, J.; Jiang, Y.; Zhang, G. Spatial-Temporal Responses of Ecosystem Services to Land Use Transformation Driven by Rapid Urbanization: A Case Study of Hubei Province, China. *Int. J. Environ. Res. Public Health* **2022**, *19*, 178. https://doi.org/10.3390/ijerph19010178

Academic Editor: Roberto Alonso González Lezcano

Received: 19 November 2021
Accepted: 22 December 2021
Published: 24 December 2021

1. Introduction

With the continuous development of the world economy, the process of global urbanization is accelerating. According to the Revised World Urbanization Prospects 2018, 55% of the world's population lives in cities, and this proportion will reach 68% by 2050 [1]. From 2015 to 2030, Asia and Africa will account for 90% of the global urban population growth (equivalent to 2.5 billion people), of which China, India and Nigeria will contribute 37% [2]. Unlike countries such as North America and Brazil, which have reached at least 80% urbanization level, most countries in Africa and Asia are experiencing rapid urbanization [3]. Rapid urbanization has brought qualitative changes to the economic, administrative, cultural and social aspects of cities, but it has also increased the pressure on the ecosystem and its components, such as natural resources environment and land use change [4]. For example, Brazil entered a period of rapid urbanization development in the 1950s, and the urbanization level increased from 36% in 1950 to 65% in 1980. However, with rapid urban development, economic, social and environmental problems also appeared, such as underemployment, urban disorder development and environmental pollution [5,6]. China has experienced the largest and fastest urbanization process. According to the data of China Bureau of statistics, the urbanization level has risen from 17.90% in 1978 to 63.89% in 2020. In this process, although the acceleration of urbanization promotes social and economic development [7], it also leads to irreversible changes in land use [7,8], mainly because the significant increase in urban land leads to a large amount of occupation of natural land such as cropland, wetland and grassland [9]. In recent decades, the pattern of land use/land cover in Mainland China has undergone significant changes [10], and urbanization is one of the most important reasons for this change.

Land use changes reflect the most direct interaction between human activities and ecosystems [11,12], and are therefore regarded as the main driving factor of ecological processes and ecosystem services [13]. Abundant research has confirmed a certain connection between land use/land cover change and ecosystem services [14,15]. For example, the replacement of forest and pasture land by cultivated land affects the soil regulation function of the ecosystem [16]. Land use change affects the food production function of the ecosystem [17–19]. The expansion of industrial and residential land has affected the water supply function of the ecosystem [20–22], resulting in water resource shortages [23]. Land use/land cover change can change the surface−atmosphere interaction in energy exchanged and have an additional effect on temperature, thus affecting the climate regulation function of ecosystem [24,25]. It also affects regional biodiversity at multiple scales and lead to changes in landscape structure [26–28]. These studies have proved that land use change causes changes in the structure and function of the ecosystem, thus changing the provision of ecosystem services.

Ecosystem services refer to the benefits obtained from ecosystems that directly or indirectly support human survival and development, including provisioning, regulation, supporting and cultural services, which are related to human life, health and well−being [29–31]. Since ecosystem services are crucial to maintaining the quality of human life, many scholars have devoted themselves to estimating and evaluating the value of ecosystem services. There are many methods to evaluate the value of ecosystem services, including monetary model, investment model [32,33], shadow engineering [34], matrix method [35], etc. Among them, the currency model evaluates the value of ecosystem services in monetary units from the perspective of economic benefits [36]. In 1997, based on the equilibrium value theory and effect to value theory, Costanza formulated the equivalent factor table of global ecosystem service value, determined the first global coefficient of ESV, and measured the ESV change caused by land use change in the perspective of monetary units [29]. On the basis of Costanza's results and a questionnaire of 500 Chinese ecologists, Chinese scholar Xie Gaodi determined the ESV equivalent factors suitable for China's terrestrial ecosystem, and based on China's national conditions through the biomass parameter tree equivalent factor table for multiple revisions to formulate "Chinese terrestrial ecosystem service value equivalent factor table" [37–39]. At present, measuring the impact of land use/cover change on the value of ecosystem services has become an important field of sustainable development science [40]. In recent years, many scholars have carried out extensive research on this in various regions, such as the world [41,42], Africa [43] OECD countries [44], Latin America and the Caribbean [45], China [46], Nigeria [14], Nepal [47], India [48], Lake Balaton in Central Europe [49], China's Hengduan Mountains [50], Qinghai−Tibet Plateau [51], the Middle Yangtze River City Group [52], Ethiopian Plateau [53], Coastal areas around the Bohai Sea [54]. These are enough to show that all regions in the world pay more and more attention to ecosystems. It is widely used to measure the health status of ecosystem through the value of ecosystem services.

In recent years, there has been considerable research on land use change and ecosystem services, which can be divided into two categories: The first type is based on different models, such as CLUE−S model [55], CA−Markov model [56], etc., based on land use conditions in different scenarios to predict the impact of future land use changes on the value of ecosystem services. These scenarios generally include three scenarios: natural growth scenario, economic development scenario, and ecological protection scenario. The other is to use land use and cover data to explore the temporal and spatial changes of the ecosystem and discover the factors that lead to this change. These factors are mostly natural and man−made factors [33,57–59] and policy factors [60]. The results of many scholars on the relationship between land use change and ecosystem services have enriched the research in the ES field. However, there are few studies on the impact of rapid urbanization on land use and ecosystem services. "Urbanization−Land Use Change−Ecosystem Services Value" is a coherent response process. In the region with rapid urbanization, this research is necessary to enhance the public's understanding of ecosystem service value and provide policy support for the government. The urbanization rate of Hubei province was 31.20% in 1995 and 56.85% in 2015. With an average annual growth rate of 1.28 percentage points in the past 20 years, the urbanization rate has increased by 25.65 percentage points, which is much faster than the urbanization development rate of developed countries and regions in Europe and the United States at the same stage. The rapid development of urbanization leads to urban expansion, non−agriculturalization of cropland, increase of transportation facilities, and reduction of lakes, all of which affect land use patterns and lead to land use/land cover change. How to assess the effects of these land use changes? The response to the value of its ecosystem services is an important evaluation path. Therefore, this research attempts: (1) To investigate the changes of LULC from 1995 to 2015 as the research basis and observe the characteristics of land use transformation in Hubei. (2) To measure the changes of ESV and ecosystem services in Hubei province from 1995 to 2015. (3) To explore the spatial response mode of ecosystem services value from the perspective of county. (4) In general, to reveal the response patterns of ecosystem services value to land use transformation driven by urbanization.

2. Materials and Methods

2.1. Study Area

Hubei province is located in central China, in the central of the Yangtze River basin, north of Dongting Lake (118°21′42″–116°07′50″ E, 29°01′53″–33°6′47″ N) and is rich in water resources. Administratively, the province has 12 prefecture−level cities, 1 autonomous prefecture, 26 county−level cities, 35 counties and 1 forest area, covering a total area of 185,900 km^2 (Figure 1). By 2020, the permanent population of Hubei had reached 59.27 million, an increase of 755,000 over 2015. Hubei province has developed industry, and equipment manufacturing industry is its important pillar industry. In recent years, it has paid attention to green environmental protection and vigorously developed tourism, low−carbon industry and the new energy industry. From the perspective of industrial structure, the proportion of tertiary industry has risen in recent years. Hubei has a variety of landforms, consisting of mountains, hills, plains and lakes. Because it is located in the transition zone of the second step to the third step of China's terrain, the terrain is high on three sides, and the middle is low and flat. Most of the region has a subtropical monsoon humid climate with an average annual temperature of 15°~17°and an average annual rainfall of 800~1600 mm. The superior natural geographical environment breeds and preserves rich and diverse biological communities, animal and plant resources, including many rare and endangered species and national key protected species. Among them, there are 1300 species of woody plants, many tree species, and precious and rare relict plants are preserved. Located in the Yangtze River basin, Hubei province has 206 species of fish [61]. The central and southern Jianghan Plain along the river is the economic center of Hubei province. The western and eastern parts of Hubei are mostly high mountains and large rivers. They are located around Hubei province with underdeveloped transportation and relatively backward economic development. During the study period, the urbanization rates in Hubei province increased from 31.20% to 56.85%. With the rapid development of urbanization in Hubei province, a series of ecological problems, such as the shortage of urban green space, environmental pollution, land shortage and biodiversity reduction, have emerged along with the transformation of land use [62].

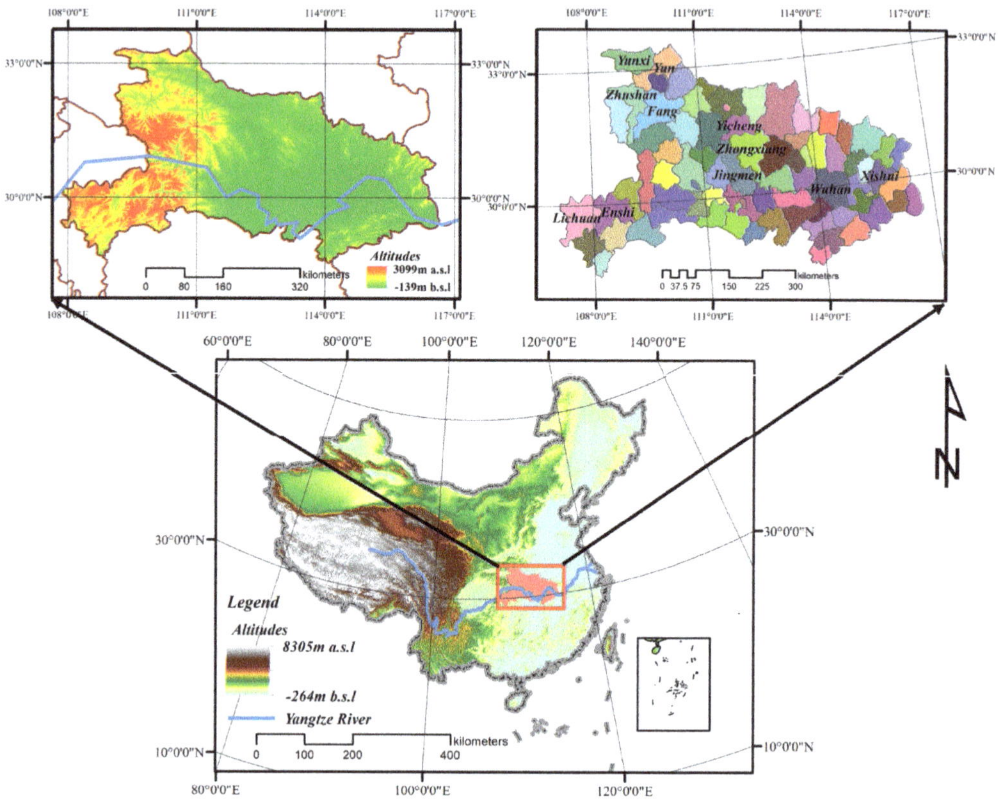

Figure 1. Location of Hubei, China. Note: Figure in top right shows the administrative area of Hubei Province. It consists of 77 administrative units, including 12 prefecture level cities, 1 Autonomous Prefecture, 26 county−level cities, 35 counties, 1 Autonomous County and 1 forest area.

2.2. Data Sources

This study used the LULC datasets from the 1995−2015 provided by the Data Center for Resources and Environmental Sciences of the Chinese Academy of Sciences (http://www.resdc.cn/, accessed on 15 December 2021). Using Landsat TM/ETM remote sensing images as the data source, the raster data onto national land use types of 1995, 2000, 2005, 2010 and 2015 with 1 km spatial resolution were generated by human–machine interactive interpretation. This paper adopted the LULC classification system and Xie Gaodi's [63] method of classifying terrestrial ecosystem in China, combines the land use characteristics of Hubei province, and divides the land use types into seven categories: cropland, forest land, grassland, water, wetland, bare land and built-up land, then adjusts and consolidates the secondary classification. The crop production, sown area and crop price data required for the study were obtained from the Hubei Statistical Yearbook 2016, the National Agricultural Product Price Survey Yearbook 2016, and the National Compilation of Information on Costs and Returns of Agricultural Products 2016.

2.3. Methods

2.3.1. Calculation of ESV

The ecosystem services classification method proposed by Costanza et al. cannot be directly applied to the calculation of ecosystem service value of China. This paper refers to the equivalent factor method and revised equivalent factor table based on Chinese ecosystem services [39], and modifies it by using grain yield correction and biomass correction methods in combination with the actual production capacity in Hubei province. With an average yield of 1 hm^2, 1/7 of the annual economic value of natural grain yields to cropland is a standard ecosystem service value equivalent factor [37].

The specific correction process is as follows: Select early rice, medium rice, late rice, japonica rice, wheat and corn as the main food crops. By consulting Hubei Statistical Yearbook in 2016 and the National Compilation of Information on Costs and Returns of Agricultural Products, the grain crops to yield, sown area and grain price and output value of Hubei province in 2015 are obtained. According to Formula (1), the equivalent value of a single ecosystem in Hubei province is 2516.20 CNY/hm^2. The ecosystem services value coefficients are shown below (Table 1).

$$E_n = \frac{1}{7}\sum_{i=1}^{n}\frac{q_i p_i}{M} \quad (1)$$

where E_n is the economic value (USD/hm^2) of 1 hm^2 ecosystem service value equivalent factor, i is the type of food crops in the study area; n is the total number of major food crops in the study area; p_i is the average price of the crop i in the study area. q_i is the average yield per unit area of type i food crop in the study area, and M is the total sown area of all food crops in the study area.

Table 1. Ecosystem services value coefficients per unit area in Hubei (USD·hm^{-2}·a^{-1}).

Top Level Ecosystem Services	Second Level of ES	Cropland	Forest	Grassland	Wetland	Bare Land	Water
Provisioning service	Food production	394.96	98.74	90.84	201.43	1.97	244.87
	Raw material produce	118.49	229.08	135.60	197.48	5.92	82.94
	Water supply	−31.60	118.49	75.04	1022.94	3.95	2812.10
Regulating service	Gas Regulation	185.63	753.38	476.58	750.42	25.67	339.66
	Climate regulation	142.18	2254.22	1259.92	1421.85	19.75	663.53
	Purifying Environment	43.45	660.57	416.02	1421.85	80.97	1129.58
	Hydrological Regulation	434.45	1475.17	922.89	9569.84	47.39	21,600.27
Supporting service	Soil conservation	233.03	917.29	580.59	912.35	29.62	185.63
	Maintaining nutrient supply	51.34	70.11	44.76	71.09	1.97	13.82
	Biodiversity	47.39	835.34	527.93	3108.32	27.65	1295.46
Cultural service	Aesthetic Landscape	23.70	366.32	233.03	1868.15	11.85	548.99
	A total of	1643.03	7778.70	4763.20	20,515.73	256.72	28,916.87

On this basis, according to the area of each land use type, the ecosystem services value of Hubei province can be calculated as follows [38,56]:

$$ESV = \sum A_i \times VC_i \quad (2)$$

$$ESV_f = \sum \left(A_i \times VC_{if}\right) \quad (3)$$

where ESV is the service value of the ecosystem in the study area, ESV_f represents the value of the service function for species f, and A_i is the area of type i land use type. VC_i is the ecosystem services value coefficient of type i land use type, and VC_{if} is the value of the fth ecological service function of the ith land use type.

2.3.2. Land Use Transfer Matrix

Land use transfer matrix is the application of Markov model in land use change. It can show the transfer direction and quantitative change of different land use types and reveal the evolution process of land use pattern. It comes from the quantitative description of system state and state transfer in system analysis. In Formula (4), $S_{(t)}$ is the system state at time t, $S_{(t+1)}$ is the system state at time t + 1, P_{ij} is the transition probability matrix in the state, and the calculation formula is as Formula (5) [64,65]:

$$S_{(t,t+1)} = P_{ij} \times S_{(t)} \tag{4}$$

$$P_{ij} = \begin{bmatrix} P_{11} & P_{12} & \cdots & P_{1n} \\ P_{21} & P_{22} & \cdots & P_{2n} \\ \vdots & \vdots & \vdots & \vdots \\ P_{n1} & P_{n2} & \cdots & P_{nn} \end{bmatrix} \left(0 \le P_{ij} \le 1\right) \tag{5}$$

where P is Markov probability matrix, P_{ij} represents the probability of transferring from the current state i to another state j in the next time period. The low conversion probability is close to 0 and the high conversion probability is close to 1.

In this research, after reclassifying the land use type grid data with ArcGIS10.2 software, import it into ENVI software, create ENVI standard classification format, edit the header file, and obtain the land use transfer matrix every 5 years through the Change Detection Statistics tool.

2.3.3. Spatial Autocorrelation Analysis

Spatial autocorrelation analysis aims to reveal the correlation and difference between the spatial distribution of a certain attribute and its neighboring regions. If the spatial correlation is positive, it indicates that the spatial distribution of the attribute has agglomeration effect. If the spatial correlation is negative, it indicates that the spatial distribution of the attribute value is significantly different. Spatial autocorrelation is divided into global spatial autocorrelation and local spatial autocorrelation. This study uses the global autocorrelation model to determine the spatial distribution pattern of ecosystem service value. The Global Moran's I index is usually used for this calculation, and the formula is as follows [66,67]:

$$I = \frac{\sum_{i=1}^{n}\sum_{j=1}^{n} W_{ij}(x_i - \overline{x})(x_j - \overline{x})}{S^2 \sum_{i=1}^{n}\sum_{j=1}^{n} W_{ij}},\ I \in [-1,\ 1] \tag{6}$$

where I is Moran index. x_i and x_j are the observed values of the ith evaluation unit and the jth ESV evaluation unit, respectively. W_{ij} is the spatial weight matrix between unit i and unit j. $\overline{x}$ is the mean of the observed values. n is the sample size, that is, the total number of ESV evaluation units at a certain scale in the study area. The Global Moran's I index is between −1 to 1. When the value is closer to −1, it indicates that the greater the difference between evaluation units, the stronger the negative correlation, and the more discrete the spatial distribution of ESV. When the Global Moran's I index value is closer to 1, it indicates that the attribute difference between evaluation units is smaller, the positive correlation is stronger, and the spatial distribution of ESV is more concentrated. When the Global Moran's I index value is close to 0, it indicates that there is no correlation between evaluation units, and the spatial distribution of ESV is random.

Hot spot analysis is a common tool to identify the spatial distribution of cold spots and hot spots. Using the Getis−Ord G^* index to analyze the local correlation between cold spots and hot spots can further study the local performance of the change of ecosystem service value in space. Hot spot analysis can determine whether there are high−value clusters (hot spots) and low−value clusters (cold spots) in the ecosystem service value of Hubei Province, as well as the spatial clustering positions of high−value and low−value regions [68]. By calculating the score Z (standard deviation) and probability P between each patch, the spatial location where the high−value elements and low−value elements gather [33].

$$G_i^* = \frac{\sum_{j=1}^{n} \omega_{ij} x_j - \overline{x}\sum_{j=1}^{n} \omega_{ij}}{S \times \sqrt{\frac{\left[n\sum_{j=1}^{n} \omega_{ij}^2 - \sum_{j=1}^{n} \omega_{ij}\right]^2}{n-1}}} \tag{7}$$

$$\overline{x} = \frac{\sum_{j=1}^{n} x_j}{n} \tag{8}$$

$$S = \sqrt{\frac{\sum_{j=1}^{n} x_j^2}{n-1} - \overline{x}^2} \tag{9}$$

x_j is plaque attribute value, and ω_{ij} is the spatial weight matrix between plaque i and plaque j. n is the total number of plaques; G_i^* is the Z score, and the Z score is a measure of statistical significance. The higher or the lower the value of G_i^*, the tighter the accumulation of hot spots or cold spots. When the ESV value is much larger than the adjacent area, a statistically significant hot spot is formed, which is called the hot spot area, that is, the area with high ESV change value. When the ESV value is much smaller than the adjacent area, a statistically significant cold spot will be formed, which is called the cold spot area, that is, the area with low ESV change value.

2.3.4. The Gravity Model

The gravity model is derived from physical concepts [69]. Later, it was widely used in trade [70], energy [71], transportation [72] and other fields. This research adopts the center of gravity shift model, which can intuitively reveal the spatial evolution characteristics of the center of gravity of ESV.

If the study area consists of n units (n represents administrative units), and (x_i, y_i) is the geometric coordinate of the ith unit (I = 1, 2, 3,..., n), then the barycenter coordinate of ESV is $(\overline{x}, \overline{y})$, it can be expressed as [73]:

$$\overline{x} = \frac{\sum_{i=1}^{n} m_i x_i}{\sum_{i=1}^{n} m_i} \tag{10}$$

$$\overline{y} = \frac{\sum_{i=1}^{n} m_i y_i}{\sum_{i=1}^{n} m_i} \tag{11}$$

The movement direction of the center of gravity can be expressed as:

$$\theta = \left[\frac{k \times \pi}{2} + \tan^{-1}\left(\frac{\overline{y_{t_2}} - \overline{y_{t_1}}}{\overline{x_{t_2}} - \overline{x_{t_1}}}\right)\right] \times \frac{180^\circ}{\pi} \tag{12}$$

The movement distance of the center of gravity is calculated by the following formula:

$$D = \sqrt{(\overline{x_{t_2}} - \overline{x_{t_1}})^2 + (\overline{y_{t_2}} - \overline{y_{t_1}})^2} \tag{13}$$

where θ represents the deflection angle of the center of gravity of ESV, (x_{t_1}, y_{t_1}) and (x_{t_2}, y_{t_2}) respectively represent the coordinates of the center of gravity at the beginning and end. t_1, t_2 represents the start time and end time, and k is the adjustment coefficient. D represents the moving distance of the center of gravity.

3. Results

3.1. Land Use Changes during the Period 1995–2015

After reclassifying land use sensing data of Hubei province in five periods from 1995 to 2015, the land use type distribution map is obtained (Figure 2). According to the results, from 1995 to 2015, forest land and cropland were the main land use types in Hubei province, and the built-up land mainly concentrated in Wuhan city and the center of each urban area in central Hubei province was in an inverted "herringbone" shape in the trend of water flow along the river at the center of Wuhan. There was an expanding trend toward wetland mainly along both sides of the Yangtze River and Han River. The water area was mainly distributed in the relatively flat Jianghan Plain.

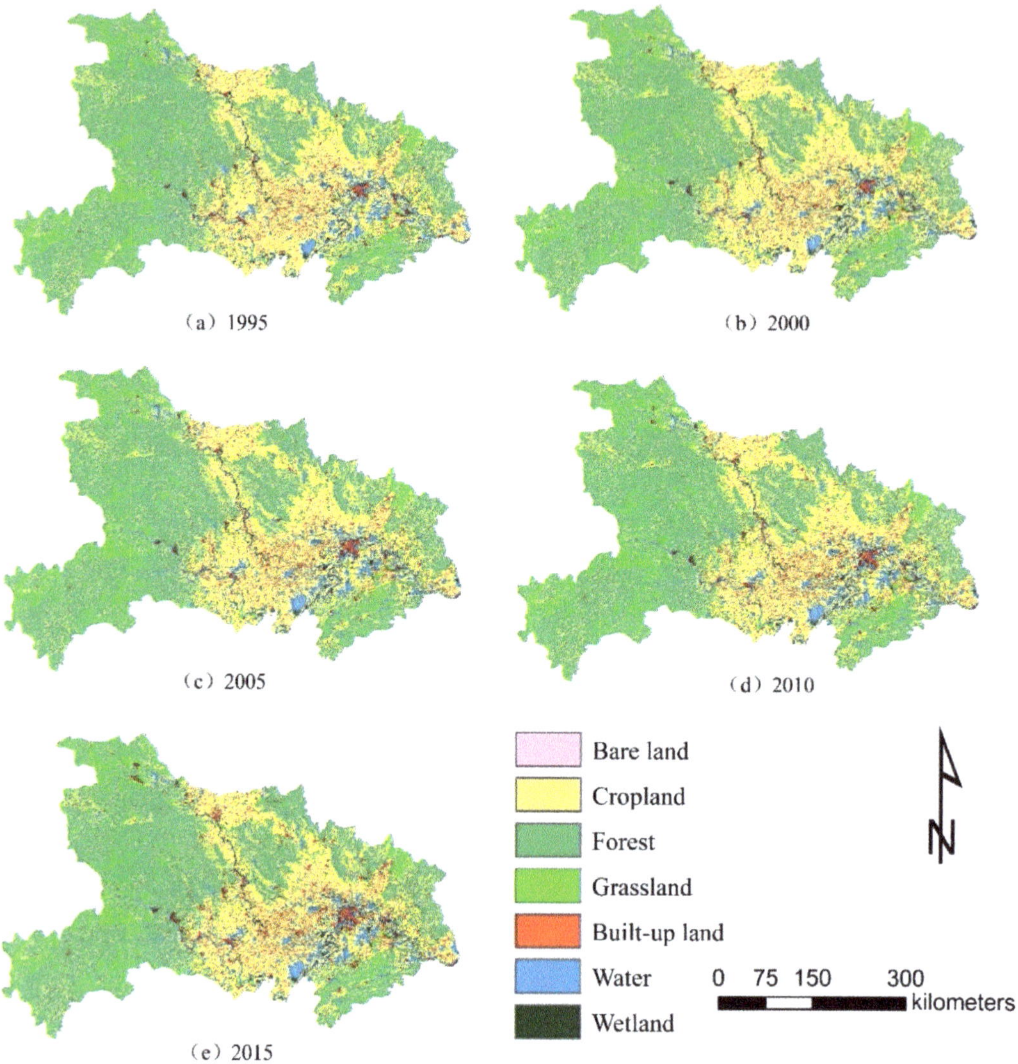

Figure 2. Land use change from 1995 to 2015.

The area and change of each land use type in the study area in five periods were obtained by zoning statistics of the reclassified data (Table 2). On the whole, the significant expansion of the built-up land and the reduction of cropland and forest were the most significant characteristics of land use change in Hubei province in the past 20 years. During the past 20 years, the area of the built-up land increased the most, which was 2148.49 km^2, and the area increased sharply from 2010 to 2015, accounting for more than 70% of the total increased area. The area of cropland decreased the most, reaching 2047.36 km^2, and the area decreased accounted for nearly 60% of the total area decreased from 2010 to 2015. Hubei province covered the largest area of forest, followed by cropland.

Table 2. Changes in the area of each category from 1995 to 2015.

Land Use Type	Periods	Cropland	Forest	Grassland	Water	Wetland	Bare Land	Built-Up
Area (km^2)	1995	69,066.83	93,458.77	7542.89	9797.99	1027.49	51.77	4954.25
	2000	69,425.60	92,660.73	7541.91	9619.07	1663.92	47.80	4940.98
	2005	68,603.72	92,591.53	7506.02	10,437.53	1513.55	46.80	5200.84
	2010	68,234.93	92,534.27	7486.07	10,435.48	1613.12	47.80	5548.33
	2015	67,019.47	92,167.33	7450.26	10,499.27	1612.13	48.79	7102.74
Area ratio (%)	1995	37.15	50.27	4.06	5.27	0.55	0.03	2.67
	2000	37.35	49.84	4.06	5.17	0.90	0.03	2.66
	2005	36.90	49.81	4.04	5.61	0.81	0.03	2.80
	2010	36.71	49.78	4.03	5.61	0.87	0.03	2.98
	2015	36.05	49.58	4.01	5.65	0.87	0.03	3.82
Variation (km^2)	1995–2000	358.76	−798.04	−0.98	−180.63	636.43	−3.98	−13.28
	2000–2005	−821.87	−69.20	−35.89	820.32	−150.37	−1.00	259.87
	2005–2010	−368.80	−57.25	−19.96	−2.00	99.57	1.00	347.49
	2010–2015	−1215.45	−366.94	−35.81	63.87	−0.99	1.00	1554.41
	1995–2015	−2047.36	−1291.43	−92.63	701.56	584.64	−2.98	2148.49
Rate of change (%)	1995–2000	0.52	−0.85	−0.01	−1.84	61.94	−7.68	−0.27
	2000–2005	−1.18	−0.07	−0.48	8.51	−9.04	−2.08	5.26
	2005–2010	−0.54	−0.06	−0.27	−0.02	6.58	2.13	6.68
	2010–2015	−1.78	−0.40	−0.48	0.61	−0.06	2.08	28.02
	1995–2015	−2.96	−1.38	−1.23	7.14	56.90	−5.76	43.37

According to the land use transfer matrix (Table 3) from 1995 to 2015, the characteristics of land use transformation in Hubei province were as follows: (1) From 1995 to 2015, the area of cropland and forest land eventually decreased. Cropland was mainly converted into forest land and the built-up land, with an area of 12,598.13 and 4323.12 km^2, respectively. Forest land was mainly converted into cropland and grassland, with an area of 12,996.31 and 3356.11 km^2, respectively. (2) Although water areas and wetlands had been developed and used for 20 years, they eventually increased. In terms of land use types occupied, waters occupied the largest area of cropland at 3450.73 km^2, and wetland also occupied the largest area of cropland at 526.92 km^2. The increase in the area of water areas and wetlands may be related to the policy of "returning farmland to lakes" implemented in the middle reaches of the Yangtze River. (3) The area of the built-up land had increased the most in 20 years, mainly occupying 4323.12 km^2 of cropland and 862.23 km^2 of forest land. The occupied land area was mainly used for urban construction. The built-up land was the land use type with the most thorough artificial transformation and the most affected by urbanization. The difference between the area transferred to the built-up land and the area transferred from the built-up land was the largest, which are 5729.23 and 3576.65 km^2, respectively. Therefore, the expansion of the built-up land was the most dramatic during the study period. The occupation of crop land and forest land while the expansion of the built-up land became a significant land use transformation feature in the period of rapid urbanization in Hubei Province. During the study period, with the rapid development of urbanization and the increase of urban and rural incomes, the demand for housing, travel and consumption has increased, and the proportion of secondary and tertiary industries in Hubei province has increased, which has promoted the occupation of urban and rural built-up land to cropland, forest land and other ecological land.

Table 3. Transition area matrix of LULC from 1995 to 2015 (km^2).

Land Use Type (km^2)		2015						
		Cropland	Forest	Grassland	Water	Wetland	Bare Land	Built-Up
1995	Cropland	47,475.51	12,598.13	743.47	3540.73	526.92	11.98	4323.12
	Forest	12,996.31	75,296.37	3356.11	1021.90	114.76	7.98	862.23
	Grassland	834.29	3307.21	3233.36	96.80	12.97	4.99	67.86
	Water	2687.48	802.35	99.80	5275.17	525.92	0.00	423.13
	Wetland	252.48	40.92	5.99	285.41	399.18	0.00	44.91
	Bare land	13.97	4.99	2.99	1.00	0.00	20.96	7.98
	Built−up	2903.04	311.36	22.95	300.38	35.93	2.99	1398.15

3.2. Temporal Response of Ecosystem Service Values to Land Use Change

3.2.1. Changes in Ecosystem Service Values of Different Land Use Types

Driven by the rapid urbanization development in Hubei province, land use transition has led to the fluctuation of ecosystem services value (Table 4). As a large amount of cropland and forest land were occupied by the built-up land expansion, the ecosystem services value of cropland and forest land showed a decreasing trend during the study period, in which the loss of forest land was the largest (USD 1.00 billion), and the loss of cropland was the largest (2.96%). From 1995 to 2015, the ESV of water area and wetland increased by USD 2.03 billion and 1.20 billion, respectively, with the largest increment of water area, but the largest increment of wetland, reaching 56.90%. Overall, the total value of ESV in Hubei province increased by USD 1.84 billion in 20 years, and the total ESV showed an increasing trend from 1995 to 2010. From 2010 to 2015, when the expansion of the built-up land invaded cropland and forest land was the most serious, the loss of ESV in Hubei province was nearly USD 320 million. The policy of returning cropland to lake in the middle reaches of the Yangtze River in 1998 may be responsible for the increase of ecosystem services value of water area and wetland, while the rapid development of urbanization may be responsible for the loss of ecosystem services value of cropland and forest land.

Table 4. ESVs for different land use types in Hubei Province from 1995 to 2015 (USD).

Ecosystem Type	Period	Cropland	Forest	Grassland	Water	Wetland	Bare Land	Total
ESV (Billion)	1995	11.35	72.70	3.59	28.33	2.11	0.00	118.08
	2000	11.41	72.08	3.59	27.82	3.42	0.00	118.31
	2005	11.27	72.02	3.58	30.18	3.11	0.00	120.16
	2010	11.21	71.98	3.57	30.18	3.31	0.00	120.25
	2015	11.01	71.69	3.55	30.36	3.31	0.00	119.93
ESV Variety (Billion)	1995–2000	0.06	−0.62	0.00	−0.52	1.31	0.00	0.23
	2000–2005	−0.14	−0.05	−0.02	2.37	−0.31	0.00	1.85
	2005–2010	−0.06	−0.04	−0.01	−0.01	0.20	0.00	0.08
	2010–2015	−0.20	−0.29	−0.02	0.18	0.00	0.00	−0.32
	1995–2015	−0.34	−1.00	−0.04	2.03	1.20	0.00	1.84

3.2.2. Changes in Individual Ecosystem Service Values

According to land use and land cover change and ESV coefficient, the contribution of each ecosystem function caused by land use transition to the overall ESV was investigated (Table 5). From the services value of each single ecosystem, hydrological regulation, climate regulation, soil conservation and biodiversity maintenance contribute the most to the overall ESV in the study area. Since 1995, with the rapid development of urbanization in Hubei province, the expansion of the built-up land has occupied a large number of cropland and forest land, and the problem of cropland conversion has intensified, which inevitably leads to the weakening of the ecosystem service function of cropland and forest land. From 2010 to 2015, food production, raw material production, climate regulation, gas regulation, soil conservation and nutrient supply, as the main ecosystem service functions of cropland and forest land, suffered losses to varying degrees, totaling USD 0.50 billion, accounting for the overall ESV losses of the main position. This indicated that the sharp decrease of cropland and forest land caused by rapid urbanization was the main source of ESV loss in the study area. From the perspective of the four service functions of the ecosystem, the largest loss was the regulation service, with a total loss of USD 270 million, followed by the supporting service, with a loss of USD 120 million, and the supply service had a relatively small loss, with a total loss of USD 110 million. In conclusion, the urbanization driven land use transition in Hubei province had the greatest impact on ecosystem regulation services, and the single ecosystem service function of the greatest impact was climate regulation. As the main ecosystem service function of waters and lakes, water supply and hydrological regulation have been increasing, with an increase of USD 250 million and 1790 million, respectively, in the past two decades. The temporal change of ecosystem services value is directly affected by land use transition. The drastic change of land use structure leads to the tightening of resources and environment in the study area, which breaks the balance of original ecosystem and leads to the decline in corresponding ecosystem service function of the region.

Table 5. ESVs for different functions in Hubei Province from 1995 to 2015 (USD).

Top Level Ecosystem Services	Second Level of ES	ESV (Billion)					ESV Variety				
		1995	2000	2005	2010	2015	95–00	00–05	05–10	10–15	95–15
Provisioning service	FP	3.98	3.99	3.98	3.96	3.91	0.01	−0.02	−0.01	−0.05	−0.07
	RMP	3.16	3.16	3.15	3.15	3.13	0.00	−0.01	0.00	−0.02	−0.04
	WS	3.81	3.81	4.03	4.04	4.05	0.00	0.22	0.01	0.02	0.25
Regulating service	GR	9.09	9.08	9.08	9.07	9.02	−0.01	−0.01	0.00	−0.05	−0.07
	CR	23.80	23.70	23.70	23.69	23.59	−0.10	0.00	−0.01	−0.10	−0.20
	PE	8.04	8.06	8.12	8.13	8.10	0.02	0.06	0.01	−0.02	0.06
	HR	39.63	39.75	41.33	41.39	41.42	0.12	1.57	0.06	0.03	1.79
Supporting service	SC	10.90	10.89	10.86	10.85	10.79	−0.01	−0.03	−0.01	−0.06	−0.11
	MNS	1.06	1.06	1.06	1.06	1.05	0.00	0.00	0.00	−0.01	−0.01
	MB	10.12	10.23	10.28	10.30	10.27	0.11	0.05	0.02	−0.03	0.15
Cultural service	AL	4.49	4.57	4.59	4.60	4.59	0.08	0.01	0.02	−0.01	0.09
	Total	118.08	118.31	120.16	120.25	119.93	0.23	1.85	0.08	−0.32	1.84

Note: FP, food production; RMP, raw material production; WS, water supply; GR, gas regulation; CR, climate regulation; PE, purifying environment; HR, hydrological regulation; SC, soil conservation; MNS, maintaining nutrient supply; MB, maintaining biodiversity; AL, aesthetic landscape.

3.3. Spatial Response of Ecosystem Service Values to Land Use Transformation

To explore the spatial response from ecosystem services value to land use transition, Global Moran's I statistic was used to measure spatial autocorrelation based on factor location and attribute to value. The spatial correlation of ecosystem services value in Hubei province in the past 20 years was analyzed. As shown in Figure 3, Moran's I values from 1995 to 2015 were greater than 0, and the county units in Hubei province were mostly in the first and third quadrants, indicating that there was a positive spatial correlation between ecosystem services value of Hubei province from 1995 to 2015. Spatial distribution had a certain spatial correlation and presented spatial aggregation distribution pattern.

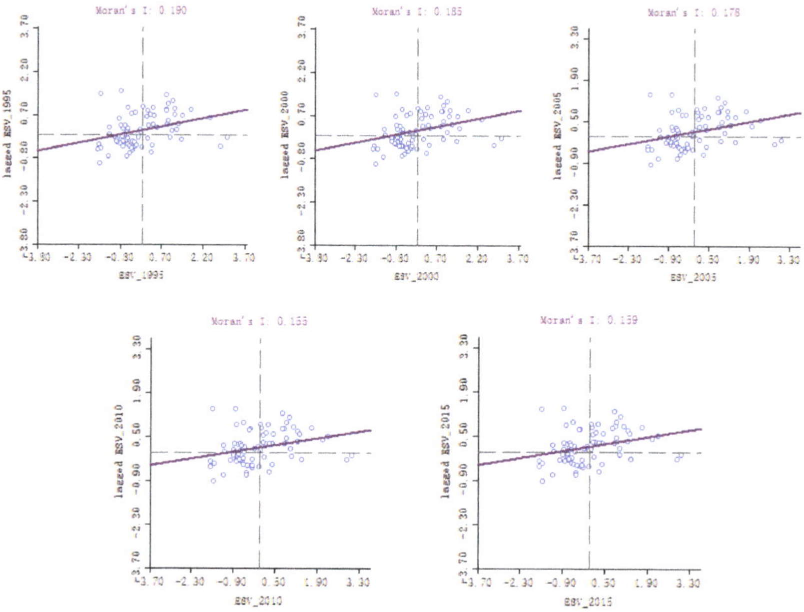

Figure 3. Global Moran's I in Hubei province from 1995 to 2015.

The hot spot analysis (Formula (7)–(9)) was used to reveal the local expression of the change of ecosystem service value in space. The hot spot analysis results (Figure 4) showed that the hot spots of ecosystem service value from 1995 to 2015 are mainly located in the western region where urbanization is relatively slow and rich in forest resources, and the distribution area is large and contiguous. Shennongjia Forestry District in the west was always a hot spot area with 99% confidence. The forest land in Shennongjia Forestry District accounts for more than 85%, the population is small, and the impact of human activities on the ecosystem is small. Fang County, Yun County, Zhushan County, Xingshan County in the northwest, and Lichuan County and Enshi City in the southwest were hot spots, with confidence levels greater than 90%, and they made a great contribution to the overall ESV. Most of these areas are mountainous areas with relatively high forest coverage and good ecosystem conditions. Xishui County in the east and Zhongxiang City and Yunmeng County in the middle were cold spots of ecosystem services value. During this period, the pace of urban construction in this area has accelerated, industry has developed rapidly, and construction land has expanded significantly.

From the number of cold spots and hot spots, from 1995 to 2005, the hot spots with 99% confidence and 95% confidence in Hubei Province decreased, and the cold spots did not change. From 2005 to 2015, the 95% confidence hot spots and 90% confidence hot spots in Hubei Province increased, and Jiangling and Gong'an counties with 90% confidence in the central region were no longer cold spots. Jiangling County and Gong'an County are close to the Yangtze River. During this period, the government paid attention to the prevention and control of water pollution and the protection of the ecological environment, so the ecosystem condition has improved. From the results of the hot spot analysis, in areas with slow urbanization development, the expansion of construction land is not obvious, and the original vegetation coverage is relatively high, so the ecosystem status is relatively stable. In addition, the Yangtze River passes through the territory of Hubei Province. Strengthening the protection of the Yangtze River will help the ecosystem in the Yangtze River Basin to improve.

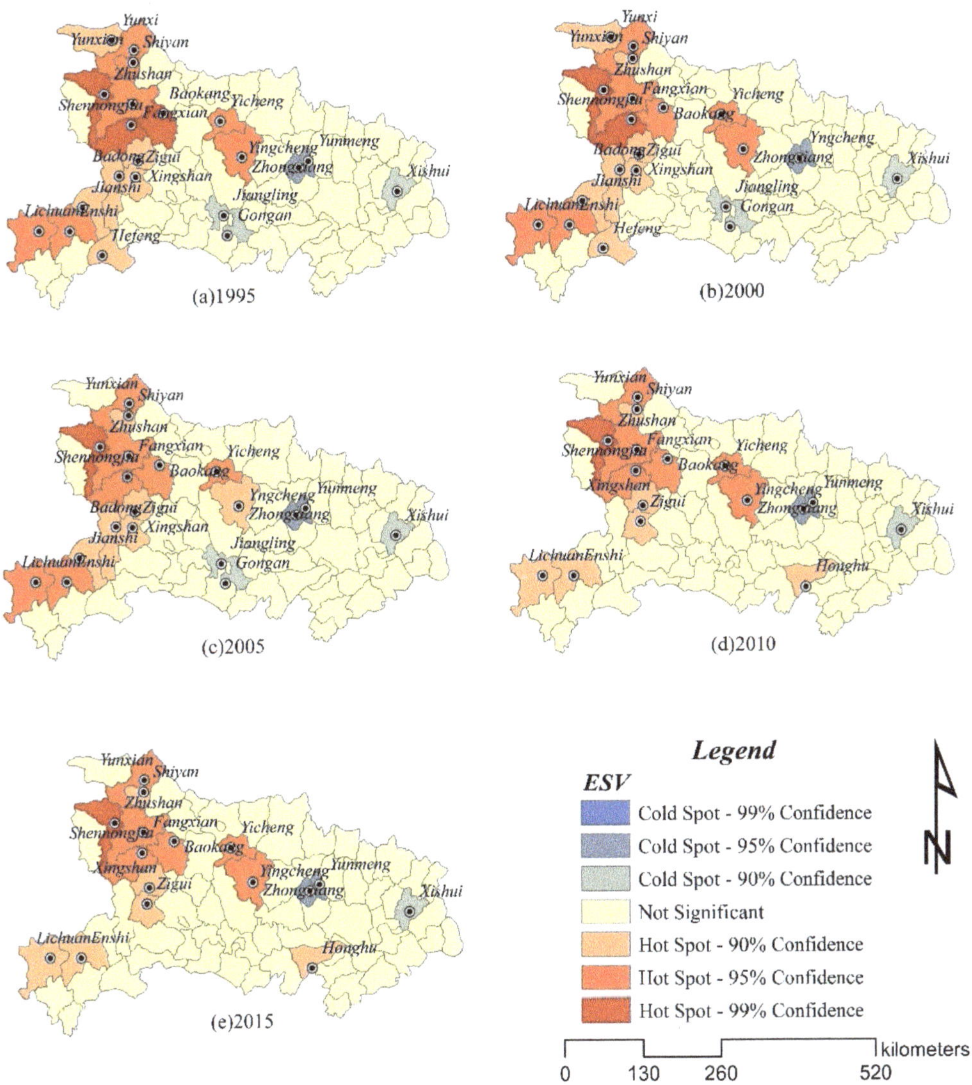

Figure 4. Hot spot analysis in Hubei province from 1995 to 2015.

The calculation of geographical gravity center can help to more accurately grasp the temporal and spatial pattern of ESV from a dynamic perspective. As shown in Figure 5, From 1995 to 2010, the gravity center of ESV shifted from northwest to southeast, with an offset angle of 23.5° and an offset distance of 5.099 km. From 2010 to 2015, the rapid development of urbanization in Hubei province led to a sharp decrease in cropland and forest land, which reduced the value of ecosystem services. The center of ecosystem services value shifted in the opposite direction, with an offset angle of 2.5°, but the deviation distance was not large. During the study period, the focus of ESV was within the boundary of Jingmen City. The results showed that the provision of ecosystem services in Hubei province showed a positive trend from 1995 to 2010, and the ecology in the eastern region was recovering. The ecosystem situation in Hubei province rebounded from 2010 to 2015, which was consistent with the change of ecosystem service values in Hubei province.

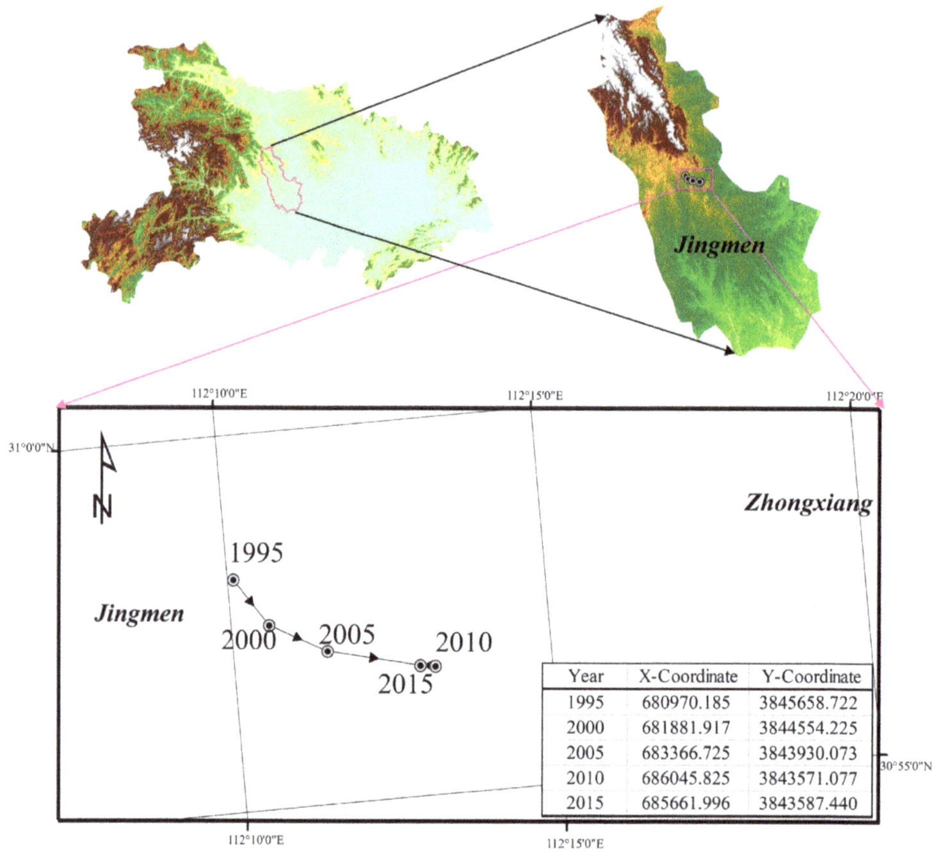

Figure 5. The trajectory of the center of gravity of ecosystem services value in Hubei province from 1995 to 2015.

4. Discussion

Under the background of rapid urbanization development in Hubei province, this study explored the characteristics of land use transformation by using land use transfer matrix and evaluated ESV of the study area. On this basis, the ways of ESV responding to land use transformation in time and space were analyzed. There has been much research on ESV responses to land use overturning changes, but little is known about ESV responses driven by rapid urbanization [33,60,74]. By constructing the analytical framework of "urbanization—land use transformation—ecosystem services value response", the study further simulates this "social economic—nature" process.

Hubei province, as an important part of China's key urban agglomeration—the middle reaches of the Yangtze River urban agglomeration, is a typical representative of China's rapid urbanization development. Under the background of rapid urbanization, a large number of labor force migrate to urban areas, regional economy develops rapidly, urban and rural income increases substantially, and demand for housing and consumption surges [75], thus promoting the occupation of urban and rural built-up land to cropland and forest land. The encroachment of the built-up land on cropland and forest land leads to the increase of the intensity and frequency of human activities' interference to the ecosystem, which directly threatens the service functions of the ecosystem [76,77]. These functions are mainly food production, climate regulation, soil conservation and so on.

As an ecological security barrier in the Shennongjia Forestry District in Hubei Province, lakes and waters in the Yangtze and Han River basins have made outstanding contributions to the overall ESV. Therefore, in future development planning, the background advantages of the ecosystem should be fully maintained and the negative impact of urbanization on land use transformation and the ecosystem should be weakened. The Yangtze River Protection Law just passed on 26 December 2020, is the first river basin law in China to protect the ecosystem of the whole Yangtze River Basin, which reflects the attention paid by the state and society to the ecological environment of the Yangtze River Basin. The tourism industry in Shennongjia Forestry District is relatively developed. While developing the tourism industry, we must always place "protecting ecological balance" first. Judging from the difference between the eastern, central and western parts of Hubei Province, the western part of Hubei Province is mostly mountainous areas, with relatively low levels of urbanization, high forest coverage, and high ecosystem security capabilities. Therefore, the ESV of each county is also high. From 1995 to 2015, the central region of Hubei Province accelerated urbanization, with rapid expansion of construction land, mostly in plain areas, with low forest coverage, so the average ESV in the central region was the lowest. The eastern region has the highest level of urbanization development, but the river system here is well−developed and contributes a lot to the overall ESV, so the average ESV in the eastern region is at a medium level. From the perspective of ESV hot spots, the distribution is relatively concentrated and the area is large in the past 20 years. Therefore, the synergistic effect of hot spots can be continued and enhanced, and ecological policies such as "encouraging social capital to participate in ecological protection and restoration policies" [78] and "ecological protection compensation policy" [79] can be used to further support the enhancement of local ecological effects. The main goal of cold spot development is to coordinate the contradiction between economic development and ecological protection. The level of urbanization in Hubei Province is still in the upgrading stage, and the built-up land is still in the expansion stage. It is a major challenge for Hubei province to ensure the economic development while maintaining the ecosystem service function and value. Hubei Province can rely on abundant higher education resources and combine its own scientific research advantages to provide intellectual support for enhancing the service functions of the ecosystem. When making plans, we should weigh various factors to avoid improper utilization of resources. We can incorporate the local index of "Ecosystem services value" into the local government performance assessment. For the cold spot area, we should first identify the reasons for the low ecosystem services value. Then, according to the degree of cropland occupied by the expansion of the built-up land, the degree of river pollution and whether the land layout is reasonable, formulate targeted plans, such as strictly controlling the building density, appropriately increasing the proportion of green space, increasing forest reserves, etc. Enhancing people's understanding of the relationship between with ecological environment and the ecological management of government departments [80] are of great significance for realizing regional sustainable development [81] and steadily improving the capability of ecosystem service assurance.

5. Conclusions

In this study, taking Hubei province in central China as the research area, we analyzed the characteristics of land use transformation driven by urbanization and the response of ecosystem service value to land use transformation from 1995 to 2015 at the county scale. The results showed that:

(1) Urbanization is an important inducement of land use transformation in Hubei province. From 1995 to 2015, with the continuous improvement of urbanization level in Hubei province, the land use structure changed constantly, and the continuous expansion of the built-up land occupying a large amount of cropland and forest land became the most significant feature of land use transformation. In addition, affected by the policy of "returning farmland to lakes" in the Yangtze River Basin, the area of water area and wetland increased during the study period, second only to construction land.

(2) The spatial and temporal distribution pattern and evolution of ecosystem services value are directly affected by land use transformation. During the study period, the value of ecosystem services in Hubei province increased from USD 118.08 billion in 1995 to USD 119.93 billion in 2015, showing an overall trend of growth. However, from 2010 to 2015, a large number of cropland and forest land in the study area were transformed into the built-up land, resulting in a total ESV loss of USD 480 million for food production, raw material production, climate regulation, gas regulation, soil conservation and other single ecological functions, which became the main reason for the ESV loss in the study area. Therefore, paying close attention to the development trend of urbanization and relevant policies, timely optimizing the land use structure and controlling the area of ecological land occupied by construction land is the focus of the work of relevant government departments in the future. The well−developed water system in Hubei province and the rich forest resources in the west have contributed greatly to the overall ESV of Hubei province. Strengthening the protection of the forest areas in the west and the waters of the Yangtze River and Han River is of great significance to maintaining the stability of the ecosystem service value in Hubei province.

(3) Affected by rapid urbanization and land use changes, the ecosystem services value in Hubei province was high in the west and low in the middle and the east. The hot spots were mainly concentrated in the western regions with slow urbanization development and high vegetation coverage, while the cold spots were mainly distributed in the central regions with strong interference from human activities. In the last five years, when the expansion of the built-up land was the most drastic, the center of gravity of ESV broke the original deviation direction, showing a rebound of migration. Using a variety of spatial analysis methods to analyze the development trend and spatial characteristics of ecosystem services value can help us formulate differentiation policies according to the actual situation of different regions, so as to help the local improve the ecological environment and enhance the ecosystem services value. In general, the response of ecosystem services value to land use transformation is the result of the interaction and synergistic development of the complex system of "society−economy−nature" driven by urbanization.

Author Contributions: Conceptualization, X.C.; Data curation, C.L.; Funding acquisition, G.Z.; Investigation, L.S., J.L., J.Z., and Y.J.; Methodology, C.L.; Project administration, X.C.; Supervision, G.Z.; Visualization, L.S.; Writing—original draft, C.L.; Writing—review and editing, X.C., L.S., J.L., J.Z., and Y.J. All authors have read and agreed to the published version of the manuscript.

Funding: National Social Science Foundation of China: 16BGL154; China Postdoctoral Science Foundation: 2019M651885; Project of Graduate Teaching and Education Reform (High−quality Teaching Cases), Zhongnan University of Economics and Law: JXAL202104.

Institutional Review Board Statement: Not applicable.

Informed Consent Statement: Not applicable.

Data Availability Statement: All data generated or analyzed during this study are included in this published article.

Conflicts of Interest: The authors declare no conflict of interest.

References

1. 2018 Revision of World Urbanization Prospects. Available online: https://www.un.org/development/desa/publications/2018$-$revision$-$of$-$world$-$urbanization$-$prospects.html (accessed on 15 December 2021).
2. World Development Indicators 2016: Featuring the Sustainable Development Goals. Available online: https://openknowledge.worldbank.org/bitstream/handle/10986/23969/9781464806834.pdf (accessed on 15 December 2021).
3. Abubakar, I.R. Predictors of Inequalities in Land Ownership among Nigerian Households: Implications for Sustainable Development. *Land Use Pol.* **2021**, *101*, 105194. [CrossRef]
4. Izakovičová, Z.; Mederly, P.; Petrovič, F. Long-Term Land Use Changes Driven by Urbanisation and Their Environmental Effects (Example of Trnava City, Slovakia). *Sustainability* **2017**, *9*, 1553. [CrossRef]
5. Ahmed, Z.; Le, H.P.; Shahzad, S.J.H. Toward Environmental Sustainability: How Do Urbanization, Economic Growth, and Industrialization Affect Biocapacity in Brazil? *Environ. Dev. Sustain.* **2021**. [CrossRef]

6. Shen, L.; Shuai, C.; Jiao, L.; Tan, Y.; Song, X. Dynamic Sustainability Performance during Urbanization Process between BRICS Countries. *Habitat Int.* **2017**, *60*, 19–33. [CrossRef]
7. Luo, Q.L.; Zhou, J.F.; Li, Z.G.; Yu, B.L. Spatial Differences of Ecosystem Services and Their Driving Factors: A Comparation Analysis among Three Urban Agglomerations in China's Yangtze River Economic Belt. *Sci. Total Environ.* **2020**, *725*, 138452. [CrossRef] [PubMed]
8. Deng, S.L. Exploring the Relationship between New−Type Urbanization and Sustainable Urban Land Use: Evidence from Prefecture−Level Cities in China. *Sustain. Comput. Inform. Syst.* **2020**, *30*, 100446. [CrossRef]
9. Hassan, M.M. Monitoring Land Use/Land Cover Change, Urban Growth Dynamics and Landscape Pattern Analysis in Five Fastest Urbanized Cities in Bangladesh. *Remote Sens. Appl. Soc. Environ.* **2017**, *7*, 69–83. [CrossRef]
10. Li, J.; Wang, Z.L.; Lai, C.G.; Wu, X.Q.; Zeng, Z.Y.; Chen, X.H.; Lang, Y.Q. Response of Net Primary Production to Land Use and Land Cover Change in Mainland China since the Late 1980s. *Sci. Total Environ.* **2018**, *639*, 237–247. [CrossRef]
11. Fu, B.L.; Li, Y.; Wang, Y.Q.; Zhang, B.; Yin, S.B.; Zhu, H.L.; Xing, Z.F. Evaluation of Ecosystem Service Value of Riparian Zone Using Land Use Data from 1986 to 2012. *Ecol. Indic.* **2016**, *69*, 873–881. [CrossRef]
12. Kusi, K.K.; Khattabi, A.; Mhammdi, N.; Lahssini, S. Prospective Evaluation of the Impact of Land Use Change on Ecosystem Services in the Ourika Watershed, Morocco. *Land Use Policy* **2020**, *97*, 104796. [CrossRef]
13. Liang, J.; Li, S.; Li, X.D.; Li, X.; Liu, Q.; Meng, Q.; Lin, A.; Li, J. Trade-off Analyses and Optimization of Water−Related Ecosystem Services (WRESs) Based on Land Use Change in a Typical Agricultural Watershed, Southern China. *J. Clean. Prod.* **2021**, *279*, 123851. [CrossRef]
14. Arowolo, A.O.; Deng, X.; Olatunji, O.A.; Obayelu, A.E. Assessing Changes in the Value of Ecosystem Services in Response to Land−Use/Land−Cover Dynamics in Nigeria. *Sci. Total Environ.* **2018**, *636*, 597–609. [CrossRef]
15. Talukdar, S.; Singha, P.; Shahfahad; Mahato, S.; Praveen, B.; Rahman, A. Dynamics of Ecosystem Services (ESs) in Response to Land Use Land Cover (LU/LC) Changes in the Lower Gangetic Plain of India. *Ecol. Indic.* **2020**, *112*, 106121. [CrossRef]
16. Aneseyee, A.B.; Elias, E.; Soromessa, T.; Feyisa, G.L. Land Use/Land Cover Change Effect on Soil Erosion and Sediment Delivery in the Winike Watershed, Omo Gibe Basin, Ethiopia. *Sci. Total Environ.* **2020**, *728*, 138776. [CrossRef] [PubMed]
17. Rutten, M.; van Dijk, M.; van Rooij, W.; Hilderink, H. Land Use Dynamics, Climate Change, and Food Security in Vietnam: A Global−to−Local Modeling Approach. *World Dev.* **2014**, *59*, 29–46. [CrossRef]
18. Sun, Z.D.; Lotz, T.; Chang, N.-B. Assessing the Long-Term Effects of Land Use Changes on Runoff Patterns and Food Production in a Large Lake Watershed with Policy Implications. *J. Environ. Manag.* **2017**, *204*, 92–101. [CrossRef] [PubMed]
19. Vliet, J.V.; Eitelberg, D.A.; Verburg, P.H. A Global Analysis of Land Take in Cropland Areas and Production Displacement from Urbanization. *Glob. Environ. Chang.* **2017**, *43*, 107–115. [CrossRef]
20. Bhattacharya, R.K.; Chatterjee, N.D.; Das, K. An Integrated GIS Approach to Analyze the Impact of Land Use Change and Land Cover Alteration on Ground Water Potential Level: A Study in Kangsabati Basin, India. *Groundw. Sustain. Dev.* **2020**, *11*, 100399. [CrossRef]
21. Huang, Y.N.; Chang, Q.R.; Li, Z. Land Use Change Impacts on the Amount and Quality of Recharge Water in the Loess Tablelands of China. *Sci. Total Environ.* **2018**, *628–629*, 443–452. [CrossRef]
22. Bonansea, M.; Bazán, R.; Germán, A.; Ferral, A.; Beltramone, G.; Cossavella, A.; Pinotti, L. Assessing Land Use and Land Cover Change in Los Molinos Reservoir Watershed and the Effect on the Reservoir Water Quality. *J. South Am. Earth Sci.* **2021**, *108*, 103243. [CrossRef]
23. Mirzaei, M.; Jafari, A.; Verrlest, J.; Haghighi, M.; Zargarnia, A.H.; Khoshnoodmotlagh, S.; Azadi, H.; Scheffran, J. Trans-Boundary Land Cover Changes and Its Influences on Water Crisis: Case Study of the Aras River. *Appl. Geogr.* **2020**, *124*, 102323. [CrossRef]
24. Dissanayake, S.; Asafu−Adjaye, J.; Mahadeva, R. Addressing Climate Change Cause and Effect on Land Cover and Land Use in South Asia. *Land Use Policy* **2017**, *67*, 352–366. [CrossRef]
25. Li, D.; Tian, P.P.; Luo, H.Y.; Hu, T.S.; Dong, B.; Cui, Y.; Khan, S.; Luo, Y. Impacts of Land Use and Land Cover Changes on Regional Climate in the Lhasa River Basin, Tibetan Plateau. *Sci. Total Environ.* **2020**, *742*, 140570. [CrossRef] [PubMed]
26. Tóth, R.; Czeglédi, I.; Kern, B.; Erős, T. Land Use Effects in Riverscapes: Diversity and Environmental Drivers of Stream Fish Communities in Protected, Agricultural and Urban Landscapes. *Ecol. Indic.* **2019**, *101*, 742–748. [CrossRef]
27. Baude, M.; Meyer, B.C.; Schindewolf, M. Land Use Change in an Agricultural Landscape Causing Degradation of Soil Based Ecosystem Services. *Sci. Total Environ.* **2019**, *659*, 1526–1536. [CrossRef] [PubMed]
28. Lira, P.K.; Tambosi, L.R.; Ewers, R.M.; Metzger, J.P. Land-Use and Land-Cover Change in Atlantic Forest Landscapes. *For. Ecol. Manag.* **2012**, *278*, 80–89. [CrossRef]
29. Costanza, R.; d'Arge, R.; de Groot, R.; Farber, S.; Grasso, M.; Hannon, B.; Limburg, K.; Naeem, S.; O'Neill, R.V.; Paruelo, J.; et al. The Value of the World's Ecosystem Services and Natural Capital. *Nature* **1997**, *387*, 253–260. [CrossRef]
30. Millennium Ecosystem Assesment Ecosystems and Human Well−Being: Synthesis. *Phys. Teach.* **2005**, *34*, 534.
31. The Economics of Ecosystems and Biodiversity: Mainstreaming the Economics of Nature—A Synthesis of the Approach, Conclusions and Recommendations of TEEB. Available online: http://teebweb.org/publications/teeb$-$for/synthesis/ (accessed on 12 May 2021).
32. Clerici, N.; Cote Navarro, F.; Escobedo, F.J.; Rubiano, K.; Villegas, J.C. Spatio-Temporal and Cumulative Effects of Land Use-Land Cover and Climate Change on Two Ecosystem Services in the Colombian Andes. *Sci. Total Environ.* **2019**, *685*, 1181–1192. [CrossRef]

33. Hu, M.; Li, Z.; Wang, Y.; Jiao, M.; Li, M.; Xia, B. Spatio-Temporal Changes in Ecosystem Service Value in Response to Land-Use/Cover Changes in the Pearl River Delta. *Resour. Conserv. Recycl.* **2019**, *149*, 106–114. [CrossRef]
34. Huang, A.; Xu, Y.Q.; Sun, P.L.; Zhou, G.Y.; Liu, C.; Lu, L.; Xiang, Y.; Wang, H. Land Use/Land Cover Changes and Its Impact on Ecosystem Services in Ecologically Fragile Zone: A Case Study of Zhangjiakou City, Hebei Province, China. *Ecol. Indic.* **2019**, *104*, 604–614. [CrossRef]
35. Juanita, A.D.; Ignacio, P.; Jorgelina, G.A.; Cecilia, A.S.; Carlos, M.; Francisco, N. Assessing the Effects of Past and Future Land Cover Changes in Ecosystem Services, Disservices and Biodiversity: A Case Study in Barranquilla Metropolitan Area (BMA), Colombia. *Ecosyst. Serv.* **2019**, *37*, 100915. [CrossRef]
36. Groot, R.D.; Brander, L.; Ploeg, S.V.D.; Costanza, R.; Bernard, F.; Braat, L.; Christie, M.; Crossman, N.; Ghermandi, A.; Hein, L.; et al. Global Estimates of the Value of Ecosystems and Their Services in Monetary Units. *Ecosyst. Serv.* **2012**, *1*, 50–61. [CrossRef]
37. Xie, G.D.; Lu, C.X.; Leng, Y.F.; Zheng, D.; Li, S.C. Ecological Assets Valuation of the Tibetan Plateau. *J. Nat. Resour.* **2003**, *18*, 189–196.
38. Xie, G.D.; Zhen, L.; Chun−Xia, L.U.; Xiao, Y.; Chen, C. Expert Knowledge Based Valuation Method of Ecosystem Services in China. *J. Nat. Resour.* **2008**, *23*, 911–919.
39. Xie, G.D.; Zhang, C.X.; Zhen, L.; Zhang, L.M. Dynamic Changes in the Value of China's Ecosystem Services. *Ecosyst. Serv.* **2017**, *26*, 146–154. [CrossRef]
40. Liu, W.; Zhan, J.; Zhao, F.; Yan, H.; Zhang, F.; Wei, X. Impacts of Urbanization-Induced Land-Use Changes on Ecosystem Services: A Case Study of the Pearl River Delta Metropolitan Region, China. *Ecol. Indic.* **2019**, *98*, 228–238. [CrossRef]
41. Song, X.P. Global Estimates of Ecosystem Service Value and Change: Taking Into Account Uncertainties in Satellite−Based Land Cover Data. *Ecol. Econ.* **2018**, *143*, 227–235. [CrossRef]
42. Costanza, R.; d'Arge, R.; de Groot, R.; Farber, S.; Grasso, M.; Hannon, B.; Limburg, K.; Naeem, S.; O'Neill, R.V.; Paruelo, J.; et al. The Value of the World's Ecosystem Services and Natural Capital. *Ecol. Econ.* **1998**, *25*, 3–15. [CrossRef]
43. Fenta, A.A.; Tsunekawa, A.; Haregeweyn, N.; Tsubo, M.; Yasuda, H.; Shimizu, K.; Kawai, T.; Ebabu, K.; Berihun, M.L.; Sultan, D.; et al. Cropland Expansion Outweighs the Monetary Effect of Declining Natural Vegetation on Ecosystem Services in Sub-Saharan Africa. *Ecosyst. Serv.* **2020**, *45*, 101154. [CrossRef]
44. Niccolucci, V.; Coscieme, L.; Marchettini, N. Benefit Transfer and the Economic Value of Biocapacity: Introducing the Ecosystem Service Yield Factor. *Ecosyst. Serv.* **2021**, *48*, 101256. [CrossRef]
45. Hernández−Blanco, M.; Costanza, R.; Anderson, S.; Kubiszewski, I.; Sutton, P. Future Scenarios for the Value of Ecosystem Services in Latin America and the Caribbean to 2050. *Curr. Res. Environ. Sustain.* **2020**, *2*, 100008. [CrossRef]
46. Li, G.; Fang, C.; Wang, S. Exploring Spatiotemporal Changes in Ecosystem-Service Values and Hotspots in China. *Sci. Total Environ.* **2016**, *545–546*, 609–620. [CrossRef] [PubMed]
47. Rimal, B.; Sharma, R.; Kunwar, R.; Keshtkar, H.; Stork, N.E.; Rijal, S.; Rahman, S.A.; Baral, H. Effects of Land Use and Land Cover Change on Ecosystem Services in the Koshi River Basin, Eastern Nepal. *Ecosyst. Serv.* **2019**, *38*, 100963. [CrossRef]
48. Sannigrahi, S.; Pilla, F.; Zhang, Q.; Chakraborti, S.; Wang, Y.; Basu, B.; Basu, A.S.; Joshi, P.K.; Keesstra, S.; Roy, P.S.; et al. Examining the Effects of Green Revolution Led Agricultural Expansion on Net Ecosystem Service Values in India Using Multiple Valuation Approaches. *J. Environ. Manag.* **2021**, *277*, 111381. [CrossRef]
49. Kertész, Á.; Nagy, L.A.; Balázs, B. Effect of Land Use Change on Ecosystem Services in Lake Balaton Catchment. *Land Use Policy* **2019**, *80*, 430–438. [CrossRef]
50. Wang, Y.; Dai, E.; Yin, L.; Ma, L. Land Use/Land Cover Change and the Effects on Ecosystem Services in the Hengduan Mountain Region, China. *Ecosyst. Serv.* **2018**, *34*, 55–67. [CrossRef]
51. Jiang, W.; Lü, Y.H.; Liu, Y.X.; Gao, W.W. Ecosystem Service Value of the Qinghai−Tibet Plateau Significantly Increased during 25 Years. *Ecosyst. Serv.* **2020**, *44*, 101146. [CrossRef]
52. Dai, X.; Wang, L.C.; Huang, C.B.; Fang, L.L.; Wang, S.Q.; Wang, L.Z. Spatio-Temporal Variations of Ecosystem Services in the Urban Agglomerations in the Middle Reaches of the Yangtze River, China. *Ecol. Indic.* **2020**, *115*, 106394. [CrossRef]
53. Kindu, M.; Schneider, T.; Teketay, D.; Knoke, T. Changes of Ecosystem Service Values in Response to Land Use/Land Cover Dynamics in Munessa–Shashemene Landscape of the Ethiopian Highlands. *Sci. Total Environ.* **2016**, *547*, 137–147. [CrossRef] [PubMed]
54. Liu, Y.B.; Hou, X.Y.; Li, X.W.; Song, B.Y.; Wang, C. Assessing and Predicting Changes in Ecosystem Service Values Based on Land Use/Cover Change in the Bohai Rim Coastal Zone. *Ecol. Indic.* **2020**, *111*, 106004. [CrossRef]
55. Peng, K.; Jiang, W.; Ling, Z.; Hou, P.; Deng, Y. Evaluating the Potential Impacts of Land Use Changes on Ecosystem Service Value under Multiple Scenarios in Support of SDG Reporting: A Case Study of the Wuhan Urban Agglomeration. *J. Clean. Prod.* **2021**, *307*, 127321. [CrossRef]
56. Akhtar, M.; Zhao, Y.Y.; Gao, G.L.; Gulzar, Q.; Hussain, A.; Samie, A. Assessment of Ecosystem Services Value in Response to Prevailing and Future Land Use/Cover Changes in Lahore, Pakistan. *Reg. Sustain.* **2020**, *1*, 37–47. [CrossRef]
57. Solomon, N.; Segnon, A.C.; Birhane, E. Ecosystem Service Values Changes in Response to Land-Use/Land-Cover Dynamics in Dry Afromontane Forest in Northern Ethiopia. *Int. J. Environ. Res. Public Health* **2019**, *16*, 4653. [CrossRef] [PubMed]
58. Li, Y.; Feng, Y.; Guo, X.; Peng, F. Changes in Coastal City Ecosystem Service Values Based on Land Use—A Case Study of Yingkou, China. *Land Use Policy* **2017**, *65*, 287–293. [CrossRef]

59. Tolessa, T.; Kidane, M.; Bezie, A. Assessment of the Linkages between Ecosystem Service Provision and Land Use/Land Cover Change in Fincha Watershed, North-Western Ethiopia. *Heliyon* **2021**, *7*, e07673. [CrossRef] [PubMed]
60. Yuan, K.; Li, F.; Yang, H.; Wang, Y. The Influence of Land Use Change on Ecosystem Service Value in Shangzhou District. *Int. J. Environ. Res. Public Health* **2019**, *16*, 1321. [CrossRef]
61. Natural Conditions. Available online: http://www.hubei.gov.cn/jmct/hbgk/202108/t20210831_3730730.shtml (accessed on 12 May 2021).
62. Jin, G.; Wu, F.; Li, Z.H.; Guo, B.S.; Zhao, X.D. Estimation and analysis of land use and ecological efficiency in rapid urbanization area. *Acta Ecol. Sin.* **2017**, *37*, 8048–8057.
63. Xie, G.D.; Zhang, C.X.; Zhang, L.M.; Chen, W.H.; Li, S.M. Improvement of the Evaluation Method for Ecosystem Service Value Based on Per Unit Area. *J. Nat. Resour.* **2015**, *30*, 1243–1254.
64. Ghalehteimouri, K.J.; Shamsodini, A.; Mousavi, M.N.; Ros, F.B.C.; Khedmatzadeh, A. Predicting Spatial and Decadal of Land Use and Land Cover Change Using Integrated Cellular Automata Markov Chain Model Based Scenarios (2019–2049) Zarriné–Rūd River Basin in Iran. *Environ. Chall.* **2021**, 100399. [CrossRef]
65. Dey, N.N.; Rakib, A.A.; Kafy, A.A.; Raikwar, V. Geospatial Modelling of Changes in Land Use/Land Cover Dynamics Using Multi-Layer Perception Markov Chain Model in Rajshahi City, Bangladesh. *Environ. Chall.* **2021**, *4*, 100148. [CrossRef]
66. Liu, J.P.; Guo, Q.B. A Spatial Panel Statistical Analysis on Cultivated Land Conversion and Chinese Economic Growth. *Ecol. Indic.* **2015**, *51*, 20–24. [CrossRef]
67. Cui, X.; Huang, S.; Liu, C.; Zhou, T.; Shan, L.; Zhang, F.; Chen, M.; Li, F.; de Vries, W.T. Applying SBM-GPA Model to Explore Urban Land Use Efficiency Considering Ecological Development in China. *Land* **2021**, *10*, 912. [CrossRef]
68. Gao, X.; Yang, L.; Li, C.; Song, Z.; Wang, J. Land use change and ecosystem service value measurement in Baiyangdian Basin under the simulated multiple scenarios. *Acta Ecol. Sin.* **2021**, *41*, 7974–7988.
69. Zhang, X.; Geng, Y.; Tong, Y.W.; Kua, H.W.; Tian, X.; Wu, R.; Zhao, X.; Chiu, A.S.F. Spatial Characteristics and Its Driving Factors of Low-Carbon Energy Technology Innovation in China: A Gravity Movement and Exploratory Spatial Data Analysis. *J. Clean. Prod.* **2021**, *295*, 126481. [CrossRef]
70. Freeman, R.; Lewis, J. Gravity Model Estimates of the Spatial Determinants of Trade, Migration, and Trade-and-Migration Policies. *Econ. Lett.* **2021**, *204*, 109873. [CrossRef]
71. Zhang, G.L.; Zhang, N.; Liao, W.M. How Do Population and Land Urbanization Affect CO2 Emissions under Gravity Center Change? A Spatial Econometric Analysis. *J. Clean. Prod.* **2018**, *202*, 510–523. [CrossRef]
72. Thompson, C.A.; Saxberg, K.; Lega, J.; Tong, D.; Brown, H.E. A Cumulative Gravity Model for Inter-Urban Spatial Interaction at Different Scales. *J. Transp. Geogr.* **2019**, *79*, 102461. [CrossRef]
73. Chai, J.; Wang, Z.Q.; Yang, J.; Zhang, L.G. Analysis for Spatial-Temporal Changes of Grain Production and Farmland Resource: Evidence from Hubei Province, Central China. *J. Clean. Prod.* **2019**, *207*, 474–482. [CrossRef]
74. Zhou, J.; Sun, L.; Zang, S.Y.; Wang, K.; Zhao, J.Y.; Li, Z.X.; Liu, X.M.; Liu, X.R. Effects of the Land Use Change on Ecosystem Service Value. *Glob. J. Environ. Sci. Manag.* **2017**, *3*, 121–130.
75. Xu, H.; Jiao, M. City Size, Industrial Structure and Urbanization Quality—A Case Study of the Yangtze River Delta Urban Agglomeration in China. *Land Use Policy* **2021**, *111*, 105735. [CrossRef]
76. Gashaw, T.; Tulu, T.; Argaw, M.; Worqlul, A.W.; Tolessa, T.; Kindu, M. Estimating the Impacts of Land Use/Land Cover Changes on Ecosystem Service Values: The Case of the Andassa Watershed in the Upper Blue Nile Basin of Ethiopia. *Ecosyst. Serv.* **2018**, *31*, 219–228. [CrossRef]
77. Ding, T.; Chen, J.; Fang, Z.; Chen, J. Assessment of Coordinative Relationship between Comprehensive Ecosystem Service and Urbanization: A Case Study of Yangtze River Delta Urban Agglomerations, China. *Ecol. Indic.* **2021**, *133*, 108454. [CrossRef]
78. Office of the State Council Opinions on Encouraging and Supporting Social Capital to Participate in Ecological Protection and Restoration. Available online: http://www.gov.cn/xinwen/2021-11/10/content_5650156.htm (accessed on 15 December 2021).
79. The General Office of the State Council Printed and Distributed the Opinions on Deepening the Reform of Ecological Protection Compensation System. Available online: http://www.gov.cn/zhengce/2021-09/12/content_5636905.htm (accessed on 15 December 2021).
80. Li, F.; Zhang, S.; Chang, N.B.; Yang, H.; Bu, K. Effects of Land Use Change on Ecosystem Services Value in West Jilin since the Reform and Opening of China. *Ecosyst. Serv.* **2018**, *31*, 12–20.
81. Ostrom, E. A General Framework for Analyzing Sustainability of Social-Ecological Systems. *Science* **2009**, *325*, 419–422. [CrossRef]

energies

MDPI

Article

Reduction Reactivity of Low Grade Iron Ore-Biomass Pellets for a Sustainable Ironmaking Process

Ariany Zulkania [1,2], Rochmadi Rochmadi [1], Muslikhin Hidayat [1] and Rochim Bakti Cahyono [1,*]

[1] Department of Chemical Engineering, Faculty of Engineering, Gadjah Mada University, Yogyakarta 55281, Indonesia; ariany.zulkania@uii.ac.id (A.Z.); rochmadi@ugm.ac.id (R.R.); mhidayat@ugm.ac.id (M.H.)

[2] Department of Chemical Engineering, Faculty of Industrial Technology, Indonesian Islamic University, Yogyakarta 55584, Indonesia

* Correspondence: rochimbakti@ugm.ac.id; Tel.: +62-813-9369-6232

Abstract: Currently, fossil fuels are still the primary fuel source and reducing agent in the steel industries. The utilization of fossil fuels is strongly associated with CO_2 emissions. Therefore, an alternative solution for green steel production is highly recommended, with the use of biomass as a source of fuel and a reducing agent. Biomass's growth consumes carbon dioxide from the atmosphere, which may be stored for variable amounts of time (carbon dioxide removal, or CDR). The pellets used in this study were prepared from a mixture of low-grade iron ore and palm kernel shells (PKS). The reducing reactivity of the pellets was investigated by combining thermogravimetric analysis (TGA) and laboratory experiments. In the TGA, the heating changes stably from room temperature to 950 °C with 5–15 °C/min heating rate. The laboratory experiments' temperature and heating rate variations were 600–900 °C and 10–20 °C/min, respectively. Additionally, the reduction mechanism was observed based on the X-ray diffraction analysis of the pellets and the composition of the reduced gas. The study results show that increasing the heating rate will enhance the reduction reactivity comprehensively and shorten the reduction time. The phase change of $Fe_2O_3 \rightarrow Fe_3O_4 \rightarrow FeO \rightarrow Fe$ increases sharply starting at 800 °C. The XRD intensities of Fe compounds at a heating rate of 20 °C/min are higher than at 10 °C/min. Analysis of the reduced gas exhibits that carbon gasification begins to enlarge at a temperature of 800 °C, thereby increasing the rate of iron ore reduction. The combination of several analyses carried out shows that the reduction reaction of the mixture iron ore-PKS pellets runs optimally at a heating rate of 20 °C/min. In this heating rate, the reduced gas contains much higher CO than at the heating rate of 10 °C/min at temperatures above 800 °C, which encourages a more significant reduction rate. In addition, the same reduction degree can be achieved in a shorter time and at a lower temperature for a heating rate of 20 °C/min compared to 10 °C/min.

Keywords: biomass; iron ore; reduction reactivity; reduction degree; pellet

Citation: Zulkania, A.; Rochmadi, R.; Hidayat, M.; Cahyono, R.B. Reduction Reactivity of Low Grade Iron Ore-Biomass Pellets for a Sustainable Ironmaking Process. *Energies* **2022**, *15*, 137. https://doi.org/10.3390/en15010137

Academic Editor: Francesco Nocera

Received: 12 November 2021
Accepted: 20 December 2021
Published: 25 December 2021

1. Introduction

The ironmaking industry is one of the largest fossil fuel-consuming industries globally. Several methods are utilized in the industry, such as the blast furnace/basic oxygen furnace (BF-BOF), direct reduction/electric arc furnace (DR-EAF), smelting reduction/basic oxygen furnace (SR-BOF), and melting of scrap in an electric arc furnace (EAF) [1]. These methods use fuel and reducing agents in coal, coke [1], natural gas, or oil derived from fossil fuels [2]. Consequently, this comprises a considerable contribution to global CO_2 emissions. Thus, renewable fuels utilization is an alternative way to reduce CO_2 emissions. Biomass is now being heavily explored, as evidenced by multiple studies indicating that biomass can help mitigate CO_2 emissions in the ironmaking process. Purwanto et al. [3] found that using charcoal obtained from oil palm empty fruit bunch for sintering low-grade iron ore potentially decreased CO_2 emission in the ironmaking process. Furthermore, utilizing torrefied biomass as an ironmaking reductant has the potential to be carbon neutral due to biomass's propensity to adsorb CO_2 during its growth phase [4]. Reducing agents required in the iron ore reduction process can be met by biomass's when thermally decomposed into carbon, CO, and H_2. This is shown in several reduction studies using charcoal from sawdust, nutshell, and waste biomass [5] and raw biomass, such as pine sawdust [6,7], coconut shell waste [8], and corn straw [9]. The use of biomass in iron ore reduction provides a good interaction between iron ore and biomass. The iron ore plays a good role as a catalyst for the pyrolysis process of biomass into the volatile matter, carbon, and gas [10,11] and, simultaneously, the pyrolysis results become reducing agents that encourage reduction reaction.

Biomass may be used as a reducing agent in various methods. The chemical vapor infiltration (CVI) method utilizes volatile matter and gas from the pyrolysis of biomass to diffuse into iron ore in different chambers. This method stimulates the formation of carbon deposits, and the reduction reaction co-occurs. The CVI method directs the formation of nanoscale distances between carbon-iron ore, which causes the reduction rate to occur faster [12]. Investigation of Cahyono et al. [13] showed that using the CVI method in a sinter plant could significantly decrease coke breeze and CO_2 emissions in the ironmaking sector. Another study indicated that the reduction rate of composites with the CVI method was higher than that of a mixture of dehydrated iron ore and coke [14]. Another way for obtaining carbon deposits as reducing agents is to impregnate iron ore with biomass tar and then carbonize it. This triggers a high reduction reactivity [15]. In addition, the biomass is also used as a composite mix with iron ore in the form of pellets or briquettes. Briquettes of a mixture of iron ore and pine sawdust, which reduced at a temperature of 1100 °C with a reaction time of 60 min, generated the reduced iron with Fe metal content up to 94.5% [16]. The investigation conducted by Guo et al. [17] showed that the pellet reduction rate with biomass was relatively higher than without biomass at the same temperature. This is caused by the increase in pellet porosity due to dehydrated and pyrolyzed biomass promoting a higher interfacial chemical reaction rate.

The biomass utilization as a reducing agent can be more efficient when it is upgraded to increase the calorific value and volumetric energy density, reduce ash, more accessible handling properties, and diminish moisture content. Several forms of upgraded biomass include a pellet form, charcoal, torrefied biomass, and others [1]. According to Yuan et al. [18], the metallization degree of the reduced iron ore-straw fiber pellets was slightly lower than those of the bamboo char-iron ore pellets and the charcoal-iron ore pellets at 600–800 °C. However, it will reach a comparable metallization value to the other two pellets at temperatures above 1000 °C. Meanwhile, another study showed slightly different things. The reduction process for iron ore-raw biomass mixture pellets provides a faster reduction rate at a relatively low temperature than composite pellets of iron ore-coke and iron ore-charcoal. In addition, it displays lower apparent activation energy than the other pellets [19]. Several reduction studies using iron ore-raw biomass mixture pellets have been carried out. Rashid et al. [20] used spherical pellets of iron ore-palm kernel shell mixture with a diameter 10–12 μm in their reduction study. The composition of PKS by 30% by weight at a temperature of 900 °C resulted in the majority content of reduced pellets being wustite (FeO). Furthermore, the study conducted by Huang et al. [6] used a cylindrical pellet mixture of iron ore-pine sawdust with a Ø 15 mm × 10 mm. The study results demonstrate that the iron ore-biomass ratio that gives the optimum degree of metallization is 1:0.6.

One of the essential parameters considered in the reduction or pyrolysis process is the heating rate. Several studies have analyzed the effect of heating rate changes on reduction reactivity through thermogravimetric analysis (TGA). The study utilized carbonized goethite ore samples [12] and iron ore-biochar pellets [21]. These studies show that increasing the heating rate on the same reducing agent will shift the initial temperature of the weight loss. However, the trend of decreasing weight loss for each heating is almost the same. Eventually, several previous studies that used biomass as a reducing agent in the iron ore-biomass pellets found it attractive to apply these for manufacturing sponge iron or direct reduction iron (DRI). Based on the analysis of Mousa et al. [1] and Suopajärvi et al. [2], one of the processes in ironmaking is with DR-EAF, which requires the supply of DRI in the process. The DRI of this iron ore-biomass pellet reduction process can be an attractive alternative.

The current study is proposed due to the promising prospects for DRI preparation in the pellets of mixture iron ore-biomass and the lack of information about the effect of the heating rate on the reduction reactivity of iron ore-biomass pellets. The purpose of this study is to find out in more detail how the reduction reactivity in pellets of low degree iron ore and palm kernel shell (PKS) mixtures at various heating rates, the mechanism of the reduction of the pellets at various temperatures and heating rates, and the effect of the temperature and heating rate on the value of the reduction and metallization degrees. Results of the thermogravimetric analysis (TGA) could inform the reduction reactivity of iron ore-PKS composites at various heating rates. The temperature and heating rate were varied during the reduction laboratory experiments. The reduction mechanism was investigated from the X-ray diffraction (XRD) analysis of the reduced composites and the composition of the reduced gas. Finally, the reduced product's degrees of reduction and metallization of the reduced product are determined.

2. Materials and Methods

2.1. Materials Specification and Preparation

PT. Meratus Jaya Iron&Steel, South Kalimantan, Indonesia, supplied raw iron ore, with a size ranging from 1 to 3 cm. Meanwhile, palm kernel shell (PKS) as the biomass utilized in the study was provided by PT. Astra Agro Lestari Tbk., South Kalimantan, Indonesia. The iron ore was finely crushed and filtered into particle sizes ranging from 53 to 149 microns. The original ore was calcined at 350 °C for 3 h in an air environment with a heating rate of 3.5 °C/min before being mixed with biomass. The heating process is designed to reduce the combined water (CW) and increase the sample surface area [9–11,22]. Additionally, biomass powder is obtained by crushing and sifting into particles with sizing of 74 to 149 μm. Eventually, molasses is used as a binder to form iron ore-biomass pellets.

Table 1 shows the composition and phase identification of the original iron ore/goethite as determined by X-ray fluorescence (XRF Epsilon 4, Malvern, UK) and X-ray diffraction (XRD-Bruker D2 Phaser, Billerica, MA, USA).

Table 1. Contexture of goethite ore.

Composition	*TFe*	Fe_2O_3	Si	Ca	Al	O	CW	C
Weight (mass%)	46.835	18.941	9.225	5.366	0.534	37.492	4.93	5.62

TFe: Total Fe; CW: combined water.

Phase identification of the dehydrated ore was also carried out by XRD analysis. N_2 adsorption-desorption measurements were used to determine the iron ore samples' BET surface area, pore-volume, and pore distribution (Quantachrome Instr. Ver. 10.01, Boynton Beach, FL, USA). Furthermore, scanning electron microscopy (SEM) was used to examine the surface structure of original and dehydrated iron ores (SEM-Jeol Jsm 6510 La, Tokyo, Japan). The reduction reactivity of dehydrated iron ore as a raw material for pellets was examined by thermogravimetric analysis (TG-Linseis STA, Selb, Germany). Additionally, components and elements of biomass and molasses were determined using the proximate analysis (Nabertherm N3/R Muffle furnace, Lilienthal, Germany; Heraeus UT 5042 EK, Burladingen, Germany) and ultimate analysis (LECO CHN/S-628/632, St. Joseph, MI, USA). The analysis results are provided in Table 2.

Table 2. Properties of the biomass and molasses.

Sample	Proximate Analysis (Mass%, Air-Dried Basis)				Ultimate Analysis (Mass%, Air-Dried Basis)				
	Fixed Carbon	Volatile Matter	Water	Ash	C	H	O	N	S
PKS	30.771	65.579	2.700	0.950	50.720	6.170	0.220	41.760	0.030
Molasses	4.968	56.441	35.191	3.430	29.690	7.730	0.560	57.400	0.260

The iron ore-biomass pellet composite is formed with an iron ore-biomass ratio of 7:3 by mass, and the binder used is 9% of the mixture. After mixed ingredients are obtained, pellets for thermogravimetric analysis (TGA) and reduction experiments are formed according to the cylinder diameter and pellet weight required. The pellets for TGA analysis are thin cylindrical pellets with a diameter of 2 mm and a composite weight of 19 mg. Pellet formation utilizes a pellet mold and a pressure of 2 kN (hydraulic pump). At the same time, the formation of cylindrical pellets for the reduction experiments uses a pellet mold with a diameter of 5 mm and a pressure of 40 kN, with a pellet weight of 0.2 g. Subsequently, they are dried in an oven at 105 °C for 3 h to expel moisture before being stored in closed storage before use.

2.2. Experimental Methods

2.2.1. Thermal Analysis

Thermal analysis of the pellets of a mixture of iron ore and biomass was carried out using thermogravimetry analysis (TG-Linseis STA, Selb, Germany). The TGA results were then used to determine the reduction reactivity of the pellets. The TGA test is executed under non-isothermal conditions from room temperature to 950 °C, with 5, 10, and 15 °C/min heating rates under N_2 gas flow.

2.2.2. Experiments on Reduction of Iron Ore-Biomass Pellets

The reduction experiments of the iron ore-biomass pellet are conducted by utilizing the apparatus, as shown in Figure 1. As a whole, the system for the lab-scale reduction process consists mainly of an electric furnace, a reduction chamber, temperature control, gas flow control, cooling circuit, effluent gas treatment, and a gas analyzer.

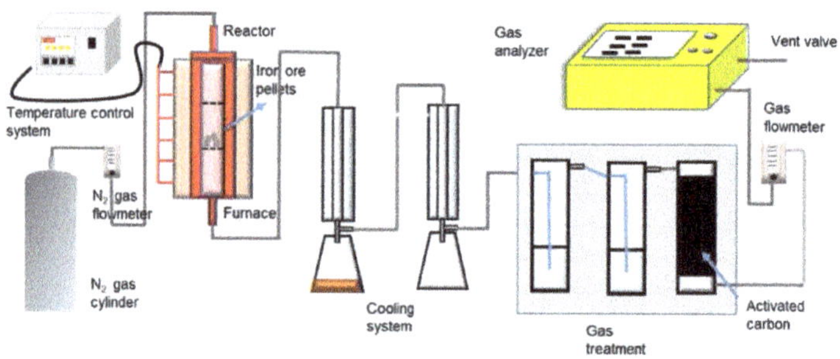

Figure 1. Scheme of apparatus for reduction experiments.

The experiment was started by inserting pellet samples weighing 16.6 g into a tubular fixed-bed reactor with a length of 20 cm and an internal diameter of 3 cm, enclosed by the furnace. After the series of cooling devices, the gas treatment, and the gas analyzer were prepared, and N_2 was flowed at 200 mL/min to ensure that oxygen was expelled from the reactor. After approximately 3 min of N_2 flow, heating began to be adjusted with a specific heating rate and reduction temperature. Temperature and heating rate variations are 600–900 °C and 10, 15, and 20 °C/min, respectively. After reaching the desired temperature, the reduction was carried out under isothermal conditions for 60 min. The N_2 flow was halted once the reactor had cooled to room temperature to avoid product re-oxidation [17]. The reduced gas from the beginning of increasing temperature until the end of the 60th minute of the reduction process was evaluated using the gas analyzer. Furthermore, the reduced pellets were weighed and subjected to be analyzed using XRD and SEM completed with energy-dispersive X-ray spectroscopy (EDS).

2.3. Determination of Reduction and Metallization Degrees

The degree of reduction identifies how much oxygen can be released from the components contained in the sample during the reduction process. Meanwhile, the degree of metallization can inform how much the iron metal content is compared to the mass total of Fe contained in the reduced sample. The reduction degree (RD) of the reduced iron ore is determined by Equation (1) [23]:

$$RD = \sum x_i \cdot RD_i \tag{1}$$

where RD_i is the reduction degree of each iron compound and x_i is the mass fraction of each iron oxide (i represents Fe_2O_3, Fe_3O_4, FeO, or Fe). The reference intensity ratio (RIR) approach [24], which is based on the intensity of the X-ray diffracted by the component's selected plane (hkl), is utilized to calculate the mass fraction of the iron oxide component [11,23]. Additionally, the value of the reduction degree of each iron oxide is approached by the following Equation (2) [23]:

$$RD_X\,(\%) = \frac{(Mr\ FeO_{1.5}) - Mr\ X}{(Mr\ FeO_{1.5}) - Mr\ Fe} \cdot 100\% \tag{2}$$

X can be $FeO_{1.5}$ (Fe_2O_3), $FeO_{1.33}$ (Fe_3O_4), FeO, or Fe. The *RDi* value in Equation (1) is calculated using Equation (2) as RD_X.

On the other hand, the metallization degree of the reduced iron ore from the reduction experiment is determined by Equation (3) [7]:

$$M = \frac{M_{Fe}}{T_{Fe}} \cdot 100\% \tag{3}$$

where *MFe* is the mass of iron metal in the reduced sample and *TFe* is the mass total of Fe in the reduced sample.

3. Results and Discussion

3.1. Effect of Dehydration Process on Iron Ore Properties

In the dehydration process, it is expected that the releasing water process from goethite occurred, as in Equation (4), leading to lessening the water content and enhancing the specific surface area of the iron ore [10,11,22].

$$2\ FeOOH \rightarrow Fe_2O_3 + H_2O \tag{4}$$

Figure 2a shows the pore size distribution, BET surface area, and pore volume of the original and dehydrated ore. It seems that both ores have nanopores at around a size of 2 nm. After dehydration, the nanopores of the dehydrated ore enhance, and the mesopores at the size of 3–8 nm slightly increase. It induces the rise of the dehydrated ore's specific surface area and pore volume.

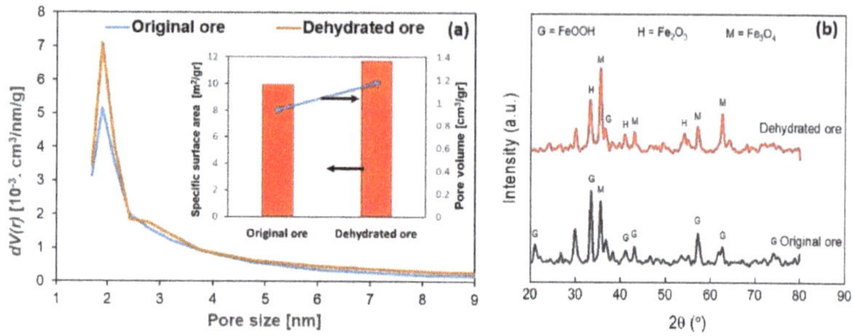

Figure 2. Alteration in (**a**) pore size distribution and S_{BET} and V_{BJH} values; (**b**) XRD patterns of original iron ore and dehydrated ore.

Furthermore, X-ray diffractometry (XRD) was used to analyze the characteristic of the ore structures before and after dehydration. Figure 2b exhibits that the goethite (FeOOH) is the dominant phase in the original sample. After heating, most of FeOOH transforms to Fe_2O_3 and subsequently partly converts to be Fe_3O_4. However, the XRD peaks also indicate that a small amount of FeOOH is still comprised in the dehydrated iron. This is conformable with the research conducted by Zhao et al. [9], where FeOOH could not be fully decomposed into Fe_2O_3 and water after being heated at a temperature of 185–400 °C. The hydroxyl and other oxygen-containing functional groups are still present in the dehydrated ore. If they do not appear as aqueous structures of the goethite, they can be the ligand and the arrangement of oxygen and hydroxide ions in the goethite with the densest hexagonal accumulation [9].

Figure 3 reflects SEM images before and after dehydration of iron ores. From Figure 3a, the goethite is abundant in the original ore sample, as evidenced by the needle-shaped bulges [25,26] and colloform texture with cavities of goethite [8], as indicated by the yellow circle lines. The needle and colloform surfaces appear smooth, with no scratches or grooves, implying that the combined water and gangues are distributed throughout the goethite samples. Figure 3b indicates how the surface shape of iron ore altered substantially after heating. Because of the elimination of water following Equation (4) and the removal of oxygen associated with iron oxide, porous structures are apparent in the heated samples. The surface appears coarse and grainy with hexagonal and cubic geometries. It suggests the presence of iron oxides, such as hematite and magnetite, respectively [27].

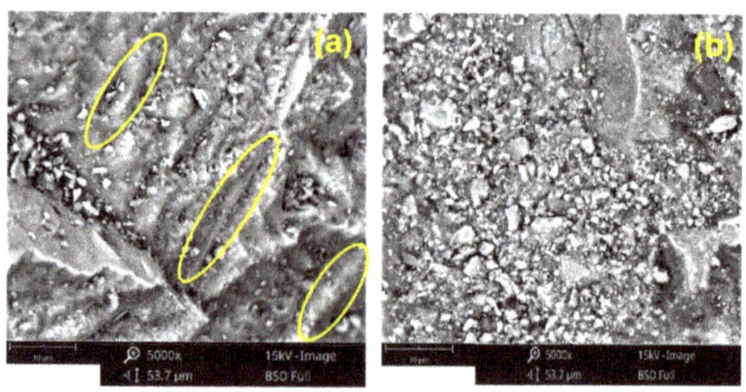

Figure 3. Images of SEM for iron ore (**a**) before and (**b**) after dehydration.

The thermogravimetric analysis and the derivative curve (*dm/dt*) of the dehydrated ore as material for the composite pellet are represented in Figure 4. For thermogravimetric analysis, dehydrated ore pellets used molasses as a binder. The curve's trend begins to decrease below the temperature of 150 °C, indicating an evaporation process of water content from the iron ore and the molasse (S1). It is also emphasized by a small maximum peak (dm/dt) at a temperature of 130 °C. The sharper weight loss occurred at 150–265 °C temperature (S2). As confirmed, dehydration, de-polymerization, and decomposition of biomass/molasses [10,20,28] by the presence of the second maximum peak occurred at a temperature of 200 °C.

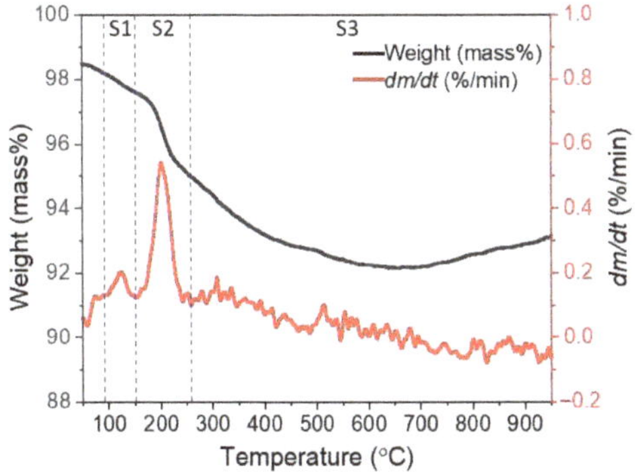

Figure 4. Weight percentage and reactivity rate curve of dehydrated iron ore at a heating rate of 10 °C/min.

Furthermore, at temperatures above 265 °C, the weight loss occurs more gently. There are processes of releasing volatile matter and reducing iron ore. There are many small peaks, indicating a continuous slow reduction process up to 900 °C. At temperatures of 180–450 °C, the gas-solid indirect reduction process may occur, since heating the iron ore-biomass composite pellets gradually produces reductive gases, such as CO and H_2 [18]. According to Cahyono et al. [10], the reduction can commence at a temperature below 560 °C by gradually following the $Fe_2O_3 \rightarrow Fe_3O_4 \rightarrow Fe$ steps. According to Zuo et al. [29], the first primary reduction reaction took place in a temperature range of 565–847 °C, which produced low valence iron oxide, such as Fe_3O_4, as the principal reduction product, while the CO gas produced might also contribute to Fe_2O_3 reduction. The reaction is as follows:

$$3\ Fe_2O_{3(s)} + C_{(s)} \rightarrow 2\ Fe_3O_{4(s)} + CO_{(g)} \quad (5)$$

3.2. Thermogravimetric Characterization of the Composite Pellet

The thermal characteristics of the composite pellets of the iron ore and PKS mixture were analyzed using the thermogravimetric. Figure 5 shows the results of the TGA analysis of pellets with a heating rate of 10 °C/min as an example. The reduction process is divided into four stages, where stage 1 (S1) occurs at 147.32–230 °C; Stage 2 (S2) occurs at 230–315 °C; Stage 3 (S3) occurs at 315–435 °C, and Stage 4 (S4) occurs at 435–950 °C.

Some of the qualitative characterization parameters used include [21]: T_i and T_f, which are the initial temperature and the final temperature for weight loss from the reduction process, respectively; $T_{max\text{-}1}$, $T_{max\text{-}2}$, $T_{max\text{-}3}$, and $T_{max\text{-}4}$, which are the peak temperatures of the reaction rate for the four stages, respectively; $dm/dt_{max\text{-}1}$, $dm/dt_{max\text{-}2}$, $dm/dt_{max\text{-}3}$, and $dm/dt_{max\text{-}4}$, which are the peak values of the reaction rate for the four stages, respectively; tr is the reaction time from T_i to T_f; and S is the comprehensive reactivity index of the iron ore-biomass pellets, where the values are according to the following Equation (1):

$$S = (dm/dt)_{mean} / \left(T_i^2 \cdot T_f\right) \quad (6)$$

where $(dm/dt)_{mean}$ denotes the decrease rate's mean value.

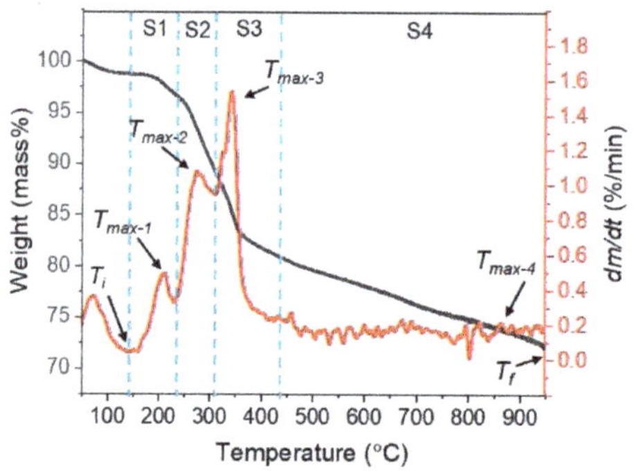

Figure 5. Weight loss and reactivity rate (*dm/dt*) curves of the iron ore-biomass pellet at a heating rate of 10 °C/min.

Figure 6 presents the TGA analysis of all samples heated to a temperature of 950 °C at a heating rate of 5–15 °C/min. The samples' weight loss and reactivity rate curves are divided into four pyrolysis/reduction temperature stages, as shown in Figure 5.

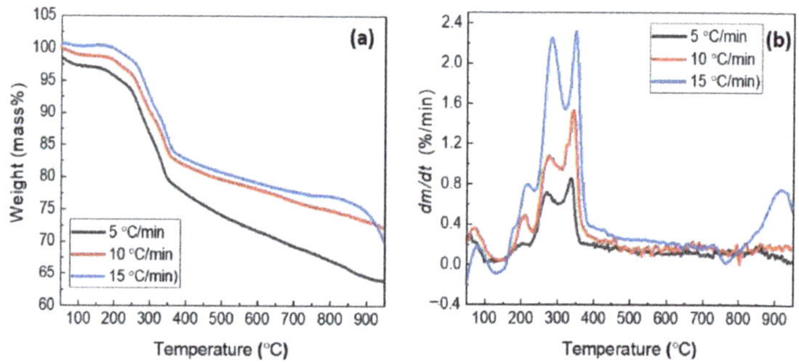

Figure 6. Thermogravimetric analysis: (**a**) weight percentage; (**b**) reactivity rate curves of composite pellet at a different heating rate.

The first to third peaks appear to be partially overlapping, while the fourth peaks are small except for the heating rate of 15 °C/min. In addition, the weight loss and reaction rate curves of the composite pellets move into the high temperature zone by enhancing the heating rates (Figure 6). This phenomenon is usually named thermal hysteresis or thermal lag. It can be induced by those individual reactions that do not have enough time to complete or reach equilibrium due to the fast heating rate. Consequently, processes at higher temperatures nearby overlap each other. On the other side, there is a temperature differential through the sample's cross-section at a high heating rate which prevents heat transfer [21]. However, the pattern of the thermal decomposition does not alter. This propensity also occurs in several studies related to pyrolysis/reduction [21,30,31].

All of the reduction characteristics described previously were computed, and the results were displayed in Table 3 to evaluate the reactivity differences of composite pellets quantitatively. From Table 3, it can be seen that the initial weight loss temperature (T_i) increases as the heating rate is increased. At same time, the total weight loss temperature (T_f) is the same at 950 °C (test temperature limit). This indicates that there is still a continuation of the reduction at temperatures above 950 °C for all samples.

Table 3. The distinctive reduction parameter of the composite pellet at three different heating rates.

Heating Rate (°C/min)	T_i (°C)	$T_{max\text{-}1}$ (°C)	$T_{max\text{-}2}$ (°C)	$T_{max\text{-}3}$ (°C)	$T_{max\text{-}4}$ (°C)	T_f (°C)	$dm/dt_{max\text{-}1}$ (%/min)	$dm/dt_{max\text{-}2}$ (%/min)	$dm/dt_{max\text{-}3}$ (%/min)	$dm/dt_{max\text{-}4}$ (%/min)	dm/dt_{mean} (%/min)	S	t_r (min)
5	109.02	200.57	269.60	336.22	847.98	950	0.21	0.72	0.86	0.19	0.17	1.5×10^{-8}	168.21
10	138.00	212.49	276.10	343.69	862.93	950	0.49	1.08	1.53	0.21	0.29	1.6×10^{-8}	82.07
15	147.32	218.44	284.05	349.66	920.00	950	0.79	2.25	2.31	0.75	0.48	2.3×10^{-8}	55.05

Further, the peak temperatures of reaction rates ($T_{max\text{-}i}$) and reaction rate peaks ($dm/dt_{max\text{-}i}$) for all stages exhibit ascent while raising the heating rate. In addition, the value of S, which is the thorough reduction reactivity, also increases with the rising heating rate. Otherwise, the reaction time (t_r) will be shorter with an increased heating rate. The tendencies are conformable with a study conducted by Wang et al. [21]. The increase in heating rate leads the rate of volatile matter/gas release to be higher than the rate of char formation in the pyrolysis process [30,31]. The produced gases, such as CO or H_2, can trigger the reduction reaction when they contact the iron ore. These cause the reactivity rate (dm/dt) to also be enhanced. Hence, the value of S also raises with the increasing heating rate. However, the analysis described previously could not explain the reduction reaction mechanism in the composite pellet sample. Therefore, the subsequent study explores the phase change and SEM analysis of the samples and analyzes the gas produced from the reduction experiments to investigate the reaction mechanism in the sample.

3.3. Reduction Behavior of Composite Pellet

Figure 7 shows the phase transformation of iron oxide due to temperature changes at two heating rates, namely 10 and 20 °C/min. From the two pictures, it can be noticed that the reduction process goes well as the temperature increases. At a temperature of 600–700 °C, it can be noted that the majority of the identified phases of iron compounds are magnetite (Fe_3O_4). In these temperatures, there has been a slow reduction reaction of $Fe_2O_3 \rightarrow Fe_3O_4$. This is reinforced by the gradual decrease in weight loss, as illustrated in Figure 6, which reveals a reduction in reactivity. In addition, based on the XRD analysis in Figure 3b for the dehydrated ore and Figure 7, it seems that FeOOH disappears after the reduction process at 600 °C. Additionally, a part of hematite (Fe_2O_3) converts into magnetite. Several studies show that slow reduction has started from around 450 °C [10,18,29]. At a temperature of 800 °C, it seems that the reduction of Fe_3O_4 to FeO is quite significant. It is indicated by the FeO phase, which appears more in Figure 7. In addition, there is also a further reaction of FeO to Fe metal at a temperature of 850–900 °C. Starting at a temperature of 800 °C, this evidences that temperature significantly influences the reduction process, which drives the reactions of $Fe_2O_3 \rightarrow Fe_3O_4 \rightarrow FeO \rightarrow Fe$ reaction. At temperatures above 800 °C, carbon gasification and CO gas reduction are essential in the iron ore reduction process [10,21,29]. In addition, Yuan et al. [18] investigated that CH_4, as one of the volatile matters yielded from the biomass pyrolysis process at ~900 °C, can be a reductive gas that plays a role in the following equation:

$$CH_4 + 4\,Fe_2O_3 \rightarrow 8\,Fe + 3\,CO_2 + 6\,H_2O \tag{7}$$

The trend of iron oxide phase transformation at both heating rates is similar. However, based on Figure 7, it can be seen that the FeO and Fe phases' intensities at the heating rate of 20 °C/min are higher than the ones at the heating rate of 10 °C/min, especially at temperatures of 850–900 °C. It signifies that the presence of FeO and Fe at the heating rate of 20 °C/min is higher than the one at the heating rate of 10 °C/min. It is conformable with the analysis of the reduction characteristics from Table 3, which indicates that increasing the heating rate enhances the thorough reduction reactivity.

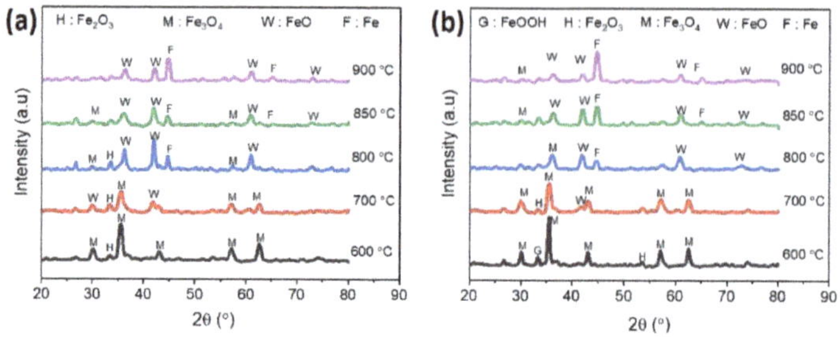

Figure 7. XRD pattern of samples after reduction process from 600–900 °C for 1 h with a heating rate of (**a**) 10 °C/min; (**b**) 20 °C/min.

The temperature effect on the gas composition (CO, CO_2, CH_4, and H_2) for the heating rates of 10 and 20 °C/min is shown in Figure 8. The graphs show the gas composition when the temperature increases (small graphs) and the isothermal reduction within 60 min for each reduction temperature. The gas profile shows that CO and H_2 are produced first, followed by CO_2 when the temperature rises at the same heating rate. At a heating rate of 10 and 20 °C/min, CO and H_2 start appearing at a temperature of about 350 and 550 °C, respectively. Continuously, they rise to 450 and 650 °C, respectively. It can be noticed that increasing the heating rate leads to a shift in the initial temperature of the decomposition. The shift is in line with the analysis of the reduction characteristics in Section 3.2. Some studies on increasing the heating rate on the reduction reactivity of iron ore show a similar phenomenon [21,32].

As shown in Figure 8a,b for the temperature increase graph, in the temperature range of 350–450 °C, the decomposition of biomass into tar, carbon, gases, and volatile compounds occurs, followed by the release of volatile compounds and gases. CO_2 gas continues to rise significantly as the temperature increases from 400 °C to 500 °C. After passing a temperature of 500 °C, it seems that the CO drops to a temperature of 700 °C (Figure S1b) while the CO_2 concentration is still above the CO levels. It indicates that there is a slow reduction between CO gas and iron oxide, as shown in the following Equation:

$$3\ Fe_2O_3 + CO \rightarrow 2\ Fe_3O_4 + CO_2 \quad (8)$$

The occurrence of the reduction reaction at temperatures below 570 °C is in accordance with several studies that have been carried out [18,29]. In addition, Zhao et al. [28] stated that carbon deposits in iron ore could induce a reduction to occur at temperatures above 500 °C. Furthermore, CO levels begin to rise above 700 °C (Figure S1b) and eventually exceed CO_2 levels at temperatures above 800 °C. This denotes that the carbon gasification process of carbon obtained from the biomass pyrolysis has occurred as the following Equation:

$$C + CO_2 \rightarrow 2\ CO \quad (9)$$

Additionally, when the temperature is raised to 800 or 900 °C (Figure S1d), there is a decrease in CH_4 and an increase in H_2. This may be due to the decomposition of CH_4 into C and H_2 [33]. Subsequently, the formed C can react with CO_2 to generate CO according to Equation (9), and then CO reacts as shown in Equation (8).

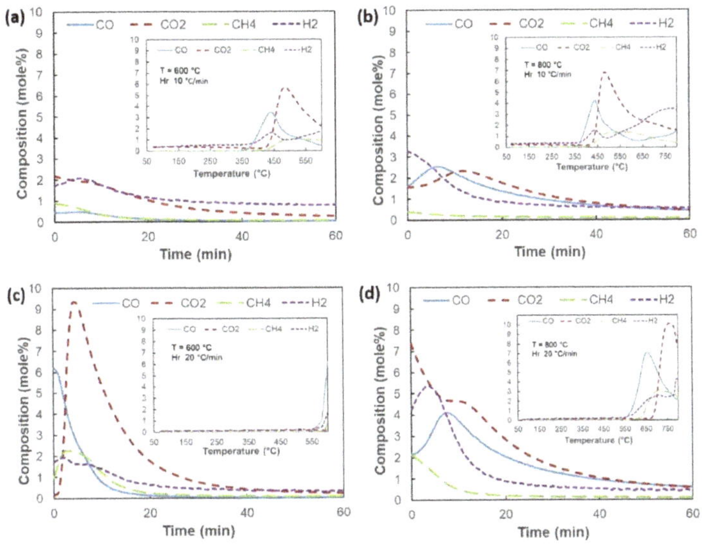

Figure 8. The temperature and heating rate effects on gas composition when the temperature rises (small graphs) and the isothermal reduction lasting 60 min for a heating rate of 10 °C/min (**a**,**b**) and 20 °C/min (**c**,**d**).

Based on Figure 8a for the isothermal reduction step lasting 60 min, it can be seen that the presence of H_2 and CO is small. This may cause the reduction to proceed slowly for the reaction of $Fe_2O_3 \rightarrow Fe_3O_4$. The reduced iron oxide phase at temperatures of 600 and 700 °C is represented in Figure 7a. At 800 °C (Figure 8b), there is an increase in CO, indicating that the carbon gasification process is beginning to expand. This enhances the reduction rate of the $Fe_2O_3 \rightarrow Fe_3O_4 \rightarrow FeO$ reactions. This occurrence corresponds to the iron oxide phase analysis in Figure 7a for a temperature of 800 °C. In addition, the reduction at a temperature of 900 °C (Figure S1d) showed that the carbon gasification process was extensive in the initial 20 min, characterized by the composition of CO, which reached 6.2% mole compared to CO_2 at 3.4% mole. Although CO then reacts further with iron oxide, the composition of CO is always higher than CO_2 until the end of the 60 min. It reveals that the carbon gasification rate is greater than the rate of CO reduction. On the other hand, the availability of excess CO triggers the reduction reaction rate. Based on Figure 7a, it can be seen that the intensity of Fe increases at a temperature of 900 °C, which means that the reaction of $FeO \rightarrow Fe$ is significant at this temperature.

According to Figure 8c,d for the temperature increase graph, it seems that when the temperature increases to 600 °C, the resultant gas concentration is minimal. This is due to a shift in the initial temperature of biomass decomposition from 350 °C to 550 °C at the heating rate of 10 °C/min to 20 °C/min, respectively. Therefore, biomass decomposition is continued at the start of isothermal heating at 600 °C. A temperature difference between the surface and the middle of the pellet is created by rapid heating [21]. It impacts the lack of heat transfer to the pellet center, leading to a small portion of FeOOH in the sample at a temperature of 600 °C not being dehydrated, as shown in Figure 7b. When the temperature rises to 700 °C (Figure S2b), it can be seen that CO, CO_2, CH_4, and H_2 gases appear. This shows a process of decomposition of biomass into volatile matter and gas. Then, the temperature rising to 800 °C causes a decrease in CO and CH_4 and an increase in CO_2 at around 800 °C. This indicates a slow CO reduction and CH_4 decomposition into C and H_2. When the temperature is raised to 900 °C (Figure S2d), a similar phenomenon to the heating rate of 10 °C/min is evident. Here, the CO and H_2 increase along with the decrease in CH_4. This is due to an intense carbon gasification process at a temperature of 900 °C, which raises the level of CO, and subsequently reacts according to Equation (4). In addition, the increase in H_2 is due to the decomposition of CH_4 into C and H_2 [33].

As shown in Figure 8c, where the isothermal heating lasts 60 min, CO and H_2 produced by biomass decomposition have little effect on the reduction process at a temperature of 600°. This is notified by the insignificant change of the iron oxide phase from the dehydrated ore (Figure 3) to the reduced ore at this temperature (Figure 7b). At a temperature of 700 °C (Figure S2b), there seems to be an increase in H_2 from the beginning, along with a decrease in CH_4. This indicates the decomposition of CH_4 into C and H_2. The presence of H_2 can influence the slow reduction that occurs. This slow reduction does not significantly change the iron oxide phase (Figures 3 and 7b). Hereafter, trends occurring at temperatures of 800 and 900 °C are similar to those observed at the heating rate of 10 °C/min. Equation (5) shows that the carbon gasification process expands at 800 °C and becomes quite substantial at 900 °C (Figure S2d). At high temperatures, endothermic carbon gasification escalates, thereby producing more CO. The exothermic reaction between iron oxide and CO, occurs more quickly. It creates a coupling reaction condition between carbon gasification and reduction of iron oxide, which controls heat transfer [34].

Further, Figure 8c,d shows that the 20 °C/min heating rate produces more CO from carbon gasification than the 10 °C/min heating rate. Consequently, the reduction rate of the reaction of $Fe_2O_3 \rightarrow Fe_3O_4 \rightarrow FeO \rightarrow Fe$ at the heating rate of 20 °C/min becomes faster than 10 °C/min. Figure 7a,b confirm that FeO and Fe peaks are more visible and higher at the heating rate of 20 °C/min than at 10 °C/min. Applying a higher heating rate in the iron-making industry will be more advantageous because it can shorten the reduction process time. In addition, the higher heating rate can provide a higher reduction rate, and more Fe metal is produced. Furthermore, the effect of the magnitude of the reduction rate can also be influenced by H_2. At temperatures above 800 °C, H_2 gas can exert a more substantial reduction reaction effect than CO gas [35]. It can be seen from Figure S2d that above a temperature of 800 °C, H_2 decreases slowly. According to Wei et al. [27], at a temperature of 900 °C, H_2 can significantly impact the reduction reaction, but if the concentration of H_2 is less than 25%, the reduction will be slow.

The results of the SEM-EDS test in Figure 9 are to see changes in the surface morphology of the reduced sample. The figure shows the difference between the reduced samples at 600 °C and 900 °C and a heating rate of 10 °C/min. From the appearance of the sample morphology, both have almost the same distribution of elements. The sample temperature of 900 °C shows a slightly higher porosity distribution, and more small basins were seen. It shows that the high temperature causes the carbon gasification process, which causes depressions to form on the surface of the reduced iron. However, in general, the final characteristics of the two reduced pellets were morphologically almost the same. This demonstrates that the temperature variation (600 and 900 °C) slightly influences the quality of the direct reduction iron product (DRI)'s surfaces but increases the pellet reduction rate, based on Figures 7 and 8. Furthermore, the sample at 900 °C has a higher Fe content and a lower carbon deposit than the sample at 600 °C, according to the results of the EDS analysis (Figure 9b,d). Compared to lower temperatures (600 °C), the carbon content of biomass decomposition at 900 °C has been converted significantly through the reduction process and carbon gasification.

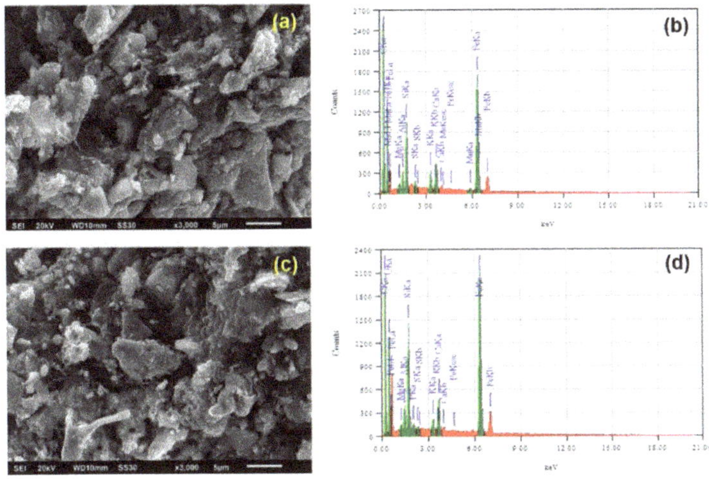

Figure 9. SEM images showing a change of iron ore surface after reduction and result of EDS analysis: (**a**,**b**) at 600 °C; (**c**,**d**) at 900 °C with heating rate 10 °C/min and reduction time 60 min.

3.4. Reduction and Metallization Degree of Composite Pellet

Figure 10 shows the degrees of reduction and metallization as a temperature and heating rate function. The figure shows that the trend of the reduction and metallization degrees' profile as a function of temperature for the three heating rates is almost the same. Increasing the temperature from 600 °C to 700 °C will cause a minimal effect on the rise of both degrees.

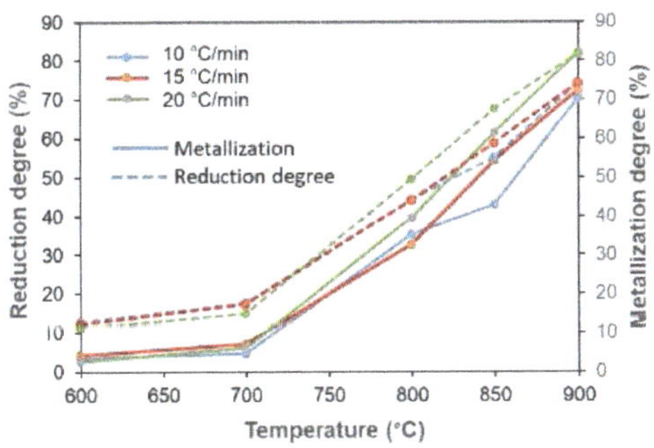

Figure 10. Reduction and metallization degrees of the iron ore-biomass pellets with temperature and heating rate variations.

Meanwhile, increasing the temperature to 800 °C begins to increase the degree of reduction and metallization significantly. This corresponds to the appearance of the phase change in Figure 7, where Fe_3O_4 commences forming into FeO significantly at a temperature of 800 °C. At 900 °C, most of the FeO is further converted into Fe. It induces both degrees to increase significantly, from 800 °C to 900 °C. In addition, at the heating rate of 20 °C/min, both degrees showed higher values starting at 800 °C compared to heating rates of 10 and 15 °C/min. Eventually, the degree of metallization values approaches the reduction degree value at a temperature of 900 °C for all heating rates as the temperature rises.

Figure 11 exhibits the comparison between the reduction degree from the current study result and the study result of Castro et al. [36] for the case of iron ore-coke in a blast furnace. There is an increase in the reduction degree from 12.90% at 600 °C to 74.14% at 900 °C in the current study results. The presence of biomass in iron ore pellets drives an increase in the porosity of the pellet so that the reaction area between the iron ore and biomass becomes large. In addition, the high porosity produced can facilitate the entry and exit of reductant gas and reduced gas, which is beneficial for the reduction of pellets and reductant gas [17]. It seems that the reduction degree at 700 °C is almost the same for both methods at about 17.50%. However, iron ore-coke in the blast furnace demonstrates that a reduction degree of 74% is achieved at temperatures above 1000 °C. This confirms that the use of iron ore-PKS by the direct reduction method can lower the reduction temperature compared to the case of iron ore-coke in a blast furnace. Therefore, using pellets of a mixture of iron ore and biomass for manufacturing direct reduced iron (DRI) in the ironmaking industry is expected to save energy.

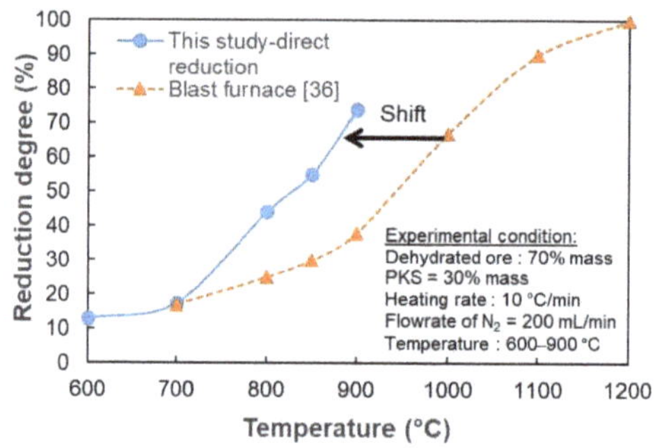

Figure 11. Reduction degree of the iron ore-biomass pellets by a direct reduction process at different temperatures compared to the blast furnace process.

4. Conclusions

The conclusions of the study are summarized as follow:

1. The dehydration process of low-grade iron ore could remove water content from the iron ore powder, which had an impact through increasing the specific surface area and the occurrence of a reduction reaction that transforms Fe_2O_3 to Fe_3O_4.
2. From thermogravimetric analysis, as the heating rate rose, the initial temperature of the weight loss shifted to a higher temperature. In addition, increasing the heating rate induces elevating the comprehensive reduction reactivity index (S) and shortening the reduction time.
3. Analysis of phase transformation based on temperature changes showed that, at a temperature of 600–700 °C, most of the formed phase was magnetite (Fe_3O_4). By increasing the temperature to 800 °C, wustite (FeO) formation was very significant. The reduction reaction at 900 °C indicated that $Fe_2O_3 \rightarrow Fe_3O_4 \rightarrow FeO \rightarrow Fe$ reaction was fast. According to the reduced gas analysis, carbon gasification significantly enhanced the reduction rate starting at 800 °C. Furthermore, a heating rate of 20 °C/min resulted in higher peak Fe intensity when compared to 10 °C/min. This could be due to the carbon gasification rate at a heating rate of 20 °C/min higher than at 10 °C/min.
4. The changing trend of the reduction and metallization degrees from 600 to 700 °C was slight. However, increasing the temperature to 800 °C showed a consistently high escalation of both degrees up to 900 °C. The degrees of reduction and metallization at a heating rate of 20 °C/min showed a more considerable increase than 10 and 15 °C/min. In addition, the current study can achieve the same degree of reduction at lower temperatures compared to the iron-coke mixture in the blast furnace method. This indicates that there is energy saving in this direct reduction process.

Supplementary Materials: The following are available online at https://www.mdpi.com/article/10.3390/en15010137/s1, Figure S1: The temperature and heating rate effects on gas composition when the temperature rises (small graphs) and the isothermal reduction lasting 60 min for a heating rate of 10 °C/min (**a**) 600 °C; (**b**) 700 °C; (**c**) 800 °C; (**d**) 900 °C. Figure S2: The temperature and heating rate effects on gas composition when the temperature rises (small graphs) and the isothermal reduction lasting 60 min for a heating rate of 20 °C/min (**a**) 600 °C; (**b**) 700 °C; (**c**) 800 °C; (**d**) 900 °C.

Author Contributions: Conceptualization, M.H., R.R., R.B.C. and A.Z.; methodology, M.H., R.R., R.B.C. and A.Z.; software, M.H., R.R. and A.Z.; validation, M.H., R.R. and R.B.C.; formal analysis, R.B.C. and A.Z.; investigation, A.Z.; resources, A.Z.; data curation, A.Z.; writing—original draft preparation, A.Z.; writing—review and editing, M.H., R.R. and R.B.C.; visualization, A.Z.; supervision, M.H., R.R. and R.B.C.; project administration, A.Z.; funding acquisition, M.H. and R.B.C. All authors have read and agreed to the published version of the manuscript.

Funding: This research and the APC were funded by "Direktorat Jenderal Penguatan Riset dan Pengembangan, Kementerian Riset, Teknologi, dan Pendidikan Tinggi" with grant number: 4504/UN1/DITLIT/DIT-LIT/PT/2021.

Institutional Review Board Statement: Not applicable.

Informed Consent Statement: Not applicable.

Data Availability Statement: The data presented in this study are available on request from the corresponding author.

Acknowledgments: The author would like to thank to "Direktorat Jenderal Penguatan Riset dan Pengembangan, Kementerian Riset, Teknologi, dan Pendidikan Tinggi" for the research funding. For additional support, the following companies are acknowledged: PT. Meratus Jaya Iron&Steel, South Kalimantan, Indonesia, and PT. Astra Agro Lestari Tbk., Jakarta, Indonesia.

Conflicts of Interest: The authors declare no conflict of interest.

References

1. Mousa, E.; Wang, C.; Riesbeck, J.; Larsson, M. Biomass applications in iron and steel industry: An overview of challenges and opportunities. *Renew. Sustain. Energy Rev.* **2016**, *65*, 1247–1266. [CrossRef]
2. Suopajärvi, H.; Kemppainen, A.; Haapakangas, J.; Fabritius, T. Extensive review of the opportunities to use biomass-based fuels in iron and steelmaking processes. *J. Clean. Prod.* **2017**, *148*, 709–734. [CrossRef]
3. Purwanto, H.; Zakiyuddin, A.M.; Rozhan, A.N.; Mohamad, A.S.; Salleh, H.M. Effect of charcoal derived from oil palm empty fruit bunch on the sinter characteristics of low grade iron ore. *J. Clean. Prod.* **2018**, *200*, 954–959. [CrossRef]
4. Ubando, A.T.; Chen, W.-H.; Ong, H.C. Iron oxide reduction by graphite and torrefied biomass analyzed by TG-FTIR for mitigating CO_2 emissions. *Energy* **2019**, *180*, 968–977. [CrossRef]
5. Cheng, Z.; Yang, J.; Zhou, L.; Liu, Y.; Guo, Z.; Wang, Q. Experimental study of commercial charcoal as alternative fuel for coke breeze in iron ore sintering process. *Energy Convers. Manag.* **2016**, *125*, 254–263. [CrossRef]
6. Huang, D.-B.; Zong, Y.-B.; Wei, R.; Gao, W.; Liu, X.-M. Direct Reduction of High-phosphorus Oolitic Hematite Ore Based on Biomass Pyrolysis. *J. Iron Steel Res. Int.* **2016**, *23*, 874–883. [CrossRef]
7. Wei, R.; Cang, D.; Bai, Y.; Huang, D.; Liu, X. Reduction characteristics and kinetics of iron oxide by carbon in biomass. *Ironmak. Steelmak.* **2016**, *43*, 144–152. [CrossRef]
8. Nayak, D.; Dash, N.; Ray, N.; Rath, S.S. Utilization of waste coconut shells in the reduction roasting of overburden from iron ore mines. *Powder Technol.* **2019**, *353*, 450–458. [CrossRef]
9. Zhao, H.; Li, Y.; Song, Q.; Liu, S.; Ma, Q.; Ma, L.; Shu, X. Catalytic reforming of volatiles from co-pyrolysis of lignite blended with corn straw over three different structures of iron ores. *J. Anal. Appl. Pyrolysis* **2019**, *144*, 104714. [CrossRef]
10. Cahyono, R.B.; Rozhan, A.N.; Yasuda, N.; Nomura, T.; Hosokai, S.; Kashiwaya, Y.; Akiyama, T. Catalytic coal-tar decomposition to enhance reactivity of low-grade iron ore. *Fuel Process. Technol.* **2013**, *113*, 84–89. [CrossRef]
11. Abe, K.; Kurniawan, A.; Ohashi, K.; Nomura, T.; Akiyama, T. Ultrafast Iron-Making Method: Carbon Combustion Synthesis from Carbon-Infiltrated Goethite Ore. *ACS Omega* **2018**, *3*, 6151–6157. [CrossRef]
12. Hosokai, S.; Matsui, K.; Okinaka, N.; Ohno, K.; Shimizu, M.; Akiyama, T. Kinetic Study on the Reduction Reaction of Biomass-Tar-Infiltrated Iron. *Energy Fuels* **2012**, *26*, 7274–7279. [CrossRef]
13. Cahyono, R.B.; Yasuda, N.; Nomura, T.; Akiyama, T. Utilization of Low Grade Iron Ore (FeOOH) and Biomass Through Integrated Pyrolysis-tar Decomposition (CVI process) in Ironmaking Industry: Exergy Analysis and its Application. *ISIJ Int.* **2015**, *55*, 428–435. [CrossRef]
14. Mochizuki, Y.; Nishio, M.; Tsubouchi, N.; Akiyama, T. Preparation of a Carbon-Containing Pellet with High Strength and High Reactivity by Vapor Deposition of Tar to a Cold-Bonded Pellet. *Energy Fuels* **2017**, *31*, 8877–8885. [CrossRef]

15. Zulkania, A.; Rochmadi, R.; Cahyono, R.B.; Hidayat, M. Investigation into Biomass Tar-Based Carbon Deposits as Reduction Agents on Iron Ore Using the Tar Impregnation Method. *Metals* **2021**, *11*, 1623. [CrossRef]
16. Luo, S.; Yi, C.; Zhou, Y. Direct reduction of mixed biomass-Fe_2O_3 briquettes using biomass-generated syngas. *Renew. Energy* **2011**, *36*, 3332–3336. [CrossRef]
17. Guo, D.; Hu, M.; Pu, C.; Xiao, B.; Hu, Z.; Liu, S.; Zhu, X. Kinetics and mechanisms of direct reduction of iron ore-biomass composite pellets with hydrogen gas. *Int. J. Hydrogen Energy.* **2015**, *40*, 4733–4740. [CrossRef]
18. Yuan, P.; Shen, B.; Duan, D.; Adweek, G.; Mei, X.; Lu, F. Study on the formation of direct reduced iron by using biomass as reductants of carbon-containing pellets in RHF process. *Energy* **2017**, *141*, 472–482. [CrossRef]
19. Yuan, X.; Luo, F.; Liu, S.; Zhang, M.; Zhou, D. Comparative Study on the Kinetics of the Isothermal Reduction of Iron Ore Composite Pellets Using Coke, Charcoal, and Biomass as Reducing Agents. *Metals* **2021**, *11*, 340. [CrossRef]
20. Rashid, R.Z.A.; Mohd-Salleh, H.; Ani, M.H.; Yunus, N.A.; Akiyama, T.; Purwanto, H. Reduction of low grade iron ore pellet using palm kernel shell. *Renew. Energy* **2014**, *63*, 617–623. [CrossRef]
21. Wang, G.; Zhang, J.; Zhang, G.; Wang, H.; Zhao, D. Experiments and Kinetic Modeling for Reduction of Ferric Oxide-biochar Composite Pellets. *ISIJ Int.* **2017**, *57*, 1374–1383. [CrossRef]
22. Saito, G.; Nomura, T.; Sakaguchi, N.; Akiyama, T. Optimization of the Dehydration Temperature of Goethite to Control Pore Morphology. *ISIJ Int.* **2016**, *56*, 1598–1605. [CrossRef]
23. Kurniawan, A.; Abe, K.; Ohashi, K.; Nomura, T.; Akiyama, T. Reduction of mild-dehydrated, low-grade iron ore by ethanol. *Fuel Process. Technol.* **2018**, *178*, 156–165. [CrossRef]
24. Hubbard, C.R.; Snyder, R.L. RIR-Measurement and Use in Quantitative XRD. *Powder Diffr.* **1988**, *3*, 74–77. [CrossRef]
25. Walter, D.; Buxbaum, G.; Laqua, W. The Mechanism of the Thermal Transformation from Goethite to Hematite. *J. Therm. Anal. Calorim.* **2001**, *63*, 733–748. [CrossRef]
26. Pradhan, N.; Nayak, R.R.; Mishra, D.K.; Priyadarshini, E.; Sukla, L.B.; Mishra, B.K. Microbial Treatment of Lateritic Ni-ore for Iron Beneficiation and Their Characterization. *World Environ.* **2012**, *2*, 110–115. [CrossRef]
27. Wei, Z.; Zhang, J.; Qin, B.; Dong, Y.; Lu, Y.; Li, Y.; Hao, W.; Zhang, Y. Reduction kinetics of hematite ore fines with H_2 in a rotary drum reactor. *Powder Technol.* **2018**, *332*, 18–26. [CrossRef]
28. Zhao, H.; Li, Y.; Song, Q.; Liu, S.; Ma, L.; Shu, X. Catalytic reforming of volatiles from co-pyrolysis of lignite blended with corn straw over three iron ores: Effect of iron ore types on the product distribution, carbon-deposited iron ore reactivity and its mechanism. *Fuel* **2021**, *286*, 119398. [CrossRef]
29. Zuo, H.-B.; Hu, Z.-W.; Zhang, J.-L.; Li, J.; Liu, Z.-J. Direct reduction of iron ore by biomass char. *Int. J. Miner. Met. Mater.* **2013**, *20*, 514–521. [CrossRef]
30. Chen, J.; Fan, X.; Jiang, B.; Mub, L.; Yao, P.; Yin, H.; Song, X. Pyrolysis of oil-plant wastes in a TGA and a fixed-bed reactor: Thermochemical behaviors, kinetics, and products characterization. *Bioresour. Technol.* **2015**, *192*, 592–602. [CrossRef]
31. Somerville, M.; Deev, A. The effect of heating rate, particle size and gas flow on the yield of charcoal during the pyrolysis of radiata pine wood. *Renew. Energy* **2020**, *151*, 419–425. [CrossRef]
32. Wu, C.; Budarin, V.L.; Gronnow, M.J.; De Bruyn, M.; Onwudili, J.A.; Clark, J.H.; Williams, P.T. Conventional and microwave-assisted pyrolysis of biomass under different heating rates. *J. Anal. Appl. Pyrolysis* **2014**, *107*, 276–283. [CrossRef]
33. Guo, D.; Li, Y.; Cui, B.; Chen, Z.; Luo, S.; Xiao, B.; Zhu, H.; Hu, M. Direct reduction of iron ore/biomass composite pellets using simulated biomass-derived syngas: Experimental analysis and kinetic modelling. *Chem. Eng. J.* **2017**, *327*, 822–830. [CrossRef]
34. Mishra, S. Review on Reduction Kinetics of Iron Ore–Coal Composite Pellet in Alternative and Sustainable Ironmaking. *J. Sustain. Metall.* **2020**, *6*, 541–556. [CrossRef]
35. Oh, J.; Noh, D. The reduction kinetics of hematite particles in H_2 and CO atmospheres. *Fuel* **2017**, *196*, 144–153. [CrossRef]
36. Castro, J.A.; Nogami, H.; Yagi, J. Transient Mathematical Model of Blast Furnace Based on Multi-fluid Concept, with Application to High PCI Operation. *ISIJ Int.* **2000**, *40*, 637–646. [CrossRef]

energies

MDPI

Article

Quantitative Risk Assessment for Aerospace Facility According to Windrose

Hee Jin Kim [1], Kyeong Min Jang [1], In Seok Yeo [2], Hwa Young Oh [2], Sun Il Kang [2] and Eun Sang Jung [1,*]

[1] Department of Bioenvironmental Energy, Pusan National University, Miryang 50463, Korea; eslab0609@pusan.ac.kr (H.J.K.); kmjang3303@gmail.com (K.M.J.)
[2] Launcher Complex Development Team, Korea Aerospace Research Institute, Daejeon 34133, Korea; yis@kari.re.kr (I.S.Y.); ohy3421@kari.re.kr (H.Y.O.); aerodol@kari.re.kr (S.I.K.)
* Correspondence: esjung@pusan.ac.kr; Tel.: +82-055-350-5433

Abstract: Wind direction and speed are the most important factors that determine the degree of damage caused by a jet fire. In this study, the metal hose used to extract/supply fuel was identified as the component with the highest risk for a jet fire occurring at an aerospace facility. A risk assessment was performed to evaluate the individual risk of a jet fire from the metal hose according to the wind direction and speed. HSE failure data was applied for calculating the jet fire probability including metal hose failure, ignition frequency, and jet fire frequency. Which was 3.0×10^{-4}. The individual risk of different fatality probabilities was calculated according to the wind rose data for the aerospace facility. The individual risk from jet fire in the aerospace facility was calculated with a maximum risk of 3.35×10^{-5} and a minimum risk of 1.49×10^{-6}. The individual risk satisfied HSE ALARP criteria. In addition, firewalls, extinguishing systems, and an emergency shut off system were enhanced, and it was thought that the risk from jet fire could satisfy acceptable criteria.

Keywords: individual risk; aerospace facility; fatality probability; jet fire; kerosene atomization; wind direction and speed

Citation: Kim, H.J.; Jang, K.M.; Yeo, I.S.; Oh, H.Y.; Kang, S.I.; Jung, E.S. Quantitative Risk Assessment for Aerospace Facility According to Windrose. *Energies* **2022**, *15*, 189. https://doi.org/10.3390/en15010189

Academic Editors: Roberto Alonso González Lezcano, Francesco Nocera and Rosa Giuseppina Caponetto

Received: 23 November 2021
Accepted: 24 December 2021
Published: 28 December 2021

1. Introduction

Fire risk is the likelihood of a fire or explosion to occur, which is affected by any unique feature or potential hazard. Increases in indoor combustibles, diverse high-rise buildings, and population density have led to increased fire risks. Fire risk assessment is necessary for maintaining the safety of buildings and designing fire safety measures. Insufficient measures can result in massive casualties and damage to property. Risk assessment considers the structure of the building, its contents, layout, wind speed, and escape routes in the event of a fire.

Fire risk assessment can be of two types: quantitative and qualitative. Quantitative assessment methods are based on frequency analysis of entities that may cause fire and explosion and a consequence analysis of the potential damage of an accident to humans or property [1–3]. Examples of quantitative assessment methods include fault tree analysis (FTA), event tree analysis (ETA), cause–consequence analysis (CCA), layer of protection analysis, risk matrix, and the frequency–number of fatalities (F–N) curve. On the contrary, qualitative assessment methods comprehensively collect the opinions of many experts and include what-if analysis, hazard and operability, and process hazard review. In Korea, fire risk assessments are generally qualitative; a quantitative assessment method has not yet been universally accepted. Quantitative fire risk assessments are needed for liquefied natural gas plants, aerospace facilities, and other facilities with major fire hazards [4,5]. Fire risk assessment for existing nuclear plants and safety-critical systems can widely vary in approaches and outcomes [6]

Recently, in order to promote national economic growth and national interest, not only government space activities, but also commercial space activities of private companies are considered as one of the key areas of activity [7]. According to the establishment and operation of space launch sites increases through the active space activities, various risks may occur in the aerospace facility, such as damage to structure and human life due to complexity and risk factors of aerospace systems. As such, a quantitative risk assessment of all parts, procedures, and operations of the aerospace facility is required [8–10]. Aerospace facilities perform various operations that pose a fire risk, such as rocket transfer and assembly, fuel and oxidant charging, and maintenance of electronics and general machinery. If a launch is rescheduled, the charged kerosene should be immediately extracted and then recharged. Due to the large amount of kerosene involved in the extraction and charging processes, as even a small leak can pose a fire risk. Jet and pool fires can be caused by fuel and oxidant leakage, tank failure, and catastrophic tank rupture. The potential of an explosion and secondary damage increases with the size of the leak. Thus, a quantitative fire risk assessment should be conducted to minimize the primary and secondary fire damage that could occur in aerospace facilities, with a special focus on the metal hose that is connected to the tank inside the rocket for supplying and extracting fuel [11,12]. Due to the metal hose posing a high risk in the event of a fuel leak, quantitative risk assessment should be performed for metal hose.

In this study, UK Health and Safety Executive (HSE) probability data was used to analyze metal hose failure and ignition frequency, and a consequence analysis was performed to analyze the fatality of jet fire. Wind rose was used to analyze the effect of wind direction and speed, which are the most important factors in the case of a jet fire. Finally, the individual risk assessment to the aerospace facility from metal hose jet fire was performed, considering the probability of failure and ignition, consequence of jet fire, wind direction and speed through comparison with the HSE risk standard.

2. Methodology

Validation for quantitative risk assessment can have several meanings that are disputable. As such, quantitative risk assessment of validation aspects, considering the objectives, expected results may be necessary [13,14]. Specifically, sampling proper data and its methods are most important to conduct quantitative risk assessment exactly. Therefore, in this study, through the validation approaches, a quantitative risk assessment was performed.

2.1. Validation Approach

Quantitative risk assessment is expressed as multiplying the frequency by consequence of a hazard factor leading to an injury or disease. In the case of frequency, it is the probability of occurrence of accidents and diseases for hazardous and dangerous work. In the case of consequence, it is the degree of exposure to human and material damage. As such, the quantitative fire risk assessment risk is a method of predicting the degree of risk for multiplying the frequency by consequence values of fire, according to the accident scenario, which are dependent on various parameters. Finally, after the quantitative risk assessment, it establishes mitigation to solve the workplace risk factors, such as installing emergency warning devices and securing a minimum safety distance [2,4,15]. Quantitative fire risk assessment consists of five methods, as shown in Figure 1 [16]. This section is introduced based on quantitative fire risk assessment to perform this research.

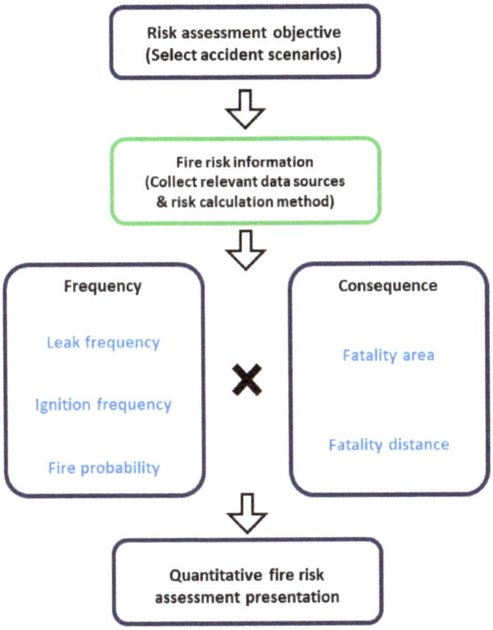

Figure 1. Quantitative fire risk assessment procedure.

2.1.1. Part 1. Risk Assessment Objective (Select Accident Scenarios)

This part means to identify hazardous source and accident scenarios that match installation specific interests. In some cases, relevant guidelines and standards could be applied for this part. Selecting proper accident scenarios is important. When a risk is calculated by considering an accident with a very low frequencies and low impact, it takes a lot of time and money to control the risk. To select the proper hazardous source, a P&ID (Piping and Instrument Diagram) and aerospace facility drawing were analyzed, and a metal hose was selected as the most dangerous source.

2.1.2. Part 2. Fire Risk Information (Collect Relevant Data Sources and Risk Calculation Method)

This part is necessary to conduct quantitative risk assessment adequately. A frequency data, which is needed to calculate fire occurrence probability, could be collected to analyze accident data from HSE, OGP (Oil and Gas Producers), NFPA (National Fire Protection Association), and HIAD (Hydrogen Incident Accident Database) [4,5]. A consequence could be calculated from various empirical equations or differential equations. Since solving differential equations is very difficult and complex, empirical equations based on various experiments are used to calculate the consequence and risk analysis. A fatality of jet fire and consequences are calculated based on the TNO Green book [17] and Han and Weng [18], considering mass release rate and probit function. An individual risk is calculated from fatality, frequency of jet fire, and weather conditions, which is made from HSE; a simplified approach to estimating individual risk [19]. A jet breakup length that is corresponded to velocity, density, surface tension, and viscosity, where the empirical equation was validated from Miesse [20]. Considering weather conditions in the Republic of Korea, wind rose data from Korea Meteorological Administration (KMA) was used.

2.1.3. Part 3. Frequency (Selecting Proper Database and Applying)

As a result of the accident probability database analysis, the specific accident probability data for a metal hose does not exist. As such HSE probability database applicable to general leak situations were selected.

In this part, the metal hose fire probability was calculated from metal hose failure and ignition probability values using the HSE and cox et al. database [21,22].

2.1.4. Part 4. Consequence

The consequence of accidents can be analyzed through fatality of overpressure, radiation intensity, and toxic gas concentration. In the case of jet fire, fatality is caused by the radiation of the flame. In this study, the fatality area and distance were calculated using the Han and Weng [18] equation based on mass release rate and probit function.

2.1.5. Part 5. Quantitative Fire Risk Assessment Presentation

Quantitative fire risk assessment can derive the final individual risk using frequency and consequence analysis. In this study, wind rose data was applied to HSE's individual risk equation [19] to consider both wind direction and speed.

2.2. Scenario and Boundary Definitions (Metal Hose)

The target scenario was set in the space launch facility at Goheung, Republic of Korea, which was operated by the Korea Aerospace Research Institute. The risk assessment focused on the metal hose, which was highly likely to cause a jet fire due to leakage, failure to switch off, cracking, or excessive flow rate. The risk of a jet fire was calculated by considering the size of the metal hose, internal temperature and pressure, flow rate, and location. Since the metal hose charges and discharges fuel, it was always exposed to danger in the event of a fire or accident. If the metal hose and rocket were separated, a larger fire may occur. Figure 2 shows the schematic of the metal hose used at the Goheung rocket launch facility, respectively. Table 1 presents the properties of kerosene [23,24]. As shown in Figure 2, the metal hose could be divided into three stages. A jet fire may occur at any stage. However, jet fires at higher stages will not result in injury to humans; thus, the fire risk assessment focused on the lowest stage (i.e., metal hose 1), since this part was most likely to cause injuries to humans.

Table 1. Properties of kerosene [23,24].

Physical Properties	Value	Physical Properties	Value
Critical temperature (°C)	321.45	Viscosity (N·s/m^2)	0.00164
Boiling point (°C)	150.82	Critical pressure (bar)	22.9
Flammable/toxic	Flammable	Surface tension (N/m)	0.0275
Molecular weight (g/mol)	128.258	Upper flammable limit (%)	5.6
Lower flammable limit (%)	0.7	Density (kg/m^3)	820
Heat of combustion (kJ/kg)	43,200	Burning velocity (mm/s)	0.07

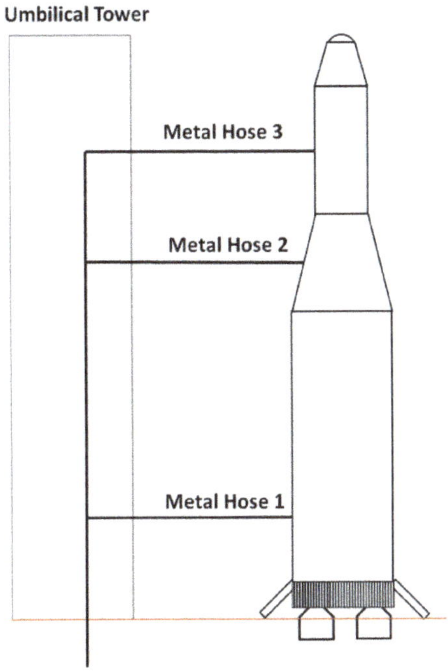

Figure 2. Schematic of metal hoses connecting the rocket to the umbilical tower.

2.3. Individual Risk

Individual risk (IR) refers to the probability of personal injury in hazardous facilities when a fire occurs near an ignition source [19,25]. It can be expressed in two ways. The first is by plotting risk contours to designate the range around a hazardous facility for the same risk level. The second is a two-dimensional profile that indicates the risk level according to distance from the hazardous facility. IR can be calculated as follows [19]:

$$IR_k = \theta_k \cdot \sum_i p_{loc,i,k} \cdot FoF_i \tag{1}$$

where IR_k is IR of population group k; θ_k is the overall fraction of time that population group k is in the area; $p_{loc,i,k}$ is the probability that population group k is at location i; FoF_i is the frequency of fatalities at location i [19,26].

FoF_i can be calculated as follows [19]:

$$FoF_i = \sum_j f_{eo,j} \cdot p_{fat,i,j} \cdot p_{weather,j} \cdot p_{direction,i,j} \tag{2}$$

where $f_{eo,j}$ is the frequency of event outcome j; $p_{fat,i,j}$ and $p_{weather,j}$ are the probabilities of fatality and weather conditions produced by event outcome j (from meteorological data, 1 for weather independent event outcomes), respectively; $p_{direction,i,j}$ is the probability of the direction required to produce event outcome i (related to the wind rose and cloud width for gas dispersion events, one for omnidirectional events). For the sake of simplicity, the following assumptions are used to calculate the individual risk [19,27,28]:

1. The wind distribution is constant, and accidents can occur in all directions.
2. Only one wind speed and climate stability degree are used.
3. Mitigation factors, such as evacuation, are not considered.
4. Leakage sources are uniformly distributed; thus, accidents can occur at any point.

2.4. Jet Fire Fatality

The fatality of a jet fire is calculated from the thermal radiation. In the case of the jet fire fatality probability function, the Equation (3) considering the thermal radiation exposure time to the target and the thermal radiation flux is used [17,29,30].

$$P_r = -14.9 + 2.56 \ln\left(t \cdot I^{\frac{4}{3}} / 10^4\right) \tag{3}$$

where t is the time that the target is exposed to radiation. The exposure time is generally assumed as 30 s in urban settings. I is the thermal radiation flux [30].

Second, if you replace the thermal radiation flux, you can use the Equation (4) using the leakage flow rate and the distance between the target and the center of the flame zone.

$$P_r = 16.61 + 3.4 \ln\left(\frac{Q}{R^2}\right) \tag{4}$$

where Q is the mass flow rate of leakage; R is the distance between the target and the center of the flame zone [30].

In the study, the probabilities of 99%, 50%, and 1% fatality can be calculated according to the radiation, while the areas and distance for these fatalities, due to a metal hose failure, can be calculated using Equation (5) with the probability values of 7.33, 5, and 2.67, respectively [17,30].

$$r_{jet,99} = 3.915\sqrt{Q},\ r_{jet,50} = 5.514\sqrt{Q},\ r_{jet.1} = 7.768\sqrt{Q} \tag{5}$$

The average fatality probability in each area can be calculated as follows [29,30].

$$\frac{\int_0^{3.915} Pdr}{\int_0^{3.915} dr} = 1,\ \frac{\int_{3.915}^{5.514} Pdr}{\int_{3.915}^{5.514} dr} = 0.805,\ \frac{\int_{5.514}^{7.768} Pdr}{\int_{5.514}^{7.768} dr} = 0.172 \tag{6}$$

Figure 3 shows a schematic of the three fatality areas around a jet fire.

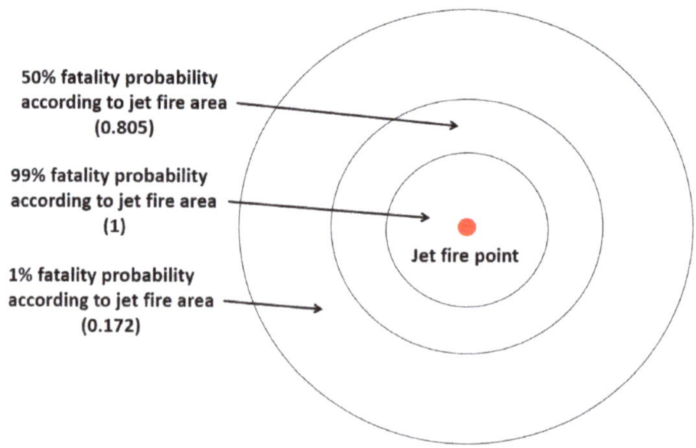

Figure 3. Schematic of fatality probability according to areas around a jet fire point.

2.5. Kerosene Atomization

During the charging process, fuel flows through the metal hose at a velocity of 4–100 m/s and a pressure of 1.5–10 bar. If the metal hose ruptures, the high velocity of the leaking fuel can cause a jet fire, where the fuel is atomized or evaporated as it combusts. At room temperature (15–20 °C), liquid propellants evaporate more slowly than liquefied propellants; thus, a pool fire is more likely to occur [31–34]. However, a jet fire can occur under high velocity and pressure conditions. Khan et al. [35] reported the combustion characteristics of kerosene droplet. Due to the research data, a kerosene droplet under the 125 μm, was immediately burned by ignitor. Therefore, atomized kerosene was sufficiently burned by ignitor, and jet fires can be generated. The size and shape of the atomization depend on *We* and *Re* of the leaking fuel. Liquid fuel frequently atomizes when the velocity was over 100 m/s [35–37]. An atomization characteristic was correlated with leakage velocity, and when the leakage velocity was increased over 100 m/s, mostly liquid fuels, which were passed atomization length (jet breakup length), were atomized and immediately vaporized, but liquefied fuels were atomized and evaporated under 100 m/s easily [31,32].

As shown in Figure 4, the atomization of the leak jet occurred at a constant breakup length. Miesse [20] had and established Equation (7) for calculating the atomization length. The Equation (7) was suitable for the density range 300 to 1500 kg/m^3, and viscosity range 0.01 to 10 cp conditions. The position where kerosene atomizes can be calculated as follows [32]:

$$L_c = 538\, d\, We^{0.5}\, Re^{-0.625} \tag{7}$$

$$We = \frac{\rho V^2 d}{\sigma} \tag{8}$$

$$Re = \rho V d/\mu \tag{9}$$

where L_c is the breakup length, d is the diameter, We is the Weber number, and Re is the Reynolds number. Table 2 presents the parameters of the metal hose according to its diameter. With the metal hose, it was impossible to meet the high-pressure conditions for kerosene atomization. Preferentially, a breakup length is calculated to consider fatality areas accurately, since the jet fire occurred after the breakup length. As show in Table 2, the minimum breakup length was 3.2 m. In this study, the accurate fatality area was described in Section 3, using the breakup length value.

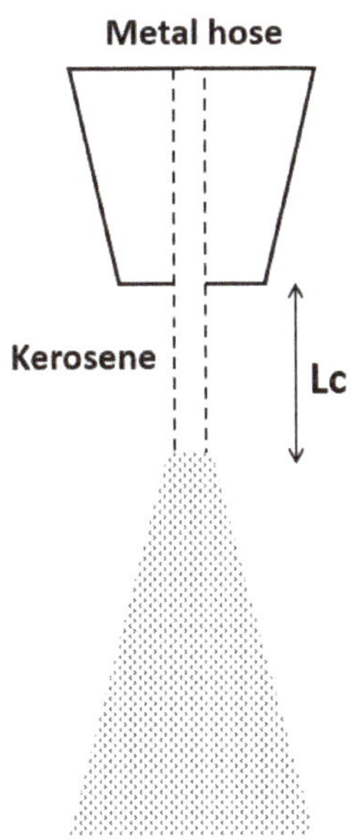

Figure 4. Kerosene atomization.

Table 2. Parameters of the metal hose.

Diameter (mm)	Velocity (m/s)	Reynolds Number	Weber Number	Breakup Length (m)
10	169.7	8.5×10^5	8.6×10^6	3.11
13	100.4	6.5×10^5	4.0×10^6	3.20
15	75.4	5.7×10^5	2.6×10^6	3.28
20	42.4	4.4×10^5	1.1×10^6	3.43
25	27.2	3.7×10^5	6.4×10^5	3.59
30	18.9	3.3×10^5	4.3×10^5	3.77
35	13.9	3.1×10^5	3.3×10^5	3.98
40	10.6	3.1×10^5	2.8×10^5	4.24

2.6. Metal Hose Ignition Probability and Wind Rose Data

Frequency analysis is a hierarchical method for calculating the probability of a fire or explosion occurring in a given structure. It can be used to identify equipment failure, faults, operating conditions, environmental conditions, and human error that contribute to fire and explosion accidents. FTA and ETA were used to calculate the failure and ignition probabilities to determine the probabilities of a pool fire, fireball, and jet fire for one year.

For FTA, the ignition probability of various flammable materials in the event of a metal hose leak was taken from the literature [38–40]. Table 3 presents the probability of a fire occurring for different release rates. The frequency analysis results for metal hoses are detailed in Section 3. Data from the UK Health and Safety Executive (HSE) were referenced to determine the failure probability of the metal hose, which was set to 1.0×10^{-2} [21,38].

Table 3. Ignition probability of a liquid according to the release rate.

Release Rate	Ignition Probability of a Liquid
<1 kg/s	1.0×10^{-2}
1–50 kg/s	3.0×10^{-2}
>50 kg/s	8.0×10^{-2}

A wind rose graphs the frequencies of the wind direction and speed at an observation point. It can be used to show the long-term average wind direction and speed [41,42], which are important factors that affect the location and extent of damage caused by a jet fire [42–44]. In this study, the wind direction was expressed as a probability, and it was combined with the frequency analysis for the fire risk assessment. Twelve wind directions were selected, and their probabilities were set according to the wind data from Goheung, which is where the aerospace facility is located. The software WPLOT [45] was used to analyze the wind rose data. Figure 5 shows the wind rose for Goheung. Table 4 presents wind data sourced from KMA from 2009 to 2018 in 12 directions according to frequency. Wind rose data is the probability data about wind direction and speed. For example, in Table 4, when the wind direction is 345 to 15 degrees, the probability of blowing with a wind speed of 0 to 1 m/s can be expressed as 26.6538%.

Wind speeds >5 m/s accounted for less than 1% of the 10 years of data and thus, were excluded from the analysis. Although a higher wind speed can lead to greater damage, the frequency was so low that the risk was negligible. The remaining wind speed data were used to quantify the probability of a jet fire in each wind direction. The total probability of a jet fire was determined by summing the probabilities in each wind direction. According to the wind rose data for this aerospace facility, the highest probability of a jet fire was at 345–15° for a wind speed of 0–1 m/s and at 315–345° for wind speeds of 1–2, 2–3, 3–4, and >4 m/s.

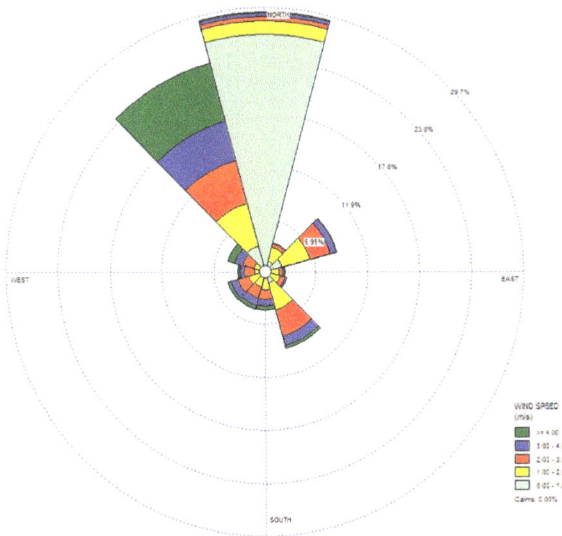

Figure 5. Wind direction and speed at the aerospace facility in Goheung (Korea Meteorological Administration).

Table 4. Probability of jet fire, according to wind direction and speed.

Direction (°)	0–1 (m/s)	1–2 (m/s)	2–3 (m/s)	3–4 (m/s)	>4 (m/s)
345–15	26.65380	1.50060	0.54358	0.32131	0.16008
15–45	1.25990	1.61807	0.44338	0.05873	0.00576
45–75	1.99926	3.33057	2.44034	0.67487	0.09213
75–105	0.71633	0.86374	0.42266	0.17620	0.09098
105–135	0.66911	1.13207	0.57237	0.14050	0.05873
135–165	1.34628	3.15206	3.00350	1.03418	0.42266
165–195	0.81537	1.23802	1.12977	0.71057	0.41575
195–225	0.64838	1.11825	1.29906	0.87871	0.45720
225–255	0.65759	1.34397	1.29791	0.83955	0.33974
255–285	0.28561	0.97084	1.19426	0.51824	0.18772
285–315	0.38465	0.96623	1.41307	0.92938	0.78773
315–345	3.02999	5.00622	4.92330	4.50871	6.79358
Total	38.46620	22.24060	18.68320	10.79100	9.81205

3. Consequence Analysis

For the consequence analysis, a kerosene jet fire was assumed to occur under the following conditions:

1. Kerosene leaks from the metal hose at a high speed.
2. Metal hose has a hole diameter of 13 mm.
3. Kerosene atomizes to form a jet fire when L_c = 3.20 m.
4. Radii from the jet fire for 99%, 50%, and 1% fatality can be determined.
5. Frequency of a jet fire can be determined for four directions, and the frequencies in each direction can be summed to obtain the total frequency.

Table 5 presents the fire probability for a metal hose with a hole diameter of 13 mm and release rate of 10.93 kg/s, while Table 6 presents the radii for 99%, 50%, and 1% fatality when a jet fire occurs with a leakage flow rate of 10.93 kg/s. According to Equations (5) and (6), the 99%, 50%, and 1% fatality areas and radii were 493.87 m^2 and 3.20~12.94 m, 518.01 m^2 and 12.94~18.23 m, and 1027.71 m^2 and 18.23~25.68 m, respectively. When the analysis of the results was performed, it was confirmed that the lower the fatality, the lower the degree of damage, but the wider the damage range.

Table 5. Metal hose fire probability.

Ignition Probability	Failure Probability	Metal Hose Fire Probability
3.0×10^{-2}	1.0×10^{-2}	3.0×10^{-4}

Table 6. Fatality area and distance from jet fire point according to metal hose release rate.

Metal Hose Release Rate	99% Fatality Area 99% Fatality Distance	50% Fatality Area 50% Fatality Distance	1% Fatality Area 1% Fatality Distance
10.93 kg/s	493.87 m^2 3.20~12.94 m	518.01 m^2 12.94~18.23 m	1027.71 m^2 18.23~25.68 m

4. Risk Analysis

IR was obtained from the results of the frequency analysis and consequence analysis, which is calculated as follows:

$$IR = \theta \cdot p_{loc} \cdot f_{mh} \cdot fat_{jet\ fire} \cdot p_{windrose} \quad (10)$$

where θ is the overall fraction of time that a person is in a given area, p_{loc} is the probability that the person is at a location, f_{mh} is the fire probability of the metal hose, $fat_{jet\ fire}$ is the fatality probability of a jet fire, and $p_{windrose}$ is the probability that the jet fire will be in one of the windrose (obtained through WPLOT).

For the risk analysis, a kerosene jet fire individual risk was assumed to occur under the following conditions:

1. θ is set to 0.33 since Korean labour standards are applied to work 8 h out of 24 h.
2. The p_{loc} was set as follows, since the person working at the space launch facility was among those working at the Korea Aerospace Research Institute located in Goheung was 0.88.

In this study, Equation (10) was created based on Equation (2). Although Equation (2) assumed to have a constant velocity distribution in all wind directions, Equation (10) used in this study that considered both wind direction and speed to calculate the individual risk result value.

Table 7 presents the values of the terms in Equation (10). Figure 5 lists the IR ranges by applying different colors to visually express the IR result values derived through Equation (10). The colors in Figure 6 are used in Figures 7–9 to visualize IR according to the wind speed and direction for each fatality probability. Figures 7–9 show the results for 99%, 50%, 1% IR. For Table 7, all probability values of the wind rose are omitted since they are listed in Section 2.5.

Table 7. Calculation of IR for different fatality probabilities.

IR (Jet Fire)	θ	p_{loc}	f_{eo}	$fat_{jet\,fire}$	$p_{wind\ rose}$
99%	0.33	0.88	3.0×10^{-4}	1	12 directions
50%	0.33	0.88	3.0×10^{-4}	0.805	12 directions
1%	0.33	0.88	3.0×10^{-4}	0.172	12 directions

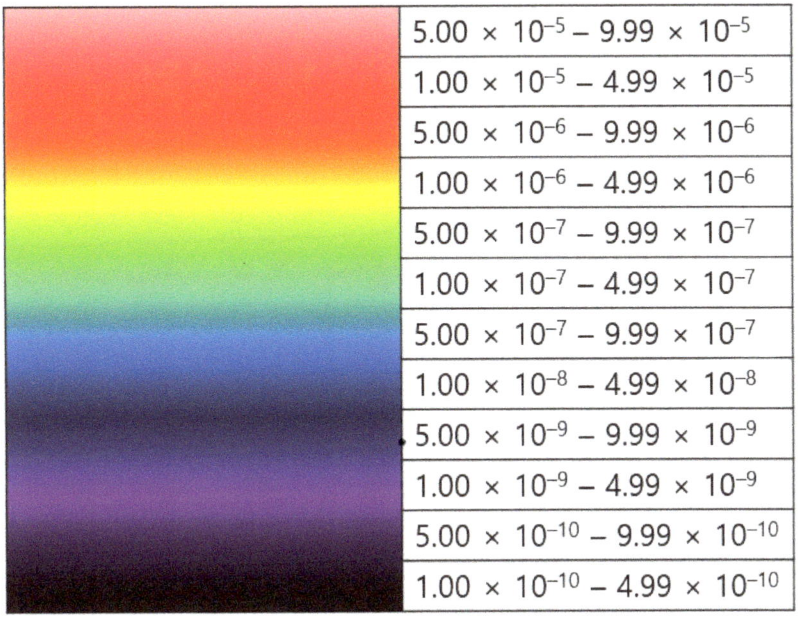

Figure 6. IR contours.

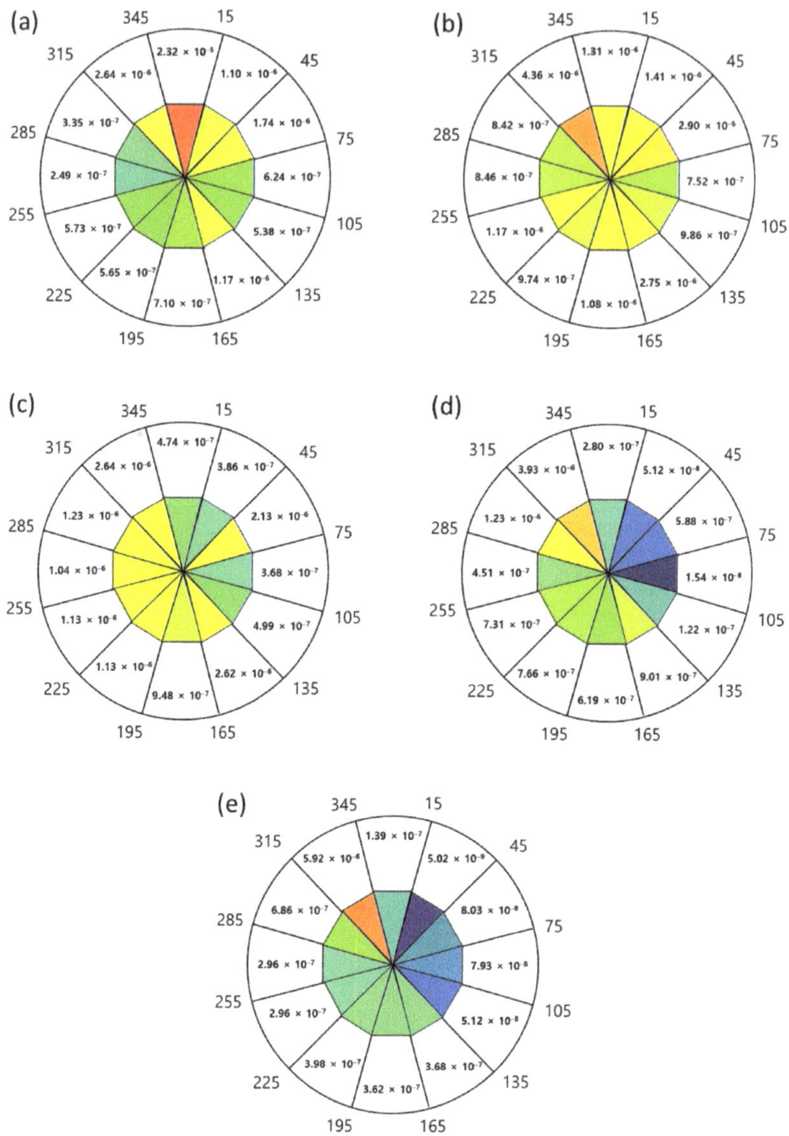

Figure 7. IR of 99% fatality at different wind directions and speeds: (**a**) 0–1 m/s, (**b**) 1–2 m/s, (**c**) 2–3 m/s, (**d**) 3–4 m/s, and (**e**) >4 m/s.

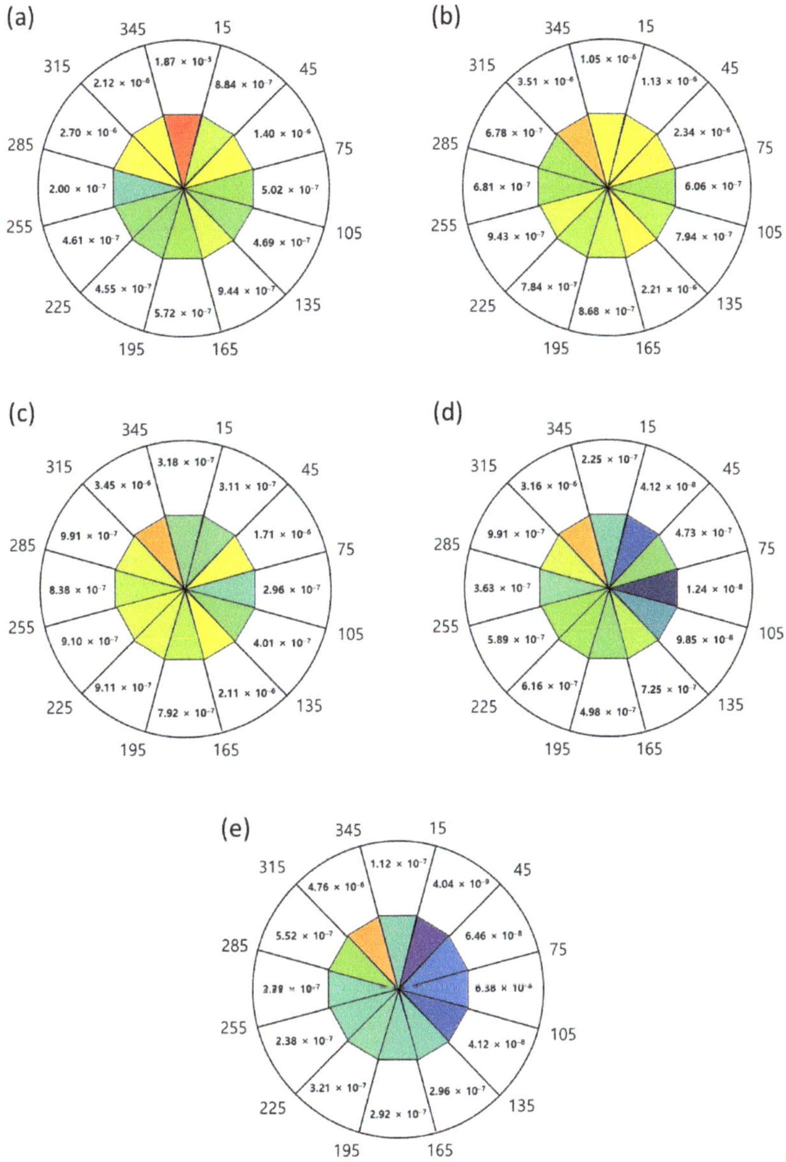

Figure 8. IR of 50% fatality at different wind directions and speeds: (**a**) 0–1 m/s, (**b**) 1–2 m/s, (**c**) 2–3 m/s, (**d**) 3–4 m/s, and (**e**) >4 m/s.

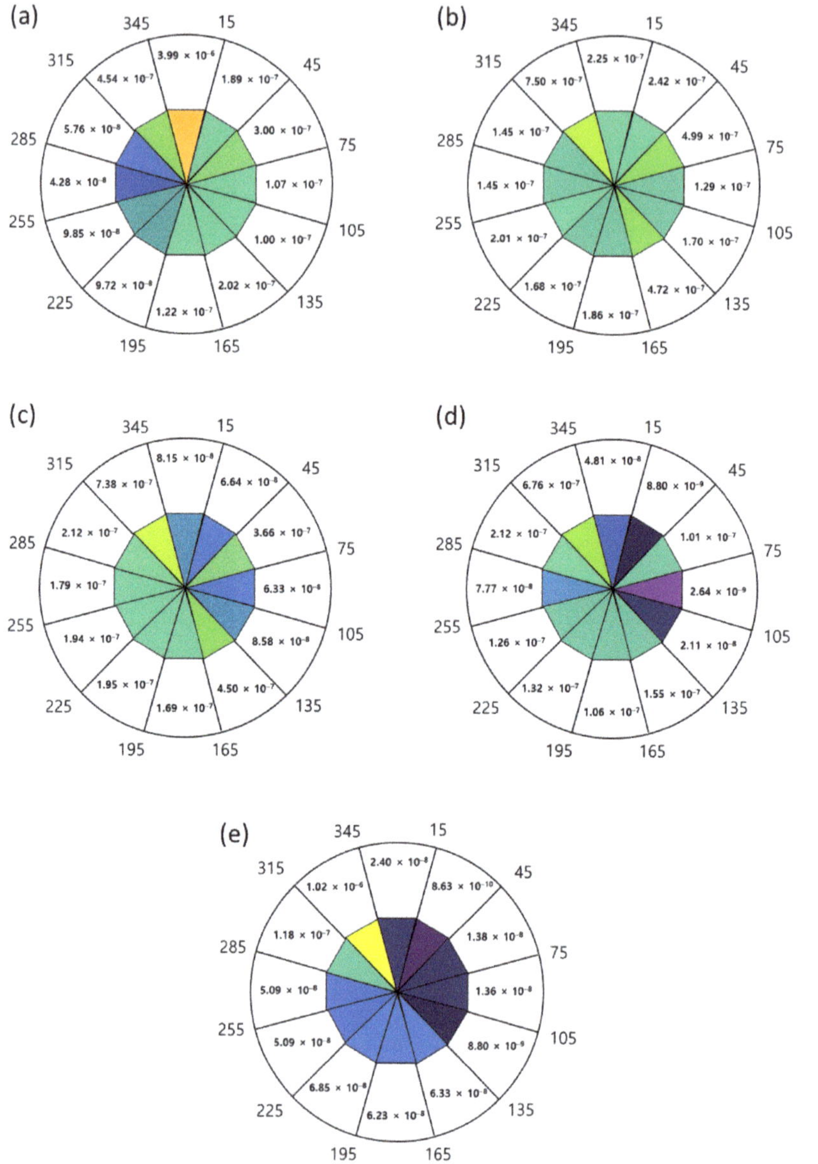

Figure 9. IR of 1% fatality at different wind directions and speeds: (**a**) 0–1 m/s, (**b**) 1–2 m/s, (**c**) 2–3 m/s, (**d**) 3–4 m/s, and (**e**) >4 m/s.

The IR results were calculated for the areas corresponding to 99%, 50%, and 1% fatality in each wind direction. The total IR was calculated for each wind speed. For the case of 99% fatality, the highest IR was at 345°–15° for a wind speed of 0–1 m/s and at 315°–345° for wind speeds >1 m/s. The lowest IR was at 255°–285° for a wind speed of 0–1 m/s, 75°–105° for wind speeds of 1–4 m/s, and 15°–45° for wind speeds >4 m/s. For the case of 50% fatality, the highest IR was at 345°–15° for a wind speed of 0–1 m/s and 315°–345° for wind speeds >1 m/s. The lowest IR was at 255°–285° for a wind speed of 0–1 m/s, 75°–105° for wind speeds of 1–4 m/s, and 15°–45° for a wind speed >4 m/s. For the case of

1% fatality, the highest IR was at 345°–15° for a wind speed of 0–1 m/s and 315°–345° for wind speeds >1 m/s. The lowest IR was at 255°–285° for a wind speed of 0–1 m/s, 75°–105° for wind speeds of 1–4 m/s, and 15°–45° for a wind speed >4 m/s. The IR showed the same tendencies at 99%, 50%, and 1% fatality. The total IR was high at 0–1 m/s, which was the most frequent wind speed; this indicates a high probability of IR when a jet fire occurs.

5. Results and Discussion

In Section 4, individual risk results were calculated by considering the 99%, 50%, and 1% fatality ranges and wind direction and speed. Furthermore, in the case of Section 4, individual risks for all wind directions, speeds, and fatality ranges were, respectively, calculated and presented. In Section 5, the total individual risk considering wind speed and fatality ranges is calculated, and the safety of the aerospace facility is confirmed when metal hose jet fire occurred through comparison with the HSE risk standard. The HSE risk standard is a criteria created to ensure plant safety from unexpected accident that does not generate damage to workers, the environment, or assets [46,47].

HSE risk standard follows the ALARP (As Low as Reasonably Practicable) standard. As shown in Figure 10, ALARP is set for the safe operation of chemical facilities and plants, and there is a difference between the risk standard for workers and for the public [48–50].

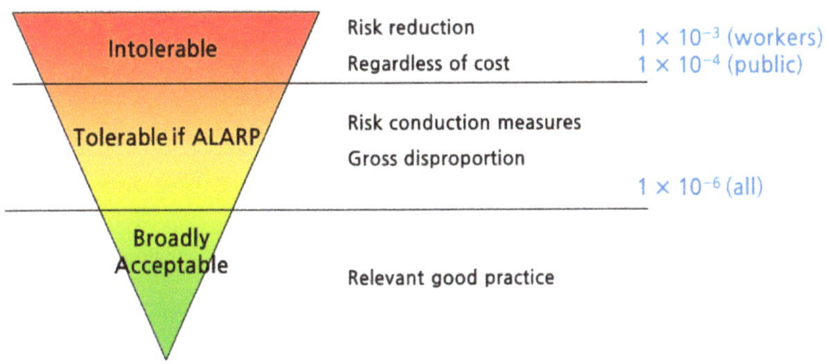

Figure 10. HSE ALARP standard.

As a result, the total individual risk result value considering fatality and wind speed was shown in Figure 11, and it was found that the individual risk decreased as the wind speed increased and the fatality decreased. In the case of wind speed, due to the probability decreasing as the wind speed was increased, the $p_{windrose}$ of Equation (10) was decreased and, consequently, the individual risk was lowered. Similarly, in the case of fatality, due to the fatality decreasing as the $fat_{jet\ fire}$ of Equation (10) was decreased, consequently, the individual risk was lowered. Finally, when compared with the ALARP standard, all individual risks were included in the ALARP standard regardless of wind speed and fatality. The individual risk from jet fire in an aerospace facility was calculated that maximum risk is 3.35×10^{-5}, minimum is 1.49×10^{-6}. According to this study's results, when a jet fire occurred from a metal hose, the risk satisfied tolerable criteria. Therefore, enhanced firewalls, extinguishing systems, and emergency shut off systems are needed to prevent jet fire accidents and to satisfy acceptable criteria. If the same accident occurs in another area, a jet fire risk assessment can be performed by implementing the same method using the wind data of the area where the rocket launch facility is located.

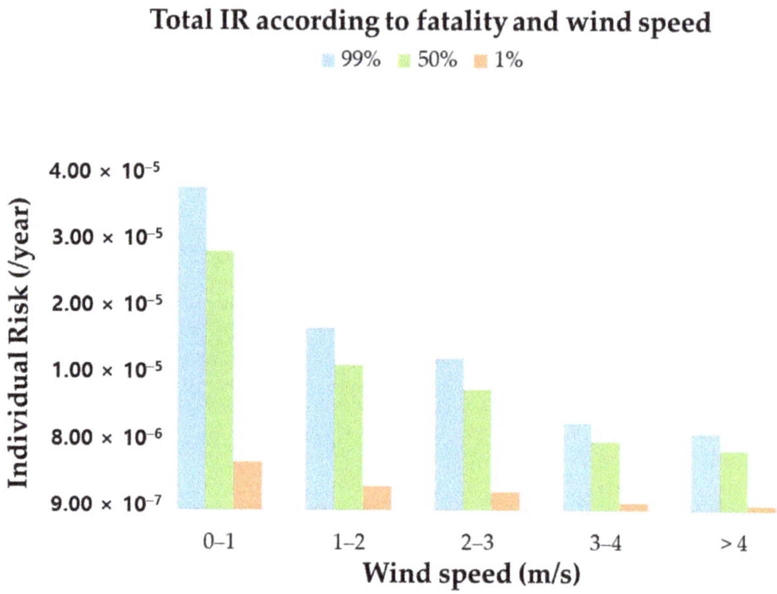

Figure 11. Total IR values according to fatality and wind speed.

In this study, the quantitative risk assessment according to the wind rose of the aerospace facility where a jet fire in a metal hose occurs was performed. Further studies should be conducted including the social risk, which is the probability of injury to the entire population in hazardous facilities when a fire occurs near an ignition source.

6. Sensitivity Analysis

Sensitivity analysis is an evaluation method that changes how the individual parameters affect the optimal solution. Sensitivity analysis was performed using p_{loc} as a parameter. As a special and high-risk facility, the aerospace facility is not required for many working people, and it was an important factor in calculating individual risk results for metal hose jet fires in aerospace facilities, as well as fire and explosion scenarios that may occur in aerospace equipment. Therefore, in this study, sensitivity analysis was calculated by considering p_{loc} among the various parameters used in the individual risk equation of metal hose jet fire according to wind direction and speed. In addition, the value of p_{loc} was the average standard of a working person in the aerospace facility, and as such sensitivity analysis was performed by selecting for higher and lower values than the average standard that was 0.88.

For the sensitivity analysis, according to the total individual risk it was assumed to occur under the following conditions:

1. The high p_{loc} value is set to 1, assuming that the working person is the maximum in the aerospace facility.
2. The high and low values are 1 and 0.5.
3. Sensitivity analysis was compared based on 99% fatality.
4. In the results and discussion, 99% fatality was selected, due to the high individual risk and sensitivity analysis was performed.

As a result, Figure 12 shows the sensitivity analysis considering the p_{loc} value. In the case of the p_{loc} value is higher than the average standard, when the maximum risk is 3.81×10^{-5} and the minimum is 9.71×10^{-6}. When the p_{loc} value is lower than the average standard, the maximum risk is 1.90×10^{-5} and the minimum is 4.86×10^{-6}. Finally, this study confirmed that individual risk satisfied the tolerable criteria even if the p_{loc} value was maximum.

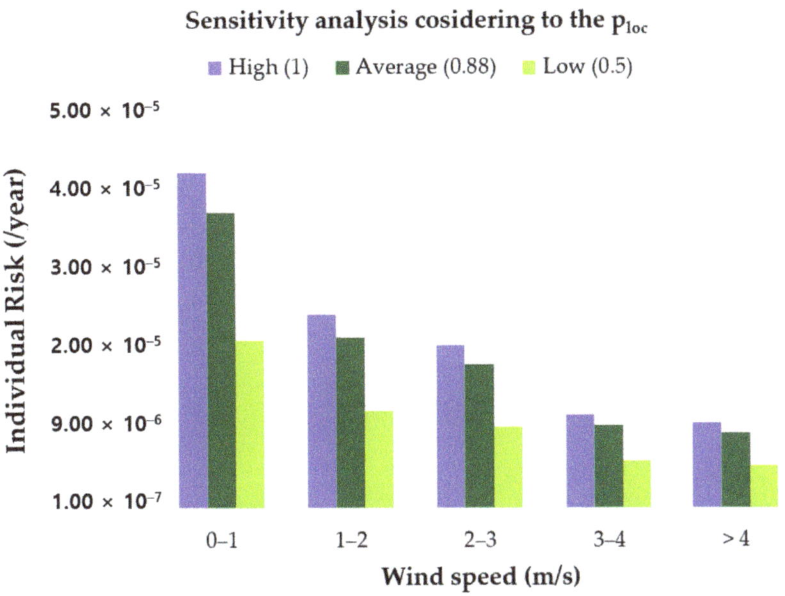

Figure 12. Sensitivity analysis considering to the p_{loc}.

7. Conclusions

In this study, a risk assessment was performed on a jet fire at an aerospace facility considering the wind direction and speed. A consequence analysis was performed based on the properties of the metal hose, kerosene, and jet fire. Next, the IR was calculated for the wind rose when a jet fire occurred in a metal hose. The following conclusions can be drawn:

1. The fire probability of a metal hose with a hole diameter of 13 mm and release rate of 10.93 kg/s is 3.0×10^{-4}.
2. In a case of jet fire occurring from a metal hose, the 99% fatality area and distance are 493.87 m^2 and 3.20~12.94 m, the 50% fatality area and distance are 518.01 m^2 and 12.94~18.23 m, and 1% fatality area and distance are 1027.71 m^2 and 18.23~25.68 m, respectively.
3. The highest IR was at 345°–15° for a wind speed of 0–1 m/s and at 315°–345° for wind speeds >1 m/s. The lowest IR was at 255°–285° for a wind speed of 0–1 m/s, 75°–105° for wind speeds of 1–4 m/s, and 15°–45° for wind speeds >4 m/s. The IR showed similar tendencies at different fatality probabilities.
4. The individual risk from jet fire in an aerospace facility was calculated that maximum risk is 3.35×10^{-5}, minimum is 1.49×10^{-6}. The highest IR of 3.35×10^{-5} is within the tolerable range according to the risk assessment criteria set by HSE ALARP standard. Furthermore, all individual risks were satisfied with the ALARP standard, regardless of wind speed and fatality. Therefore, the risk of metal hose jet fire was tolerable.
5. As a result of sensitivity analysis according to p_{loc}, which is an important factor in considering individual risk results for metal hose jet fire, this study appeared that all individual risks satisfy the tolerable criteria, even if the p_{loc} value is maximum.

To summarize the results of this study, the major risk component is the metal hose, and the maximum IR in aerospace facility satisfies HSE ALARP standard. Further, using these results, it is possible to strengthen safety by applying additional firewalls, extinguishing systems, and emergency shut off systems.

Author Contributions: Conceptualization: I.S.Y. and E.S.J.; methodology: H.J.K. and K.M.J.; formal analysis: H.J.K.; data curation: H.J.K. and K.M.J.; writing-original draft preparation: H.J.K., K.M.J. and E.S.J.; writing-review and editing: H.Y.O. and S.I.K.; visualization: H.J.K.; supervision: E.S.J. All authors have read and agreed to the published version of the manuscript.

Funding: This research did not receive any specific grant from funding agencies in the public, commercial, or not-for-profit sectors.

Institutional Review Board Statement: Not applicable.

Informed Consent Statement: Not applicable.

Data Availability Statement: Data is contained within the article.

Acknowledgments: This work was supported by the Korea Space Launch Vehicle (KSLV-II) funded by the Ministry of Science and ICT (MSIT, Republic of Korea).

Conflicts of Interest: The authors declare no conflict of interest.

Nomenclature

IR_k	IR of population group k (1/year)
θ_k	Overall fraction of time that population group *k* is in the area (-)
$p_{loc,i,k}$	Probability that population group k is at location *i* (-)
FoF_i	Frequency of fatalities at location *i* (-)
$f_{eo,j}$	Frequency of event outcome *j* (1/year)
$p_{fat,i,j}$	Probabilities of fatality produced by event outcome *j* (-)
$p_{weather,j}$	Probabilities of weather conditions produced by event outcome *j* (-)
$p_{direction,i,j}$	Probability of the direction required to produce event outcome *i* (-)
t	Time that the target is exposed to radiation (s)
I	Thermal radiation flux (W/m^2)
Q	Mass flow rate of leakage (kg/s)
R	Distance between the target and the center of the flame zone (m)
L_c	Jet breakup length (m)
We	Weber number
Re	Reynolds number
ρ	Density (kg/m^3)
V	Jet velocity (m/s)
d	Diameter of nozzle or hole (m)
σ	Surface tension (N/m)
μ	Viscosity (kg/m/s)
θ	Overall fraction of time that a person is in a given area (-)
p_{loc}	Probability that the person is at a location (-)
f_{mh}	Fire probability of the metal hose (1/year)
$fat_{jet\ fire}$	The fatality probability of a jet fire (-)
$p_{windrose}$	Probability that the jet fire will be in one of the wind rose (-)

References

1. West Yorkshire Fire & Rescue Service (WYFRA). Methods of Fire Risk Assessment (Fire Safety Training), West Yorkshire Fire & Rescue Service Procedure & Guidance Fire Safety, UK. 2011. Available online: https://www.westyorksfire.gov.uk/your-safety/work/fire-risk-assessments/ (accessed on 15 June 2020).
2. Burt, B.A. Definitions of Risk. *J. Dent. Educ.* **2001**, *65*, 1007–1008. [CrossRef] [PubMed]
3. Alp, E.; Eng, P.; Atkinson, D.; Beatty, R.; De Gagne, D.; Gagner, V.; Gulbinas, E.; Hilber, M.; Hyatt, N.; Kelly, B.; et al. *Risk Assessment—Recommended Practices for Municipalities and Industry*; Canadian Society for Chemical Engineering: Ottawa, ON, Canada, 2004; Available online: https://www.cheminst.ca/about/about-csche/ (accessed on 7 September 2018).
4. Uijt de Haag, P.A.M.; Ale, B.J.M. Guidelines for quantitative risk assessment, CPR 18E. In *TNO Purple Book*; Netherlands Or-ganisation for Applied Scientific Research: The Hague, The Netherlands, 2005.

5. CCPS (Center for Chemical Process Safety). Event Probability and Failure Frequency Analysis. In *Guidelines for Chemical Process Quantitative Risk Analysis*, 2nd ed.; American Institute of Chemical Engineers: New York, NY, USA, 2010.
6. Cummings, M.L. Factors that Influence the Acceptance of New Aerospace Risk Assessment Techniques. *AIAA Scitech Forum* **2020**. [CrossRef]
7. Gonzales, E.; Murray, D. FAA's Approaches to Ground and NAS Separation Distances for Commercial Rocket Launches. In Proceedings of the 48th AIAA Aerospace Sciences Meeting Including the New Horizons Forum and Aerospace Exposition, Orlando, FL, USA, 4–7 January 2010; pp. 1–12.
8. Altavilla, A.; Garbellini, L. Risk assessment in the aerospace industry. *Saf. Sci.* **2002**, *40*, 271–298. [CrossRef]
9. Padiha, D.; Butt, C.; Tisato, J.; Wilson, S. The Australian approach to ground population modelling and risk assessment. In Proceedings of the 4th IAASS Workshop on Launch and Re-entry Safety, Chincoteague, VA, USA, 18 September 2012; pp. 1–6.
10. Lariviere, M.; Kezirian, M.T. Preliminary safety assessment of the DLR SpaceLiner vehicle. *J. Space Saf. Eng.* **2019**, *6*, 15–23. [CrossRef]
11. Coccorullo, I.; Russo, P. Jet fire consequence modeling for high-pressure gas pipelines. *AIP Conf. Proc.* **2016**, *1790*, 110007. [CrossRef]
12. Jo, Y.-D.; Ahn, B.J. A method of quantitative risk assessment for transmission pipeline carrying natural gas. *J. Hazard. Mater.* **2005**, *123*, 34. [CrossRef]
13. Lee, S.; Landucci, G.; Reniers, G.; Paltrinieri, N. Validation of Dynamic Risk Analysis Supporting Integrated Operations Across Systems. *Sustainability* **2019**, *11*, 6745. [CrossRef]
14. Goerlandt, F.; Khakzad, N.; Reniers, G. Validity and validation of safety-related quantitative risk analysis: A review. *Saf. Sci.* **2017**, *99*, 127–139. [CrossRef]
15. Tixier, J.; Dusserre, G.; Salvi, O.; Gaston, D. Review of 62 risk analysis methodologies of industrial plants. *J. Loss Prev. Process. Ind.* **2002**, *15*, 291–303. [CrossRef]
16. Lee, S. Quantitative risk assessment of fire & explosion for regasification process of an LNG-FSRU. *Ocean Eng.* **2020**, *197*, 106825. [CrossRef]
17. Roos, A.J. Methods for the Determination of Possible Damage, CPR 16E. In *TNO Green Book*; Netherlands Organisation for Applied Scientific Research: The Hague, The Netherlands, 1992.
18. Han, Z.; Weng, W. An integrated quantitative risk analysis method for natural gas pipeline network. *J. Loss Prev. Process. Ind.* **2010**, *23*, 428–436. [CrossRef]
19. Franks, A. A Simplified Approach to Estimating Individual Risk, Health & Safety Executive, UK. 2017. Available online: https://www.hse.gov.uk/research/misc/vectra300-2017-r03.pdf (accessed on 23 June 2019).
20. Miesse, C.C. Correlation of Experimental Data on the Disintegration of Liquid Jets. *Ind. Eng. Chem.* **1955**, *47*, 1690–1701. [CrossRef]
21. Washington, J. Failure Rate and Event Data for Use within Risk Assessments. Health & Safety Executive, UK. 2012. Available online: https://wwwhsegovuk/landuseplanning/failure-ratespdf (accessed on 6 February 2018).
22. Cox, A.W.; Lees, F.P.; Ang, M.L. *Classification of Hazardous Locations*; IChemE: London, UK, 1990; pp. 56–61.
23. Magee, J.W.; Bruno, T.J.; Friend, D.G.; Huber, M.L.; Laesecke, A.; Lemmon, E.W.; McLinden, M.O.; Perkins, R.A.; Baranski, J.; Widegren, J.A. Thermophysical Properties Measurements and Models for Rocket Propellant RP-1: Phase I, National Institute of Standards and Technology (NIST), USA. 2007. Available online: https://nvlpubs.nist.gov/nistpubs/Legacy/IR/nistir6646.pdf/ (accessed on 10 December 2021).
24. Vukadinovic, V.; Habisreuther, P.; Zarzalis, N. Influence of pressure and temperature on laminar burning velocity and markstein number of kerosene jet A-1: Experimental and numerical study. *Fuel* **2013**, *111*, 401–410. [CrossRef]
25. Franks, A.; Maddison, T. A Simplified Method for the Estimation of Individual Risk. *Process. Saf. Environ. Prot.* **2006**, *84*, 101–108. [CrossRef]
26. Shao, H.; Duan, G. Risk Quantitative Calculation and ALOHA Simulation on the Leakage Accident of Natural Gas Power Plant. *Procedia Eng.* **2012**, *45*, 352–359. [CrossRef]
27. Kim, S.B.; Kim, Y.H.; Lee, C.; Um, S.I.; Ko, J.W.; Baek, J.B. A study on the individual and societal risk estimation for the use and storage facility with toxic materials. *J. Korean Soc. Saf.* **1997**, *12*, 51–59. Available online: https://www.koreascience.or.kr/article/JAKO199711922390725.page (accessed on 23 May 2021).

28. Renjith, V.R.; Madhu, G. Individual and societal risk analysis and mapping of human vulnerability to chemical accidents in the vicinity of an industrial area. *Int. J. Appl. Eng. Res.* **2010**, *1*, 135–148. Available online: https://www.semanticscholar.org/paper/Individual-and-societal-risk-analysis-and-mapping-RenjithV-Madhu/af09801ce0302f54fd67740704a1b36c1486d654 (accessed on 19 October 2021).
29. Skřínský, J.; Sluka, V.; Senčík, J.; Pražáková, M.; Maly, S. Application of emergency planning criteria for the control of major accident hazards—Calculation of the consequences of fire accidents. *Saf. Reliab. Risk Anal.* **2013**, *2013*, 135–142. [CrossRef]
30. Ma, L.; Li, Y.; Liang, L.; Li, M.; Cheng, L. A novel method of quantitative risk assessment based on grid difference of pipe-line sections. *Saf. Sci.* **2013**, *59*, 219–226. [CrossRef]
31. Bayvel, L.; Orzechowski, Z. *Liquid Atomization*, 1st ed.; Taylor & Francis: Milton Park, FL, USA, 1993.
32. Lefebvre, H.; McDonell, V.G. *Atomization and Sprays*, 2nd ed.; CRC Press: Boca Raton, FL, USA, 2017.
33. Bremond, N.; Clanet, C.; Villermaux, E. Atomization of undulating liquid sheets. *J. Fluid Mech.* **2007**, *585*, 421–456. [CrossRef]
34. Chen, X.; Ma, D.-J.; Yang, V.; Popinet, S. High-fidelity simulations of impinging jet atomization. *At. Sprays* **2013**, *23*, 1079–1101. [CrossRef]
35. Khan, O.S.; Baek, S.W.; Hojat, G. On the autoignition and combustion characteristics of kerosene droplets at elevated pressure and temperature. Combust. *Sci. Technol.* **2007**, *179*, 2437–2451.
36. Inoue, C.; Watanabe, T.; Himeno, T. Numerical Analysis on Dynamics and Inner Structures of Liquid Jet in Pinch-Off. In Proceedings of the 43rd AIAA/ASME/SAE/ASEE Joint Propulsion Conference & Exhibit, Cincinnati, OH, USA, 8–11 July 2007.
37. Wang, T.-S. Thermophysics Characterization of Kerosene Combustion. *J. Thermophys. Heat Transf.* **2001**, *15*, 140–147. [CrossRef]
38. Daycock, J.H.; Rew, P.J. *Development of a Method for the Determination of On-Site Ignition Probabilities*; Health & Safety Executive: Bootle, UK, 2004. Available online: https://www.hse.gov.uk/research/rrhtm/rr226.htm (accessed on 22 May 2019).
39. Zhu, C.; Jiang, J.; Yuan, X. Study on Ignition Probability of Flammable Materials after Leakage Accidents. *Procedia Eng.* **2012**, *45*, 435–441. [CrossRef]
40. Rew, P.J.; Spencer, H. A framework for ignition probability of flammable gas clouds. *Icheme. Symp. Ser.* **2005**, *141*, 151–162. Available online: https://wwwsemanticscholarorg/paper/A-FRAMEWORK-FOR-IGNITION-PROBABILITY-OF-FLAMMABLE-Rew-Spencer/3c0e49153a49710d3e448ef62af2aaa371406153 (accessed on 23 August 2018).
41. Applequist, S. Wind Rose Bias Correction. *J. Appl. Meteorol. Clim.* **2012**, *51*, 1305–1309. [CrossRef]
42. Slusser, W. Wind Rose Maps of the United States. *Weather* **1965**, *18*, 260–263. [CrossRef]
43. Varma, S.A.K.; Srimurali, M.; Varma, S.V. Evolution of wind rose diagrams for RTPP. Kadapa, AP, India. *Int. J. Innovat. Res. Dev.* **2013**, *2*, 2278. Available online: https://wwwsemanticscholarorg/paper/Evolution-of-Wind-Rose-Diagrams-for-RTPP%2C-KADAPA%2C-Varma-Srimurali/652d3848683cd8f43fe46f0b2df85915b1db1752 (accessed on 13 January 2021).
44. Bharani, R.; Sivaprakasam, A. Meteorosoft: A excel function for wind data processing and rose diagram. *Earth Sci. Inform.* **2019**, *13*, 965–971. [CrossRef]
45. Thé, J.L.; Thé, C.L.; Johnson, M.A. *WRPLOT View Release Notes*; Lakes Environmental: Waterloo, ON, Canada, 2018.
46. Amir-Heidari, P.; Maknoon, R.; Taheri, B.; Bazyari, M. Identification of strategies to reduce accidents and losses in drilling industry by comprehensive HSE risk assessment—A case study in Iranian drilling industry. *J. Loss Prev. Process. Ind.* **2016**, *44*, 405–413. [CrossRef]
47. Brookes, K.; Limbert, C.; Deacy, C.; O'Reilly, A.; Scott, S.; Thirlaway, K. Systematic review: Work-related stress and the HSE Management Standards. *Occup. Med.* **2013**, *63*, 463–472. [CrossRef]
48. Baybutt, P. The ALARP principle in process safety. *Process. Saf. Prog.* **2014**, *33*, 36–40. [CrossRef]
49. Melchers, R. On the ALARP approach to risk management. *Reliab. Eng. Syst. Saf.* **2001**, *71*, 201–208. [CrossRef]
50. Maselli, G.; Macchiaroli, M.; Nesticò, A. ALARP Criteria to Estimate Acceptability and Tolerability Thresholds of the Investment Risk. *Appl. Sci.* **2021**, *11*, 9086. [CrossRef]

energies

MDPI

Article

Performance Evaluation of a Full-Scale Fused Magnesia Furnace for MgO Production Based on Energy and Exergy Analysis

Tianchi Jiang, Weijun Zhang * and Shi Liu

School of Metallurgy, Northeastern University, Shenyang 110819, China; 1910595@stu.neu.edu.cn (T.J.); liu_s@163.com (S.L.)
* Correspondence: zhangwj@smm.neu.edu.cn

Abstract: A three-electrode alternating current fused magnesia furnace (AFMF) with advanced control technology was evaluated by combined energy and exergy analysis. To gain insight into the mass flow, energy flow and exergy efficiency of the present fused magnesia furnace, the exergy destruction was analysed to study the energy irreversibility of the furnace. Two different production processes, the magnesite ore smelting process (MOP) and light-calcined magnesia process (LMP), are discussed separately. Two methods were carried out to improve LMP and MOP; one of which has been applied in factories. The equipment consists of an electric power supply system, a light-calcined system and a three-electrode fused magnesia furnace. All parameters were tested or calculated based on the data investigated in industrial factories. The calculation results showed that for LMP and MOP, the mass transport efficiencies were 16.6% and 38.3%, the energy efficiencies were 62.2% and 65.5%, and the exergy destructions were 70.5% and 48.4%, respectively. Additionally, the energy efficiency and exergy efficiency of the preparation process of LMP were 39.4% and 35.6%, respectively. After the production system was improved, the mass transport efficiency, energy efficiency and exergy destruction were determined.

Keywords: fused magnesia; exergy efficiency; energy efficiency; energy saving; alternating current furnace

Citation: Jiang, T.; Zhang, W.; Liu, S. Performance Evaluation of a Full-Scale Fused Magnesia Furnace for MgO Production Based on Energy and Exergy Analysis. *Energies* **2022**, *15*, 214. https://doi.org/10.3390/en15010214

Academic Editor: Lyes Bennamoun

Received: 22 November 2021
Accepted: 25 December 2021
Published: 29 December 2021

Publisher's Note: MDPI stays neutral with regard to jurisdictional claims in published maps and institutional affiliations.

1. Introduction

Refractory materials are widely used in high-temperature industrial environments, such as the aerospace, steel and construction industries. Magnesia oxide plays an irreplaceable role in refractory material production because of its resistance to oxidation, deoxidation and thermal decomposition. An electric arc furnace (EAF) was first used to produce fused magnesia in 1991 to facilitate high-quality magnesia oxide production in China [1]. In the industrial process of MgO production, the main equipment used to produce fused magnesia oxide is a fused magnesia furnace, and the heat resource of the furnace consists of arc heat generation (40%) and resistance heat generation (60%) [2]. With a rapid increase in MgO requirement in several industries, over 90% of electrically fused magnesia oxide has been produced in a low energy efficiency EAF, which is a serious waste of electrical energy [3–6]. There are two common electric fused systems that are used to produce electrically fused magnesia oxide: the two-electrode direct current magnesia furnace (DFMF) and three-electrode alternating current fused magnesia furnace (AFMF). The researchers' research focuses mainly on power supply systems and automation control. Wang et al. estimated the electrical system losses of electric arc furnaces, and Fu et al. studied the common blow-out phenomenon in electric magnesia furnaces and gave a predictive model that can predict the occurrence of the phenomenon of blasting furnaces in magnesia fusion furnaces [7,8]. Compared with the DFMF system, the AFMF system is a widely used method because of its mature technology and good production ability; however, the DFMF system is also used in some plants due to its higher energy efficiency and low equipment cost. Qin improved the basic structural parameters and operation methods of the two-electrode DC electric arc furnace and described the energy-saving characteristics of the two-electrode DC electric arc furnace. In addition, Kong et al. improved the control method of a three-electrode AC electric arc furnace and summarised the advantages of a three-phase electric arc furnace [9,10]. Furthermore, it is also clear that substantial energy consumption and large numbers of byproducts exist in both the AFMF system and DFMF system. As the requirement of high-quality MgO increases, AFMF systems play an important role in high-quality MgO production, and the improvement in the energy efficiency of AFMF systems has received much attention in the past decade. Li et al. conducted a series of studies on the cleaner production of magnesium oxide in Liaoning Province, analysed the production process from the perspective of the urban environment and production environment and gave the best production process for refractory materials using magnesium oxide [5,11]. Based on the metallurgical system, Chai et al. carried out a comparative modelling of the fused magnesia production process, applied the CPS system to the fused magnesia production process and gave the basic realisation route of the fused magnesia CPS system [12]. The AFMF system can also be divided into two processes, namely, the magnesite ore smelting process (MOP) and light-burned magnesia process (LMP), due to different raw material preparation methods.

The raw materials of the MOP process are produced in an ore-crushing plant, and magnesite ores are mined from the magnesite mines and are transported to be crushed. The main raw material of the LMP process is light calcinated magnesia. Light calcinated magnesia powder is generally produced in a light-burning plant, where the raw material ore is sent to the light-calcinating equipment for calcination at a temperature of 900–1000 K [13]. Inside, the ore decomposes and generates light calcinated magnesia. During the light calcination process, the main heat source is the combustion of the gas by the gas producer. After the light calcinated magnesia powder is produced, it is placed for cooling to room temperature.

After cooling, light-calcined magnesia powder can be pressed to pellets and sent to an electric-fused plant. In addition to the equipment used in light-calcined plants, the basic equipment of MOPs and LMPs are almost the same in electric fused plants.

The light-calcined system is the main equipment in the LMP. Unlike in the MOP, a light-calcined system is used to pretreat the raw materials by heating them at a temperature between 800 K and 1000 K. In the temperature range from 800–1000 K, the $MgCO_3$ in magnesite ores decompose into CO_2 and MgO. Longo et al. provided several chemical reaction equations for $MgCO_3$ decomposition production at different temperature ranges, and studies have shown that the production of MgO presents different states at different temperature ranges [14]. Jie Y. et al. summarised the research directions in the field of fused magnesia as optimisation, control, modelling and experimental constraints and also summarised the main problems in the field of fused magnesia and the intelligent technologies that can be applied [15].

The three-electrode alternating current fused magnesia furnace (AFMF) system plays the most important role in both MOPs and LMPs, and the system in electric fused plants mainly consists of a high-voltage transformer (HVT), material transport equipment (MTE) and an AFMF. High-voltage electrical power is translated into standard electricity with a regime of 2800 kVA through a multistage coil in the HVT. A mathematical model used to calculate the electric loss of HVTs was developed by Gutiérrez et al. considering multistage coil loss (copper loss), wire loss (iron loss) and reactive power [16]. The electrical loss assessment of an HVT was discussed by Zhou's group with respect to source-load power uncertainty and electricity price fluctuations [17]. An MTE system consists of material feeders and material setters; a complex control system was designed by Chai based on a cyber-physical system (CPS) system, and an integrated optimal operation control algorithm was proposed [18]. Liu designed and modelled all of the equipment to lay magnesite ores, and the structural strength and stability were studied based on ANSYS workbench 17.0. At the same time, a control program compiled by a ladder diagram was also developed [19]. The AFMF is the most important equipment in both MOPs and LMPs; raw materials are preheated at the upper part of the furnace, and a smelting process occurs in the lower part of the furnace [7]. Shan explained the mechanism of ore preheating and surface heat transfer and discussed the influencing factors of the resultant heat transfer. The equipment used to heat water, which is needed for use in industrial parks, was designed and applied in Don-xing refractory company to avoid wasting heat [20]. Fu. et al. performed some research on the prediction of eruptions occurring in the AFMF, and a software and hardware set that can accurately identify the vibration frequency of raw material eruptions was developed together [21]. Li established a mathematical model to describe phenomena that occurs in furnaces, i.e., the magnetic field, fluid flow field and heat transfer; at the same time, the combustion enthalpy change was also considered in the model [22]. Although researchers have performed many studies on the control system of AFMF systems and affiliated equipment to achieve better energy efficiency, few studies have provided a clear comparison of MOPs and LMPs with respect to energy performance.

Exergy analysis has been widely used to evaluate the energy efficiency of industrial processes, and the efficiency and rationality of the exergy concept has been proven in metallurgical systems. Rong et al. applied exergy analysis to the rotary kiln-electric furnace (RKEF) system, investigated the potential for energy savings, and used waste heat to preheat the raw materials [23]. Yu et al. presented comprehensive exergy and energy analyses to compare the energy performance of RKEF systems and sintering-preheating-submerge arc furnace (SPSF) systems and concluded that SPSF systems are more environmentally friendly than RKEF systems and that waste gas could be recycled and show a better energy saving effect [24]. Zhang et al. studied the exergy loss of each component of electric vehicles, and an exergy analysis was carried out on the heat pump air conditioning system (HPACS) of electric vehicles with a battery thermal management system. The results show that under all operating conditions, the compressor is the main source of system exergy losses [25–29]. Harmed K. also carried out corresponding research in the field of seawater desalination. This article focuses on the recovery of sewage as the research object and uses electric energy as the energy supply for evaporation treatment to provide good environmental protection. Energy-exergy loss was evaluated. In addition, the researchers also conducted corresponding evaluations and studies on the reverse osmosis seawater desalination process based on geothermal energy [30–32]. Mahmoudan A. proposed a new type of integrated energy system based on a geothermal heat source and LNG radiator and carried out energy, exergy and exergy economic evaluations of the system. At the same time, parameter research was carried out on different decision variables, and finally, the TOPSIS method specified the optimal control scheme [31]. Although many exergy analyses have been applied in several industrial systems, exergy analyses of MOP and LMP in AFMF systems have not been discussed in previous studies. The preparation process of MgO requires large amounts of electricity, and the energy saving potential urgently needs to be evaluated.

In the present work, energy, exergy, and environmental analyses of a real-scale magnesite smelting process were applied to evaluate the energy efficiency, exergy efficiency and performance with respect to environmental protection of MOP and LMP. In the circumstances of a reduction in carbon emissions, the importance of evaluating the energy and exergy efficiency and eco-friendliness of energy-intensive enterprises is obvious. This study provides a series of key parameter analyses in magnesite smelting process systems and shows the tremendous potential of environmental protection, energy savings and exergy savings

2. System Description

Figure 1 shows the main equipment of the MOP and LMP systems. The two parts in the picture were taken on the top and side of the mould, showing the electrode, the mould and the finished product of fused magnesia waiting to be broken after the production process. The three-phase magnesia smelting furnace is located at No. 1 Magnesite Plant of Hai-cheng Magnesite Group Corporation. The furnace provides experimental data used in the text. The equipment mainly consists of three carbon electrodes, servo motors and crystallisers.

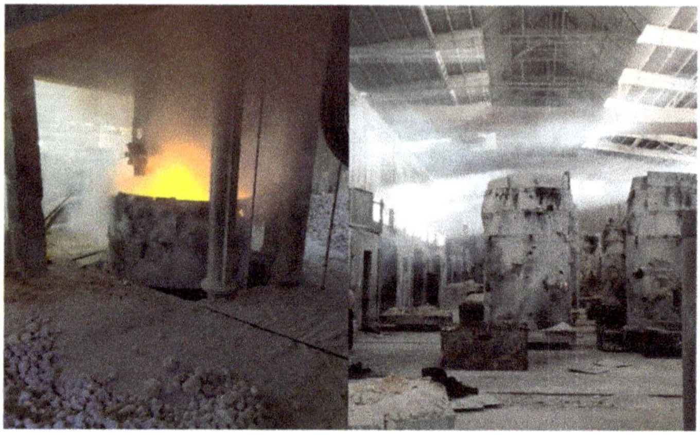

Figure 1. Fused Magnesium Furnace.

Figure 2 shows the total process of MOP and LMP. The arrows in the map show the translation of materials and directions of energy and mass flow. LMP and MOP utilise different pretreatments of materials of different purities. Ores were first mined from a magnesite mine and transported to a sorting centre in which the mass fraction of different batch ores can be tested and divided into three ranges. The raw materials with mass fraction of $MgCO_3$ between 0.7 and 0.8 are referred to as inferior ores; these raw materials must be floated in a flotation kiln first to filter out the materials with a mass fraction lower than 0.75 based on the standards summarised from production experience. Materials with a mass fraction lower than 0.75 were used to treat pollution gas. Other materials were sent to a light-calcined warehouse and were mixed with raw materials with a mass fraction between 0.8 and 0.9 (named premium ores). The materials were sent to a light-calcined bed, and after the light-calcined process, the pre-production materials were transported to the electric fused furnace. This total process is referred to as LMP. In addition to the materials mentioned above, ores with mass fractions higher than 0.9 are named excellent ores. These ores are only crushed in crushing plants first and then are transported to electric fused furnaces. This process is named MOP.

Figure 3a shows the specific production process under the two different processes of LMP and MOP, as well as the boundary division when calculating the mass–energy–exergy balance. First, regarding the mass balance, in the MOP route, ore, electrodes, combustion air and refractory materials are considered input items of the process flow. After the smelting is completed, the fused magnesia, flue gas, remaining ore and byproducts are considered outputs. In the LMP route, the ore is processed in the light calciner and then sent to AFMF to complete smelting. The decomposition process of the ore is completed in the light calciner. The mass input and output items are the same as in the MOP route. In the light calciner, less attention has been given to the flue gas emission of the calcination process because the preparation process of the raw materials is not the focus of this article. The article only calculates the mass output of its light calcinated magnesia powder. Second, regarding the energy balance, in the MOP route, Figure 3a cannot explain the preheating of the ore or the incomplete solidification of molten magnesium oxide. As a supplement, the detailed flow of internal energy is given in Figure 3b. Combining the two figures, the information on the energy balance, input items, output items, and loss items of the energy balance are all marked. Unlike the MOP process, the LMP process involves the light calcination process. To make the calculation more detailed, the electrical system, the light calcinating system and the AFMF are divided into several calculation domains. The sum of the results of each calculation domain can obtain the energy balance of the overall LMP process, and the production unit consumption of the two process routes are calculated. Finally, regarding the analysis of exergy balance, the exergy input of the MOP process mainly includes ore, electrodes, reaction air, etc., and the output items mainly include fused magnesia, auxiliary products, etc., unlike MOP, exergy loss also exists in the light calcination process, and the exergy loss is also calculated separately. Figure 3c shows the distribution of refractory materials, byproducts and fused magnesia after smelting and cooling. The main component of the byproducts is heavy calcinated magnesia. Although its market value is lower than that of fused magnesia, it is also a useful product, so some attention should be given to the output of byproducts.

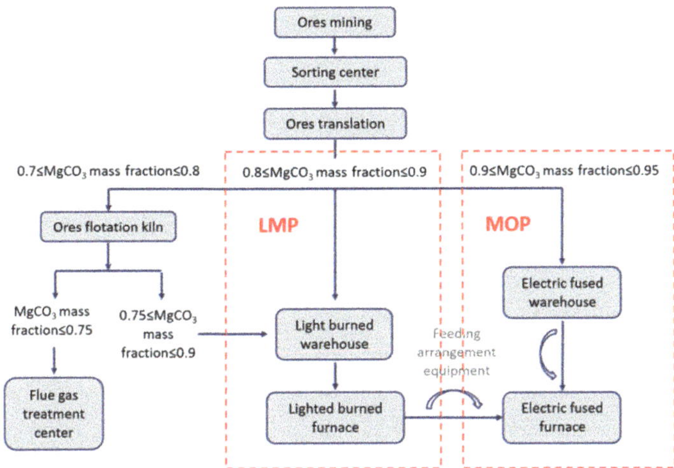

Figure 2. Magnesite oxide production industrial process diagram.

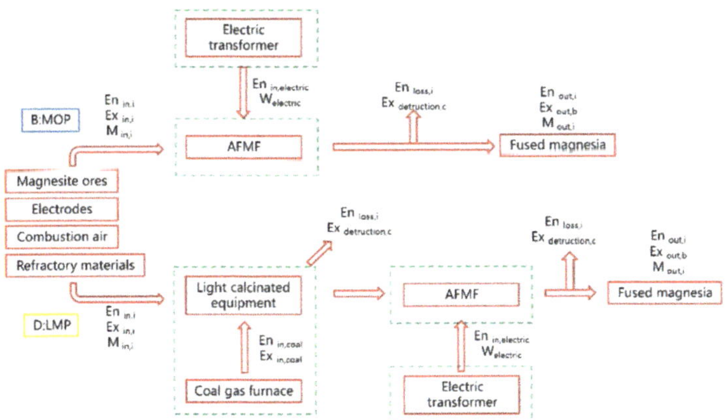

(a)

Figure 3. *Cont.*

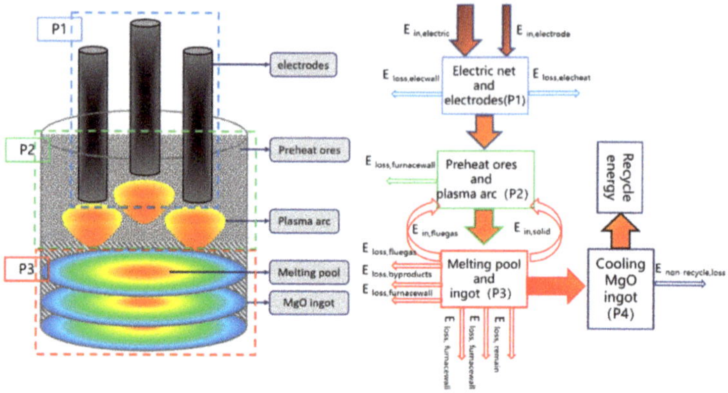

(**b**)

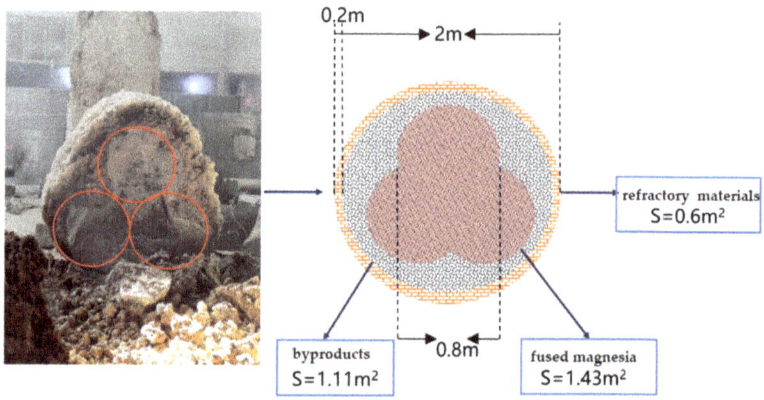

(**c**)

Figure 3. Process flow diagram and mass–energy–exergy flow. (**a**) Process flow diagram; (**b**) the internal energy transmission diagram of AFMF; (**c**) the difference between fused magnesia and byproducts.

3. System Modelling

3.1. Reactions Mechanism

Several different reactions occurred in both the LMP and MOP, and details of the reactions are tabulated in Tables 1 and 2.

Table 1. Reactions occurred in MOP.

Reactions	Equations	Abbreviations of Reactions
Combustion of carbon electrodes	$C + O_2 = CO_2$	MOP-ELET-1
	$2C + O_2 = 2CO$	MOP-ELET-2
Decomposition of raw materials	$MgCO_3 = MgO + CO_2$	MOP-RM-1
	$CaCO_3 = CaO + CO_2$	MOP-RM-2
Reduction reaction	$C + CO_2 = 2CO$	MOP-SAF-1
Reduction reaction	$C + MgO = Mg + CO$	MOP-SAF-2
Slagging reaction	$SiO_2 + CaO = CaO{\cdot}SiO_2$	MOP-SAF-3
Slagging reaction	$SiO_2 + MgO = MgO{\cdot}SiO_2$	MOP-SAF-4

Table 2. Reactions occurred in LMP.

Reactions	Equations	Abbreviations of Reactions
Combustion of carbon electrodes	$C + O_2 = CO_2$	LMP-ELET-1
	$2C + O_2 = 2CO$	LMP-ELET-2
Decomposition of raw materials	$MgCO_3 = MgO + CO_2$	LMP-RM-1
	$CaCO_3 = CaO + CO_2$	LMP-RM-2
Reduction reaction	$C + CO_2 = 2CO$	LMP-SAF-1
Reduction reaction	$C + MgO = Mg + CO$	LMP-SAF-2
Reduction reaction	$C + SiO_2 = Si + CO$	LMP-SAF-3
Reduction reaction	$C + Fe_2O_3 = 2FeO + CO$	LMP-SAF-4
Reduction reaction	$C + FeO = Fe + CO$	LMP-SAF-5
Slagging reaction	$SiO_2 + CaO = CaO{\cdot}SiO_2$	LMP-SAF-6
Slagging reaction	$SiO_2 + MgO = MgO{\cdot}SiO_2$	LMP-SAF-7

3.2. Mass Balance Analysis

According to the combustion equations of the production process, the input mass flows consist of carbon electrode mass loss, preheated raw ores, combustion air and prefilled refractory materials. Fused magnesite oxide ingots, byproducts, remaining ores, flue gas and dust mixed in high-temperature gas are considered output mass flows. The mass balance equation can be written as follows:

$$\begin{aligned} &M_{in,ce} + M_{in,ho} + M_{in,ca} + M_{in,fm} = \\ &M_{out,mi} + M_{out,fg} + M_{out,bp} + M_{out,ro} + M_{out,fm} \end{aligned} \quad (1)$$

The symbols in the above equation represent the mass of carbon electrodes (*ce*), heated raw ores (*ho*), combustion air (*ca*), filled refractory materials (*fm*), magnesite oxide ingot (*mi*), byproducts (*bp*), flue gas loss (*fg*), and remaining ores (*ro*).

In the process, the mass flow transfer efficiency is calculated by [27]:

$$\eta_{mt} = \frac{M_{out,mi}}{M_{in,ce} + M_{in,ho} + M_{in,ca} + M_{in,fm}} \times 100\% \quad (2)$$

M_{ce}, M_{ho}, M_{fm}, M_{mi}, M_{bp} and M_{ro} can be obtained through experiments in a factory. M_{ca} can be calculated as:

$$M_{ca} = 10.5 \times M_{ce} \quad (3)$$

M_{fg} can be calculated as:

$$M_{fg} = \frac{44}{40} \times M_{mi} + M_{ca} + M_{ce} \quad (4)$$

3.3. Energy Analysis

According to the actual production, the energy analysis is different from the traditional calculation of energy balance. First, at the end of the smelting process, part of the magnesia oxide is not completely solidified, and the latent heat of fusion during the smelting process is not completely released in the form of solidification heat. Because the process is submerged arc smelting, part of the heat in the high-temperature flue gas from the furnace is used to preheat the ore. To study the heat solidification heat release and flue gas preheating in more detail, they are regarded as heat income items. The energy analysis of the paper mainly consists of equations on all energy sources, energy expenditures and energy efficiency of the process. The energy balance equation is as follows:

$$\sum_i E_{in,i} = \sum_i E_{out,i} + \sum_i E_{loss,i} \quad (5)$$

$$\sum_i E_{in,i} = E_{in,electrode} + E_{in,electic} + E_{in,solid} + E_{in,fluegas} \quad (6)$$

$$\sum_i E_{out,i} = E_{out,oresheat} + E_{out,mgoheat} + E_{out,oresdecom} \tag{7}$$

$$\begin{aligned}\sum_i E_{loss,i} = & E_{loss,elecwall} + E_{loss,furnacewall} + E_{loss,gas} + E_{loss,melting} + E_{loss,byproducts} \\ & + E_{loss,electricity} + E_{loss,refractory} + E_{loss,remain} + E_{loss,elecheat} + E_{loss,other}\end{aligned} \tag{8}$$

$$\eta_{et} = \frac{\sum_i E_{out,i}}{\sum_i E_{in,i}} \tag{9}$$

where $E_{in,i}$, $E_{out,i}$ and $E_{loss,i}$ are the input, output and loss energy flows, respectively. The subscripts show the different input, output and loss energy flows.

The energy calculation equations are listed in Table 3.

Table 3. Basic energy equations of energy balance.

	Item	Calculation Equation
Energy balance	Heat	$E = C_p \times (T - T_0)$
	Combustion	$E = m \times LHV$
	Wall loss	$E = \lambda \times (T - T_0)$
	Solid/melt potential	$E = m \times \Delta H_f$

3.4. Exergy Analysis

Exergy analysis means calculating the exact exergy value of every part in the MOP and LMP systems based on the reasonable assumptions mentioned above, every items of exergy were shown in Table 4.

Table 4. The exergy process of every part.

Inlet Exergy	Outlet Exergy	Destruction Exergy
Ores	Flue gas	Combustion
Combustion electrode	Fused magnesium	Dissociation reaction
Reaction air	Potential heat of byproducts	Heat transfer
-	Potential heat of soot	-

According to the Szargut study in 1988 [30], the exergy balance equations are as follows:

$$\sum_a Ex_{in,a} + W_{electric} = \sum_b Ex_{out,b} + \sum_c Ex_{destruction,c} \tag{10}$$

$$\sum_a Ex_{in,a} = Ex_{in,ores} + Ex_{in,air} + Ex_{in,electrode} \tag{11}$$

$$\sum_b Ex_{out,b} = Ex_{out,gas} + Ex_{out,fused} + Ex_{out,byproducts} + Ex_{out,soot} \tag{12}$$

$$\sum_c Ex_{destruction,c} = Ex_{destruction,combustion} + Ex_{destruction,dissociation} + Ex_{destruction,heat} \tag{13}$$

$$W_{electric} = 4800 \times N_{num} \tag{14}$$

where every variable in Equations (11)–(14) is shown in Table 3, and $W_{electric}$ and N_{num} are the electric energy input through the grid and the electricity indicator number change, respectively.

The exergy flow consists of physical exergy and chemical exergy, and the exergy balance equation can be written as:

$$Ex = Ex_{ph} + Ex_{ch} \tag{15}$$

where Ex is the total exergy in the process, Ex_{ph} is the physical exergy and Ex_{ch} is the chemical exergy.

$$Ex_{ph} = (H - H_0) + T_0(S_0 - S) + Ex_{ch} \tag{16}$$

where $(H - H_0)$ and $(S_0 - S)$ represent the enthalpy and entropy change, respectively. T_0 refers to the reference temperature in the reference environment. In Equation (18), $(H - H_0)$ can be calculated as follows:

$$H - H_0 = m \cdot c_p(T) \cdot (T - T_0) \tag{17}$$

$(S_0 - S)$ can be calculated by Equations (19) and (20), and Equation (19) can be used to calculate the entropy change in materials whose properties cannot be influenced by pressure.

$$S_0 - S = m \int_T^{T_0} \frac{c_p(T)}{T} dT \tag{18}$$

Equation (20) calculates the entropy change in materials whose properties can be influenced by pressure through the addition of an amendment [19,29].

$$S_0 - S = m \left(\int_T^{T_0} \frac{c_p(T)}{T} dT - R \ln \frac{P_0}{P} \right) \tag{19}$$

where R is the ideal gas constant and $c_p(T)$ is the specific heat of materials at different temperatures. The equations to calculate R and $c_p(T)$ are as follows [29]:

$$c_p(T) = A_0 + A_1 T + A_2 T^2 + A_3 T^3 \tag{20}$$

$$R = \frac{PV}{nT} \tag{21}$$

$$n = \frac{m}{M} \tag{22}$$

where n is the mole number of the gas, T is the temperature of the gas, M is the relative molecular mass, m is the mass of the gas, and V is the volume of the gas.

Chemical exergy is another important part of the total exergy; in this paper, solid fuels should be calculated as follows:

$$Ex_{ch} = m \cdot \mu \cdot q_{LHV} \tag{23}$$

where μ is the chemical exergy coefficient and q_{LHV} is the low caloric value. The chemical exergy of gas generated in MOP and LMP can be calculated as:

$$Ex_{ch} = m \cdot (\sum_i f_i \cdot Ex_{ch,i} + RT_0 \sum_i f_i \cdot \ln f_i) \tag{24}$$

In Equation (25), f_i is the mole fraction of i, and $Ex_{ch,i}$ is the normal chemical exergy of i. The chemical exergy of the fused magnesia ingot and byproducts can be calculated as:

$$Ex_{ch} = m \cdot \sum_j f_j \cdot Ex_{ch,j} \tag{25}$$

The exergy of heat loss is given by [24,29]:

$$Ex_{loss} = (1 - \frac{T_0}{T})Q \tag{26}$$

$$Q = \frac{\lambda_{\text{trans}}(T_{w,in} - T_{w,out})S}{l} \tag{27}$$

where λ_{trans} is the coefficient of heat transfer, $T_{w,in}$ and $T_{w,out}$ represent the temperature of the steel wall inside and outside, respectively, l is the equivalent length of heat transfer and S is the heat transfer area of heat transfer.

In MOP and LMP systems, the processes are irreversible, and several researchers have defined the exergy efficiency to evaluate the minimum energy value required for the production process of fused magnesia; thus, the exergy efficiency can be calculated as the ratio of total exergy and demanded exergy in the production process:

$$\delta = \frac{Ex_{demand}}{Ex_{total}} \times 100\% \tag{28}$$

where δ is the efficiency of exergy and Ex_{demand} is the exergy demanded in MOP and LMP.

To explore ways to improve the efficiency of exergy more conveniently, chemical exergy and physical exergy can be divided into avoidable exergy and inevitable exergy:

$$Ex_{destruction} = Ex_{destruction,avoidable} + Ex_{destruction,inevitable} \tag{29}$$

Corner mark has explained the implication of terms.

4. Results Analysis

The data in the following calculation results were tested on the 4th AFMF at Hai-cheng Magnesia Group Corporation during 20 July 2021 and 31 July 2021.

4.1. Mass Balance Results

4.1.1. Mass Conservations

The mass fraction of the MOP and LMP can be calculated as follows. First, the total mass balance is shown in Figure 3a. The mass input includes the flow of ores, carbon electrodes and combustion air; similarly, the output flows were fused magnesia ingot, flue gas soot, byproducts, remaining ores and additional materials. The mass balance equation is shown in Equation (1). The weights of ores, carbon electrodes, fused magnesia, byproducts, remaining ores and additional materials were tested in a factory. These amounts are weighed by a floor scale, where the raw material part is measured before being added into the furnace, and the product part is measured after the product is cooled and sorted. The total mass balance results are shown in Tables 5 and 6.

Table 5. MOP system mass flow balance.

Input Flows	Amount (kg/h)	per (%)	Output Flows	Amount (kg/h)	per (%)
M_{ho}	3800	13.1	M_{mi}	907.6	16.3
M_{ce}	65.3	1.2	M_{fg}	2909.7	13.2
M_{ca}	714.3	71.5	M_{bp}	720.5	1.6
M_{fm}	776.1	14.2	M_{ro}	100	2.5
			M_{fm}	776.1	14.2
Total	5455.7	100	Total	5455.7	100

Table 6. LMP system mass flow balance.

Input Flows	Amount (kg/h)	per (%)	Output Flows	Amount (kg/h)	per (%)
M_{ho}	3800	71.6	M_{mi}	2031	38.3
M_{ce}	62.7	1.2	M_{fg}	730.7	13.7
M_{ca}	668	12.6	M_{bp}	1669	31.5
M_{fm}	776.1	14.6	M_{ro}	100	1.9
			M_{fm}	776.1	14.6
Total	5306.8		Total	5306.8	100

4.1.2. The Properties of the Flue Gas

Due to a government policy, CO_2 emission is an important limitation, and monitoring carbon dioxide emission is very important, but in normal operation, it is impractical to obtain the emission of CO_2 exactly. In the present study, it is assumed that the sources of CO_2 emission were the combustion of carbon electrodes and the decomposition of ores. The main composition of ores was $MgCO_3$ (85–90%) and $CaCO_3$ (5–8%), the composition of combustion air was assumed to consist of O_2 (21%), N_2 (78.7%) and CO_2 (0.3%), and the composition of carbon electrodes was mainly graphite. The results were calculated based on Equations (1)–(4) and are shown in Tables 5 and 6. In addition, in the LMP route, due to the few mass loss during the light burning process is, the mass transfer efficiency can generally reach more than 95% in actual production. In this section, the mass flow of the light burning process is not analysed separately.

4.1.3. Mass Conversion Rate

The magnesia carbonate content in the ores was significant in comparison to the calcium carbonate content; the lowest temperature in the furnace reached at least 900 K, and the magnesia carbonate and calcium carbonate were totally decomposed in fused magnesia and byproducts range which can be seen in Figure 3c. The mass conversion rate was calculated as follows:

$$\eta_{mc} = \frac{M_{mi}}{M_{ho} + M_{ce} + M_{ca} + M_{fm}} \tag{30}$$

η_{mc} is the mass conversion rate of the process. The maximum theoretical mass conversion rates of MOP and LMP were 34% and 71.6%, the actual mass conversion rates of MOP and LMP were 16.6% and 38.3% and the difference between the actual results and theoretical results was 17.4% and 33.3%, respectively. The quality conversion rate has considerable room for improvement.

In addition, in order to better analyse the output of magnesia per ton of raw materials, the different qualities of fused magnesia produced per ton of ore have also been counted.

In Table 7, the output mass and output ratio of fused magnesia with different purity under the two routes are shown respectively. The output ratio is the ratio of different purity fused magnesia and raw materials. It is obvious that under the LMP route, the ratio of raw materials converted into magnesia with 97.5% purity is 0.055, and the ratio of raw materials converted into magnesia 97% is 0.074, which are 0.009 and 0.012 higher than those under the MOP route, respectively. The results show that the LMP route has more advantages in preparing high-quality fused magnesia than MOP. In addition, under the LMP route, the output ratio of byproducts is 0.199, which still has great potential for fused magnesia quality improvement.

Table 7. Proportion of products.

	Raw Materials	Fused Magnesia (97.5%)	Fused Magnesia (97%)	Fused Magnesia (96%)	Fused Magnesia (95%)	Byproducts
MOP	3900 kg/h	175 kg/h (0.046)	236 kg/h (0.062)	341 kg/h (0.089)	155 kg/h (0.041)	720.5 kg/h (0.180)
LMP	8400 kg/h	465 kg/h (0.055)	621 kg/h (0.074)	533 kg/h (0.063)	412 kg/h (0.049)	1669 kg/h (0.199)

4.2. Energy Balance Results

In MOP systems, the input energy flow mainly consists of the combustion of carbon electrodes, electricity power, preheating power of flue gas and solidification exotherm energy. The output energy flow consists of the following: the potential energy of carbon electrodes, the decomposition energy of ores, the melting potential energy of MgO at 3073 K, the potential energy of byproducts when the temperature increased from 973 K–1673 K, the heat loss of the flue gas and refractory materials, the potential energy of byproducts when the temperature increased from 973 K–3073 K and the energy loss of electric system. Therefore, the energy balance can be expressed as Equations (6)–(8). In addition, since the raw materials of the LMP must be light calcined, and the reason for the energy balance calculation in different regions has been explained in the previous section, in this section, the energy balance of the electrical system, the preparation process of raw materials and AFMF involved in the LMP and MOP are separately evaluated for energy, and the unit consumption of the product is comprehensively analysed at the end.

4.2.1. Energy Balance of Electric System

The structure of the electric system of the fused magnesia furnace is shown in Figure 4. It generally includes electric blockers, electric reactors, electric transformers, carbon electrodes and arc zones. Generally, the factory voltmeter is connected after the reactor and before the transformer, which is equivalent to the circuit shown in the figure above. In the electrical system of this article, the impedance loss caused by the blocker and the reactor is not calculated because the single furnace meter cannot accurately reflect the corresponding power consumption. At the same time, due to the special structure of the three-phase EAF, the three electrodes forming the three-phase electric arc need to be connected in a star shape.

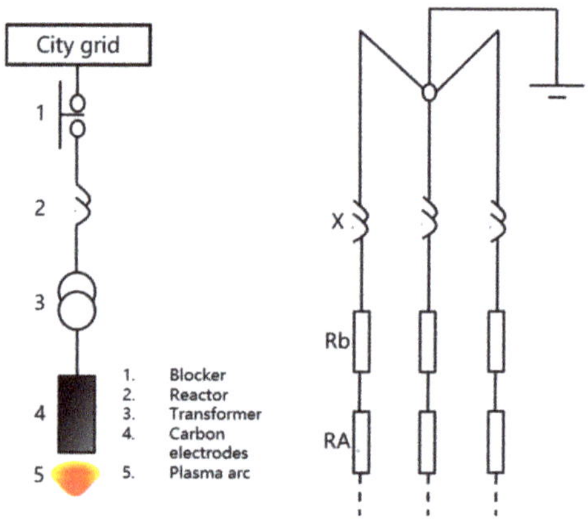

Figure 4. Electric system of MOP and LMP system.

Figure 5 shows the load equivalent circuit from the primary side of the transformer to the secondary side of the transformer and finally to the arc zone. In this process, the circuit on the left represents the primary side, and the circuit on the right represents the secondary side. Each component area has a corresponding reactance and impedance. Due to the extremely high voltage on the primary side, the circuit impedance and inductance loss are small, so they are omitted in the equivalent change process. On the secondary side, the impedance and inductive reactance of the transformer's secondary coil (corner mark 2) and the impedance and inductance of the short network part (corner mark b) are mainly considered. In addition, RA is the arc resistance. Therefore, the reactance in the simplified circuit is recorded as the total reactance X, and the total impedance in the circuit is recorded as the impedance R.

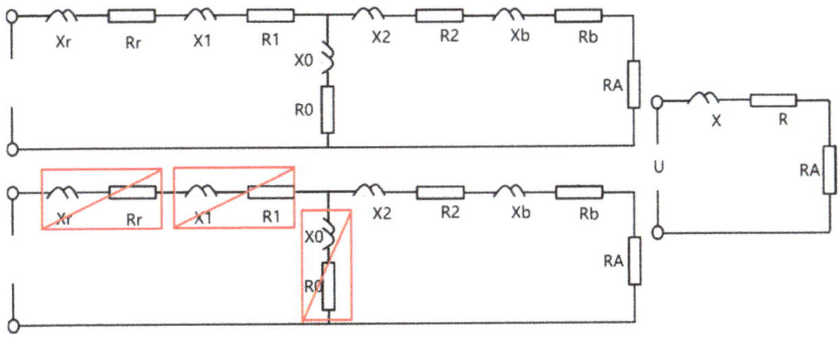

Figure 5. Equivalent circuit of electrical system.

The energy loss of the electric system can be calculated based on GB/T 19212.3-2012, and the equation follows:

$$E_{elecloss} = \sqrt{(R^2 + X^2)} \cdot I^2 + E_{transloss} \tag{31}$$

where $E_{elecloss}$ is the total energy loss of the electric system, $R = 0.00056\ \Omega$ is the resistance of the electric short net, $X = 0.0042\ \Omega$ is the reactance of the electric short net, $I = 8151$ A is the current of the electric short net, and $E_{transloss} = 25.5$ kW, which was demanded based on the industry standard in China "GB/T 19212.3-2012".

4.2.2. Raw Materials Preparation Energy Balance of LMP

As the raw material of the LMP system was light-calcined magnesia oxide, the preparation process of this material was also analysed in this section. The basic equations of the process were almost the same as the equations above. The calculation results were listed in Table 8.

Table 8. Energy calculation results of the preparation process.

Input Energy	per	Amount (kWh/t)	Output Energy	per	Amount (kWh/t)
Coal chemistry	100	1929.1	Gas loss		109.1
			Cooling air loss		124.8
			MgO heat		14.7
			Ores decomposition		634.4
			Vaporisation		161.5
			Wall loss		148.1
			Other loss		736.5
total	100	1929.1	total		1929.1

The preparation process was divided into two processes, gas preparation and light-calcined magnesia oxide preparation. All calculation results are listed in Table 8, and the total efficiency of gas preparation was 81.6%. During the light-calcined magnesia oxide preparation process, gas combustion was the main energy source of the process, accounting for approximately 80.8%, the preheated ores brought a 16.4% energy input, and the energy consumption per ton was 6,944,000 kJ (1929.1 kWh). In the output energies, the physical heat of flue gas and magnesia oxide was 43,027,875 kJ (1195.2 kWh) per ton. The calculation in this section provides a basis for the following analysis. The coefficients specific heat capacity equations are shown in Table 9.

Table 9. The coefficients specific heat capacity equation.

Materials	A0	A1	A2	A3	Range
CO	28.16	0.168×10^{-2}	0.537×10^{-5}	-2.222×10^{-9}	273 K–1800 K
CO_2	22.26	5.981×10^{-2}	-3.501×10^{-5}	7.469×10^{-9}	273 K–1800 K
O_2	25.48	1.520×10^{-2}	-0.716×10^{-5}	1.312×10^{-9}	273 K–1800 K
H_2O	32.24	0.192×10^{-2}	1.055×10^{-5}	-3.595×10^{-9}	273 K–1800 K
N_2	28.90	-0.157×10^{-2}	0.808×10^{-5}	-2.873×10^{-9}	273 K–1800 K

4.2.3. Energy Balance of MOP and LMP

In Equation (21), the constants A0–A3 are listed in Table 6. The specific heat capacity of flue gas was the average of all components, and the calculation equation was as follows [31]:

$$C_{p,average} = \frac{1}{n}\sum_{1}^{n} C_{p,i} \tag{32}$$

where $C_{p,i}$ is the specific heat of i and $C_{p,average}$ is the average specific heat of all components.

The basic equations applied to the calculation of Tables 10 and 11 are given in the initial part of Section 4. All the calculation results are given in Tables 10 and 11 and are summarised in Figures 6 and 7. It is not difficult to see that in MOP, similar to the LMP system (Figure 8), the main energy source is electric energy, which accounts for 61% and 50% of the total energy input, i.e., 2826 kWh/t and 1182.3 kWh/t, respectively. At the same time, there are considerable byproducts as a result of the two processes. The economic value of byproducts is much lower than that of fused magnesia, and the product quality has substantial room for improvement. The difference is that there is a large amount of preheating of flue gas during the MOP process. This part of the energy accounts for 19.7% of the total energy input. Compared with an open EAF, the energy efficiency is improved. In addition, when the molten magnesia oxide solidifies, a large amount of heat will be released, accounting for 10.1% of the energy input. The actual product unit consumption is 2803 kWh/t, and the theoretical product unit consumption is 1600 kWh/t. In addition, in the LMP, since the raw material was light burnt magnesia powder, the amount of flue gas generated during the reaction process was not large, which led to a poor preheating effect of the ore, but the output of fused magnesia was much higher than that in the MOP. This situation led to 39.1% of the total energy of the solidification exotherm in the LMP. This calculation result clearly shows that the MOP process is affected by the lower output, the LMP is affected by the lack of a preheating process, and both have great potential for product quality improvement and energy efficiency improvement.

Table 10. Energy calculation results of MOP.

Input Energy	per	Amount (kWh/t)	Output Energy	per	Amount (kWh/t)
Electrode comb	9.1	421.3	Electrodes wall loss	0.1	4.3
Electricity	60.9	2826	Potential heat of electrodes	1	45.6
Solidification	10.3	479	Decomposition ores	17.5	811.9
Flue gas preheat	19.7	909.6	Ores heating	15.6	721.2
-			Magnesium oxide heating	17.5	813.4
-			Byproducts heating	4.4	205.4
-			Melting potential heat	11.6	538.3
			Wall loss	4.4	202.2
			Flue gas	16.3	757
			Remained ores	0.3	11.7
			Electricity loss	7.3	341.1
			Refractory materials	3.5	161.9
			Other loss	0.5	21.9
Total	100	4635.9	Total	100	4635.9

Table 11. Energy calculation results of LMP.

Input Energy	per	Amount (kWh/t)	Output Energy	per	Amount (kWh/t)
Electrode comb	7.6	179.4	Electrodes wall loss	0.1	1.9
Electricity	50.2	1182.3	Potential heat of electrodes	0.9	20.2
Solidification	39.1	920.3	Magnesium oxide heating	42.8	1008.8
Flue gas preheat	3.1	74	Byproducts heating	17.3	406.9
			Melting potential heat	22.7	534
			Wall loss	3.8	89.7
			Flue gas	2.7	63.4
			Remained ores	0.2	4.9
			Electricity loss	6.4	151.2
			Refractory materials	3	71.8
			Other loss	0.1	3.2
Total	100	2356	Total	100	2356

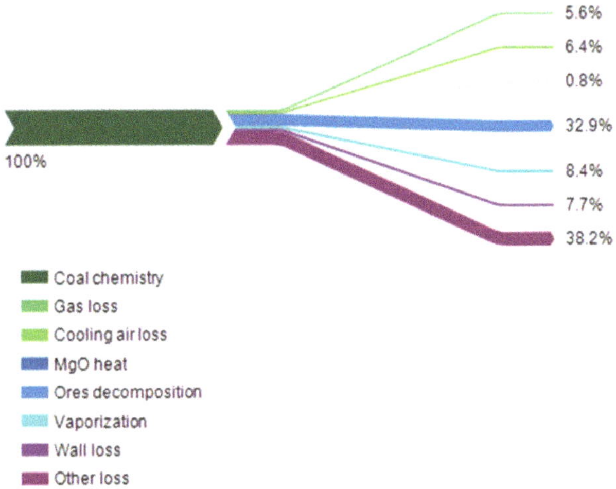

Figure 6. Energy flow of preparation process.

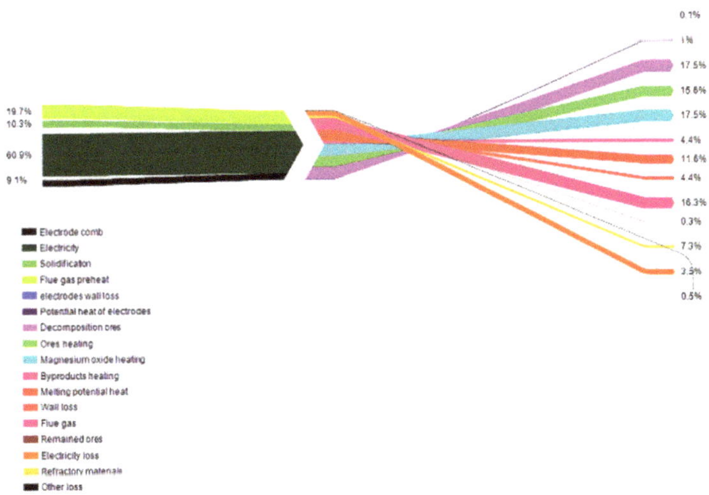

Figure 7. Energy flow of MOP.

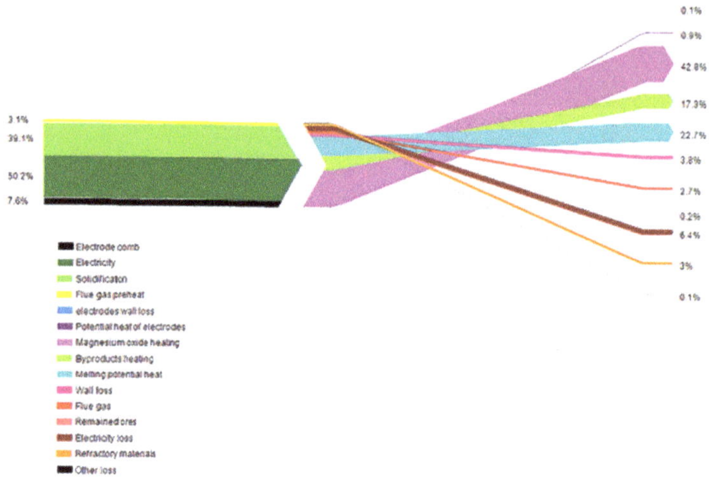

Figure 8. Energy flow of LMP.

To more scientifically reflect the effects of the two process routes, the comprehensive energy consumption of the two process routes is calculated and compared. In the MOP route, the energy consumption per ton of magnesium oxide is 2826 kWh/t. In the LMP route, the energy consumption per ton is 2826 kWh/t. The energy consumption per ton of magnesium oxide is 3111.4 kWh/t, of which the energy consumption of the light burning part is 1929.1 kWh/t, and the energy consumption of the AFMF part is 1182.3 kWh/t. In general, the unit consumption of the LMP process is slightly higher than that of the MOP process. However, from another point of view, in the LMP process, the residual energy of the fused magnesia is 1415.7 kWh/t, and the energy of the residual fused magnesia in the MOP process is 1018.8 kWh/t, which shows that the LMP process has greater energy-saving potential.

4.3. Exergy Balance Results

4.3.1. Exergy Balance

Through the energy analysis in the previous section, the input and output channels of the energy flow and their values are determined. The energy quality and rationality can be discussed through exergy analysis. The exergy input items of MOP and LMP include carbon electrodes, combustion air, ores, electric energy and the exergy output items include magnesia ingot, byproducts, flue gas and heat loss through walls. The main exergy loss methods were as follows: decomposition exergy loss, wall heat transfer exergy loss, exergy loss of refractory materials and gas heat transfer (see also in Table 3 and Figure 3c).

The main exergy balance equation is shown in Equation (11). $Ex_{electric}$ was determined to be 2544 kW based on Equation (15). Ex_{ores}, Ex_{fused} and $Ex_{byproducts}$ can be calculated based on Equation (26). As the main element of the byproducts was MgO, Ex_{MgO} consisted of Ex_{fused} and $Ex_{byproducts}$, and the value was 573.7 kW. During the combustion process of electrodes, compressible gas was generated and can be calculated based on Equations (16)–(25). The exergy output of flue gas was 279.4 kW, and the thermal exergy caused by heat loss through the walls was determined by Equations (27) and (28). Standard chemical exergy values are listed in Table 12. All calculation results can be seen in Tables 13–15.

Table 12. Standard chemical exergy values of ores, fused magnesium ingot, and byproducts.

Species	Standard Chemical Exergy (kJ/kmol)
$CaCO_3$	1000
$MgCO_3$	37,900
MgO	66,800
C	410,534
O_2	3933
CO_2	20,125
CaO	110,200
SiO_2	1900
Fe_2O_3	16,500
$MgO{\cdot}SiO_2$	198,960
$CaO{\cdot}SiO_2$	275,400
$Fe_2O_3{\cdot}SiO_2$	18,400

Table 13. Exergy calculation results of preparation.

Input Exergy	kWh/t	Output Exergy	kWh/t	Exergy Destruction	kWh/t
		Gas preparation			
Ex_{coals}	1937.1	$Ex_{gas,}$	1461.3	Heat and mass transfer	475.8
Total	1937.1	Total	1461.3	Total	475.8
		Light calcined magnesium oxide preparation 0.11			
Gas chemistry	1450.5	MgO physical	146.4	Heat and mass transfer	371.6
gas physical	128.7	Flue gas	544.1	Combustion	390.8
Ores physical	10.9			Ores dissociation	137.2
Total	1590.1	Total	690.5	Total	899.6

Table 14. Exergy calculation results of MOP.

Input Exergy	kWh/t	Output Exergy	kWh/t	Exergy Destruction	kWh/t
Ores	522.1	Magnesia chemical	355.3	Combustion	46.2
Electrodes	688.8	Magnesia physical	504.2	Dissociation	1385
Combustion air	10.6	Flue gas chemical	335.7	Heat and mass transfer	576.8
Leaking air	1.1			Byproduct chemical	282.1
Electric	2826.7			Byproduct physical	177.9
				Prefilled materials	47.9
				Wall loss	339.1
Total	4050.2	Total	1195.2	Total	2855

Table 15. Exergy calculation results of LMP.

Input Exergy	kWh/t	Output Exergy	kWh/t	Exergy Destruction	kWh/t
Ores	583.9	Magnesia chemical	352.6	Combustion	23.8
Electrodes	293.3	Flue gas chemical	16.1	Heat and mass transfer	248.5
Combustion air	4.5	Magnesia physical	733.7	Byproducts chemical	289.8
Leaking air	0.5			Byproducts physical	331.6
Electric	1253.2			Prefilled materials	21.0
				Wall loss	122.8
Total	2139.9	Total	1102.4	Total	1037.5

The calculation results of preparation process were shown in Figure 9 and Table 13. During the gas preparation process, the exergy input was coal chemistry exergy, with a value of 1937.1kWh/t, the exergy destruction was 475.8kWh/t and the exergy efficiency of gas preparation was 75.4%.

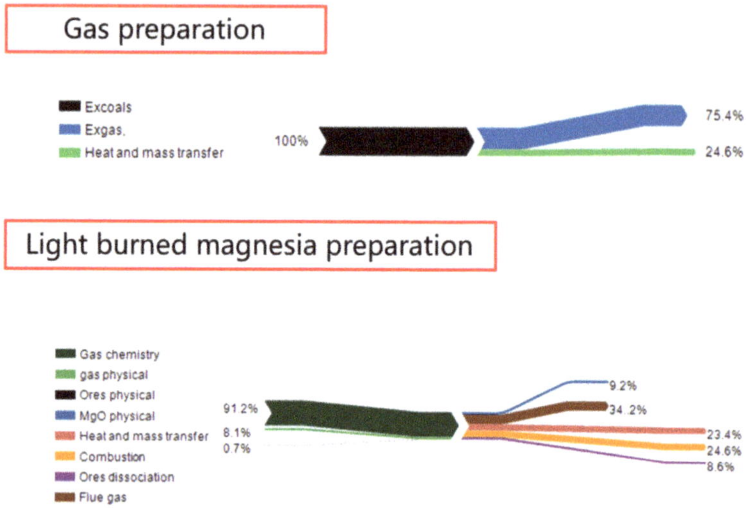

Figure 9. Exergy flow of raw materials preparation.

In the LMP process, the exergy calculation results were determined in the same manner as above. In addition, as the main raw material was light-calcined magnesia, the exergy flow of the preparation of the LMP process was determined as follows:

In the light-calcined magnesia oxide preparation process, the main exergy input was gas exergy, with a value of 1450.5kWh/t. The exergy output consisted of the physical exergy of magnesia oxide and flue gas, i.e., 146.4kWh/t and 544.1kWh/t, respectively. The exergy destruction methods were heat and mass transfer, combustion and ore dissociation, and the total exergy destruction was 899.6kWh/t.

Tables 14 and 15, Figures 10 and 11 show the exergy balance calculation results of MOP and LMP. In MOP, the exergy input items are electric energy exergy, electrode chemical exergy, and ore chemical exergy, the values of which are 2826.7 kWh/t, 688.8 kWh/t, 522.1 kWh/t. The main exergy output item is the chemical exergy and physical exergy of fused magnesia the values of which are respectively 355.3 kWh/t and 335.7 kWh/t, the exergy efficiency is 29.5%. In LMP, the exergy input items are also electric energy exergy, electrode chemical exergy, the values are 583.9 kWh/t, 293.3 kWh/t, 1253.2 kWh/t. The exergy output items are the chemical exergy and physical exergy of fused magnesia. The values are respectively 352.6 kWh/t, 733.7 kWh/t, the exergy efficiency is 51.5%. Exergy loss and other calculations are shown later.

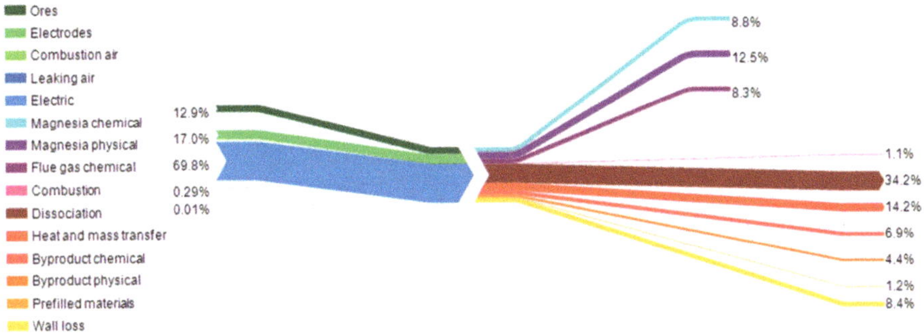

Figure 10. Exergy flow of MOP.

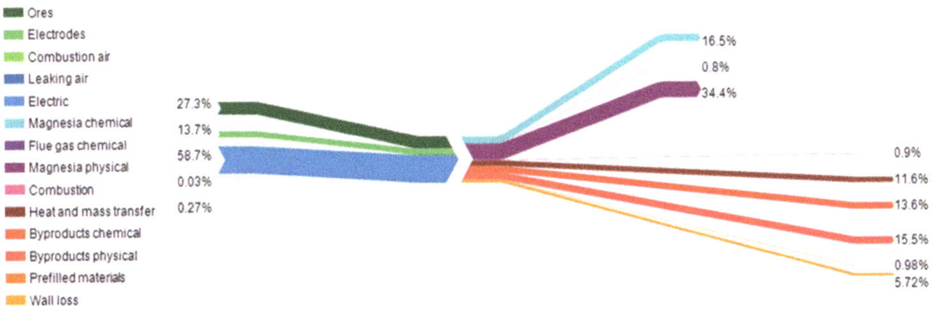

Figure 11. Exergy flow of LMP.

4.3.2. Exergy Destruction

Generally, an exergy reduction process is always accompanied by an entropy increase process which was shown in Table 16. Entropy production is always an irreversible process, such as friction heat generation, electrothermal effects, chemical reactions, and limited temperature difference heat transfer. For MOP and LMP processes, the irreversible process is roughly divided into three types: electrode combustion, ore decomposition and heat and component transfer in the overall process. In Equations (17)–(20), the basic entropy change calculation formula is given. In the MOP process, according to Equations (17)–(20), in order to evaluate the exergy destruction, the following series of equations are proposed to calculate the entropy production value:

$$S_0 - S = (\Delta S_{combustion} - S_{combustion}) + (\Delta S_{discomp} - S_{discomp}) \tag{33}$$

where ΔS is the entropy change, $S_{combustion}$ is the entropy transfer during the electrode combustion process and $S_{dissociate}$ is the entropy transfer during the ore dissociation process. The entropy changes of the combustion process and dissociation process are named $\Delta S_{combustion}$ and $\Delta S_{combustion}$, respectively, for the electrode combustion process:

$$\Delta S_{combustion} = S_{prod} - S_{react} \tag{34}$$

where subscripts prod and react stand for production and reactants. The entropy values used to calculate the entropy change are listed in Table 13. The entropy change in electrode combustion was determined to be 40.7 kW.

Table 16. Entropy of reactions.

	T (K)	Mass (kg/s)	N (kmol/s)	S (kj/kmol*k)	x_i
		Combustion of electrodes			
C	315	0.018	0.0014	5.694	0.097
O_2	315	0.047	0.0014	205.138	0.254
N_2	315	0.12	0.0043	191.598	0.649
CO_2	973	0.065	0.0014	213.76	0.351
N_2	973	0.12	0.0043	191.598	0.649
		Dissociation of ores			
$MgCO_3$	973	1.04	0.0122	147.32	0.934
$CaCO_3$	1173	0.073	0.00073	214.76	0.066
MgO	973	0.45	0.012	64.315	0.436
CO_2	973	0.512	0.012	250.635	0.497
CaO	1173	0.041	0.00073	102.67	0.040
CO_2	1173	0.032	0.00073	278.03	0.031

The entropy transfer caused by heat transfer can be calculated as follows [32]:

$$S_{combustion} = \frac{m_{elec} \cdot q_{carbon} - m_{elec} \cdot c_{pelec} \cdot T_{elec}}{T_{elec}} \tag{35}$$

where T_{elec} is the combustion temperature of the electrodes and combustion air. In this study, because the actual combustion temperature cannot be tested directly, the value was assumed to be 700 °C. During the electrode combustion process, the entropy transfer equals 3.75 kW, and the total entropy generation through the combustion process is 36.9 kW.

The exergy destruction of the decomposition of ores consists of two parts: the exergy destruction of the decomposition of ores and the mass transfer of CO_2. Similar to the calculation process above, the exergy destruction of the decomposition of ores can also be calculated, and the results are shown in Table 13. The reactions considered in the decomposition process were endothermic reactions, and the entropy transfer can be calculated as:

$$S_{discomp} = -\frac{Q_{discomp}}{T_{ediscomp}} \tag{36}$$

According to the energy balance results, the entropy transfers of $MgCO_3$ and $CaCO_3$ dissociation are -60.56 kJ/kmol·K and -116 kJ/kmol·K, respectively, and the exergy destruction of this part is 707 kW; thus, the total exergy destruction of the ore decomposition process is 1246.5 kW.

Another part of the exergy destruction of ores decomposition process was the generation of CO_2, according to the Equation (20), the exergy destruction caused by the mass transfer of the system is equal to 183.1 kW, during the MOP process, the mass and heat transfer exergy destruction of prefilled refractory materials are determined as follows:

$$Exd^{others}_{heat\ and\ mass\ transfer} = Ex_{input} - Ex_{output} - Exd_{combustion} - Exd_{decomposition} - Exd^{CO_2}_{heat\text{ and mass transfer}} \tag{37}$$

Because the mass and heat transfer boundary of prefilled refractory materials and other materials can hardly be defined, the value of exergy destruction was determined by the difference among the results of exergy input, exergy output and other exergy destruction methods.

4.3.3. Analysis of Exergy Balance

Four processes were discussed above: LMP, MOP, light-calcined preparation and gas preparation. The calculation results were shown in Figures 9–11 and Tables 13–15. Large amounts of exergy were wasted during the processes; thus, the exergy recycling potential will be discussed.

For the MOP process, the exergy destruction of ore dissociation was light-calcined magnesia, which is a pretreated raw material. Therefore, its preparation process is also considered in this article, including the preparation of fuel gas and light-calcined magnesia in the raw material preparation process. In the gas preparation process, the coal-gas conversion process is realised. In this process, coal and water vapour undergo an oxidation-reduction reaction, and part of the exergy is lost in the heat and mass transfer process. The overall transfer efficiency of the process is 75.4%. In the preparation process of light-calcined magnesia, a large amount of carbon dioxide is generated, which leads to complicated air flow in the equipment. The mixing of high-temperature carbon dioxide and room temperature air produces a large amount of exergy loss. This part of the loss is 3378.5 kW. At the same time, during the fuel combustion process, a large amount of chemical reaction exergy losses (43.4%) are produced. In theory, improving the quality of fuel can effectively reduce this part of the loss. In the LMP system, the products of the above preparation process are used as raw materials for production. The main inevitable exergy loss in the production process is heat and mass transfer loss, which accounts for 35.9% of the total exergy loss. The physical exergies of the byproducts and magnesia product are 673.2 kW and 1489.4 kW, respectively, and these two parts can be used for ore preheating or other recovery methods. The total exergy efficiency of the process was 12.7%, and the value was at a low level.

According to the exergy and energy balance calculation above, the reasons for the low efficiencies of MOP and LMP are summarised as follows. First, the MOP production equipment is not completely closed, causing a large amount of gas generated during the smelting process to overflow and carry a large amount of energy. Relying only on the accumulation of materials in the furnace body cannot fully recover this part of the energy. Second, in the products of MOP and LMP, the output of byproducts due to the low furnace temperature is close to 50%. Excessively high byproducts reduce the production efficiency of the furnace, indicating that the energy input of the furnace body is not enough to completely decompose and melt the raw materials in the furnace. Finally, in the LMP raw material preparation process, the high-temperature light-calcined magnesia powder is not directly used in LMP. A large amount of physical heat of the light-calcined magnesia powder is wasted in the storage and transport process, and the light-calcined magnesia needs to be reheated in LMP. For the above reasons, the improvement methods are proposed in the next section.

4.4. *Analysis of Improving Methods*

The analysis of the improved methods is mainly aimed at the MOP and LMP processes. Optimisation research on the gas preparation process and the preparation process of light burnt magnesia will continue in future research. This section divides the improvement measures into three parts in response to the problems summarised above. The first is to seal the furnace body to reduce the flue gas emissions and recover the heat taken away by the high-temperature magnesia ingot at the same time. The second is to increase smelting power, improve product quality and reduce energy loss caused by byproducts.

4.4.1. The Energy Saving Potential of Energy Saving Recycling

Preheat treatment of decomposed ore is often proposed in production processes such as submerged arc furnaces. Therefore, this article refers to the existing waste heat recovery research content and the energy balance calculation results and proposes a closed furnace body and heat recovery equipment. Based on this method, the heat carried by the flue gas in the LMP process and the heat of the high-temperature magnesia oxide lumps in the

MOP process can be recovered for material production, where the energy conversion rate is set to 1 to determine the potential for energy-saving recycling.

The energy recycling potential and efficiency are shown in Figure 12. The avoidable energy loss of preparation was the most of three processes due to the energy loss of a large amount of flue gas during the preparation process. The avoidable energy loss of the LMP process was the second of the processes. Due to the physical energy of the magnesia ingot and flue gas, the energy loss of wall heat transfer and the electric system cannot be avoided. The energy loss recycling potential of LMP was the least of the processes as a result of the energy loss of ore dissociation that occurred in the preparation process. The proportions of avoidable energy loss of the LMP, MOP and preparation were 20.7%, 19.8% and 53.2%, respectively; only the recovery potential was estimated in this section. The actual recovery path and equipment design were not studied, but will be investigated in future research.

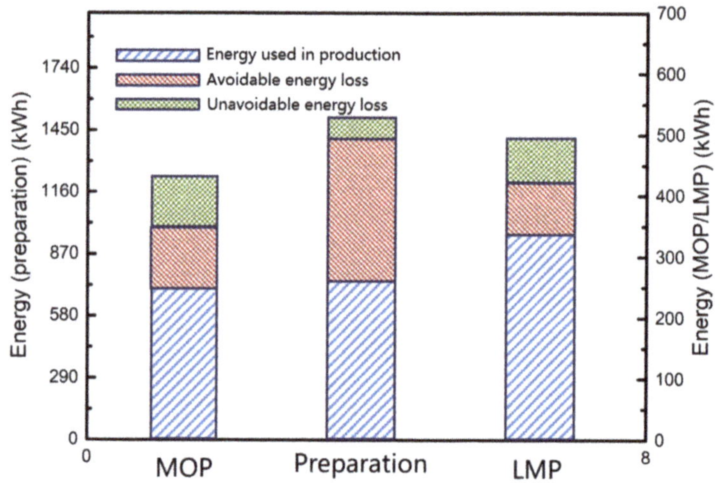

Figure 12. Energy recycling potential.

4.4.2. The Replacement of Different Electric Transformer

According to the previous calculation results, it is not difficult to see that the high proportion of byproducts in the product due to an insufficient furnace temperature is an important cause of low energy efficiency. Therefore, under the premise that other factors do not change, transformers with ratings of 3500 kVA and 4200 kVA are used. Using the factory production data, the calculation evaluation of the energy efficiency and exergy efficiency were carried out.

According to the calculation results in Figure 13, the high output of byproducts has led to a large amount of energy loss and exergy loss. At the same time, the production of byproducts is due to the small volume of the high-temperature zone of the molten pool. The energy loss of byproducts accounts for 4.4% and 17.3%. The maximum temperature of the molten pool and the volume of the molten pool can be increased by increasing the power of the transformer. The calculation results are shown in Figure 13. The energy and exergy efficiency of the LMP was higher than that of the MOP. After increasing the transformer power, the energy efficiency of MOP and LMP increased to 52.5% and 71.2%, and the exergy efficiency increased to 32.5% and 53.7%, respectively.

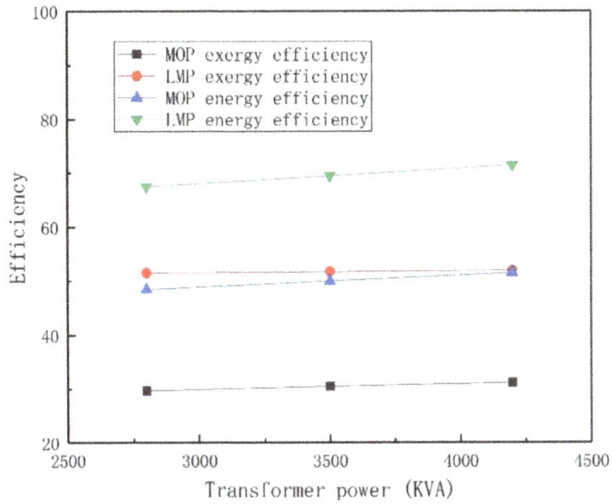

Figure 13. Energy and exergy efficiency at different transformer power.

5. Conclusions

Based on the energy and exergy analysis of the LMP, MOP, and preparation process, the main conclusions are described as follows:

1. The energy efficiencies of LMP, MOP, and the preparation process were 65.5%, 46.7%, and 39.4%, respectively, and the calculation consisted of all processes in the fused magnesia production process. The results show that the fused magnesia production process has great potential for energy savings in electric systems, raw material preparation and AFMFs.
2. The exergy efficiencies of the LMP, MOP, and the preparation process were 51.6% 29.5% and 35.6%, respectively, and the exergy destruction mainly consisted of heat and mass transfer, byproduct physical and chemical exergy and decomposition of ores.
3. The energy recycling potential of the three processes was calculated to ensure the value of avoidable energy loss, and the proportions of avoidable energy loss of the LMP, MOP and preparation process were 20.7%, 19.8% and 53.2%, respectively. Another energy saving method was carried out to improve the energy efficiency of LMP and MOP. As the electrical transformer power increased, the energy efficiency of LMP and MOP increased to 52.5% and 71.2%, respectively, and the exergy efficiency of LMP and MOP slightly increased to 32.5% and 53.7%, respectively.

Author Contributions: Conceptualization, T.J.; methodology, T.J.; software, T.J.; validation, T.J. and S.L.; formal analysis, T.J.; investigation, W.Z.; resources, W.Z.; data curation, T.J.; writing—original draft preparation, T.J.; writing—review and editing, T.J.; visualization, T.J.; supervision, W.Z.; project administration, W.Z.; funding acquisition, W.Z. All authors have read and agreed to the published version of the manuscript.

Funding: This research was funded by National Science Foundation of China grant number 2017YFA070030[illegible]

Institutional Review Board Statement: Not applicable.

Informed Consent Statement: Not applicable.

Data Availability Statement: Not applicable.

Acknowledgments: The authors are grateful to the National Science Foundation of China (Grant No. 2017YFA0700300) and Northeastern University-Magnesium Group Co-construction Laboratory Fundamental Fund.

Conflicts of Interest: The authors declare no conflict of interest.

References

1. Wang, H.; Zhang, W. Study on fusion synthesis of magnesium aluminum spinel and its application. *J. Wuhan Inst. Iron Steel* **1991**, *14*, 379–384.
2. Guo, M. *Industrial Electric Furnace*; Metallurgical Industry Press: Beijing, China, 2002.
3. Qi, G.C.; Shan, F.J.; Li, Q.; Yu, J.Y. Analysis of Fused Magnesia Production Process with 3000kVA Electric Arc Furnace. *Appl. Mech. Mater.* **2013**, *275*, 2143–2147. [CrossRef]
4. Ghosh, C.; Singh, S.K.; Sinhamahapatra, S. Fused magnesia aggregate from Indian magnesite through plasma processing. *Indoceram AIPMA* **2016**, *4*, 33–36.
5. Li, J.; Zhang, Y.; Shao, S.; Zhang, S.; Ma, S. Application of cleaner production in a Chinese magnesia refractory material plant. *J. Clean. Prod.* **2016**, *113*, 1015–1023. [CrossRef]
6. Dai, Y.; Bin, L.; Chao, F. China's total energy consumption control and energy conservation during the 13th Five-Year Plan period. *J. Beijing Inst. Technol. Soc. Sci. Ed.* **2015**, *1*, 1–7. [CrossRef]
7. Wang, D.; Guo, M. Research on the electric heating power and furnace type of magnesia fused furnace. *Energy Metall. Ind.* **1997**, *1*, 36–39.
8. Zhen, W.; Ninghui, W.; Tie, L.; Yong, C.A.O. 3D Numerical Analysis of the Arc Plasma Behavior in a Submerged DC Electric Arc Furnace for the Production of Fused MgO. *Plasma Sci. Technol.* **2012**, *14*, 321–326. [CrossRef]
9. Qin, Q.; Yue, Q.; Gu, G.; Guo, M. Two-electrode direct current melting magnesium submerged arc furnace. *J. Northeast. Univ.* **2003**, *7*, 685–688. [CrossRef]
10. Kong, W. *Research on the Optimization Decision-Making Method of the Electricity Consumption per Ton of Magnesia Smelting Furnace*; Northeastern University: Shenyang, China, 2013.
11. Li, J.; Zhang, Y.; Shao, S.; Zhang, S. Comparative life cycle assessment of conventional and new fused magnesia production. *J. Clean. Prod.* **2015**, *91*, 170–179. [CrossRef]
12. Chai, T.; Zhang, J.; Yang, T. Demand Forecasting of the Fused Magnesia Smelting Process With System Identification and Deep Learning. *IEEE Trans. Ind. Inform.* **2021**, *17*, 8387–8396. [CrossRef]
13. Oates, J. *Lime and Limestone: Chemistry and Technology, Production and Uses*; John and Wiley and Sons: Hoboken, NJ, USA, 1998. [CrossRef]
14. Longo, G.M.; Longo, S. Thermal decomposition of $MgCO_3$ during the atmospheric entry of micrometeoroids. *Int. J. Astrobiol.* **2017**, *16*, 368–378. [CrossRef]
15. Yang, J.; Lu, S.; Wang, L. Fused magnesia manufacturing process: A survey. *J. Intell. Manuf.* **2020**, *31*, 327–350. [CrossRef]
16. Gutiérrez, A.S.; Martínez, J.B.C.; Vandecasteele, C. Energy and exergy assessments of a lime shaft kiln. *Appl. Therm. Eng.* **2013**, *51*, 273–280. [CrossRef]
17. Zhou, X.; Gu, Z.; Huang, W. Research on transformer loss calculation method. *Power Demand Side Manag.* **2013**, *15*, 11–14. [CrossRef]
18. Chai, T.-Y.; Wu, Z.-W.; Wang, H. A CPS Based Optimal Operational Control System for Fused Magnesium Furnace. *IFAC-PapersOnLine* **2017**, *50*, 14992–14999. [CrossRef]
19. Liu, B. *Research and Development of Automatic Distributing Device for Electric Smelting Magnesium Furnace*; Liaoning University of Science and Technology: Anshan, China, 2019.
20. Shan, Q. *Research on a New Process of Recovery and Utilization of Fused Magnesium Waste Heat Based on Field Temperature Measurement Experiment*; Northeastern University: Shenyang, China, 2012.
21. Fu, Y.; Wang, Z.; Wang, Z.; Wang, N.; Wang, X. Splattering Suppression for a Three-Phase AC Electric Arc Furnace in Fused Magnesia Production Based on Acoustic Signal. *IEEE Trans. Ind. Electron.* **2017**, *64*, 4772–4780. [CrossRef]
22. Li, L. *Numerical Simulation and Optimization of the Temperature Field of Magnesia Smelting Furnace*; Northeastern University: Shenyang, China, 2015.
23. Rong, W.; Li, B.; Qi, F.; Cheung, S.C. Energy and exergy analysis of an annular shaft kiln with opposite burners. *Appl. Therm. Eng.* **2017**, *119*, 629–638. [CrossRef]
24. Yu, Y.; Li, B.; Fang, Z.; Wang, C. Energy and exergy analyses of pellet smelting systems of cleaner ferrochrome alloy with multi-energy supply—ScienceDirect. *J. Clean. Prod.* **2020**, *285*, 124893. [CrossRef]
25. Zhang, K.; Li, M.; Yang, C.; Shao, Z.; Wang, L. Exergy Analysis of Electric Vehicle Heat Pump Air Conditioning System with Battery Thermal Management System. *J. Therm. Sci.* **2020**, *29*, 408–422. [CrossRef]
26. George, P.A.O.; Gutiérrez, A.S.; Martínez, J.B.C.; Vandecasteele, C. Cleaner production in a small lime factory by means of process control. *J. Clean. Prod.* **2010**, *18*, 1171–1176. [CrossRef]
27. Szargut, J. *Exergy in Thermal Systems Analysis*; Springer Netherlands: Dordrecht, The Netherlands, 1999.
28. ÇENGEL; Yunus, A.; Boles, M.A. Thermodynamics: An Engineering Approach. *McGraw-Hill Ser. Mech. Eng.* **1989**, *33*, 1297–1305. [CrossRef]
29. Bes, A. Dynamic Process Simulation of Limestone Calcination in Normal Shaft Kilns. Ph.D. Thesis, Otto-von-Guericke University Magdeburg, Magdeburg, Germany, 2006.
30. Kariman, H.; Hoseinzadeh, S.; Heyns, P.S. Energetic and exergetic analysis of evaporation desalination system integrated with mechanical vapor recompression circulation—ScienceDirect. *Case Stud. Therm. Eng.* **2019**, *16*, 100548. [CrossRef]

31. Mahmoudan, A.; Samadof, P.; Hosseinzadeh, S.; Garcia, D.A. A Multigeneration Cascade System Using Ground-source Energy with Cold Recovery: 3E Analyses and Multi-objective Optimization. *Energy* **2021**, *233*, 121185. [CrossRef]
32. Hoseinzadeh, S.; Heyns, S. Advanced Energy, Exergy and Environmental (3E) Analyses and Optimization of a Coal-Fired 400 MW Thermal Power Plant. *J. Energy Resour. Technol.* **2021**, *143*, 082106. [CrossRef]

buildings

MDPI

Article

Current Status of Old Housing for Low-Income Elderly Households in Seoul and Green Remodeling Support Plan: Economic Analysis Considering the Social Cost of Green Remodeling

Jaemoon Kim [1,2], Seunghoon Nam [1] and Duhwan Lee [1,*]

1 Technology Research Institution, SAMOOCM Architect and Engineers, Seoul 05556, Korea; jaem0216@snu.ac.kr (J.K.); nshwow1@samoocm.com (S.N.)
2 Graduate School of Environmental Studies, Seoul National University, Seoul 08826, Korea
* Correspondence: ldhex@samoocm.com; Tel.: +82-10-8921-3517

Abstract: In this study, the economic feasibility of green remodeling (GR), which could improve the health, safety, and energy of elderly households considering social cost, was analyzed. As a result, the net present value of GR was '−10,267 USD (49.7%)', which was found to be uneconomical compared to the total construction cost (20,981 USD, 100%) despite benefits of energy saving, carbon reduction, and air pollutant reduction. Based on this result, in order to expand GR for low-income elderly households, who cannot afford to perform GR, a GR support measure linked to the currently implemented energy conversion and old-age housing support policies was proposed. It allows the government to perform GR for low-income elderly households with 1/4 of the total construction cost. This result could revitalize GR to reduce greenhouse gas and contribute to housing stability for low-income elderly households who are vulnerable to COVID-19 and climate change.

Keywords: old housing; sick building syndrome; green remodeling; social cost; energy transition; housing stability policy

Citation: Kim, J.; Nam, S.; Lee, D. Current Status of Old Housing for Low-Income Elderly Households in Seoul and Green Remodeling Support Plan: Economic Analysis Considering the Social Cost of Green Remodeling. *Buildings* **2022**, *12*, 29. https://doi.org/10.3390/buildings12010029

Academic Editors: Roberto Alonso González Lezcano, Francesco Nocera and Rosa Giuseppina Caponetto

Received: 22 November 2021
Accepted: 28 December 2021
Published: 31 December 2021

1. Introduction

1.1. Background and Purpose

The World Health Organization (WHO) has pointed out the aging generation problem, where the global population over the age of 60 is expected to increase from 900 million in 2015 to 2 billion in 2050 [1]. Korea has become an aging society, with an aging rate of 14% as of 2017, and it is expected to reach 20% by 2025, at which point it will become a super-aging society. Recently, Statistics Korea predicted that this trend of aging in Korea will be accelerated more and more [2]. Due to the global COVID-19 pandemic from the end of 2019, "untact", non-face-to-face society (business, education, shipping, etc.), and non-face-to-face services (food, goods, drive-thru shopping, etc.) have quickly been established in Korea as the New Normal [3]. These social changes increase the staying time of residents in buildings, and they emphasize the importance of indoor environment (temperature/humidity/ventilation) and air quality, which directly affect human health [4]. In this regard, the housing condition of an aged house is affected by the indoor environment and air quality, and it is closely related to the health of the residents [5]. For example, high or low temperature indoors (summer/winter) causes cardiovascular diseases, high blood pressure, and respiratory problems [6]. Specifically, an imbalance in room temperature or humidity leads to mold growth, which may cause respiratory disease and lung cancer [7]. In addition, the problem of noise from the outside intruding into the house may also cause cardiovascular diseases, sleep problems, and cognitive impairment [8]. Improving the energy efficiency of old houses is known to be a good strategy for enhancing the housing condition of a house in the long term [9]. For example, improving building envelope insulation, windows, and heating-cooling equipment may enhance the indoor thermal environment, and making high-performance window improvements using sealing materials (airtight tape, etc.) may reduce the external noise problem [10]. The total heat exchange ventilation system improves the indoor air quality by introducing purified outside air [11]. Insulation, windows, high-efficiency air conditioning systems (boiler/EHP), and total heat exchange ventilation systems are actively used as the elementary technologies of GR (Green Remodeling) for improving the energy performance of old buildings. These measures for improving the energy efficiency of old buildings are referred to using various terms such as energy retrofit and green renovation, but in this paper, the term 'GR' is used. Further, 'GR' in this paper includes deep energy retrofitting, such as improving insulation, windows, air condition, ventilation, etc., rather than a single measurement for performance improvement.

In April 2019, in a report on the perspective of the clean energy transition, the IEA highlighted the importance of energy transition through GR of old buildings [12]. The GR is used as a core energy saving policy in the building sector for energy conversion and greenhouse gas reduction. However, there are several barriers to applying GR policy for reducing greenhouse gas emissions, so many countries are using various measures to overcome these barriers [13,14].

The most representative barriers are economic feasibility, such as high initial construction cost and low subsidy. Technical skill level, information imbalance, uncertainty, and rebound effect have also been mentioned as barriers [13–15]. To alleviate these barriers and implement GR, many countries are using construction cost support, low-interest loans, technical support, and various types of promotional support according to the energy improvement performance of old buildings as auxiliary policies [13,14]. Many other research papers involving GR suggest an optimal GR planning direction by approving the energy effect of GR and analyzing economic feasibility to alleviate the aforementioned policy barriers. First, simple remodeling action (insulation replacement, windows replacement or air conditioning replacement) can bring about lower results than expected in terms of energy and cost effectiveness as compared to GR (insulation + windows + HVAC + ventilation) [16]. These relationships can be confirmed from empirical GR analysis cases in Europe and the United States [17–19]. The cause of this is that using a simple measure that is not coordinated with other aging elements (such as walls, roofs, windows, ventilation, and air conditioning) can lead to a lower energy saving effect than expected, due to the deteriorated quality of thermal bridges and elements that were not improved after construction [20]. By contrast, the GR provides energy performance to new construction levels by examining the deterioration of the target building in advance and planning all elements that require improved consideration of the latest legislations (insulation, thermal bridges, air tightness and ventilation, and mechanical and electrical installations). Accordingly, the EU Commission also recommends GR in consideration of reliable energy efficiency improvement and economic feasibility for the owners and investors of old buildings [21].

However, this GR is not a measure that can be adopted by all owners of old buildings, because of the high initial construction cost which requires about 10 years (relatively long term) to recover the construction cost [22]. This is particularly true for low-income elderly households who experience a relatively large impact on energy bill burden, indoor environment, and air pollution. Although elderly households desperately need GR, it will be difficult to improve energy, indoor environment, and air quality without government support.

This paper investigated the aging status of buildings as well as the energy performance and usage status of nine old houses for low-income elderly households in Seoul, Korea. Among them, one old house was selected, and the total construction cost required for GR and energy savings before and after GR were analyzed. Based on the results of these analyses, an economic analysis was conducted in consideration of social costs. Then, to activate GR for low-income elderly households, a GR support plan that links the current energy transition with the low-income old housing support policy was proposed by utilizing the health, safety, and energy improvement effects of GR. This support plan is expected to contribute to an improved residential environment along with activation of the GR from the GR support for low-income elderly households who are vulnerable to COVID-19 and climate change.

The unique features of this study are that when planning the GR of old housing for low-income elderly households, energy, health, and safety factors that were considered as housing characteristics of elderly households were all reflected in the construction cost to analyze economic feasibility. Therefore, an effective housing stabilization plane was proposed by integrating the old housing support policy for low-income elderly households with the direct and indirect effect of GR.

1.2. Procedure and Method

The research procedure was divided into four stages: Section 2 describes the literature review, Section 3 details the target selection and GR plan, Section 4 discusses the economic analysis, and Section 5 presents the GR support concept proposal. In the literature review in Section 2, previous studies were reviewed to derive health problems and the causes for the residents of old houses, and architectural methods that could be used to improve these issues were summarized. Then, factors for safety improvement were investigated in consideration of the residential characteristics of elderly households, which may be the most vulnerable group among residents of old houses. Finally, the scope of energy elements and performance level of improvement for old houses were investigated, and the improvement scope and performance level of buildings and facilities that were suitable for the characteristics of old houses in Korea were summarized. The GR range of this study based on the review includes health, safety, and energy performance improvements in consideration of the residential characteristics of low-income elderly households.

In Section 3, the status of aging houses of low-income elderly households in Seoul, Korea was investigated, and target buildings were selected for GR analysis. First, the aging status of the houses in which the vulnerable class (such as elderly households) with less than 70% income reside among the old single houses and multi-family houses that have been in Seoul for more than 30 years was investigated and analyzed. Next, GR target buildings were selected, and the scope and methods for GR improvement were summarized based on the results of a literature review and on-site investigations. This GR plan includes building and facility elements applied in terms of health, safety, and energy. The performance level of these elements was planned in consideration of regulations and construction costs.

In Section 4, the economic analysis considering social costs was described. First, the total construction cost was derived by calculating the construction costs of each element in the GR plan. For energy analysis, the annual energy and reduced amounts of the greenhouse gas (CO_2) for the target building before and after GR were calculated using ECO-2 (Korean Building Energy Efficiency Rating Program). To analyze the economic feasibility, the annual energy saving cost (benefit of residence) was calculated by converting the amount of the energy into the electricity rates for houses. The social cost was calculated by converting the reduction amount of greenhouse gas (Social Benefit-(1)) and the reduction effect of the air pollutant (Social Benefit-(2)) into cost [23]. For the economic feasibility analysis, the residence benefit and the social benefit according to the GR of the old house compared to the total construction cost of the GR were analyzed and compared using the Net Present Value (NPV) method. The NPV method was used to analyze economic feasibility, because it can suggest the present value of future accrued benefits, and the results of its analyses can be used for other analyses [24].

In Section 5, a GR support plan was proposed in which the housing stability policy and the energy conversion policy for low-income elderly households were mixed based on the analysis results. Figure 1 shows a flowchart of the research contents according to the research procedure.

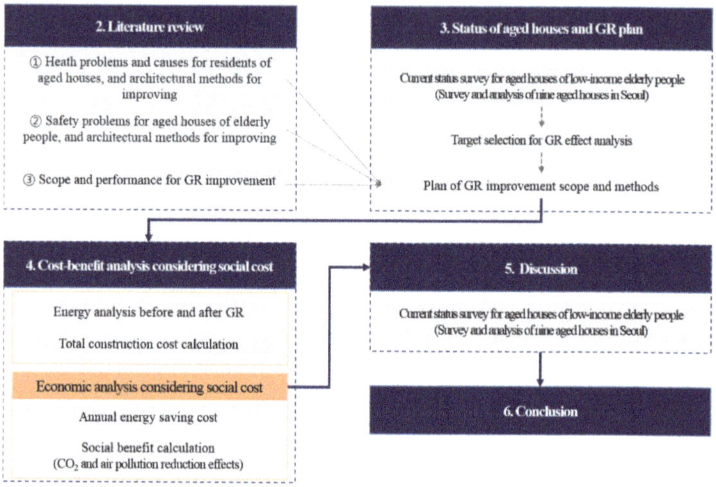

Figure 1. Research flowchart.

2. Literature Review

In the literature review of previous studies, three aspects of old housing were investigated. First, the causes of health problems in old houses and architectural methods to improve them were investigated; second, using the 2017 Seoul housing situation survey data, factors for improving the safety aspect of the elderly households who are vulnerable groups were derived; and third, GR factors and performance levels in terms of energy were summarized. The results of this survey will be used as basic data when planning the GR of old housing for low-income elderly households.

2.1. Causes of Health Problems in Old Houses and Methods of Architectural Improvement

Sick Building Syndrome refers to a phenomenon wherein the indoor air quality and indoor environment can adversely affect the health of the residents [25]. Outside air polluted by PM2.5 and PM10 enters the room without being purified, which can cause respiratory diseases in the residents [26,27]. In addition, various damages may be caused to residents due to damp wallpaper and mold growing inside the wall, various harmful gases leaking from the grain pipe, and VOCs (volatile organic compounds) that may be present after interior construction [8,25,28].

First, the unexpected inflow of polluted outdoor air by particle materials (PM2.5, PM10) into the room is largely affected by the quality of the aged windows [27]. The inflow of polluted outdoor air can be reduced by replacing old windows and sealing window edges. Mold growing indoors mainly occurs on the side walls (where the outside and the wall come into contact) according to the temperature difference between the inside and outside, and this difference worsens when the indoor air is not ventilated. The vulnerable areas to indoor dewing and mold are mainly the space between furniture (closets, etc.) and the wall and/or in the space between the wallpaper and the wall. The main cause of this problem may be the wall heat bridging and lack of indoor ventilation. For an architectural method to improve this problem, an insulation construction without thermal bridges (external insulation) and a total heat exchange ventilation system suitable for the purpose may be applied [29,30]. The leakage of methane gas, ammonia gas, carbon monoxide, and carbon dioxide from old drains or gas pipes may cause headaches or dizziness. To solve these problems, old pipes should be regularly cleaned and replaced [30]. Specifically, it is necessary to properly manage and replace the trap protecting the water seal which can block the backflow of odors to facilitate drainage and manage aging vent pipes to protect the water seal. There is a possibility of causing chronic diseases such as headaches and allergies due to organic compounds such as acetone, benzene, and formaldehyde generated from materials and furniture that is newly installed due to repair activities, such as interior construction and furniture replacement, while maintaining the building. This problem may be improved by regular ventilation and the use of environment friendly materials [31,32].

According to the Health and Home Upgrades research report by DOE (U.S. Department of Energy) in February 2017, housing environment has a significant impact on resident health, and improving the energy performance and ventilation facilities of old buildings also enhances the energy and health of residents [28]. As an empirical case of health improvement by GR, Beysse et al. analyzed the health improvement effect of 40 elderly households after GR in the US. As a result, respiratory diseases, overall health problems, indoor environment (temperature/humidity), indoor air quality, and musty smell from pipes were all improved [33]. Ahrentzen et al. performed GR (including eco-friendly finishing material and furniture) for 57 aged houses of low-income elderly citizens in the United States. As a result, the indoor environment (temperature/humidity) and indoor air quality (formaldehyde, particle matter, etc.) were improved, and the overall health of residents was enhanced as well [34]. In addition, in the analysis of a number of GR empirical cases, the resident health was enhanced from the improvement of the indoor environment and indoor air quality after GR [35–37].

In summary, energy saving and improvements in both indoor environment and indoor air quality are some of the expected benefits of reforming insulation, windows, heating and cooling, and ventilation facilities which are general elements of GR. Further, the results showed that it can help improve the indoor environment to enhance the health of residents by applying eco-friendly materials and furniture, as well as proper management and replacement of old pipes when improving the interior space.

2.2. Review of Housing Improvement Factors for Elderly Households among the Vulnerable Classes

To capture the housing situation survey in Seoul in 2017, the factors necessary for housing improvement were investigated by reflecting the characteristics of elderly households [38]. A survey was conducted that covered a total of 10 items, as shown in Figure 2. In the results of a study comparing owned houses to rented houses, 'Nonslip Floor Materials', 'Indoor Emergency Bell', 'Door Knobs', and 'Support Knobs' appeared at high proportions. Among 10 items, except for the 'Indoor Emergency Bell' and 'Safety Knobs', these items are optional items which can be reflected in a GR plan without affecting the cost and the plan. Therefore, when planning a GR improvement model in this study, the items of 'Indoor Emergency Bell' and 'Safety Knobs' were included in consideration of the characteristics of elderly households of aged houses, and they were reflected in the construction cost.

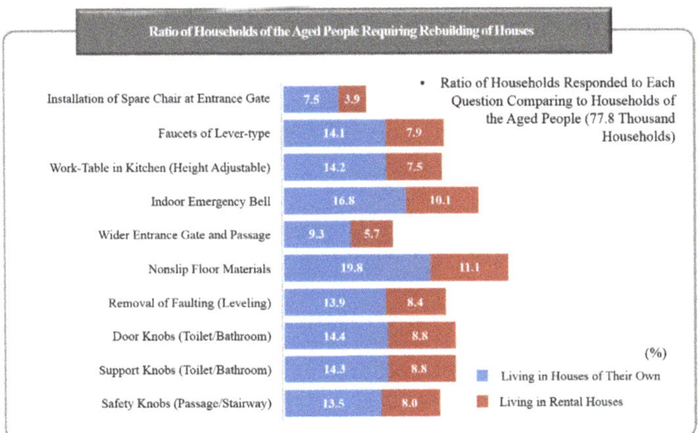

Figure 2. Ratio of items required for rebuilding houses of elderly households.

2.3. Investigation of Energy Performance Improvement (GR) Factors and Performance Level of Aged Houses

Recently, the research on energy performance improvements of aged buildings has mainly focused on energy saving by total GR or the cost efficiency of zero-energy GR, rather than the energy efficiency of individual items. In particular, to increase the utilization of GR research, various studies have examined GR strategies for apartment houses, school facilities, and business facilities, which are in high demand [10,39–41]. The improvement scopes and performances of these precedent studies have differences in climate by region, technology level, and residential environment, so care should be taken when adopting the applied technology for use in various settings. Accordingly, in this study, the performance of the improvement scope was considered by referring to the GR guidelines issued by the Korean government.

In 'Guidelines for the Establishment and Implementation of Urban Renewal Revitalization Plan for Urban Renewal New Deal Projects' published in August 2018, the Korean government disclosed GR cases, scope of technical elements, and recommended performance of aged houses [41]. The scope of improvement in the guidelines includes the replacement of roof/exterior wall insulation, windows (including entrance doors), air conditioning equipment, indoor LED lightening, and renewal of façade design. These need to be additionally reflected when planning the GR improvement model, because the literature review does not include the consideration of a ventilation system or sealing system for resident's health. This guideline provides performance improvement standards for each GR item, and it can be used to determine the performance level. Table 1 presents the improvement in factors and performance for each item. 'Bad' refers to the performance of the aged building, 'Good' refers to the performance of a passive house in Germany, and 'Recommended' refers to the performance level of each item of the GR plan considered in this study.

Table 1. Improvement in factors and performance in terms of energy consumption [41].

Locations	Level of Performance/Location		
	Bad	**Recommended**	**Good**
Insulation of Roof (W/m^2·K)	0.33	0.15	0.08
Insulation of Exterior Wall (W/m^2·K)	0.45	0.22	0.13
Insulation of Window (W/m^2·K)	2.9	1.41	0.75
Lighting Density (W/m^2)	17.29	9.46	3.40
Heating/Cooling	-	A Product of Class I of the Energy Consumption Efficiency	
Amount of Energy Consumption (kWh/m^2·y)	228.10	167.43	55.0
Amount of Primary Energy Consumption (kWh/m^2·y)	267.20	214.43	150.7

Finally, the use of IoT-based smart home technology for small elderly households is spreading [29]; however, the GR plan described in this study minimizes the automatic control facilities and applies only the items related to safety (emergency bell linked to mobile phone) while considering the cost aspect.

Figure 3 summarizes the problems in health, safety, and energy aspects and the direction of architectural improvement considering the characteristics of residents of aged houses from the literature research. Figure 3 shows that the architectural method for enhancing the health problems of aged houses and the method for improving the building energy performance have many items in common. Based on this, it is clear that performing the GR described in the literature review has the effect of enhancing the health problems of residents. However, the GR scope of this study considering the health and safety of elderly households should be additionally applied to the material selection and replacement of sanitary piping, and the additional installation of various knobs, non-slip pads, and emergency bells, along with the removal of faulting should be considered based on the fact that the residents are elderly people. The results of this survey will be used in a GR plan considering health, safety, and energy after investigating the status of aged houses of low-income elderly households.

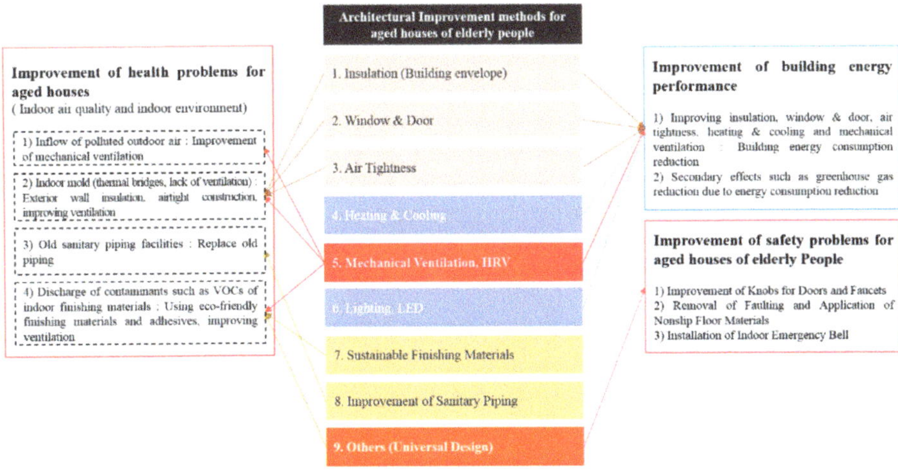

Figure 3. Issues associated with aged people in households of the old houses and the orientation of improvement in parts of the GR.

3. Current Status Survey and GR Plan for Aged House of Elderly Households in Seoul, Korea (Scope of Improvement and Performance)

To investigate the current status of aged houses of elderly households in Seoul, the sites were surveyed with the project implementer for about two months with the cooperation of the 'Hope home repair project' of Seodaemun-gu, Seoul and the 'Structural safety status survey project' of Dongjak-gu, Seoul. More than 20 aged houses were investigated, and nine households were found to be suitable for this study.

Accordingly, in this section, common characteristics were derived by summarizing the aging status and problems of nine buildings of low-income elderly households. Among them, buildings that could be used to analyze the improvement effect by GR were selected as the target sites.

3.1. Survey on Current Status of Aged Houses for Elderly Households in Seoul

Table 2 summarize the building status, resident information, and building energy performance of aged self-owned houses or aged multi-family houses in which elderly households reside. As shown in the survey results, most elderly households living in aged houses for around 30 years were women over 70 years old, and they often lived on the lower floors (1st floor) with inconvenient movement and relatively insufficient ventilation and light.

Table 2. Results of survey on sites of old houses of households of aged people.

Items		Results of Survey on Each Household									Common Feature
		Household #1	Household #2	Household #3	Household #4	Household #5	Household #6	Household #7	Household #8	Household #9	
	Selected House	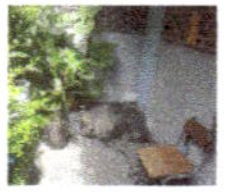	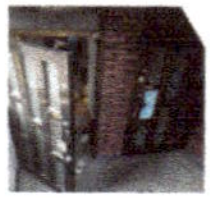	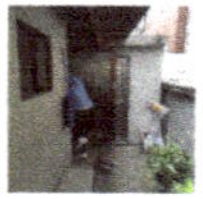	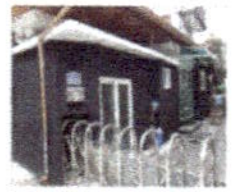	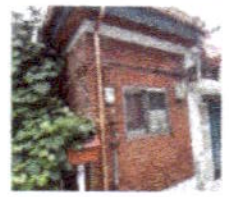	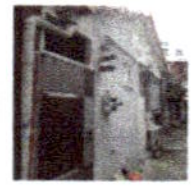	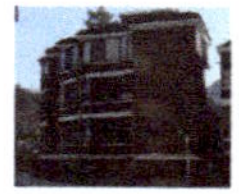	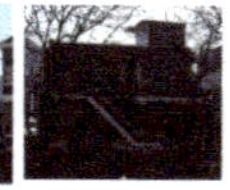	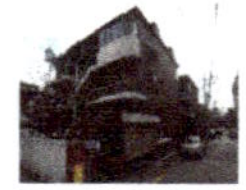	Single house and lower floor of multi-family house
Building Information	Location	Hong-je Dong 304-25	Hong-je Dong 287-72	Hong-je Dong 285-34	Sadang-Dong 275-15, 1	Sadang-Dong 275-15, 2	Sadang-Dong 249-45	#4 Ganho-Avenue 37, 301	Ganho-Avenue 28-4 Ground Floor (Semi-Basement)	Pobangteo-Road 18, 101	Hongje-dong and Sadang-dong
	Year of Completion	1991	1990	1987	February, 1972	February, 1972	March, 1972	April, 1991	March, 1993	January, 1992	Average service life of more than 30 years
	Structure	Brick	Brick	Brick and reinforced concrete	Brick	Brick	Brick	Brick	Brick	Brick	Brick
	Exterior Finishing	Face brick	Face brick	Face brick	Face brick and partial painting	Face brick and partial painting	Brick and painting	Face brick and painting	Face brick and painting	Face brick	Painted brick (efflorescence and crack)
	Interior Finishing	Wallpaper (Good)	Wallpaper (Moderate)	Wallpaper (Moderate)	Wallpaper (Good)	Wallpaper (Poor)	Wallpaper (Moderate)	Wallpaper (Moderate)	Wallpaper (Moderate)	Wallpaper (Moderate)	Wallpaper
	Remarks	Blistered wallpaper, Toilet threshold: 500 mm, (Disordered behavior of occupant)	Mold/dewing on side walls and boiler room observed	Mold/dewing in common-use toilet (Disordered behavior of occupant)	Windows, exterior finishing, and entrance gate require complementary works	Dewing and mold on side walls were observed	Partial remodeling works completed	Boiler and windows in main living room became obsolescent	Boiler and windows in main living room became obsolescent	Windows in all rooms became obsolescent	Immediate renewal due to mold, and dewing due to aging of building
Residential Information	Occupied Floor	Ground floor (House of two stories)	Second floor (House of three stories)	Ground floor (House of three stories)	Ground floor (One-story house)	Ground floor (One-story house)	Ground floor (One-story house)	Third floor (House of three stories; 8 households)	Ground floor (House of three stories; 4 households)	Second floor (House of three stories)	Lower floor
	Area of Occupation	-	-	-	28 m^2	32.93 m^2	27.37 m^2	30 m^2	15 m^2	32 m^2	Avg.: around 25 m^2
	Type of Residence	Rental (Monthly)	Rental (Monthly)	Rental (Monthly)	One's own house	One's own house	Rental (monthly)	Rental (Monthly)	Rental (Monthly)	Rental (Monthly)	Monthly rent
	Resident	Female (Age 70)	Female (-)	Female (Age 79)	Male (age 75) and a daughter	Female (age 65) and a son	Female (Age 73)	Female (Age 70)	Female (Age 60) and another one, husband	Male (Age 86)	Avg.: 70 years or more
Performance of Energy Consumption of Building	Insulation	EPS (Expanded Polystyrene) 50 mm	EPS 50 mm	EPS 50 mm	EPS 50 mm	- (None, the domestic regulations pertinent to insulation were stipulated after 1979)		EPS 50 mm	EPS 50 mm	EPS 50 mm	Dewing/mold
	Windows	Wood 3 mm and Aluminum 3 mm	Wood 3 mm and Al 3 mm	Wood 3 mm and Al 3 mm	Replaced—with PVC (Polyvinyl Chloride) double window	Wood 3 mm and Al 3 mm	Replaced—with PVC double window	Wood 3 mm and Al 3 mm	Wood 3 mm and Al 3 mm	Wood 3 mm and Al 3 mm	Sealing deterioration and dewing/mold
	Main Entrance Gate	No windbreak structure									Deterioration of sealing and energy performance
	Cooling	PAC (Package Air Conditioner)	PAC	PAC	PAC	PAC	PAC	PAC	PAC	PAC	Cooling: air-conditioner Heating: floor heating
	Heating	Gas boiler	Gas boiler	Gas boiler	Gas boiler	Gas boiler	Gas boiler	Gas boiler (Replacement needed due to obsolescence)	Gas boiler (Replacement needed due to obsolescence)	Gas boiler	
	Hot Water Supply	Electric water heater	Electric water heater	Electric water heater		Electric water heater					
	Ventilation	None									Vulnerable to PM
	Others	Requested rental apartment	-	Requested subsidy for housing expense	Requested installation of the main gate of house	-	-	Improvement of boiler and windows was planned			No safety knobs such as handrails

Dewing and mold, both of which have substantial effects on the health of residents in terms of building function and age, were found in all except the two remodeled houses (No. 4 and 6). There was a household (No. 3) with a public restroom and a household (No. 1) with an indoor rest room that had thresholds higher than 500 mm, despite the inconvenience of mobility. In terms of building energy and indoor air quality, all households had very poor insulation. Regarding the windows, all except two households were equipped with a combination of wooden single windows and AL single windows, so the insulation performance was less than 1/3 of the current legal standard performance. As the window frames have been used for more than 20 years, the air tightness performance was very weak. In addition, the front doors of all households were not equipped with a windproof structure, and there were no ventilation facilities at all. This was expected to have a significant negative impact on the health of elderly people, who are relatively vulnerable to particle matters and indoor air pollutants. Finally, regarding the heating and cooling facilities, all households were equipped with wall mounted air conditioners for cooling and boilers for heating using urban gas. Some households had outdated cooling/heating equipment, but there was no problem in usage. Table 3 presents images of major defects such as dewing and mold, a restroom in need of improvement, old window sets, and household front doors.

Table 3. Survey cases of defects in aged houses.

Dewing and Mold	Poor Toilet Threshold	Obsolete Set of Windows	Front Gate of Households
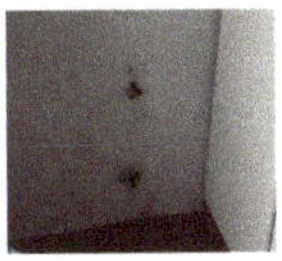 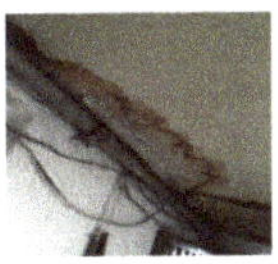	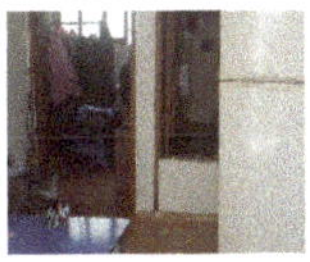 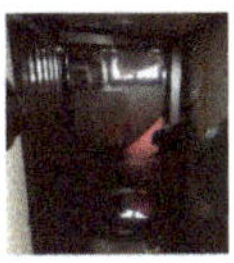	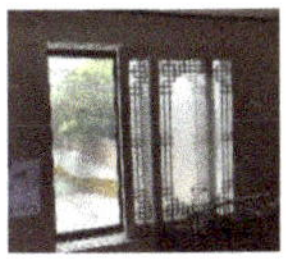 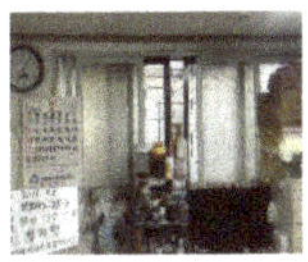	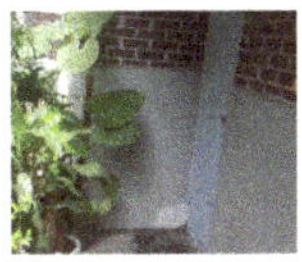 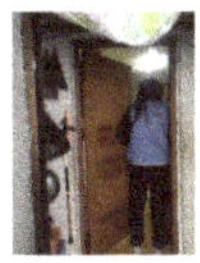
(Above): Household #2 (Below): Household #3	(Above): Household #1 (Below): Household #3	(Above): Household #6 (Below): Household #7	(Above): Household #2 (Below): Household #3
Interior Finish: Wallpaper Flutter	**Water Leakage**	**Safety (Electricity)**	**Others (Thermal Bridge and Airtightness)**
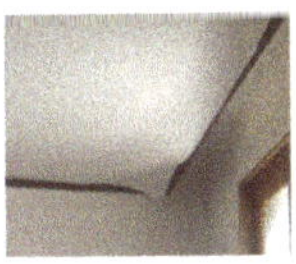 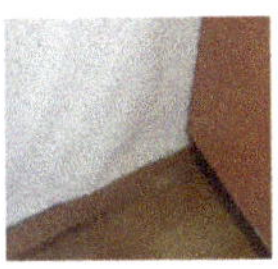	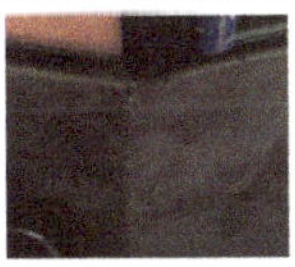 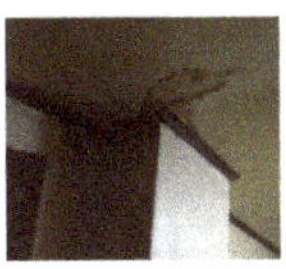	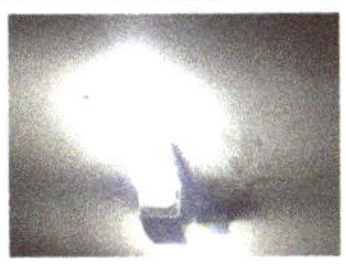 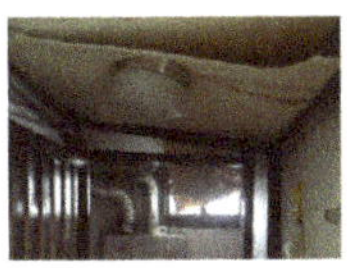	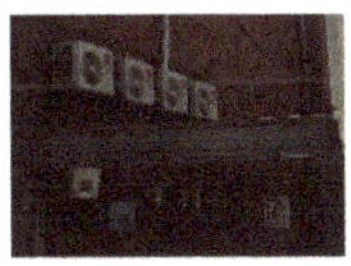 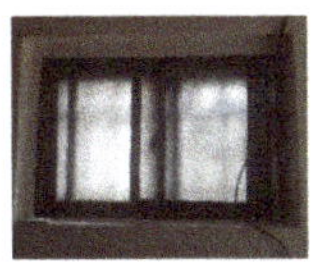
(Above/Below): five households	(Above): two households (Below): seven households	(Above/Below): three households	(Above): three households (Below): two households

3.2. Selection and Status of Target Sites for GR Effect Analysis

According to the site survey, the low-income elderly households were living on the lower floors of single-family or multi-family houses with monthly rent or that they owned themselves. Among them, residents of multi-family houses that were paying monthly rent requested relocation to a public rental apartment or housing cost support rather than facility improvement. By contrast, residents in their own aged house wanted subsidies for facility improvement or full facility improvement. In the case of owned single-family households, there was a problem in new construction and sale because the site area was small (less than 33 m^2) and it was located in a dead-end alley. To solve this problem, it may be an option to proceed with the remodeling by consulting with the neighbor of the adjacent site, but this is not easy.

Although all households surveyed require housing stability by facility improvement, by considering problems such as (1) self-ownership or rental, (2) relocation of residential households after facility remodeling, and (3) the scope of facility remodeling, the houses with clear land and architectural boundaries among self-owned houses were selected as the target buildings for GR analysis of aged houses. From the households surveyed, three households were single-family houses, and among them, No. 4 and 5 were candidates. No. 4, which has a relatively clear boundary of the building area on the site, was selected for analysis. Even though No. 4 was renewed by some facility improvements such as a window renewal and interior-exterior finishing renewal project in July 2019, there were no improvements in building energy, indoor air quality, or safety, except for windows. Table 4 presents the status of No. 4 after facility improvement.

Table 4. Cases of the survey on defects of old houses.

Land and Plan of an Old House	Exterior/Interior Improvement in Finishes		Improvement of Window
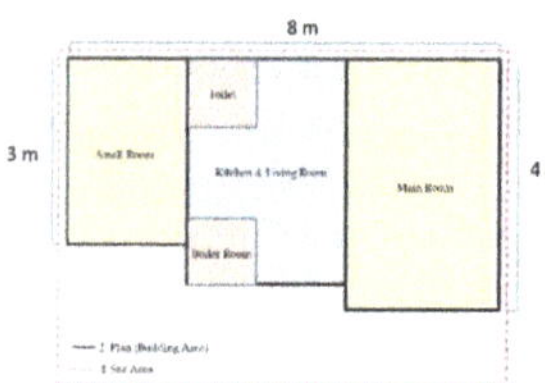	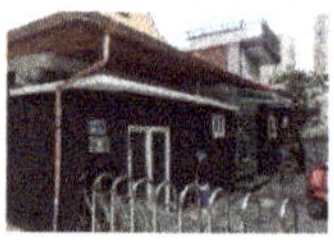 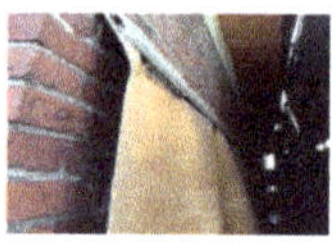	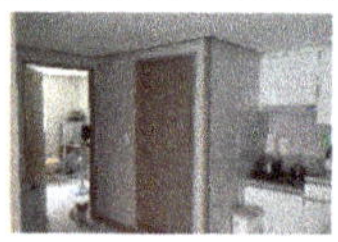 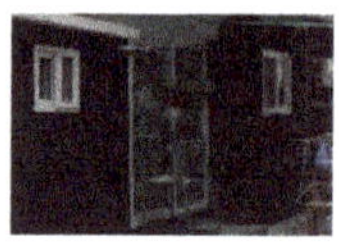	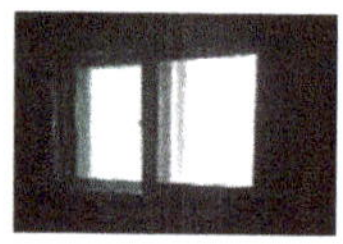 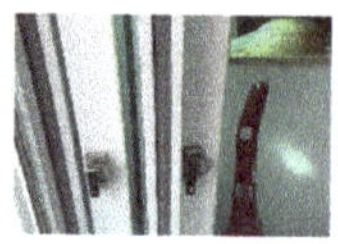
Formation of house plan via actual measurement at site	(Above): Front view (Below): Back view Paint finish (only for main entrance)	(Above): Indoor view (Below): Main gate	PVC(Polyvinyl Chloride) Double window

3.3. GR Scope and Planning Direction of the Selected Building

Considering the utilization of the analysis results and the wide-ranging maintenance statuses of aged houses, the site and building type were based on the No. 4 case, but the aging performance of each item was analyzed as the aging performance with the highest ratio among the aging status survey results of the nine households. Table 5 (1) summarizes the average aging performance in terms of the building envelope (insulation, windows, doors), facility performance, indoor air quality, and user (elderly household) safety of the investigated buildings, (2) summarizes the problems in energy, air quality, and safety according to the aging performance of each item, and (3) explains the scope of improvement and method of remodeling for each item in terms of building envelope performance, interior and exterior finishing, facility performance, indoor air quality, and safety.

Table 5. Energy performance of aged houses, health problems of residents, and improvement directions according to the site survey.

Items	Location	(1) Average Performance Result from the Survey	(2) Health Issues of Occupants and Energy Consumption of Houses According to Respective Performances of Houses	(3) Targets for Improvement
Performance of building envelope	Insulation	None	Deteriorated indoor heating environment Caused dewing and appearance of mold Caused energy loss Caused health problems of aged people in winter	Exterior insulation (reinforcement of heat bridging performance): To improve indoor dewing and heating environment Works for improved air tightness of windows and window frames: to improve energy consumption Performance and heating environment Planning of windbreaker structure for frequently used doors
	Windows	Wood 3 mm and AL 3 mm		
	Air tightness	Frames of window became obsolete		
	Doors	No windbreak structure		
Interior and exterior finishing	Interior	Wallpaper	Mold appearing between wallpaper and furniture	Replacement with wallpaper with ecofriendly materials
	Exterior	Face brick and paint	Poor appearance of blushing and cracks	Improvement of finishing according to improved insulation
Equipment performance	Cooling	Air conditioner exclusively used for cooling	Caused by the consumption of more energy than actually required due to deteriorated performance of building	Replace with equipment of efficient energy consumption (Class I) to improve the performance of energy consumption
	Heating	Gas boiler		
	hot water supply			
Indoor air quality	Ventilation	None	Poorly ventilated fumes from cooking and micro-particulates that caused health problems in bronchus of mold	Installation of ventilator needs to be obligatory for households with aged people
Safety	Others	None	Convenience in use of toilet for aged people; handrails or emergency bells are not installed	Space planning without step Installation of handrails in toilet and emergency bells

4. Economic Analysis Considering Social Cost

4.1. Analytical Procedures and Methods

Regarding the analysis procedure and method, first, the energies before and after GR were analyzed by considering the spatial characteristics of the target building and the aging performances of the nine aged houses. The analysis tool was ECO-2, a Korean building energy efficiency rating program. For weather data of ECO-2, standard profiles were brought in from ECO-2 central server to allow selection of average data for 66 regions in Korea. Essentially, Korea has distinct climatic characteristics of four seasons: spring, summer, fall, and winter. Weather data of ECO-2 provide monthly average values calculated based on TMY (typical meteorological year data) weather data, which provides monthly average ambient temperature and monthly average solar intensity according to the incident angle by bearing. The target building of this study was located in Seoul. Accordingly, in ECO-2, Seoul was set out of 66 areas in Korea and analysis was conducted.

For the existing model (=building to be analyzed) and the improved model (=GR plan), the energy consumption was analyzed by preparing an improvement plan based on the aging performance and the renewal direction for each of items (1) and (3) in Figure 3 and Table 5. Second, the total construction cost was calculated per each item by dividing the aging performance (demolition cost, interior and exterior finishing, rest room renewal, etc.), health, safety, and energy performance of the improved model. Third, by comparing the energy and carbon generation of the existing model to the improved model in terms of ECO-2 analysis, the annual energy savings, greenhouse gas (CO_2) savings, and air pollutant savings were derived, then converted into costs to calculate the annual benefits. Next, by calculating the benefits ((1) energy saving cost (resident benefit—1), (2) greenhouse gas reduction (social cost—1) and (3) air pollutant reduction (social cost—2)) of the improved model compared to the total construction cost (cost), the economic feasibility was analyzed using the net present value method (NPV). Based on this, in the discussion section of Section 5, a GR support policy concept for low-income elderly households was proposed by mixing the 'housing stability policy for low-income elderly people' and the 'urban energy transition policy' of Korea Government. Figure 4 depicts a schematic diagram of the analysis procedure detailing each step and method of the target building (existing model).

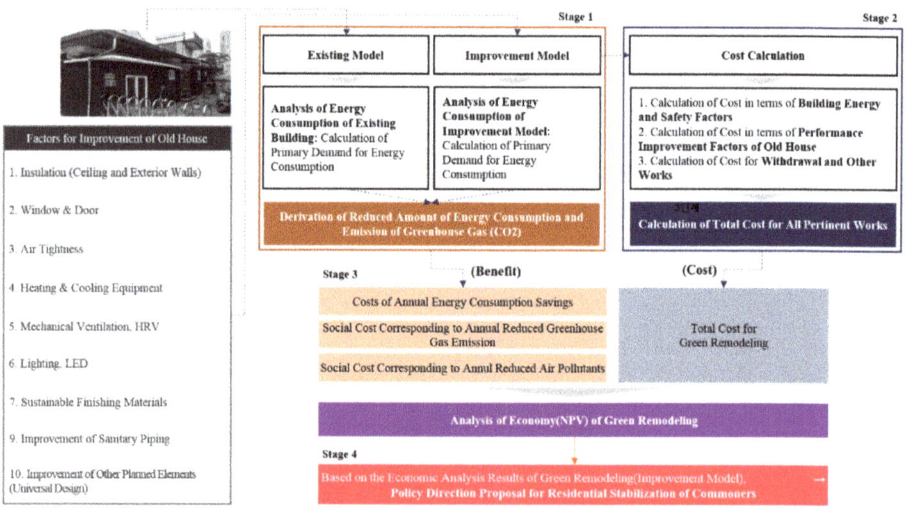

Figure 4. Problems considering elderly households in aged houses and improvement directions for each GR item.

4.2. Primary Energy Consumption Analysis for Existing and Improved Models

4.2.1. Primary Energy Consumption Analysis for Existing Model

As mentioned above, the primary energy consumption analysis for the existing model was conducted based on the architectural spatial properties (actual area and height) of the No. 4 case and the average aging performances of the nine aged houses. Tables 6 and 7 lists the key input values for energy performance analysis of the existing model as well as the reference notices and the energy performance result value output from ECO-2.

4.2.2. Improved Model Analysis

The energy performance of the improved model was set at the recommended level of the GR technical reference notices [41], and external insulation (adding 100 mm of mineral wool and dry finish) was applied for insulation remodeling in consideration of thermal bridge improvement and fire safety. Further, to improve the airtight performance, by applying a first-grade window set with airtight performance as well as applying airtight tape to the window frame (wall joint) and hole portions of the ventilation device, the building's airtight performance was analyzed by assuming grade 3 (based on ACH 50). Tables 8 and 9 shows the key input value for ECO-2 and the analysis results for the improved model.

4.2.3. Calculation of Annual Energy and Greenhouse Gas Reduction from the Energy Analysis Results

ECO-2 (Energy) Result Analysis: Comparison before to after GR

The heating energy requirement of the existing model was 173.9 kWh/m^2·y, and the heating energy requirement of the improved model was 60.4 kWh/m^2·y, which represents a reduction to 1/3 of the original value. In terms of cooling, it slightly increased from 31.4 kWh/m^2·y to 34.4 kWh/m^2·y. This is an analysis result that is generally acquired in residential buildings with improved insulation, as the heat exchange of the indoor heat generating load becomes difficult as the building's thermal insulation and airtight performance are improved.

The primary energy consumption of the existing model was the lowest grade (grade 7) for the building energy efficiency of 413.1 kWh/m^2·y, which indicated very poor energy performance. The primary energy consumption of the improved model was slightly lower than grade 3 for the building energy efficiency of 246.2 kWh/m^2·y, which was similar to the level of a newly constructed building. Improvements could be made to a higher level than this. However, as the level of improvement was judged to be appropriate in consideration of the construction cost, the current legal standards, and recommended standards of the Ministry of Land, Infrastructure and Transport, no additional energy performance improvement was conducted.

Comparison of Annual Energy Consumption and CO_2 Emission

The annual energy consumption and CO_2 emission were calculated based on ECO-2 analysis, and the energy consumption was calculated by converting it into the used amount of energy. It is necessary to understand the terms of primary energy consumption and the energy consumption. Energy consumption refers to the actual amount of energy required for equipment (cooling and heating equipment, hot water supply, ventilation and lighting equipment). The value calculated by converting the energy consumption into the primary energy is the primary energy consumption (= energy consumption × primary energy conversion factor for each source). Tables 10 and 11 present comparisons of the annual energy consumption and CO_2 emission for the existing model and the improved model, respectively.

Table 6. Key input values for 'ECO-2'—Existing model.

Items	Location	Investigation Results	Performance Corresponding to Survey Results	Sources and Assumptions
Usage	Usage profile	Residential space	-	Refer to [Attached Table 2] of the "Guidelines for Certification of the Class of Energy Consumption Efficiency of Buildings" [42]
Performance of building envelope	Exterior wall	Brick	0.611 ($W/m^2{\cdot}K$)	Calculation of Thermal Transmittance: 1.0 B + EPS(Expanded Polystyrene) 50 mm + 0.5 B
	Ceiling	Shed roof	0.631 ($W/m^2{\cdot}K$)	Calculation of Thermal Transmittance: Finishing + EPS(Expanded Polystyrene) 50 mm + Wood
	Windows	Wood 3 mm and AL 3 mm	4.0 ($W/m^2{\cdot}K$)	Refer to [Attached Table 4] of the "Design Standards to Save the Energy Consumption in Buildings" [43]
	Doors	Ordinary door (of no windbreak structure)	2.70 ($W/m^2{\cdot}K$)	
	Air tightness	Obsolete window frames	Six times (ACH50)	Educational Materials Prepared for the Program to Determine the Class of Energy Consumption Efficiency (In ECO-2, a domestic building energy evaluation program, for air tightness of residential buildings, ACH50 6.0 times is to be applied in the preliminary certification. Field measurement result is to be applied in the main certification. For this building, the preliminary certification standard was applied.)
Equipment performance	Cooling	PAC for exclusive cooling	(Cooling Capacity) 2.3 kW (Power Consumption) 0.67 kW	Performance of air conditioner installed at Household #4
	Heating Domestic hot water (DHW)	Gas boiler	(Heating Output) 24.4 kW (Thermal Efficiency) 83.4%	Performance of gas boiler for heating and hot water supply installed at the Household #4

Table 7. 'ECO-2' results of analysis—Existing model.

Category	Heating	Cooling	DHW	Lighting	Ventilation	Total
Energy Demand ($kWh/m^2{\cdot}y$)	173.9	31.9	30.7	28.0	0	264.4
Energy Consumption ($kWh/m^2{\cdot}y$)	379.5	8.3	36.8	28.0	0	452.6
Primary Energy Consumption ($kWh/m^2{\cdot}y$)	425.6	22.9	40.6	76.9	0	566.0
CO_2 Emission ($kgCO_2$)	78.0	3.9	7.5	13.1	0	102.5
Primary Energy Consumption ($kWh/m^2{\cdot}y$) for class	286.3	22.9	26.9	76.9	0	413.0

Table 8. Key input values for 'ECO-2'—Improved model.

Items	Location	Performance Improvement of Model	Details of Performance Improvement with Applied Materials	Remarks
Usage	Usage profile	Residential space	-	Equal to Table 8
Performance of building envelope	Insulation of exterior wall	0.23 (W/m²·K)	Added with 100 mm of mineral wool (Dryvit)	Exterior insulation: minimization of costs for finishing and works against fire occurrence
	Insulation of floor	-	Added with the specially extruded heating plate (70 mm)	Preservation of heating energy and absorptivity of insulators were taken into account
	Insulation of ceiling	0.19 (W/m²·K)	Added with 100 mm of rigid urethane foam	Application of inner insulation works by taking into account the Existing Framework
	Windows	1.41 (W/m²·K)	PVC(Polyvinyl Chloride) and low-e double glazing duplicated window	Application of PVC(Polyvinyl Chloride) by taking into account the insulation and pertinent cost
	Doors	1.7 (W/m²·K)	Insulated aluminum entrance door	Application of AL by taking into account of insulation and durability of entrance door
	Air tightness	Three times (ACH50)	Application of Airtight Tape to Windows and Parts joining with Doors	Materials for "air tightness" are applied to installation works for window frame and ventilator for three times (ACH50), the phrase of air tightness of ACH50 3.0 times that is generally applied after replacing windows in Korea is to be applied [10,44]
Equipment performance	Cooling	Replaced	(Capacity) 3.2 kW, (Power Consumption) 0.96 kW	A Product of Class I of the Energy Consumption Efficiency
	Heating / Hot water supply	Replaced	(Capacity) 13,000 Kcal, (Efficiency) 86.3%	A Product of Class I of the Energy Consumption Efficiency
	Ventilation	Additional equipment	(Capacity) 90 m²/h, (Efficiency) Heating 71%, Cooling 56%	A Product Certified as the Equipment of High-efficiency in Energy Consumption

Table 9. 'ECO-2' results of analysis—Improved model.

Category	Heating	Cooling	DHW	Lighting	Ventilation	Total
Energy Demand (kWh/m^2·y)	60.4	34.4	30.7	19.1	0	144.5
Energy Consumption (kWh/m^2·y)	172.1	9.2	35.6	19.1	3.1	239.2
Primary Energy Consumption (kWh/m^2·y)	196.0	25.4	39.3	52.5	8.6	321.9
CO_2 Emission (kgCO_2)	35.8	4.3	7.2	9.0	1.5	57.8
Primary Energy Consumption (kWh/m^2·y) for class	133.5	25.4	26.1	52.5	8.6	246.2

Table 10. Comparison of annual energy consumption and savings.

Items	Annual Energy Consumption per Area	Area of Use	Annual Energy Consumption
Existing Model	452.6 kWh/m^2·y	28 m^2	12,672.8 kWh/y
Improvement Model	239.2 kWh/m^2·y	28 m^2	6697.6 kWh/y
Amount of Saving	-	-	5975.2 kWh/y
Rate of Saving (%)			47.2%

Table 11. Comparison of annual CO_2 emission.

Items	Annual CO_2 Emission per Area	Area of Use	Annual CO_2 Emission
Existing Model	106.3 kgCO_2/m^2·y	28 m^2	2976.4 kgCO_2/y
Improvement Model	57.8 kgCO_2/m^2·y	28 m^2	1618.4 kgCO_2/y
Amount of Saving	-	-	1358 kgCO_2/y
Rate of Saving (%)			45.7%

The energy consumption and CO_2 emission results in Tables 10 and 11 may have varied depending on the usage profile of ECO-2 (Regulations on Operation of Energy Efficiency Rating in Buildings, Annex 2) [42] and the actual building usage time and pattern, equipment efficiency, etc. However, ECO-2 is currently the only officially approved building energy performance evaluation tool in Korea, and it is generally used to estimate building energy performance and energy usage in the building planning stage and related research fields.

4.3. Calculation of Total Construction Cost (Cost) and Annual Benefit (Benefit) for Economic Analysis

4.3.1. Calculation of Total Construction Cost (Cost)

The calculation of the total construction cost of the improved model was entrusted to a construction cost expert. For the energy performance improvement, the performance level satisfying the "recommendation" of the GR technical reference [41] was applied. The mechanical equipment, the total heat exchange ventilation system (health improvement), and safety were separately quoted and applied. In addition, the aging performance improvement cost is the construction cost calculated based on the performance applied to a general house. The total construction cost came to about 20,000 USD; the construction cost per area is 714.2 USD/m^2. Considering that the new construction cost of an aged facility in Korea is 2100 USD/m^2 [45], it is possible to improve the energy performance of aged houses to the level of new constructions with a construction cost of about 33% compared to the cost of new construction.

Further, in the process of calculating the construction cost, it can be recognized that the energy performance and aging performance improvement should be carried out simultaneously instead of separately, while including the replacement of interior finishing (aging performance improvement) for window construction (energy performance improvement), and including the replacement of floor finishing for the improvement of floor heating, etc. This shows that the efficiency is high when the energy performance policy for aged houses and the housing stability policy for the people are implemented as a combined policy rather than as separate policies. Details of the total construction cost of the improved model are shown in Table 12 below.

Table 12. Calculation of construction cost for improved model.

No.	Location	Items	Area	Unit	Unit Cost (USD)	Total Cost (USD)	Remarks
1	Removal works	Interior removal, Waste disposal, Cleaning	28	m^2	35	980	Performance improvement of old house
2	Floor works	Water proofing, Panel heating, Specially extruded heating plate (70 mm)	27	m^2	45	1215	Improvement of energy consumption
3		Replacement of papered floor	28	m^2	25	700	Performance improvement of old house
4		Mop board (floor)	31	m	2.5	77.5	
5	Indoor walls	Finishing and papering of indoor walls	77	m^2	10,000	770	
6	Ceiling	Installation of wooden ceiling	27	m^2	15	405	
7		Gypsum boarding	27	m^2	7	189	
8		Papering	27	m^2	7	189	
9		Molding	35	m	4	140	
10		Ceiling insulation (rigid urethane foam 100 mm)	28	m^2	22	616	Performance improvement in energy consumption
11	Toilet	Replacement of tiles, Caulking, Water proofing	10	m^2	50	490	Performance improvement of old house
12		Toilet ceiling	2	m^2	60	120	
13		Washstand	1	ea	200	200	
14		Toilet bowl	1	ea	300	300	
15		Bath (shower) taps	1	ea	100	100	
16		Closet in toilet (for towels) including mirror	1	ea	300	300	
17		Hangers in toilet (towels and toilet papers)	1	ea	70	70	
18	Furniture	Installation of kitchen sink including taps	1	set	700	700	
19		Shoe closet	1	set	250	250	

Table 12. *Cont.*

No.	Location	Items	Area	Unit	Unit Cost (USD)	Total Cost (USD)	Remarks
20	Windows works	Replacement of inside doors	4	ea	250	1000	
21		Replacement of windows (PL window), Cracks	2	ea	350	700	Performance improvement in energy consumption
22		Ironware of windows for crime prevention	2	ea	150	300	
23		Replacement of entrance door and hardware	1	ea	550	550	
24	Miscellaneous works	Miscellaneous ironware (curtain box, floor frame)	1	sum	150	150	
25	Exterior works	Dryvit 100 mm (exterior wall)	72	m^2	70	5040	
26	Electrical works	Replacement of lighting (LED) of ceiling	3	ea	150	450	
27		Switches, socket outlets	1	sum	250	250	
28	Equipment	Installation of boiler and flue (Model: PRO135KS, N00)	1	sum	1000	1000	
29		Air conditioner on wall Attachment type (Model: SQ08S9JWAS, L00)	1	ea	1090	1090	
30		Total heat exchanging ventilator (Model: THE-80, L00)	1	ea	600	600	Health promotion (respiratory diseases, etc.)
31	Safety works	Emergency bells (living room 1, toilet 1) and in association with mobile phone	1	ea	380	380	Improvement in safety
32		Guide rails in toilet and living room	10	m	15	150	
33	Others	Other maintenance cost	1	sum	500	500	-
34	Overhead costs	Overhead cost for construction management	5	days	200	1000	
Sum of costs for works of improvement performance in health, safety and energy consumption (USD)					12,491		(59%)
		Sum of costs of works for performance improvement of old facilities (USD)			8,490		(41%)
		Total cost for all pertinent works (USD)			20,981		(100%)

4.3.2. Annual Benefit Calculation

Generally, social cost refers to the cost born from the activities of producers on the public and society as a whole. Social cost may include the external costs as a basic factor, and it may include or exclude private costs depending on the particular definition [46]. External costs are the costs incurred in removing public harms such as soot, odor, and noise. The external costs are not internalized by producers, but they are very important from a social point of view. As environmental problems grow, the importance of the external cost on social costs increases.

The social cost concept used in this study focused on external costs while excluding the private costs incurred from the generation of electricity. The external costs in terms of power generation can occur regardless of the size of the project, such as carbon emission reduction, air pollutant emission reduction, avoidance of distribution line construction cost, and avoidance of measuring cost [47]. However, it was excluded due to the limitation of social cost data, such as the avoidances of the distribution line construction cost and the measuring cost. Accordingly, the benefits of economic analysis considering the social cost in this study were set with the effects from (1) energy consumption cost reduction, (2) carbon emission reduction, and (3) air pollutant emission reduction.

Benefit from Annual Energy Saving

The annual energy cost savings were calculated by converting the annual energy consumption savings in Table 10 into costs. The annual electricity rate per kWh was calculated by applying 'the electricity rates for house in Korea (low voltage)' + '0.093 USD per kWh of electricity rate for the section below 300 kWh'. The calculation method is the same as that shown in Equation (1).

$$\text{Annual Energy Saving (USD/y)} = (\text{Energy Consumption } [(\text{kWh}/(\text{m}^2{\cdot}\text{y})) \times \text{Area } (\text{m}^2)] \times \text{Electricity Rate (USD/kWh)} \quad (1)$$

Benefit from Annual Carbon Emission Reduction

The benefits of reducing carbon emissions are the social benefits resulting from the reduced consumption of electricity and energy.

The social benefits of the annual carbon emission (CO_2) reduction were calculated by converting the annual carbon savings in Table 11 into costs. To convert carbon emission reduction into cost, it was calculated by applying the average annual price of carbon credits in 2019 on the Korea Exchange (KAU 19), 22.8 USD per tCO_2. The calculation method is the same as that shown in Equation (2) [47].

$$\text{Benefit of annual carbon emission reduction (USD/y)} = (\text{Annual carbon emission reduction amount } [(\text{tCO}_2/(\text{m}^2{\cdot}\text{y})) \times \text{Area } (\text{m}^2)] \times \text{Price of carbon credits } (\text{USD/tCO}_2) \quad (2)$$

Benefit from Annual Air Pollutant Material Reduction

The benefit of air pollutant material reduction is also a social benefit generated by the reduced consumption of electricity and energy. The calculation method is the same as that shown in Equation (3) [22]. The social cost of air pollutants was referred to as the social cost per MWh for nitrogen oxide, sulfur oxide, and dust by air pollutants in the preliminary feasibility report of "Smart Grid Expansion Project (2015)" of KDI. The benefit of nitrogen oxide was applied with 6.92 USD/MWh, that of sulfur oxide was applied with 3.97 USD/MWh, and that of dust was applied with 0.71 USD/MWh [47]. Table 13 provides the results of calculating the annual air pollutant reduction benefits according to the annual electricity savings.

$$\text{Annual air pollutant reduction benefit (USD/y)} = [(\text{Annual electricity savings (kWh/(m}^2\cdot\text{y))} \times \text{Area (m}^2)] \times \sum[(\text{Social cost of air pollutant (USD/kWh)}] \tag{3}$$

Table 13. Social cost according to the air pollutant reduction from the electricity saving.

Contents			Remarks
Annual amount of reduced energy consumption (MWh)		5975.2	Table 8 Results of analysis
Social cost corresponding to reduced emission of air pollutants	Nitrogen Oxides (USD/MWh)	6.92	[47]
	Sulfur Oxides (USD/MWh)	3.97	
	Dust (USD/MWh)	0.71	
Total benefit corresponding to annual amount of reduction of air pollutants (USD)		69.29	-

Table 14 shows the calculation of the total cost and benefit for economic analysis.

Table 14. Comparison of annual energy consumption and savings.

Items	Total Cost (USD)	Annual Amount of Total Benefit (USD)		
		Cost Corresponding to Reduced Annual Consumption of Energy	Social Cost Corresponding to Reduced Annual CO_2 Emission	Social Cost Corresponding to Reduced Emission of Air Pollutants
Total construction cost (Cost)	20,981.50	-	-	-
Annual amount of reduction cost (Benefit)		557.49	31.99	69.29

4.4. *Economic Analysis Considering Social Cost*

4.4.1. Economic Analysis Criteria

For economic analysis, the net present value (NPV) method was applied instead of the commonly used CBA (cost–benefit analysis). This was performed because the present value of future accrued benefits can be provided, and this can be used for other analyses in consideration of the analyzed net present value [24]. In addition, for the economic analysis criteria for public policies and buildings, the revision and supplementary studies of the general guidelines for conducting preliminary feasibility studies for public corporations and quasi-governmental institutions of the Korea Development Institute (KDI) were conducted while referring to [23]. The social discount rate was calculated as 4.5%, and the analysis period was set to 30 years, as was the case for building. The calculation method is the same as that shown in Equation (4). As a result of the analysis, when the net present value is greater than "0", it is judged to be economical. Here, Bt refers to the benefit of 't' period, Ct refers to the cost of 't' period, r refers to the social discount rate (interest rate), and t refers to the number of years of use.

$$\text{Net Present Value(NPV)} = \sum_{t=0}^{n} \frac{Bt}{(1+r)^t} - \sum_{t=0}^{n} \frac{Ct}{(1+r)^t} \tag{4}$$

4.4.2. Economic Analysis Result

As the result of the GR economic analysis of the aged house, the net present value was found to be "−10,267.15 USD (49.7%)", indicating that it is not economical, despite the effects of carbon reduction and air pollutant reduction applied. The amount of government support for the GR of low-income elderly households is not the total construction cost of "20,981.50 USD (100%)", but it may instead be estimated to be "10,267.15 USD (49.7%)" corresponding to the amount of support excluding residents net benefits (annual energy consumption reduction cost) and the social benefits from carbon and air pollutant reduction (see Table 15).

Table 15. Economic analysis result (net present value, NPV).

NPV	Total Cost (USD)	Total Benefit for Period of Operation (USD)		
		Cost Corresponding to Reduced Consumption of Energy (A)	Social Cost Corresponding to Reduced CO_2 Emission (B)	Social Cost Corresponding to Reduced Emission of Air Pollutants (C)
−10,267.15 (49% of Total Cost)	20,981.50 (100%)	9080.83 (43.2%)	504.85 (2.4%)	1128.67 (5.3%)
		10,714.35 (Sum of Benefit A, B, C; 51% of Total Cost)		

5. Discussion

According to the analysis results, among the total construction cost of GR, which has the effect of improving the health of residents of aged houses and reducing greenhouse emission, the ratio of construction cost for health, safety, and energy saving was 59%, and the ratio of construction cost for improving aging performance was 41%, as presented in Table 12.

From the 59% of health, safety, and energy saving construction cost, the energy saving cost incurred during the operation period is 43.2%, which is directly returned to the resident as a benefit generated while the resident continues to live in the property after GR. From the remaining 15.8%, 7.7% (2.4% + 5.3%) can be offset by the social benefits stemming from the carbon and air pollutant reduction effect according to the reduction in electricity consumption. That is, 15.8% of the actual cost is supported by the government for health, safety, and energy saving construction costs, but 7.7% is offset by the environmental improvement effect (effect of reducing carbon and air pollutants), so it can be estimated that only 8.1% would be supported. Seoul, Korea achieved a reduction of 4.7 million TOE of GHG emissions from December 2019 to April 2021 with the One Less Nuclear Power Plant Project, an energy transition policy [48]. Of the project budget, 89% was invested in the installation of new and renewable energy including solar power [49]. However, solar power is mainly installed in existing buildings, so there may be a difference between the installation efficiency of the system and the actual production efficiency due to climate influences such as surrounding buildings, maintenance, and the rainy seasons [50]. In areas with high building density, such as Seoul, there is a limitation to the quantitative expansion of energy conversion that can be achieved by installing solar power, so it is necessary to diversify the energy conversion policies rather than continuously increase the installation of solar power. As of 2021, 10 years have passed since this support policy was started, Seoul Metropolitan Government is still providing subsidies for solar power installation as part of the energy transition policy, which total 8.38 billion USD per year [48]. Some of this subsidy may be changed to support GR policy by linking it with energy conversion policy considering the energy saving effect (reduction of carbon and air pollutants) according to GR. Figure 5 presents the ratio of the energy saving construction cost support amount of GR as part of the energy conversion policy linked with the energy saving effect of GR.

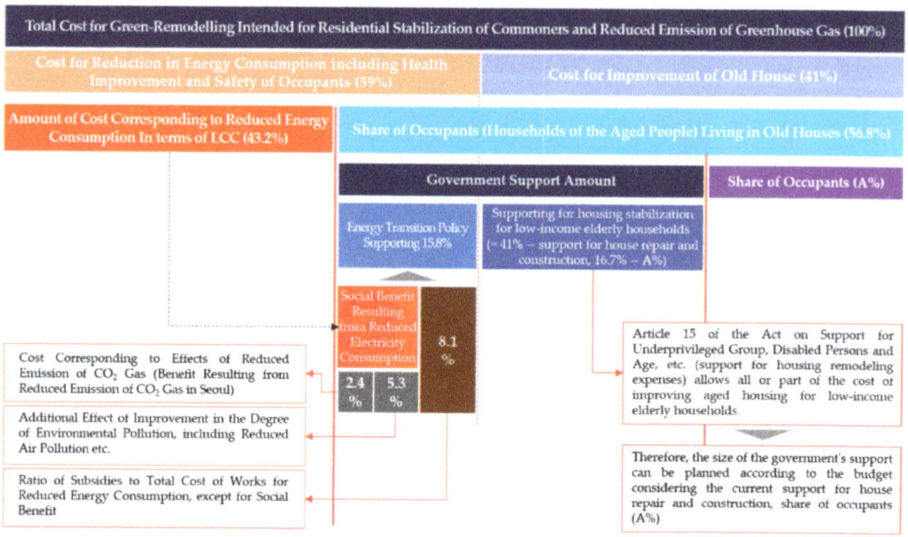

Figure 5. Concept of policy for supporting low-income housing stability from GR linked with the energy transition policy.

From the total construction cost of GR, the construction cost for aging performance improvement (41%) can be supported by the home repair and construction support policies for self-owned or rental households among low-income households with less than 60% of the median income in Seoul [51]. The scope of support is wallpaper, flooring, insulation, sanitary equipment (wash basin/toilet), lighting, etc., the scale of support is up to 1200 USD per household, and the support can reach up to 3200 USD by linking with the energy efficiency improvement project of the Korea Energy Foundation [52]. In addition, the Korean Government is subsidizing all or part of the cost of improving aged housing for low-income elderly households based on Article 15 of the Act on Support for Underprivileged Group, Disabled Persons and Age, etc. (support for housing remodeling expenses) [53]. From this study, the government can determine the amount of support by investigating the maximum payable dead amount to each households share amount (A%), calculating the "subsidy for the housing stabilization policy for elderly households (= 41%−(support for house repair and construction, 16.7%)−(resident share (A%)) by considering the size of the city and county unit budget secured, and establishing a plan to support each year depending on the number of supported households. Therefore, the size of the GR subsidy per households can be adjusted at a maximum of 24.4% of the total construction cost, according to the resident's share (A%).

Accordingly, it is possible to reduce the burden of construction cost for the GR implementation of low-income elderly households, and to increase the effect of improving facilities in aged houses from GR. It is expected that if the government utilizes the direct/indirect effects of GR, then the low-income elderly households can perform GR with support of a 1/4 of the GR construction cost, and the burden of the amount of support can be reduced as a result.

6. Conclusions

In this study, the economic feasibility of GR was analyzed while considering health, safety, and energy by investigating the status and characteristics of aged houses of low-income elderly people in Seoul. From the literature review, problems in the health, safety, and energy aspects of aged houses and architectural improvement directions were derived. Further, the aging status and energy performance of nine single-family and multi-family houses in which low-income elderly people in Seoul reside were investigated. A GR project was planned to improve health, safety, and energy performance by selecting one aged house where GR analysis was possible among the nine aged houses surveyed. Based on this plan, the total construction cost and energy performance before and after GR were analyzed, and the economic analysis was conducted in consideration of the social cost. As a result of the economic analysis of the GR for aged houses in which low-income elderly people live, the net present value was "−10,267.15 USD (49.7%)", indicating that there was no economic effect even though energy saving (9080.83 USD, 43.2%) as well as carbon (504.85 USD, 2.4%) and air pollutant reduction (1128.67 USD, 5.3%) effects were applied.

Nevertheless, from the analysis result, we propose a GR support plan linking with the current energy transition policies and the aged housing support policies for the low-income people, in an attempt to expand the GR of low-income people who are vulnerable to the health and safety of the aged houses and unable to implement GR. Of the total GR construction cost, the energy saving construction cost (59%) can be offset by 15.8% by linking with the energy transition support policy and by the energy consumption reduction amount of residents (43.2%). In addition, of the total construction cost of GR, the construction cost for improvement of aging performance (41%) was partially offset in Seoul by housing repair and construction support, and it was possible to secure a budget according to the Act on Support for Underprivileged Groups, Disabled Persons and Age, etc. of the Korean Government. Therefore, it is possible to calculate the subsidy for the housing stabilization policy for low-income households (=41%−support for house repair and construction, 16.7%−resident share, A%). Accordingly, it would be possible to establish policies at the city or county level to provide support each year according to the total supported households of low-income elderly people and the size of the budget secured.

Finally, in this study, the concept of a support policy was suggested through GR to improve old housing of small-scale low-income elderly people. However, this study has a limitation, in that the analysis was made only for detached houses. It is necessary to increase the reliability of the analysis result by increasing the number of buildings to be analyzed in the future. In addition, to improve housing of the poor, according to various housing types and ages in Korea, more diverse types of measures to improve housing for the general population are needed in the future. In the analysis process, ECO-2 was used to analyze the energy consumption of an aged house, but for the usage profile, the housing type of a general family, which is the default value of the program, is reflected, so it may differ from the housing patterns of elderly households and ordinary people. This value is the default value set by the government. Therefore, it is necessary to modify it or to revise the study so that more practical results can be derived by adding supplementary data.

Author Contributions: J.K., conceptualization, energy audit, energy simulation, green remodeling model development, and cost–benefit analysis, project administration; S.N., writing—original draft preparation, writing—review and editing, methodology, energy audit, proposal for improving green remodeling; D.L., energy audit, data collection and analysis, writing—original draft preparation, writing—review and editing. All authors have read and agreed to the published version of the manuscript.

Funding: This research was supported by a grant (code 22AUDP-C151639-04) from Urban Architecture Research and Development Project Program funded by the Ministry of Land, Infrastructure, and Transport of the Korean government.

Institutional Review Board Statement: Not applicable.

Informed Consent Statement: Informed consent was obtained from all subjects in-volved in the study.

Data Availability Statement: The data presented in this study are available on reasonable request from the corresponding author.

Conflicts of Interest: The authors declare no conflict of interest.

References

1. World Health Organization. WHO Study on Global Ageing and Adult Health. 2018. Available online: http://www.who.int/news-room/facts-in-pictures/detail/ageing (accessed on 30 June 2021).
2. Statistics Korea. 2017 Population and Housing Survey Total Results. 2018. Available online: https://www.kostat.go.kr/portal/korea/kor_nw/1/2/2/index.board?bmode=read&bSeq=&aSeq=370326&pageNo=2&rowNum=10&navCount=10&currPg=&searchInfo=&sTarget=title&sTxt= (accessed on 30 June 2021).
3. Kim, M. A study on architectural approaches corresponding to the Post-COVID era-proposal of prevention of infectious disease through environmental design. *J. Archit. Inst. Korea* **2021**, *37*, 67–75. [CrossRef]
4. Pietrogrande, M.C.; Casari, L.; Demaria, G.; Russo, M. Indoor air quality in domestic environments during periods close to Italian COVID-19 lockdown. *Int. J. Environ. Res. Public Health* **2021**, *18*, 4060. [CrossRef]
5. Mosalam, K.M.; Casquero-Modrego, N. Sunlight permeability of translucent concrete panels as a building envelope. *J. Archit. Eng.* **2018**, *24*, 04018015. [CrossRef]
6. Vandentorren, S.; Bretin, P.; Zeghnoun, A.; Mandereau-Bruno, L.; Croisier, A.; Cochet, C.; Ledrans, M. August 2003 heat wave in France: Risk factors for death of elderly people living at home. *Eur. J. Public Health* **2006**, *16*, 583–591. [CrossRef]
7. Bonnefoy, X. Inadequate housing and health: An overview. *Int. J. Environ. Pollut.* **2007**, *30*, 411–429. [CrossRef]
8. World Health Organization. WHO Environmental Health Inequalities in Europe Health. 2019. Available online: https://apps.who.int/iris/bitstream/handle/10665/325176/9789289054157-eng.pdf?sequence=1&isAllowed=y (accessed on 30 June 2021).
9. Ortiz, J.; Casquero-Modrego, N.; Salom, J. Health and related economic effects of residential energy retrofitting in Spain. *Energy Policy* **2019**, *130*, 375–388. [CrossRef]
10. Kim, J.M.; Nam, S.H. IEQ and energy effect analysis according to empirical full energy efficiency retrofit in South Korea. *Energy Build.* **2021**, *235*, 110629. [CrossRef]
11. Marsik, T.; Johnson, R. Use of simulink to evaluate the air-quality and energy performance of HRV-equipped residences in Fairbanks, Alaska. *Energy Build.* **2008**, *40*, 1605–1613. [CrossRef]
12. International Energy Agency. Perspectives for the Clean Energy Transition-The Critical Role of Buildings. Available online: https://www.iea.org/reports/the-critical-role-of-buildings (accessed on 30 December 2021).
13. Kim, J.; Lim, S. A direction to improve EER (Energy Efficiency Retrofit) policy for residential buildings in South Korea by means of the recurrent EER policy. *Sustain. Cities Soc.* **2021**, *72*, 103049. [CrossRef]
14. Asdrubali, F.; Venanzi, D.; Evangelisti, L.; Guattari, C.; Grazieschi, G.; Matteucci, P.; Roncone, M. An evaluation of the environmental payback times and economic convenience in an energy requalification of a school. *Buildings* **2021**, *11*, 12. [CrossRef]
15. Liu, G.; Li, X.; Tan, Y.; Zhang, G. Building green retrofit in China: Policies, barriers and recommendations. *Energy Policy* **2020**, *139*, 111356. [CrossRef]
16. Liu, Y.; Liu, T.; Ye, S.; Liu, Y. Cost-benefit analysis for Energy Efficiency Retrofit of existing buildings: A case study in China. *J. Clean. Prod.* **2018**, *177*, 493–506. [CrossRef]
17. Zhivov, A.M.; Lohse, R. Deep Energy Retrofit-A Guide for Decision Makers, Annex 61, Subtask D, IEA EBC. 2017. Available online: https://iea-annex61.org/files/results/Subtask_D_Guide_Final_Version_2017-11-06.pdf (accessed on 30 June 2021).
18. Polly, B.; Gestwick, M.; Bianchi, M.; Anderson, R.; Horowitz, S.; Christensen, C.; Judkoff, R. *Method for Determining Optimal Residential Energy Efficiency Retrofit Packages (No. NREL/TP-5500-50572; DOE/GO-102011-3261)*; National Renewable Energy Lab. (NREL): Golden, CO, USA, April 2011. [CrossRef]
19. Leinartas, H.A.; Stephens, B. Optimizing whole house deep energy retrofit packages: A case study of existing chicago-area homes. *Buildings* **2015**, *5*, 323–353. [CrossRef]
20. Streicher, K.N.; Mennel, S.; Chambers, J.; Parra, D.; Patel, M.K. Cost-effectiveness of large-scale deep energy retrofit packages for residential buildings under different economic assessment approaches. *Energy Build.* **2020**, *215*, 109870. [CrossRef]
21. Castellazzi, L.; Zangheri, P.; Paci, D.; Economidou, M.; Labanca, N.; Ribeiro Serrenho, T.; Broc, J. *Assessment of Second Long-Term Renovation Strategies under the Energy Efficiency Directive*; Publications Office of the European Union: Luxembourg, 2019; Volume 10, p. 973672. [CrossRef]
22. Nam, S.; Kim, J.; Lee, D. Current status of aged public buildings and effect analysis prediction of green remodeling in South Korea. *Sustainability* **2021**, *13*, 6649. [CrossRef]
23. Lee, J.; Jung, D.; Cho, M.; Kim, Y. Revised General Guidelines for Conducting Preliminary Feasibility Studies on Public Enterprises and Quasi-Governmental Institutions (Second Edition). KDI Public Investment Management Center. 2018, p. 247. Available online: https://www.kdi.re.kr/research/subjects_view.jsp?pub_no=15989 (accessed on 30 June 2021).
24. Kim, J.M. Economic analysis of zero energy building in South Korea-focusing on Cost-Benefit analysis considering social cost. *J. Archit. Inst. Korea Struct. Constr.* **2020**, *36*, 147–157. [CrossRef]
25. Rostron, J. Sick building syndrome: A review of causes, consequences and remedies. *J. Retail. Leis. Prop.* **2008**, *7*, 291–303. [CrossRef]
26. Alves, C.; Nunes, T.; Silva, J.; Duarte, M. Comfort parameters and particulate matter (PM10 and PM2.5) in school classrooms and outdoor air. *Aerosol Air Qual. Res.* **2013**, *13*, 1521–1535. [CrossRef]
27. Ścibor, M.; Balcerzak, B.; Galbarczyk, A.; Targosz, N.; Jasienska, G. Are we safe inside? Indoor air quality in relation to outdoor concentration of PM10 and PM2.5 and to characteristics of homes. *Sustain. Cities Soc.* **2019**, *48*, 101537. [CrossRef]

28. Jacobs, D.; Wilson, J.; Tohn, E. Health and home upgrades. *ASHRAE J.* **2017**, *59*, 66–68.
29. Park, S.J.; Kim, M.J. A framework for green remodeling enabling energy efficiency and healthy living for the elderly. *Energies* **2018**, *11*, 2031. [CrossRef]
30. Kwon, Y.P. *Mechanical Facilities for Building*; DAEGA Books: Gyeonggi-do, Korea, 2013; pp. 267–313.
31. Zender-Świercz, E. Review of IAQ in premises equipped with façade–ventilation systems. *Atmosphere* **2021**, *12*, 220. [CrossRef]
32. Sun, Y.; Hou, J.; Cheng, R.; Sheng, Y.; Zhang, X.; Sundell, J. Indoor air quality, ventilation and their associations with sick building syndrome in Chinese homes. *Energy Build.* **2019**, *197*, 112–119. [CrossRef]
33. Breysse, J.; Dixon, S.L.; Jacobs, D.E.; Lopez, J.; Weber, W. Self-reported health outcomes associated with green-renovated public housing among primarily elderly residents. *J. Public Health Manag. Pract.* **2015**, *21*, 355–367. [CrossRef] [PubMed]
34. Ahrentzen, S.; Erickson, J.; Fonseca, E. Thermal and health outcomes of energy efficiency retrofits of homes of older adults. *Indoor Air* **2016**, *26*, 582–593. [CrossRef]
35. Jacobs, D.E.; Breysse, J.; Dixon, S.L.; Aceti, S.; Kawecki, C.; James, M.; Wilson, J. Health and housing outcomes from green renovation of low-income housing in Washington, DC. *J. Environ. Health* **2014**, *76*, 8–17. [PubMed]
36. Breysse, J.; Jacobs, D.E.; Weber, W.; Dixon, S.; Kawecki, C.; Aceti, S.; Lopez, J. Health outcomes and green renovation of affordable housing. *Public Health Rep.* **2011**, *126*, 64–75. [CrossRef] [PubMed]
37. Colton, M.D.; Laurent, J.G.C.; MacNaughton, P.; Kane, J.; Bennett-Fripp, M.; Spengler, J.; Adamkiewicz, G. Health benefits of green public housing: Associations with asthma morbidity and building-related symptoms. *Am. J. Public Health* **2015**, *105*, 2482–2489. [CrossRef] [PubMed]
38. The Seoul Institute. A Study on the Residential Status Survey in Seoul, Seoul Metropolitan City. 2017, pp. 35–51. Available online: https://sca.seoul.go.kr/front/reference/rsReport/view.do?board_sn=456&searchCondition=&searchKeyword=&sBbs_group_code=B09 (accessed on 30 June 2021).
39. Irulegi, O.; Ruiz-Pardo, A.; Serra, A.; Salmerón, J.M.; Vega, R. Retrofit strategies towards net zero energy educational buildings: A case study at the University of the Basque Country. *Energy Build.* **2017**, *144*, 387–400. [CrossRef]
40. Fotopoulou, A.; Semprini, G.; Cattani, E.; Schihin, Y.; Weyer, J.; Gulli, R.; Ferrante, A. Deep renovation in existing residential buildings through façade additions: A case study in a typical residential building of the 70s. *Energy Build.* **2018**, *166*, 258–270. [CrossRef]
41. Ministry of Land, Infrastructure and Transport. *Guidelines for Green Remodeling Planning and Implementation of Urban Regeneration New Deal*; MOLIT: Sejong, Korea, 2018.
42. Korea Energy Agency. Regulations on Operation of Energy Efficiency Rating in Building, Residential Usage Profile. 2016. Available online: http://www.kemco.or.kr/web/kem_home_new/info/news/notice/kem_view.asp?q=19882 (accessed on 30 June 2021).
43. Ministry of Land, Infrastructure and Transport. Energy Saving Design Standards for Buildings, Annex 2, 4. 2018. Available online: https://www.law.go.kr/admRulSc.do?menuId=5&subMenuId=41&tabMenuId=183&query=%EA%B1%B4%EC%B6%95%EB%AC%BC%20%EC%97%90%EB%84%88%EC%A7%80%EC%A0%88%EC%95%BD%EC%84%A4%EA%B3%84%EA%B8%B0%EC%A4%80#liBgcolor0 (accessed on 30 June 2021).
44. Korean Institute of Architectural Sustainable Environment and Building Systems. Building Airtightness Criteria, 4p. 2013. Available online: http://www.kiaebs.org/servlet/Aik_FileDownload?filecode=06&filename=kiaebs157476659.pdf&filename2=01%20KIAEBS%20C-1(2013)%20%B0%C7%C3%E0%B9%B0%C0%C7%20%B1%E2%B9%D0%BC%BA%B4%C9%20%B1%E2%C1%D8.pdf (accessed on 23 December 2021).
45. Public Procurement Service. An Analysis of Construction Cost by Public Building Type in 2017. 2018. Available online: https://www.korea.kr/news/pressReleaseView.do?newsId=156278350 (accessed on 30 June 2021).
46. Shin, D.; Song, Y.M.; Kim, S.A. Social costs estimation to evaluate urban trip activity-An application of student housing and social costs analysis for urban planning. *J. KIBIM* **2016**, *6*, 19–28. [CrossRef]
47. Lee, S.; Lee, H.; Kim, T.; Cho, S. Smart Grid Spread Business, Korea Development Institute Preliminary Feasibility Study Report. 2015, pp. 13–50. Available online: https://www.kdi.re.kr/research/subjects_view.jsp?pub_no=14204 (accessed on 30 June 2021).
48. Seoul Metropolitan City. Performance and Effectiveness of Reducing One Nuclear Power Plant. 2018. Available online: https://news.seoul.go.kr/env/environment/climate-energy/one-less-nuclear-power-plant (accessed on 30 June 2021).
49. Choi, S.; Choi, G. A study on the activation of photovoltaic power generation for energy conversion: Focusing on seoul metropolitan government. *J. Korean Urban Manag. Assoc.* **2016**, *29*, 275–295.
50. Kim, H.; Jung, H. A study on power generation efficiency through the post evaluation of photovoltaic panels in complex type buildings-focused on annual generation performance of S-university. *Korean J. Constr. Eng. Manag.* **2017**, *18*, 11–19. [CrossRef]
51. Seoul Metropolitan City. Seoul Hope House Repair Project. 2019. Available online: https://housing.seoul.go.kr/site/main/content/sh01_070701 (accessed on 30 June 2021).
52. Korea Energy Foundation. Energy Efficiency Improvement Project. 2017. Available online: https://www.koref.or.kr/web/intropage/intropageShow.do?page_id=37840ebcd7004927bbb095d0a1dd58d6 (accessed on 30 June 2021).
53. Ministry of Land, Infrastructure and Transport. Act on the Support for Housing Disadvantaged Persons Including Persons with Disabilities and the Aged, Article 15 (Subsidization for Cost of Remodeling Housing Units). 2019. Available online: https://www.law.go.kr/LSW/lsInfoP.do?lsiSeq=208483&chrClsCd=010203&urlMode=engLsInfoR&viewCls=engLsInfoR#0000 (accessed on 30 June 2021).

buildings

MDPI

Review

Machine Learning Techniques Focusing on the Energy Performance of Buildings: A Dimensions and Methods Analysis

Maria Anastasiadou [1,*], Vítor Santos [1] and Miguel Sales Dias [2]

[1] NOVA Information Management School, Universidade Nova de Lisboa, 1070-312 Lisbon, Portugal; vsantos@novaims.unl.pt
[2] Department of Information Science and Technology, Instituto Universitário de Lisboa (ISCTE-IUL), ISTAR, 1649-026 Lisbon, Portugal; miguel.dias@iscte-iul.pt
* Correspondence: manastasiadou@novaims.unl.pt

Abstract: The problem of energy consumption and the importance of improving existing buildings' energy performance are notorious. This work aims to contribute to this improvement by identifying the latest and most appropriate machine learning or statistical techniques, which analyze this problem by looking at large quantities of building energy performance certification data and other data sources. PRISMA, a well-established systematic literature review and meta-analysis method, was used to detect specific factors that influence the energy performance of buildings, resulting in an analysis of 35 papers published between 2016 and April 2021, creating a baseline for further inquiry. Through this systematic literature review and bibliometric analysis, machine learning and statistical approaches primarily based on building energy certification data were identified and analyzed in two groups: (1) automatic evaluation of buildings' energy performance and, (2) prediction of energy-efficient retrofit measures. The main contribution of our study is a conceptual and theoretical framework applicable in the analysis of the energy performance of buildings with intelligent computational methods. With our framework, the reader can understand which approaches are most used and more appropriate for analyzing the energy performance of different types of buildings, discussing the dimensions that are better used in such approaches.

Keywords: energy performance certificate (EPC); machine learning (ML); energy-efficient retrofitting measures (EERM); energy performance of buildings (EPB); energy efficiency (EE)

Citation: Anastasiadou, M.; Santos, V.; Dias, M.S. Machine Learning Techniques Focusing on the Energy Performance of Buildings: A Dimensions and Methods Analysis. *Buildings* **2022**, *12*, 28. https://doi.org/10.3390/buildings12010028

Academic Editors: Roberto Alonso González-Lezcano, Francesco Nocera and Rosa Giuseppina Caponetto

Received: 3 December 2021
Accepted: 23 December 2021
Published: 31 December 2021

1. Introduction

Considering that buildings account for 40% of the primary energy consumption (EC) in the European Union [1], reducing the EC of buildings has become a necessity. The European Union, considering the increasing urbanization and climate change trends, defined the objective to reduce EC by 32.5% until 2030, from the baseline year of 2007, as a key priority in the EU's strategy and Green deal [2] to increase EE and decrease the energy performance (EP) of existing buildings [2–4]. This goal is aligned with the United Nations' seventh Sustainable Development Goal (SDG): "Ensure access to affordable, reliable, sustainable and modern energy for all" [5].

Buildings are responsible for the second largest portion of the final EC in the European Union [1,6,7], with households on 26.3% and public buildings on 28.8%, just after the transport sector (with 30.9%). Their refurbishment and energy-efficient retrofitting is a priority for many countries to reduce EC and decrease the EP of existing buildings as part of the EU Green deal [2,8]. In the current state of the art, data science and machine learning are available to analyze, predict and improve energy efficiency (EE) in buildings in meaningful ways. Such computer science approaches can be used to forecast and minimize energy consumption, design energy-efficient buildings, define strategies for mitigating impacts on the environment and climate, and predict and propose useful and cost-effective retrofit measures to increase the EE of buildings to provide a comfortable indoor living environment [9,10]. By measuring, monitoring, and improving the EE in buildings, we can reduce the amount of energy consumed while maintaining or even enhancing the quality of services provided by those buildings, a "double the global rate of improvement in EE"—SDG7.8 [5,11].

This paper proposes a conceptual and theoretical framework applicable in the analysis of literature papers that tackle the problem of the EPB with machine learning or statistical methods. In more detail, this work aims to add to the improvement of the EP of existing buildings, one of the core goals of the EU Green deal [2], by identifying and analyzing the latest and most appropriate machine learning or statistical techniques, as a baseline for future research by building a conceptual and theoretical framework based on a systematic literature review using PRISMA guidelines. Our approach helps the researcher find which methods are most used and more appropriate for analyzing the EP of different types of buildings.

Moreover, our framework addresses the dimensions and factors extracted from available data sources such as building energy certification data, EC data, wheatear and climate data, and others. Our proposal will help the community foster innovation on enhanced buildings' energy performance (EP) and predict energy-efficient retrofit measures (EERM).

In this context, our study adopts a well-established systematic literature review (SLR) method, the Preferred Reporting Items for Systematic Reviews and Meta-Analyses (PRISMA [12]), to identify the most relevant literature contributions to the energy performance of buildings (EPB) and the prediction of EERM, using machine learning (ML) or statistical methods. Furthermore, we used a visualization bibliometric tool, VOSviewer [13], to find the most used terms in the literature related to the EPB with machine learning or statistical methods.

Some literature review papers tackle similar problems, mostly related to EC [14–18]. The main innovation and novelty of the study is how we present and group the data, focusing on the building types and addressing the dimensions and methods for each type. We believe that our study will help the community foster innovation on the enhanced EPB and predict energy-efficient retrofit measures. We present and visualize our results using the bibliometric network software tool VOSviewer. This tool allows creating and visualizing bibliometric networks based on text data and keyword co-occurrence, and authors' co-authorship networks of terms. This allows us to visualize and identify the most important terms and authors co-authorship respective relations for quantitative analysis.

Considering the stated intentions of this paper, we raised the following research questions:

- RQ1: What are the most relevant machine learning or statistical approaches that automatically evaluate buildings' EP using EPC data?
- RQ2: What are the most relevant machine learning or statistical approaches for predicting energy-efficient retrofit measures to improve buildings' EP?

The research questions focus on two objectives (1) automatic clustering—classification of the EPC of a building, and (2) prediction of energy-efficient retrofit measures, using ML and EPC data. Additionally, as mentioned, our approach brings a clear contribution to the EU Green deal and SDG7 of the United Nations [5].

Our paper is organized as follows. Section 2 presents the adopted systematic literature review technique (PRISMA) and our overall methodology. Section 3 describes the application of PRISMA and details the collected data from the survey, whereas in Section 4, we present and analyze such results using the visualization and bibliometric tool. Section 5 discusses our findings, aligned with our research questions, while in Section 6, we present our conclusions.

2. Methodology

The SLR analysis was performed by adopting a well-established systematic literature review and meta-analysis method (PRISMA). In our methodology, we combined this method with data visualization techniques, ending up with 4 main phases: (1) data selection, (2) results and analysis: survey results, categorization and dimensions analysis, visualization and bibliometric analysis, (3) discussion, (4) conclusions [19], as depicted in Figure 1.

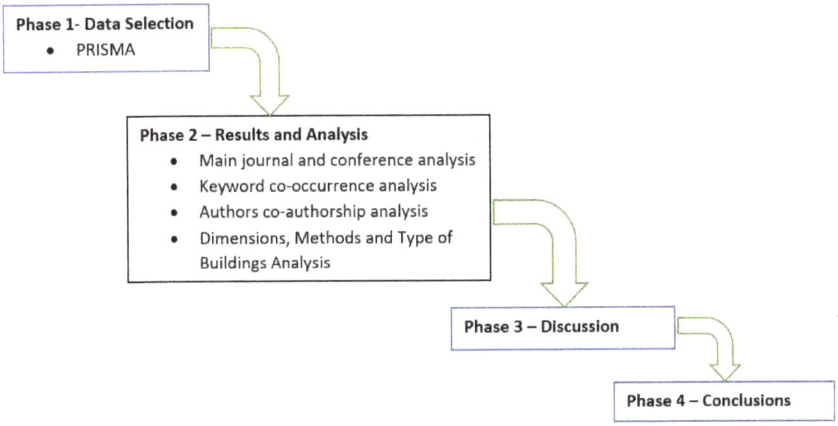

Figure 1. Methodology.

Phase 1—Data Collection: Following PRISMA guidelines [12], we conducted an evidence-based systematic review to select the best basis for reporting systematic reviews. Our adoption of PRISMA follows the literature trend of using such a method as a basis for reporting systematic reviews, especially evaluations of interventions [12]. The PRISMA guidelines consist of a flow diagram and a checklist. The flow diagram of conducting a PRISMA survey has four phases: identification, screening, eligibility, and inclusion, as depicted in Figure 2. The checklist proposes a pre-defined structure for a survey with different sections. In addition, there are precise guidelines to be followed and described in more detail in Section 3 [12]. As mentioned, we focused our analysis on ML or statistical approaches using the public build, residential, and office buildings.

Phase 2—Results and Analysis: In this phase, we present the analysis of our PRISMA results. We analyze the main journals and conferences, the keyword co-occurrence, and the authors' co-authorship. We present and visualize our results using the bibliometric network software tool VOSviewer. This tool allows creating and visualizing bibliometric networks based on text data, particularly keyword co-occurrence and authors' co-authorship networks of terms. This analysis illustrates the relationships and connections between the network's elements (nodes), corresponding to the most used terms, allowing the identification of networks characteristics, such as node and cluster centrality. VOSviewer calculates the node links and weight, demonstrating each node's importance in the network. This allows us to visualize and detect the most important terms and authors' co-authorship individual relations for quantitative analysis. The size of nodes presents the degree of centrality: the larger the node, the more times it is reported in the text data. The thickness of edges presents the number of times two linked nodes are reported, showing their significance; by default, the networks are allocated from the largest to the smallest [13]. With this approach, we could summarize and critically analyze the most used dimensions, clustering and classification techniques, EP retrofitting prediction techniques, and the most used building types in each study. This method allowed us to find, accurately and efficiently, the best literature modeling practices and techniques for achieving enhanced EP.

Phase 3—Discussion: In this phase, we discuss the previous phases' findings by following the research questions. We specifically address the identified knowledge gaps and our study limitations.

Phase 4—Conclusion: We sum up and present the conclusion of our study.

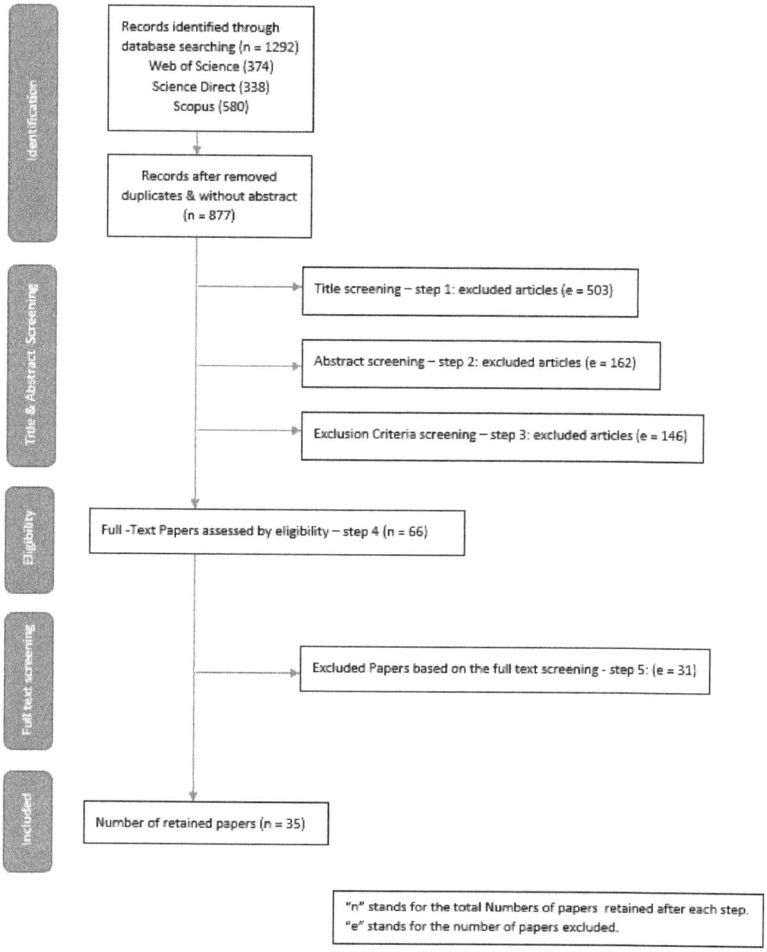

Figure 2. PRISMA Flowchart.

3. Data Collection

3.1. PRISMA Method

By adopting the PRISMA guidelines, the SLR was performed as follows. First, a search process was conducted to detect publications that have in their titles, abstract or keywords the following Boolean expressions:

> *("energy retrofit*" OR "energy performance" OR "energy analysis" AND ("artificial intelligence" OR "artificial neural networks" OR "machine learning" OR "genetic algorithms" OR "classification" OR "clustering analysis") OR "certificat*" OR "hypercube" OR "k-means")*

The literature search was performed in April 2021 using the following data repositories: Science Direct, Web of Science, and Scopus. Using 'OR,' and 'AND' statements, we include all papers published between the periods 1st January 2016–27th of April 2021. The analyzed topics were integrative, including computer science, mathematics, engineering, environmental, and data science. While all sources were used, the analysis indicated that most of the publications from Science Direct were also in Web of Science and Scopus.

The final set of SLR papers for qualitative and quantitative analysis was organized using the Mendeley references manager open-source tool [20]. This step permitted us to extract metadata, remove duplicates, and obtain precise figures on the relative importance of the author of a particular keyword. The obtained metadata were: authors, publication metadata, references, and citations.

3.2. PRISMA Results

The following PRISMA flow diagram presents the SLR data collection process for our quantitative and qualitative analyses (Figure 2). The initial step in this approach identified published papers through a database search, resulting in 1292 publications (Web of Science 374; Science Direct 338; Scopus 580). The inclusion criteria were original research papers written in English and published in Q1–Q2 peer-reviewed journals (based on scimago rank) and related conferences in the said period. We focused only on papers with studies within the EU, given the applicability of EU directives and regulations and building energy certification, which differs for countries outside the EU. Moreover, even within the EU, there is variation in the methods used to identify and assess EC and building energy certification [21]. Additionally, review, position, and reports papers were excluded.

Subsequently, we removed duplicates (e = 415). Then, we performed title and abstract screening. Step 1 excluded all the papers whose title was not relevant to the scope and objectives of this study (e = 503). Step 2 excluded all the papers without an abstract or whose abstract was not relevant to the scope and objectives of this study (e = 162). Finally, step 3 excluded all the papers according to the outlined inclusion and exclusion criteria (e = 146) as mentioned in the previous paragraph. Next, the full texts of the remaining 66 papers were read, assessed, and fitted on the scope of the research. Thirty-one papers were excluded, given that they did not use ML or statistical techniques. Finally, the remaining 35 papers were considered eligible for further analysis. Thirty-three were published in scientific journals, whereas two were published in conference proceedings.

4. Results and Analysis

4.1. Journals and Conferences Analysis

In the study of a total of 33 literature papers, we analyzed 13 journal papers, including from Applied Energy (9), Energy & Buildings (7), Sustainable Cities & Society (4), Energies (3), Energy (2), Sustainability (1), IEEE Transactions on Automation Science & Engineering (1), Renewable & Sustainable Energy Reviews (1), Measurement (1), Croatian Review of Economic, Business & Social Statistics (1), Journal Electronics (1), Energy Policy (1) and Neural Computing & Applications (1). Table 1 shows the summary of the journals with their information, that most journals are Q1-quartile ranked (9), representing 90%, (2) are Q2-quartile-ranked, and the remaining (1) is not yet classified by the quartile-ranked [22], although the quartile rank can change over time.

The five major research areas found in the analysis were energy, engineering, environmental science, mathematics, and social sciences. The 33 selected papers' publishers originate from five countries, with most of them from the United Kingdom (6) and The Netherlands (2), followed by Switzerland (2), the United States of America (1), Croatia (1), and China (1). The top publishers found are Elsevier BV (5), Elsevier Ltd. (4), Taylor and Francis Ltd. (2), MDPI Multidisciplinary Digital Publishing Institute (1), MDPI AG (1), Institute of Electrical and Electronics Engineers Inc (1), Croatian Statistical Association (1), Science Press (1) and Springer London (1).

Table 1. Journals details.

Journals	No.	Publisher	Country	Field Publisher
Applied Energy	9	Elsevier BV	United Kingdom	Energy, Engineering, Environmental Science
Energy and Buildings	7	Elsevier BV	Netherlands	Engineering
Sustainable Cities & Society	4	Elsevier BV	Netherlands	Energy, Engineering, Social Sciences
Energies	3	MDPI Multidisciplinary Digital Publishing Institute	Switzerland	Energy, Engineering, Mathematics
Energy	2	Elsevier Ltd.	United Kingdom	Energy, Engineering, Environmental Science, Mathematics
Sustainability	1	MDPI AG	Switzerland	Energy, Environmental Science, Social Sciences
IEEE Transactions on Automation Science and Engineering	1	Institute of Electrical & Electronics Engineers Inc.	United States	Engineering
Renewable & Sustainable Energy Reviews	1	Elsevier Ltd.	United Kingdom	Energy
Measurement	1	Taylor & Francis Ltd.	United Kingdom	Mathematics, Social Sciences
Croatian Review of Economic, Business & Social Statistics	1	Croatian Statistical Association	Croatian	Statistics
Journal Electronics	1	Science Press	China	Engineering
Energy Policy	1	Elsevier BV	United Kingdom	Energy, Environmental Science
Neural Computing & Applications	1	Springer London	United Kingdom	Computer Science

The conferences found in this study were IEEE International Conference on Internet of Things and Green Computing & Communications and Cyber, Physical & Social Computing and Smart Data (2017), and IOP Conference Series: Earth & Environmental Science (2019). Table 2 presents that the major research areas of the conference are computer and environmental science in the United Kingdom and Indonesia.

Table 2. Conferences details.

Conference	No.	Publisher Country	Field
IEEE International Conference on Internet of Things and Green Computing and Communications & Cyber, Physical and Social Computing and Smart Data (2017)	1	United Kingdom	Computer Science
IOP Conference Series: Earth and Environmental Science (2019)	1	Indonesia	Environmental Science

4.2. *Keyword Co-Occurrence Analysis*

Term co-occurrence analysis was conducted utilizing the mentioned text mining tool for network analysis, VOSviewer. The analysis was conducted utilizing a full counting method, encompassing 143 screened terms, with a minimum threshold of two co-occurrences. Of the total 143, only 21 terms were chosen for the analysis (Table 3).

Table 3. Keywords co-occurrence ranked by the link strength.

Keywords	Occurrence	Total Link Strength
Energy Efficiency	7	10
Building Energy Retrofit	4	8
Machine Learning	4	8
Office Buildings	3	8
Building Energy Performance	5	7
Energy Performance Certificate	5	7
Energyplus	3	7
Multi-Objective Optimization	3	7
Genetic Algorithm	2	6
Sensitivity Analysis	2	6
Artificial Neural Networks	2	5
Building Retrofit	3	5
Cluster Analysis	2	5
Energy Simulation	3	5
Energy Retrofitting	2	4
Energy Savings	2	4
Genetic Algorithm (Nsga-Ii)	2	4
Reference Buildings	2	4
Dell'olmo, Jacopo	2	4
Piscitelli, Marco Savino	2	4
Salata, Ferdinando	2	4
Energy Performance Certificates	2	3
Building Sampling	2	2
Fernández Bandera, C	2	2
Ramos Ruiz, G	2	2
Data Exploration	2	1

Most of the analyzed keywords were related to energy efficiency (EE), building energy retrofit, ML, and building energy performance. The top five found keywords were EE (7 occurrences, 10 total link strength), building energy retrofit (4 occurrences, 8 total link strength), ML (4 occurrences, 8 total link strength), office buildings (3 occurrences, 8 total link strength) and building EP (5 occurrences, 7 total link strength).

In keywords of co-occurrence analysis, four clusters (Figure 3) were found with 21 keywords and 50 links. The biggest nodes of each cluster were identified as EE (blue), building EP and EPC (red), office buildings (green), and energy simulation (yellow).

Focusing on the interrelated network of Figure 3 (21 items, 4 clusters, and 50 links), the energy simulation term (yellow cluster) has a connection only with the term energy efficiency (EE) (blue cluster). The building energy performance term (red cluster) has a connection only with the term EE (blue cluster), and the energy performance certificate (EPC) term (red cluster) has a connection with the terms building retrofit (blue cluster) and energy retrofitting (green cluster). The office buildings term (green cluster) relates to all the clusters, namely with the term's sensitivity analysis (yellow cluster), building energy retrofit and artificial neural networks (ANN) (red cluster), EE, and building retrofit (blue cluster). Finally, the EE term (blue cluster) relates to all the clusters too, namely with the term's energy simulation (yellow cluster), ANN, building energy performance and ML (red cluster), office buildings, and clustering analysis (green cluster).

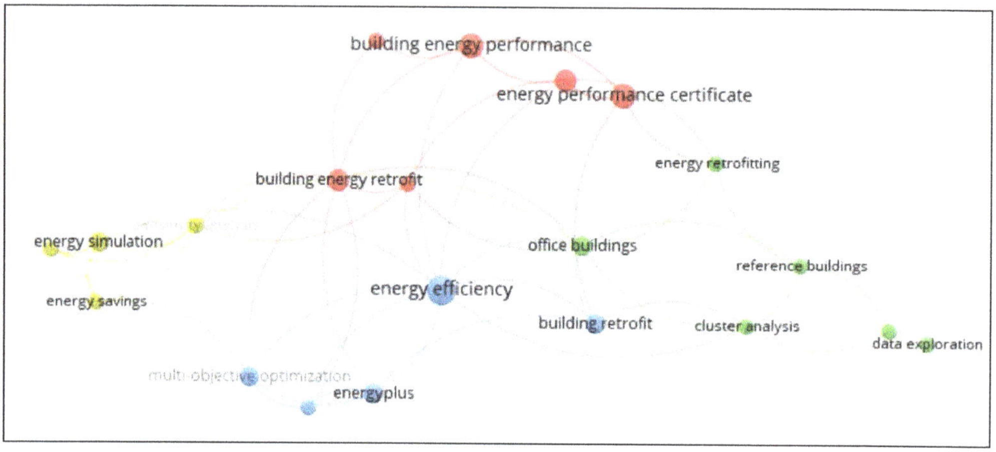

Figure 3. Keyword occurrence network visualization.

An extensive, connected network of keywords and groups of keywords occurs in individual articles, mostly between 2018 and 2020 (Figure 4). The keyword analysis indicated research fields emphasizing ML and EE and found ML techniques, such as clustering analysis, energy simulation, and ANN.

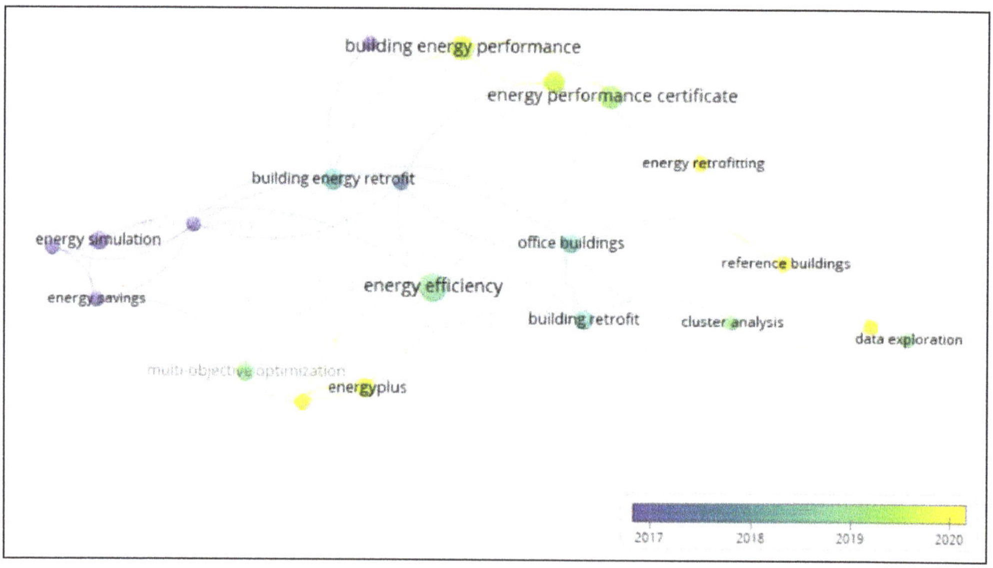

Figure 4. Keyword co-occurrence by year overlay visualization.

4.3. Authors' Co-Authorship Analysis

An authors' occurrence analysis was conducted using the reported text mining tool for network and bibliometric analysis, VOSviewer. The analysis was conducted applying the full count method, choosing 15 maximum number of authors per document and a minimum threshold of 2, resulting in a total of 154 authors meeting this threshold, of which 28 authors were analyzed (Figure 5).

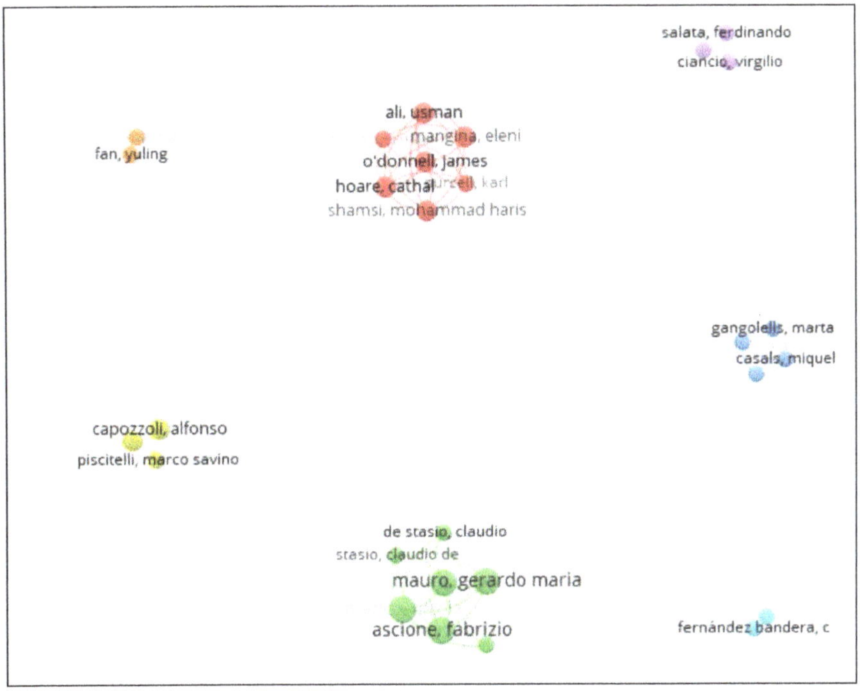

Figure 5. Authors' co-authorship network visualization analysis.

The top 10 found authors were Ascione Fabrizio with a link strength of 21 [23–27], Bianco Nicola with a link strength of 21 [23–27], Mauro Gerardo Maria with a link strength of 21 [23–27], Vanoli Giuseppe Peter with a link strength of 21 [23–27], Ali Usman with a link strength of 16 [28–30], Hoare Cathal with a link strength of 16 [28–30], Mangina Eleni with a link strength of 16 [28–30], O'Donnell James with a link strength of 16 [28–30], Shamsi Mohammad Haris with a link strength of 16 [28–30], and Bohacek Mark with a link strength of 12 [28,29].

In the authors' co-authorship analysis, seven clusters were found with 28 items and 54 links. Cluster 1 (green) relates to the top four author co-authorships ranked by link strength. For De Stasio Claudio with a link strength of 9 [23–25] and De Masi Rosa Francesca with a link strength of 8 [26,27] (Table 4), Cluster 2 (red) has seven items and found Ali Usman and Bohacek Mark. For Hoare Cathal, Mangina Eleni, O'Donnell James, Purcell Karl, Shamsi Mohammad Haris [28–30], Cluster 3 (yellow) has four items and found Casals Miquel, Ferré-Bigorra Jaume, Gangolells Marta, and Macarulla Marcel [31,32]. Cluster 4 (blue) has three items and found Capozzoli Alfonso, Cerquitelli Tania and Piscitelli Marco Savino [33–35], and Cluster 5 (cyan) has three items and found Ciancio Virgilio, Dell'olmo Jacopo and Salata Ferdinando [36,37]. Cluster 6 (purple) has two items: Fernández Bandera C and Ramos Ruiz G [38].

Table 4. Authors' co-authorship ranked by link strength.

Authors	Documents	Total Link Strength
Ascione, Fabrizio	5	21
Bianco, Nicola	5	21
Mauro, Gerardo Maria	5	21
Vanoli, Giuseppe Peter	5	21
Ali, Usman	3	16
Hoare, Cathal	3	16
Mangina, Eleni	3	16
O'Donnell, James	3	16
Shamsi, Mohammad Haris	3	16
Bohacek, Mark	2	12
Purcell, Karl	2	12
De Stasio, Claudio	3	9
De Masi, Rosa Francesca	2	8
Casals, Miquel	2	6
Ferré-Bigorra, Jaume	2	6
Gangolells, Marta	2	6
Macarulla, Marcel	2	6
Capozzoli, Alfonso	3	5
Cerquitelli, Tania	3	5
Ciancio, Virgilio	2	4
Dell'olmo, Jacopo	2	4
Piscitelli, Marco Savino	2	4
Salata, Ferdinando	2	4
Fernández Bandera, C	2	2
Ramos Ruiz, G	2	2

Clusters 2, 3, and 5 relate to authors' published articles in 2020–2021. Cluster 4 relates to authors with publications in 2019, and cluster 7 corresponds to authors with publications in 2018; for the remaining authors, articles were published in 2017. Figure 6 indicates that the top 10 author co-authorships were published in 2017, demonstrating that the academic community had a strong connection in 2017. Finally, the most relevant papers were published from 2017 to 2020, demonstrating that the academic community has increased.

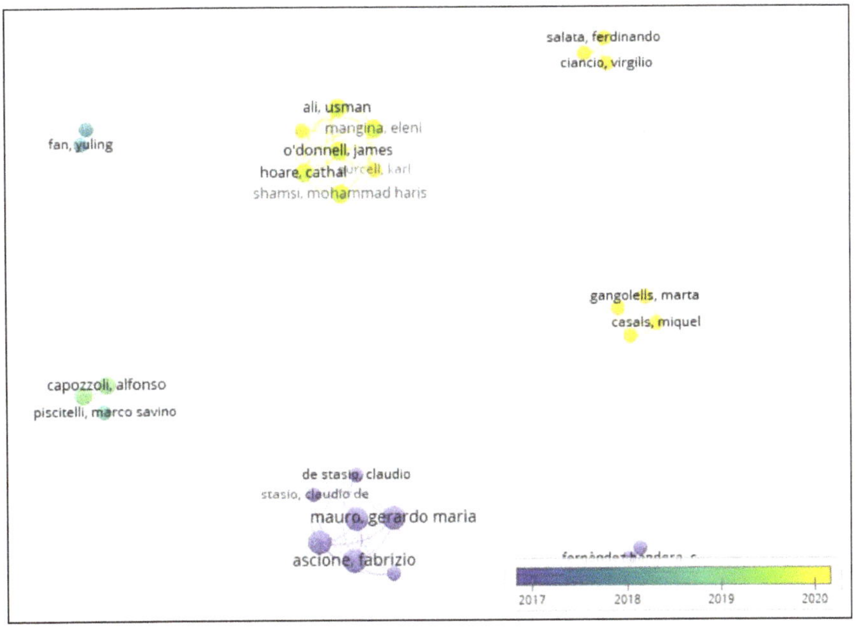

Figure 6. Authors' co-authorship visualization by year.

4.4. Most Cited Publications

Analysis of the most-cited publications helped us to detect the important research topics in the literature. The most cited and chosen publications were searched using Science Direct, Scopus and Web of Science datasets. The study detected publications that have been cited between 84 times and 0 times. Table 5 shows this process's resulting conceptual and theoretical framework with each paper's dimensions, intelligent computing methods, and type of buildings.

The top five found publications are from the following authors: Ascione, Bianco, Stasio et al. [23] with 84 citations (the most cited), followed by Ramos Ruiz et al. [38] with 44 citations, Ascione, Bianco, De Masi et al. [27] with 44 citations, Niemelä, Kosonen, and Jokisalo [39] with 39 citations and Beccali et al. [40] with 37 citations. These results (Table 5) are coherent with previous analyses described above. These papers are the most cited and present the central concepts in the field.

The top five cited papers present in Table 5 were published in Q1-ranked journals and mostly in Energy and Buildings and Applied Energy journals. Furthermore, and coherent to the analysis, the most cited article is also emphasized in the authors' co-authorship analysis (Section 4.3). Cluster 1 (green) in Figure 5 groups the most cited author co-authorship Ascione, Bianco, Stasio et al. [23] and cluster 6 (purple) groups most of the author co-authorships of the second most-cited article Ramos Ruiz et al. [38]. In keyword co-occurrence analysis (Section 4.3), the term ANN was outstanding and is one of the techniques used by the most cited publication of Beccali et al. [40].

Table 5. Publications ranked by the number of citations.

N	Ref.	Publication	Dimension Category	Methods	Building Type	No. of Citations
1	[16]	Applied Energy	-Thermo-physical characteristics -Building envelope -HVAC systems -Weather -Energy use	-Simulation -Latin hypercube sampling -Pareto—sensitive Analysis -Genetic Algorithm	Hospital	84
2	[31]	Applied Energy	-Climatic location -Geometry -Construction elements -Building properties -Internal temperature measures	-Genetic Algorithm NSGA-II -Simulation -Parametric analysis -Sensitivity analysis -Uncertainty analysis: fi, CV(RMSE)	University	44
3	[20]	Energy & Buildings	-Building envelope -Building operation -HVAC systems -Financial attributes	-Genetic algorithms -Transient energy simulations	University	44
4	[32]	Energy & Buildings	-Building Envelope -HVAC systems -Internal heat gains -Weather -Cost of different renovation measures	-Simulation-based Optimisation methods -Pareto-Archive NSGA-II Genetic algorithm	Residential	39
5	[33]	Energy	-Thermophysical parameters -HVAC plants -Typology -Building characteristics -Climate -Geometry -Energy consumption	-Artificial neural networks (ANN)	School	37
6	[34]	Energy	-Climatic location -Building materials -Financial attributes	-Life-Cycle Cost method -Monte Carlo simulation -Discount rate	Residential	35
7	[35]	Energy & Buildings	-Design variables -Climate (Thermal zone) -Cooling and heating	-Pareto front -Simulation -Non-dominated Sorting Genetic Algorithm-II (NSGA-II)	Residential	30

Table 5. *Cont.*

N	Ref.	Publication	Dimension Category	Methods	Building Type	No. of Citations
8	[36]	Applied Energy	-Geometry -Weather -Construction materials	-Energy Simulation -Residual network model	Residential	27
9	[30]	Applied Energy	-Climate -Building location -Energy sources (gas and electricity) -Building characteristics -Installation systems -Photovoltaic -Thermal solar panels -Building geometry	-Simulations -Active Archive Non-Dominated Sorting Genetic Algorithm (aNSGA-II type). -Pareto frontier	Residential	22
10	[37]	Applied Energy	-Weather -Building Envelope -HVAC systems -Energy use	-Latin-hypercube sampling -Joint mutual information maximization -Energy conservation measure	Residential and offices	21
11	[38]	Measurement	-Building envelope -Orientation -Heating load -Cooling load	-Estimation Maximization algorithm -Adaptive Neuro-Fuzzy Inference System method -Principal Component Analysis	Residential	14
12	[22]	Applied Energy	-Building geometry -Energy performance index -Building shape -Dwelling type -Building envelope -Number of floors; walls, and windows -Envelope U-values -Construction assemblies -HVAC systems	-Crude statistical analysis -Visual analysis of statistical representation (Box plots) -Local Outlier Factor (LOF) algorithms -Deep Learning -Rule Induction -Neural Network -Naïve Bayes -Decision Tree -Random Forest -Gradient Boosted Trees -Learning Vector Quantization (LVQ) -9 k-Nearest Neighbors (kNN).	Residential	14

Table 5. *Cont.*

N	Ref.	Publication	Dimension Category	Methods	Building Type	No. of Citations
13	[29]	Energy & Buildings	-Geometry -Envelope -Useful floor area (m^2) -Building shape -Climate zone Window -Glazing type -Wall insulation -Heating system Heating -Energy source -Cooling system Cooling	-Sorting genetic algorithm (aNSGA-II) -Optimal solution in the R 4 space -Pareto frontier -Simulation	Residential	14
14	[39]	Sustainable Cities & Society	-Building Envelope -Heating systems -HVAC systems -Electricity consumption	-REVIT -Simulation -Genetic algorithm	Residential	13
15	[18]	Sustainability	-Geometry -Building envelope -Building operation -HVAC systems -Climate	-Latin hypercube sampling technique -Simulation-based large-scale uncertainty/sensitivity Analysis of Building EP	Residential, Offices and Schools	12
16	[40]	Energies	-Weather -Building age -Construction year -Building envelope -Heating/ Cooling systems	-Group by building age -Simulation Monte Carlo -Genetic Algorithm NSGA-II	Residential	12
17	[41]	Journal IEEE Transactions on Automation Science & Engineering	-Building intrinsic properties -Occupancy patterns -Environmental conditions	-Artificial neural network -Genetic algorithm -Multi regression analysis -Principal component analysis	Care home	9
18	[28]	Energies	-Geometry -Envelope -Construction year -Average global efficiency for space heating	-Artificial Neural Network -Support Vector Machine -Reduced Error Pruning Tree -Random Forests	Residential	8

Table 5. *Cont.*

N	Ref.	Publication	Dimension Category	Methods	Building Type	No. of Citations
19	[42]	Applied Energy	-Building envelope -Indoor facilities	-Manual grouping method and 'notch test' data -Generic Algorithm -Mathematics	Offices	7
20	[43]	Renewable & Sustainable Energy Reviews	-Thermophysical properties -Building envelope	-Artificial neural network (ANN) -K-means clustering -Geographic information systems (GIS)	School	7
21	[44]	Applied Energy	-Hot water -Internal heat gain and lighting -Wall to floor and window -Standard Emission Rate -Air infiltration rate -Terminal unit energy -Demand and cooling system efficiency. -Roof wall ratio -Solar radiation on the roof	-Simplified Building Energy Model (SBEM) tool -Sensitivity analysis -Gradient boosted regression trees (GBRT) -Cross-validation -Standard statistical re-sampling method, -Sequential Model-based Algorithm Configuration (SMAC)	Commercial, School	7
22	[45]	Croatian Review of Economic, Business & Social Statistics	-Geospatial -Construction shape -Heating characteristics -Cooling characteristics -Meteorological characteristics -Occupational characteristics -Energetic characteristics	-Artificial neural network (ANN) -K-means clustering -Correlation Analysis -Chi-square tests -Symmetric mean average percentage error -DBSCAN algorithm	Residential, Offices and Schools	6
23	[21]	Applied Energy	-Geometric data: building shape, building type, building fabric, number of floors, window-wall ratios -Non-geometric building: envelope U-values, construction assemblies, Heating Ventilation, Air Conditioning (HVAC) systems properties -EPC data -Building footprint -Building height data	-GIS -Decision Analysis (MCDA) approach -Fuzzy string algorithms -Jaro -Jaro–Winkler -Levenshtein -JaccnaïveNaive Bayes Generalized Linear Model -Logistic Regression -Deep Learning -Decision Trees -Random Forest -Gradient Boosted Trees -Support Vector Machine	Residential	6

Table 5. *Cont.*

N	Ref.	Publication	Dimension Category	Methods	Building Type	No. of Citations
24	[46]	Sustainable Cities & Society	-Geometrical -Thermophysical features	-Wrapper Feature Selection -Random Forests -K-means Clustering	Schools	5
25	[25]	Energy & Buildings	-Building norm -Window glazing -Climate zone -Cooling system -Useful floor area -Shape factor -Domestic hot water energy source -Heating energy source -Existence of thermal insulation in building envelopes	-K-means Clustering -Correlation analysis -Stepwise regression analysis -Root-mean-square standard deviation -Elbow method	Offices industrial—residential	5
26	[47]	Sustainable Cities & Society	-Climate zone -Building layout -Seasonal efficiency Heat delivery efficiency -Average water inlet temperature Hot water supply temperature -Mechanical ventilation Infiltration -Maximum power consumption -Luminous energy conversion efficiency Schedule -Occupants Lighting	-Dynamic simulation tool -IES Virtual Environment (VE) -Combination packages -Energy Limiting Difference (ELD) assessment factor	Residential	4
27	[48]	Energy & Buildings	-Construction age -Building size -Heating and hot water systems -Heat loss through the building fabric -Climatic location -Operation & occupancy pattern -Heating demand	-Statistical approach -Synthetical Average Building (SyAv) approach identifies	Residential	4

Table 5. *Cont.*

N	Ref.	Publication	Dimension Category	Methods	Building Type	No. of Citations
28	[23]	Energy & Buildings	-Geometric data -Envelope U-values -HVAC systems -Construction year -Climate zone	-Local Outlier Factor algorithm -K-means clustering -Weighting coefficients -Building national statistics -Building EP Simulation -Geographical Information System (GIS) visualization maps	Residential	2
29	[26]	IEEE International Conference on Internet of Things and Green Computing & Communications & Cyber, Physical & Social Computing & Smart Data (2017)	-Buildings Characteristics -Efficiency of the subsystems for space heating -System efficiency -EP (Normalized primary energy demand for space heating [kWh/m^2], etc.)	-Pearson correlation analysis -Principal component analysis -K-means clustering -Classification and Regression Tree algorithm -Silhouette based indices -Singular value decomposition -Statistics -Boxplot distributions -Generalized association rule	Residential	2
30	[49]	Energy Policy	-Dwelling type -Year of construction -Dwelling size -Occupancy status -Energy class -Surface coefficient of heat exchange -Real energy consumption -Systematic energy source -Heating system type -Region Climatic zone -Urban size -Renovation changes	-Statistical approach -Cost–benefit analysis. -Monte Carlo simulation -Sensitivity analysis -Hierarchical Classification (Ward's criterion)	Residential	2
31	[50]	IOP Conference Series: Earth & Environmental Science	-HVAC systems -Envelope U-values	-ENERFUND tool -Geographical Information System (GIS) visualization	Commercial and Residential	1

Table 5. *Cont.*

N	Ref.	Publication	Dimension Category	Methods	Building Type	No. of Citations
32	[27]	Electronics	-Aspect ratio -Surface area -Floor area -Average u-value of the vertical opaque envelope -Average u-value of the windows -Heating system global efficiency -Construction year	-Density-based spatial clustering of application with noise algorithm (dbscan) -Pearson correlation -Max–min binormalization -Elbow method -K-means -Spatial constrained k-nn -Geospatial maps	Residential	1
33	[51]	Energies	-Building type -Number of stories -Construction year -Heated space per story -Area code -Number of stairwells per Apartment	-Google Street View -ANN -Image recognition -Stepwise regression -Logistic regression (LR) -Support vector machines (SVM)	Residential	1
34	[24]	Sustainable Cities & Society	-Useful floor area (m^2) -Building shape -Climate zone Window -Glazing type -Wall insulation -Heating system Heating -Energy source -Cooling system Cooling	-Statistical approach -Life-cycle energy impact: Calculate the global energy savings -Life-cycle economic impact -Calculate life environmental impact	Offices	1
35	[52]	Neural Computing & Applications	-Useful surface (m^2) -Thermal power (kW) -CO^2 emissions -Primary energy consumption -Opaque enclosures -Holes and skylights	-Statistical approach -Bayesian Gaussian process regression (GPR) -Genetic algorithms (GAs) -Limited-memory Broyden–Fletcher–Goldfarb– Shanno (L-BFGS) optimizers	Residential	0

Likewise, several ML and statistical methods were used for energy applications on SLR papers. The 10 top most-cited papers used a combination of methods, namely simulation techniques, Pareto front, genetic algorithm NSGA-II, and ANN (Table 5). As input in those methods, these top 10 papers used the following dimensions extracted from the data: climate and weather, building thermo-physical characteristics, building envelope, building geometry, HVAC systems, EC, and building typology. In the case studies, most of them used residential buildings (6), offices (1), universities (2), schools (1), and hospitals (1), refs. [23,27,37–44]. The remaining SLR papers used similar dimensions: building geometry, building envelope, other building properties, climate and weather, HVAC systems, and energy consumption (EC) [16,18,20,21,28–48]. A total of 19 out of 35 papers used a residential building as the case study [28–30,33–37,39,41–43,45–47,53–57]. Some of them combine different types of buildings. Five papers combined residential and commercial buildings—offices and schools [25,32,44,52,58], two papers addressed offices [31,49] and six analyzed schools and universities [27,38,40,50,51,59]. Only one addressed a hospital [23] and one a care home [48].

Furthermore, only the most recent papers utilized building EPC data for their analysis [28,29,31,34,50–54,56,57,60,61]. This aspect is surprising since the first directive on building energy performance, "the Energy Performance of Building Directive (EPBD)," was introduced by the European Parliament in 2002. Additionally, improvements to the EPBD were performed in 2010 [60,61]. The remaining papers use energy building audits analysis and reference buildings for their research.

The most-used techniques for predicting EP and retrofitting were energy performance simulation techniques, statistical-based approaches, genetic algorithms, and ANN. Few studies use only ML methods, namely (13) studies [28,29,31,33–35,40,45,48,50,52,56,59]. The most common clustering and classification techniques were K-means (7), statistical methods (6), Latin hypercube sampling (2), other manual groupings (2), decision tree (2), and probability density function (1) [23,25,28–34,47,50–52,54,55,57,59].

4.5. Type of Buildings, Dimensions, and Methods Analysis

A conceptual and theoretical framework was built to evaluate this survey's building types, dimensions, and computational intelligence methods in more detail; see Tables 6 and 7. This framework seeks to understand the most-used ML and statistical approach according to each SLP study's dimensions and building types resulting from the previous analysis (Table 5). It focuses on research inputs, goals, and outcomes to create the basis for our research evaluation criteria.

Table 6. Analysis of the used Dimensions by Type of Buildings.

No.	Building Type	Dimension Category	Reference
1	Hospital	-Thermo-physical characteristics -Building envelope -HVAC systems -Weather -Energy use	[16]
3	University/School	-Building envelope -Building operation -HVAC systems -Financial attributes -Thermophysical parameters -Typology -Climate -Geometry -Energy consumption -Hot water -Internal heat gain and lighting -Standard Emission Rate -Air infiltration rate Terminal unit energy -Demand and cooling system efficiency. -Roof wall ratio -Solar radiation on the roof	[20,31,33,43,44,46]

Table 6. *Cont.*

No.	Building Type	Dimension Category	Reference
4	Residential	-Building Envelope -Geometry -HVAC systems -Internal heat gains -Weather -Building materials -Financial attributes -Cost data of different renovation measures -Building–location–orientation -Photovoltaic -Energy performance index -Envelope U-values -Construction assemblies -Thermal solar panels -Electricity consumption -Building age -Construction year -Average global efficiency for space heating -EPC -Construction age -EP (Normalized primary energy demand for space heating [kWh/m^2], etc.) -Occupancy status -Energy class -Renovation changes -CO_2 emissions -Primary energy consumption	[21–23,26–30,32,34–36,38–40,47–49,51,52]
4	Residential and offices	-Weather -Building Envelope -HVAC systems -Energy use -Envelope U-values	[37,50]
5	Residential, Offices and Schools	-Geometry -Building envelope -HVAC systems -Climate -Geospatial -Construction shape -Occupational characteristics -Energetic characteristics -Building Insulation	[18,25,45]
6	Care homes	-Building intrinsic properties -Occupancy patterns -Environmental conditions	[41]
7	Offices	-Building envelope -Indoor facilities -Useful floor area (m2) -Building shape -Climate -Glazing type -Wall insulation -Heating system -Energy source -Cooling system	[24,42]

Table 4 presents our findings on dimensions by building types to implicate new knowledge, which helps energy experts to learn and use the most critical dimensions for particular building types in their modeling and research work.

The SLR analysis suggests that the dimensions extracted from the data sources, can be grouped in the following way:

- Climate: location, weather, building orientation.
- Building geometry: building shape, building type, building fabric, number of floors, window-wall ratios.
- Non-geometric building data: envelope U-values, construction assemblies, heating ventilation, air conditioning (HVAC) systems properties, building age.
- Energy consumption: electricity consumption, energy use, average global efficiency for space heating, HVAC systems, internal heat gain, and lighting.

- Energy performance: standard emission rate, CO_2 emissions, terminal unit energy, energy performance index, the efficiency of the subsystems for space heating.
- Financial attributes: cost data of different renovation measures
- Occupational characteristics.

Table 7 presents our inference which may help data scientists understand the right method to employ for further research.

Table 7. Methods by Dimensional Analysis.

No.	Computational Intelligence Method	Dimension Category	Reference
1	Simulation	-Climate -Building geometry -Non-geometric building data -Energy consumption -Energy performance	[16,18,20,23,29–32,34,37,39,40,47,49]
2	Genetic Algorithm	-Climate -Geometric building -Non-geometric building data -Energy consumption -Energy performance -Financial attributes	[16,20,29–32,35,39–42,52]
3	Sensitivity analysis	-Climate -Building geometry -Non-geometric building data -Energy consumption -Energy performance -Financial attributes	[31,44,49]
4	Artificial neural networks (ANN)	-Climate -Building geometry -Non-geometric building data -Energy consumption -Energy performance -Occupational characteristics	[28,33,41,43,45,51]
5	K-means clustering	-Climate -Building geometry -Non-geometric building data -Energy consumption -Energy performance -Occupational characteristics	[23,25–27,43,45,46]
6	Geographic information systems (GIS)	-Climate -Building geometry -Non-geometric building data -Energy consumption -Energy performance	[21,23,27,43,50,51]
7	DBSCAN algorithm	-Climate -Building geometry -Non-geometric building data -Energy consumption -Energy performance -Occupational characteristics	[27,45]
8	Correlation analysis	-Climate -Building geometry -Non-geometric building data -Energy consumption -Energy performance -Occupational characteristics	[23,25–27,45]

Table 7. *Cont.*

No.	Computational Intelligence Method	Dimension Category	Reference
9	Statistical approach	-Climate data -Building geometry -Non-geometric building data -Energy consumption -Energy performance	[22–26,29,30,35,41,42,44,48,49,51,52]
10	Cost-Benefit analysis	-Climate data -Building geometry -Non-geometric building data -Energy consumption -Energy performance -Financial attributes	[24,34,49]
11	Principal Component Analysis	-Climate -Building geometry -Non-geometric building data -Energy consumption	[38,41]

The above analysis allows us to use the most common dimension categories of building to find an adequate method to evaluate the energy performance according to the building type we are interested in. As the results demonstrated, most studies have common dimensions no matter the building type and methods.

5. Discussion

Our research aimed to highlight and detect the literature on machine learning (ML) and statistical techniques that tackle the EPB and create a systematic, organized view of those literature studies.

Following, we discuss how our study answers the posed research questions, namely:

- RQ1: What are the most relevant machine learning or statistical approaches that automatically evaluate buildings' energy performance using EPC data?
- RQ2: What are the most relevant ML or statistical approaches for predicting energy-efficient retrofit measures to improve buildings' energy performance?

5.1. Research Questions Discussion

Our analysis indicates that the two problems discussed by the proposed machine learning or statistical approaches are clustering (classification) and prediction in the energy performance of buildings.

Regarding the first question (RQ1), 13 studies used the EPC dataset [30,32–35,52,58] as explained in Sections 4.4 and 4.5. This kind of data is multi-dimensional, given that each energy certificate has many attributes. The exploitation of a given data mining algorithm on such data (such as cluster analysis) is challenging due to the high variability and dimensionality of the data [33]. As for data classification and clustering techniques, most studies applied the K-means clustering algorithm to characterize the cluster sets with given energy performance, as explained in Sections 4.4 and 4.5. Some studies used a density-based spatial clustering of application with noise algorithm (DBSCAN) to handle outliers and correlation analysis to identify the best input demission for their clustering analysis [32–34,52]. A few studies referring to RQ1 used GIS and geospatial maps to visualize their clustering results [30,58]. Finally, (5) papers of similar studies answered RQ1, namely [30,33–35,58].

Regarding RQ2, most approaches to predicting energy-efficient retrofit measures used simulation tools such as EnergyPlus [62] or TRNSYS [63] to model the energy consumption (EC) of a 3D model of the building. They understudy and then use GA to perform multi-objective optimization, obtaining a good solution for the different criteria defined as important in their studies [46]. The strategy of using precomputed 3D models requires a large database of models and the accuracy depends on how close those models match real-world buildings. Although the most common algorithm for multi-objective optimization is the non-dominated sorting GA II (NSGA-II), it is possible to improve the algorithm by customizing it for energy retrofitting scenarios [64]. NSGA-II is a GA and customizing it for the specific field of energy retrofit would yield more efficient computations. Additionally, the more recent NSGA-III is not used by researchers [65]. The improved version will be more efficient computationally when finding optimal solutions. The simulation's quality depends on having a good model representation of the building and using other environmental factors such as weather data and orientation of the building/solar exposition [44].

The environmental characteristics that impact the building EP are also important criteria to determine what retrofitting measures are cost-effective. It is also essential to describe the building materials in terms of their heat loss/gain rating by the thicknesses (U-value) of features, namely roof, wall, floor, ceiling, and window, as well as identify the type of heating and cooling systems, renewable energy systems being used, occupation density, and others that might affect the building's energy consumption. It can be considered that the more extreme the weather conditions are in the region of the building, the more critical it is to include it in the modeling of EP [44].

Moreover, referring to the RQ2, several authors used GA (7) [23,27,38,39,42,48] to predict cost-optimal energy retrofit solutions. Some approaches used artificial neural networks (ANN) [35,40,48,50,52,56]. Most papers in this category are case studies using a single building or a representative building sample to collect the necessary data to serve their experiments. No study referring to RQ2 used GIS and geospatial maps to visualize. Finally, (15) papers of similar studies answered the RQ2, namely [23,25,27,29,36–39,41,42,44,46,48,55].

Some studies (8) answer both research questions; two such approaches are an excellent example of using K-means clustering and ANN with public EPC databases to predict EERM [50,52]. Other approaches focusing only on predicting energy consumption (EC) show that it is possible to use a data-driven urban energy simulation to predict the hourly, daily, and monthly energy consumption. In addition, models are used as a baseline for EC and then apply a residual network ML model to predict the EC on the various scales [43].

The primary objectives of the studies in this category (8 studies) are the prediction of EP, potential for energy savings, and cost-optimal retrofitting solutions [40,43,45,47,49,50,52,59]. As data classification and clustering techniques, some studies (6) adopted K-means [28,32,50,52,57,59]. Ultimately, some (2) applied manual classification [47,49]. As a prediction of EP and cost-optimal retrofit solutions techniques, some approaches (7) employed ANN and GA [40,47,49,50,52,56,57]. Others implemented different ML algorithms, such as random forest (RF) [59]. Lastly, some of the approaches executed simulations and mathematical techniques, such as a multiple linear regression, Pearson's correlation, principal component analysis, Monte Carlo, Gaussian process regression model, Gaussian mixture regression model, and deep learning algorithms [28,49,56]. Finally, some studies (3) use geographical information systems (GIS) and geospatial maps to visualize their results [28,50,56].

5.2. Knowledge Gap

Our analysis concluded that the research gap is related to identifying and testing ML approaches that are best fitted and have better performance in targeting automatic evaluation of buildings' energy performance using EPC data. Moreover, most of the studies use statistical and audit approaches at a multilevel scope [15,17,19,22,24,25,27–41,45,48,49]. However, some studies (13) use the EPC dataset for their analysis [28,29,31,34,50–54,56,57,60,61]. Furthermore, most studies apply simulation techniques and GA for prediction, targeting multi-objective cost-optimal solutions, a promising approach.

We conclude that more research is needed to validate and improve future modeling strategies using EPC datasets and different features. These gaps have shown an opportunity for future research.

5.3. Study Limitations

Although we tried to guarantee the quality of this review and, particularly, the data selection, this study has limitations. Specifically, we would like to highlight the dependency on the keywords and the selected data repositories, since additional data repositories could be used and only English papers were included, neglecting publications written in other languages. Finally, another important limitation of this study is the time frame, given that we focused on papers published in the last five years, between early 2016 and April 2021.

6. Conclusions

The PRISMA methodology summarized the SLR analysis and generated a systematic view of ML and statistical approaches applied in improving the EPB which can be used for future research. This study showed that after 2019, most studies used, processed, and analyzed EPC datasets, adopting ML or statistical approaches. Clustering analysis is applied to find similar patterns in buildings' EPC data. Simulation techniques and K-means clustering are the most used approaches to group buildings with similar characteristics. Box plot statistical analysis and dbscan are robust techniques used to eliminate outliers and noise due to their ability to deal with complex and high-dimensional data. Correlation analysis showed that the best approach is to estimate the importance of each analyzed input dimension. Additionally, the literature indicated that the best and most used evaluation method of the performance of the proposed algorithm was the accuracy of the ML-based solution.

Our research findings aim to fulfill identified knowledge gaps and open a methodological agenda that will help the reader identify effective combinations of ML and statistical approaches, addressing EPB and EERM in the future, providing a good starting point for further research.

Author Contributions: M.A.: Conceptualization, Methodology, Formal analysis, Literature Review, Investigation, Data curation, Writing—Original Draft, Writing—Review and Editing, Visualization, Project administration. V.S.: Conceptualization, Methodology, Formal analysis, Writing—Review and Editing, Supervision, Project administration, Funding acquisition. M.S.D.: Conceptualization, Methodology, Formal analysis, Writing—Review and Editing, Supervision, Project administration, Funding acquisition. All authors have read and agreed to the published version of the manuscript.

Funding: This work was supported by a Ph.D. Scholarship of NOVA IMS supported by project POCI-05-5762-FSE 000223, and its scope lies in the context of Simplex #109 "Consumo SMART". This work is partially funded by national funds through FCT—Foundation for Science and Technology, I.P., under the project FCT UIDB/04466/2020.

Informed Consent Statement: Not applicable.

Acknowledgments: We would like to thank Ricardo Pinto and Vitória Albuquerque [66] for their help reviewing the paper. The authors would also like to thank the reviewers and the editorial team who offered edifying and useful remarks to enhance the quality of the paper.

Conflicts of Interest: The authors declare no conflict of interest. The sponsors had no role in the design, collection, analysis, or interpretation of data, or writing of the study, nor in the decision to publish the results.

References

1. Rocha, P.; Kaut, M.; Siddiqui, A.S. Energy-efficient building retrofits: An assessment of regulatory proposals under uncertainty. *Energy* **2016**, *101*, 278–287. [CrossRef]
2. A European Green Deal. Available online: https://ec.europa.eu/info/strategy/priorities-2019-2024/european-green-deal_en (accessed on 1 May 2021).
3. Eurostat. *Shedding Light on Energy in the EU—A Guided Tour of Energy Statistics*, 2021st ed.; Eurostat: Luxembourg, 2021. [CrossRef]
4. Canevari, C. *How the EU Built the 2030 Energy Efficiency Target*; European Commission DG Energy: Vienna, Austria, 2018.
5. United Nations. Transforming Our World: The 2030 Agenda for Sustainable Development. 2020. Available online: https://sdgs.un.org/2030agenda (accessed on 13 May 2020).
6. European. Final Energy Consumption by Sector and Fuel in Europe. 2020. Available online: https://www.eea.europa.eu/data-and-maps/indicators/final-energy-consumption-by-sector-10/assessment (accessed on 10 February 2020).

7. Eurostat. Energy Statistics—An Overview. 2021. Available online: https://ec.europa.eu/eurostat/statistics-explained/index.php?title=Energy_statistics_-_an_overview#Final_energy_consumption (accessed on 30 November 2021).
8. Koo, C.; Hong, T. Development of a dynamic operational rating system in energy performance certificates for existing buildings: Geostatistical approach and data-mining technique. *Appl. Energy* **2015**, *154*, 254–270. [CrossRef]
9. Mehmood, M.U.; Chun, D.; Zeeshan; Han, H.; Jeon, G.; Chen, K. A review of the applications of artificial intelligence and big data to buildings for energy-efficiency and a comfortable indoor living environment. *Energy Build.* **2019**, *202*, 109383. [CrossRef]
10. Molina-Solana, M.; Ros, M.; Ruiz, M.D.; Gómez-Romero, J.; Martin-Bautista, M. Data science for building energy management: A review. *Renew. Sustain. Energy Rev.* **2017**, *70*, 598–609. [CrossRef]
11. Vaquero, P. Buildings Energy Certification System in Portugal: Ten years later. *Energy Rep.* **2019**, *6*, 541–547. [CrossRef]
12. Moher, D.; Liberati, A.; Tetzlaff, J.; Altman, D.G.; The PRISMA Group. Preferred reporting items for systematic reviews and meta-analyses: The PRISMA Statement. *PLoS Med.* **2009**, *6*, e1000097. [CrossRef]
13. VOSviewer—Visualizing Scientific Landscapes. Available online: https://www.vosviewer.com// (accessed on 23 January 2021).
14. Fathi, S.; Srinivasan, R.; Fenner, A.; Fathi, S. Machine learning applications in urban building energy performance forecasting: A systematic review. *Renew. Sustain. Energy Rev.* **2020**, *133*, 110287. [CrossRef]
15. Wei, Y.; Zhang, X.; Shi, Y.; Xia, L.; Pan, S.; Wu, J.; Han, M.; Zhao, X. A review of data-driven approaches for prediction and classification of building energy consumption. *Renew. Sustain. Energy Rev.* **2018**, *82*, 1027–1047. [CrossRef]
16. Wang, Z.; Srinivasan, R. A review of artificial intelligence based building energy use prediction: Contrasting the capabilities of single and ensemble prediction models. *Renew. Sustain. Energy Rev.* **2016**, *75*, 796–808. [CrossRef]
17. Seyedzadeh, S.; Rahimian, F.; Glesk, I.; Roper, M. Machine learning for estimation of building energy consumption and performance: A review. *Vis. Eng.* **2018**, *6*, 5. [CrossRef]
18. Grillone, B.; Danov, S.; Sumper, A.; Cipriano, J.; Mor, G. A review of deterministic and data-driven methods to quantify energy efficiency savings and to predict retrofitting scenarios in buildings. *Renew. Sustain. Energy Rev.* **2020**, *131*, 110027. [CrossRef]
19. Pickering, C.; Byrne, J. The benefits of publishing systematic quantitative literature reviews for PhD candidates and other early-career researchers. *High. Educ. Res. Dev.* **2014**, *33*, 534–548. [CrossRef]
20. Mendeley, Elsevier. 2019. Available online: https://www.mendeley.com/?interaction_required=true (accessed on 10 January 2017).
21. Semple, S.; Jenkins, D. Variation of energy performance certificate assessments in the European Union. *Energy Policy* **2019**, *137*, 111127. [CrossRef]
22. Scimago Lab. Scimago Journal & Country Rank, Scimago J. Ctry. Rank. 2021. Available online: https://www.scimagojr.com/ (accessed on 10 July 2021).
23. Ascione, F.; Bianco, N.; De Stasio, C.; Mauro, G.M.; Vanoli, G.P. Multi-stage and multi-objective optimization for energy retrofitting a developed hospital reference building: A new approach to assess cost-optimality. *Appl. Energy* **2016**, *174*, 37–68. [CrossRef]
24. Ascione, F.; Bianco, N.; De Stasio, C.; Mauro, G.M.; Vanoli, G.P. A Methodology to Assess and Improve the Impact of Public Energy Policies for Retrofitting the Building Stock: Application to Italian Office Buildings. *Int. J. Heat Technol.* **2016**, *34*, S277–S286. [CrossRef]
25. Ascione, F.; Bianco, N.; De Stasio, C.; Mauro, G.M.; Vanoli, G.P. Addressing Large-Scale Energy Retrofit of a Building Stock via Representative Building Samples: Public and Private Perspectives. *Sustainability* **2017**, *9*, 940. [CrossRef]
26. Ascione, F.; Bianco, N.; De Masi, R.F.; Mauro, G.M.; Vanoli, G.P. Resilience of robust cost-optimal energy retrofit of buildings to global warming: A multi-stage, multi-objective approach. *Energy Build.* **2017**, *153*, 150–167. [CrossRef]
27. Ascione, F.; Bianco, N.; de Masi, R.F.; Mauro, G.M.; Vanoli, G.P. Energy retrofit of educational buildings: Transient energy simulations, model calibration and multi-objective optimisation towards nearly zero-energy performance. *Energy Build* **2017**, *144*, 303–319. [CrossRef]
28. Ali, U.; Shamsi, M.H.; Bohacek, M.; Purcell, K.; Hoare, C.; Mangina, E.; O'Donnell, J. A data-driven approach for multi-scale GIS-based building energy modeling for analysis, planning and support decision making. *Appl. Energy* **2020**, *279*, 115834. [CrossRef]
29. Ali, U.; Shamsi, M.H.; Bohacek, M.; Hoare, C.; Purcell, K.; Mangina, E.; O'Donnell, J. A data-driven approach to optimize urban scale energy retrofit decisions for residential buildings. *Appl. Energy* **2020**, *267*, 114861. [CrossRef]
30. Ali, U.; Shamsi, M.H.; Hoare, C.; Mangina, E.; O'Donnell, J. A data-driven approach for multi-scale building archetypes de-velopment. *Energy Build* **2019**, *202*, 109364. [CrossRef]
31. Gangolells, M.; Gaspar, K.; Casals, M.; Ferré-Bigorra, J.; Forcada, N.; Macarulla, M. Life-cycle environmental and cost-effective energy retrofitting solutions for office stock. *Sustain. Cities Soc.* **2020**, *61*, 102319. [CrossRef]
32. Gangolells, M.; Casals, M.; Ferré-Bigorra, J.; Forcada, N.; Macarulla, M.; Gaspar, K.; Tejedor, B. Office representatives for cost-optimal energy retrofitting analysis: A novel approach using cluster analysis of energy performance certificate databases. *Energy Build.* **2019**, *206*, 109557. [CrossRef]
33. Di Corso, E.; Cerquitelli, T.; Piscitelli, M.S.; Capozzoli, A. Exploring Energy Certificates of Buildings through Unsupervised Data Mining Techniques. *IEEE Xplore* **2017**, 991–998. [CrossRef]
34. Cerquitelli, T.; Di Corso, E.; Proto, S.; Bethaz, P.; Mazzarelli, D.; Capozzoli, A.; Baralis, E.; Mellia, M.; Casagrande, S.; Tamburini, M. A Data-Driven Energy Platform: From Energy Performance Certificates to Human-Readable Knowledge through Dynamic High-Resolution Geospatial Maps. *Electronics* **2020**, *9*, 2132. [CrossRef]

35. Attanasio, A.; Piscitelli, M.S.; Chiusano, S.; Capozzoli, A.; Cerquitelli, T. Towards an Automated, Fast and Interpretable Estimation Model of Heating Energy Demand: A Data-Driven Approach Exploiting Building Energy Certificates. *Energies* **2019**, *12*, 1273. [CrossRef]
36. Rosso, F.; Ciancio, V.; Dell'Olmo, J.; Salata, F. Multi-objective optimization of building retrofit in the Mediterranean climate by means of genetic algorithm application. *Energy Build.* **2020**, *216*, 109945. [CrossRef]
37. Salata, F.; Ciancio, V.; Dell'Olmo, J.; Golasi, I.; Palusci, O.; Coppi, M. Effects of local conditions on the multi-variable and multi-objective energy optimization of residential buildings using genetic algorithms. *Appl. Energy* **2019**, *260*, 114289. [CrossRef]
38. Ruiz, G.R.; Bandera, C.F.; Temes, T.G.-A.; Gutierrez, A.S.-O. Genetic algorithm for building envelope calibration. *Appl. Energy* **2016**, *168*, 691–705. [CrossRef]
39. Niemelä, T.; Kosonen, R.; Jokisalo, J. Cost-effectiveness of energy performance renovation measures in Finnish brick apartment buildings. *Energy Build.* **2017**, *137*, 60–75. [CrossRef]
40. Beccali, M.; Ciulla, G.; Brano, V.L.; Galatioto, A.; Bonomolo, M. Artificial neural network decision support tool for assessment of the energy performance and the refurbishment actions for the non-residential building stock in Southern Italy. *Energy* **2017**, *137*, 1201–1218. [CrossRef]
41. Copiello, S.; Gabrielli, L.; Bonifaci, P. Evaluation of energy retrofit in buildings under conditions of uncertainty: The prominence of the discount rate. *Energy* **2017**, *137*, 104–117. [CrossRef]
42. Bre, F.; Fachinotti, V. A computational multi-objective optimization method to improve energy efficiency and thermal comfort in dwellings. *Energy Build.* **2017**, *154*, 283–294. [CrossRef]
43. Nutkiewicz, A.; Yang, Z.; Jain, R.K. Data-driven Urban Energy Simulation (DUE-S): A framework for integrating engineering simulation and machine learning methods in a multi-scale urban energy modeling workflow. *Appl. Energy* **2018**, *225*, 1176–1189. [CrossRef]
44. Shen, P.; Braham, W.; Yi, Y. The feasibility and importance of considering climate change impacts in building retrofit analysis. *Appl. Energy* **2018**, *233-234*, 254–270. [CrossRef]
45. Nilashi, M.; Dalvi-Esfahani, M.; Ibrahim, O.; Bagherifard, K.; Mardani, A.; Zakuan, N. A soft computing method for the prediction of energy performance of residential buildings. *Measurement* **2017**, *109*, 268–280. [CrossRef]
46. Eskander, M.; Reyes, M.E.S.; Silva, C.A.S.; Vieira, S.; Sousa, J.M.C. Assessment of energy efficiency measures using multi-objective optimization in Portuguese households. *Sustain. Cities Soc.* **2017**, *35*, 764–773. [CrossRef]
47. Hirvonen, J.; Jokisalo, J.; Heljo, V.J.; Kosonen, R. Towards the EU Emission Targets of 2050: Cost-Effective Emission Reduction in Finnish Detached Houses. *Energies* **2019**, *12*, 4395. [CrossRef]
48. Hosseini, M.; Lee, B.; Vakilinia, S. Energy performance of cool roofs under the impact of actual weather data. *Energy Build.* **2017**, *145*, 284–292. [CrossRef]
49. Fan, Y.; Xia, X. Building retrofit optimization models using notch test data considering energy performance certificate compliance. *Appl. Energy* **2018**, *228*, 2140–2152. [CrossRef]
50. Cecconi, F.R.; Moretti, N.; Tagliabue, L. Application of artificial neutral network and geographic information system to evaluate retrofit potential in public school buildings. *Renew. Sustain. Energy Rev.* **2019**, *110*, 266–277. [CrossRef]
51. Seyedzadeh, S.; Pour Rahimian, F.; Oliver, S.; Rodriguez, S.; Glesk, I. Machine learning modelling for predicting non-domestic buildings energy performance: A model to support deep energy retrofit decision-making. *Appl. Energy* **2020**, *279*, 115908. [CrossRef]
52. Zekić-Sušac, M.; Scitovski, R.; Has, A. Cluster analysis and artificial neural networks in predicting energy efficiency of public buildings as a cost-saving approach. *Croat. Rev. Econ. Bus. Soc. Stat.* **2018**, *4*, 57–66. [CrossRef]
53. Qu, K.; Chen, X.; Ekambaram, A.; Cui, Y.; Gan, G.; Økland, A.; Riffat, S. A novel holistic EPC related retrofit approach for residential apartment building renovation in Norway. *Sustain. Cities Soc.* **2019**, *54*, 101975. [CrossRef]
54. Ahern, C.; Norton, B. A generalisable bottom-up methodology for deriving a residential stock model from large empirical databases. *Energy Build.* **2020**, *215*, 109886. [CrossRef]
55. Belaïd, F.; Ranjbar, Z.; Massié, C. Exploring the cost-effectiveness of energy efficiency implementation measures in the residential sector. *Energy Policy* **2021**, *150*, 112122. [CrossRef]
56. Von Platten, J.; Sandels, C.; Jörgensson, K.; Karlsson, V.; Mangold, M.; Mjörnell, K. Using Machine Learning to Enrich Building Databases—Methods for Tailored Energy Retrofits. *Energies* **2020**, *13*, 2574. [CrossRef]
57. García-Nieto, P.J.; García-Gonzalo, E.; Paredes-Sánchez, J.P.; Sánchez, A.B. A new hybrid model to foretell thermal power efficiency from energy performance certificates at residential dwellings applying a Gaussian process regression. *Neural Comput. Appl.* **2020**, *33*, 6627–6640. [CrossRef]
58. Geissler, S.; Androutsopoulos, A.; Charalambides, A.G.; Escudero, C.J.; Jensen, O.M.; Kyriacou, O.; Petran, H. ENERFUND—Identifying and rating deep renovation opportunities. *IOP Conf. Ser. Earth Environ. Sci.* **2019**, *323*, 012174. [CrossRef]
59. Pistore, L.; Pernigotto, G.; Cappelletti, F.; Gasparella, A.; Romagnoni, P. A stepwise approach integrating feature selection, regression techniques and cluster analysis to identify primary retrofit interventions on large stocks of buildings. *Sustain. Cities Soc.* **2019**, *47*, 101438. [CrossRef]
60. European Commission. Directive 2002/91/EC of the European Parliament and of the Council of 16 December 2002 on the energy performance of buildings. 2002. Available online: https://eur-lex.europa.eu/legal-content/EN/TXT/PDF/?uri=%0ACELEX:32002L0091&from=IT (accessed on 10 March 2019).

61. *Directive 2010/31/EU of the European Parliament and of the Council of 19 May 2010 on the Energy Performance of Buildings (Recast)*; European Union: Brussels, Belgium, 2010.
62. EnergyPlus. Available online: https://energyplus.net/ (accessed on 2 March 2019).
63. TRNSYS. Transient System Simulation Tool. Available online: http://www.trnsys.com (accessed on 2 March 2019).
64. Tadeu, S.F.; Alexandre, R.F.; Tadeu, A.J.; Antunes, C.H.; Simões, N.A.; da Silva, P.P. A comparison between cost optimality and return on investment for energy retrofit in buildings—A real options perspective. *Sustain. Cities Soc.* **2016**, *21*, 12–25. [CrossRef]
65. Ciro, G.C.; Dugardin, F.; Yalaoui, F.; Kelly, R. A NSGA-II and NSGA-III comparison for solving an open shop scheduling problem with resource constraints. *IFAC PapersOnLine* **2016**, *49*, 1272–1277. [CrossRef]
66. Albuquerque, V.; Dias, M.S.; Bacao, F. Machine Learning Approaches to Bike-Sharing Systems: A Systematic Literature Review. *ISPRS Int. J. Geo Inf.* **2021**, *10*, 62. [CrossRef]

energies

Article

Numerical Investigation of Single-Row Double-Jet Film Cooling of a Turbine Guide Vane under High-Temperature and High-Pressure Conditions

Jin Hang, Jingzhou Zhang *, Chunhua Wang * and Yong Shan

Key Laboratory of Thermal Management and Energy Utilization of Aircraft, College of Energy and Power Engineering, Nanjing University of Aeronautics and Astronautics, Nanjing 210016, China; hjhangjin@163.com (J.H.); nuaasy@nuaa.edu.cn (Y.S.)
* Correspondence: zhangjz@nuaa.edu.cn (J.Z.); chunhuawang@nuaa.edu.cn (C.W.)

Abstract: Single-row double-jet film cooling (DJFC) of a turbine guide vane is numerically investigated in the present study, under a realistic aero-thermal condition. The double-jet units are positioned at specific locations, with 57% axial chord length (C_x) on the suction side or 28% C_x on the pressure side with respect to the leading edge of the guide vane. Three spanwise spacings (Z) in double-jet unit (Z = 0, 0.5d, and 1.0d, here d is the film hole diameter) and four spanwise injection angles (β = 11°, 17°, 23°, and 29°) are considered in the layout design of double jets. The results show that the layout of double jets affects the coupling of adjacent jets and thus subsequently changes the jet-in-crossflow dynamics. Relative to the spanwise injection angle, the spanwise spacing in a double-jet unit is a more important geometric parameter that affects the jet-in-crossflow dynamics in the downstream flowfield. With the increase in the spanwise injection angle and spanwise spacing in the double-jet unit, the film cooling effectiveness is generally improved. On the suction surface, DJFC does not show any benefit on film cooling improvement under smaller blowing ratios. Only under larger blowing ratios does its positive potential for film cooling enhancement start to show. Compared to the suction surface, the positive potential of the DJFC on enhancing film cooling effectiveness behaves more obviously on the pressure surface. In particular, under large blowing ratios, the DJFC plays dual roles in suppressing jet detachment and broadening the coolant jet spread in a spanwise direction. With regard to the DJFC on the suction surface, its main role in film cooling enhancement relies on the improvement of the spanwise film layer coverage on the film-cooled surface.

Keywords: double-jet film cooling; turbine guide vane; pressure surface; suction surface; numerical simulation

Citation: Hang, J.; Zhang, J.; Wang, C.; Shan, Y. Numerical Investigation of Single-Row Double-Jet Film Cooling of a Turbine Guide Vane under High-Temperature and High-Pressure Conditions. *Energies* **2022**, *15*, 287. https://doi.org/10.3390/en15010287

Academic Editors: Roberto Alonso González Lezcano, Francesco Nocera and Rosa Giuseppina Caponetto

Received: 19 November 2021
Accepted: 27 December 2021
Published: 1 January 2022

1. Introduction

Film cooling has been widely applied to the highly-efficient thermal protection of guide vanes in modern gas turbines [1]. As the gas turbines advance, the turbine inlet temperature will be progressively elevated such that the thermal-protection requirement becomes more critical. To ensure the guide vanes work reliably under crucial aero-thermal conditions without significant deterioration, developing more efficient film cooling schemes is a necessity.

Researchers have devoted tremendous efforts to explore effective strategies for enhancing film cooling performance, either in passive or active mode [2,3]. The innovation of shaped holes is regarded as the most inspiring advancement [4]. Through shaped film cooling holes, the jet injection is modified and subsequently, the flow dynamics of jet-in-crossflow, which is attributed to the cancellation of the kidney vortex pair or counter-rotating vortex pair (CVP) that originates from the mutual interaction of the ejecting jet with oncoming crossflow. It is well known that the earlier exploration of shaped holes was initialized in the middle of the 1970s. The preliminary investigation of Goldstein et al. [5]

demonstrated that a fan-shaped hole could produce a marked film cooling improvement on the immediate downstream surface. Following this acceptance, fan-shaped hole film cooling attracted much attention during the past decades. For instance, Thole et al. [6] presented a detailed flowfield measurement for the coolant injection from shaped holes with expanded exits. Gritsch et al. [7,8] experimentally investigated the geometric influence of fan-shaped holes on film cooling performances. Lee and Kim [9] conducted a single-objective geometric optimization study of fan-shaped hole film cooling with the aim of increasing cooling effectiveness. Saumweber and Schulz [10] researched the effect of the geometric parameters of fan-shaped holes on the film cooling performance. These further investigations illustrated clearly the dominate dynamic flow features of fan-shaped hole film cooling, including less coolant-mainstream shear mixing, less coolant-jet penetration into the mainstream, and wider coolant-jet lateral spread relative to the conventional hole. Despite the widespread use in practical, the challenging subjects in multi-parameter influence and multi-objective optimization of fan-shaped hole film cooling remain unexamined so far. More recently, Huang et al. [11] performed a multi-objective optimization of the laidback fan-shaped hole as applied to the turbine guide suction surface by taking the film cooling effectiveness and the discharge coefficient into consideration. Lenzi et al. [12] revealed the unsteady flowfield characterization of a shaped-hole effusion system in the swirling mainstream from detailed experimental tests. Kim et al. [13] investigated the influence of fan-shaped hole position and jet-to-crossflow density ratio on the film cooling performance. Baek et al. [14] performed a numerical study to deeply reveal the inherent flow dynamics of fan-shaped hole film cooling by using the large eddy simulation methodology. Lee et al. [15] optimized the fan-shaped hole using experimental methods, wherein the influence of primary flow velocity on the optimization was examined. Based on the fan-shaped holes, many innovative film cooling holes were suggested in recent years (e.g., arrowhead hole [16], NEKOMIMI hole [17], crescent hole [18], dumbbell hole [19], ridge hole [20], tripod hole [21], slot-similar hole [22], etc.), aiming at the possible solutions to approach the ideal art of film cooling. Although these innovative shaped holes have been confirmed to indeed play positive roles in improving film cooling effectiveness, they generally face fabrication and feasibility problems in engineering application due to their complex geometries. From this viewpoint, apparently, developing more realistic film cooling enhancement configurations is of more practical significance.

The double-jet film cooling configuration, referred as DJFC, is a simply constructed combined-hole configuration, wherein two film cooling holes with opposite orientation angles are integrated in a unit. On account of its realistic fabrication, DJFC gained much attention recently. Kusterer and his partners conducted a succession of investigations on the DJFC. Initially, they tried different spanwise spacings of the DJFC holes under a series of blowing ratios [23,24] and proved that the DJFC has the potential to produce an anti-kidney vortex pair. However, at this stage, some of the structures they tried were unsuccessful. For example, a "negative" spanwise spacing would significantly reduce the cooling effectiveness. Soon they discovered the reasonable double-jet structures and conducted further research with the use of these structures under both low and high blowing ratios [25,26]. They concluded that the DJFC with an appropriate design could form an anti-CVP structure to effectively alleviate the adverse CVP effect. As the double jets were arranged with opposite orientation angles, the compound injection angle was identified to be a crucial geometric parameter that affected the film cooling characteristics. Wang et al. [27] investigated the influence of streamwise spacing in a double-jet unit on film cooling performance. It was found that a larger streamwise spacing helps the formation of the anti-CVP structure and thus the improvement of film cooling effectiveness. Han et al. [28] studied the DJFC by using pressure sensitive paint technology and numerical simulation. It was demonstrated that the anti-CVP structure formed in the DJFC was tightly associated with the double-jet pitch and the compound injection angle, wherein the former affected the interaction and the latter affected the strength of each branch of the anti-kidney vortexes. Choi et al. [29] and Lee et al. [30] carried out an optimization of the DJFC configurations by selecting four variables (spanwise and streamwise distances between film-hole centers, and respective spanwise injection angles) as design variables. The cooling performance was optimized with the increase in the spanwise injection angle, attributed to a wider spanwise spreading of coolant coverage. Khalatov et al. [31] experimentally studied the influence of primary flow turbulence and pressure gradient on the DJFC. From the test results, they concluded that the double-jet scheme is superior to the traditional two-row scheme. An increase of about 20% of the averaged cooling effectiveness could be achieved under low and moderate blowing ratios. In general, the primary flow turbulence had a weak influence on the average cooling effectiveness of the DJFC, but the favorable streamwise pressure gradient could reduce the average film cooling effectiveness by about 25%. Graf and Kleiser [32] performed an LES study to determine the influence of the coolant injection condition and yaw angle on the thermal and aerodynamic performances of the DJFC. They identified that the increase in the yaw angle helped to improve the spanwise spread of the coolant jet. However, the far downstream film cooling effectiveness was reduced and the mixing loss increased. It should be noted that their research was mainly carried out under the double-jet layout with zero spanwise spacing. Yao et al. [33,34] performed experimental studies to determine the influence of spanwise spacing and streamwise spacing of double-jet unit on the film cooling performance. They reported that the spanwise distance greatly influenced the range of lateral coverage. Under moderate spanwise distances, the anti-kidney vortex effect more clearly dominated, whereas this anti-kidney vortex effect was weaker under a larger spanwise distance. Furthermore, the influence of streamwise spacing on the DJFC was tightly associated with the spanwise spacing. He et al. [35] studied the influence of the primary flow attack angle on the DJFC. It was found that larger negative attack angles of primary flow generally had an adverse influence on double-jet film cooling because of the limited lateral coverage. Liao et al. [36] performed an investigation to determine the surface curvature influence on the DJFC. Compared to the flat surface, the film cooling effectiveness of the DJFC on a convex surface increased, but the situation was opposite on a concave surface under low blowing conditions. The appropriate blowing ratio varied in accordance with the surface curvature. In general, in the DJFC, the main geometric parameters that significantly affected film cooling performance were the compound injection angle and spanwise and streamwise pitches of the double-jet unit.

As far as we know, most of the previous investigations on the DJFC were performed on a flat surface. However, the film cooling performance is significantly influenced by the surface curvature and pressure gradient of the primary flow passage. Apparently, the assessment of shaped-hole film cooling on its potential use in real gas turbines is an obligatory issue. Although the effects of major variables in the DJFC have been extensively investigated, little attention has been paid to DJFC application in gas turbine vanes. Aiming at this issue, a numerical investigation is conducted in the current study to provide more detailed insight into the DJFC roles in the application of a turbine guide vane under the high-temperature and high-pressure conditions of gas turbines. From this work, the influence of the blowing ratio, spanwise injection angle, and spanwise spacing in a double-jet unit on film cooling performance is illustrated. Of particular, the different influential roles of the DJFC on the suction and pressure surfaces of a specific guide vane are identified.

2. Computational Procedures

2.1. Brief Description of the Physical Model

The simulated turbine guide vane was simply treated as a linear two-dimensional vane without considering its complicated contours. Its sectional profile was extracted from the mid-span of a real gas turbine guide vane, referring to Zhu et al. [37], as schematically displayed in Figure 1a. The main geometric parameters are listed in Table 1, including the chord length (C), axial chord length (C_x), cascade pitch (P_{vane}), inflow angle (φ), orientation angle (θ), and segment height in the computational domain. In this study, the baseline case was set by positioning a single row of cylindrical holes at specific streamwise locations, with 57% C_x on the suction side or 28% C_x on the pressure side with respect to the leading edge of guide vane, as displayed in Figure 1a. With regard to the DJFC, the cylindrical hole was replaced by the double-jet unit, wherein the streamwise location of the rear-hole outlet was kept the same with the baseline case, as displayed in Figure 1b.

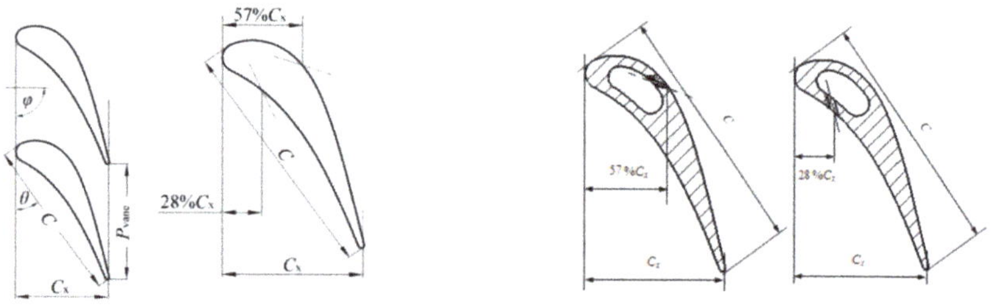

(a) **(b)**

Figure 1. Schematic of the turbine guide vane and coolant injection position. (**a**) turbine guide vane, (**b**) coolant injection position on the vane surface.

Table 1. Main parameters of the turbine guide vane.

Parameters	Symbol	Value
chord length	C	74.4 mm
axial chord length	C_x	42.3 mm
cascade pitch	P_{vane}	53.6 mm
inflow angle	φ	90°
orientation angle	θ	35.7°
segment height	H	4 mm

Figure 2 shows the schematic layout of the double-jet unit, wherein the double jets are arranged with opposite orientation angles. The geometric parameters in the DJFC configuration include the hole diameter (d), hole height (t), streamwise injection angle (α) and spanwise injection angle (β) with respect to each hole, streamwise spacing (X) and spanwise spacing (Z) between staggered holes, and the hole-to-hole pitch of adjacent double-jet units (P). In this work, two key geometric parameters (β and Z) were selected as the variable parameters for consideration, as they have been well demonstrated to be the main influential parameters in the DJFC. The other geometric parameters were kept constant, such as d = 0.8 mm, t/d = 2.5, P/d = 3, X/d = 3, and α = 30°. All of the geometric parameters in the DJFC are summarized in Table 2, wherein four spanwise injection angles (β = 11°, 17°, 23°, and 29°) and three spanwise spacings (Z/d = 0, 0.5, and 1.0) were taken into consideration. For the purpose of comparison, the film-hole diameter in the baseline case was set to $\sqrt{2}\,d$ to ensure that it had the same equivalent film-hole outlet area as that of the double-jet unit. As displayed in Figure 2, the coordinate system originated at the crossing point between the line linking the centers of rear-hole outlets (related to the leading edge of the guide vane) and the middle line of the spanwise spacing. This origin was the center of cylindrical hole in the baseline case. The x-direction (also s-direction along the respective surface) denoted the streamwise direction; y- and z- directions denoted the normal direction and spanwise direction, respectively.

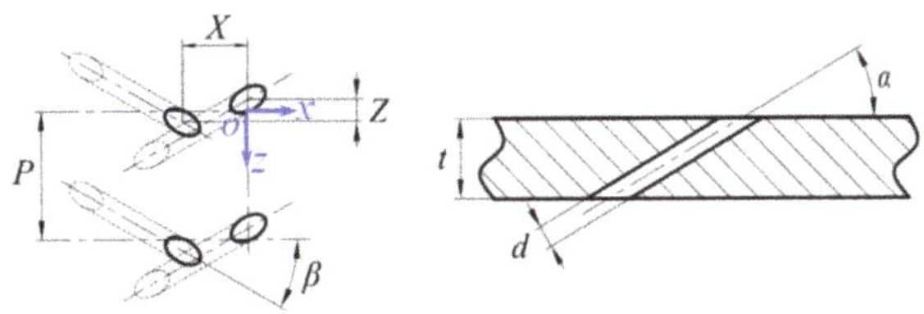

Figure 2. Schematic layout of the DJFC holes.

Table 2. Main geometric parameters in the DJFC.

Parameters	Symbol	Value
film-hole diameter	d	0.8 mm
film-hole height	t	2.5d
row pitch	P	3d
streamwise injection angle	α	30°
streamwise spacing	X	3d
spanwise injection angle	β	11°, 17°, 23°, 29°
spanwise spacing	Z	0, 0.5d, 1.0d

2.2. Computational Model

On account that the cascade flow was of periodicity, one cascade pitch was considered, as schematically shown in Figure 3. In addition, a segment of guide vane was selected as the spanwise size of computational domain, wherein one pitch of adjacent double-jet units was included, by defining the spanwise-end sections as the periodic boundaries. The plenum-fed mode was adopted to supply cooling air for coolant jet injection. In accordance with the current computational domain, the boundary conditions included the inlet and outlet of cascade flow, inlet of coolant flow, film-cooled surface, and the periodic boundaries that enclose the computational domain. They are briefly summarized as follows.

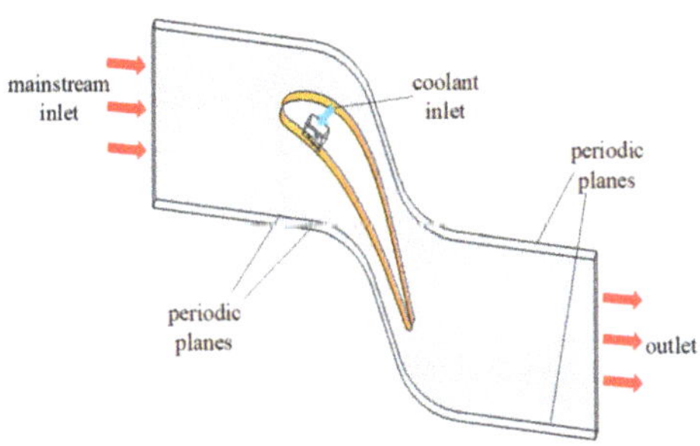

Figure 3. Schematic diagram of the computational domain.

Cascade channel: the cascade inlet that was located at a position 1.0 C_x upstream of the guide vane leading edge. At the cascade inlet, a velocity-inlet condition was applied, corresponding to a specified mainstream Reynolds number of Re_∞ = 425,000, as defined in Equation (1). The total inlet temperature of the mainstream ($T_{t,\infty}$) was 2100 K. Referring to Ragab and El-Gabry [38], the turbulence intensity level was selected as 8% under engine-representative conditions. The cascade outlet was set downstream the guide vane trailing edge, with an axial distance of 1.5 C_x. At the cascade outlet, a constant static pressure (p_{out}) of 1.3 MPa was applied.

$$Re_\infty = \frac{\rho_\infty u_\infty C}{\mu_\infty} \quad (1)$$

where ρ_∞ is the mainstream density, u_∞ is the mainstream inlet velocity, and μ_∞ is the mainstream dynamic viscosity.

Coolant plenum: the coolant-plume inlet was set as the mass-flow inlet condition. It was set in accordance with the required blowing ratio (M), as defined in Equation (2). The coolant had a total temperature ($T_{t,c}$) of 900 K and a turbulence intensity level of 5%. In the present study, four blowing ratios were considered. They were 0.5, 1.0, 1.5, and 2.0.

$$M = \frac{\rho_c u_c}{\rho_\infty u_\infty} \tag{2}$$

where ρ_c is the coolant density, and u_c is the bulk-average coolant jet injection velocity.

Periodic planes: on the periodic planes that enclosed the computational domain, the periodic boundary condition was applied.

Film-cooled surface: on the film-cooled surface, both the adiabatic thermal boundary condition and the no-slip flow boundary condition were applied.

2.3. Computational Methodology and Validation

Numerical simulations were conducted with the use of Fluent-CFD solver [39], wherein 3-D steady-state Reynolds-average N-S equations together with turbulence transport equations were solved. The SIMPLEC algorithm was adopted for the treatment of pressure-velocity coupling. The second-order upwind scheme and the central differencing scheme were used for the spatial discretization of convection terms and diffusion terns in the governing equations, respectively. On account of a compressible effect, an ideal air approach was applied for the working fluid, with the uses of ideal-gas-based density, Sutherland law-based viscosity, Kinetic theory-based specific heat, and thermal conductivity in the computations. Referring to previous works (e.g., Ely and Jubran [40], Silieti et al. [41], Balasubramaniyan and Jubran [42], Zhu et al. [43]), the realizable k-ε turbulence model was adopted in the present study. The computation process was regarded to be convergent when the residual descended to five orders of magnitude.

Based on the computed film-cooled surface temperature under thermally adiabatic film-cooled conditions (T_{aw}), the adiabatic film cooling effectiveness was determined as:

$$\eta_{ad} = \frac{T_\infty - T_{aw}}{T_\infty - T_c} \tag{3}$$

where T_∞ and T_c are the respective static temperatures of primary flow and coolant flow at their respective inlets.

In the entire computational domain, multi-block meshes were generated in different computational zones, such as the cascade channel, coolant chamber, and film holes. Figure 4a shows the local meshes in the film-hole center-line section and in the vicinity of the double-jet unit. Viscous clustering was applied to the near-wall zone of the guide vane to ensure that y^+ was less than unity. In the present study, the grid independence and numerical uncertainty were evaluated in advance with the use of the grid convergence index method (GCI) [44] by applying three sample grid systems (coarse, intermediate, and fine). Figure 4b displays the center-line η_{ad} distributions with the uses of three sets of grids and the extrapolated curve. Figure 4c presents the discretization error bars along with the intermediate-grid solution. When the grid number exceeded 3.0 million, the numerical simulation was not sensitive to the grid number. Therefore, the final computational mesh set was selected with approximately 3.0 million grids. In this situation, the maximum discretization error was less than 5%.

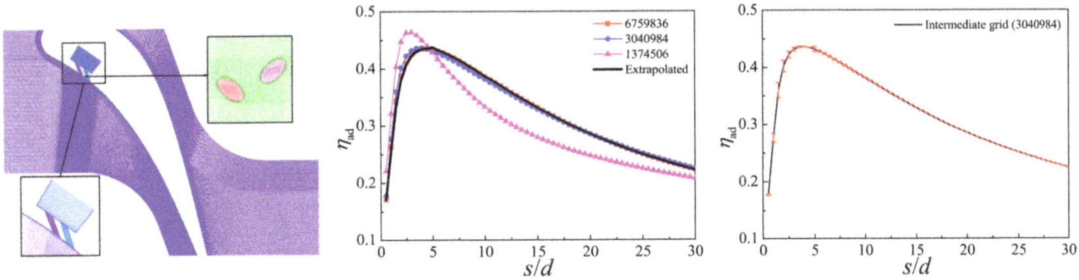

(a) (b) (c)

Figure 4. Representative meshes and grid independence test. (**a**) computational meshes, (**b**) adiabatic film cooling effectiveness along the centerline, (**c**) intermediate grid solution with discretization error bars.

Three examples were selected to validate the computational scheme in advance against the published experimental results. The first example was selected to validate the static pressure distribution simulation against a scaled turbine guide vane model test performed by Dees et al. [45], as displayed in Figure 5a. The static pressure coefficient is defined as $c_p = (p_s - p_{t\infty})/(0.5\rho_\infty u_\infty^2)$, where p_s and $p_{t\infty}$ are the static pressure on the guide vane surface and the total pressure of the mainstream at the entrance. It was found that the simulation agreed well with the experimental result. The second example was selected to validate the simulation of η_{ad} against a scaled fan-shaped-hole film-cooled guide vane test model presented by Dittmar et al. [46], as displayed in Figure 5b. The last example was the DJFC on a flat plat presented by Yao et al. [47], as displayed in Figure 5c. It was confirmed that the current simulation with the use of a realizable *k*-ε turbulence model presented a better prediction of the film cooling performance. In comparison with the experimental results, the relative deviation of numerical prediction was generally less than 7%.

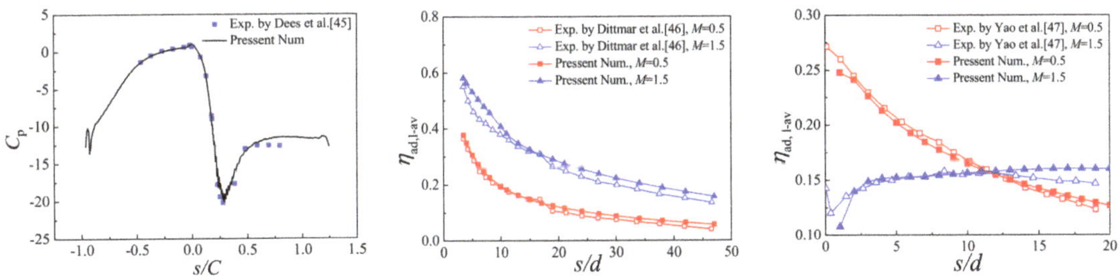

(a) (b) (c)

Figure 5. Validation of the computational scheme. (**a**) static pressure coefficient distribution, (**b**) fan-shaped hole film cooling on the pressure side, (**c**) DJFC on a flat surface.

3. Results and Discussion

3.1. DJFC on the Pressure Surface

Figure 6 presents local η_{ad} contours on the pressure surface downstream film cooling holes, for a specific double-jet layout with β = 29° and Z/d = 1.0. For the DJFC, local η_{ad} distribution immediately behind the front-hole (relative to the leading edge of the turbine guide vane) was very similar to the single compound-angle hole film cooling before the front jet interacted with the rear jet. When two coolant jets merged together in the downstream flow field, the cooling film coverage in the spanwise direction broadened rapidly, taking on a "branched" feature along the streamwise direction. At M = 0.5, the local film cooling effectiveness in the vicinity of film cooling holes was higher, as found Figure 6a. As the ejecting jets with a small blowing ratio have a weaker normal penetration momentum, they would remain closer to the downstream surface nearby the film cooling holes, as displayed in Figure 7a with the use of definition of $\Theta = (T - T_c)/(T_\infty - T_c)$. At this blowing ratio, only one pair of vortices was observed on the left side of $z/d = 0$ (negative z-direction), corresponding to the rear jet of double jets. On the right side (positive z-direction) in the DJFC, the kidney-like vortex was seriously destroyed due to the interaction between double jets. At $M = 1.5$, as the coolant jets had stronger injection momentum, a stronger normal penetration would occur in the double-jet film cooling. As displayed in Figure 8a, two pairs of counter-rotating vortices were clearly observed in the immediate downstream section of $s/d = 3$. Each individual pair of vortices retained a kidney-vortex feature, but took on an asymmetric distribution. It was also seen that the scale of the kidney-vortex on the left side of $z/d = 0$ was distinct from that on the right side in the DJFC. As the kidney-like vortex on the right side was generated from the front jet of the double-jet unit, in the same streamwise location, it developed with a longer distance compared to the rear jet. Farther downstream the film cooling holes, two pairs of counter-rotating vortexes gradually coupled together to form a single pair of counter-rotating vortices, as displayed in Figure 8b–d. Interestingly, although these central vortices in the DJFC were similar to the conventional kidney vortices of a single jet, their rotational directions were completely opposite with respect to the conventional kidney vortices originating from a baseline cylindrical hole (as displayed in Figure 9). For the cylindrical hole with compound injection angles, the flow field will not form a symmetric kidney vortex pair. Due to the existence of the compound angle, the branch of the vortex facing the mainstream will be weakened upon the impact of the mainstream. At the same time, the branch facing away from the mainstream will be strengthened by the mainstream, thus forming an asymmetric vortex pair. The flow field of the DJFC coolant jet can be considered the combination of flow fields caused by two 'individual' cylindrical holes with opposite compound angles. It was composed of two asymmetric vortex pairs, and the outer branches of these two vortex pairs quickly disappeared upon the impact of mainstream. As a result, only one anti-kidney-shaped vortex pair was left in the far downstream flow field. By observing the secondary flow field of the anti-kidney vortex pair on a series of cross-sections along the mainstream direction, it can be seen that in the middle area of the anti-kidney vortex pair, the cooling air flowed towards the surface. At the bottom of anti-kidney vortex pair, the cooling air was pushed towards the outside of the vortex pair, which not only prevented the high-temperature mainstream from moving to the bottom of the anti-kidney vortex pair, but also increased the coverage area of the film layer on the wall surface. Therefore, dominated by these anti-kidney vortices, the normal penetration of coolant jets in the far downstream position was suppressed effectively. Even at a large blowing ratio, the detachment of coolant jet from the film-cooled surface could be eliminated in the DJFC, by comparing Figures 8d and 9d. At the same time, as the coolant jets with a higher blowing ratio had a stronger injection momentum, so their downward spreading capacity was enhanced. As a consequence, among the current range of blowing ratios, the film layer coverage on the far downstream surface increased with the increase in the blowing ratio in the DJFC, as demonstrated in Figure 6.

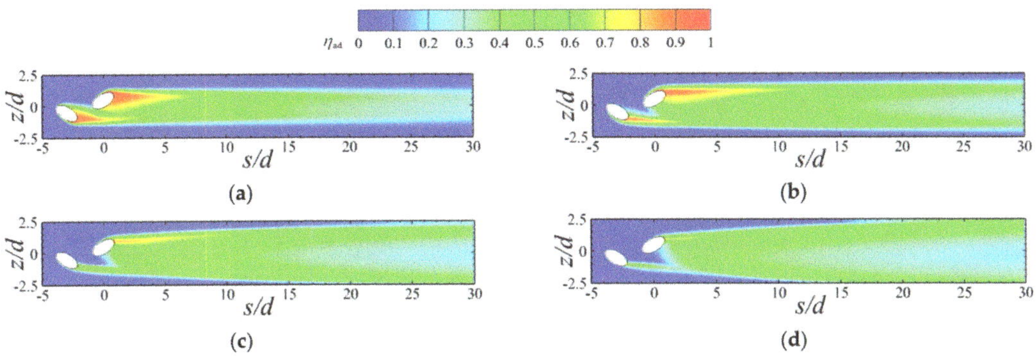

Figure 6. Local film cooling effectiveness distribution on the pressure surface for DJFC with $\beta = 29^{\circ}$ and $Z/d = 1.0$. (**a**) $M = 0.5$, (**b**) $M = 1.0$, (**c**) $M = 1.5$, (**d**) $M = 2.0$.

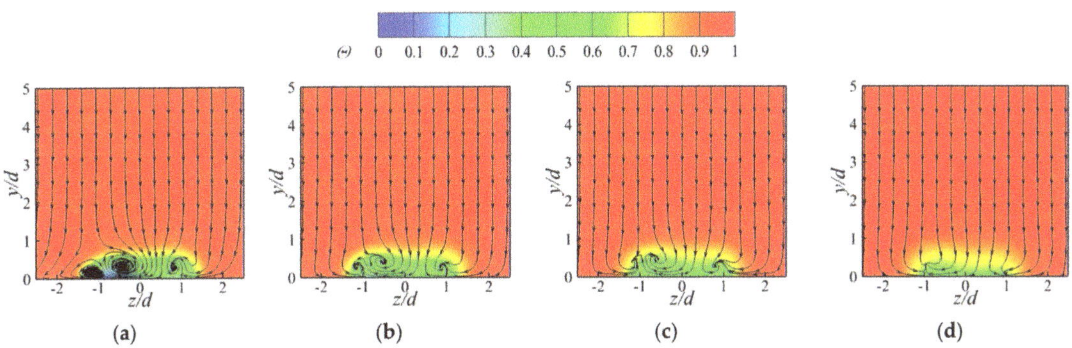

Figure 7. Dimensionless temperature contours and streamlines in downstream normal sections on the pressure side for DJFC under $M = 0.5$. (**a**) $s/d = 3$, (**b**) $s/d = 6$, (**c**) $s/d = 9$, (**d**) $s/d = 15$.

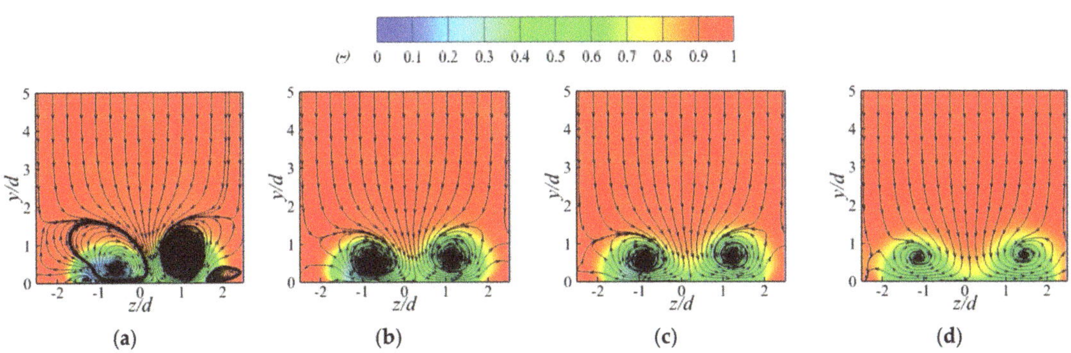

Figure 8. Dimensionless temperature contours and streamlines in downstream normal sections on the pressure side for DJFC under $M = 1.5$. (**a**) $s/d = 3$, (**b**) $s/d = 6$, (**c**) $s/d = 9$, (**d**) $s/d = 15$.

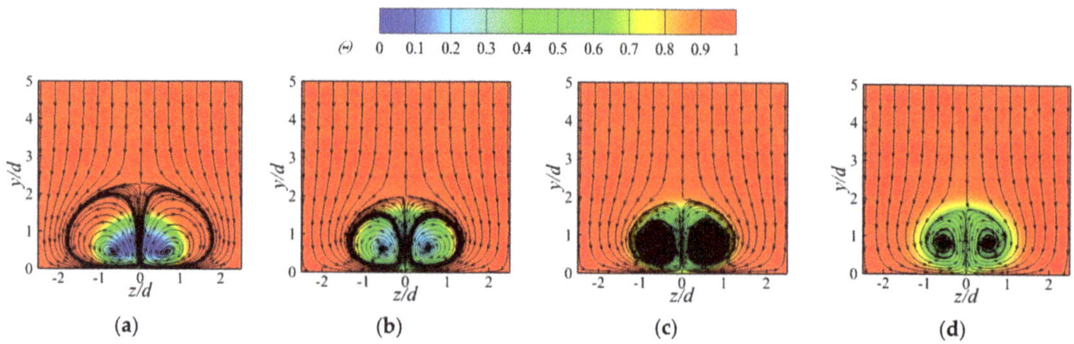

Figure 9. Dimensionless temperature contours and streamlines in downstream normal sections on the pressure side for cylindrical holes under $M = 1.5$. (**a**) $s/d = 3$, (**b**) $s/d = 6$, (**c**) $s/d = 9$, (**d**) $s/d = 15$.

For the DJFC, because of the additional interaction between double jets, the flow dynamics of jet-in-crossflow are tightly affected by the layout of double jets. To illustrate the effects of the spanwise injection angle and spanwise spacing in a double-jet unit, Figure 10 displays the streamlines and dimensionless temperature contours in the specified downstream normal sections of $s/d = 3$ and $s/d = 6$ for two typical double-jet units under $M = 1.5$. Combined with Figure 8, it is distinctly demonstrated that vortical structures of the DJFC behind the film cooling holes varied significantly in accordance with the spanwise injection angle and spanwise spacing. When the double jets were aligned with zero spanwise spacing ($Z/d = 0$), the development of the vortical structure originated from the front jet would be more seriously affected by the rear jet. On the contrary, the coolant jet ejected from the rear hole would also be affected seriously by the front jet. For this cause, in this situation, the near field behind the film cooling holes was mainly dominated by a single central vortex, as displayed in Figure 10a. Seen from Figure 11 wherein the streamwise vortices distributions are displayed, this single central vortex dominated nearly the entire downstream flow field (as demonstrated in Figure 11b). With the increase in spanwise spacing in the double-jet unit, the interaction between double jets would be alleviated such that the anti-kidney vortices are able to generate. As displayed in Figure 11c, in the situation of $Z/d = 0.5$ and $\beta = 29°$, the anti-kidney vortices were identified. When compared to the situation of $Z/d = 1.0$ and $\beta = 29°$ (as seen in Figure 11d), the scale of vortices in situation of $Z/d = 0.5$ and $\beta = 29°$ was smaller. In general, when the double jets were arranged with a spanwise spacing of $Z/d = 1.0$, two pairs of counter-rotating vortices would form at the near field behind the film cooling holes, regardless of the coolant injection angle. However, if the spanwise injection angle is small, these two pairs of counter-rotating vortices cannot easily merge together along the streamwise direction, as displayed in Figures 10b and 11e.

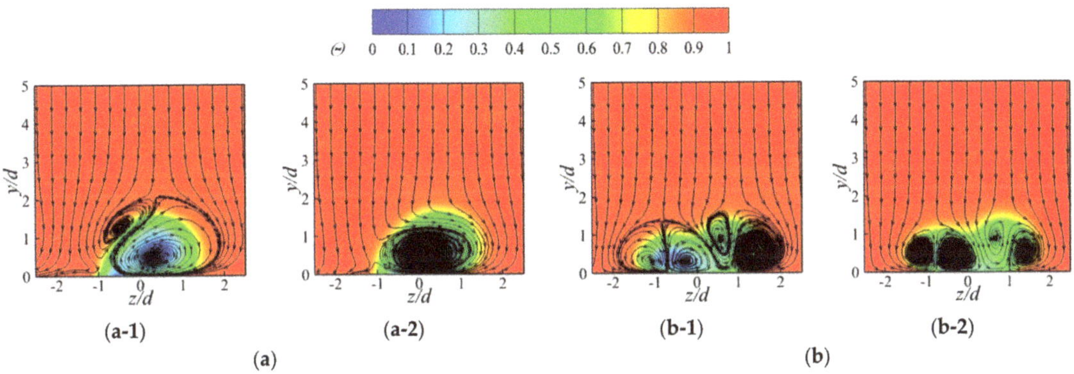

Figure 10. Dimensionless temperature contours and streamlines in downstream normal sections on the pressure side for two typical situations under $M = 1.5$. (**a**) $Z/d = 0$, $\beta = 29°$, (**a-1**) $s/d = 3$, (**a-2**) $s/d = 6$; (**b**) $Z/d = 1.0$, $\beta = 11°$, (**b-1**) $s/d = 3$, (**b-2**) $s/d = 6$.

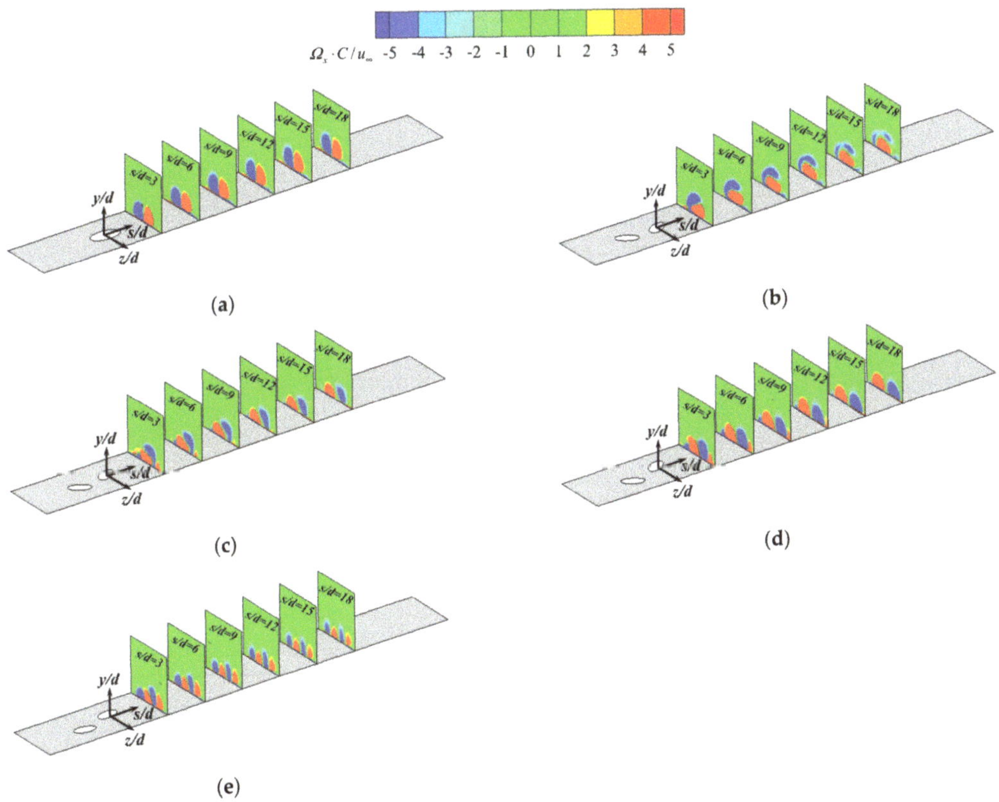

Figure 11. Streamwise vorticity distributions in downstream normal sections for some situations under $M = 1.5$. (**a**) cylindrical hole, (**b**) $Z/d = 0$, $\beta = 29°$, (**c**) $Z/d = 0.5$, $\beta = 29°$, (**d**) $Z/d = 1.0$, $\beta = 29°$, (**e**) $Z/d = 1.0$, $\beta = 11°$.

From the flow dynamics of jet-in-crossflow in the DJFC as mentioned above, it is conjectured that the layout of double jets would significantly affect the DJFC performance. Figure 12 displays the dimensionless temperature contours in downstream normal sections as well as film-cooled surface on the pressure side under $M = 0.5$. At a small blowing ratio, the coolant jet ejecting from cylindrical hole generally demonstrated good attachment on the downstream surface, as displayed in Figure 12a. Therefore, the positive role of the DJFC on suppressing coolant-jet detachment was conjectured to be weakly reflected, although the vortical structures were altered. For the DJFC, when the spanwise spacing in double-jet unit was zero, the coolant jet spreading in spanwise direction as well the film layer coverage was nearly the same as that in the cylindrical hole film cooling, as seen in Figure 12b. With the increase in spanwise spacing in the double-jet unit, the coolant jet spreading in the spanwise direction as well as the film layer coverage on the downstream surface broadened gradually, as demonstrated in Figure 12c,d, so that the positive potential of the DJFC on film cooling enhancement could be realized. Under a large blowing ratio, the single cylindrical hole coolant jet showed a serious detachment on the downstream surface, as displayed in Figure 13a. The DJFC provided dual roles on film cooling enhancement, as demonstrated in Figure 13b–d. On the first aspect, the coolant jet detachment was effectively suppressed. On the second aspect, the cooling film coverage in the lateral direction broadened. In particular, for the double-jet with a larger spanwise spacing, these positive roles were more pronounced due to the significant alteration of vortical structures.

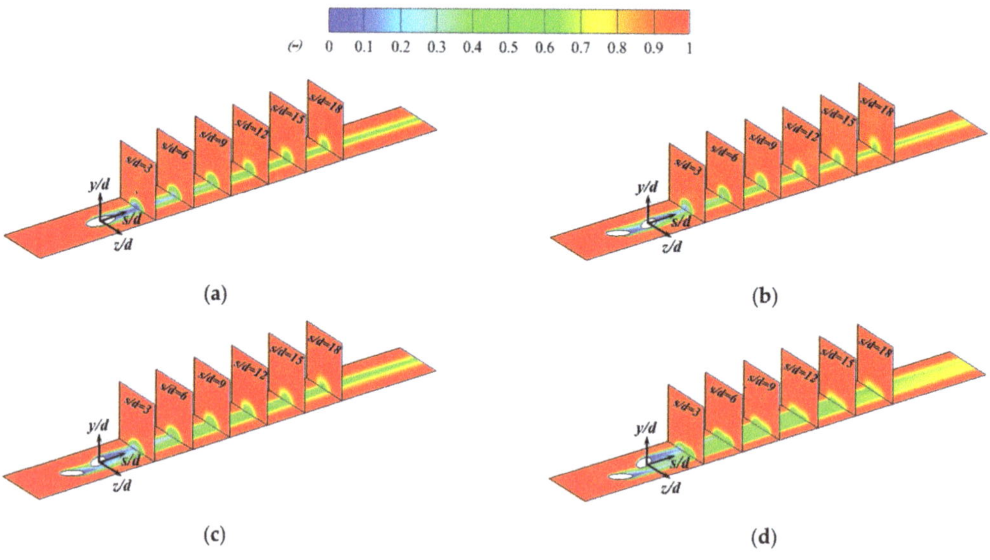

Figure 12. Dimensionless temperature contours in downstream normal sections on the pressure side under $M = 0.5$. (**a**) cylindrical hole, (**b**) $Z/d = 0$, $\beta = 29°$, (**c**) $Z/d = 0.5$, $\beta = 29°$, (**d**) $Z/d = 1.0$, $\beta = 29°$.

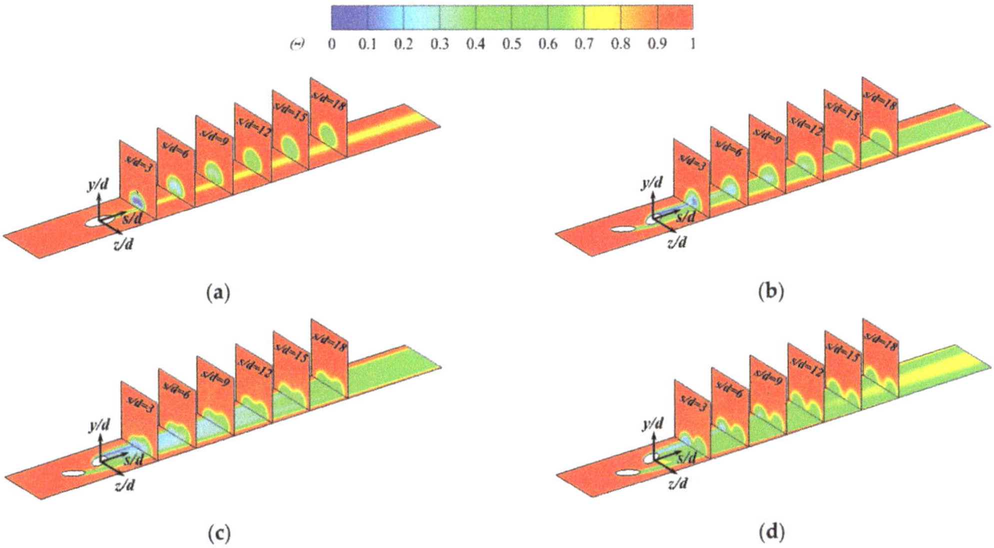

Figure 13. Dimensionless temperature contours in downstream normal sections on the pressure side under $M = 1.5$. (**a**) cylindrical hole, (**b**) $Z/d = 0$, $\beta = 29°$, (**c**) $Z/d = 0.5$, $\beta = 29°$, (**d**) $Z/d = 1.0$, $\beta = 29°$.

Figure 14 presents the effects of spanwise spacing in a double-jet unit on $\eta_{\text{ad,l-av}}$ distribution at the pressure surface, at a specified spanwise injection angle of $\beta = 29°$. Seen from Figure 14, the spanwise spacing in double-jet unit was confirmed to be an extremely important geometric parameter that affects the DJFC performance. At $M = 0.5$, as seen in Figure 14a, an unreasonable layout of double jets would reduce the film cooling effectiveness compared to the cylindrical hole, such as the $Z/d = 0$ case. Under larger blowing ratios, the advantage of double-jet film cooling behaves significantly when compared to the cylindrical hole, owing to its positive roles on preventing the coolant jet detachment from the film-cooled surface and broadening the coolant jet spreading in a spanwise direction. It is also found from Figure 14a that a larger spanwise spacing in the double-jet unit is more favourable under a smaller blowing ratio, by comparing the $Z/d = 0.5$ case and $Z/d = 1.0$ case, but under large blowing ratios, the $Z/d = 0.5$ layout produces stronger film cooling enhancement than the $Z/d = 1.0$ case, as seen in Figure 14c,d. In general, a certain spanwise spacing in the double-jet unit is needed to ensure the formation of anti-vortexes in the downstream flow field. As previously mentioned in Figure 11c,d, the scale of vortices in the situation of $Z/d = 0.5$ and $\beta = 29°$ was smaller than that in the situation of $Z/d = 1.0$ and $\beta = 29°$. Therefore, the film layer in the downstream position was more stable to be weakly destroyed by the hot primary flow invasion in the situation of $Z/d = 0.5$ and $\beta = 29°$ compared to the situation of $Z/d = 1.0$ and $\beta = 29°$, as demonstrated in Figure 15.

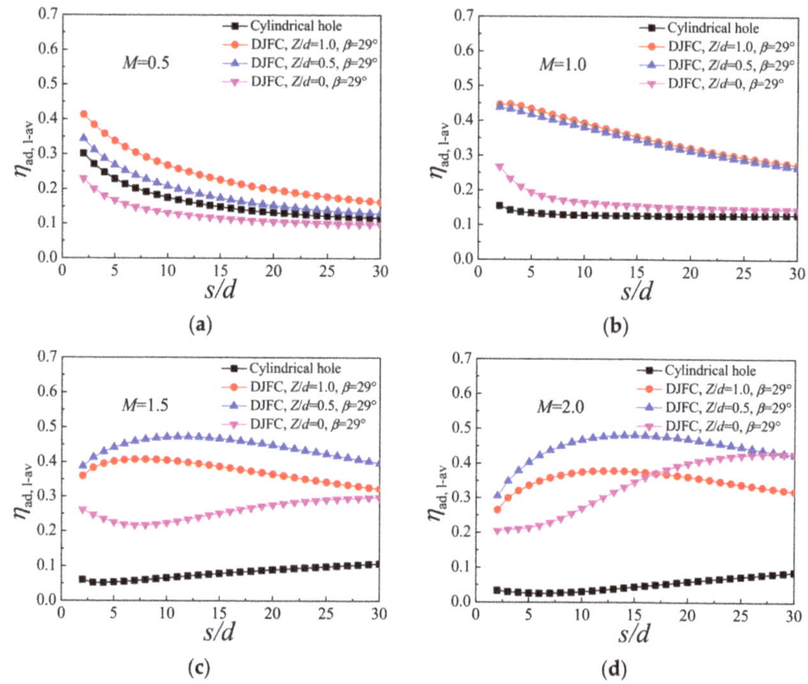

Figure 14. Effect of spanwise spacing on laterally averaged film cooling effectiveness on the pressure surface. (**a**) $M = 0.5$, (**b**) $M = 1.0$, (**c**) $M = 1.5$, (**d**) $M = 2.0$.

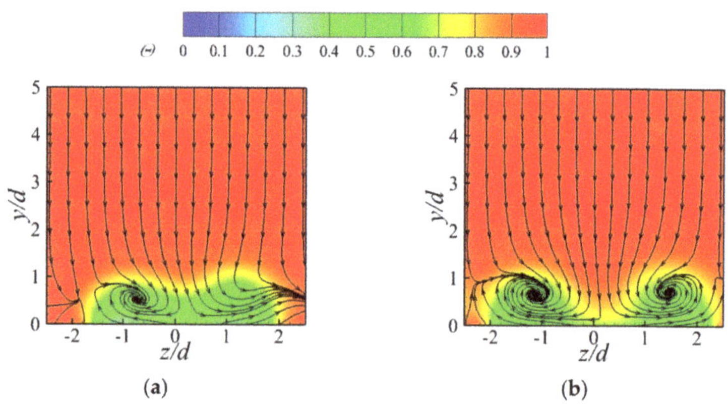

Figure 15. Dimensionless temperature contours and streamlines on a normal section of $s/d = 18$ on the pressure side under $M = 1.5$. (**a**) $Z/d = 0.5$ and $\beta = 29°$, (**b**) $Z/d = 1.0$ and $\beta = 29°$.

Figure 16 shows the influence of spanwise injection angle on $\eta_{ad,l\text{-}av}$ distribution on the pressure surface at a specified spanwise spacing of $Z/d = 1.0$ in the double-jet unit. It was confirmed that η_{ad} was certainly enhanced when the double jets were arranged with a spanwise spacing of $Z/d = 1.0$, regardless of the coolant injection angle. With the increase in the spanwise injection angle in the current range, $\eta_{ad,l\text{-}av}$ increased in general. It was also noted that when the spanwise injection angle increased from $\beta = 23°$ to $\beta = 29°$, the film cooling effectiveness barely improved.

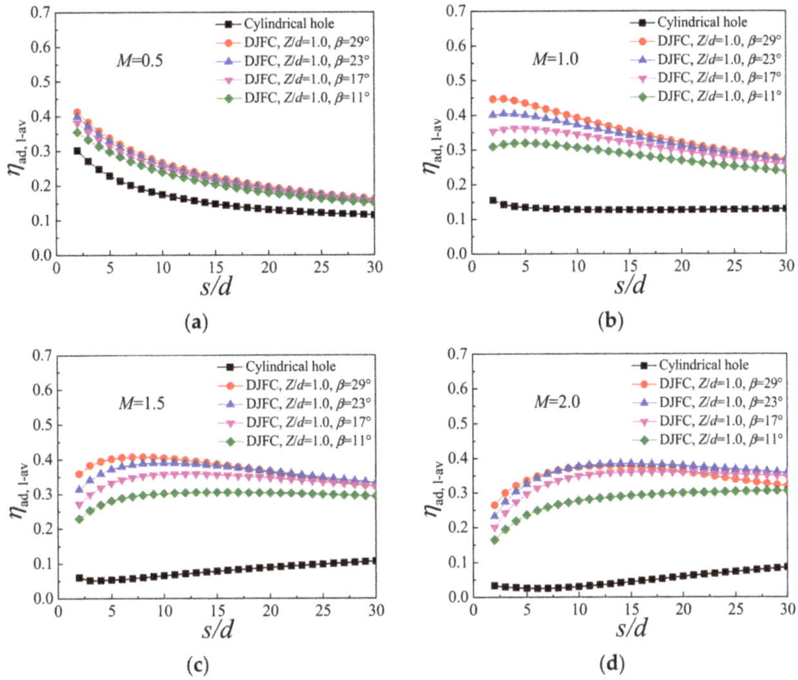

Figure 16. Effect of the spanwise injection angle on laterally averaged film cooling effectiveness on the pressure surface. (**a**) $M = 0.5$, (**b**) $M = 1.0$, (**c**) $M = 1.5$, (**d**) $M = 2.0$.

3.2. DJFC on the Suction Surface

On the suction surface, the DJFC did not show any benefit on film cooling improvement under smaller blowing ratios. Only under larger blowing ratios did its positive potential on film cooling enhancement start to show, as displayed in Figure 17. When compared to Figure 14, it was confirmed that the effect of the double-jet layout on $\eta_{ad,l\text{-}av}$ distribution on the suction surface was similar to that on the pressure surface. That is, a larger spanwise spacing in the double-jet unit generally produced a higher film cooling enhancement. Evaluated under the spatially averaged film cooling effectiveness ($\eta_{ad,s\text{-}av}$) over a specified zone between $s/d = 0$ and $s/d = 30$, a direct comparison is presented here to illustrate the different roles of the DJFC on the suction side and pressure side by selecting the most favourable layout of double jets ($Z/d = 1.0$ and $\beta = 29°$). On the suction side, according to Figure 17, the $\eta_{ad,s\text{-}av}$ for this double-jet film cooling was nearly the same as the baseline cylindrical hole under $M = 0.5$. Under large blowing ratios ($M = 1.5$ and $M = 2.0$), the $\eta_{ad,s\text{-}av}$ increased by about 11–15% by using the double-jet scheme with respect to the baseline cylindrical hole. On the pressure side, according to Figure 14, the $\eta_{ad,s\text{-}av}$ increased by about 12.5% under $M = 0.5$ by using this double-jet layout with respect to the cylindrical hole. This value could reach nearly 300% under large blowing ratios.

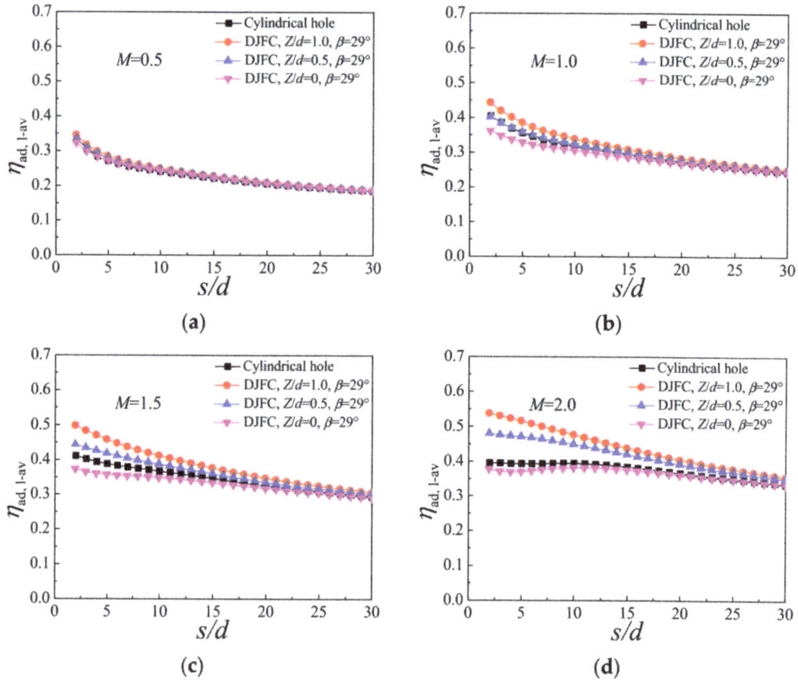

Figure 17. Laterally averaged film cooling effectiveness on the suction surface. (**a**) $M = 0.5$, (**b**) $M = 1.0$, (**c**) $M = 1.5$, (**d**) $M = 2.0$.

It is well known that at the suction side, the mainstream experiences a significant acceleration from the leading edge to the middle chord of the turbine guide vane. Due to this strong acceleration process, the static temperature of oncoming primary flow is reduced and the oncoming flow velocity is increased. Regarding the flow dynamics of jet-in-crossflow for the film cooling hole positioned under such a flow-accelerated circumstance, the normal penetration of coolant jet injection is effectively suppressed. As a consequence, the mutual interaction between double jets would be altered compared to that on the pressure side. Figure 18 displays temperature contours and streamlines in downstream normal sections on the suction side for the DJFC ($Z/d = 1.0$ and $\beta = 29°$) under $M = 1.5$. In the immediate downstream section of $s/d = 3$, only a single pair of counter-rotating vortices is observed, as displayed in Figure 18a. Comparing with Figure 8, wherein the appearance of dual counter-rotating vortex pairs are clearly observed on the pressure side, it is suggested that the merger of vortical structures that originated from double jets would be stronger on the suction side. Figure 19 displays temperature contours and streamlines in downstream normal sections on the suction side for DJFC ($Z/d = 0$ and $\beta = 29°$) under $M = 1.5$. When compared to Figure 18, the main feature of vortical development nearly remained, but the coolant layer was more concentrated in the central zone around $z = 0$ at a small spanwise spacing.

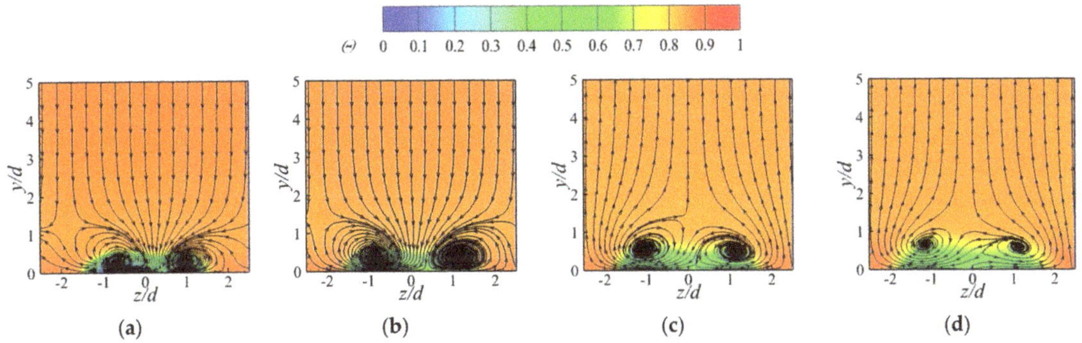

Figure 18. Dimensionless temperature contours and streamlines in downstream normal sections on the suction side for DJFC (Z/d = 1.0 and β = 29°) under M = 1.5. (**a**) s/d = 3, (**b**) s/d = 6, (**c**) s/d = 12, (**d**) s/d = 18.

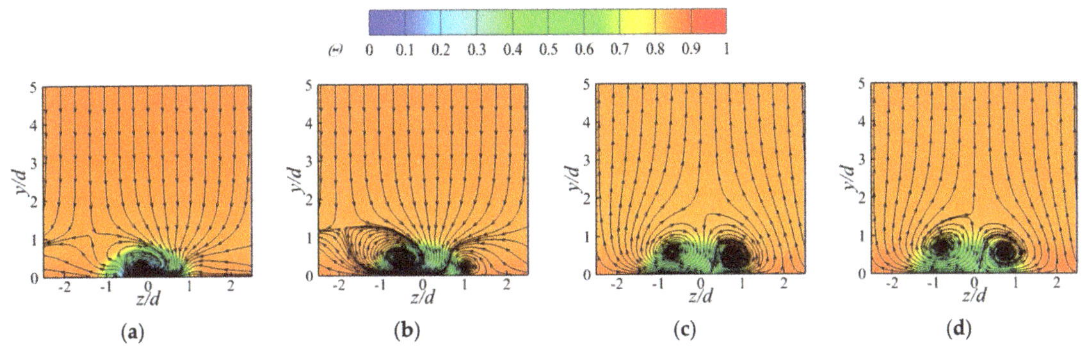

Figure 19. Dimensionless temperature contours and streamlines in downstream normal sections on the suction side for DJFC (Z/d = 0 and β = 29°) under M = 1.5. (**a**) s/d = 3, (**b**) s/d = 6, (**c**) s/d = 12, (**d**) s/d = 18.

Figure 20 displays the dimensionless temperature contours in downstream normal sections as well as the film-cooled surface on the suction side under M = 1.5. As seen in Figure 20a, the cylindrical hole the film layer is well attached to the downstream surface, without the appearance of serious detachment as occurred on the pressure side. This is the main reason for the positive potential of the DJFC in improving film-cooling behavior more significantly on the pressure surface when compared to the suction surface. In particular, as the coolant jet detachment could be suppressed well on the suction side, the main role of the DJFC on film cooling enhancement should rely on the improvement of the spanwise spreading of coolant jets and subsequent film layer coverage in the spanwise direction. For the DJFC, when the spanwise spacing in double-jet unit was zero, the film layer coverage was nearly the same as that in the cylindrical hole film cooling, as seen in Figure 20b. With the increase in spanwise spacing in the double-jet unit, the film layer coverage on downstream surface broadened, as demonstrated in Figure 20d, so that the positive potential of the DJFC on film cooling enhancement was realized.

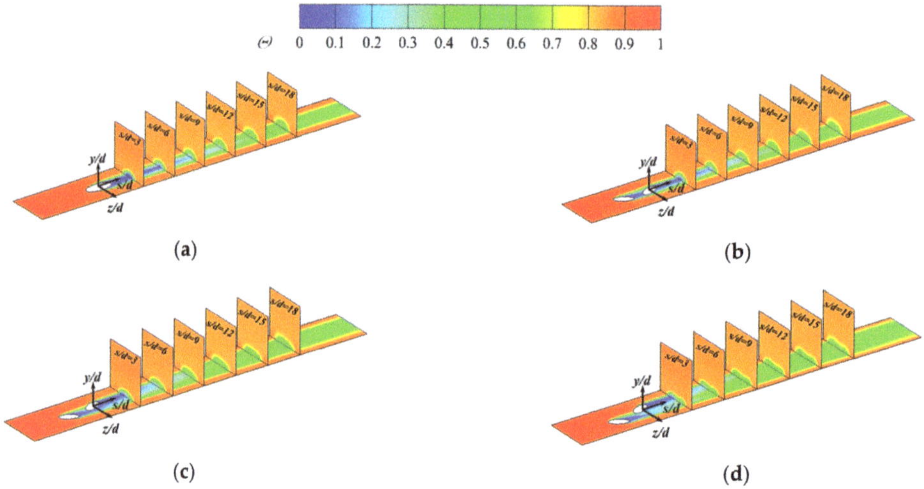

Figure 20. Dimensionless temperature contours in downstream normal sections on the suction side under $M = 1.5$. (**a**) cylindrical hole, (**b**) $Z/d = 0$, $\beta = 29°$, (**c**) $Z/d = 0.5$, $\beta = 29°$, (**d**) $Z/d = 1.0$, $\beta = 29°$.

Figure 21 presents the local η_{ad} distribution on the guide vane surface for a specific double-jet layout with $\beta = 23°$ and $Z/d = 1.0$. While the blowing ratio increases, the coverage of the cooling jet on film-cooled surface expands in the spanwise direction, either on the pressure surface or suction surface. By comparing the η_{ad} on the turbine surfaces, it can be seen that the coolant jet ejecting from DJFC holes had a stronger downward tracing capacity on the pressure surface compared to the suction surface.

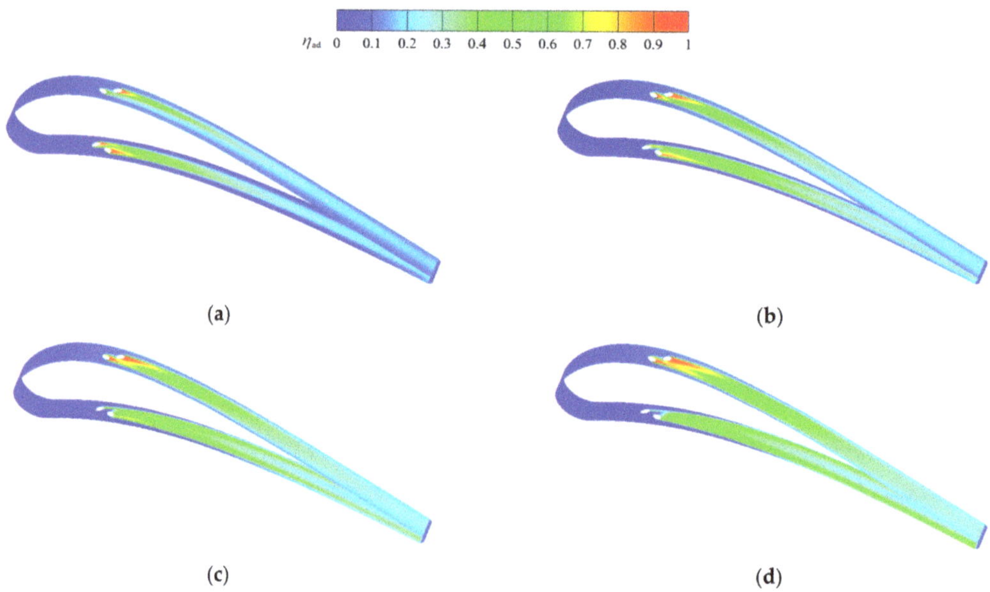

Figure 21. Local film cooling effectiveness distribution on the guide vane surface for DJFC with $\beta = 23°$ and $Z/d = 1.0$. (**a**) $M = 0.5$, (**b**) $M = 1.0$, (**c**) $M = 1.5$, (**d**) $M = 2.0$.

4. Conclusions

This paper presents a numerical study to research the film cooling performance of a single line double-jet unit on a turbine guide vane under high-temperature and high-pressure conditions. The double-jet unit was positioned at an axial location of 57% C_x on the suction surface or 28% C_x on the pressure surface apart from the leading edge of guide vane. Four spanwise injection angles ($\beta = 11°, 17°, 23°$, and 29°) and three spanwise spacings in the double-jet unit ($Z/d = 0, 0.5$, and 1.0) were taken into consideration. According to the current research, the conclusions are deduced as the follows.

(1) The layout of double jets affects the mutual interaction between adjacent jets and subsequently changes the jet-in-crossflow dynamics. Relative to the spanwise injection angle, the spanwise spacing in the double-jet unit is a more important geometric parameter that affects the vortical structures in the downstream flow field. In particular, a certain spanwise spacing in the double-jet unit is needed for producing stronger anti-kidney vortices and better film cooling performance. By increasing the spanwise injection angle and spanwise spacing in double-jet unit, the film cooling effectiveness is improved in general.

(2) On the suction surface, the DJFC does not show any benefit on film cooling improvement under smaller blowing ratios. Only under larger blowing ratios does its positive potential on film cooling enhancement start to show. When compared to the suction surface, the positive potential of the DJFC on improving film cooling behaves significantly on the pressure surface, especially under large blowing ratios. In the viewing of spatially-averaged film cooling effectiveness over a specified zone between $s/d = 0$ and $s/d = 30$, an increase of about 11~15% is achieved by the most favorable double-jet layout on the suction surface with respect to the cylindrical hole under large blowing ratios, while on the pressure side, this value could reach nearly 300%.

(3) On the pressure side, dual roles of the DJFC on film cooling enhancement are identified under large blowing ratios. On the first aspect, the coolant jet detachment is effectively suppressed. On the second aspect, the coolant jet spread in a spanwise direction is broadened, while under small blowing ratios, the film cooling enhancement with the use of the DJFC on the pressure side mainly relies on the second role. With regard to the DJFC on the suction surface, its main role in film cooling enhancement relies on the improvement of the spanwise film layer coverage on the film-cooled surface

Author Contributions: Computation and writing—original draft preparation, J.H.; methodology and formal analysis, funding acquisition, C.W.; supervision, Y.S.; funding acquisition, J.Z. All authors have read and agreed to the published version of the manuscript.

Funding: This research was funded by the Fundamental Research Funds of the Central Universities, grant number NS2020013; the National Natural Science Foundation of China, grant number U1508212; the National Science and Technology Major Project, grant number J2019-III-0019-0063.

Conflicts of Interest: The authors declare no conflict of interest.

Nomenclature

C	chord length (m)
C_p	static pressure coefficient
C_x	axial chord length (m)
d	film hole diameter (m)
H	segment height of guide vane (m)
M	nominal blowing ratio
m	mass flow-rate (kg/s)
P	hole-to-hole pitch (m)
P_{vane}	cascade pitch (m)
p	static pressure (Pa)
Re	Reynolds number
s	streamwise direction
T	temperature (K)

t	film hole height (m)
u	velocity (m/s)
X	streamwise spacing between double jets (m)
x	axial direction
y	normal direction
Z	spanwise spacing between double jets (m)
z	lateral or spanwise direction
Greek Letters	
α	streamwise injection angle (°)
β	lateral injection angle (°)
η	film cooling effectiveness
ϕ	inflow angle of vane (°)
μ	dynamic viscosity ($N \cdot s/m^2$)
θ	orientation angle of vane (°)
ρ	density (kg/m^3)
ω	vorticity (1/s)
Θ	dimensionless temperature
Subscripts	
ad	adiabatic
aw	adiabatic wall
c	coolant or secondary flow
l-av	laterally-averaged
s-av	spatially-averaged
s	static condition
t	total condition
∞	primary flow

References

1. Bogard, D.G.; Thole, K.A. Gas turbine film cooling. *AIAA J. Propul. Power* **2006**, *22*, 249–269. [CrossRef]
2. Acharya, S.; Kanani, Y. Advances in film cooling heat transfer. *Adv. Heat Transfer* **2017**, *49*, 91–156.
3. Zhang, J.Z.; Zhang, S.C.; Wang, C.H.; Tan, X.M. Recent advances in film cooling enhancement: A review. *Chin. J. Aeronaut.* **2020**, *33*, 1119–1136. [CrossRef]
4. Bunker, R.S. A review of turbine shaped film cooling technology. *ASME J. Heat Transfer* **2005**, *127*, 441–453. [CrossRef]
5. Goldstein, R.J.; Eckert, E.R.G.; Burggraf, F. Effects of hole geometry and density on three-dimensional film cooling. *Int. J. Heat Mass Transfer* **1974**, *17*, 595–607. [CrossRef]
6. Thole, K.A.; Gritsch, M.; Schulz, A.; Wittig, S. Flowfield measurements for film-cooling holes with expanded exits. *ASME J. Turbomach.* **1998**, *120*, 327–336. [CrossRef]
7. Gritsch, M.; Schulz, A.; Wittig, S. Adiabatic wall effectiveness measurements of film-cooling holes with expanded exit. *ASME J. Turbomach.* **1998**, *120*, 549–556. [CrossRef]
8. Gritsch, M.; Colban, W.; Schar, H. Effect of hole geometry on the thermal performance of fan-shaped film cooling holes. *ASME J. Turbomach.* **2005**, *127*, 718–725. [CrossRef]
9. Lee, K.D.; Kim, K.Y. Shape optimization of a fan-shaped hole to enhance film-cooling effectiveness. *Int. J. Heat Mass Transfer* **2010**, *53*, 2996–3005. [CrossRef]
10. Saumweber, C.; Schulz, A. Effect of geometry variations on the cooling performance of fan-shaped cooling holes. *ASME J. Turbomach.* **2012**, *134*, 061008. [CrossRef]
11. Huang, Y.; Zhang, J.Z.; Wang, C.H.; Zhu, X.D. Multi-objective optimization of laidback fan-shaped film cooling hole on turbine vane suction surface. *Heat Mass Transfer* **2019**, *55*, 1181–1194. [CrossRef]
12. Lenzi, T.; Picchi, A.; Bacci, T.; Andreini, A.; Faccini, B. Unsteady flow field characterization of effusion cooling systems with swirling main flow: Comparison between cylindrical and shaped holes. *Energies* **2020**, *13*, 4993. [CrossRef]
13. Kim, Y.S.; Jeong, J.Y.; Kwak, J.S.; Chung, H. The effects of hole arrangement and density ratio on the heat transfer coefficient augmentation of fan-shaped film cooling holes. *Energies* **2021**, *14*, 186. [CrossRef]
14. Baek, S., II; Ryu, J.; Ahn, J. Large eddy simulation of film cooling with forward expansion hole: Comparative study with LES and RANS simulations. *Energies* **2021**, *14*, 2063. [CrossRef]
15. Lee, S.I.; Jung, J.Y.; Song, Y.J.; Kwak, J.S. Effect of mainstream velocity on the optimization of a fan-shaped film-cooing hole on a flat plate. *Energies* **2021**, *14*, 3573. [CrossRef]
16. Okita, Y.; Nishiura, M. Film effectiveness performance of an arrowhead-shaped film-cooling hole geometry. *ASME J. Turbomach.* **2007**, *129*, 331–339. [CrossRef]

17. Kusterer, K.; Elyas, A.; Bohn, D.; Sugimoto, T.; Tanaka, R.; Kazari, M. The NEKOMIMI cooling technology: Cooling holes with ears for high-efficient film cooling. In Proceedings of the ASME Turbo Expo 2011, GT2011-45524, Vancouver, BC, Canada, 6–10 June 2011.
18. Dai, P.; Lin, F. Numerical study on film cooling effectiveness from shaped and crescent holes. *Heat Mass Transfer* **2011**, *47*, 147–154. [CrossRef]
19. Kim, S.M.; Lee, K.D.; Kim, K.Y. A comparative analysis of various shaped film-cooling holes. *Heat Mass Transfer* **2012**, *48*, 1929–1939. [CrossRef]
20. Yang, C.F.; Zhang, J.Z. Experimental investigation on film cooling characteristics from a row of holes with ridge-shaped tabs. *Exp. Therm. Fluid Sci.* **2012**, *37*, 113–120. [CrossRef]
21. Ramesh, S.; Ramirez, D.G.; Ekkad, S.V.; Alvin, M.A. Analysis of film cooling performance of advanced tripod hole geometries with and without manufacturing features. *Int. J. Heat Mass Transfer* **2016**, *94*, 9–19. [CrossRef]
22. Zhang, J.Z.; Zhu, X.D.; Huang, Y.; Wang, C.H. Investigation on film cooling performance from a row of round-to-slot holes on flat plate. *Int. J. Therm. Sci.* **2017**, *118*, 207–225. [CrossRef]
23. Kusterer, K.; Bohn, D.; Sugimoto, T.; Tanaka, R. Double-jet ejection of cooling air for improved film cooling. *ASME J. Turbomach.* **2007**, *129*, 809–815. [CrossRef]
24. Kusterer, K.; Bohn, D.; Sugimoto, T.; Tanaka, R. Influence of blowing ratio on the double-jet ejection of cooling air. In Proceedings of the ASME Turbo Expo 2007, GT2007-27301, Montreal, QE, Canada, 14–17 May 2007.
25. Kusterer, K.; Elyas, A.; Bohn, D.; Sugimoto, T.; Tanaka, R. Double-jet film-cooling for highly efficient film-cooling with low blowing ratios. In Proceedings of the ASME Turbo Expo 2008, GT2008-50073, Berlin, Germany, 9–13 June 2008.
26. Kusterer, K.; Elyas, A.; Bohn, D.; Sugimoto, T.; Tanaka, R.; Kazari, M. A parametric study on the influence of the lateral ejection angle of double-jet holes on the film cooling effectiveness for high blowing ratios. In Proceedings of the ASME Turbo Expo 2009, GT2009-59321, Orlando, FL, USA, 8–12 June 2009.
27. Wang, Z.; Liu, J.J.; An, B.T.; Zhang, C. Effects of axial row spacing for double-jet film-cooling on the cooling effectiveness. In Proceedings of the ASME Turbo Expo 2011, GT2011-46055, Vancouver, BC, Canada, 6–10 June 2011.
28. Han, C.; Ren, J.; Jiang, H.D. Multi-parameter influence on combined-hole film cooling system. *Int. J. Heat Mass Transfer* **2012**, *55*, 4232–4240. [CrossRef]
29. Choi, D.W.; Lee, K.D.; Kim, K.Y. Analysis and optimization of double-jet film-cooling holes. *J. Thermophy. Heat Transfer* **2013**, *27*, 246–254. [CrossRef]
30. Lee, K.D.; Choi, D.W.; Kim, K.Y. Optimization of ejection angles of double-jet film-cooling holes using RBNN model. *Int. J. Therm. Sci.* **2013**, *73*, 69–78. [CrossRef]
31. Khalatov, A.A.; Borisov, I.I.; Dashevsky, Y.J.; Panchenko, N.A.; Kovalenko, A.S. Flat-plate film cooling from a double jet holes: Influence of free-stream turbulence and flow acceleration. *Thermphy. Aeromech.* **2014**, *21*, 545–552. [CrossRef]
32. Graf, L.; Kleiser, L. Film cooling using antikidney vortex pairs: Effects of blowing conditions and yaw angle on cooling and losses. *ASME J. Turbomach.* **2014**, *136*, 011008. [CrossRef]
33. Yao, J.X.; Xu, J.; Zhang, K.; Lei, J.; Wright, L.M. Interaction of flow and film-cooling effectiveness between double-jet film-cooling holes with various spanwise distances. *ASME J. Turbomach.* **2018**, *140*, 121011. [CrossRef]
34. Yao, J.X.; Zhang, K.; Wu, J.M.; Lei, J.; Fang, Y.; Wright, L.M. An experimental investigation on streamwise distance and density ratio effects on double-jet film-cooling. *Appl. Therm. Eng.* **2019**, *156*, 410–421. [CrossRef]
35. He, J.H.; Yao, J.X.; Yang, X.; Duan, J.T.; Lei, J.; Xie, G.N. Effects of mainstream attack angle on film cooling effectiveness of double-jet film-cooling. *Int. J. Therm. Sci.* **2020**, *149*, 106183. [CrossRef]
36. Liao, G.L.; Wang, J.J.; Li, J.; Zhang, F. Effects of curvature on the film cooling effectiveness of double-jet film cooling. In Proceedings of the ASME Turbo Expo 2014, GT2014-26263, Dusseldorf, Germany, 16–20 June 2014.
37. Zhu, X.D.; Zhang, J.Z.; Tan, X.M. Numerical assessment of round-to-slot film cooling performances on a turbine blade under engine representative conditions. *Int. Commun. Heat Mass Transfer* **2019**, *100*, 98–110. [CrossRef]
38. Ragab, K.E.; El-Gabry, L. Heat transfer analysis of the surface of nonfilm-cooled and film-cooled nozzle guide vanes in transonic annular cascade. In Proceedings of the ASME Turbo Expo 2017, GT2017-64982, Charlotte, NC, USA, 26–30 June 2017.
39. ANSYS. *Fluent 14.0 User's Guide*; ANSYS Inc.: Canonsburg, PA, USA, 2012.
40. Ely, M.J.; Jubran, B.J. A numerical evaluation on the effect of sister holes on film cooling effectiveness and the surrounding flow filed. *Heat Mass Transfer* **2009**, *45*, 1435–1446. [CrossRef]
41. Silieti, M.; Kassab, A.J.; Divo, E. Film cooling effectiveness: Comparison of adiabatic and conjugate heat transfer CFD models. *Int. J. Therm. Sci.* **2009**, *48*, 2237–2248. [CrossRef]
42. Balasubramaniyan, S.; Jubran, B.A. Numerical analysis of film cooling from micro-hole. *Heat Mass Transfer* **2015**, *51*, 1277–1285. [CrossRef]
43. Zhu, R.; Simon, T.W.; Xie, G.N. Influence of secondary hole injection angle on enhancement of film cooling effectiveness with horn-shaped or cylindrical primary holes. *Num. Heat Transfer Part A* **2018**, *74*, 1207–1227. [CrossRef]
44. Celik, I.B.; Ghia, U.; Roache, P.J.; Freitas, C.J.; Coleman, H.; Raad, P.E. Procedure for estimation and reporting of uncertainty due to discretization in CFD applications. *ASME J. Fluids Eng.* **2008**, *130*, 0780011.
45. Dees, J.E.; Bogard, D.G.; Laskowski, G.M. Experimental measurements and computational predictions for an internally cooled simulated turbine vane. *ASME J. Turbomach.* **2012**, *134*, 061003. [CrossRef]

46. Dittmar, J.; Schulz, A.; Wittig, S. Adiabatic effectiveness and heat transfer coefficient of shaped film cooling holes on a scaled guide vane pressure side model. *Int. J. Rotating Mach.* **2004**, *10*, 345–354. [CrossRef]
47. Yao, J.X.; Su, P.F.; He, J.H.; Wu, J.M.; Lei, J.; Fang, Y. Experimental and numerical investigations on double-jet film-cooling with different mainstream incidence angles. *Appl. Therm. Eng.* **2020**, *166*, 114737. [CrossRef]

buildings

Article

Investigation of the Mechanical, Microstructure and 3D Fractal Analysis of Nanocalcite-Modified Environmentally Friendly and Sustainable Cementitious Composites

Mahmoud Ziada [1], Yosra Tammam [2], Savaş Erdem [1,*] and Roberto Alonso González Lezcano [3,*]

1 Avcilar Campus, School of Civil Engineering, Istanbul University-Cerrahpasa, Istanbul 34200, Turkey; m.ziada@ogr.iu.edu.tr
2 Civil Engineering Department, Avcilar Campus, Istanbul Gelisim University, Istanbul 34200, Turkey; yosra.tammam@ogr.iu.edu.tr
3 Architecture and Design Department, Escuela Politécnica Superior, Universidad CEU San Pablo, 28668 Madrid, Spain
* Correspondence: savas.erdem@iuc.edu.tr (S.E.); rgonzalezcano@ceu.es (R.A.G.L.)

Abstract: Unlike conventional concrete materials, Engineered Cementitious Composites (ECC) use a micromechanics-based design theory in the material design process. Recently, the use of nanoparticles in various concretes and mortars has increased. This study used nanocalcite to investigate the mechanical, microstructural fractal analysis of environmentally friendly nanocalcite-doped ECC (NCa-ECC). This paper investigated the effects of nanocalcite (NCa) with different contents (0.5, 1, and 1.5% by mass of binder) on the mechanical properties of engineered cementitious composites (ECC). For this purpose, compressive strength, ultrasonic pulse velocity (UPV), and flexural strength tests were conducted to investigate the mechanical properties of the ECC series. In addition, SEM analyses were carried out to investigate the microstructural properties of the ECC series. The content of nanocalcite improved the mechanical and microstructural properties of the nanocalcite-modified ECC series. In addition, the 1 NCa series (1% nanocalcite modified to the mass of the binder) had the best performance among the series used in this study.

Keywords: nanocalcite; environmentally friendly cementitious composite; mechanical properties; microstructure analysis; 3D fractal analysis; sustainability; fly ash

Citation: Ziada, M.; Tammam, Y.; Erdem, S.; Lezcano, R.A.G. Investigation of the Mechanical, Microstructure and 3D Fractal Analysis of Nanocalcite-Modified Environmentally Friendly and Sustainable Cementitious Composites. *Buildings* **2022**, *12*, 36. https://doi.org/10.3390/buildings12010036

Academic Editor: Chiara Bedon

Received: 19 November 2021
Accepted: 22 December 2021
Published: 2 January 2022

1. Introduction

Cementitious materials perform a necessary part in the construction sector and are therefore of paramount importance to improve their durability and mechanical characteristics [1–5]. Because of recent characterization technology progress, the characteristics of all these synthetic structures may be examined on a variety of length scales ranging from nano to macro [6–8]. Thus, cement materials' structure and behavior patterns at the sub-micrometer scale are better understood, which has improved their macro-properties [9]. For example, the durability can be improved by reducing the cement paste's total porosity by inserting additives in a range of pores primarily present at a micrometer length scale [10–12]. The studies performed on environmentally friendly and sustainable composites recently have gained importance. Tosee et al. [13] investigated the compressive strength of environmentally friendly concrete modified with eggshell powder using the hybrid ANN-SFL optimization algorithm. They found that the highest compressive strength was obtained for the samples containing 7–9% of eggshell powder and it was 55% higher than their control samples. Ziada et al. [14] produced environmentally friendly fly ash-based and basalt powder waste-filled sustainable geopolymer mortar with basalt fiber. They found that the produced sustainable mortar had high strength and durability properties and the use of 1.2% of basalt fiber increased samples' compressive strength by up to 18%

and flexural strength by up to 44%. Şahmaran et al. [15] produced ECC mixes with various FA/PC ratios (1.2, 2.2, and 4.2). They found that the increase of FA content in ECC specimens exhibit more ductile behavior.

Ultra-high-molecular-weight polyethylene, carbon, and high-modulus polyvinyl alcohol (PVA) fibers are now used in cement-based products. PVA fibers are widely used because the first two fibers are too costly to be commonly used [16–18]. The modification of fibers in cement-based materials focuses on increasing toughness [19,20]. Overall, using fiber improves interfacial adhesion. However, this enhances the bridging result between such fiber and the interface, and it overlooks the influence of sliding friction on fracture energy. When fibers are detached, the increased bond strength at the interface causes a large amount of fracture energy to be generated quickly, raising the potential of brittle fracture [21]. Previous articles had improved the toughness of concrete by altering the content of cementitious composites, such as micro compounding, in which certain microscale particles are added to the concrete mix to increase the toughness of the concrete [22,23].

Unlike conventional concrete materials, Engineered Cementitious Composites (ECC) use a micromechanics-based design theory in the material design process. In a single tensile loading, PVA-ECC has tight and multiple cracking behaviors. The intrinsically cracking width of less than 100 mm is high ductility and improved durability [24]. The tensile strain capacity for PVA-ECC over five percent was demonstrated using commonly available materials and equipment in the concrete manufacturing sector [25]. Li et al. [26] found that the fiber volume should not be more than 2% to ensure good performance in ECC blends. Due to their composite performance and economic considerations, PVA fibers are among the types of fibers used by ECC and the other high performance cementitious composites [27–31].

Nanomaterials have been demonstrated to enhance the interfacial transition area of structures by speeding up the hydration reaction, considerably improving the porosity and durability of the hardened cement-based mixtures [32]. Furthermore, the addition of nanoparticles generally increase the matrix fracture toughness due to the shielding effect on the crack tip and improves the multiple cracking behavior of engineered cementitious composites by making the fiber distribution more homogenous [25]. Among the nanoparticles, nano-$CaCO_3$ is one of the most used nanoparticles in cementitious composites [33]. The most stable shape of naturally abundant inorganic Calcium Carbonate ($CaCO_3$) material in nature is nanocalcite. Calcium Carbonate ($CaCO_3$) is immaculate, crystalline, and highly transparent. Nanocalcite offers advantages in addition to its excellent functions, such as enhancing resilience and rigidity, providing perfect stability and insulation in electricity.

The fracture surface morphology of cementitious materials resulting from crack propagation under loading would explain the differences in the mechanical behavior and the corresponding failure mode [34,35]. It is well established that several parameters control the roughness and texture of the fracture surface of the cementitious composite. The meandering of main crack (for example, tortuous or much less tortuous fracture surfaces) is considerably influenced by the use of micro and nano additives, properties of aggregate particles, and the concrete mix design [36]. Beginning with the pioneering work by Mandelbrot [37], the concept of fractal geometry and fractal dimension has become popular in construction technology and associated materials to better understand the relationship between the flexural response and the tortuosity of fracture surface in ECC [33] and for the design multiscale reinforcing fibers of composite materials [38].

The literature review above clearly indicates that research in this field has generally focused on evaluating strength properties, durability-related behavior, and thermo-mechanical performance at a macro level. However, research conducted thus far is still less to comprehensively evaluate the microstructure-associated mechanical and fracture characterization of engineered cementitious mixes modified with nanocalcite and 3D fractal characterization. This leads to the aim of this study, which is to analyze the mechanical performance and micro-structural damage characteristics of nano-modified ECC mixes and to improve the toughness, the multiple cracking behavior and the strength of the strain hardening ECC composites for the development of super infrastructures, which are driven to attain higher strength and higher toughness. In this study, the effects of nanocalcite on ECC's mechanical and microstructural properties are investigated by modifying nanocalcite with 0%, 1%, and 1.5% mass of binder. Compressive strength, flexural tensile strength, and ultrasonic pulse velocity (UPV) tests were performed to investigate nano-modified ECC mixtures' mechanical and physical properties. In addition, scanning electron microscopy (SEM) and 3D fractal analysis were performed to examine the microstructural and crack analysis of the samples.

2. Materials and Methods

2.1. Materials and Mixing Procedures

CEM I 42.5N Portland cement, fly ash (Class F), silica sand, water, high-range water-reducing admixture (HRWRA), and polyvinyl alcohol (PVA) fibers were used to prepare the ECC samples. The chemical and physical properties of the binder (Portland cement and fly ash) and filler (silica sand) are listed in Tables 1 and 2, respectively. In addition, the mixing ratios of the blends are listed in Table 3. Ding et al. [39] replaced the NCa material with Portland cement by 0%, 1%, 2%, 3% ratios to obtain nano-$CaCO_3$ modified ultra-high performance engineered cementitious composites mixes. In this study, the NCa was replaced with the binder by 0%, 0.5%, 1%, 1.5% ratios. Figure 1 shows the used nanocalcite materials and PVA fibers. In the mixing phase, the Portland cement (PC), fly ash (FA), and silica sand were dry blended for 3 min in a mixer. After that, HRWRA and dissolved water were added and mixed for another 5 min. Then, PVA fibers were added into the fresh mortar until it was homogeneous. Finally, nanocalcite was added with 0.5, 1, and 1.5 ratios and mixed homogeneously. The nanocalcite used in this study is white, with a purity of 99.9% and an average particle size of 900 nm. The freshly prepared mixture was poured into 15 × 50 × 350 mm molds and 50 × 50 × 50 mm cubic molds, and then these molds were covered with a plastic sheet. The specimens were cured at 23 °C. Figure 2 shows poured fresh nanocalcite-doped ECC samples.

Table 1. Chemical properties of binder and filler materials (% by weight).

Binder and Filler Materials Used	Na_2O	K_2O	MgO	CaO	Fe_2O_3	SiO_2	Al_2O_3	LOI
FA	0.7	1.9	1.7	3.5	5.5	61.1	21.8	1.58
PC	0.2	0.8	2.5	61.3	3.34	20.80	5.50	2.22
Sand	0.021	0.011	0.011	0.022	0.022	99.80	0.062	0.075

Table 2. Physical properties of binder and filler materials.

Binder and Filler Materials Used	Specific Gravity	BF (m^2/kg)
FA	2.11	292
PC	3.065	326
Sand	2.65	-

Table 3. Mixture ratios of nanocalcite-doped ECC series.

Mixture ID.	PC	W/B [1]	PVA (vol.%)	FA/PC	NCa/B [1] (%)	Sand/PC	HRWRA (kg/m^3)
0 NCa	1	0.25	2	1.25	-	0.82	5.50
0.5 NCa	1	0.25	2	1.25	0.5	0.82	5.55
1 NCa	1	0.25	2	1.25	1	0.82	5.60
1.5 NCa	1	0.25	2	1.25	1.5	0.82	5.65

[1] B: Binder materials (PC + FA).

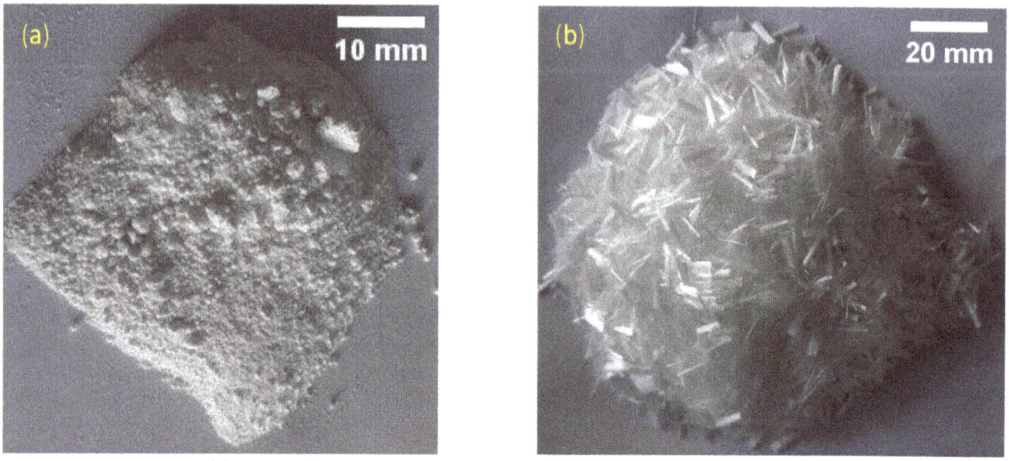

(a) (b)

Figure 1. (**a**) Nanocalcite materials (**b**) PVA fiber.

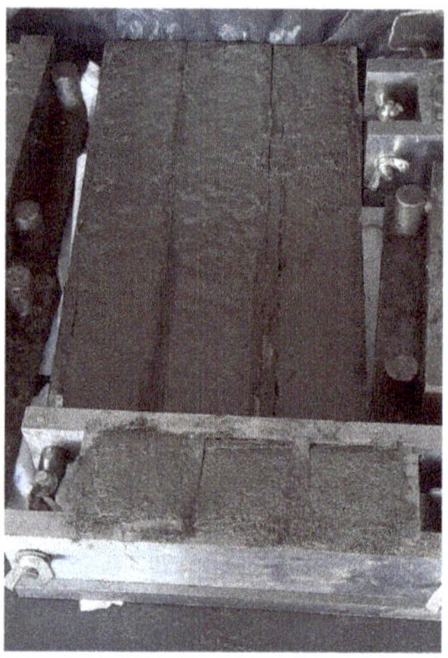

Figure 2. Poured fresh nanocalcite-doped ECC samples.

2.2. Performed Tests and Specimens

In this study, compressive strength, flexural strength, and UPV tests were performed on NCa-ECC specimens. Then, 3D fractal analysis was conducted. Finally, the microstructure of the specimens was investigated using SEM analysis. First, the ultrasonic pulse velocity (UPV) was tested according to ASTM C 597 to determine the UPV values of three 50 × 50 × 50 mm cube samples for each series after 28 days [40]. Then, 50 × 50 × 50 mm cube specimens were placed in a compressive strength testing machine with a capacity of 2000 kN and subjected to compression at a rate of 0.602 MPa/s. Factors such as loading speed, size, and age of the samples were entered into the pressure machine before loading to obtain compressive strength values automatically. Thus, the compressive strength test was performed on three cubes of each series according to ASTM C109 [41]. The flowability of the fresh mixtures was tested according to ASTM C230 [42]. The spreading diameter of the mixtures obtained from this experiment was equal and measured approximately 210 mm. Thus, the fresh mixtures given in Table 3 showed good fluidity without segregation.

In this study, the flexural strength test was performed on 15 × 50 × 350 mm samples to obtain flexural strength, mid-span displacement, strain, and stress-deflection curves according to ASTM C348 [43]. For this proposal, a closed-loop controlled universal testing machine (Figure 3) with a loading rate of 0.003 mm/s was used. Three samples were used for each series, and the average results of the samples were obtained. The flexural stress-deflection curves were obtained using flexural strength values and deflections, recorded by the computer data recording system on the testing machine. Erdem and Gurbuz [44] performed a similar test on hybrid fiber reinforced engineered cementitious specimens.

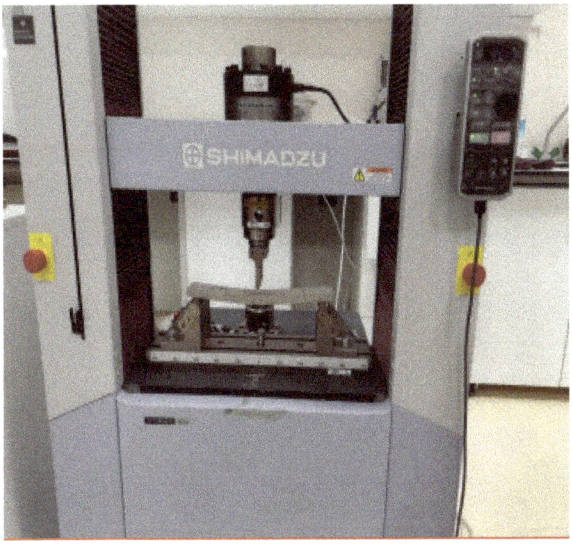

Figure 3. The flexural test set-up.

Figure 4 shows the multiple cracks formed in the samples subjected to the flexural strength test. The crack of the prismatic sample was obtained using a 40× magnification microscope to observe the PVA inside the crack. Figure 5. shows the crack of the sample subjected to the flexural test at 40× magnification. After the strength tests, small pieces of the specimen were taken and subjected to SEM. The microstructure of the samples was studied using SEM analysis.

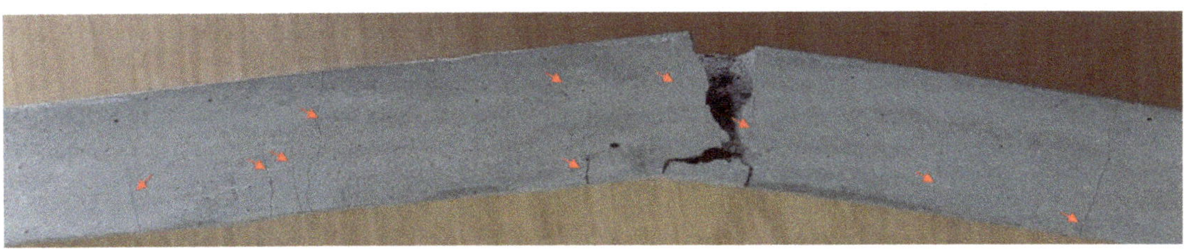

(a)

Figure 4. *Cont.*

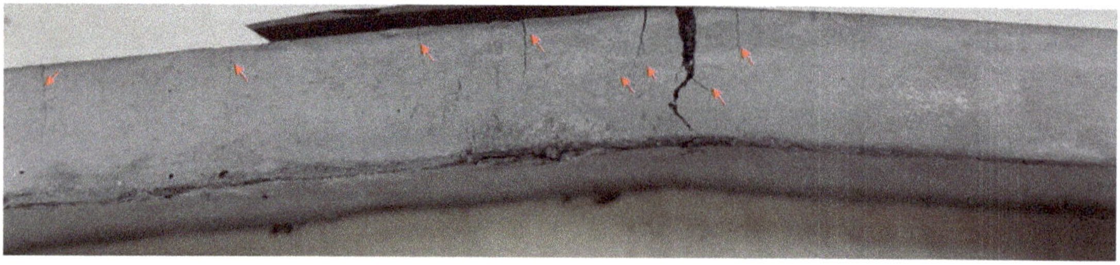

(b)

Figure 4. The specimens were subjected to the flexural strength test. (a) 0 NCa; (b) 1 NCa.

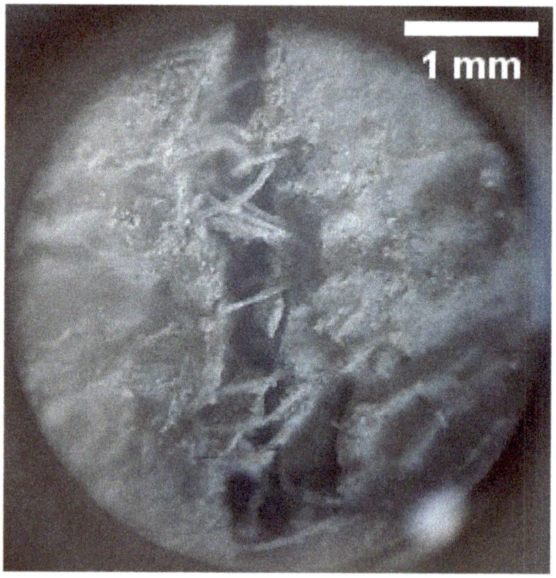

Figure 5. The appearance of a crack in a specimen subjected to the flexural test at 40× magnification.

In addition, following the flexural tensile tests, the fractal dimensions of cracks were determined. Images of the samples after the flexural testing were firstly captured using a high-resolution camera. Then, these images were converted from RGB mode to an 8 bytes greyscale and scaled up to reflect the actual dimensions. The main flexural bending moment-induced cracks at the same point for all the samples were digitized for thresholding using open-access digital image analysis software called Image J. Then, these were covered by imaginary meshes with rectangular box sizes containing the number of pixels of the crack image (Figure 6). Next, the number of grid squares to cover the cracks was counted for the plot of In (box count) versus In (box size), which were used to compute the average value of fractal dimension that is the slope of the line joining the logarithm of the number of grid squares encountered by the crack and the logarithm of the square grid dimension.

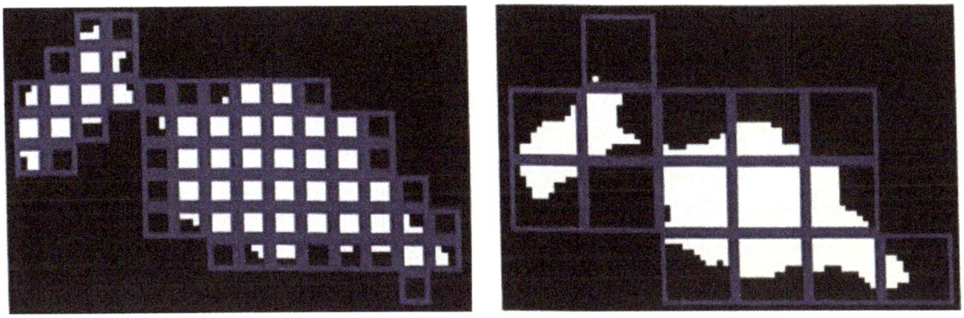

(a) (b)

Figure 6. Example of crack analysis with different box sizes using Image-J software. (**a**) Boxing size of 1 unit (**b**) Boxing size of 4 unit.

Then, using the formula established by Guo et al. [45], the composites' dissipated fracture energy (Ws/Gf) was approximated at the macro scale as a function of the surface macro-cracks. The ratio of energy (Ws) produced by crack propagation to fracture energy (Gf) is shown by the value of Ws/Gf.

$$Ws/Gf = a \times (\delta/a)\ D^{1-d} \quad (1)$$

where a denotes the Euclidean length (equal to the diameter of the tested composite), and D^{1-d} denotes the fractal dimension of the crack.

3. Results and Discussion

3.1. Compressive Strength and Ultrasonic Pulse Velocity (UPV) Results

The compressive strength and UPV tests after 28 days of the fabricated series with three different ratios of nanocalcite are shown in Figures 7 and 8. Compressive strength results were obtained by averaging three 50 × 50 × 50 mm cubic samples for each series. The maximum increase in compressive strength and UPV values were obtained for 1 NCa (1% by mass of binder) specimens. When the NCa content was increased from 0.5 to 1 percent, the compressive strength of NCa-ECC increased steadily by 2.17 to 6.92 percent compared to the 0 NCa series. When the NCa content was increased to 1.5 percent, the enhancement of compressive strength decreased to 4.64 percent. The increased strength could be attributed to both the filling effect and the chemical effect associated with NCa. NCa can react with C3A to form mono-carbonate, which has a unique structure with strong hydrogen bonds between oxygen atoms and interlayer waters in carbonate groups [46]. In addition, $CaCO_3$ can increase the stability and nature of ettringite [47]. The difficulty of uniform distribution may be the reason for the less apparent positive effect of NCa at higher dosage on compressive strength [39]. As a result, increasing the nanocalcite content in the mixes increased the compressive strength values. These increases were 50.17, 51.26, 53.64, and 52.50 MPa for 0, 0.5, 1, and 1.5 NCa series. When the content of Nano-$CaCO_3$ increased from 1% to 1.5%, the improvement of strengths was reduced. Because excessive NCa addition led to poor dispersion of the matrix, insufficient hydration, and limited the improvement of the strength of the samples [48]. In addition, The matrix had an agglomeration effect due to the increase of nano-materials. In addition, free water cannot reach the cement particles, which reduces hydration and reduces the strength of the concrete [49].

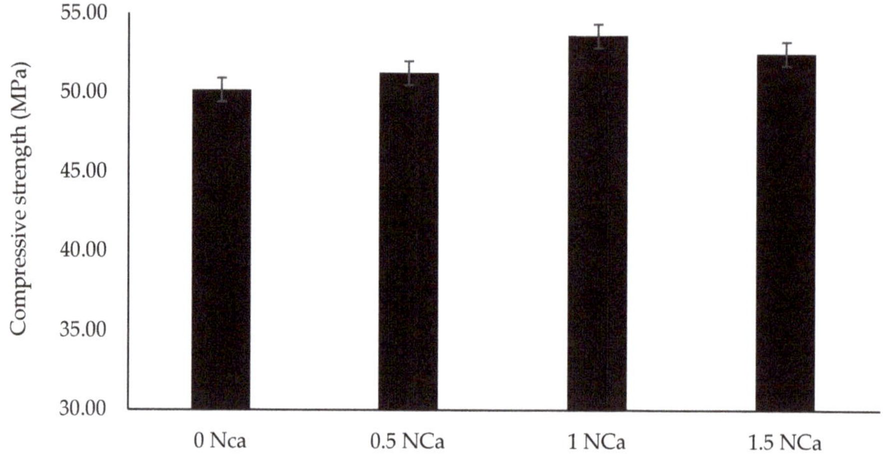

Figure 7. Compressive strength results of NCa-ECC.

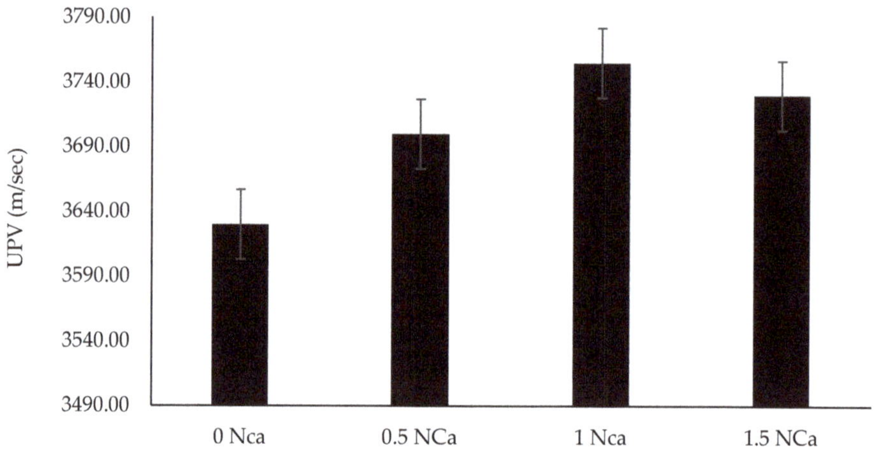

Figure 8. UPV results of NCa-ECC.

Figure 8 shows the ultrasonic pulse velocity (UPV) testing of NCa-ECC samples with different mixtures. Looking at the UPV results, it is observed that the result has a parallel relationship with the compressive strength results. The UPV increased with increasing nanocalcite content in the mixes by 3630.06, 3700, 3755, and 3630 m/sec for 0, 0.5, 1, and 1.5 NCa series. Adesina and Das [50] investigated the UPV values of 50 × 50 × 50 mm cubic ECC samples by replacing crumb rubber with silica sand. They found that the UPV value of ECC samples without adding crumb rubber was 3689 m/s, while the UPV value decreased to 2976 m/s when they used 100% crumb rubber. The UPV result of ECC without the addition of crumb rubber obtained in their study was consistent with the UPV result of the ECC without the addition of NCa obtained in this study. In addition, the correlation between compressive strength and UPV for all the mixes is shown in Figure 9. Figure 9 shows that the R coefficient is 0.9264. This R coefficient indicates a strong relationship between UPV and the compressive strength of the specimens.

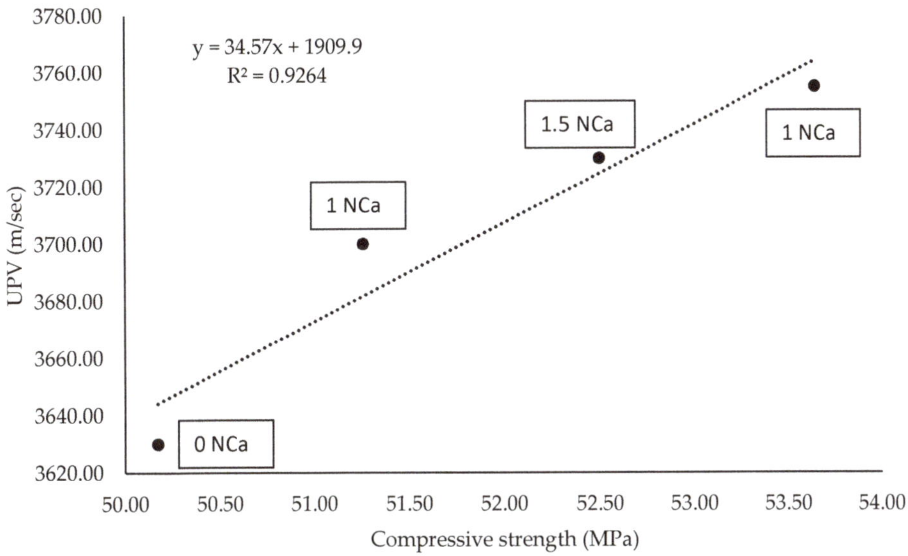

Figure 9. Correlation between compressive strength and UPV.

3.2. Flexural Performance

Test results of 15 × 50 × 350 mm specimens subjected to flexural test after 28 days are shown in Figure 10. The results were obtained by averaging the flexural results of three samples for each series. The maximum increase in flexural strength was obtained for 1 NCa specimen. Accordingly, the increase in the nanocalcite content in the mixes increased the flexural strength values. Sun et al. [51] found that the content of nano-$CaCO_3$ improved the flexural performance of ECC. In addition, increasing the nanocalcite content in the blends increased the flexural strength values to 13.1, 14.31, 16.9, and 15.31 MPa for 0, 0.5, 1, and 1.5 NCa series, respectively. In general, the increase in the flexural strength values with the addition of the nanomaterials would be further beneficial for applying ECC-steel bar reinforced composite beams. In this case, the ECC with higher flexural strength could carry developing tensile stress under flexural loading and the steel reinforcement rebar after cracks. This, in turn, results in a much higher load-carrying capacity for the composite.

Moreover, mid-span displacement, strain, and stress-deflection curves were obtained from the flexural strength test. The strain, mid-span displacement, flexural toughness, and ductility index results obtained from the stress-deflection curves are shown in Table 4. This table indicates that 1 NCa samples have the highest strain and mid-span displacement values. Thus, the increase in the content of nanocalcite increased the flexural performance and compressive strength of the samples. In addition, by examining the stress-deflection curves of 15 × 50 × 350 mm specimens shown in Figure 11, the content of NCa improved the flexural performance. The maximum deflection values (deflection capacity) of the samples subjected to the flexural strength test were obtained from the endpoints of the flexural stress-deflection curves. The increases in the deflection capacity of the 0.5 NCa (11.74 mm), 1 NCa (12.88 mm), and 1.5 NCa (12.51 mm) series were 46.70%, 61.01%, and 56.39%, respectively, compared to the 0 NCa (8 mm) series. Furthermore, the flexural strength increases of 0.5, 1, and 1.5 NCa series were 8.68%, 31.55%, and 18.68, respectively, compared to the 0 NCa series. Thus, series 1 NCa exhibited the best flexural properties, having the highest flexural stress and deflection values. Ding et al. [39] found that the content of nano-$CaCO_3$ increased the strength of UHP-ECC, and an NC content of three percent (by mass of cement) was considered ideal. In their study, they replaced the NC material with PC only, but if they had replaced the NC material with a binder (FA and PC), the ratio they used would have been approximately 1–1.5% by mass of the binder. Thus, their conclusion was close to the conclusion of this study.

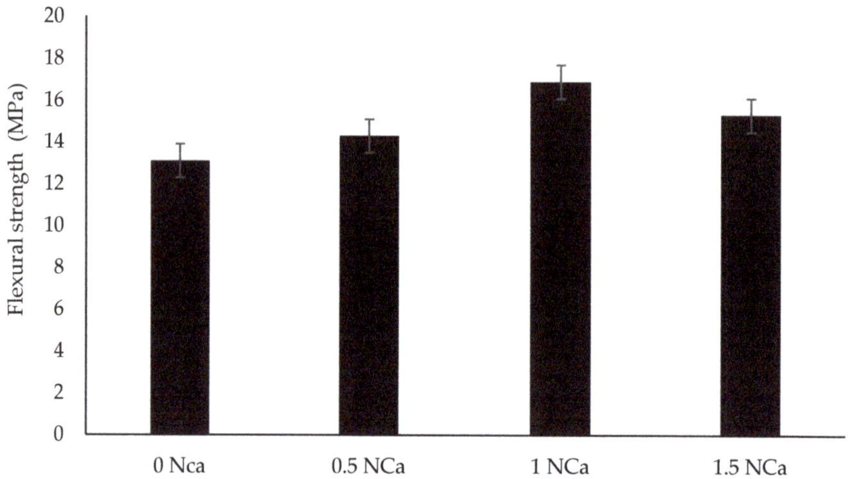

Figure 10. Flexural strength results of NCa-ECC.

Table 4. Strain, mid-span displacement, flexural toughness, and ductility results.

Mix ID	0 NCa	0.5 NCa	1 NCa	1.5 NCa
Mid-span displacement (mm)	3.50	3.48	8.45	5.57
Strain (%)	0.39	0.38	0.84	0.56
Flexural Toughness (MPa.mm)	74.7	75	161	99.2
Ductility index increase (%)	0	0.21	98.20	39.44

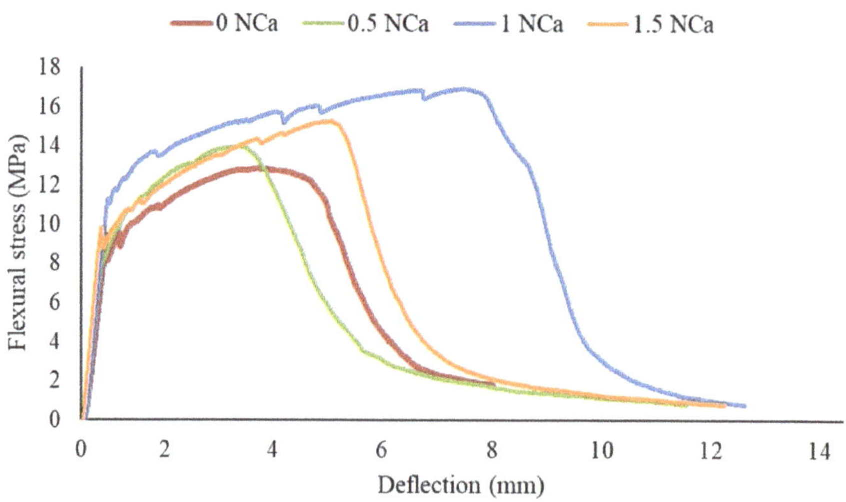

Figure 11. Flexural stress–deflection curves of the specimens.

Ductility and flexural toughness can be evaluated using flexural load-deflection curves, as indicated in the literature [52,53]. The area under the whole load-deflection curve is used to compute flexural toughness, and the load–deflection curves were also used to calculate ductility. The ductility index (μ) calculated using the formula;

$$\mu = \delta u/\delta y \quad (2)$$

where δu is the ultimate displacement and δy is the yield displacement. After calculating the ductility indexes of the samples, the percent increases of the ductility indexes of the samples compared to the 0 NCa series were calculated and given in Table 4. NCa-containing mixtures exhibit considerably greater deflections in the ultimate state and higher loads when compared to the 0 NCa mixture. This results in a greater area under the load-deflection curves, which may indicate increased toughness. In addition, it can be concluded that adding NCa to the ECC mixes improves the ductility and flexural toughness of the mixes. In this study, the highest flexural toughness and ductility were obtained for 1 NCa specimen. Yeşilmen et al. [54] used nano-silica and nano-$CaCO_3$ in ECC mixtures, and they found that the nano- $CaCO_3$ contained ECC mixtures had the highest ductility. The higher fracture toughness and improved multiple cracking behavior associated with the nano-particle reinforced mix can make ECC effectively improve the unstable crack propagation caused by the surrounding concrete or old/new concrete interface. This, in turn, reduces the common early damage types in repair structures such as spalling and interlaminar fracture [55].

3.3. Fractal Analysis

In the literature, there are various methods (cube counting, variance methods, etc.) for extracting and then calculating the cracking map and fractal dimension of surface cracks at the fractured 15 × 50 × 350 mm samples shown in Figure 12. Box-counting is the most preferred and practical technique for measuring the borders of a form by measuring the distances between points on it using square boxes. Erdem and Blankson [36] described the techniques in depth in prior research.

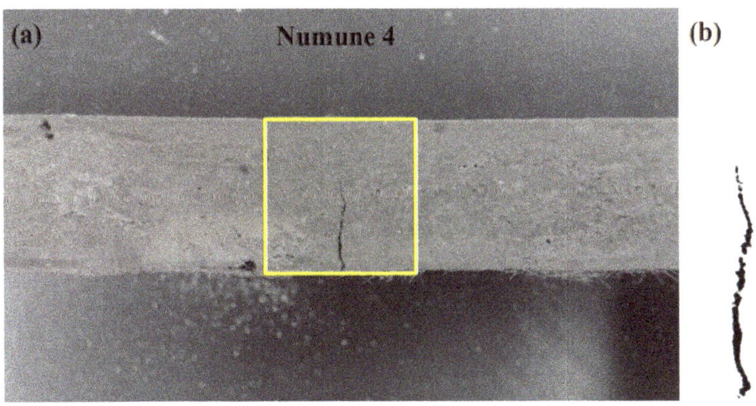

Figure 12. (**a**) An example of the crack on the studied sample (**b**) the extracted map of the crack.

The fractal dimension values of the surface cracks provided by the Image J program are illustrated in Figure 13. The results clearly show that the ECC mix with 1% nanocalcite particles (1 NCa) has the highest fractal dimension value among the NCa-ECC series. In addition, the other nanocalcite dopped ECC samples had a fractal dimension higher than the control ECC series (0 NCa). The greater fractal dimension of the 1 NCa mixture resulted in higher fracture energy dissipation at the macro scale level, as verified by the findings shown in Table 5. The greater fractal dimension values with the adding nanoparticles most likely indicate that the filling effect of nanocalcite particles refines the pore structures and reduces unsaturated bonds, resulting in improved bondability between and creating the deformation hardening method along the fracture front and voids. However, using more than 1% nanocalcite particles decreases fractal dimension and fractural energy. In general, the previous studies [37,55] show that the fractal of general cementitious materials has a value of 1 and 2. The results of this study are consistent with the existing literature.

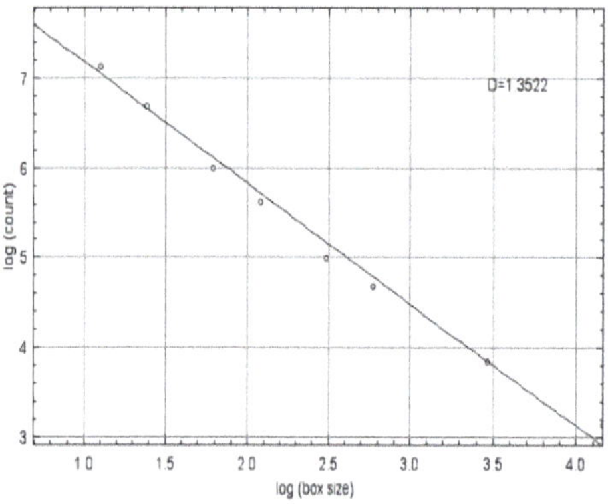

(a)

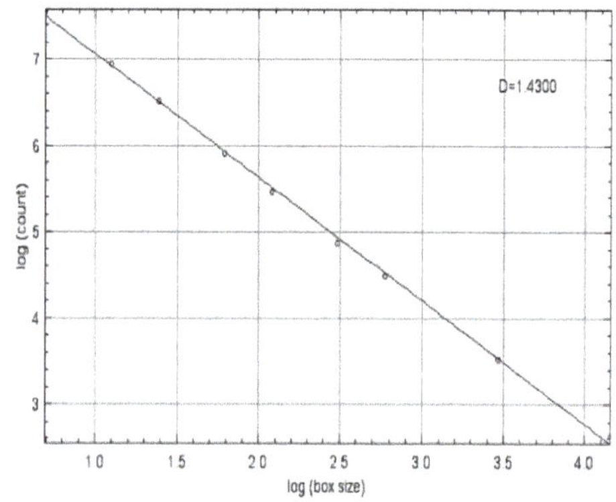

(b)

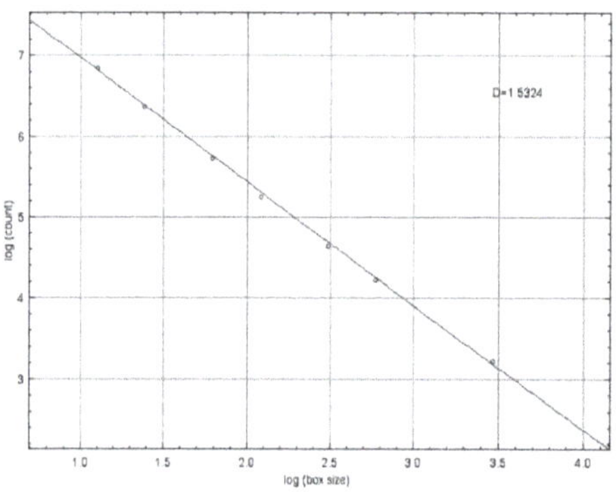

(c)

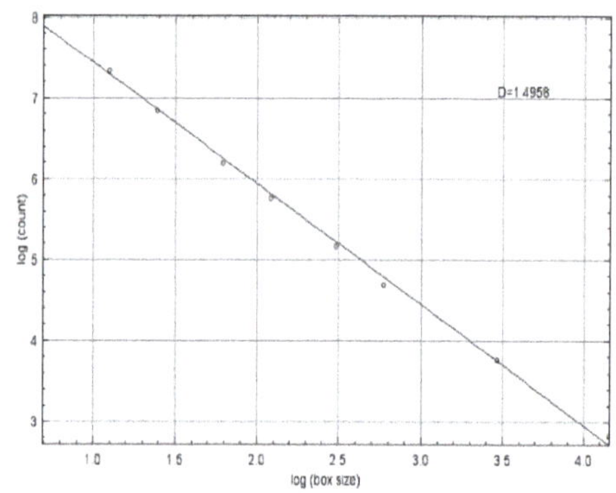

(d)

Figure 13. Fractal dimensions of the (**a**) 0 NCa, (**b**) 0.5 NCa, (**c**) 1 NCa, and (**d**) 1.5 NCa samples.

Table 5. The summary of the fractal analysis of the mixtures.

Mix ID	Fractal Dimension -D	Ws/Gf (mm)
0 NCa	1.352	113.58
0.5 NCa	1.430	158.68
1 NCa	1.532	246.40
1.5 NCa	1.495	210.53

Figure 14 illustrated 3D views of the cracked surfaces' crack surface roughness. According to the findings, the sample containing 1% nanocalcite particles had the greatest energy value during fracture initiation and propagation. The 3D surfaces curves of the mixtures corresponding with the depth of the sample locations are shown in Figure 14. The findings showed that the more fibers associated with, the larger surface area would be available to bridge cracks during the crack propagation process under flexural loading. This would, in turn, result in much higher fiber bridging complementary energy in terms of the micromechanical principles. In general, the strong bridging ability could confirm the excellent deflection capacity with the increase in the content of the NCa particles.

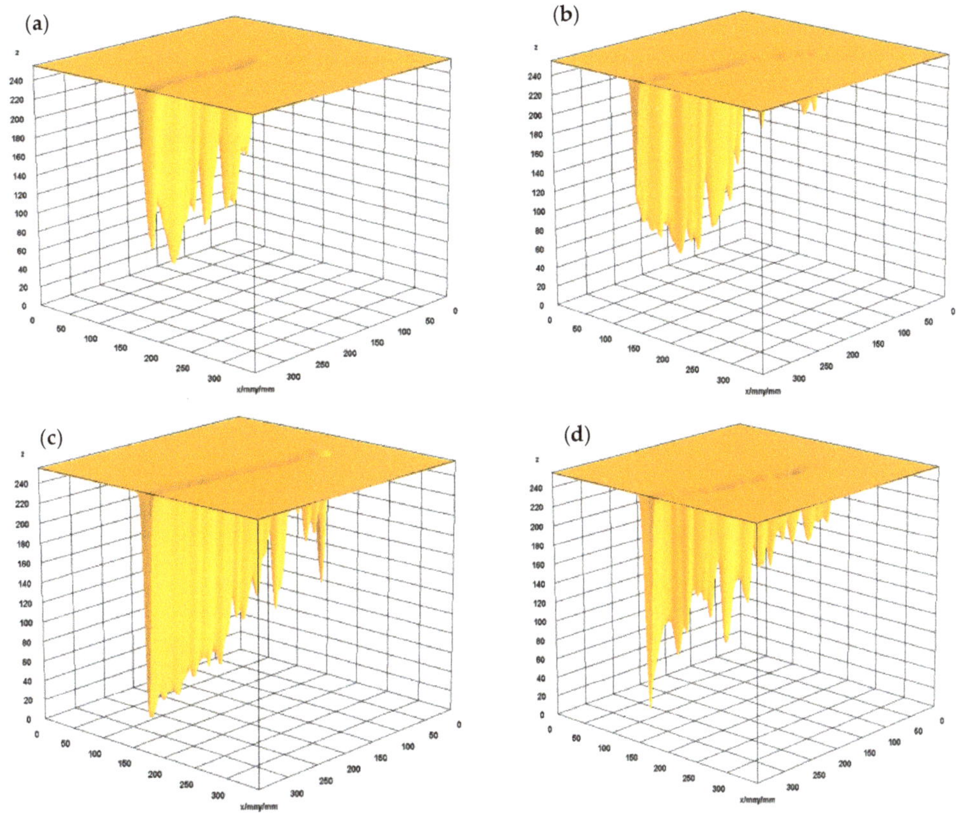

Figure 14. 3D surface graphs of the fracture surfaces of the (**a**) 0 NCa, (**b**) 0.5 NCa, (**c**) 1 NCa, and (**d**) 1.5 NCa samples.

3.4. SEM Analysis

The ECC matrix without nanomaterials is shown in Figure 15. The micrograph in Figure 15 indicates that the composites were relatively loose, with unhydrated fly ash particles clustered with distinct interfaces. It consists of dense calcium silicate hydrate (CSH) gel, unhydrated FA particles, amorphous and crystallized calcium hydroxide (CH). The micromorphology of a modified ECC sample matrix with nanocalcite (1 NCa) is shown in Figure 16. The matrix compactness improved after nanomaterials were added, and although unhydrated fly ash particles were retained, their distribution was uniform and had no clear interfaces. The main explanation for this was that the nanoparticles have a similar particle size to hydrated calcium silicate [56]. In addition, the newly formed hydration products slightly increased the density of the matrix, which improved the mechanical properties.

Conversely, the matrix did not exhibit visible micro-cracks. This, in turn, indicates that the addition of NCa particles can increase the fracture toughness of the matrix. The improvement of the matrix fracture toughness would be attributable to the shielding effect on crack tips [57]. As found in the Due et al. [58] study, the active ingredients of FA in 28-day samples prepared in this study reacted together with $Ca(OH)_2$. This reaction effectively improves the growth rate of matrix strength and imparts good strength to NCa-ECC.

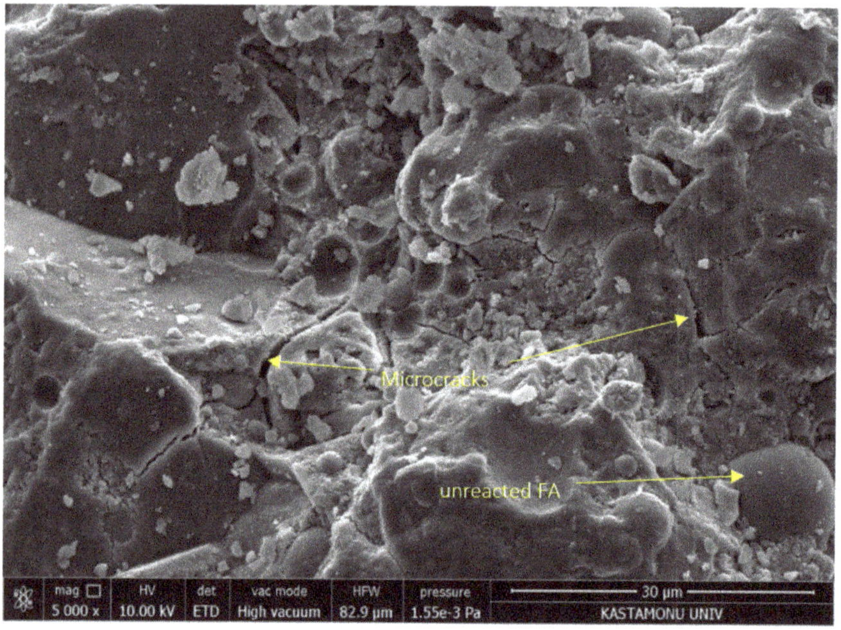

Figure 15. SEM of the 0 NCa sample magnified at 5000 times.

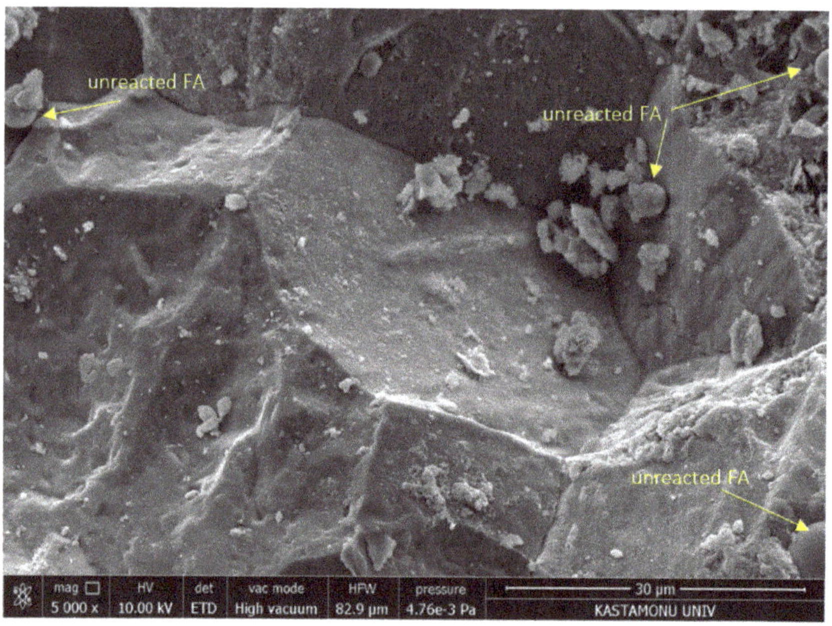

Figure 16. SEM of the 1 NCa sample magnified at 5000 times.

4. Conclusions

In this study, NCa-ECC blends were prepared by replacing 0.5, 1, and 1.5 proportions of nanocalcite in the binder of the prepared blends. Compressive strength, flexural strength, and UPV tests were carried out to investigate the mechanical properties of the NCa-ECC mixes. In addition, SEM analyses were carried out to investigate the microstructural properties of the specimens. As a result of these tests, the following results were obtained:

- Increasing the nanocalcite content in NCa-ECC mixtures increased the compressive strength. The increase in compressive strength was 2.17%, 6.92%, and 4.64% for 0.5, 1, and 1.5 NCa, respectively, compared to the 0 NCa blend.
- The increase in nanocalcite content in NCa-ECC blends increased flexural strength values. The increase in flexural strength values was 9.24%, 29.01%, and 16.87% for 0.5, 1, and 1.5 NCa, respectively, compared to the 0 NCa blend.
- Increasing the nanocalcite content in NCa-ECC blends increased the UPV. The increases in UPV were 1.93%, 3.44%, and 2.75% for 0.5, 1, and 1.5, respectively, compared to the 0 NCa blend.
- The use of nanocalcite increased the fractal dimension of the NCa-ECC samples. These increases were 5.77%, 13.31%, and 10.57% for 0.5, 1, and 1.5 NCa, respectively, compared to the 0 NCa blend.
- In general, the nanocalcite content improved the mechanical and microstructural properties of NCa-ECC mixtures.
- The addition of nanocalcite particles into the ECC mixes can increase the compressive strength. Adding more NCa particles seems to have had a negative effect on enhancing the compressive strength due to poor dispersion and a more significant air-entraining effect beyond some limit. In this experimental work, adding 1% of NCa can obtain the optimal quasi-static compressive strength.
- The deflection capacity under flexure of the ECC mixes had a significant increase after adding the NCa particles. Moreover, the strain hardening behavior associated with multiple cracks was enhanced after adding the NCa particles. Based on this experimental work, the NCa is suitable for improving the strain hardening behavior of the ECC mixes.
- This study enables producing the high toughness and high strength ECC products with the nano-particle inclusion. Nanomodified ECC, with larger Poission's effect than concrete, may be used in concrete-filled-steel-tube column that decrease the imperfect interface bonding between concrete and steel, and to produce a more ductile composite for the development of super infrastructure.

Author Contributions: Conceptualization, M.Z., S.E., Y.T. and R.A.G.L.; methodology, M.Z., S.E. and Y.T.; formal analysis, M.Z., S.E. and Y.T.; investigation, M.Z., S.E. and Y.T.; resources, M.Z., S.E., Y.T. and R.A.G.L.; data curation, M.Z. and S.E.; writing—original draft preparation, M.Z., S.E. and Y.T.; writing—review and editing, M.Z., S.E. and R.A.G.L.; visualization, M.Z., S.E. and Y.T.; supervision, R.A.G.L.; project administration, M.Z., S.E., Y.T. and R.A.G.L.; funding acquisition, R.A.G.L. All authors have read and agreed to the published version of the manuscript.

Funding: The authors wish to thank CEU San Pablo University Foundation for the funds dedicated to the project ref. MCP21V12 provided by CEU San Pablo University.

Institutional Review Board Statement: Not applicable.

Informed Consent Statement: Not applicable.

Data Availability Statement: The data presented in this study are available on request from the corresponding author.

Conflicts of Interest: The authors declare no conflict of interest.

References

1. Balapour, M.; Ramezanianpour, A.; Hajibandeh, E. An investigation on mechanical and durability properties of mortars containing nano and micro RHA. *Constr. Build. Mater.* **2017**, *132*, 470–477. [CrossRef]
2. Joshaghani, A.; Balapour, M.; Ramezanianpour, A.A. Effect of controlled environmental conditions on mechanical, microstructural and durability properties of cement mortar. *Constr. Build. Mater.* **2018**, *164*, 134–149. [CrossRef]
3. Joshaghani, A.; Moeini, M.A.; Balapour, M. Evaluation of incorporating metakaolin to evaluate durability and mechanical properties of concrete. *Adv. Concr. Constr.* **2017**, *5*, 183–199. [CrossRef]
4. Karein, S.M.M.; Balapour, M.; Karakouzian, M. Improving the hardened and transport properties of perlite incorporated mixture through different solutions: Surface area increase, nanosilica incorporation or both. *Constr. Build. Mater.* **2019**, *209*, 187–194. [CrossRef]
5. Ramezanianpour, A.; Ghoreishian, S.; Ahmadi, B.; Balapour, M.; Ramezanianpour, A. Modeling of chloride ions penetration in cracked concrete structures exposed to marine environments. *Struct. Concr.* **2018**, *19*. [CrossRef]
6. Balapour, M.; Joshaghani, A.; Althoey, F. Nano-SiO_2 contribution to mechanical, durability, fresh and microstructural characteristics of concrete: A review. *Constr. Build. Mater.* **2018**, *181*, 27–41. [CrossRef]
7. Balapour, M.; Zhao, W.; Garboczi, E.J.; Oo, N.Y.; Spatari, S.; Hsuan, Y.G.; Billen, P.; Farnam, Y. Potential use of lightweight aggregate (LWA) produced from bottom coal ash for internal curing of concrete systems. *Cem. Concr. Compos.* **2020**, *105*, 103428. [CrossRef]
8. Wang, X.Q.; Chow, C.L.; Lau, D. A review on modeling techniques of cementitious materials under different length scales: Development and future prospects. *Adv. Theory Simul.* **2019**, *2*, 1900047. [CrossRef]
9. Chae, S.R.; Moon, J.; Yoon, S.; Bae, S.; Levitz, P.; Winarski, R.; Monteiro, P.J.M. Advanced nanoscale characterization of cement based materials using X-ray synchrotron radiation: A review. *Int. J. Concr. Struct. Mater.* **2013**, *7*, 95–110. [CrossRef]
10. Ardalan, R.B.; Jamshidi, N.; Arabameri, H.; Joshaghani, A.; Mehrinejad, M.; Sharafi, P. Enhancing the permeability and abrasion resistance of concrete using colloidal nano-SiO_2 oxide and spraying nanosilicon practices. *Constr. Build. Mater.* **2017**, *146*, 128–135. [CrossRef]
11. Joshaghani, A.; Moeini, M.A. Evaluating the effects of sugar cane bagasse ash (SCBA) and nanosilica on the mechanical and durability properties of mortar. *Constr. Build. Mater.* **2017**, *152*, 818–831. [CrossRef]
12. Mukhopadhyay, A.K. Next-generation nano-based concrete construction products: A review. *Nanotechnol. Civ. Infrastruct.* **2011**, 207–223. [CrossRef]
13. Tosee, S.V.; Faridmehr, I.; Bedon, C.; Sadowski, Ł.; Aalimahmoody, N.; Nikoo, M.; Nowobilski, T. Metaheuristic Prediction of the Compressive Strength of Environmentally Friendly Concrete Modified with Eggshell Powder Using the Hybrid ANN-SFL Optimization Algorithm. *Materials* **2021**, *14*, 6172. [CrossRef] [PubMed]
14. Ziada, M.; Erdem, S.; Tammam, Y.; Kara, S.; Lezcano, R.A. The Effect of Basalt Fiber on Mechanical, Microstructural, and High-Temperature Properties of Fly Ash-Based and Basalt Powder Waste-Filled Sustainable Geopolymer Mortar. *Sustainability* **2021**, *13*, 12610. [CrossRef]
15. Sahmaran, M.; Lachemi, M.; Hossain, K.M.A.; Ranade, R.; Li, V.C. Influence of aggregate type and size on ductility and mechanical properties of engineered cementitious composites. *ACI Mater. J.* **2009**, *106*, 308.
16. Banthia, N.; Gupta, R. Influence of polypropylene fiber geometry on plastic shrinkage cracking in concrete. *Cem. Concr. Res.* **2006**, *36*, 1263–1267. [CrossRef]
17. Han, T.C.; Wang, F.J.; Dou, H.Q. Application of ultra high toughness cementitious composites to tunnel lining. *Appl. Mech. Mater.* **2013**, *256*, 1226–1229. [CrossRef]
18. Nyström, U.; Gylltoft, K. Comparative numerical studies of projectile impacts on plain and steel-fibre reinforced concrete. *Int. J. Impact Eng.* **2011**, *38*, 95–105. [CrossRef]
19. Cai, X.H.; He, Z.; Liu, W. Experimental study on Impact Resistance of PVA Fiber Reinforced Cement-based Composite. *Appl. Mech. Mater.* **2014**, *584*, 1630–1634. [CrossRef]
20. Manikandan, V.; Jappes, J.T.W.; Kumar, S.M.S.; Amuthakkannan, P. Investigation of the effect of surface modifications on the mechanical properties of basalt fibre reinforced polymer composites. *Compos. Part B Eng.* **2012**, *43*, 812–818. [CrossRef]
21. Jalal, A.; Shafiq, N.; Nikbakht, E.; Kumar, R.; Zahid, M. Mechanical properties of hybrid basalt-polyvinyl alcohol (PVA) fiber reinforced concrete. *Key Eng. Mater.* **2017**, *744*, 3–7. [CrossRef]
22. Chaipanich, A.; Nochaiya, T.; Wongkeo, W.; Torkittikul, P. Compressive strength and microstructure of carbon nanotubes–fly ash cement composites. *Mater. Sci. Eng. A* **2010**, *527*, 1063–1067. [CrossRef]
23. Luo, Z.; Li, W.; Gan, Y.; He, X.; Castel, A.; Sheng, D. Nanoindentation on micromechanical properties and microstructure of geopolymer with nano-SiO_2 and nano-TiO_2. *Cem. Concr. Compos.* **2021**, *117*, 103883. [CrossRef]
24. Li, V. On Engineered Cementitious Composites (ECC) A Review of the Material and Its Applications. *J. Adv. Concr. Technol.* **2011**, *1*, 215–230. [CrossRef]
25. Lepech, M.D.; Li, V.C. Large-scale processing of engineered cementitious composites. *ACI Mater. J.* **2008**, *105*, 358.
26. Li, V.C. *Engineered Cementitious Composites-Tailored Composites through Micromechanical Modeling, Fiber Reinforced Concrete*; Banthia, N., Bentur, A., Mufti, A., Eds.; Present and the Future, Canadian Society of Civil Engineers: Montreal, QC, Canada, 1997; p. 38.
27. Ekaputri, J.; Limantono, H.; Triwulan, T.; Susanto, T.; Abdullah, M.M.A.B. Effect of PVA Fiber in Increasing Mechanical Strength on Paste Containing Glass Powder. *Key Eng. Mater.* **2015**, *673*, 83–93. [CrossRef]

28. Kunieda, M.; Rokugo, K. Recent progress on HPFRCC in Japan. *J. Adv. Concr. Technol.* **2006**, *4*, 19–33. [CrossRef]
29. Li, V.C.; Wang, S.; Wu, C. Tensile strain-hardening behavior of polyvinyl alcohol engineered cementitious composite (PVA-ECC). *Mater. J.* **2001**, *98*, 483–492.
30. Ling, Y.; Zhang, P.; Wang, J.; Taylor, P.; Hu, S. Effects of nanoparticles on engineering performance of cementitious composites reinforced with PVA fibers. *Nanotechnol. Rev.* **2020**, *9*, 504–514. [CrossRef]
31. Topič, J.; Prošek, Z.; Indrová, K.; Plachý, T.; Nežerka, V.; Kopecky, L.; Tesarek, P. Effect of PVA modification on the properties of cement composites. *Acta Polytech.* **2015**, *55*, 64–75. [CrossRef]
32. Yan, H.; Ran, Q.; Yang, Y.; Shu, X.; Zhang, Q.; Zhang, J.; Liu, J. Investigation on the Effect of Hydroxyapatite Nanorod on Cement Hydration and Strength Development. *J. Nanosci. Nanotechnol.* **2021**, *21*, 1578–1589. [CrossRef] [PubMed]
33. Zhang, P.; Zheng, Y.; Wang, K.; Zhang, K. Combined influence of nano-$CaCO_3$ and polyvinyl alcohol fibers on fresh and mechanical performance of concrete incorporating fly ash. *Struct. Concr.* **2020**, *21*, 724–734. [CrossRef]
34. Ficker, T.; Martišek, D. Digital fracture surfaces and their roughness analysis: Applications to cement-based materials. *Cem. Concr. Res.* **2012**, *42*, 827–833. [CrossRef]
35. Ficker, T.; Martišek, D.; Jennings, H.M. Roughness of fracture surfaces and compressive strength of hydrated cement pastes. *Cem. Concr. Res.* **2010**, *40*, 947–955. [CrossRef]
36. Erdem, S.; Blankson, M.A. Fractal–fracture analysis and characterization of impact-fractured surfaces in different types of concrete using digital image analysis and 3D nanomap laser profilometery. *Constr. Build. Mater.* **2013**, *40*, 70–76. [CrossRef]
37. Farhan, A.H.; Dawson, A.R.; Thom, N.H. Characterization of rubberized cement bound aggregate mixtures using indirect tensile testing and fractal analysis. *Constr. Build. Mater.* **2016**, *105*, 94–102. [CrossRef]
38. Farina, I.; Goodall, R.; Hernández-Nava, E.; di Filippo, A.; Colangelo, F.; Fraternali, F. Design, microstructure and mechanical characterization of Ti6Al4V reinforcing elements for cement composites with fractal architecture. *Mater. Des.* **2019**, *172*, 107758. [CrossRef]
39. Ding, Y.; Liu, J.-P.; Bai, Y.-L. Linkage of multi-scale performances of nano-$CaCO_3$ modified ultra-high performance engineered cementitious composites (UHP-ECC). *Constr. Build. Mater.* **2020**, *234*, 117418. [CrossRef]
40. *ASTM C597*; Standard Test Method for Pulse Velocity Through Concrete. ASTM International: West Conshohocken, PA, USA, 2016.
41. *ASTM C109/C109M*; Standard Test Method for Compressive Strength of Hydraulic Cement Mortars (Using 2-in. or [50 mm] Cube Specimens). ASTM International: West Conshohocken, PA, USA, 2021.
42. *ASTM C230*; Standard Specification for Flow Table for Use in Tests of Hydraulic Cement. ASTM International: West Conshohocken, PA, USA, 2008.
43. *ASTM C348*; Standard Test Method for Flexural Strength of Hydraulic-Cement Mortars. ASTM International: West Conshohocken, PA, USA, 2021.
44. Erdem, S.; Gürbüz, E. Influence of microencapsulated phase change materials on the flexural behavior and micromechanical impact damage of hybrid fibre reinforced engineered cementitious composites. *Compos. Part B Eng.* **2019**, *166*, 633–644. [CrossRef]
45. Guo, L.-P.; Sun, W.; Zheng, K.-R.; Chen, H.-J.; Liu, B. Study on the flexural fatigue performance and fractal mechanism of concrete with high proportions of ground granulated blast-furnace slag. *Cem. Concr. Res.* **2007**, *37*, 242–250. [CrossRef]
46. Moon, J.; Oh, J.E.; Balonis, M.; Glasser, F.P.; Clark, S.M.; Monteiro, P.J.M. High pressure study of low compressibility tetracalcium aluminum carbonate hydrates 3CaO· Al2O3· $CaCO_3$· 11H_2O. *Cem. Concr. Res.* **2012**, *42*, 105–110. [CrossRef]
47. Lothenbach, B.; Le Saout, G.; Gallucci, E.; Scrivener, K. Influence of limestone on the hydration of Portland cements. *Cem. Concr. Res.* **2008**, *38*, 848–860. [CrossRef]
48. Ariyagounder, J.; Veerasamy, S. Experimental Investigation on the Strength, Durability and Corrosion Properties of Concrete by Partial Replacement of Cement with Nano-SiO_2, Nano-$CaCO_3$ and Nano-$Ca(OH)_2$. *Iran. J. Sci. Technol. Trans. Civ. Eng.* **2021**. [CrossRef]
49. Camiletti, J.; Soliman, A.M.; Nehdi, M.L. Effect of nano-calcium carbonate on early-age properties of ultra-high-performance concrete. *Mag. Concr. Res.* **2013**, *65*, 297–307. [CrossRef]
50. Adesina, A.; Das, S. Performance of engineered cementitious composites incorporating crumb rubber as aggregate. *Constr. Build. Mater.* **2021**, *274*, 122033. [CrossRef]
51. Sun, M.; Zhu, J.; Sun, T.; Chen, Y.; Li, X.; Yin, W.; Han, J. Multiple effects of nano-$CaCO_3$ and modified polyvinyl alcohol fiber on flexure–tension-resistant performance of engineered cementitious composites. *Constr. Build. Mater.* **2021**, *303*, 124426. [CrossRef]
52. Jastrzebski, Z.D.; Komanduri, R. The Nature and Properties of Engineering Materials. *J. Eng. Mater. Technol.* **1988**, *110*, 294. [CrossRef]
53. Low, N.M.P.; Beaudoin, J.J. The flexural toughness and ductility of portland cement-based binders reinforced with wollastonite micro-fibres. *Cem. Concr. Res.* **1994**, *24*, 250–258. [CrossRef]
54. Yeşilmen, S.; Al-Najjar, Y.; Balav, M.H.; Şahmaran, M.; Yıldırım, G.; Lachemi, M. Nano-modification to improve the ductility of cementitious composites. *Cem. Concr. Res.* **2015**, *76*, 170–179. [CrossRef]
55. Erdem, S.; Dawson, A.R.; Thom, N.H. Impact load-induced micro-structural damage and micro-structure associated mechanical response of concrete made with different surface roughness and porosity aggregates. *Cem. Concr. Res.* **2012**, *42*, 291–305. [CrossRef]

56. Ren, Z.; Liu, Y.; Yuan, L.; Luan, C.; Wang, J.; Cheng, X.; Zhou, Z. Optimizing the content of nano-SiO_2, nano-TiO_2 and nano-$CaCO_3$ in Portland cement paste by response surface methodology. *J. Build. Eng.* **2021**, *35*, 102073. [CrossRef]
57. Chen, Z.; Yang, Y.; Yao, Y. Effect of nanoparticles on quasi-static and dynamic mechanical properties of strain hardening cementitious composite. *Adv. Mech. Eng.* **2019**, *11*, 1687814019846776. [CrossRef]
58. Du, Q.; Cai, C.; Lv, J.; Wu, J.; Pan, T.; Zhou, J. Experimental Investigation on the Mechanical Properties and Microstructure of Basalt Fiber Reinforced Engineered Cementitious Composite. *Materials* **2020**, *13*, 3796. [CrossRef] [PubMed]

energies

MDPI

Article

Energy-Optimal Structures of HVAC System for Cleanrooms as a Function of Key Constant Parameters and External Climate

Mieczysław Porowski * and Monika Jakubiak

Institute of Environmental Engineering and Building Installations, Poznan University of Technology, Pl. M. Sklodowskiej-Curie 5, 60-965 Poznan, Poland; monika.ja.mackowiak@doctorate.put.poznan.pl
* Correspondence: mieczyslaw.porowski@put.poznan.pl

Abstract: This article presents approximating relations defining energy-optimal structures of the HVAC (Heating, Ventilation, Air Conditioning) system for cleanrooms as a function of key constant parameters and energy-optimal control algorithms for various options of heat recovery and external climates. The annual unit primary energy demand of the HVAC system for thermodynamic air treatment was adopted as the objective function. Research was performed for wide representative variability ranges of key constant parameters: cleanliness class—C_s (ISO5÷ISO8), unit cooling loads—$\dot{q}_j$ (100 ÷ 500) W/m^2 and percentage of outdoor air—α_o (5 ÷ 100)%. HVAC systems are described with vectors $\bar{x}$ with coordinates defined by constant parameters and decision variables, and the results are presented in the form of approximating functions illustrating zones of energy-optimal structures of the HVAC system $\bar{x}^* = f(C_s, \dot{q}_j, \alpha_o)$. In the optimization procedure, the type of heat recovery as an element of optimal structures of the HVAC system and algorithms of energy-optimal control were defined based on an objective function and simulation models. It was proven that using heat recovery is profitable only for HVAC systems without recirculation and with internal recirculation (savings of 5 ÷ 66%, depending on the type of heat recovery and the climate), while it is not profitable (or generates losses) for HVAC systems with external recirculation or external and internal recirculation at the same time.

Keywords: cleanrooms; ventilation; air conditioning; energy consumption; optimization

Citation: Porowski, M.; Jakubiak, M. Energy-Optimal Structures of HVAC System for Cleanrooms as a Function of Key Constant Parameters and External Climate. *Energies* **2022**, *15*, 313. https://doi.org/10.3390/en15010313

Academic Editors: Roberto Alonso González Lezcano and Fabrizio Ascione

Received: 24 November 2021
Accepted: 27 December 2021
Published: 3 January 2022

Publisher's Note: MDPI stays neutral with regard to jurisdictional claims in published maps and institutional affiliations.

1. Introduction

HVAC systems for cleanrooms generate very high energy consumption for thermodynamic treatment and forcing through air. The literature provides a lot of data confirming this thesis. According to Kircher et al. [1], the energy consumption of HVAC systems for cleanrooms in the USA is 30 ÷ 50% times higher than for commercial buildings. According to Tschudi et al. [2], as well as Zhuang et al. [3], this range is wider and equals 10 ÷ 100%. Shan and Wang [4], as well as Tsao et al. [5,6], report that the percentage of energy consumption by HVAC systems in factories with advanced technologies equals 30 ÷ 65%, while, according to Hu et al. [7] and Zhao et al. [8], the percentage for cleanrooms with semiconductor manufacturing equals 40 ÷ 50% of the total energy consumption. High-energy inputs for air conditioning for cleanrooms inspire research aimed to reduce the energy consumption. Such studies address two issues: the optimization of the structure of the HVAC system or the optimization of control algorithms according to the energy criterion. The support tool here is software for determining energy consumption by the HVAC system of cleanrooms; significant results of work in this area were obtained by Hu et al. [9–11]. In Reference [9], the authors presented a validated FES (Fab Energy Simulation) simulation tool to determine energy consumption in an application for a semiconductor manufacturing fab. The mathematical model for the HVAC system was based on the energy balance equations for the individual components. In relation to the commercial comparable program "CleanCalc II", the FES program allowed for the definition of a few additional parameters by the user while showing excellent consistency of the results (2.33%). The study [10] developed a new ECF (energy conversion factor) calculator in an application for high-tech factories, including HVAC systems. In turn, in article [11], the authors presented the integration of both tools: the FES program and the ECF calculator in order to optimize energy consumption by HVAC systems in technologically advanced factories (high-tech fabs).

Research on optimizing structures of the HVAC system for cleanrooms was performed by Lin et al. [12], who modified a classic MAU (Make-up Air Unit) + FFU (Filter Fan Unit) + DCC (Dry Cooling Coil) in the recirculation channel, replacing the DCC with FDCU (Fan Dry Cooling Unit) modules in the ceiling of a cleanroom. As a result of elimination of under pressure above the suspended ceiling and air infiltration, as well as the reduction of forcing through losses, they achieved a reduction in energy consumption of the HVAC system with FDCU by 4.3% compared to the system with the DCC. Hu and Tsao [13] investigated five cases of structures of HVAC system of semiconductor manufacturing rooms. The HVAC structures were different combinations of elements: RCU (Recirculation Air Unit), MAU, FCU (Fan Coil Unit), FFU and DCC. The authors compared the annual electricity consumption in each of these systems, calculating the "Energy Consumption Evaluation" coefficient with values of 1.08, 1.12, 1.19 and 3.80 in relation to the optimal system—MAU + DCC + FFU.

Shan and Wang [4] presented simulation results for three typical options of the structure of the HVAC system for cleanrooms in the pharmaceutical industry: "Interactive option", "Partially decoupled option" and "Fully decoupled option". They proved, for the chosen application, that using the "Partially decoupled option" made it possible to reduce the consumption of electricity and gas for cooling and heating by 69.8% and 87.8%, respectively.

Tsao et al. [14] presented simulation results for eight different combinations of a structure of the HVAC system of a semiconductor manufacturing room. These combinations included: the location of a fan in MAU (push-through vs. draft-through), one or two temperature levels of cooling water from chillers and using condensation heat recovery in chillers for reheating in MAU. They proved the possibility of reducing electricity consumption by 38.65% compared to the standard option.

Additionally, Kim et al. [15] simulated the operation of a HVAC system for cleanrooms for four options: Variable Air Volume (VAV), AIR WASHer System (AIRWASH), Dedicated Outdoor Air System (DOAS) and Integrated with Indirect and Direct Evaporative Coolers (IDECOAS). The simulation tool used was the EES (f-chart Software 2009) program. The scope of the simulation included two types of systems (type 1—percentage of outdoor air $\alpha = 100\%$ and type 2—$\alpha \neq 100\%$) and six types of climates. The simulation results proved that DOAS and IDECOAS applications make it possible to reduce the annual demand for cold and heat by 67.5% and 59.5%, respectively, compared to a VAV system. Yin et al. [16,17] energetically optimized a classic HVAC system: MAU + FFU + DCC, in which, as part of the modification, only part of the recirculation air was cooled in the DCC, and reheating in MAU was replaced by a mixing operation in a space above the suspended ceiling. Eventually, the demand for cold in the DCC was decreased by $40 \div 52\%$ compared to the classic system [17]. Similarly, Ma et al. [18] optimized the heat exchanger system in the MAU unit by resigning from reheating and achieving energy savings for pumping in the MAU unit in the range of 10.7–17.2%. The mentioned authors also optimized the structure of the filtration system by filtering the return and outdoor air separately. They proved that, by replacing the HEPA filters on the return with fine filters, the energy consumption could be reduced from 25.8% to 45% due to the lower air flow resistance [19].

Additionally, Yin et al. [20] optimized an existing classic HVAC system (MAU + FFU + DCC) in a semiconductor manufacturing factory. Based on the results of the measurements and numerical simulations for a HVAC system upgrade option, they proved that, by implementing high-temperature chillers, heat recovery from DCC to MAU and resigning from reheating, the energy consumption can be reduced by 20.2% compared to the existing HVAC system.

Chen et al. [21] analyzed the possibilities and energy effects of the application of adiabatic humidification for HVAC systems of selected cleanrooms. They indicated the system "spray nozzles using high-pressure water atomization" as the most advantageous in the case of adiabatic humidification. Xu et al. [22] presented the results of research on the efficiency of FFU fans. The evaluation criteria were the TPE (total pressure efficiency) and EPI (energy performance index) values. They proved that greater energy efficiency is usually associated with larger fans. Energy consumption for the various HVAC system structures of operating theaters was one of the criteria for multicriteria evaluating these systems presented by Fan et al. [23]. By solving the MCDM (multicriteria decision-making) problem, the authors proved a relationship between energy consumption, ventilation effectiveness and user satisfaction. Research in this area, especially with regards to recirculation and heat recovery, was also carried out by Ozyogurtcu et al. [24], who analyzed the energy consumption of four different HVAC systems in hospital operating rooms. They proved that the optimal energy is the HVAC system with a recuperator and regulated air recirculation.

The research on the optimization of the structure of the cooling system for HVAC systems of cleanrooms was conducted by Jia et al. [25]. The authors investigated two free cooling systems integrated with the central cooling system: tap water and cooling tower. They proved that the COP coefficients of a tap water free cooling system were about 7.4 and 2.2 times higher than that of mechanical cooling and tower cooling systems. In turn, the results of research on the optimization of an integrated cooling and heat generation system for HVAC systems in an electronics factory were presented by Zheng and Li [26]. The authors developed the GMEL (Grade Match Between Energy and Load) method that allows for the optimal use of cold and waste heat for the mutual compensation of loads. For the case study, they achieved energy savings of 26.7/52.4% in the summer and winter, respectively.

Research on the optimization of the control of HVAC systems of cleanrooms with the structure MAU + DCC was led by Wang et al. [27], demonstrating savings of 7.09% compared to the classic PDI controller. In turn, Zhuang et al. [28] developed and implemented an energy-optimized control strategy for multizone HVAC systems in a pharmaceutical plant on a simulation platform, achieving 20% energy savings compared to the standard control strategy.

A series of papers dedicated to research concerning the energy-optimal control of a HVAC system for cleanrooms, mainly in the pharmaceutical industry, was published by Zhuang, Wang and Shan [3,29–31].

In paper [29], the authors presented a probabilistic method of optimal control of HVAC systems based on the ADV strategy ("Adaptive Full-Range Decoupled Ventilation Strategy"). They proved that the implementation of this strategy makes it possible to reduce the annual average energy cost compared to the DV (Dedicated Outdoor Air Ventilation), PD (Partially Decoupled Control) and IC (Interactive Control) strategies by 18.2%, 13.6% and 6.5%, respectively.

In another study [31], the authors showed savings of 6.8 ÷ 40.8% as a result of the implementation of the ADV over IC strategy.

Using a simulation platform, Zhuang et al. [30] also tested and implemented the ADV strategy for a HVAC system for cleanrooms of a pharmaceutical factory in Hong Kong. In this case, they proved that the implementation of this strategy makes it possible to reduce the annual energy consumption by 21.64%, 15.63% and 7.77%, respectively, compared to the PD, IC and DV strategies.

In paper [3], the authors addressed solving the problem of energy-optimal control of a multizone HVAC system of a classic structure (MAU + AHU) and different loads in individual zones (rooms). They proposed the Coordinated Demand—Controlled Ventilation (CDCV) strategy, the implementation of which made it possible to reduce the demand for reheating by 89.6% and to reduce the total energy demand by 63.3%.

In turn, Chang et al. [32] investigated six strategies for controlling a cleanroom HVAC system, indicating the energy-optimal variant. They proved that the setting of the required room temperature is of key importance here; increasing this temperature by 1 °C resulted in a reduction of energy consumption by 1%. Loomans et al. [33,34] and Molnaar [35], on the other hand, simulated and experimentally tested three ventilation strategies in pharmaceutical cleanrooms: Fine-tuning, DCF (Demand Controlled Filtration) and Optimizing airflow pattern. They proved that, using the DCF strategy, it is possible to reduce the energy consumption of fans by up to 70% and 93.6% in the case studies under consideration.

Shao et al. [36] investigated experimentally the effect of airflow reduction as a factor of reducing energy consumption on the relative concentration of particles in a cleanroom. The obtained results and correlations allowed for optimal energetic determination of the air stream as a function of the cleanliness class of the room.

To summarize the current state of research concerning the optimization of HVAC system for cleanrooms, the following can be stated:

- until now, researchers have mainly focused on case studies in pharmaceutical and semiconductor industries;
- optimal structures of the HVAC system are calculated by performing simulations for several predetermined acceptable variants and indicating the variant for which the annual energy consumption is minimal;
- there is no global approach to calculating the optimal structures of the HVAC system as a function of key constants parameters being the input data and describing the HVAC system.

Therefore, there is a methodological gap at the stage of determining the set of acceptable structures of HVAC systems of cleanrooms fulfilling the functional function described by: cleanliness class, temperature, relative humidity, air velocity, degree of turbulence, overpressure, concentration of pollutants and share of outside air.

At the same time, there is a need to undertake research on support tools in order to determine, from a set of acceptable variants, the optimal structure and algorithms of HVAC system control.

Therefore, for the needs of the application, methods and tools are sought that allow, at the starting point, to define a set of acceptable structures of HVAC systems on the basis of output data—the standard parameters defining the utility function, decision variables and limiting conditions. Next, relationships are sought on the basis of which optimal structures and algorithms for controlling HVAC systems can be determined. In applications, it is important that the arguments in these relations are constant parameters constituting the output data in the optimization procedure.

The aim of the presented paper is to calculate approximating functions describing optimal structures of the HVAC system for cleanrooms depending on key constant parameters (arguments): cleanliness class (C_s), percentage of outdoor air (α_o) and unit cooling load (q_j) and determination of the energy-optimal control algorithms for heat recovery options and the outdoor climate. The annual unit primary energy demand of the HVAC system for thermodynamic air treatment was adopted as the objective function.

The proposed method is an original approach, both from the scientific and the application points of view.

2. Research Problem, General Algorithm

Every HVAC system can be described by a vector with coordinates defined by constant parameters and decision variables. With regards to cleanrooms, the constant parameters are primarily temperature, relative humidity, cleanliness class, percentage of outdoor air, unit cooling load and pressure gradients.

For determined combinations of constant parameters values of a HVAC system, a single optimization problem can be defined concerning calculating the optimal HVAC system for which the annual energy demands (final, primary) reach the minimum values.

The constant parameters of a HVAC system for cleanrooms are within realistic value ranges. In general, one can define a set of combinations of constant parameter values in which each constant parameter takes values representing the entire range of variability.

The research problem comes down to calculating the set of optimal structures of a HVAC system assigned to combinations of values of constant parameters representing realistic ranges of variability of these parameters in cleanrooms.

On this basis, it is possible to calculate approximating relations defining structures of HVAC systems as a function of combinations of constant parameter values.

The general algorithm of the optimization procedure partly based on the methodology presented earlier by the authors of References [37,38] is presented in Figure 1. The algorithm includes:

- calculating the set of constant parameters $\overline{x}_i$ and the set of decision variables x_j;
- two phases of analysis: calculating the matrix of all possible variants of limiting conditions and of acceptable variants, respectively, for:
  - combinations of decision variables values x_j for normalizing constant parameters (matrices $\mathbf{W}_i$, $\mathbf{W}$, $\mathbf{G}_i$, $\mathbf{G}_j$ and $\mathbf{W}_g$) and
  - the HVAC system (matrices $\mathbf{X}^J$, $\mathbf{G}$ and $\mathbf{X}$);
- calculating the optimal structures of HVAC systems $\overline{x}^*_{ngk}$ for combinations of values of key constant parameters (arguments): cleanliness class (C_{sk}), percentage of outdoor air (αok) and unit cooling load (q_{jk}), k = 1 ... K;
- defining approximation relations $\overline{x}^*_{ngk} = f(C_{sk}, \alpha_{ok}, q_{jk})$;
- defining algorithms of energy-optimal control for optimal structures of HVAC systems $\overline{x}^*_{ngk}$ based on the objective function;
- calculating the optimal variant $\overline{x}^*$.

Constant parameters are by definition invariant in the optimization procedure, but in general, they can be functions of both time and space. The decision variables change during the optimization procedure and are the arguments of the $\overline{x}$ describing the HVAC system, the constraint conditions and the objective function. The fragment of the procedure in Figure 1, leading to the determination of the set of acceptable HVAC system structures, the **X** matrix, is based on the methodology described in detail in Reference [37]. After determining the **X** matrix, in the next step of the optimization procedure, the real required ranges for the variability of key fixed parameters in cleanroom applications, are determined: cleanliness class (C_{sk}), share of outside air (α_{ok}) and unit cooling load (q_{jk}). Then, on this basis, a representative set of combinations of the values of the key parameters of the HVAC system constants is determined, and for each of these combinations, the optimal structure of the HVAC system $\overline{x}^*_{ngk}$ is determined based on an algorithm from the set of permissible structures (**X** matrices). In the next step, on the basis of the obtained results, the general algorithm assumes the development of approximating relations defining energy-optimal structures of HVAC systems as a function of key constant parameters $\overline{x}^*_{ngk} = f(C_{sk}, \alpha_{ok}, q_{jk})$. In the final stage of the optimization procedure, the objective function is determined—the minimum annual demand for primary energy for thermodynamic treatment, the optimal type of heat recovery for various outdoor climate options and the energy-optimal control algorithms.

The algorithm structure of the general optimization procedure includes three basic steps:

- determination of a set of permissible HVAC system structures—X matrix, based on the utility function (normalized constants and limiting conditions);
- determination of the optimal structure of the HVAC system—$\overline{x}^*_{ng}$ based on the key constants: C_s—cleanliness class, $\dot{q}_j$—unit heat load and α_o—percentage of outside air;
- determination of the energy-optimal variant of the HVAC system—vector $\overline{x}^*$, taking into account the optimal structure and the optimal type of heat recovery.

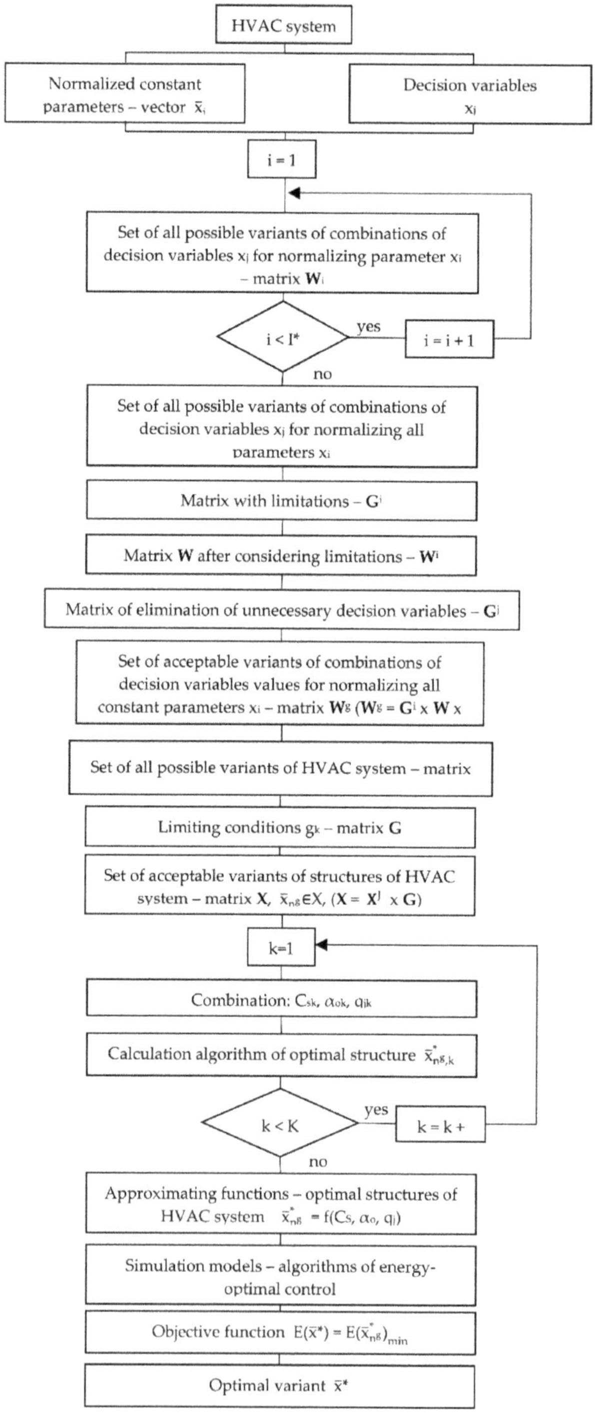

Figure 1. Optimization procedure—general algorithm.

3. Acceptable Structures of HVAC System

The starting point in determining the permissible structures of the HVAC system is the determination of a set of parameters standardized by this system. A wide range of normalized constant parameters in a cleanroom was used:

- temperature, t_R
- relative humidity $\varphi_R \in (\varphi_{R1}, \varphi_{R2})$
- acceptable concentration of contaminants, k_d
- cleanliness class, C_S
- overpressure, Δp
- percentage of outdoor air, α_o

The procedure leading to the determination of acceptable structures of the HVAC system based on the methodology previously developed by the authors of Reference [37] is presented in Appendix A. This procedure uses system analysis and matrix calculus. The forms of the determined matrices are listed in Appendix A; these matrices are described in the following order:

- normalized constant parameters;
- a set of all possible variants of a combination of decision variables for the normalization of each individual and all constant parameters together;
- limiting conditions for variants of combinations of decision variables for the standardization of constant parameters;
- set of eliminated decision variables;
- a set of all possible variants of the HVAC system for the standardization of constant parameters;
- limiting conditions for possible variants of the HVAC system;
- set of acceptable HVAC system structures.

Acceptable variants $\overline{x}_{ng}$ of the structure of the HVAC system for cleanrooms are presented synthetically in a form of a general model in Figure 2.

$\dot{V}_o$,$\dot{V}_c$, $\dot{V}$, $\dot{V}_e$, $\dot{V}_1$, $\dot{V}_2$, $\Delta\dot{V}$—volume stream of outdoor air, processing air, supply air, exhaust air, external recirculation air, internal recirculation air and balance sheet difference.

$\alpha_o = \frac{\dot{V}_o}{\dot{V}}$, $\alpha_c = \frac{\dot{V}_c}{\dot{V}}$, $\alpha_1 = \frac{\dot{V}_1}{\dot{V}}$, $\alpha_2 = \frac{\dot{V}_2}{\dot{V}}$—percentage of outdoor air, processing air, external recirculation air and internal recirculation air;

E_1, E_2, E_3—filtration efficiency of the 1°, 2° and 3° stages;

HR—heat recovery.

Acceptable variants $\overline{x}_{ng}$ of the HVAC system include:

$\overline{x}_1$—CAV air system without recirculation:

a. AHU—thermodynamic treatment: heat recovery, primary heater, cooler, secondary heater and steam humidifier;
b. hygienic standard: three stages of filtration, 3rd stage filter integrated with a supply diffuser, hygienic design;
c. installation: variable flow regulators.

$\overline{x}_2$—CAV air system with external recirculation:

a. two air handling units in cascade at the supply: MAU + AHU;
b. MAU of outdoor air with heat recovery;
c. AHU—thermodynamic treatment: primary heater, cooler, secondary heater and steam humidifier;
d. hygienic standard: as with $\overline{x}_1$ point b;
e. installation: as with $\overline{x}_1$ point c.

$\overline{x}_3$—CAV air system with internal recirculation (room):

a. two air handling units in cascade at the supply: AHU + RU (RDCU);
b. AHU—thermodynamic treatment: heat recovery, primary heater, cooler, secondary heater and steam humidifier;

c. RU (Recirculation Unit) or RDCU (Recirculation Dry Cooling Unit)—recirculation (recirculation with dry cooling);
d. hygienic standard: as with $\overline{x}_1$ point b;
e. installation: as with $\overline{x}_1$ point c.

$\overline{x}_4$—CAV system with external and internal recirculation (room):

a. three air handling units in cascade at the supply: MAU + AHU + RU (RDCU);
b. MAU of outdoor air with heat recovery;
c. AHU—thermodynamic treatment: primary heater, cooler, secondary heater and steam humidifier;
d. RU or RDCU—recirculation (recirculation with dry cooling);
e. hygienic standard: as with $\overline{x}_1$ point b;
f. installation: as with $\overline{x}_1$ point c.

In variants $\overline{x}_3$ and $\overline{x}_4$, alternatives to internal recirculation RU (RDCU) are: FFU (FFU + DCC) or FFU + FDCU.

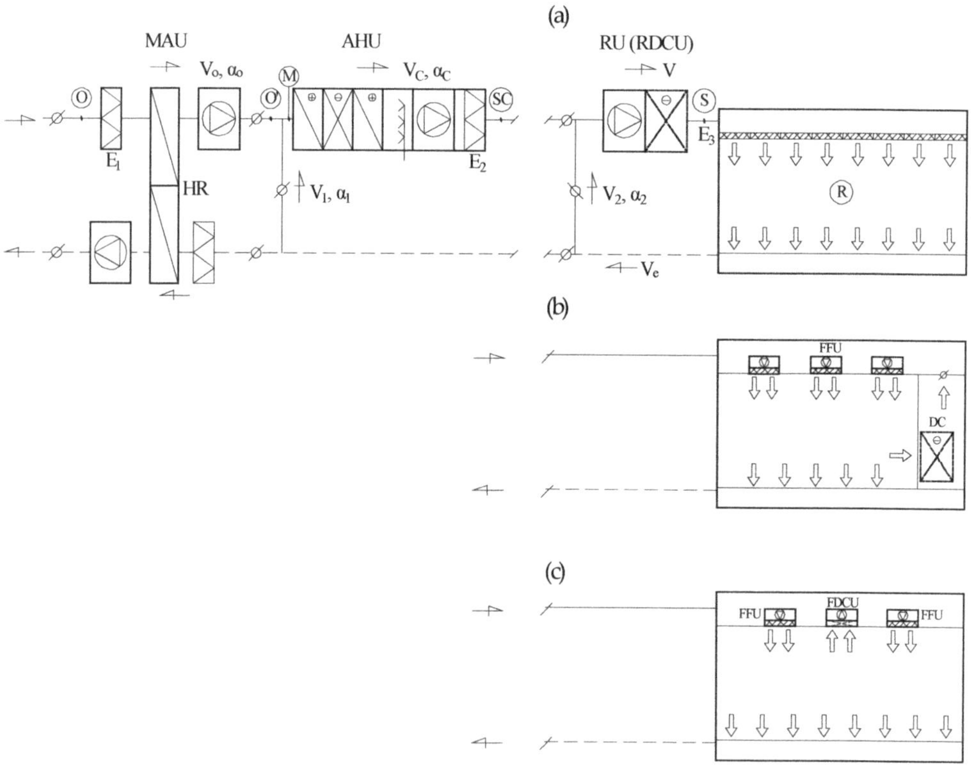

Figure 2. General model of the acceptable variants of structures of the HVAC system for cleanrooms: $\overline{x}_1$—without recirculation ($\alpha_1 = 0$, $\alpha_2 = 0$, $\alpha_o = 1$); $\overline{x}_2$—with external recirculation ($\alpha_1 \neq 0$, $\alpha_2 = 0$); $\overline{x}_3$—with internal recirculation ($\alpha_1 = 0$, $\alpha_2 \neq 1$); $\overline{x}_4$—with external and internal recirculation ($\alpha_1 \neq 0$, $\alpha_2 \neq 0$). Variants of internal recirculation ($\alpha_2 \neq 0$): (**a**) RU or RDCU, (**b**) FFU or FFU + DCC, (**c**) FFU + FDCU.

4. Optimal Structures of HVAC System

4.1. Optimal Structure Selection Algorithm

The calculation algorithm of the optimal structure of the HVAC system is shown in Figure 3. The starting point includes constant parameters of the HVAC system and set of acceptable variants $\bar{x}_{ng} \in X$. Selection of the optimal structure of the HVAC system is a permissibility function of recirculation (hygienic function) and values of three air streams:

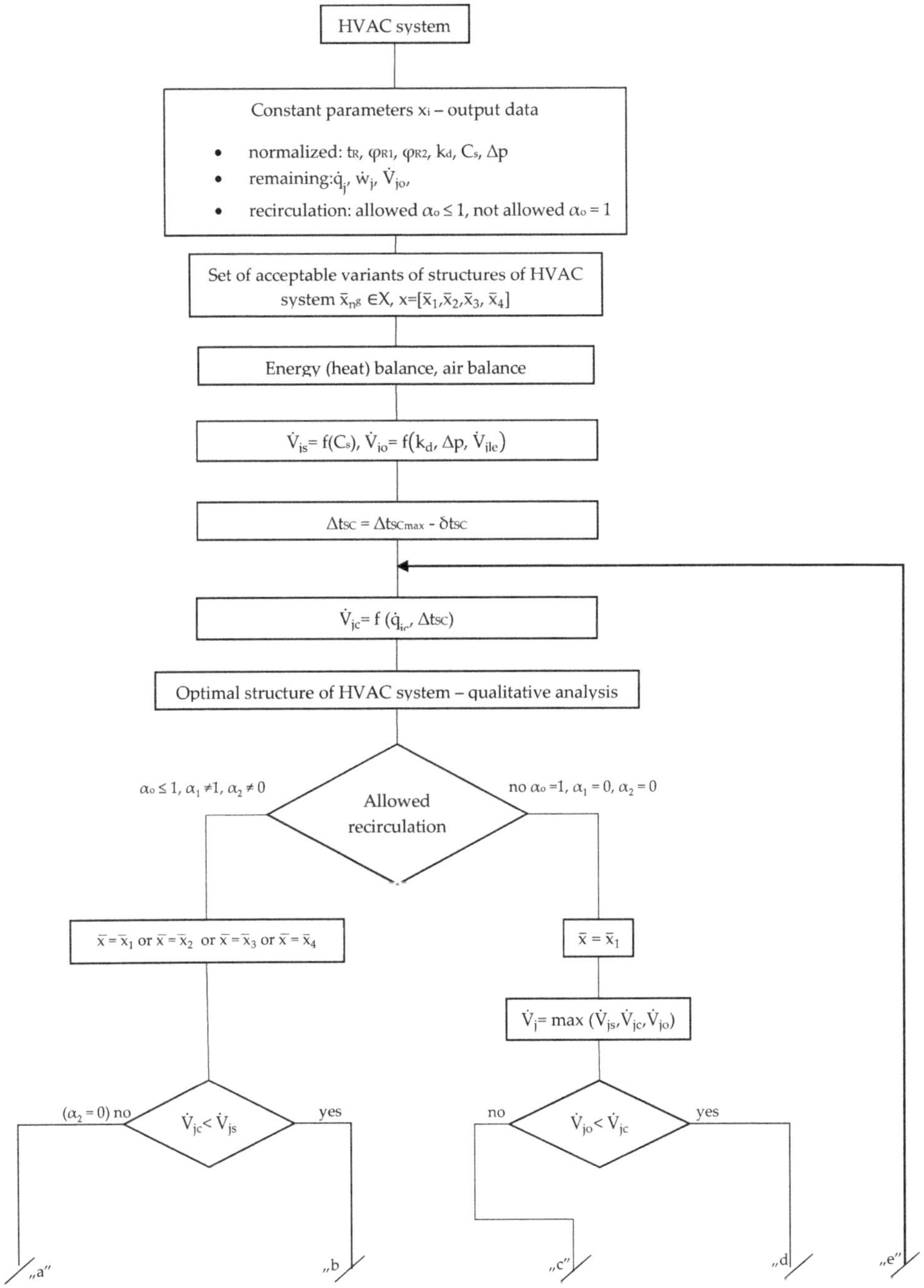

Figure 3. *Cont.*

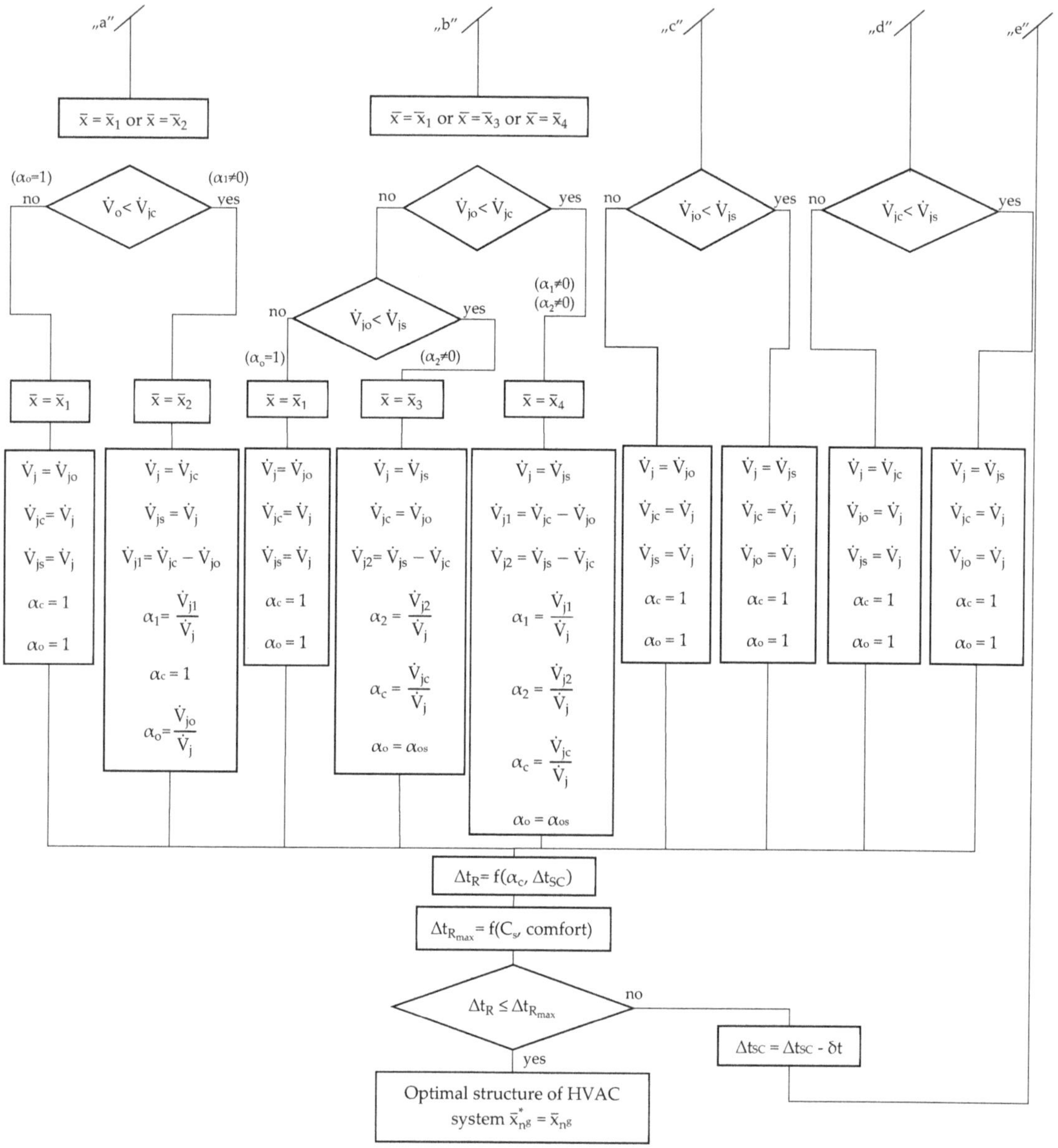

Figure 3. Calculation algorithm of the optimal structure of the HVAC system.

- $\dot{V}_{jo} = f(kd, \Delta p, \dot{V}_{jle})$—unit outdoor air stream as a function of hygiene requirements (the concentration of pollutants—k_d), overpressure (Δp) or compensation of exhaust air from local exhausts ($\dot{V}_{jle}$);
- $\dot{V}_{js} = f(C_S)$—unit air stream as a function of the room cleanliness class;
- $\dot{V}_{jc} = \dot{V}_{jc_{min}} = f\left(\dot{q}_j\right)$—unit air stream as a function of the cooling loads discharged using AHU.

In case recirculation is not allowed, the only system acceptable is $\overline{x}_1$; if allowed, all systems are possible: $\overline{x}_1$, $\overline{x}_2$, $\overline{x}_3$ and $\overline{x}_4$.

Unit stream of outdoor air $\dot{V}_{jo}$, depending on the conditions, is within the range corresponding to the percentage of outdoor air $\alpha_o = 5 \div 100\%$.

Unit air stream as a function of the cleanliness class $\dot{V}_{js}$ is calculated based on the average air speed from the range (w_{min}, w_{max}) required for a specific room cleanliness class according to ASHRAE [39]. Unit air stream for discharging cooling loads using AHU is calculated—taking into consideration the designations in Figure 4—using relation:

$$\dot{V}_{jc} = \frac{\dot{q}_{jc}}{\rho c_p \Delta t_{SC}}, \tag{1}$$

whereby:

$$\dot{q}_{jc} = q_j - q_{jDC} \tag{2}$$

with:

q_j—unit cooling loads;
q_{jc}—unit cooling load discharged using AHU;
q_{jDC}—unit cooling load discharged by dry coolers in the recirculation circuit (DCC, RDCU and RCU).

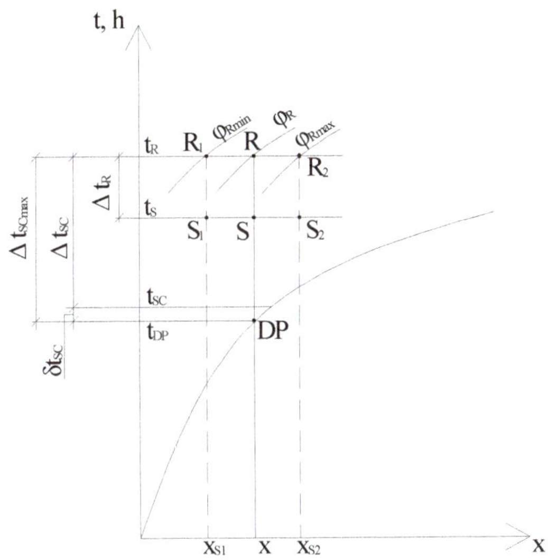

Figure 4. Isotherms characteristic for calculating the $\dot{V}_{jc}$ (AHU) air stream.

In a specific case, when $\dot{q}_{jDC} = 0$

$$\dot{q}_{jc} = \dot{q}_j \tag{3}$$

In the first step, requirement $\dot{V}_{jc}$ = min (corresponding to the minimum energy consumption) implies relation:

$$\Delta t_{SC} = \Delta t_{SCmax} - \delta t_{SC} = (t_R - t_{DP}) - \delta t_{SC} \tag{4}$$

which means that

$$t_{SC} = t_{SCmin} = t_{DP} + \delta t_{SC} \tag{5}$$

where:

δt_{SC}—realistic tolerance range with temperature t_{SC} in relation to temperature t_{DP}, $\delta t_{SC} = (0 \div 1)$ °C
t_{DP}—dew point temperature.

In the physical interpretation, this requirement means that the minimum air flow to dissipate cooling loads $\dot{V}_{jc}$ is determined assuming the maximum possible temperature difference Δt_{SC} between the air in the room and the supply air. In turn, the minimum supply air temperature t_{SCmin} is theoretically equal to the dew point temperature t_{DP}; in practice, it should be slightly higher (here, the real tolerance range δt_{SC} was adopted).

Then, on the basis of the values of air flows $\dot{V}_{js}$, $\dot{V}_{jc}$ and $\dot{V}_{jo}$, which are comparative terms, the algorithm determines the optimal structure of the HVAC system $\overline{x}_1$, $\overline{x}_2$, $\overline{x}_3$ or $\overline{x}_4$, and the resulting temperature difference Δt_R and the supply temperature t_S are calculated according to the relations:

- system $\overline{x}_1$ ($\alpha_1 = 0$, $\alpha_2 = 0$, $\alpha_c = 1$):

$$\Delta t_R = \Delta t_{SC} \tag{6}$$

$$t_S = t_{SC} \tag{7}$$

- system $\overline{x}_2$ ($\alpha_1 \neq 0$, $\alpha_2 = 0$, $\alpha_c = 1$):

$$\Delta t_R = \Delta t_{SC} \tag{8}$$

$$t_S = t_{SC} \tag{9}$$

- system $\overline{x}_3$ ($\alpha_1 = 0$, $\alpha_2 \neq 0$, $\alpha_c \neq 0$):

$$\Delta t_R = \alpha_c \cdot \Delta t_{SC} = (1 - \alpha_2) \cdot \Delta t_{SC} \tag{10}$$

$$t_S = \alpha_c \cdot t_{SC} + (1 - \alpha_c)\, t_R \tag{11}$$

$$t_{SC} = \frac{1}{\alpha_c} \cdot t_S + (1 - \frac{1}{\alpha_c}) \cdot t_R \tag{12}$$

- system $\overline{x}_4$ ($\alpha_1 \neq 0$, $\alpha_2 \neq 0$, $\alpha_c \neq 0$):

$$\Delta t_R = \alpha_c \cdot \Delta t_{SC} = (1 - \alpha_2)\, \Delta t_{SC} \tag{13}$$

$$t_S = \alpha_c \cdot t_{SC} + (1 - \alpha_c)\, t_R \tag{14}$$

$$t_{SC} = \frac{1}{\alpha_c} \cdot t_S + (1 - \frac{1}{\alpha_c}) \cdot t_R \tag{15}$$

whereby:

$$\alpha_c = 1 - \alpha_2 = \alpha_o + \alpha_1 \tag{16}$$

In the next step, a significant limitation is the relationship resulting from the air distribution system required in the room:

$$\Delta t_R \leq \Delta t_{SC} \tag{17}$$

indirectly related to relation:

$$t_{SC} \leq t_S \tag{18}$$

and a comparative section:

$$\Delta t_R \leq \Delta t_{Rmax} \tag{19}$$

It should be noted that the maximum value of the temperature difference

$$\Delta t_{Rmax} = t_R - t_{Smin} \tag{20}$$

is the result of comfort limitations (air supply system) and, indirectly, of the room cleanliness class.

At this stage, it may turn out that the determined temperature difference Δt_{SC}, which corresponds to the air stream $\dot{V}_{jc}$ = min, is greater than the permissible temperature difference Δt_{Rmax} for comfort or technological reasons. In such a case, the algorithm assumes a decrease in the value of the temperature difference Δt_{SC} according to the relation:

$$\Delta t_{SC} \equiv \Delta t_{SC} - \delta t \tag{21}$$

with:

$\delta t = (0.5 \div 1.0)$ °C—iterative temperature jump, and the procedure is repeated.

Based on the algorithm (Figure 3), the optimal variants of the HVAC system structure of cleanrooms were determined as a function of the relationship between the streams $\dot{V}_{js}$, $\dot{V}_{jc}$ and $\dot{V}_{jo}$; these variants are summarized in Table 1.

Table 1. Optimal variants of the HVAC structure $\overline{x}^*_{ng}$ of clean air as a function of the relation of streams $\dot{V}_{js}$, $\dot{V}_{jc}$ and $\dot{V}_{jo}$.

Optimal Variant of the HVAC Structure $\overline{x}^*_{ng}$	Relations: $\dot{V}_{js}, \dot{V}_{jc}$ and $\dot{V}_{jo}$	Air Streams
$\overline{x}_1$	$\alpha_o = 1$ i $\alpha_1 = 0$ i $\alpha_2 = 0$ $\dot{V}_{jo} \geq \dot{V}_{js}, \dot{V}_{jo} \geq \dot{V}_{jc}$	$\dot{V}_j = \dot{V}_{jo}$ $\dot{V}_{jc} = \dot{V}_j$
$\overline{x}_2$	$\dot{V}_{jo} < \dot{V}_{jc}, \dot{V}_{jc} \geq \dot{V}_{js}$	$\dot{V}_j = \dot{V}_{jc}$ $\dot{V}_{js} = \dot{V}_j$
$\overline{x}_3$	$\dot{V}_{jo} < \dot{V}_{js}, \dot{V}_{jo} \geq \dot{V}_{jc}, \dot{V}_{jc} < \dot{V}_{js}$	$\dot{V}_j = \dot{V}_{js}$ $\dot{V}_{jc} = \dot{V}_{jo}$
$\overline{x}_4$	$\dot{V}_{jo} < \dot{V}_{jc}, \dot{V}_{jc} < \dot{V}_{js}$	$\dot{V}_j = \dot{V}_{js}$

4.2. Optimal Structure Selection Algorithm

By analyzing realistic required ranges of variability of the key constant parameters in applications for cleanrooms, the following conclusions can be made:

- dry bulb temperature changes in a narrow range of +21 ÷ +23 °C; on average, t_R = +22 °C;
- relative humidity usually changes in the range of (50 ± 5)% (sometimes, the range is wider);
- the most common cleanliness classes are ISO5 classes (M3.5—cl. 100), ISO7 (M5.5—cl. 10,000) and ISO8 (M6.5—cl. 100,000) [39];
- unit cooling loads are $q_j = (100 \div 500)$ W/m^2 [40];
- the required percentage of outdoor air is $\alpha_o = (5 \div 100)\%$.

Therefore, further analyses include variants of combinations of key constant parameters of a HVAC system, in which each constant parameter takes values representing the mentioned variability ranges.

4.3. Approximating Functions

Optimal structures of the HVAC system for cleanrooms are calculated based on the algorithm in Figure 3 for representative variants of combinations of key constant parameters: cleanliness class C_s, unit cooling load q_j ($q_j = q_{jc}$) and percentage of outdoor air α_o are shown in Table 2. The analyses were performed with the temperature of t_R = +22 °C and relative humidity φ_R = (50 ± 5)%.

Table 2. Optimal structures of the HVAC system for cleanrooms $\overline{x}^{*}_{ng}$.

Variant of Constant Parameters	Cleanliness Class ISO(US.FSd.209e)	q_j /6 W/m^2	α_{os} /4 %	$\dot{V}_{js}$ m^3/hm^2	$\dot{V}_{jo}$ m^3/hm^2	$\dot{V}_{js}$ /7 m^3/hm^2	Optimal Structure of HVAC System					
							$\overline{x}_{ng}$	$\dot{V}_j$ m^3/hm^2	α_o /5 %	α_c %	α_1 %	α_2 %
1.1.1	ISO Class 5 1/ (M3.5—cl. 100)	100	5	900	45	27.1	$\overline{x}_3$	900	5	5	-	95
1.1.2			10	900	90	27.1	$\overline{x}_3$	900	10	10	-	90
1.1.3			30	900	270	27.1	$\overline{x}_3$	900	30	30	-	70
1.1.4			50	900	450	27.1	$\overline{x}_3$	900	50	50	-	50
1.1.5			100	900	900	27.1	$\overline{x}_1$	900	100	100	-	-
1.2.1		300	5	900	45	81.4	$\overline{x}_4$	900	5	9	4	91
1.2.2			10	900	90	81.4	$\overline{x}_3$	900	10	10	-	90
1.2.3			30	900	270	81.4	$\overline{x}_3$	900	30	30	-	70
1.2.4			50	900	450	81.4	$\overline{x}_3$	900	50	50	-	50
1.2.5			100	900	900	81.4	$\overline{x}_1$	900	100	100	-	-
1.3.1		500	5	900	45	135.7	$\overline{x}_4$	900	5	15	10	85
1.3.2			10	900	90	135.7	$\overline{x}_4$	900	10	15	5	85
1.3.3			30	900	270	135.7	$\overline{x}_3$	900	30	30	-	70
1.3.4			50	900	450	135.7	$\overline{x}_3$	900	50	50	-	50
1.3.5			100	900	900	135.7	$\overline{x}_1$	900	100	100	-	-
2.1.1	ISO Class 7 2/ (M5.5—cl.10 000)	100	5	216	10.8	27.1	$\overline{x}_4$	216	5	12.5	7.5	87.5
2.1.2			10	216	21.6	27.1	$\overline{x}_4$	216	10	12.5	2.5	87.5
2.1.3			30	216	64.8	27.1	$\overline{x}_3$	216	30	30	-	70
2.1.4			50	216	108	27.1	$\overline{x}_3$	216	50	50	-	50
2.1.5			100	216	216	27.1	$\overline{x}_1$	216	100	100	-	-
2.2.1		300	5	216	10.8	81.4	$\overline{x}_4$	216	5	37.7	32.7	62.3
2.2.2			10	216	21.6	81.4	$\overline{x}_4$	216	10	37.7	27.7	62.3
2.2.3			30	216	64.8	81.4	$\overline{x}_4$	216	30	37.7	7.7	62.3
2.2.4			50	216	108	81.4	$\overline{x}_3$	216	50	50	-	50
2.2.5			100	216	216	81.4	$\overline{x}_1$	216	100	100	-	-
2.3.1		500	5	216	10.8	135.7	$\overline{x}_4$	216	5	62.8	57.8	37.2
2.3.2			10	216	21.6	135.7	$\overline{x}_4$	216	10	62.8	52.8	37.2
2.3.3			30	216	64.8	135.7	$\overline{x}_4$	216	30	62.8	32.8	37.2
2.3.4			50	216	108	135.7	$\overline{x}_4$	216	50	62.8	12.8	37.2
2.3.5			100	216	216	135.7	$\overline{x}_1$	216	100	100	-	-
3.1.1	ISO Class 8 3/ (M6.5—cl.100 000)	100	5	90	4.5	27.1	$\overline{x}_4$	90	5	30	25	70
3.1.2			10	90	9	27.1	$\overline{x}_4$	90	10	30	20	70
3.1.3			30	90	27	27.1	$\overline{x}_3$	90	30	30	-	70
3.1.4			50	90	45	27.1	$\overline{x}_3$	90	50	50	-	50
3.1.5			100	90	90	27.1	$\overline{x}_1$	90	100	100	-	-
3.2.1		300	5	90	4.5	81.4	$\overline{x}_4$	90	5	90	85	10
3.2.2			10	90	9	81.4	$\overline{x}_4$	90	10	90	80	10
3.2.3			30	90	27	81.4	$\overline{x}_4$	90	30	90	60	10
3.2.4			50	90	45	81.4	$\overline{x}_4$	90	50	90	40	10
3.2.5			100	90	90	81.4	$\overline{x}_1$	90	100	100	-	-
3.3.1		500	5	90	4.5	135.7	$\overline{x}_2$	135.7	3.3	100	96.7	-
3.3.2			10	90	9	135.7	$\overline{x}_2$	135.7	6.6	100	93.4	-
3.3.3			30	90	27	135.7	$\overline{x}_2$	135.7	19.9	100	80.1	-
3.3.4			50	90	45	135.7	$\overline{x}_2$	135.7	33.2	100	66.8	-
3.3.5			100	90	90	135.7	$\overline{x}_1$	135.7	100	100	-	-

1/ w = 0.25 m/s (300 1/h, H = 3 m), 2/ w = 0.06 m/s (72 1/h, H = 3 m), 3/ w = 0.025 m/s (30 1/h, H = 3 m) [39], 4/ $\alpha_{os} = \dot{V}_{jo}/\dot{V}_{js}$, 5/ $\alpha_o = \dot{V}_{jo}/\dot{V}_j$, 6/ $q_j = q_{jc}$ and 7/ $\Delta t_{SCmax} = 11\ ^\circ C$.

The unit air stream $\dot{V}_{js}$ as a function of the cleanliness class C_s was determined by assuming the average air velocities from the compartments assigned to the ASHRAE cleanliness classes [39].

For cleanliness classes with optimal structures of the HVAC system $\overline{x}_3$ or $\overline{x}_4$ based on the results in Table 2, limit percentages of the outdoor air α_{og} were calculated (equal to the percentages of air of an AHU for discharging cooling loads). Value α_{og} is calculated using:

$$\alpha_{og} = \frac{\dot{V}_{jc}}{\dot{V}_{js}} \tag{22}$$

These values represent the selection criterion of the optimal structure of the HVAC system according to relation:

$$\alpha_o \geq \alpha_{og} \text{optimal structure } \overline{x}_3 \tag{23}$$

$$\alpha_o < \alpha_{og} \text{optimal structure } \overline{x}_4 \tag{24}$$

For cleanliness classes that include the optimal HVAC structures $\overline{x}_2$, $\overline{x}_3$ and $\overline{x}_4$ (here, ISO Class 8)—based on the results in Table 2—an additional limit unit cooling load $\dot{q}_{jg}$ was calculated using relation:

$$\dot{q}_{jg} = \dot{V}_{js} \rho c_p \Delta t SC_{max} \tag{25}$$

In the physical interpretation, parameter $\dot{q}_{jg}$ is the maximum cooling load that can be discharged by the air flow $\dot{V}_{jc} = \dot{V}_{js}$ resulting from the room cleanliness class.

Values $\dot{q}_{jg}$ represent the selection criteria of the optimal structure of the HVAC system according to relation:

$$\dot{q}_j \geq \dot{q}_{jg} \text{optimal structure } \overline{x}_2 \tag{26}$$

$$\dot{q}_j < \dot{q}_{jg} \text{optimal structure } \overline{x}_3 \text{ or } \overline{x}_4 \tag{27}$$

The parameter calculation results α_{og} and $\dot{q}_{jg}$ are shown in Table 3.

Table 3. Limit percentages of the outdoor air α_{og} and limit unit cooling load $\dot{q}_j$ for optimal structures of the HVAC system.

Cleanliness Class ISO 14644-1 (USFStd 209e)	$\dot{q}_j$ W/m^2	$\dot{V}_{js}$ m^3/hm^2	$\dot{V}_{jc}$ m^3/hm^2	α_{og} %	$\dot{q}_{jg}$ W/m^2
ISO Class 5 (M 3.5—cl. 100)	100	900	27.1	3	3300 */
	300		81.4	9	
	500		135.7	15	
ISO Class 7 (M 5.5—cl. 10,000)	100	216	27.1	12.5	796 */
	300		81.4	37.7	
	500		135.7	62.8	
ISO Class 8 (M 6.5—cl. 100,000)	100	90	27.1	30	332
	300		81.4	90	
	500		135.7	- **/	

*/ in applications $\dot{q}_j < \dot{q}_{jg}$, **/ is not calculated, because the optimal structure of the HVAC system is $\overline{x}_2\left(\dot{V}_j = \dot{V}_{jk}\right)$.

Based on the calculation results presented in Tables 2 and 3, the authors calculated the approximating functions in the form of diagrams illustrating zones of optimal structures of the HVAC system for cleanrooms.

These functions, in coordinate system $\overline{x}^*_{ng} = f(C_S, \alpha_o, q_j)$ for cleanliness classes ISO Class 5, ISO Class 7 and ISO Class 8, are shown in Figure 5.

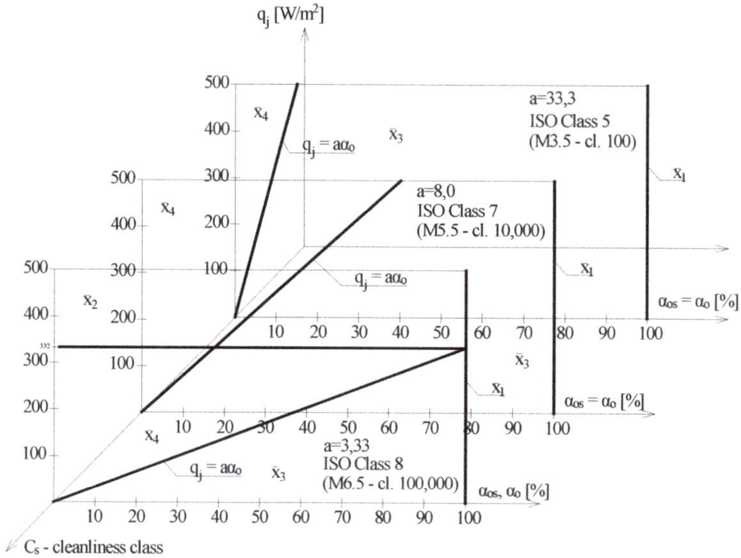

Figure 5. The function $\overline{x}^*_{ng}$ = f(C_S, α_o, q_j) of the zone of optimal structures of the HVAC system for cleanrooms ISO Class 5 (M3.5—cl. 100), ISO Class 7 (M5.5—cl. 10,000) and ISO Class 8 (M6.5—cl. 100,000).

Directional coefficients of limit lines equations between zones of the optimal structures $\overline{x}_3$ and $\overline{x}_4$ in Figure 5 were calculated based on the data in Table 3 and relation:

$$a = \frac{\Delta\dot{q}_j}{\Delta\alpha_{og}} \tag{28}$$

$\Delta\dot{q}_j$—difference in values of the unit cooling loads in Table 3;

$\Delta\alpha_{og}$—difference of the limit value of the percentage of outdoor air in Table 3 assigned to a defined difference $\Delta\dot{q}_j$.

Based on calculation results (Tables 2 and 3) illustrated by the approximating functions $\overline{x}^*_{ng}$ = f(C_S, α_o, q_j) in Figure 5, the following conclusions can be made:

1. The dominant optimal structures of HVAC system for cleanrooms with acceptable recirculation are systems with internal recirculation $\overline{x}_3$ and systems with internal and external recirculation $\overline{x}_4$.
2. Directional coefficients of the limit lines $\dot{q}_j = a\alpha_o$ dividing zones of optimal structures of the HVAC system HVAC $\overline{x}_3$ and $\overline{x}_4$ are inversely proportional to the cleanliness classes of rooms and equal:
    - a = 33.3—for ISO Class 5 (M3.5—cl.100);
    - a = 8.0—for ISO Class 7 (M5.5—cl.10,000);
    - a = 3.33—for ISO Class 8 (M6.5—cl.100,000),
3. Systems with internal recirculation $\overline{x}_3$ are optimal HVAC system structures for rooms with low cooling loads $\dot{q}_j$ and relatively high percentages of outdoor air α_o.
4. Systems with internal and external recirculation $\overline{x}_4$ are optimal HVAC system structures for rooms with high cooling loads $\dot{q}_j$ and relatively low percentages of outdoor air α_o.
5. Systems with external recirculation $\overline{x}_2$ are optimal HVAC system structures for rooms with high cooling loads $\dot{q}_j$ and low requirements regarding cleanliness of high cleanli-

ness classes. The limit line in system $\dot{q}_j = f(\alpha_o)$ between the zone of optimal structures $\overline{x}_2$ and $\overline{x}_3$ or $\overline{x}_2$ and $\overline{x}_4$ is ordinate $\dot{q}_{jg}$ (horizontal line). For cleanliness classes ISO Class 8 (M6.5—cl. 100,000) the limit unit cooling load equals $\dot{q}_{jg} = 332\ \mathrm{W/m^2}$. For unit cooling loads $\dot{q}_j \geq \dot{q}_{jg}$, the optimal structure of the HVAC system is a system with external recirculation $\overline{x}_2$, while, for $\dot{q}_j < \dot{q}_{jg}$, optimal structures are systems with internal recirculation $\overline{x}_3$ or systems with internal and external recirculation $\overline{x}_4$. The limit of division of optimal zones $\overline{x}_3$ and $\overline{x}_4$ is line $\dot{q}_j = a\alpha_o$.

6. Approximating functions in the form of a graph $\overline{x}^*_{ng} = f(C_S, \alpha_o, q_j)$ with zones of optimal structures of the HVAC system for cleanrooms in Figure 5 are of great application significance at the stage of selecting and designing energy-efficient HVAC systems of such rooms. Based on cleanliness class C_s of unit cooling loads $\dot{q}_j$ and the percentage of outdoor air α_o, they make it possible to unambiguously calculate an energy-optimal structure of a HVAC system for a cleanroom. For "middle" cleanliness classes between ISO5 and ISO7, zones of optimal HVAC structures can be calculated using interpolation.

5. Heat Recovery, Energy-Optimal Control

5.1. Objective Function, Simulation Models

For each HVAC system with energy-optimal structure $\overline{x}^*_{ng}$, where heat recovery occurs as a cumulative variable, it is possible to calculate an objective function defining the quantitative optimization criterion.

Based on this criterion, the energy-optimal type of the heat recovery and energy-optimal control algorithms are determined.

The objective function defines the annual primary energy demand of the HVAC system, which is possible to calculate using relation [37]:

$$E_p = \frac{w_H}{\eta_{H,t}} \cdot Q_{H,n} + \frac{w_{el}}{\eta_{el,t}} \cdot Q_{el,n} + \frac{w_C}{\eta_{C,t}} \cdot Q_{C,n} + \frac{w_B}{\eta_{B,t}} \cdot Q_{B,n} + w_{el} E_{el,pom} \tag{29}$$

or

$$E_p = w_H Q_{K,H} + w_{el} Q_{K,H_{el}} + w_C Q_{K,C} + w_B Q_{K,B} + w_{el} E_{el,pom} \tag{30}$$

whereby:

$$Q_{K,H} = \frac{1}{\eta_{H,t}} Q_{H,n} \tag{31}$$

$$Q_{K,H_{el}} = \frac{1}{\eta_{H_{el},t}} Q_{H_{el},n} \tag{32}$$

$$Q_{K,C} = \frac{1}{\eta_{C,t}} Q_{C,n} \tag{33}$$

$$Q_{K,B} = \frac{1}{\eta_{B,t}} Q_{B,n} \tag{34}$$

with:

$Q_{H,n}$ ($Q_{Hel,n}$)—annual heat demand (net) of water heaters (electric heaters), kWh/ym^2;
$Q_{C,n}$—annual cold demand (net) of cooler, kWh/ym^2;
$Q_{B,n}$—annual heat demand (net) of steam humidifiers, kWh/ym^2;
$Q_{K,H}$ ($Q_{K,Hel}$)—annual final energy demand of water heaters (electric heaters)—final heat kWh/ym^2;
$Q_{K,C}$—annual final energy demand of coolers—final cold, kWh/ym^2;
$Q_{K,B}$—annual final energy demand of steam humidifiers—final heat of humidifiers, kWh/ym^2;
$E_{el,pom}$—annual demand for final electrical energy for the drive of auxiliary devices, kWh/ym^2;

$\eta_{H,t}$—seasonal average total efficiency of a heating system with water air heaters, $\eta_{H,t} = \eta_{H,g}\ \eta_{H,s}\ \eta_{H,d}\ \eta_{H,e}$, with $\eta_{H,t} = 0.81$ ($\eta_{H,g} = 0.90$—generation, $\eta_{H,s} = 1.0$—accumulation, $\eta_{H,d} = 0.94$—distribution and $\eta_{H,e} = 0.95$—regulation and control);
$\eta_{Hel,t}$—seasonal average total efficiency of a heating system with electric heaters, with $\eta_{Hel,t} = 0.95$;
$\eta_{C,t}$—seasonal average total efficiency of a system with air coolers; $\eta_{C,t}$ = ESEER $\eta_{C,s}\ \eta_{C,d}\ \eta_{C,e}$, with $\eta_{C,t} = 3.0$ (ESEER = 3.5—European Seasonal Energy Efficiency Ratio, $\eta_{C,s} = 0.95$—accumulation, $\eta_{C,d} = 0.94$—distribution and $\eta_{C,e} = 0.97$—regulation and control);
$\eta_{B,t}$—seasonal average total efficiency of a heating system for supplying steam humidifiers, $\eta_{B,t} = \eta_{B,g}\ \eta_{B,d}\ \eta_{B,e}$ ($\eta_{B,g}$—generation, $\eta_{B,d}$—distribution and $\eta_{H,e}$—regulation and control), with $\eta_{B,t} = 0.95$;
w_i—input coefficient of nonrenewable primary energy for generation and providing the final energy carrier (or energy) (w_H—concerns heat, w_C—concerns cold, w_B—concerns steam, w_{el}—concerns electrical energy) with $w_H = 1.1$—gas/oil boiler, $w_C = 3.0$—chiller with electrical drive and $w_B = 3.0$—electric steam generator).

The energy demand (net) of heaters, coolers and steam humidifiers is calculated using algorithms of energy-optimal thermodynamic air treatment according to the following criterion:

$$f_c = \sum_{i=1}^{n} \dot{m}_i \left|\Delta h_i\right| = \min \tag{35}$$

where:

$\dot{m}_i$—mass stream in i-operation;
Δh_i—change of the specific enthalpy in i-operation.

Tools for calculating the objective function are simulation models of the operations of HVAC systems throughout the year. Algorithms of these models were presented in papers [37,38], while, for the presented application, the general algorithm of the simulation model is shown in Figure 6.

The starting point of the general algorithm are the output data on the basis of which the family of characteristic boundary isotherms is determined. Then, for each acceptable variant of the HVAC structure, algorithms for optimal air treatment are determined and the annual demand for net energy, auxiliary energy and primary energy corresponding to these algorithms. In conclusion, the optimal variant is determined.

5.2. Objective Function, Simulation Models

The objective functions were defined for representative variants of the HVAC system for cleanrooms with energy-optimal structures $\overline{x}_1^*$, $\overline{x}_2^*$, $\overline{x}_3^*$ and $\overline{x}_4^*$ (Figure 2), respectively; the variants are shown in Table 4.

As decision variables, the optimization algorithm includes: p—the type of heat recovery and q—external climate.

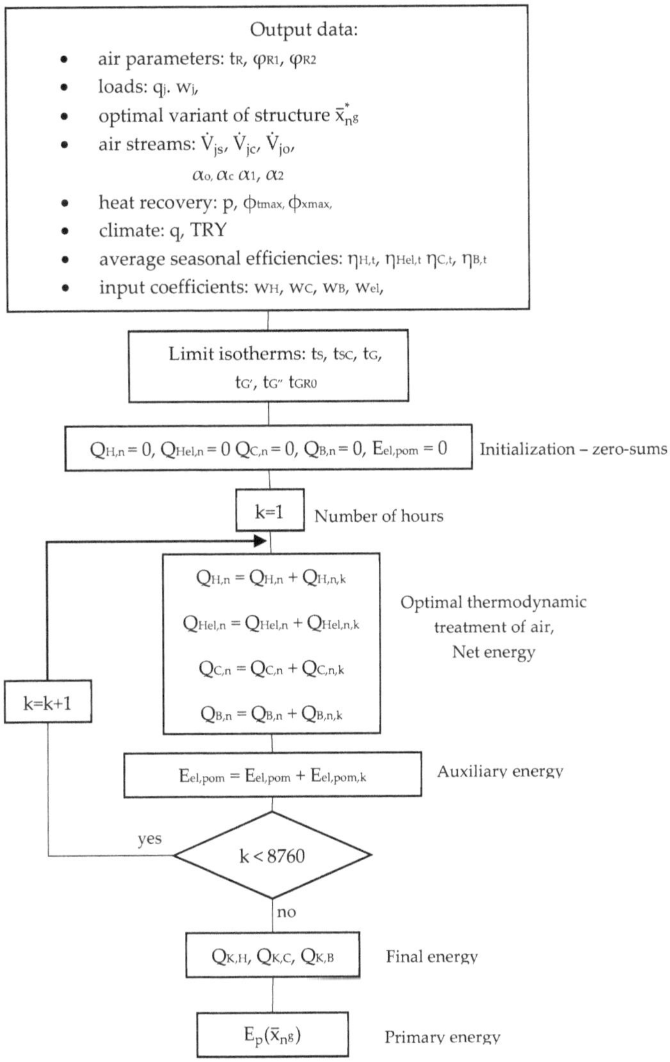

Figure 6. General algorithm of the simulation model for $\bar{x}^*_{ng}$ of the HVAC system.

Table 4. Representative variants of the HVAC system for cleanrooms with optimal structures.

Optimal Structure of HVAC System $\bar{x}^*_{ng}$	Variant Designation ISO N $\bar{x}^*_{ngpq}$		Variant of Constant Parameters [1/]	q_j	α_o	Heat Recovery			External Climate
				W/m [2]	%	p [2/]	ϕ_t, %	ϕ_x, %	q [3/]
$\bar{x}^*_1$	ISO8	$\bar{x}^*_{11q}$	3.1.5	100	100	1	70	0	1,2,3
		$\bar{x}^*_{12q}$				2		60	
		$\bar{x}^*_{13q}$				3		0	
		$\bar{x}^*_{14q}$				4		0	
		$\bar{x}^*_{15q}$				5	0	0	

Table 4. *Cont.*

Optimal Structure of HVAC System $\overline{x}^{*}_{ng}$	Variant Designation ISO N $\overline{x}^{*}_{ngpq}$		Variant of Constant Parameters [1/]	q_j	α_o	Heat Recovery			External Climate
				W/m [2]	%	p [2/]	ϕ_t, %	ϕ_x, %	q [3/]
$\overline{x}^{*}_{2}$	ISO8	$\overline{x}^{*}_{21q}$	3.3.3	500	19.9	1	70	0	1,2,3
		$\overline{x}^{*}_{22q}$				2		60	
		$\overline{x}^{*}_{23q}$				3		0	
		$\overline{x}^{*}_{24q}$				4		0	
		$\overline{x}^{*}_{25q}$				5	0	0	
$\overline{x}^{*}_{3}$	ISO 5	$\overline{x}^{*}_{31q}$	1.2.3	300	30	1	70	0	1,2,3
		$\overline{x}^{*}_{32q}$				2		60	
		$\overline{x}^{*}_{33q}$				3		0	
		$\overline{x}^{*}_{34q}$				4		0	
		$\overline{x}^{*}_{35q}$				5	0	0	
$\overline{x}^{*}_{4}$	ISO7	$\overline{x}^{*}_{41q}$	2.2.2	300	10	1	70	0	1,2,3
		$\overline{x}^{*}_{42q}$				2		60	
		$\overline{x}^{*}_{43q}$				3		0	
		$\overline{x}^{*}_{44q}$				4		0	
		$\overline{x}^{*}_{45q}$				5	0	0	

[1/] According to Table 2; [2/] p = 1—rotary energy regenerator (RR_t), $\phi_t \neq$ const. (stepless regulation), p = 2—rotary enthalpy regenerator (RR_x), $\phi_t \neq$ const., $\phi_x \neq$ const. (stepless regulation), p = 3—cross-flow or countercurrent exchanger with bypass (R+ bypass), $\phi_t = \phi_{tmax}$ or $\phi_t = 0$, p = 4—crossflow or countercurrent exchanger with bypass and electric preheater (H_{el}+ R + bypass) and p = 5—no heat recovery and [3/] q = 1, 2, 3—continental climate, subarctic and subtropical [41].

In calculations based on the simulation models [37], the following assumptions and output data were considered:

1. Air parameters in the room equal: $t_R = +22\ °C$, $\varphi_R = (50 \pm 5)\%$—$\varphi_{R1} = 45\%$, $\varphi_{R2} = 55\%$. Further parameters are included in Table 4.
2. It is assumed that the gains in room humidity w_j in relation to the air stream $\dot{V}_j$ are negligible ($x_S = x_R$).
3. The surface temperature of the cooler was assumed to be equal to $t_D = t_{DP} - 1K$.
4. For HVAC systems $\overline{x}_{13}$ and $\overline{x}_{14}$, $\overline{x}_{23}$ and $\overline{x}_{24}$, $\overline{x}_{33}$ and $\overline{x}_{34}$ and $\overline{x}_{43}$ and $\overline{x}_{44}$ (with a crossflow or countercurrent exchanger), the outdoor air temperature at which frost occurs, equal to $t_{GR0} = 0\ °C$, was used.
5. The calculations were performed for three representative types of external climates according to Köppen [41]: continental with warm summer (q = 1), subarctic (q = 2) and subtropical (q = 3).
6. Continuous operation of the HVAC system is assumed—$\tau = 24/7$ with constant air streams.
7. Final and primary energy demands for forcing through air (fans) are neglected, except for heat recovery exchangers, for which a realistic pressure loss of $\Delta p_{HR} = 150$ Pa and a total efficiency of forcing through $\eta_W = 80\%$ are used.

As a result, component $E_{el,pom}$ in Equations (29) and (30) is defined as:

$$E_{el,pom} = \Delta E_R = \frac{\dot{V}_o \Delta p_{HR}}{\eta_W} \cdot \tau \cdot 10^{-3},\ \mathrm{kWh/y/m^2} \quad (36)$$

with:

ΔE_R—final energy demand for forcing through by heat recovery exchangers.

Considering energy inputs for forcing through air by heat recovery exchangers is necessary for evaluating the energy profitability of applying such exchangers.

Omission of the energy demand for fans as a component of the objective function (29) can be justified as follows:

- the objective function (29) is determined for each optimal structure of the HVAC system $\overline{x}^*_{ng}$ in which the location of the fans is specified; the energy demand of these fans does not therefore affect the selection of the optimal structure;
- determining the energy demand for fans would require assuming system pressure losses, which is not an objective parameter (such a possibility is provided for a case study);
- the purpose of the research at this stage is to determine the optimal type of heat recovery; to achieve this purpose, it is not necessary to determine the energy demand for the fans.

8. Annual demand for the final energy for the drive of auxiliary devices is neglected.
9. The following values of physical constants were used: air density $\rho = 1.2$ kg/m^3, specific heat of air $c_p = 1.005$ kg/kgK, specific heat of steam $c_{pp} = 1.86$ kg/kgK, heat of vaporization of water with temperature 0 °C, $r_o = 2500.8$ kJ/kg and atmospheric pressure $p_a = 105$Pa.
10. Thermodynamic parameters of humid air were calculated based on Reference [42].

5.3. Algorithms of Energy-Optimal Control

For representative variants of the HVAC system shown in Table 4, the structures of which are shown in Figure 2, algorithms of energy-optimal control were defined in accordance with criterion (35). The algorithms are shown in Figures 7–10.

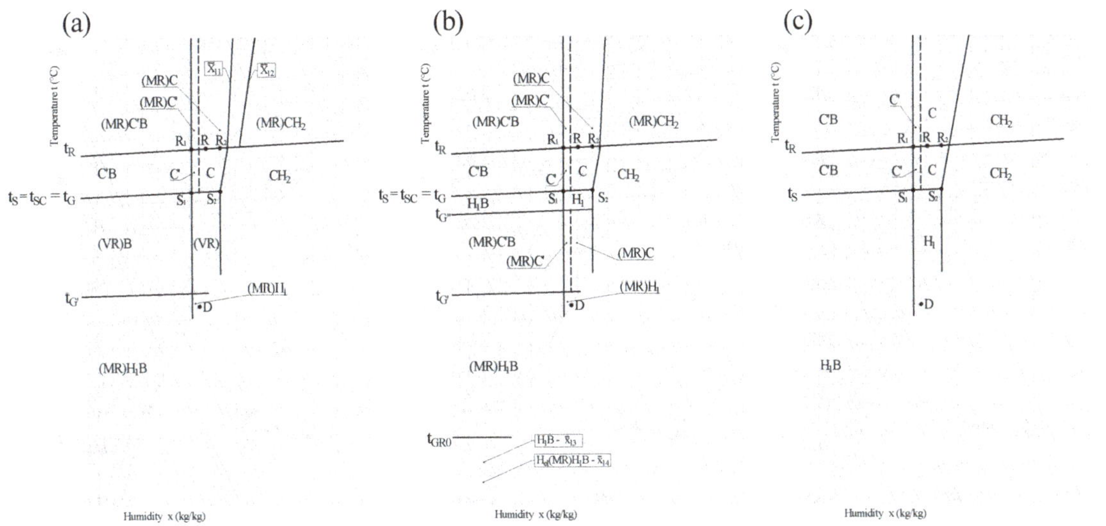

Figure 7. ISO8 variant (**a**) $\overline{x}^*_{11} - \overline{x}^*_{12}$, (**b**) $\overline{x}^*_{13} - \overline{x}^*_{14}$, (**c**) $\overline{x}^*_{15}$ (without recirculation).

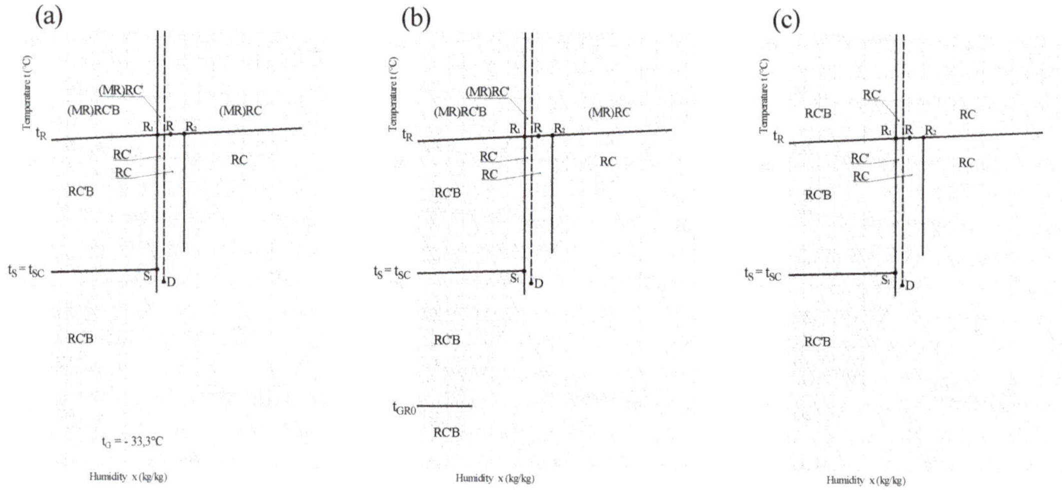

Figure 8. ISO8 variants (**a**) $\overline{x}_{21}^{*} - \overline{x}_{22}^{*}$, (**b**) $\overline{x}_{23}^{*} - \overline{x}_{24}^{*}$ and (**c**) $\overline{x}_{25}^{*}$ (external recirculation).

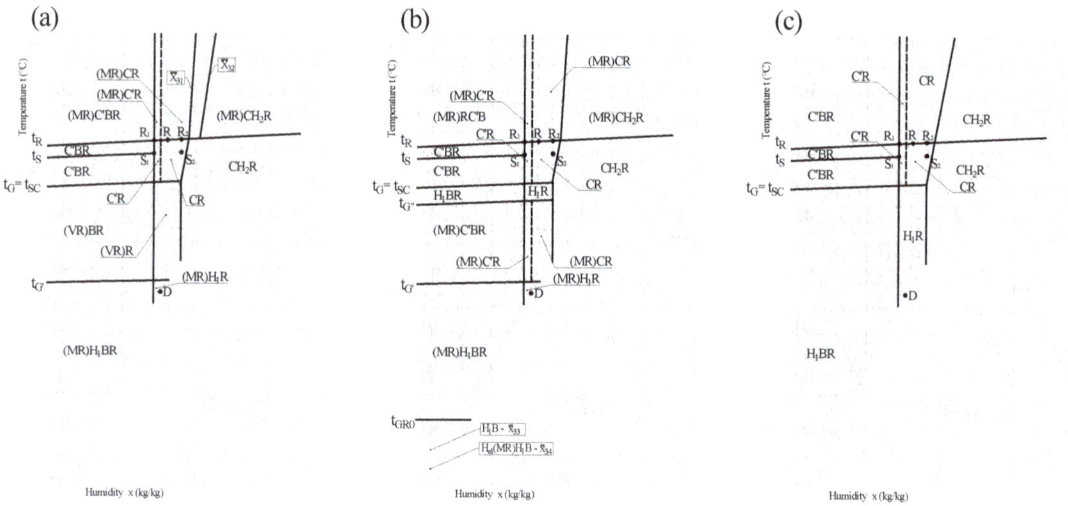

Figure 9. ISO5 variants (**a**) $\overline{x}_{31}^{*} - \overline{x}_{32}^{*}$, (**b**) $\overline{x}_{33}^{*} - \overline{x}_{34}^{*}$ and (**c**) $\overline{x}_{35}^{*}$ (internal recirculation).

For the identification of zones of optimal thermodynamic treatment of air in Figures 7–10 h–x, the following designations are used:

(MR)—maximum heat recovery, (VR)—regulated heat recovery, H_1—heating (preheater), H_2—heating (secondary heater), H_{el}—heating (electric heater), C′—sensible cooling (without drying), C—cooling with drying, B—steam humidification and R—recirculation.

At the same time, the following designations of the characteristic points are used (Figure 2):

R—air condition in the room, S—condition of air supplied to the room, SC—air condition downstream AHU and D—air condition at the cooler surface.

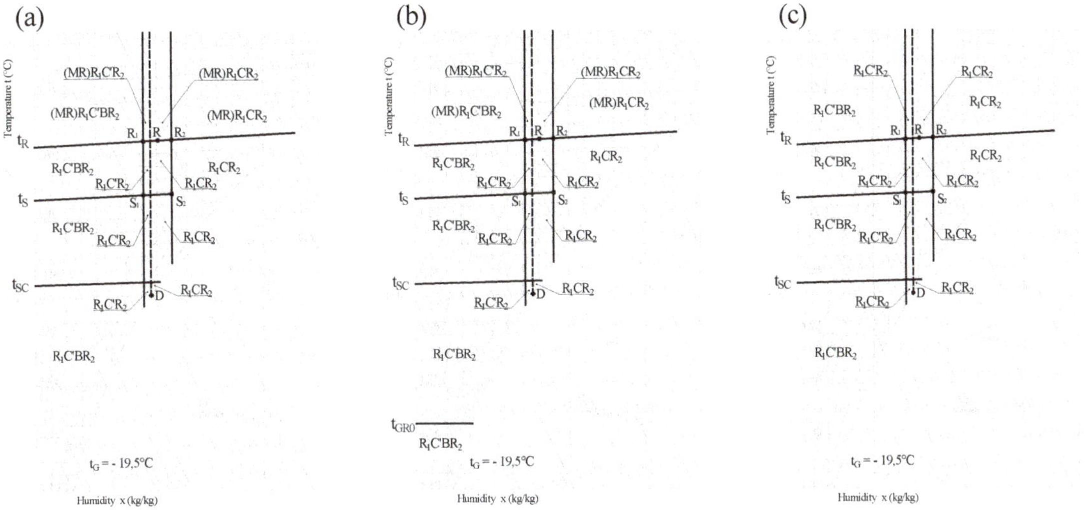

Figure 10. ISO7 variants (**a**) $\overline{x}^*_{41} - \overline{x}^*_{42}$, (**b**) $\overline{x}^*_{43} - \overline{x}^*_{44}$ and (**c**) $\overline{x}^*_{45}$ (external and internal recirculation).

Equations of the limit isotherms and limit lines between the zones of optimal thermodynamic treatment of air in Figures 7–10 h–x take the following form:

- isotherm t_S

$$t_S = t_R - \frac{q_j}{\dot{V}_j \rho c_p} \tag{37}$$

- isotherm t_{SC}

$$t_{SC} = t_R - \frac{q_j}{\dot{V}_{jc} \rho c_p} \tag{38}$$

- isotherm t_G

$$t_G = t_R - \frac{1}{\alpha_\upsilon}(t_R - t_S) \tag{39}$$

- isotherm $t_{G'}$

$$t_{G'} = t_R - \frac{t_R - t_S}{\alpha_o(1 - \phi_{t_{max}})} \tag{40}$$

- isotherm $t_{G''}$

$$t_{G''} = \frac{t_G\left(\frac{w_H}{\eta_{H,t}} + \frac{w_C}{\eta_{C,t}}\right) - \frac{w_C}{\eta_{C,t}}\phi_t t_R}{\frac{w_H}{\eta_{H,t}} + \frac{w_C}{\eta_{C,t}}(1-\phi_t)} \tag{41}$$

- limit line (MR)C/(MR)CH$_2$—$\overline{x}_{11}$

$$t_{zg} = \frac{1}{1-\phi_t}\left(\frac{x - x_D}{x_{S_2} - x_D} t_S - \frac{x - x_{S_2}}{x_{S_2} - x_D} t_D\right) - \frac{\phi_t}{1-\phi_t} t_R \tag{42}$$

- limit line (MR)C/(MR)CH_2—$\overline{x}_{12}$

$$t_{zg} = \frac{(t_S - t_D)\left[x - \phi_x\left(x - x_{R_2}\right) - x_D\right] - (\phi_t t_R - t_D)\left(x_{S_2} - x_D\right)}{(1 - \phi_t)\left(x_{S_2} - x_D\right)} \tag{43}$$

- limit line C/CH_2

$$t_{zg} = t_D + (t_S - t_D)\frac{x - x_D}{x_{S_2} - x_D} \tag{44}$$

- limit line (MR)C/(MR)CH_2R—$\overline{x}_{31}$

$$t_{zg} = \frac{1}{1 - \phi_t}\left(\frac{x - x_D}{x_{R_3} - x_D}t_R - \frac{x - x_{R_3}}{x_{R_3} - x_D}t_D\right) - \frac{\phi_t}{1 - \phi_t}t_R \tag{45}$$

$$x_{R_3} = x_D + \left(x_{S_2} - x_D\right)\frac{t_R - t_D}{t_{SC} - t_D} \tag{46}$$

- limit line (MR)C/(MR)CH_2R—$\overline{x}_{32}$

$$t_{zg} = \frac{(t_{SC} - t_D)\left[x - \phi_x\left(x - x_{R_2}\right) - x_D\right] - (\phi_t t_R - t_D)\left(x_{R_2} - x_D\right)}{(1 - \phi_t)\left(x_{R_2} - x_D\right)} \tag{47}$$

- limit line CR/CH_2R

$$t_{zg} = t_D + \frac{t_{SC} - t_D}{x_{S_2} - x_D}(x - x_D) \tag{48}$$

5.4. Calculation Results, Interpretation

Results of the calculations of the annual demands for primary energy for the representative HVAC systems shown in Table 4 are presented in Table 5.

Table 5. Primary energy demand for the representative HVAC systems $\overline{x}^*_{ng}$.

	Optimal Structure of HVAC System $\overline{x}^*_{ng}$	Heat Recovery (p)	Primary Energy E_p, kWh/m^{2}y		
			Continental Climate (Poland) q = 1	Subarctic Climate (Russia) q = 2	Subtropical Climate (Brazil) q = 3
$\overline{x}_{11}$	ISO8	RO_t (p = 1)	6354.0	9554.0	4877.0
$\overline{x}_{12}$		RO_x (p = 2)	3464.0	5013.0	3915.0
$\overline{x}_{13}$		R + by-pass (p = 3)	7643.0	13,693.0	4921.0
$\overline{x}_{14}$		H_{el} + R + by-pass (p = 4)	6901.0	13,943.0	4921.0
$\overline{x}_{15}$		Without heat recovery (p = 5)	9426.0	14,733.0	5118.0

Table 5. *Cont.*

Optimal Structure of HVAC System $\overline{x}^{*}_{ng}$		Heat Recovery (p)	Primary Energy E_p, kWh/m^{2}y		
			Continental Climate (Poland) q = 1	Subarctic Climate (Russia) q = 2	Subtropical Climate (Brazil) q = 3
$\overline{x}_{21}$	ISO8	RO_t (p = 1)	4965.0	5078.0	5118.0
$\overline{x}_{22}$		RO_x (p = 2)	4930.0	5055.0	4945.0
$\overline{x}_{23}$		R + by-pass (p = 3)	4965.0	5078.0	5118.0
$\overline{x}_{24}$		H_{el} + R + by-pass (p = 4)	4965.0	5078.0	5118.0
$\overline{x}_{25}$		Without heat recovery (p = 5)	4898.0	5010.0	5091.0
$\overline{x}_{31}$	ISO5	RO_t (p = 1)	19,053.0	28,656.0	14,634.0
$\overline{x}_{32}$		RO_x (p = 2)	10,382.0	15,014.0	11,747.0
$\overline{x}_{33}$		R + by-pass (p = 3)	22,883.0	41,033.0	14,686.0
$\overline{x}_{34}$		H_{el} + R + by-pass (p = 4)	20,703.0	41,830.0	14,686.0
$\overline{x}_{35}$		Without heat recovery (p = 5)	28,278.0	44,198.0	15,354.0
$\overline{x}_{41}$	ISO7	RO_t (p = 1)	3071.0	3203.0	3159.0
$\overline{x}_{42}$		RO_x (p = 2)	3040.0	2950.0	3000.0
$\overline{x}_{43}$		R + by-pass (p = 3)	3070.0	3477.0	3159.0
x_{44}		H_{el} + R + by-pass (p = 4)	3070.0	3477.0	3159.0
$\overline{x}_{45}$		Without heat recovery (p = 5)	3018.0	3322.0	3134.0

A percentage comparison of the unit annual demand for the primary energy of variants of the HVAC system for various external climates and types of heat recovery, compared to variants without heat recovery, are shown in Figures 11–14. The subject of the assessment is the impact of the type of heat recovery and the external climate—as decision variables—for the selection of the energy-optimal variant.

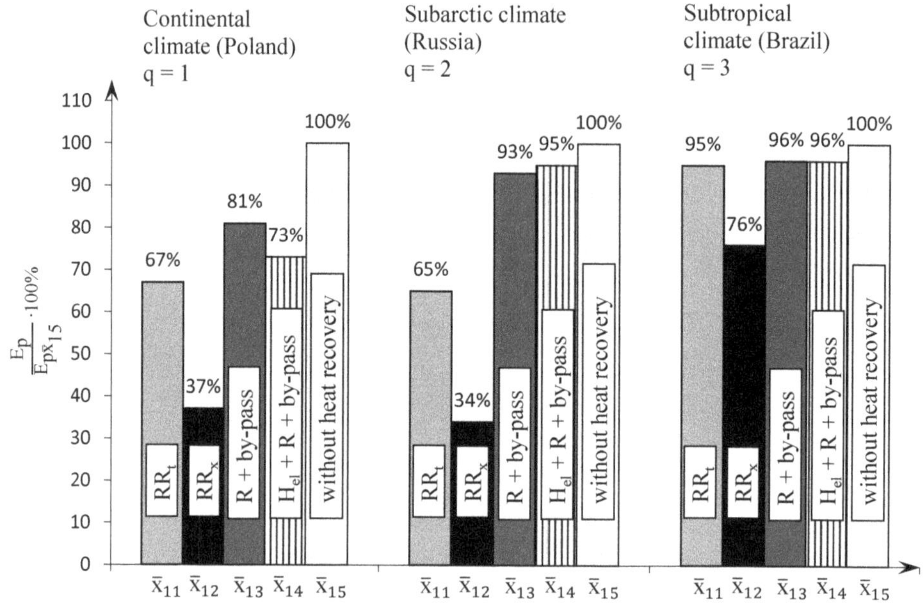

Figure 11. Annual relative demand for the primary energy of the variants of HVAC system ISO8 $\bar{x}_{1_{pq}}$ (without recirculation) for various external climates and types of heat recovery compared to the variants without heat recovery.

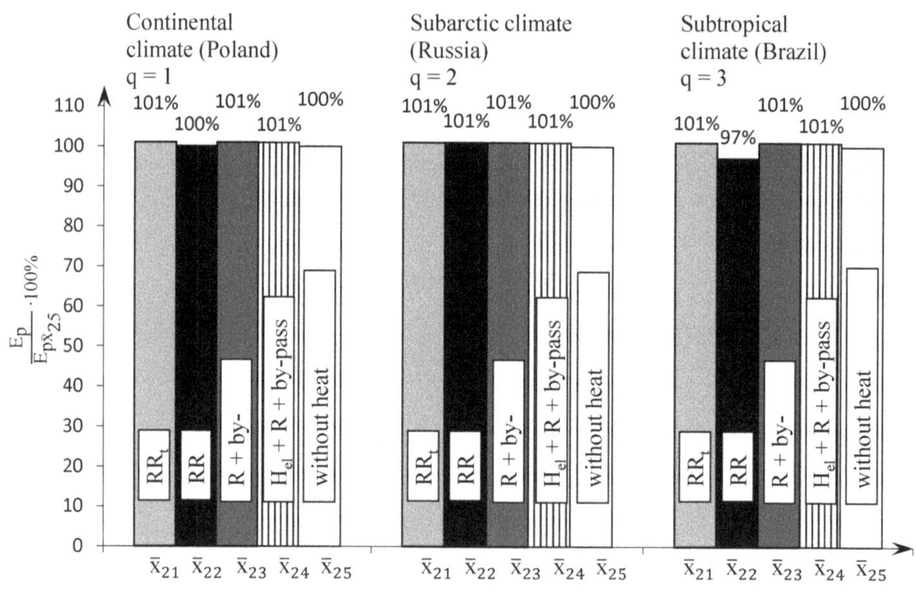

Figure 12. Annual relative demand for the primary energy of the variants of HVAC system ISO8 $\bar{x}_{2_{pq}}$ (external recirculation) for various external climates and types of heat recovery compared to the variants without heat recovery.

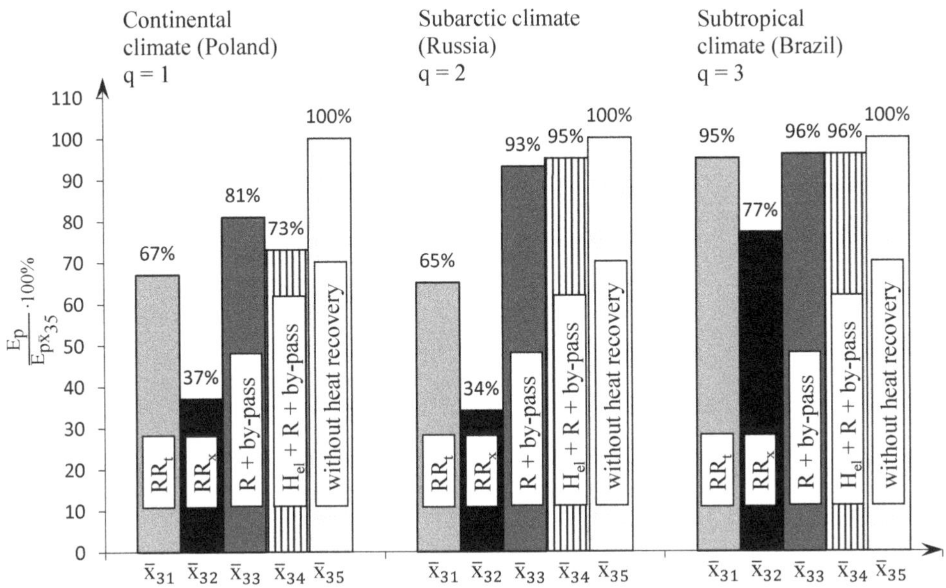

Figure 13. Annual relative demand for the primary energy of the variants of HVAC system ISO8 $\bar{x}_{3_{pq}}$ (internal recirculation) for various external climates and types of heat recovery compared to the variants without heat recovery.

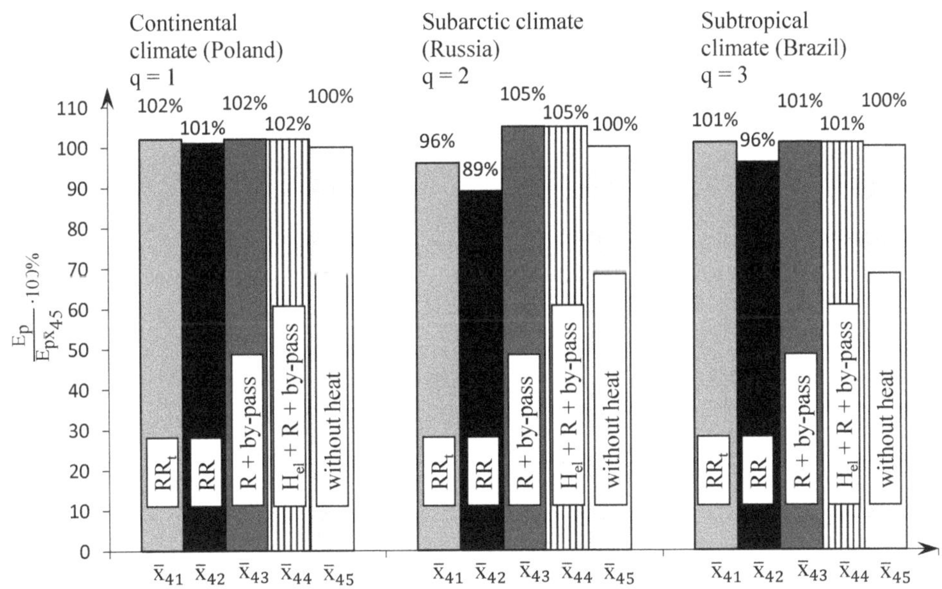

Figure 14. Annual relative demand for the primary energy of the variants of HVAC system ISO8 $\bar{x}_{4_{pq}}$ (external and internal recirculation) for various external climates and types of heat recovery compared to the variants without heat recovery.

Based on the analysis of the calculation results, the following can be stated:

1. For HVAC systems without air recirculation $\bar{x}_1$ the optimal device for heat recovery is a rotary sorption regenerator (p = 2) and, then, an energy regenerator (p = 1) and a crossflow exchanger (p = 3 or p = 4). The obtained energy savings are here a function of climate—Figure 11 and Table 5. Using the rotary sorption regenerator in the analyzed HVAC system ISO8 $\bar{x}_1$ makes it possible to decrease the annual primary energy demand by 63%, 64% and 24% in relation to the system without heat recovery, respectively, for continental (q = 1), subarctic (q = 2) and subtropical (q = 3) climates. For the rotary energy regenerator, the values are lower and equal 33%, 35% and 5%, respectively. For the crossflow exchanger, the savings are significantly lower and equal 19 ÷ 27% for the continental climate, 5 ÷ 7% for the subarctic climate and 4% for the subtropical climate. Therefore, in the subtropical climate, the only rational device for heat recovery is the rotary sorption regenerator, and the savings effect is mainly achieved by drying air.

The representative percentages of the annual primary energy demand for thermodynamic air treatment for individual components and optimal variant ISO8 $\bar{x}_{12}$ (with a rotary sorption regenerator) are shown in Figure 15.

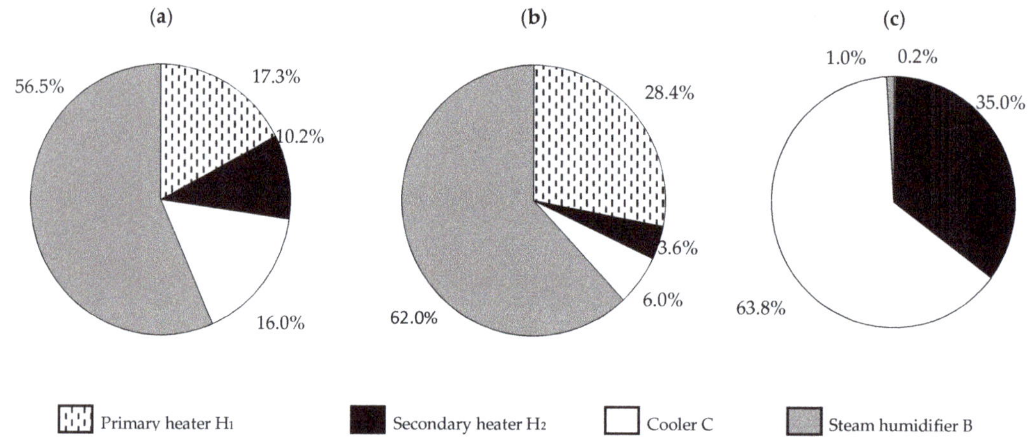

Figure 15. Percentages of the annual primary energy demand for thermodynamic air treatment for individual components and optimal variant ISO8 $\bar{x}_{12}$ (without recirculation, rotary sorption regenerator): (**a**) continental climate (q = 1), (**b**) subarctic climate (q = 2) and (**c**) subtropical climate (q = 3).

For the continental climate (q = 1) and subarctic climate (q = 2), the dominant is the percentage of the demand for air humidification—56.5% and 62.0%, respectively; then, for heating air—27.5% and 32%, respectively, and cooling—16.0% and 6.0%, respectively. While, for the subtropical climate (q = 3), the dominant is the percentage of cooling—63.8%, then heating at 35.2%, including 35% of reheating after drying and, marginally, humidification—1%. The conclusions resulting from the results of the calculations of representative shares of the annual primary energy demand for thermodynamic air treatment correlate directly with the conclusions concerning the optimal type of heat recovery.

2. For HVAC systems with external recirculation $\bar{x}_2$ (optimal for cleanrooms with high unit cooling loads q_j and relatively low requirements of cleanliness class C_s), using additional heat recovery has no energy justification for any of the considered devices and external climates (savings between 1 ÷ 3% for ISO8 $\bar{x}_2$)—Figure 12 and Table 5.
3. For systems with internal recirculation $\bar{x}_3$ (optimal for cleanrooms with low cooling loads q_j and relatively large percentages of outdoor air α_o), using devices for heat recovery is definitely energetically justified, especially for the continental climate (q = 1) and the subarctic climate (q = 2)—Figure 13 and Table 5. The optimal device

for heat recovery is, similar to the system without recirculation, a rotary sorption regenerator and, then, an energy regenerator and a crossflow exchanger. For the considered system ISO5 $\overline{x}_3$ energy savings related to a system without heat recovery, primary energy and using the sorption regenerator equal 63%, 66% and 23%, respectively, for the continental, subarctic and subtropical climates—Figure 13. Lower savings are obtained by using an energy regenerator: 33%, 35% and 5% or a crossflow exchanger: 19 ÷ 27%, 5 ÷ 7% and 4%, respectively, for the continental, subarctic and subtropical climates. The percentages of the annual primary energy demand for thermodynamic air treatment for individual components (heaters, cooler and steam humidifier) of optimal variant ISO5 $\overline{x}_{32}$ (with a sorption regenerator) and external climates are practically identical as for HVAC system $\overline{x}_{12}$ (Figure 15).

4. For HVAC systems with external and internal recirculation $\overline{x}_4$ (optimal for cleanrooms with high cooling loads q_j and relatively low percentages of outdoor air α_o), additionally using heat recovery is energetically justified only for the subarctic climate and concerns only the rotary sorption regenerator—Figure 14 and Table 5. Savings in the primary energy demand for the analyzed HVAC system ISO7 $\overline{x}_{42}$ (with a sorption regenerator) and the subarctic climate equal 11% related to a system without heat recovery.

It should be noted that, in the other analyzed use cases of devices for heat recovery, especially the crossflow exchanger, the energy effect was opposite to what was expected; the primary energy demand increased 1 ÷ 5%, because the heat or cold recovery was lower than the inputs for forcing through by heat recovery exchangers.

5.5. Validation of the Calculation Results

Validation of the calculation results with the existing energy simulation tools is possible under the following conditions:

- it must be possible to implement the system structure in the program (in the case under consideration, four variants: $\overline{x}_1$, $\overline{x}_2$, $\overline{x}_3$ and $\overline{x}_4$);
- it must be possible to implement various types of heat recovery along with control options: two-position control (maximum efficiency/0) and smooth control (variable energy-optimal efficiency);
- it must be possible to implement control algorithms (open code).

In this article, a simulation model was developed for each HVAC system structure. In these models, for each hour of the comparative year TRY (est. Reference Year), the optimal course of thermodynamic air treatment was determined, and on this basis, the energy consumption was obtained—after summing (8760 h), the annual energy consumption. The available energy simulation programs are universal, but also limited, among others:

- no possibility to implement any HVAC system structure;
- no possibility to implement any control algorithms;
- frequently closed program code.

The validation of the calculation results in this article was carried out by taking into account the above-mentioned limitations and the available other tool for energy simulation—the HAP (Hourly Analysis Program) program developed by the CARRIER company. It is a closed-source program.

The possible scope of the simulation included CAV systems (constant air volume) with heat recovery (excluding the option of a recuperator with an electric preheater before the recuperator—$\overline{x}_{14}$ and $\overline{x}_{24}$) with or without external recirculation ($\overline{x}_1$ and $\overline{x}_2$ in the article). The calculation results are presented in Table 6.

Table 6. Primary energy demand for the representative HVAC systems $\overline{x}^*_{ng}$ calculation results according to the HAP program (Hourly Analysis Program).

Optimal Structure of HVAC System $\overline{x}^*_{ng}$		Heat Recovery (p)	Primary Energy E_p, kWh/m²y — External Climate (q)								
			Continental Climate (Poland) q = 1			Subarctic Climate (Russia) q = 2			Subtropical Climate (Brazil) q = 3		
			Simulation	HAP Carrier	Difference */ %	Simulation	HAP Carrier	Difference */ %	Simulation	HAP Carrier	Difference */ %
$\overline{x}_{11}$	IOS8	RO_t (p = 1)	6354.0	6402.0	+0.75	9554.0	10,408.0	+8.2	4877.0	4466.0	−8.4
$\overline{x}_{12}$		RO_x (p = 2)	3464.0	3212.0	−7.3	5013.0	4623.0	−7.8	3915.0	3656.0	−6.6
$\overline{x}_{13}$		R + by-pass (p = 3)	7643.0	7231.0	−5.3	13,693.0	14,530.0	+5.7	4921.0	4466.0	−9.2
$\overline{x}_{15}$		Without heat recovery (p = 5)	9426.0	9408.0	−0.2	14,733.0	15,961.0	+7.7	5118.0	4819.0	−6.0
$\overline{x}_{21}$	IOS8	RO_t (p = 1)	4965.0	5231.0	+5.0	5078.0	4849.0	−4.5	5118.0	5106.0	−0.2
$\overline{x}_{22}$		RO_x (p = 2)	4930.0	5178.0	+4.8	5055.0	4592.0	−9.2	4945.0	4533.0	−8.3
$\overline{x}_{23}$		R + by-pass (p = 3)	4965.0	5244.0	+5.3	5078.0	4849.0	−4.5	5118.0	5106.0	−0.2
$\overline{x}_{25}$		Without heat recovery (p = 5)	4898.0	5170.0	+5.3	5010.0	4886.0	−2.5	5091.0	5084.0	−0.1

*/ Related to own simulation.

Taking into account the above-mentioned conditions and limitations, it can be concluded that the obtained results of the calculations are satisfactory, and the differences in the annual energy demand according to our own calculations and the HAP program, related to the values obtained in our own calculations, are acceptable. These differences range from −9.2% to +8.2% (minimal differences: −0.2% to +0.75%). The mean absolute percentage of the differences in the results of these calculations is 5.1%. Taking into account that the simulation models of the other systems included in the article ($\overline{x}_3$—with internal recirculation and $\overline{x}_4$—with internal and external recirculation) are a modification of the models for the validated systems $\overline{x}_1$ and $\overline{x}_2$, it can be assumed that the obtained calculation results are also acceptable.

6. Conclusions

This article presents the original results of research on the optimization of HVAC systems for cleanrooms. The HVAC systems were described by vectors with coordinates defined by constant parameters and decision variables. Then, the authors defined, based on limitations, a set of acceptable variants covering the following structures of HVAC system: $\overline{x}_1$—without recirculation, $\overline{x}_2$—with external recirculation, $\overline{x}_3$—with internal recirculation and $\overline{x}_4$—with external and internal recirculation.

In the next stage, based on the optimization algorithm, the authors defined a set of energy-optimal structures of the HVAC system for cleanrooms as a function of key constant parameters and wide representative variability ranges of these parameters: cleanliness classes C_s—ISO5, ISO7 and ISO8; u nit cooling loads $q_j = (100 \div 500)$ W/m^2 and percentage of outdoor air $\alpha_o = (5 \div 100)$%.

The original achievement of the research, which constitutes a new cognitive quality, is the development of relations approximating $\overline{x}^*_{ng} = f(C_S, \alpha_o, q_j)$ defining the zones of energy-optimal structures of cleanroom HVAC systems; the equations derived the boundary lines separating these zones.

It was proven that HVAC systems with external recirculation ($\overline{x}_2$) are optimal structures for rooms with high cooling loads q_j and low requirements concerning keeping the cleanliness class, HVAC systems with internal recirculation ($\overline{x}_3$) are optimal for rooms with low cooling loads q_j and relatively high percentages of outdoor air α_o, while HVAC systems with external and internal recirculation ($\overline{x}_4$) are optimal structures for rooms with high cooling loads q_j and relatively low percentages of outdoor air α_o.

The obtained results, due to the used wide ranges of variability of key constant parameters, are general in nature and have great application value.

An important result of the research was defining energy-optimal control algorithms and the type of heat recovery as an element of optimal structures of the HVAC system. At this stage, the equations of the boundary lines between the zones of optimal thermodynamic air treatment were determined, which is of great application importance.

In the optimization procedure based on simulation models, the objective function was defined as the minimum unit annual primary energy demand for thermodynamic air treatment of the HVAC system ($E_p(\overline{x}^*_{ng}$ = min). The algorithms take into account the energy demand for forcing through by heat recovery exchangers.

Summarizing the results of the analyses and calculations concerning the energetic profitability of using heat recovery in optimal structures of HVAC systems for cleanrooms, it can be stated that:

- it is energetically profitable to use heat recovery, especially for HVAC systems without recirculation ($\overline{x}_1$) or with internal recirculation ($\overline{x}_3$), whereby the biggest energy savings are achieved for the continental climate (Poland) and the subarctic climate (Russia).
- in any case, the biggest savings in primary energy demand are the result of using, as heat recovery, a rotary sorption regenerator and, then, an energy regenerator and a crossflow (or countercurrent) exchanger.
- quantitatively, using a sorption regenerator in the energy-optimal structures of HVAC system ISO8 $\overline{x}_1$ (without recirculation) and ISO5 $\overline{x}_3$ (with internal recirculation) resulted in a decrease in the primary energy demand for thermodynamic treatment by 63%, 64 ÷ 66% and 23 ÷ 24%, respectively, for the continental, subarctic and subtropical climates. For an energy regenerator and a crossflow exchanger, these savings were significantly lower and equaled about 33%, 35% and 5%, respectively.
- for energy-optimal structures of HVAC systems with external recirculation $\overline{x}_2$ or with external and internal recirculation $\overline{x}_4$, using devices for heat recovery is generally energetically not justified and, in all cases, causes an increase in the energy demand (heat or cold recovery is lower than the energy inputs for forcing through by the heat recovery exchanger). The only debatable exception is the application of a sorption regenerator in the HVAC system $\overline{x}_4$ for the subarctic climate—primary energy savings for thermodynamic air treatment of 11% in the ISO7 application $\overline{x}_{42}$.

Author Contributions: Conceptualization, M.P.; methodology, M.P.; software, M.J.; validation, M.P. and M.J.; formal analysis, M.P. and M.J.; investigation, M.P. and M.J.; resources, M.P. and M.J.; data curation, M.P.; writing—original draft preparation, M.P.; writing—review and editing, M.J.; visualization, M.P.; supervision, M.P.; project administration, M.P. and funding acquisition, M.P. All authors have read and agreed to the published version of the manuscript.

Funding: This research was funded by the Polish Ministry of Education and Science, grant number 504101/0713/SBAD/0948.

Institutional Review Board Statement: Not applicable.

Informed Consent Statement: Not applicable.

Data Availability Statement: Not applicable.

Conflicts of Interest: The authors declare no conflict of interest.

Abbreviations

The following abbreviations are used in this manuscript:

AHU	Air-Handling Unit
MAU	Make-up Air-Handling Unit
RU (RDCU)	Return Unit (Return Dry Cooling Unit)
FFU (FDCU)	Filter Fan Unit (Fan Dry Cooling Unit)
DCC	Dry Cooling Coil

The following contractual values are used in this manuscript:

C_s	cleanliness class
E_1, E_2, E_3	efficiency of air filter of 1st, 2nd and 3rd stage
$E_{el,pom}$	annual demand for final electrical energy for the drive of auxiliary devices of HVAC system
E_P	annual primary energy demand of HVAC system
$g_{()_k}(x_j)$	k-limitation (T)—technological, (H)—hygienic, (A)—acoustic, (E)—energetic, (M) material, (AK)—architectural and constructional and (BN)—concerning safety and reliability [37]
G	binary matrix of limitation conditions for matrix $\mathbf{X}^J$
$\mathbf{G}^i$	binary matrix of limitation conditions for matrix **W**
$\mathbf{G}^j$	binary matrix of elimination of unnecessary decision variables for matrix ($\mathbf{G}^i \times \mathbf{W}$)
k_d	acceptable concentration of contaminants in room
$\dot{m}$	air mass stream
$\dot{q}_j$	unit cooling load of room, W/m^2
$\dot{q}_{jc}$	unit cooling load discharged using AHU, W/m^2
$\dot{q}_{j_{DC}}$	unit cooling load of room discharged by the dry cooler in the internal recirculation circuit, W/m^2
$Q_{H,n}$, $Q_{Hel,n}$, $Q_{C,n}$, $Q_{B,n}$	net annual energy demand of heaters, electric heaters, coolers and steam humidifiers
$Q_{K,H}$, $Q_{K,C}$, $Q_{K,B}$	annual final energy demand of heaters (final heat), coolers (final cold) and steam humidifiers (final heat for humidifiers)
t	temperature, °C
t_{DP}	dew point temperature
t_G	outdoor air temperature (with percentage α_o) for which the sensible heat gains are transferred without heat recovery ($\phi_t = 0$), heating or cooling in AHU
$t_{G'}$	outdoor air temperature (with percentage α_o) for which the sensible heat gains are transferred at maximal efficiency of heat recovery $\phi_t = \phi_{tmax}$ but without heating air or cooling in AHU
$t_{G''}$	outdoor air temperature at which primary energy demand for the option of maximal heat and cold recovery ($\phi_t = \phi_{tmax}$) is equal to this demand for the heating-only option
t_{GR0}	outdoor air temperature limit below which the recuperator freezes
t_S	air supply temperature
t_{SC}	air supply temperature downstream AHU for which sensible heat gains are discharged from room as a result of mixing this air (with percentage α_o) with internally recirculated air
t_R	air temperature in room
Tu	turbulence degree
$\dot{V}_j$	unit calculation ventilation air stream for cleanroom, m^3/hm^2
$\dot{V}_{js}$	unit required air stream as function of room cleanliness class, m^3/hm^2
$\dot{V}_{jc}$	unit required air stream as function of cooling loads discharged using AHU, m^3/hm^2
$\dot{V}_{jo}$	unit required outdoor air stream, m^3/hm^2
w	average air speed in room

w_i	input coefficient of nonrenewable primary energy for generation and supply of final energy carrier (or energy)—for balance boundary of building (w_H—concerns heat for heaters, w_C—concerns cold for coolers, w_B—concerns heat for steam humidifiers and w_{el}—concerns electrical energy)
$\mathbf{W}_i$	binary matrix of all possible variants of combinations of decision variables values x_j for normalizing constant parameter x_i
$\mathbf{W}(\mathbf{W}^g)$	binary matrix of all possible variants (of acceptable variants) of combinations of decision variables values x_j for normalizing all constant parameters x_i of a HVAC system
x_i	constant parameter of a HVAC system
x_j	decision variable of a HVAC system
$\overline{x}$	vector of a HVAC system
$\overline{x}_{n^g}$	binary vector defining the n-variant (n^g-acceptable variant) of structure of a HVAC system used for normalizing all constant parameters
$\overline{x}^*$	vector of the optimal variant of HVAC system
$\mathbf{X}^J(\mathbf{X})$	binary matrix of all possible variants (of acceptable variants) of a HVAC system for normalizing constant parameters
α_o (α_{os})	percentage of outdoor air compared to unit calculation air stream supplied to cleanroom $\dot{V}_j$ (of unit required air stream as function of cleanliness class—$\dot{V}_{js}$)
α_c	percentage of air being thermodynamically treated in AHU in air stream supplied to room—$\dot{V}_j$
α_1, α_2	percentage of air under external recirculation, internal recirculation in air stream supplied to room—$\dot{V}_j$
ε_{sdop}	relative concentration of microorganisms
$\eta_{H,t}$, $\eta_{Hel,t}$, $\eta_{C,t}$, $\eta_{B,t}$	seasonal average total efficiency of heating system for water heaters, heating system for electric heaters, cold system for coolers and heating system for steam humidifiers
φ_R	relative air humidity in room
Δp	differential pressure (overpressure and underpressure in a room)
Δh	change in specific enthalpy of the air
ϕ_t, ϕ_x	efficiency of sensible heat recovery, humidity

The following indices are used in this manuscript:

i	index of constant parameter of HVAC system
I	number of constant parameters of HVAC system
I*	number of normalized constant parameters of HVAC system
J	number of decision variables of HVAC system
k	index of k-combination of values of key constant parameters of HVAC system
K	number of combinations of values of key constant parameters of HVAC system
K	k-hour of reference year (TRY—Test Reference Year, k = 1 : 8760)
k_d	permissible concentration of pollutants
N	number of all possible variants of HVAC system for normalizing constant parameters

Appendix A. Procedure for Determining the Matrix of Acceptable Variants of the HVAC System

The matrix of normalized constant parameters is defined as:

$\mathbf{X}^{I^*} =$ (A1)

i	x_i	$\overline{x}_i$
1	t_R	1
2	φ_R	1
3	k_d	1
4	C_s	1
5	ε_{sdop}	0
6	$T_u^{1/}$	0
7	Δp	1
8	α_o	1

where:

$^{1/}$—correlation with cleanliness class CS applies to special cases (DIN 1946-4:2018-09 [43]).

$\mathbf{X}^{I^*}$—binary matrix of normalized constant parameters x_i of HVAC system,

$i = 1 \ldots I^*$—number of normalized constant parameter,

I^*—number of normalized constant parameters of HVAC system,

x_i—constant parameter of HVAC system,

$\bar{x}_i$—vector of normalized constant parameters of HVAC system.

Matrix **W** of all possible variants of combinations of decision variables for normalizing all constant parameters of HVAC system is defined as:

W = Variants $\overline{w}_{r(i,m_i)} = \overline{w}_{m_i}$ (Decision variables x_j, $j \equiv j^*$) (A2)

i	m_i	$r(i, m_i)$	1.1	1.6	1.24	1.25	1.26	1.28	1.30	1.32	1.35	1.37	1.38	1.39	1.41	1.42	1.43	1.51	1.57a	1.57b	1.57c	1.64	1.68	1.81	1.85	1.111	1.112	1.115	2.14
			1	2	3	4	5	6	7	8	9	10	11	12	13	14	15	16	17	18	19	20	21	22	23	24	25	26	27
1	1	1	1	1	0				0	1	1	0		0	1	1	1	1	0										0
	2	2	1	1	0				0	1	1	0			0	1	1	1	0										0
2	1	3	1	0	1	1	0	1	1	0	1	0			0	1	1	0											0
	2	4	1	0	1	0	1	1	1	0	1	0			0	1	1	0											0
3	1	5	0																		0	1	1	1	1	1	1	1	0
4	1	6	0	0	1	1	0														0	1	1	1	1	1	1	1	0
	2	7	0	0	1	0	1	0													0	1	1	1	1	1	1	1	0
7	1	8	0								0	1	0															0	1
	2	9										0	1	0														0	1
	3	10											0	1	0													0	1
8	1	11	0								0	1	0						0	1	0								0
	2	12	0									0	1	0					0	1	0								0
	3	13	0									0	1	0				0	1	0									0
	4	14	0										0	1	0			0	1	1	0								0
	5	15	0								0	1	0							0	1	0							0

where:

W—binary matrix of all possible variants of combinations of decision variables values x_j for normalizing all constant parameters x_i of HVAC system,

x_j—decision variable of HVAC system,

j—index of decision variable of HVAC system,

j*—index of decision variable of HVAC system from a universal set in Tables A2 and A3 [37],

m_i or $r(i,m_i)$—index of m_i- or $r(i,m_i)$-variant of combinations of decision variables values x_j for normalizing x_i-constant parameter of HVAC system,

M_i—number of all possible variants of combinations of decision variables values x_j for normalizing x_i-constant parameter of HVAC system,

$\overline{w}_{m_i}$ or $\overline{w}_{r(i,m_i)}$—binary vector defining m_i- or $r(i, m_i)$-variant of combinations of decision variables values x_j for normalizing x_i-constant parameter of HVAC system (matrix element **W**).

$m_i = 1 \ldots M_i$

$$r(i, m_i) = \begin{cases} m_i, \ i = 1 \\ \sum_{k=1}^{i=1} (M_k) + m_i, \ i = 2 \ldots I^* \end{cases} \quad \text{(A3)}$$

whereby:

$r(i, m_i) = 1 \ldots M$

$$M = r(I^*, M_i) = \sum_{i=1}^{I^*} M_i \quad \text{(A4)}$$

The rows of the **W** matrix are variants (m_i or $r(i,m_i)$) of combinations of decision variables for the normalization of successive of the constants parameters included in the matrix $\mathbf{X}^{I^*}$:

($i = 1, x_1 \equiv t_R$)—two variants including the CAV (Constant Air Volume) system with AHU with heat recovery (1.51—here cumulative variable), primary heater (option), cooler and secondary heater.

($i = 2, x_2 \equiv \varphi_R$)—two variants including AHU with cooler, secondary heater and steam humidifier in the unit or in the duct (option),

($i = 3, x_3 \equiv k_d$)—one variant with the hygienic design of AHU, three stages of filtration at the supply, 3rd stage filter integrated with a supply diffuser,

($i = 4, x_4 \equiv C_s$)—two variants as for ($i = 3, x_3 \equiv k_d$) and a steam humidifier in the AHU unit or in the duct,

($i = 5, x_5 \equiv \alpha$)—five variants depending on the number of units in the cascade (one, two or three) and the recirculation option:

$x_{1.57a}$—internal (room) recirculation, cumulative variable,

$x_{1.57b}$—external recirculation (in front of the AHU),

$x_{1.57c}$—without recirculation,

Matrix **W** is of type (15,27). Matrix with limitations $\mathbf{G}^i$ for matrix **W** is of type (15,15) and is defined as:

$G^i =$

	1	2	3	4	5	6	7	8	·	·	15
1	1										
2		0									
3			1								
4				0							
5					1						
6						1					
7							0				
8								1			
·									·		
·										·	
15											1

(A5)

where:

$\mathbf{G}^i$—binary matrix of limitation conditions for matrix **W**,

$g_{r(i,m_i)r(i,m_i)}$—binary value in matrix of elimination of unnecessary decision variables $\mathbf{G}^i$ for $r(i,m_i)$—variant of combinations of decision variables values x_j for normalizing x_i-constant parameter defined by vector $\overline{w}_{r(i,m_i)}$ in matrix **W**.

The words $g_{r(i,m_i)r(i,m_i)}$ correspond to the eliminated variants in matrix W and result from limitations. Taking into account the notations in the table of restrictions A9 [37], the assignment here is as follows: $r(i,m_i) = 2 - g_{T6}, g_{T19}$, $r(i,m_i) = 4 - g_{T11}, g_{T28}$, $r(i,m_i) = 7 - g_{T1}1, g_{T28}$.

Interpretation of elements $g_{r(i,m_i)r(i,m_i)} = 0$—of eliminated variants in matrix W is shown in Table A1.

After taking into account the constraints, redundant decision variables can be identified, which in the adopted methodology are eliminated in order to reduce the description of the mathematical problem.

Table A1. Interpretation of elements $g_{r(i,m_i)r(i,m_i)} = 0$ in matrix **G**.

$r(i,m_i)$	Limitations $g_{()k(xj)}$ */	Comments
2	g_{T6}	lack of a primary heater, with a large power differentiation for summer and winter, prevents the optimal selection of k_V output coefficients of control valves for the secondary heater—and as a consequence causes unstable operation of control valves and extends the range of tolerance of the supply air temperature
	g_{T19}	lack of a primary heater poses a risk of freezing of the water cooler
4	g_{T11} g_{T28}	steam humidifier with lance in channel does not provide easy operational access to the humidification block for control and disinfection—difficulties in maintenance and decrease in safety
7	g_{T11} g_{T28}	steam humidifier with lance in channel does not provide easy operational access to the humidification block for control and disinfection—difficulties in maintenance and decrease in safety

*/ Designation of restrictions according to [37].

Matrix G^j of type (27,27) of elimination of unnecessary decision variables is defined as:

$G^i =$ (A6)

	1	2	3	4	5	6	7	8	·	·	15
1	1										
2		0									
3			1								
4				0							
5					1						
6						1					
7							0				
8								1			
·									·		
·										·	
15											1

where:

$\mathbf{G}^j$—binary matrix of elimination of unnecessary decision variables for matrix ($\mathbf{G}^i \times \mathbf{W}$),

Matrix W^g—after considering limitations and eliminating unnecessary decision variables is obtained as the product of matrices defined as:

$$\mathbf{W}^g = \mathbf{G}^i \times \mathbf{W} \times \mathbf{G}^j \tag{A7}$$

After eliminating zero rows and columns—matrix $\mathbf{W}^g$ is defined as:

$W^g =$ (A8)

Variants $\overline{w}_{r(i,m_i^g)} = \overline{w}_{m_i^g}$	i	m_i	m_i^g	$r(i, m_i^g)$	Decision variables x_j, j = j* 1.1	1.6	1.24	1.25	1.28	1.30	1.32	1.35	1.37	1.38	1.39	1.41	1.42	1.43	1.51	1.57a	1.57b	1.57c	1.64	1.68	1.81	1.85	1.111	1.112	1.115	2.14
					1	2	3	4	5	6	7	8	9	10	11	12	13	14	15	16	17	18	19	20	21	22	23	24	25	26
	1	1	1	1	1	1	0			0	1	1	0		0	1	1	1	1	0										0
	2	1	1	2	1	0	1	1	1	1	0	1	0			0	1	1	0											0
	3	1	1	3	0																	0	1	1	1	1	1	1	1	0
	4	1	1	4	0	0	1	1	0													0	1	1	1	1	1	1	1	0
		1	1	5	0							0	1	0															1	0
	7	2	2	6	0								0	1	0														0	1
		3	3	7	0									0	1	0													0	1
		1	1	8	0							0	1	0						0	1	0								0
		2	2	9	0								0	1	0					0	1	0								0
	8	3	3	10	0								0	1	0				0	1	0	0								0
		4	4	11	0									0	1	0			0	1	1	0								0
		5	5	12	0							0	1	0							0	1	0							0

where:

W^g—binary matrix of acceptable variants of combinations of decision variables values x_j for normalizing all constant parameters x_i of HVAC system,

$\overline{w}_{m_i^g}$ or $\overline{w}_{r(i,m_i^g)}$—binary vector defining m_i- or r(i, m_i)-variant $r(i,m_i^g)$-acceptable variant) of combinations of decision variables values x_j for normalizing x_i-constant parameter of HVAC system (matrix element W^g),

m_i^g or $r(i,m_i^g)$—index of m_i^g- or $r(i,m_i^g)$-variant of combinations of decision variables values x_j for normalizing x_i-constant parameter of HVAC system, after considering limitations.

Matrix X^J of all possible variants of HVAC system is defined as:

$X^J =$ (A9)

Variants $\overline{w}_{r(i,m_i^g)} = \overline{w}_{m_i^g}$	i	m_i	m_i^g	$r(i, m_i^g)$	Variants $\overline{x}_n$, n: 1	2	3	4	5	6	7	8	9	10	11	12	13	14	15
	1	1	1	1	1	1	1	1	1	1	1	1	1	1	1	1	1	1	1
	2	1	1	2	1	1	1	1	1	1	1	1	1	1	1	1	1	1	1
	3	1	1	3	1	1	1	1	1	1	1	1	1	1	1	1	1	1	1
	4	1	1	4	1	1	1	1	1	1	1	1	1	1	1	1	1	1	1
		1	1	5	1	1	1	1	1	0									0
	7	2	2	6	0				0	1	1	1	1	1	0				0
		3	3	7										0	1	1	1	1	1
		1	1	8	1	0			0	1	0			0	1	0			0
		2	2	9	0	1	0			0	1	0			0	1	0		0
	8	3	3	10	0	0	1	0			0	1	0			0	1	0	0
		4	4	11	0		0	1	0			0	1	0			0	1	0
		5	5	12	0			0	1	0			0	1	0			0	1

where:

X^J—binary matrix of acceptable variants of HVAC system for normalizing constant parameters,

$\overline{x}_n$—binary vector defining the n-variant of structure of HVAC system used for normalizing all constant parameters,

$x_{m_i^g n}$ or $x_{r(i,m_i^g)n}$—binary value in the n-variant structures of HVAC system for m_i^g- or $r(i,m_i^g)$-variant of combinations of decision variables values for normalizing x_i-constant parameter defined by vector $\overline{w}_{m_i^g}$ or $\overline{w}_{r(i,m_i^g)}$ in matrix $\mathbf{W}^g$, matrix element $\mathbf{X}^J$,
M_i^g—number of all possible variants of combinations of decision variables values x_j for normalizing xi-constant parameter of HVAC system, after considering limitations.

Vector $\overline{x}_n$ is created by selecting from matrix $\mathbf{W}^g$ a single variant of combinations of decision variables $\overline{w}_{r(i,m_i^g)} = \overline{w}_{m_i^g}$ from ranges $m_i^g = 1 \ldots M_i^g$ for each of normalized constant parameters x_i, I = 1 ... I^* and by assigning this variant value $x_{r(i,m_i^g)} = 1$, and by assigning the remaining variants from range $m_i^g = 1 \ldots M_i^g$ each of normalized constant parameters x_i value $x_{r(i,m_i^g)} = 0$.

The number of all, defined in this particular way, possible vectors $\overline{x}_n$—of all possible variants of HVAC system for cleanroom equals:

$$N = \prod_{i=1}^{8} M_i^g = 1 \cdot 1 \cdot 1 \cdot 1 \cdot 3 \cdot 5 = 15 \quad (A10)$$

By identifying the values of the words of the vector $\overline{x}_n$ (column of the $\mathbf{X}^J$ matrix), the structure of the HVAC system is identified for the normalization of successive constant parameters.

Limiting Conditions, Set of Acceptable Variants

Matrix **G** of type (15,15) of limiting conditions for matrix $\mathbf{X}^J$ of all possible variants of HVAC system for cleanroom is defined as:

G = (A11)

	1	2	3	4	5	6	7	8	9	10	11	12	13	14	15
1	0														
2		0													
3			0												
4				0											
5					1										
6						0									
7							1								
8								1							
9									0						
10										0					
11											0				
12												0			
13													0		
14														1	
15															0

where:

G—binary matrix of limitation conditions for matrix $\mathbf{X}^J$,
g_{nn}—binary value in matrix with limitations **G** for the n-variant of structure of HVAC system defined by vector $\overline{x}_n$ in matrix $\mathbf{X}^J$,

The words $g_{n,n} = 0$ correspond to eliminating variants (vectors $\overline{x}_n$) in the matrix $\mathbf{X}^J$. Variants that are internally inconsistent or identical to other variants are eliminated.

Interpretation of elements $g_{n,n} = 0$—of eliminated vectors $\overline{x}_n$ in matrix $\mathbf{X}^J$—is shown in Table A2.

Table A2. Interpretation of vectors $g_{n,n} = 0$ in matrix $\mathbf{X}^J$.

n	Comments
1	Variant thermodynamically identical to variant $\overline{x}_7$ (n = 7), variant $\overline{x}_7$ more favorable for the regulation of overpressure in the room
2	No consistency—Δp regulation—one air handling unit, α regulation—two air handling units
3	No consistency—Δp regulation—one air handling unit, α regulation—two air handling units
4	No consistency—Δp regulation—one air handling unit, α regulation—three air handling units
6	No consistency—Δp regulation—two air handling units in cascade, α regulation—one air handling unit
9	No consistency—Δp regulation—two air handling units in cascade, α regulation—three air handling units
10	Irrational variant—two air handling units (fans) in cascade in a system without recirculation
11	No consistency—Δp regulation—three air handling units, α regulation—one air handling unit
12	No consistency—Δp regulation—three air handling units, α regulation—two air handling units
13	No consistency—Δp regulation—three air handling units, α regulation—two air handling units
15	Irrational variant—three air handling units (fans) in cascade in a system without recirculation

Matrix **X** of acceptable variants of the structure of HVAC system $\overline{x}_{n^g}$ for cleanroom is the product of:

$$\mathbf{X} = \mathbf{X}^J \times \mathbf{G} \quad \text{(A12)}$$

after eliminating zero columns.

Matrix **X** is defined as:

X = (A13)

Variants $\overline{w}_{r(i,m_i^g)} = \overline{w}_{m_i^g}$	i	m_i	m_i^g	$r(i, m_i^g)$	Variants $\overline{x}_n$, $\overline{x}_{n^g}$: n = 5, n^g = 1	n = 7, n^g = 2	n = 8, n^g = 3	n = 14, n^g = 4
	1	1	1	1	1	1	1	1
	2	1	1	2	1	1	1	1
	3	1	1	3	1	1	1	1
	4	1	1	4	1	1	1	1
	7	1	1	5	1	0	0	0
		2	2	6	0	1	1	0
		3	3	7	0	0	0	1
	8	1	1	8	0	0	0	0
		2	2	9	0	1	0	0
		3	3	10	0	0	1	0
		4	4	11	0	0	0	1
		5	5	12	1	0	0	0

where:

X—binary matrix of acceptable variants of HVAC system for normalizing constant parameters,

($x_{m_i^g n^g}$ or $x_{r(i,m_i^g)n^g}$)—binary value in the ng-acceptable variant structures of HVAC system for m_i^g- or $r\left(i, m_i^g\right)$—variant of combinations of decision variables values for nor-malizing x_i-constant parameter defined by vector $\overline{w}_{m_i^g}$ or $\overline{w}_{r(i,m_i^g)}$ in matrix W^g, matrix element X^J,

$\overline{x}_{n^g}$—binary vector defining the n^g-acceptable variant of structure of HVAC system used for normalizing all constant parameters,

$n(n^g)$—index of the n-variant (of the n^g-acceptable variant) of HVAC system.

By analyzing and interpreting backwards values of elements of subsequent matrices X, X^J and W^g defining a function of constant parameters and decision variables, it is possible to identify the full structure of acceptable variants of HVAC system.

References

1. Kircher, K.; Shi, X.; Patil, S.; Zhang, K.M. Cleanroom energy efficiency strategies: Modeling and simulation. *Energy Build.* **2010**, *42*, 282–289. [CrossRef]
2. Tschudi, W.; Xu, T. Cleanroom Energy Benchmarking Results. *ASHREA Trans.* **2003**, *109*, 733–739.
3. Zhuang, C.; Shan, K.; Wang, S. Coordinated demand-controlled ventilation strategy for energy-efficient operation in multi-zone cleanroom air-conditioning systems. *Build. Environ.* **2021**, *191*, 107588. [CrossRef]
4. Shan, K.; Wang, S. Energy efficient design and control of cleanroom environment control systems in subtropical regions—A comparative analysis and on-site validation. *Appl. Energy* **2017**, *204*, 582–595. [CrossRef]
5. Tsao, J.-M.; Hu, S.-C.; Xu, T.; Chan David, Y.L. Capturing energy-saving opportunities in make-up air systems for cleanrooms of high-technology fabrication plant in subtropical climate. *Energy Build.* **2010**, *42*, 2005–2013. [CrossRef]
6. Tsao, J.J.M.; Hu, S.-C.; Kao, W.-C.; Chien, L.-H. Clean Room Exhaust Energy Recovery Optimization Design. *ASHRAE Trans.* **2010**, *116*, 81–86.
7. Hu, S.-C.; Chuah, Y.K. Power consumption of semiconductor fabs in Taiwan. *Energy-Int. J.* **2003**, *28*, 895–907. [CrossRef]
8. Zhao, Y.; Li, N.; Tao, C.; Chen, Q.; Jiang, M. A comparative study on energy performance assessment for HVAC systems in high-tech fabs. *J. Build. Eng.* **2021**, *39*, 102188. [CrossRef]
9. Hu, S.-C.; Lin, T.; Fu, B.-R.; Chang, C.-K.; Cheng, I.-Y. Analysis of energy efficiency improvement of high-tech fabrication plants. *Int. J. Low-Carbon Technol.* **2019**, *14*, 508–515. [CrossRef]
10. Hu, S.-C.; Tsai, Y.-W.; Fu, B.-R.; Chang, C.-K. Assessment of the SEMI energy conversion factor and its application for semiconductor and LCD fabs. *Appl. Therm. Eng.* **2017**, *121*, 39–47. [CrossRef]
11. Hu, S.-C.; Lin, T.; Huang, S.-H.; Fu, B.-R.; Hu, M.-H. Energy savings approaches for high-tech manufacturing factories. *Case Stud. Therm. Eng.* **2020**, *17*, 100569. [CrossRef]
12. Lin, T.; Hu, S.-C.; Xu, T. Developing an innovative fan dry coil unit (FDCU) return system toimprove energy efficiency of environmental control for missioncritical cleanrooms. *Energy Build.* **2015**, *90*, 94–105. [CrossRef]
13. Hu, S.-C.; Tsao, J.-M. A comparative study on energy consumption for HVAC systems of high-tech FABs. *Appl. Therm. Eng.* **2007**, *27*, 2758–2766. [CrossRef]
14. Tsao, J.-M.; Hu, S.-C.; Chan, D.Y.L.; Hsu, R.T.C.; Lee, J.C.C. Saving Energy in the make-up unit (MAU) for semiconductor clean rooms in subtropical areas. *Energy Build.* **2007**, *40*, 1387–1393. [CrossRef]
15. Kim, M.-H.; Kwon, O.-H.; Jin, J.-T.; Choi, A.-S.; Jeong, J.-W. Energy Saving Potentials of a 100% Outdoor Air System Integrated with Indirect and Direct Evaporative Coolers for Clean Rooms. *J. Asian Archit. Build. Eng.* **2012**, *405*, 1279–1285. [CrossRef]
16. Yin, J.; Liu, X.; Guan, B.; Zhang, T. Performance and improvement of cleanroom environment control system related to cold-heat offset in clean semiconductor fabss. *Energy Build.* **2020**, *224*, 110294. [CrossRef]
17. Yin, J.; Zhang, T.; Ma, Z.; Liu, X. Feasibility analysis of canceling reheating after condensation dehumidification in semiconductor cleanrooms. *J. Build. Eng.* **2021**, *43*, 102589. [CrossRef]
18. Ma, Z.; Liu, X.; Zhang, T. Measurement and optimization on the energy consumption of fans in semiconductor cleanrooms. *Build. Environ.* **2021**, *197*, 107842. [CrossRef]
19. Ma, Z.; Guan, B.; Liu, X.; Zhang, T. Performance analysis and improvement of air filtration and ventilation process in semiconductor clean air-conditioning system. *Energy Build.* **2020**, *228*, 110489. [CrossRef]
20. Yin, J.; Liu, X.; Guan, B.; Ma, Z.; Zhang, T. Performance analysis and Energy saving potential of air conditioning system in semiconductor cleanrooms. *J. Build. Eng.* **2021**, *37*, 102158. [CrossRef]
21. Chen, J.; Hu, S.-C.; Chien, L.-H.; Tsao, J.J.M.; Lin, T. Humidification of Large-Scale Cleanrooms by Adiabatic Humidification Method in Subtropical Areas: An Industrial Case Study. *ASHRAE Trans.* **2009**, *115*, 299–305.
22. Xu, T.; Lan, C.-H.; Jeng, M.-S. Performance of large fan-filter units for cleanroom applications. *Build. Environ.* **2007**, *42*, 2299–2304. [CrossRef]
23. Fan, M.; Cao, G.; Pedersen, C.; Lu, S.; Stenstad, L.-I.; Skogås, J.G. Suitability evaluation on laminar airflow and mixing airflow distribution strategies in operating rooms: A case study at St. Olavs Hospital. *Build. Environ.* **2021**, *194*, 107677. [CrossRef]
24. Ozyogurtcu, G.; Mobedi, M.; Ozerdem, B. Economical assessment of different HVAC systems for an operating room: Case study for different Turkish climate regions. *Energy Build.* **2011**, *43*, 1536–1543. [CrossRef]
25. Jia, L.; Liu, J.; Wei, S.; Xu, J. Study on the performance of two water-side free cooling methods in a semiconductor manufacturing factory. *Energy Build.* **2021**, *243*, 110977. [CrossRef]
26. Zheng, G.; Li, X. Construction method for air cooling/heating process in HVAC system based on grade match between energy and load. *Int. J. Refrig.* **2021**, *131*, 10–19. [CrossRef]
27. Wang, K.-J.; Dagne, T.B.; Lin, C.J.; Woldegiorgis, B.H.; Nguyen, H.-P. Intelligent control for energy conservation of air conditioning system in manufacturing systems. *Energy Rep.* **2021**, *7*, 2125–2137. [CrossRef]
28. Zhuang, C.; Wang, S. Risk-based online robust optimal control of air-conditioning systems for buildings requiring strict humidity control considering measurement uncertainties. *Appl. Energy* **2020**, *261*, 114451. [CrossRef]
29. Zhuang, C.; Wang, S.; Shan, K. Probabilistic optimal design of cleanroom air-conditioning systems facilitating optimal ventilation control under uncertainties. *Appl. Energy* **2019**, *253*, 113576. [CrossRef]
30. Zhuang, C.; Wang, S.; Shan, K. Adaptive full-range decoupled ventilation strategy and air-conditioning systems for cleanrooms and buildings requiring strict humidity control and their performance evaluation. *Energy* **2019**, *168*, 883–896. [CrossRef]

31. Zhuang, C.; Wang, S. An adaptive full-range decoupled ventilation strategy for buildings with spaces requiring strict humidity control and its applications in different climatic conditions. *Sustain. Cities Soc.* **2020**, *52*, 101838. [CrossRef]
32. Chang, C.-K.; Lin, T.; Hu, S.-C.; Fu, B.-R.; Hsu, J.-S. Various Energy-Saving Approaches to a TFT-LCD Panel Fab. *Sustainability* **2016**, *8*, 907. [CrossRef]
33. Loomans, M.G.L.C.; Molenaar, P.C.A.; Kort, H.S.M.; Joostenb, P.H.J. Energy demand reduction in pharmaceutical cleanrooms through optimization of ventilation. *Energy Build.* **2019**, *202*, 109346. [CrossRef]
34. Loomans, M.G.L.C.; Ludlage, T.B.J.; van den Oever, H.; Molenaar, P.C.A.; Kort, H.S.M.; Joosten, P.H.J. Experimental investigation into cleanroom contamination build-up when applying reduced ventilation and pressure hierarchy conditions as part of demand controlled filtration. *Build. Environ.* **2020**, *176*, 106861. [CrossRef]
35. Molenaar, P. Ventilation Efficiency Improvement in Pharmaceutical Cleanrooms for Energy Demand Reduction. Master's Thesis, Eindhoven University of Technology, Eindhoven, The Netherlands, 2017. Available online: https://research.tue.nl/en/studentTheses/ventilation-efficiency-improvement-in-pharmaceutical-cleanrooms-f (accessed on 7 October 2021).
36. Shao, X.; Liang, S.; Zhao, J.; Wang, H.; Fan, H.; Zhang, H.; Cao, G.; Li, X. Experimental investigation of particle dispersion in cleanrooms of electronic industry under different area ratios and speeds of fan filter units. *J. Build. Eng.* **2021**, *43*, 102590. [CrossRef]
37. Porowski, M. The optimization method of HVAC system from a holistic perspective according to energy criterion. *Energy Convers. Manag.* **2019**, *181*, 621–644. [CrossRef]
38. Porowski, M. Energy optimization of HVAC system from a holistic perspective: Operating theater application. *Energy Convers. Manag.* **2019**, *182*, 461–496. [CrossRef]
39. ASHRAE. Chapter 18—Clean space. In *ASHRAE Application Handbook*; American Society of Heating, Refrigerating and Air-Conditioning Engineers Inc.: Atlanta, GA, USA, 2011.
40. Xu, T. Characterization of minienvironments in a cleanroom: Assessing energy performance and its implications. *Build. Environ.* **2008**, *43*, 1545–1552. [CrossRef]
41. Chen, D.; Chen, H. Using the Köppen classification to quantify climate variationand change: An example for 1901–2010. *Environ. Dev.* **2013**, *6*, 69–79. [CrossRef]
42. Szczechowiak, E. Analityczne obliczanie parametrów powietrza wilgotnego. *Chłodnictwo* **1985**, *20*, 8.
43. DIN 1946-4:2018-09 Ventilation and Air Conditioning—Part 4: Ventilation in Buildings and Rooms of Health Care. Available online: https://standards.globalspec.com/std/13389630/DIN1946-4 (accessed on 10 October 2021).

International Journal of
Environmental Research and Public Health

MDPI

Article

Relations among Pro-Environmental Behavior, Environmental Knowledge, Environmental Perception, and Post-Materialistic Values in China

Jinchen Xie and Chuntian Lu *

Department of Sociology, Xi'an Jiaotong University, Xi'an 710049, China; jinchenxie@stu.xjtu.edu.cn
* Correspondence: luchuntian@xjtu.edu.cn

Abstract: During the economic boom, China's government was mainly concerned with economic development; however, numerous environmental problems have arisen. Evidence suggests that Chinese individuals' pro-environmental behavior (PEB) is at a low level in Asia. However, it does not match their high-quality environmental knowledge. In this paper, the database of the Chinese General Social Survey was used to explore the correlation between environmental knowledge and PEB in a broader context. Subsequently, environmental perception and post-materialistic values (PMV) were taken as the mediator and moderator into structural equation modeling, and every variable kept robust and consistent through exploratory factor analysis. The empirical results indicated that: (i) individuals with higher environmental knowledge always show higher passion to PEB; (ii) environmental perception plays a partially mediating role between environmental knowledge and PEB; (iii) PMV moderate the formation of environmental behavior systematically; and (iv) compared with public counterpart, the relation between environmental knowledge and PEB is significantly higher in private environmental behavior. The study results could become the basis for the Chinese government and environmental NGOs to effectively spread environmental knowledge, advocate a post-materialistic lifestyle, and improve the authenticity of online media reports on environmental issues.

Keywords: pro-environmental behavior; environmental knowledge; environmental perception; post-materialistic values

Citation: Xie, J.; Lu, C. Relations among Pro-Environmental Behavior, Environmental Knowledge, Environmental Perception, and Post-Materialistic Values in China. *Int. J. Environ. Res. Public Health* **2022**, *19*, 537. https://doi.org/10.3390/ijerph19010537

Academic Editors: Roberto Alonso González Lezcano, Francesco Nocera and Rosa Giuseppina Caponetto

Received: 9 December 2021
Accepted: 31 December 2021
Published: 4 January 2022

Publisher's Note: MDPI stays neutral with regard to jurisdictional claims in published maps and institutional affiliations.

1. Introduction

With the rapid development of China's economy and the continuous advancement of urbanization [1], a series of environmental problems are becoming increasingly worse, including the greenhouse effect, water pollution, acid rain, and desertification [2]. This is attributed to the decline in Chinese pro-environmental behavior (PEB). Recently, evidence has suggested that Chinese residents' PEB is nearly the last among Asians, which is inconsistent with their economic situation [3]. However, according to several large-scale comprehensive surveys, Chinese individuals' environmental knowledge is at the highest level in the world [4]. In other words, Chinese individuals' environmental knowledge has not been effectively transformed into PEB, and this needs to be paid special attention.

Recently, abundant literature has tried to fill this correlation gap between environmental knowledge and environmental behavior, and found that environmental knowledge affects PEB mainly through two systematic methods [5]. On the one hand, according to the theory of planned behavior, environmental knowledge can directly stimulate environmental behavior [6], and this viewpoint is supported by abundant of literature. Furthermore, researchers have found that this positive effect exists in East Asia, the United States, and Europe, simultaneously. For a specific country, the relevance between environmental knowledge and environmental behavior might change with individual demographic characteristics. More specific, compared with men and the poor, women and the rich are more likely to transform environmental knowledge into environmental behavior.

On the other hand, environmental knowledge indirectly affects PEB through some mediating factors. This viewpoint attracts extensive attention of researchers. For example, the typical normal activation model indicated that pro-environmental conceptual schema played a mediating role between the environmental knowledge and PEB [7]. Meanwhile, environmental perception can significantly explain the indirect effect between environmental knowledge and PEB, especially in Europe and the United States [8–10]. However, it should be pointed out that almost all researchers ignore that environmental perception can be divided into different categories, which lead to the heterogeneous mediating effects. In addition, some Chinese researchers believe that the media usage is a potential mediating variable between environmental knowledge and PEB [11]. Although, more researchers used environmental knowledge as a control variable in their empirical research.

However, based on the above analysis, with respect to the Chinese context, a fundamental factor must be taken into consideration, namely, post-materialist values. Because Chinese individuals are always regarded as the following contradictory characteristics: rich but lacking environmental morality. However, a few studies have mentioned that post-materialistic values (PMV) may moderate the relationship between environmental knowledge and PEB among Chinese individuals. In addition, whether or not the mediating effects of environmental perception is still significant in China is worth discussing, because environmental perception usually arises from media rather than direct perception. However, China's media tend to cover up the truth of environmental issues for economic purposes. Additionally, a few studies have noticed that environmental behavior and environmental knowledge contain different types [12,13]. For example, environmental knowledge about water pollution may have a positive impact on public environmental behavior, but not on private behavior. Therefore, this paper tried to set up systematic correlations between environmental knowledge and PEB, and took environmental perception and PMV as the mediator and/or moderator, respectively.

2. Basic Concepts: Pro-Environmental Behavior, Environmental Knowledge, Environmental Perception, Post-Materialistic Values

At present, China's government is confronted with the challenge of greenhouse gas emission reduction, which is highly connected with the reverse of the environmentally unfriendly lifestyles. At the same time, China has become the largest garbage producer and greenhouse gas emitter country in the word since about 2005 [14]. Chinese residents' perception of environmental pollution in their daily life is much higher than the international average level. In addition, as the second largest economic entity, China has achieved modernization as a whole. Therefore, it is very important to investigate the impact of PMV on environmental behavior. Furthermore, in order to accurately obtain the relevant mechanism, it is of vital necessity to focus on the correlation between environmental knowledge and PEB with the moderating or mediating of environmental perception and PMV.

Pro-environmental behavior (PEB): PEB is usually defined as behavior that individuals spontaneously undertake in their daily life and contribute to the improvement of environmental quality. In this study, PEB was divided into public PEB and private PEB, and they are conceptually distinct. Private PEB can be conceptualized as the PEB that is generated from an individuals' daily life, such as recycling plastic bags. Public PEB is the process by which individuals participate in public environmental protection in response to the call of the government or social organizations, such as participating in environmental debates.

Environmental knowledge: Environmental knowledge refers to the cognition of the environmental problems, environmental science, and environmental governance. Generally speaking, environmental knowledge is divided into daily environmental knowledge and professional environmental knowledge. Daily environmental knowledge can be conceptualized as the environmental knowledge related to the common environmental pollution in life, such as harmful noise. Professional environmental knowledge usually occurs in specialized fields (e.g., chemical pharmacy, industrial production, and soil research), which are little known to the public, such as a single species of forest being susceptible to diseases.

Environmental perception: Environmental perception is conceptualized as the subjective judgment and direct feeling of the individuals facing objective environmental risks, such as an environmental phenomenon directly perceived by the residents, which will have a significant impact on environmental protection behavior. Capaldi et al. (2014) divided environmental perception into two systematically and different kinds: ecological environmental perception and daily environmental perception [15]. An individuals' perception of all natural, social, or cultural environments of human life is usually defined as ecological environmental perception, and the perception of daily environmental problems is defined as daily environmental perception.

Post-materialistic values (PMV): PMV can be defined as the cultural concepts of social groups, which get rid of the "materialism" that focuses on meeting basic survival needs, and turns to the pursuit of high-quality life security. Ronald and Inglehart (1995) believed that after the material needs are met, post-materialistic behaviors such as environmental protection, democratic consciousness, political participation, and gender equality will systematically appear in society [16].

The existing literature rarely considers the above four factors in a specific model, especially where this relationship is positioned in a broader context of institutions and their effects. Thus, we took environmental perception as a mediator because the existing literature proved that environmental knowledge could stimulate environmental perception, and environmental perception will affect environmental behavior. Meanwhile, we took PMV as a moderator, to investigate whether PMV can positively impact the generation of residents' PEB. The added value of our research is threefold. First, PMV was taken into our research, and answered whether it played a part in the formation of Chinese PEB; second, we classified environmental knowledge, PEB, and environmental perception into different types, and discussed the correlation among them, respectively; third, we tried to position the correlation between these four factors into a specific model, so as to construct a moderated mediating model and further discussion. Appropriate research questions were formulated as below:

1. For Chinese residents, is there a significant relationship between environmental knowledge and PEB? Is the relationship between different types of environmental knowledge and behavior consistent?
2. Does environmental perception play a role in the above process as a mediator? Is the mediating effect complete or partial?
3. Does PMV participate in the above process as a moderator? Is the moderating effect positive or negative?

3. Methodology

3.1. Data

We collected data from the Chinese General Social Survey (CGSS), which was jointly conducted by Renmin University of China and relevant academic institutions. The respondents were adults in Mainland China, including over 10,000 samples from 31 provinces/municipalities in China. Since the first round of survey in 2003, CGSS had completed ten rounds of annual survey, which fully reveals the characteristics of Chinese individuals. It is worth noting that the focus of each round of CGSS is significantly different, just like the World Value Survey. The environmental issues concerned in this paper are the main focus of CGSS in 2013. Therefore, we chose the survey data in CGSS in 2013. After dropping the invalid respondents, the final sample size was 11,438.

3.2. Measures

3.2.1. Dependent Variable

PEB is the dependent variable to which we paid attention. Exploratory factor analysis (EFA) was conducted on ten related PEBs of CGSS in 2013. Two common factors, public PEB and private PEB, were obtained (KMO = 0.826, Bartlett < 0.001). The private PEB contains (a) garbage classification, (b) rarely use plastic bags, (c) pay attention to environmental news, and (d) discuss environmental issues with others. The public PEB contains (a) donate for environmental protection, (b) actively participate in public environmental affairs, (c) actively participate in environmental NGOs, (d) protect trees or green space spontaneously, and (e) complaints for environmental protection. (KMO = 0.826, Bartlett < 0.001) PEB was coded 1–3 as "never participate", "generally" and "always participate".

3.2.2. Independent Variable

Environmental knowledge is the main independent variable in our research. The conceptual framework of Bradley and Waliczek (1999) was referred to extract variables from CGSS in 2013. After conducting EFA, two common factors were extracted. The former contains three elements: (a) overuse of chemical fertilizer is harmful, (b) fluorine destroys the ozone layer, and (c) using coal leads to acid rain. The latter contains: (a) every species is important in the biological chain, (b) a single species of forest is susceptible to diseases, and (c) carbon dioxide causes air warming. (KMO = 0.816, Bartlett < 0.001). It should be noted that the former three factors are generally recognized in China, while the latter three factors are less understood. Thus, we conceptualized these two factors as general environmental knowledge and professional environmental knowledge, respectively. Every variable was assessed by a binary scale (0 = no 1 = yes), each question has a standard answer, and the data we used were also expressed by binary variables, 0 and 1 denotes wrong or right, respectively.

3.2.3. Mediating Variable

According to theoretical analysis, environmental perception was taken as a mediating variable among the correlation of different environmental knowledge and different PEB. We conducted EFA on the twelve related factors of environmental perception in CGSS in 2013, and finally extracted two common factors: daily environmental perception and ecological environment perception. The former contains the following seven elements: (a) air pollution, (b) water pollution, (c) noise, (d) industrial garbage, (e) daily garbage, (f) lack of green space, and (g) food pollution. The latter contains: (a) forest destruction, (b) cultivated land degradation, (c) lack of fresh water, (d) desertification, and (e) reduction in wildlife (KMO = 0.913, Bartlett < 0.001). All factors were rated as the 5-point Likert scale (1 = lightly perceive; 5 = strongly perceive).

3.2.4. Moderating Variable

We focused on the process that PMV shapes the PEB of Chinese residents; thus, we took PMV as the moderating variable. EFA was conducted to extract five common factors representing PMV from CGSS in 2013, which included (a) government needs democracy, (b) the people must have a voice of public affairs, (c) representatives should express public opinion, (d) people's benefits are more important than the national, and (e) people should participate in national decision-making (KMO = 0.801, Bartlett < 0.001). All factors were binary (0 = disagree and 1 = agree), and we added them up and obtained a continuous variable, a higher score meant more positive in post materialist values.

3.3. *Analysis*

Structural Equation Modeling (SEM) has been widely applied to estimate the structural correlations among the latent variables. SEM was chosen in this study because of the following two reasons. First, we paid more attention to the correlation among latent variables, which are difficult to achieve in the traditional regression method. While SEM is an appropriate analytical approach to discuss the correlation among latent variables. Second, we constructed a mediation model, and SEM is more effective to reveal the relationship among variables in the complex model. The following procedures were conducted in our research: (i) the EFA of four latent variables was firstly conducted, including PEB, environmental knowledge, environmental perception, and PMV; (ii) descriptive analysis of all variables was reported; (iii) SEM was conducted to identify the correlation among the environmental knowledge and PEB, describing the correlation of between these two factors preliminarily; and (iv) mediator and moderator were added to draw the systematically correlations between these four factors.

4. Results

4.1. Descriptive Statistics

The comprehensive information of the whole variables (e.g., correlations, mean, and standard deviation) are listed, as shown in Table 1. The correlations between each adjacent variable are statistically significant, except the correlation between materialistic-value and public PEB, which indicated that our data highly support the subsequent SEM model. The normality assumption of all the variables were well met, where the skewness values were less than 3 and kurtosis values were less than 10.

Table 1. Correlations and descriptive statistics for study variables.

	Item	Factor Loading	Mean	SD
Public environmental behavior	Garbage classification	0.544	1.57	0.701
	Rarely use plastic bags	0.609	1.57	0.632
	Pay attention to environmental news	0.546	2.15	0.78
	Discuss environmental issues with others	0.636	1.63	0.700
Private environmental behavior	Donate for environmental protection	0.654	1.20	0.444
	Actively participate in public environmental affairs	0.768	1.27	0.525
	Actively participate in environmental NGOs	0.760	1.19	0.450
	Protect trees or green space spontaneously	0.488	1.19	0.479
	Complaints for environmental protection	0.587	1.11	0.357
Daily environmental knowledge	Overuse of chemical fertilizer is harmful	0.423	0.70	2.504
	Fluorine destroys the ozone layer	0.490	0.79	0.405
	Using coal leads acid rain	0.743	0.44	0.496
Professional Environmental knowledge	Every species is important in the biological chain	0.776	0.47	0.499
	A single species of forest is susceptible to diseases	0.666	0.42	0.493
	Carbon dioxide causes air warming	0.754	0.49	0.500
Daily environmental perception	Air pollution	0.839	3.44	1.888
	Water pollution	0.805	3.51	1.864
	Noise	0.810	3.68	1.906
	Industrial garbage	0.733	4.13	2.057
	Daily garbage	0.671	4.10	1.743
	Lack of green space	0.539	3.60	1.965
	Food pollution	0.705	3.44	2.080
Ecological environmental perception	Forest destruction	0.707	4.65	2.033
	Cultivated land degradation	0.624	4.26	2.084
	Lack of fresh water	0.713	4.29	2.072
	Desertification	0.678	5.44	1.976
	Reduction of wildlife	0.610	4.91	2.177
Post-materialistic value	Government needs democracy	0.597	0.79	0.406
	The people must have a voice of public affairs,	0.735	0.68	0.465
	Representatives should express public opinion,	0.624	0.78	0.417
	People's benefits are more important than national's	0.498	0.79	0.404
	People should participate in national decision-making	0.524	0.71	0.453

Table 1. *Cont.*

Pearson correlation test	1.	2.	3.	4.	5.	6.	7.
1. Public environmental behavior	1.00						
2. Private environmental behavior	0.23 ***	1.00					
3. Daily environmental knowledge	0.15 ***	0.13 ***	1.00				
4. Professional environmental knowledge	0.19 ***	0.23 ***	0.53 ***	1.00			
5. Daily environmental perception	−0.09 ***	−0.13 ***	−0.18 ***	−0.19 ***	1.00		
6. Ecological environment perception	−0.05 ***	−0.18 ***	−0.04 ***	−0.10 ***	0.56 ***	1.00	
7. Post-materialistic values	0.01	−0.10 ***	0.13 ***	0.09 ***	0.101 ***	0.08 ***	1.00
Means	6.81	5.95	1.99	1.73	25.83	24.23	3.76
SD	0.36	0.02	0.09	0.15	0.13	0.11	0.14

*** significant at $p < 0.001$.

4.2. SEM Model

The whole model was highly acceptable (chi square = 3170.97, CFI = 0.924, TLI = 0.879, RMSEA = 0.057, 90% C.I. = (0.056, 0.058)). To display the outcome clearly, the model was divided into four groups, respectively(shown as Figure 1). Firstly, we focused on the correlation between daily environmental knowledge and public environmental behavior, the direct coefficient of these two factors was positive and significant ($\beta = 0.496$, $p < 0.001$). The result also showed that the indirect relationship between these two factors via daily environmental perception and ecological environment perception was significant (indirect effect = 0.074, 95% CI (0.054, 0.095)) and significant (indirect effect = 0.002, 95% CI (−0.003, 0.006)), respectively. Our result indicated that the daily environmental knowledge of Chinese residents can effectively stimulate the generation of public PEB. For example, when Chinese residents have understood that automobile exhaust emissions are harmful to health (Daily environmental knowledge), they would call for public transport instead of driving (Public environmental behavior). Additionally, the daily environment perception partially mediates the above process. Such conclusion is consistent with the extent literature [17,18].

Secondly, the net effects between professional environmental knowledge and public PEB was identified, and the coefficient was significantly positive ($\beta = 0.333$, $p < 0.001$). The indirect relationship between these two factors through daily/ecological environmental perception was significant (indirect effect = 0.039, 95% CI (0.029; 0.050)) and non-significant (indirect effect < 0.001, 95% CI (−0.004; 0.004)), respectively. Compared with daily environmental knowledge, professional environmental knowledge showed systematically disadvantage in stimulating public PEB, whether directly or indirectly. These conclusions are rarely found in previous literature because the previous studies rarely divided environmental behavior and environmental knowledge into different types nor discussed the relationship between them in-depth [19,20].

Thirdly, the correlation of daily environmental knowledge and private PEB was positive statistically ($\beta = 0.15$, $p < 0.001$). It should be pointed out that the indirect correlation is totally different from the mentioned above. Compared with daily counterpart (indirect effect < 0.001, 95% CI (−0.004, 0.004)), the ecological environment perception significantly mediated the relationship between daily environmental knowledge and private PEB (indirect effect = 0.039, 95% CI (0.029, 0.050)). More specific, Chinese residents may be more concerned about the public environmental crisis, rather than pollution in daily life. This conclusion is inconsistent with the literature describing the characteristics of the Chinese as lacking public morality [21,22]. The reason is that in China, individual benefits are far less important than public benefits.

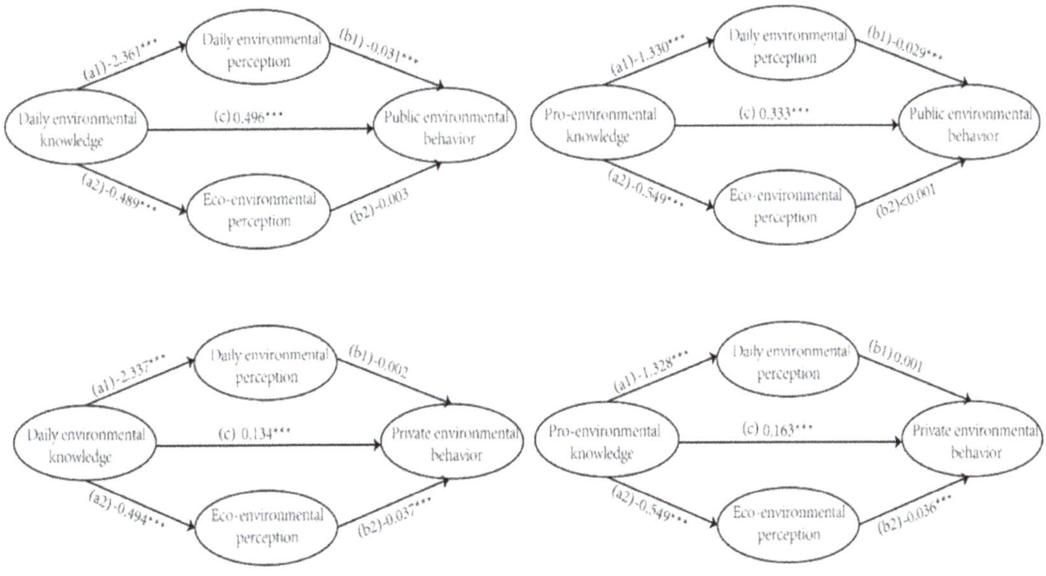

Figure 1. Final model estimations with standardized beta weight (SE). Note. *** $p < 0.05$.

Fourth, a positive correlation between professional environmental knowledge and private PEB was obtained ($\beta = 0.16$, $p < 0.001$). Comprehensively speaking, environmental knowledge was better at stimulating the generation of public PEB (the direct relation in model 1,2) rather than private PEB (the direct relation in model 3,4). This also supports the conclusion that we refuted the Chinese people's lack of public morality in the previous paragraph. Meanwhile, the indirect correlation between these two factors through daily/ecological environment perception showed non-significant (indirect effect = −0.001, 95% CI (−0.008, 0.007)) and significant (indirect effect = 0.020, 95% CI (0.013, 0.027)), respectively.

Lastly, as suggested in theoretical analysis, the PMV may moderating the formation of PEB. So, we added the PMV into SEM, and the moderating effects were obtained, as shown in Table 2. A panoramically positive moderating effects indicated that PMV was systematically benefit for the formation of PEB, whether through environmental knowledge or environmental perception. The results showed that when people's values shift from materialism to post-materialism, Chinese residents' PEB will be systematically improved, as shown in Table 3.

Table 2. Mediating coefficients for the explanatory model pathways.

Effects	Daily Knowledge to Public Behavior		Pro-Knowledge to Public Behavior		Daily Knowledge to Private Behavior		Pro-Knowledge to Private Behavior	
	Effect	95%CI	Effect	95%CI	Effect	95%CI	Effect	95%CI
C′	0.496 ***	0.429; 0.563	0.333 ***	0.299; 0.367	0.134 ***	0.074; 0.195	0.165 ***	0133;0.195
b1	−0.031 ***	−0.038; −0.025	−0.029 ***	−0.036; −0.023	−0.002	−0.007; 0.004	0.001	−0.005; 0.006
b2	−0.003	−0.011; 0.005	<0.001	−0.008; 0.008	−0.037 ***	−0.044; −0.030	−0.036 ***	−0.043; −0.029
a1	−2.361 ***	−2.712; −2.009	−1.330 ***	−1.512; −1.147	−2.337 ***	−2.688; −1.985	−1.328 ***	−1.511; −1.145
a2	−0.489 ***	−0.774; −0.204	−0.549 ***	−0.695; −0.398	−0.494 ***	−0.779; −0.208	−0.549 ***	−0.698; −0.401
Effects from environmental knowledge to environmental behavior								
Total	0.571 ***	0.505; 0.637	0.372 ***	0.338; 0.406	0.158 ***	0.097; 0.218	0.184 ***	0.152–0.214
Ind. Total	0.075	0.057–0.095	0.039 ***	0.031; 0.049	0.023 ***	0.007; 0.039	0.019 ***	0.011; 0.027
Ind1(a1 × b1)	0.074 ***	0.054; 0.095	0.039 ***	0.029; 0.050	0.005	−0.009; 0.181	−0.001	−0.008; 0.007
Ind2(a2 × b2)	0.002	−0.003; 0.006	<0.001	−0.004; 0.004	0.018 ***	0.008; 0.030	0.020 ***	0.013; 0.027

*** significant at $p < 0.001$.

Table 3. Moderating effects of post-materialistic value on the coefficients.

	Public Environmental Behavior			Private Environmental Behavior		
	β	SE	p	β	SE	p
Daily environmental knowledge	0.025 ***	0.011	0.019	0.046 ***	0.016	0.005
Professional environmental knowledge	0.024 ***	0.012	0.042	0.036 ***	0.013	0.006
Daily environmental perception	0.029 ***	0.012	0.014	0.053 ***	0.014	0.000
Ecological environment perception	0.024 ***	0.012	0.042	0.036 ***	0.013	0.006

*** significant at $p < 0.001$.

5. Discussion

The results indicated that daily/professional environmental knowledge positively predicts the formation of public PEB, which means that enhancing Chinese residents' environmental knowledge will significantly improve their public PEB. Meanwhile, the indirect correlation among these three factors through environmental perception showed significantly positive consistence, except that ecological environment perception partially mediated the formation of PEB. Such results revealed that environmental perception (whether public or ecological) plays a part of active mediation in the process of transforming environmental knowledge into public PEB.

It is worth mentioning that the private PEB has a comparatively mild positive relationship between environmental knowledge and environmental perception compared with the public counterpart. The result is consistent with conventional view that Chinese individuals pay more attention to the cleanliness of their private environment and lack public awareness of environmental protection. The direct correlation among daily/professional environmental knowledge and private PEB significantly positive, respectively. Based on the above conclusions, if we want to change the current situation of weak PEB of Chinese residents, it is of vital necessity to increase environmental knowledge (whether daily or professional). The indirect correlation among these three factors through environmental perception showed systematically insignificant, except the mediating of ecological environment perception in the correlation between professional environmental knowledge and private PEB. Thus, we conclude that daily/ecological environmental perception is more likely to mediate the formation of pubic PEB than private PEB.

Of interest, such conclusions are consistent with several extent literature about Chinese individuals' PEB, which indicated a positive correlation between environmental knowledge and PEB [23,24]. However, Chinese residents are systematically insensitive to the mediating role of environmental perception in this correlation. While several European and American researchers found that environmental perception significantly mediated the generation of PEB [25,26]. Our result showed that Chinese individuals may be less sensitive to environmental issues.

As for the moderating effects of PMV into the formation of PEB, Chinese residents showed statistically positive significance. Our results indicated that it is still applicable for the PMV theory in China context, which is in line with the content literature [27,28]. Data showed that there is a mismatch between the lack of PEB and the high-quality economic of China. According to our empirical analysis, when people with materialistic values are gradually replaced by people with PMV, Chinese residents' PEB will be systematically improved.

In summary, environmental knowledge and PMV are attributed to the formation of Chinese residents' PEB significantly, while environmental perception played a partial role. A conceivable explanation for the outcomes is that Chinese residents are insensitive to environmental issues. Generally speaking, individual environmental perception is obtained mainly from network media rather than daily experience. However, China's media have been criticized for a long time, and they usually hide the truth of environmental problems for commercial purposes. Therefore, the environmental perception of Chinese residents is generally not as abundant as it should be, and it is difficult for environmental perception to participate in the formation of PEB. The above conclusions also inspire researchers to pay more attention to the correlation between network media, environmental perception, and PEB, especially in Western countries.

In the context of policy, these results underpin several supporting to ongoing environmental investments in China. During the economic boom, China's government has paid the majority of its attention to economic development, which has led to numerous environmental problems. It not only threatens the health and prospects of current and future generations, but also undermines the sustainability of long-term growth. While, since 2020, every Chinese individual has basically met their material needs, the government and environmental NGOs have made great efforts to improve residents' environmental consciousness. Our empirical results indicate that it is of vital necessity for China's government to strengthen the policy of spreading environmental knowledge and advocating a post-materialistic lifestyle.

There are several limitations to be interpreted carefully as follows: (i) non-random distribution of environmental attributes may lead to endogenous problems, which means that our empirical results only describe the correlation; (ii) our results were generally based on respondents' self-reported surveys, which means that this article only partially revealed the individuals' objective environmental attributes; and (iii) last but not least, the year of this survey is another important limitation, which needs to be carefully addressed. Despite these limitations, our research provided a relatively perfect framework to explore the formation of individuals' PEB, and to discuss the heterogeneous situation of PEB. Accordingly, this study is of vital importance both theoretically and empirically.

6. Conclusions

This paper revealed a potential mechanism among PEB, environmental knowledge, environmental perception, and PMV in China. The main contribution of this paper is to construct the SEM including the four factors listed below, simultaneously, and to discuss the structural relationship among them. Meanwhile, the mediating and moderating model was used to discuss the potential mechanism of the generation of Chinese residents' PEB. Additionally, we discussed the heterogeneity of correlation coefficients between different environmental attributes, so as to enrich the research conclusions.

The important conclusions of this study can be summarized as follows: Firstly, individuals with higher environmental knowledge always show higher passion to PEB. Similar conclusions have been found in the United States, India, New Zealand, and other countries. It indicates that improving environmental knowledge is a feasible way to promote Chinese residents' PEB. Secondly, environmental perception plays a partially mediating role in the above relationship, but it is not always significant. More specifically, daily environmental perception indirectly impacts the generation of public PEB, whereas ecological environmental perception significantly mediates the formation of private PEB. These conclusions are important, and have not been revealed in previous studies. Thirdly, PMV moderated the formation of PEB systematically. Furthermore, the moderating effect remains positive on each related path. This conclusion indicates that the promotion of PMV is of vital necessity to stimulate Chinese residents' PEB. It is also consistent with PMV theory proposed by Professor Ingelhart.

This study has a practical value in assessing the formation of Chinese individuals' PEB. Our results could become the basis for China's government and environmental NGOs to spread environmental knowledge, advocate a post-materialistic lifestyle, and improve the authenticity of online media reports on environmental issues. More notably, our empirical research provides some meaningful insights for future research works. Environmental perception has been shown to participate in the generation of PEB as a mediator, so other factors affecting PEB (like environmental perception) may also exist, such as government trust or media contact, which may mediate the generation of PEB as well. Future researchers might use the above elements proposed by this study to design a serial multiple-mediator SEM.

Author Contributions: Conceptualization, J.X.; data curation, J.X.; methodology, C.L.; supervision, C.L.; writing—original draft, J.X. and C.L.; writing—review and editing, J.X. and C.L. All authors have read and agreed to the published version of the manuscript.

Funding: This work was supported by Basic business expenses of Central Universities of China, grant number SK2018048.

Informed Consent Statement: Informed consent was obtained from all subjects involved in the Study.

Data Availability Statement: Data are obtained from the Official website of Chinese General Social Survey. All data permission has been obtained and there is no copyright issue for all the figures in the paper.

Acknowledgments: We would like to thank RenMin university and the relevant academic institutions who provided data support, and all relevant individuals who helped to improve our paper.

Conflicts of Interest: The authors declare no conflict of interest.

References

1. Guo, H.; Liu, J.; Wei, J. Ambient Ozone, PM1 and Female Lung Cancer Incidence in 436 Chinese Counties. *Int. J. Environ. Res. Public Health* **2021**, *18*, 10386. [CrossRef]
2. Grao-Cruces, A.; Segura-Jiménez, V.; Conde-Caveda, J.; García-Cervantes, L.; Martínez-Gómez, D.; Keating, X.D.; Castro-Piñero, J. The role of school in helping children and adolescents reach the physical activity recommendations: The UP&DOWN study. *J. Sch. Health* **2019**, *89*, 612–618. [PubMed]
3. Organization for Economic Co-Operation and Development. Available online: https://www.oecd-ilibrary.org/environment/oecd-environmental-outlook-to-2030_9789264040519-en (accessed on 8 December 2021).
4. World Value Survey. Environmental Findings and Insights. Available online: https://www.worldvaluessurvey.org/WVSContents.jsp (accessed on 8 December 2021).
5. Kim, M.S.; Stepchenkova, S. Altruistic values and environmental knowledge as triggers of pro-environmental behavior among tourists. *Curr. Issues Tour.* **2020**, *23*, 1575–1580. [CrossRef]
6. Azjen, I. *Understanding Attitudes and Predicting Social Behavior*; Prentice-Hall: Hoboken, NJ, USA, 1980; pp. 202–277.
7. De Groot, J.I.; Steg, L. Morality and prosocial behavior: The role of awareness, responsibility, and norms in the norm activation model. *J. Soc. Psychol.* **2009**, *149*, 425–449. [CrossRef] [PubMed]
8. Kautish, P.; Sharma, R. Determinants of pro-environmental behavior and environmentally conscious consumer behavior: An empirical investigation from emerging market. *Bus Strategy Dev.* **2020**, *3*, 112–127. [CrossRef]
9. Aldieri, L.; Makkonen, T.; Vinci, C.P. Environmental knowledge spillovers and productivity: A patent analysis for large international firms in the energy, water and land resources fields. *Resour. Policy* **2020**, *69*, 101877. [CrossRef]
10. Gkargkavouzi, A.; Paraskevopoulos, S.; Matsiori, S. Public perceptions of the marine environment and behavioral intentions to preserve it: The case of three coastal cities in Greece. *Mar. Policy* **2020**, *111*, 103727. [CrossRef]
11. Yang, X.; Chen, L.; Wei, L.; Su, Q. Personal and media factors related to citizens' pro-environmental behavioral intention against haze in China: A moderating analysis of TPB. *Int. J. Environ. Res. Public Health* **2020**, *17*, 2314. [CrossRef]
12. Indriani, I.A.D.; Rahayu, M.; Hadiwidjojo, D. The influence of environmental knowledge on green purchase intention the role of attitude as mediating variable. *Int. J. Multicult. Multireligious Underst.* **2019**, *6*, 627. [CrossRef]
13. Grúňová, M.; Brandlová, K.; Svitálek, J.; Hejcmanová, P. Environmental education supports conservation action by increasing the immediate and long-term environmental knowledge of children in West Africa. *Appl. Environ. Educ. Commun.* **2017**, *16*, 3–16. [CrossRef]
14. Globe Carbon Project. Ten Years of Advancing Knowledge on the Global Carbon Cycle and Its Management. 2010. Available online: https://www.globalcarbonproject.org/products/reports.htm (accessed on 5 December 2021).
15. Capaldi, C.A.; Dopko, R.L.; Zelenski, J.M. The relationship between nature connectedness and happiness: A meta-analysis. *Front. Psychol.* **2014**, *5*, 976. [CrossRef]
16. Abramson, P.R.; Inglehart, R.F. *Value Change in Global Perspective*; University of Michigan Press: Ann Arbor, MI, USA, 2009; pp. 67–143.
17. Otto, S.; Pensini, P. Nature-based environmental education of children: Environmental knowledge and connectedness to nature, together, are related to ecological behaviour. *Glob. Environ. Chang.* **2017**, *47*, 88–94. [CrossRef]
18. Sun, H.; Teh, P.L.; Linton, J.D. Impact of environmental knowledge and product quality on student attitude toward products with recycled/remanufactured content: Implications for environmental education and green manufacturing. *Bus Strategy Environ.* **2018**, *27*, 935–945. [CrossRef]
19. Ogbeide, O.A.; Ford, C.; Stringer, R. The environmental benefits of organic wine: Exploring consumer willingness-to-pay premiums? *J. Food Prod. Mark.* **2015**, *21*, 482–502. [CrossRef]

20. Liu, P.; Teng, M.; Han, C. How does environmental knowledge translate into pro-environmental behaviors?: The mediating role of environmental attitudes and behavioral intentions. *Sci. Total Environ.* **2020**, *728*, 138126. [CrossRef] [PubMed]
21. Zhao, L.; Ding, X.; Yu, F. Public moral motivation during the COVID-19 pandemic: Analysis of posts on Chinese social media. *Soc. Behav. Personal. Int. J.* **2020**, *48*, 1–14. [CrossRef]
22. Baum, T.J. The responsibility of power: Shifts in Chinese conceptualisation of the legitimacy of overseas intervention to protect nationals abroad. *Glob. Chang. Peace Secur.* **2020**, *32*, 259–273. [CrossRef]
23. Duan, W.; Sheng, J. How can environmental knowledge transfer into pro-environmental behavior among Chinese individuals? Environmental pollution perception matters. *J. Public Health* **2018**, *26*, 289–300. [CrossRef]
24. Tong, Q.; Anders, S.; Zhang, J.; Zhang, L. The roles of pollution concerns and environmental knowledge in making green food choices: Evidence from Chinese consumers. *Food Res. Int.* **2020**, *130*, 108881. [CrossRef]
25. Schweiker, M.; Ampatzi, E.; Andargie, M.S.; Andersen, R.K.; Azar, E.; Barthelmes, V.M.; Zhang, S. Review of multi-domain approaches to indoor environmental perception and behaviour. *Build. Environ.* **2020**, *176*, 106804. [CrossRef]
26. Shafiei, A.; Maleksaeidi, H. Pro-environmental behavior of university students: Application of protection motivation theory. *Glob. Ecol. Conserv.* **2020**, *22*, e00908. [CrossRef]
27. Henn, M.; Sloam, J.; Nunes, A. Young cosmopolitans and environmental politics: How postmaterialist values inform and shape youth engagement in environmental politics. *J. Youth Stud.* **2021**, *1*, 1–21. [CrossRef]
28. Babula, M.; Muschert, G. Post-Materialist Waste: A Study of Turkey's Importation of Rubbish. *Open J. Sociol. Stud.* **2020**, *4*, 2. [CrossRef]

energies

MDPI

Article

A Win-Win Scheme for Improving the Environmental Sustainability of University Commuters' Mobility and Getting Environmental Credits

Laura Cirrincione [1], Salvatore Di Dio [2], Giorgia Peri [1], Gianluca Scaccianoce [1], Domenico Schillaci [3] and Gianfranco Rizzo [1,*]

1 Dipartimento di Ingegneria, Università degli Studi di Palermo, Viale delle Scienze Ed. 9, 90128 Palermo, Italy; laura.cirrincione@unipa.it (L.C.); giorgia.peri@unipa.it (G.P.); gianluca.scaccianoce@unipa.it (G.S.)
2 Dipartimento di Architettura, Università degli Studi di Palermo, Viale delle Scienze Ed. 14, 90128 Palermo, Italy; salvatore.didio@unipa.it
3 PUSH Design Lab, Piazza Sant'Anna n. 3, 90133 Palermo, Italy; d.schillaci@wepush.org
* Correspondence: gianfranco.rizzo@unipa.it

Citation: Cirrincione, L.; Di Dio, S.; Peri, G.; Scaccianoce, G.; Schillaci, D.; Rizzo, G. A Win-Win Scheme for Improving the Environmental Sustainability of University Commuters' Mobility and Getting Environmental Credits. *Energies* **2022**, *15*, 396. https://doi.org/10.3390/en15020396

Academic Editor: Shi-Jie Cao

Received: 17 December 2021
Accepted: 4 January 2022
Published: 6 January 2022

Publisher's Note: MDPI stays neutral with regard to jurisdictional claims in published maps and institutional affiliations.

Abstract: European Union Member States are called upon to meet internationally proposed environmental goals. This study is based, in particular, on the recommendation of the European Union (EU), which encourages Member States to pursue effective policies to reduce greenhouse gas (GHGs) emissions, including through appropriate changes in the behavioral habits of citizens. In this respect, among the main sectors involved, transport and mobility should certainly be mentioned. National institutions should be adequately involved in order to achieve the objectives set; in this regard, universities must certainly be considered for their educational value. These latter, for instance, could commit to improving the environmental performance of the mobility of their commuter students (to a not insignificant extent), since commuting modes are often the cause of high CO_2 emissions; indeed, they still largely involve the use of internal combustion engines based on fossil fuels. In this paper, the effectiveness of a smartphone-app-based method to encourage commuter students to adopt more sustainable transport modes is evaluated. In more detail, starting from a statistical analysis of the status quo of mobility habits of a sample of students at the University of Palermo (Italy), an improvement of current habits toward a more sustainable path is encouraged through a new application (specifically created for this purpose) installed on students' smartphones. Then, the daily and annual distances traveled by commuters with the new mobility modes are calculated, and the resulting savings in energy and CO_2 emissions are estimated. Finally, it is proposed that the reduced emissions could be converted into energy-efficiency credits that the University could use to enter the emission trading system (ETS), here contextualized within the Italian "TEE" ("Energy Efficiency Credits") scheme, while the benefits for students participating in the program could consist of reduced fees and free access to university services. The results obtained show the feasibility of the proposal. This approach can be considered a useful model that could be adopted by any other public institutions—not only universities—to facilitate their path toward decarbonization.

Keywords: sustainable mobility; universities; commuter students; efficiency credits; smartphone's social-game-based app; mobility behavior

1. Introduction

Freight transportation and people mobility represent an important part of the tertiary sector (that aims to provide services to citizens) in advanced societies, not only from an economic point of view but also in relation to both the amount of energy required and the rate of associated pollutant emissions attributable to them [1]. According to a 2020 report of the International Energy Agency (IEA) (these figures refer to twenty-four countries—Australia, Austria, Belgium, Canada, Czech Republic, Denmark, Finland, France, Germany,

Greece, Hungary, Italy, Japan, Korea, Luxembourg, the Netherlands, New Zealand, Poland, Portugal, Slovak Republic, Spain, Switzerland, the United Kingdom and the United States—of the IEA that account for about 92% of the total IEA final energy consumption of the considered year), the transport sector accounts for 36% of total energy consumption, of which 21% is ascribable to passenger cars and 15% to freight roads (i.e., cargo transport) and other transportations [2]. On the other hand, these two segments of the transport sector are also responsible for a significant amount of CO_2 emissions related to human activity; specifically, quotas of 20% and 10% have been indicated that affect passenger cars and freight roads [2], respectively. Referring to Italy, energy-consumption rates are comparable with those of other IEA countries. In fact, the most recent figures [3] show that energy consumption in the transportation sector accounts for 39.4 Mtoe, or for 33.8% of the total final energy consumption of the country (116 Mtoe).

This is the reason why, in recent years, the transport sector has been affected by interventions aimed at limiting its energy burden and the amount of fossil fuels required for its operations [4]. These limitations are imposed by the European Union (EU), with very stringent targets: in fact, greenhouse gases (GHGs) emissions are required to be reduced by 40% by 2030 compared to 1990 levels.

Unfortunately, EU Member States are missing their targets. In fact, national projections show that the EU emissions' reductions could actually achieve a reduction of only 30%, which is far from the 40% target and, more importantly, well below the potential target of 50% [5].

However, it should be noted that the COVID-19 pandemic emergency has been inducing major trend changes in energy demand and pollutant emissions from the transport sector. The consequences of such an unpredictable situation could lead to a twofold scenario [6]. On the one hand, the dramatic collapse of public and freight transportation during the lockdown (or semi-lockdown) period certainly resulted in a decrease in energy consumption and GHGs emissions from the sector [7]. On the other hand, it is hoped that measures taken by governments, aimed at modifying mobility modalities of people (pushing in the direction of electric and hybrid vehicles, among others) can trigger a faster transition of the sector toward more sustainable paths [8]. As already pointed out, the role of local governments and authorities in the implementation, governance and promotion of less impactful transport practices can facilitate the transition toward a more sustainable and smart urban mobility [9–11]. Moreover, attention to the changes imposed by the COVID-19 emergency in the transportation sector now seems to be of paramount importance for institutions and international organizations. The G7 group, for example, is deeply interested in this issue, particularly with regard to transportation safety and health-related aspects.

Several studies have been conducted [12,13] in order to make the operation of transport smoother from a structural point of view, thus making the whole sector more efficient and effective [14,15]. On the other hand, less attention has been paid to the behavioral patterns that characterize user mobility (that represent the focus of the present analysis), although some studies have focused on possible changes in mobility modalities in urban contexts. Indeed, the impacts related to a mixed use of different modes of mobility [16], such as single-occupant vehicles, transit and walking, and the so-called real-time human perception [17], have been questioned for a long time, in the belief that the people's awareness is a crucial element to improve the efficiency and the environmental performances of an urban mobility system. Moreover, it has been emphasized that the features of built environments and urban landscapes [18,19] should be properly considered as key elements that can deeply influence people's propensity to adopt less environmentally impactful and healthier modes of mobility [20]. Among these key elements, the physical characteristics of urban contexts, the role of structural configurations (such as the streets' network and width, connectivity and land-use mix), travel distances in relation to the travel task [21,22] and population density [23,24] have been considered important elements in both facilitating walking at neighborhood scale [25] and inducing a delay in traffic flow [26].

Clearly, commuters are an important part of urban mobility, and, at the same time, growing awareness of climatic threats, along with health considerations, have further oriented people toward more sustainable ways of commuting to and from cities in order to effectively counteract the general worsening of the environmental quality of cities and limit the congestion problems currently affecting urban areas [27]. Specifically, because urban design variables are recognized as crucial points in determining commuters' travel behavior, these characteristics have been associated with the active population traveling to/from work and educational facilities. Specifically, it has been shown how, once socioeconomic and demographic characteristics are suitably accounted for, improved roadway infrastructure would support the transport-related physical activities, regardless of the geographical area considered [28,29].

Students represent a relevant component among commuters worldwide. That is why learning about students' mobility behaviors and teaching about sustainable transportation (at different levels of education) by using new participatory educational solutions are key elements [30].

In light of this, specific attention has long been paid to sustainable-transportation planning on large campuses [31,32] in order to identify best practices that could help students transition to more effective travel modes [33], while also taking into account the correlation between psychosocial and environmental issues [34,35]. In addition, other studies have investigated the positive effects of active commuting on physical activity and students' overweight [36], as well as comparisons of walking, biking and motorcycle riding [37].

Researchers' attention on students' attitude in assuming active mobility practices has been and still is quite active both in terms of analyzing mode's preferences [38] and the potential for active commuting [39,40], based on demographics, psychological and environmental variables [41]. Other factors could usefully enhance the effectiveness and the environmental performance of commuting. Some other actions seem, in fact, particularly promising, such as the adoption of appropriate student-housing policies and the improvement of bicycle networks [42]. In any case, the analysis of individual factors [43] and the structural elements [44,45] remains an important field of research currently investigated in order to provide exhaustive answers on what drives university students toward a sweeter sustainable mobility [46].

In fact, in relation to both the global-climate-change scenario [47] and the role that active travel has in mitigating mobility related CO_2 emissions [48], university campuses, being educational facilities that shape the minds and behaviors of present and future generations of students, represent crucial places where attention toward low-carbon development strategies that include greener and healthier lifestyles can be raised [49]. In this regard, student involvement has generally been considered within the evaluation of green strategies and initiatives implemented by higher education institutions on their path toward sustainability [50], fostering sustainable practices in curricula and research programs [51] and integrating different dimensions of the university system: education, research, governance and campus operation [52].

Therefore, the idea arises of enhancing these practices that improve mobility and its environmental performance by including them in the procedures that institutions, industrial plants, and companies can activate to receive benefits (credits) for the energy requalification actions implemented. These procedures have been recognized and formalized by the European Union—as part of the new policies and objectives aimed at the decarbonization of production systems—by including these benefits in a market of credits where the most virtuous institutions and production sites can sell them to companies whose practices are less sustainable. This exchange market is called Emission Trading System (ETS). Several documents have been released on this issue, i.e., "EU revision for the time period 2021–2030" (phase 4), https://ec.europa.eu/clima/policies/ets/revision_en, (accessed on 16 December 2021); "DIRECTIVE 2003/87/EC"; and "DIRECTIVE (EU) 2018/410 OF THE EUROPEAN PARLIAMENT AND OF THE COUNCIL", https://eur-lex.europa.eu/eli/dir/2018/4

10/oj, (accessed on 16 December 2021). Specifically, according to this trading scheme, efficiency measures that can provide energy savings in terms of tons of oil equivalent (toe) would allow companies to obtain certificates that could be traded on the pertinent public platform through bi-lateral negotiations. The effectiveness of the market trading scheme is based on the commitment made by companies to obtain a number of credits corresponding to the amount of their annual emissions; on the other hand, virtuous companies can keep their credits in order to balance possible future emissions.

In this context, given that a more environmentally conscious mobility system could generally imply a reduction in the energy consumption of the involved transport means, it would then be reasonable for institutions pursuing such practices to be eligible for energy efficiency or environmental sustainability credits under the existing trading schemes. Referring to Italian institutions, this hypothesis would be further supported by the circumstance that the national trading system for energy-efficiency credits (whose acronym is "TEE") contemplates the inclusion of behavioral patterns among the modalities and projects to which credits are awarded [53], the so-called white certificates. The question that arises here is whether, among the positive effects induced by a more sustainable mobility system, there are additional benefits for institutions that enable such sustainable practices.

A possible inclusion of these behavioral practices among those eligible for the white certificates would lead to a win-win scheme, such as the one described in Figure 1, where it is graphically depicted how an improvement in the environmental (and energy) performance of the commuter mobility could translate into a tangible benefit to the university through the acquisition of white certificates, which could be traded by the university governance in the existing credits market.

Figure 1 outlines the structure of this article and the steps through which the work was carried out. In detail, the study begins with a statistical analysis (based on a questionnaire) of the status quo of student mobility and the ways in which it is carried out (Step 1); it then continues with the direct involvement (of a sample) of students, who are encouraged to change their commuting habits toward more sustainable modes, which are detected through a new application (specifically created for this purpose) installed on their smartphones (Step 2). Following this, the daily and annual distances covered by commuters with the new modes of mobility are calculated, and the resulting savings in energy and CO_2 emissions are estimated (Step 3); finally, the energy efficiency credits resulting from these savings and attributable to the university are estimated, and some benefits for the students that have generated these improvements are suggested (Step 4).

In other words, a twofold goal is therefore pursued with this paper: on the one hand, to show the strong potential of an action regarding the change of students' mobility habits (entailing the benefits previously described), and on the other hand, to propose to entitle universities to enter environmental credit markets. In particular, Section 2 addresses the application of a smartphone-app-based ICT method aimed at enhancing the sustainability of the commuter's mobility, while Section 3 advances the hypothesis that the university could get environmental credits as a result of such a mobility-improvement initiative.

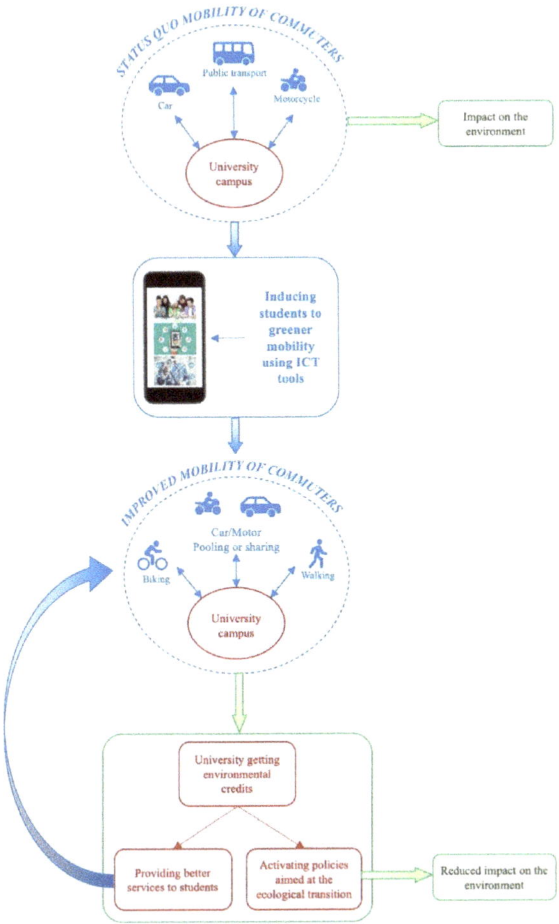

Figure 1. Visual sketch of the win-win proposal for the mobility of the commuter students.

2. Toward a More Sustainable Mobility of Commuter Students

The evaluation and promotion of a sustainable mobility related to university campuses, as a mean of transition toward more environmentally conscious and low carbon cities, has been a topic of interest within the scientific community in recent years [15,54,55].

Within this conceptual framework, a study and application involving commuter students who daily reach the campus of the University of Palermo in Southern Italy are presented here.

The Sicilian University of Palermo, encompassing 16 Departments, 134-degree courses and 23 Ph.D. courses, represents one of the largest Italian Universities, counting more than 42,000 enrolled students, with a rising trend in the last two years, and approximately 10,000 new freshmen in the 2020/2021 academic year only [56]. Most of the services offered by the University of Palermo take place on the campus sited in Viale delle Scienze, also known as "Cittadella" (meaning "small city"), given its large extension—about 37 hectares—characterized by the presence of large avenues and wide green areas and, in addition to that, various parking lots and buildings (Figure 2). Obviously, the circles in Figure 2 have the sole purpose of providing a draft visual representation of the distance between the different areas from which commuters originate and their target.

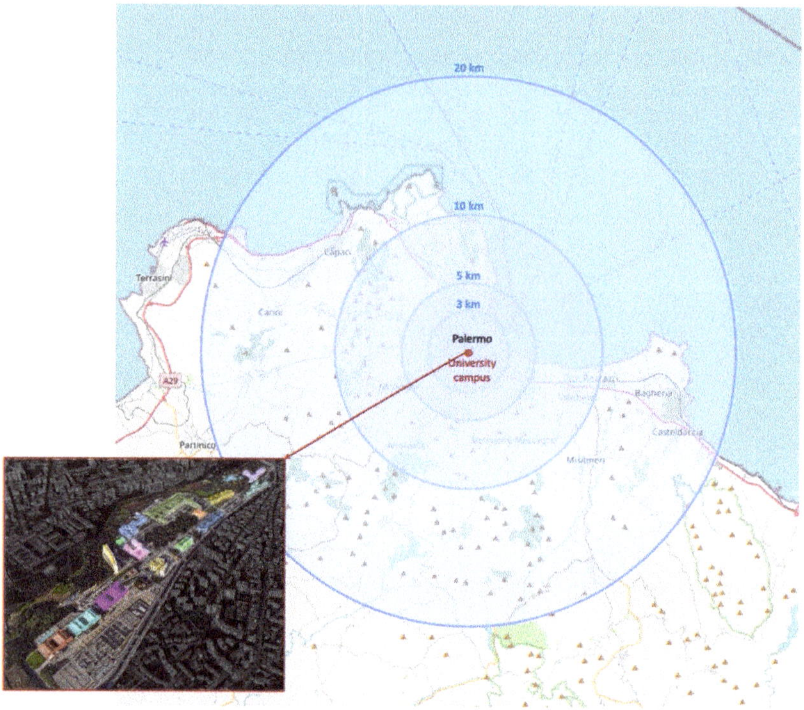

Figure 2. Campus and the circular distances from where commuters originate.

In order to reduce the use of carbon-related primary energy sources, and with the aim of contributing to the fulfillment of the target proposed by the EU [57,58] and the United Nations' Sustainable Development Goals (SDGs) [59], the University of Palermo has undertaken an effective path of energy saving since 2010. Specifically, SDGs numbers 7 [60] and 11 [61], regarding the promotion of concepts and technologies able to pursue energy efficiency, environmental sustainability, safety and resilience, were taken as a guide, as they seem to be of utmost relevance to the university sector. Among these actions, the mobility of students who reach the campus on a daily basis is considered by the university administration.

2.1. *The Actual Structure of the Commuter Students' Mobility*

Most students at the University of Palermo do not live near the campus (within walking distance); thus, they must travel daily to attend classes, and, usually, most of the commuting is accomplished by traditional polluting mobility modalities. Therefore, abandoning the use of private and highly polluting transportation in favor of more sustainable alternatives (i.e., walking, biking, public transport and vehicle pooling and/or sharing) would lead to a significant reduction in polluting emissions [62].

Clearly, the first step in any greener policy must start with an understanding of the actual structure of the commuters' mobility, pertinent to the modality of transportation, in relation to their distance from the campus. Approximately 25,000 daily commuters can be located in circular areas that are nearly 3, 5, 10 and 20 km far from the campus. The remaining part of them lives more than 20 km far from the university campus: for these students, a mean daily trip of 60 km has been found (students that live at greater distances are not commuters but usually stay in rented rooms that are relatively close to the university) [63].

We started with a survey conducted by the university on the origin of the paths of students arriving at the campus daily to attend classes (Table 1).

Table 1. Distribution of the commuter students by distances from the campus.

Parameter	Distance (D) of Origins from the Campus					
	$D \leq 3$ km	$3 < D \leq 5$ km	$5 < D \leq 10$ km	$10 < D \leq 20$ km	$D > 20$ km	TOT
Average round-trip daily path, L_{zc} (km/commuter)	3	8	15	30	60	
Sample share by distance, MS_z (%)	30	26	27	9	8	100
Number of commuters by zone, NC_z (-)	7500	6500	6750	2250	2000	25,000
Total distances by zones, $TL_z = NC_z \times L_{zc}$ (km)	22,500	52,000	101,250	67,500	120,000	363,250

Based on this distribution, a sample campaign was conducted [64] from May 2013 to June 2015, involving a total number of 311 university students who were distributed by distance, as reported in the survey provided. The purpose of this campaign was to single out, by distances class, the percentage share of students' preferred mobility modalities to reach the campus daily (columns MS_{zm} of Table 2).

Table 2. Share of commuters (MS_{zm}) and related numbers (NC_{zm}) per zone and per modality.

Modalities of Mobility	Distance (D) of Origins from the Campus									
	$D \leq 3$ km		$3 < D \leq 5$ km		$5 < D \leq 10$ km		$10 < D \leq 20$ km		$D > 20$ km	
	MS_{zm} (%)	NC_{zm}	MS_{zm} (%)	NC_{zm}	MS_{zm} (%)	NC_{zm}	MS_{zm} (%)	NC_{zm}	MS_{zm} (%)	NC_{zm}
Walking	62	4,650	32	2080	0	0	0	0	0	0
Biking	12	900	20	1300	4	270	0	0	0	0
Public transportation	10	750	13	845	25	1688	19	428	34	680
Car	5	375	9	585	34	2295	35	788	35	700
Motorcycle	0	0	14	910	12	810	9	203	3	60
Carpooling	6	450	8	553	17	1148	25	574	25	500
Moto-pooling	5	375	4	228	8	540	12	259	3	60
Car sharing	0	0	0	0	0	0	0	0	0	0

Such a breakdown has been attributed to the total number of commuters (NC) in order to obtain the number of daily commuters (NC_{zm}) by mode of transport and by travel distance to the campus, as reported in Table 2.

Subsequently, starting from the total distances by zones, TL_z (Table 1), using the pertinent MS_{zm} shares, the total daily trip lengths per zone and modality, TL_{zm}, can be calculated as follows:

$$TL_{zm} = TL_z \times MS_{zm} \tag{1}$$

At this point, it is easy to estimate the daily CO_2 emissions (tons of CO_2), Ezm, by zone and mobility modality (for the average vehicle occupation), as reported in Table 3:

$$E_{zm} = TL_{zm} \times E_m/OR_m \tag{2}$$

where OR_m represents the mean occupation rate (pass/vehicle) of the transportation means used to make the daily round-trips path from home to university and vice versa, and E_m refers to the emission rate (g CO_2/km) for the carbon dioxide of the involved transportation means. Despite the fact that these parameters are available in recent technical reports [65], due to the average age of the Italian passenger mobility fleet, in the present application, we refer to the previously released values of CO_2 emission factors [66,67].

Table 3. *SCENARIO 0*—daily CO_2 emissions per zone and mobility modality and per vehicle occupation for all commuters, E_{zm} (tons of CO_2).

Modalities of Mobility	CO_2 Emissions per Distance (D) of Origins from the Campus					Total (Tons of CO_2)
	$D \leq 3$ km	$3 < D \leq 5$ km	$5 < D \leq 10$ km	$10 < D \leq 20$ km	$D > 20$ km	
Walking	0.0000	0.0000	0.0000	0.0000	0.0000	**0.0000**
Biking	0.0000	0.0000	0.0000	0.0000	0.0000	**0.0000**
Public transportation	0.0013	0.0038	0.0143	0.0072	0.0230	**0.0496**
Car	0.2240	0.9317	6.8534	4.7033	8.3615	**21.0740**
Motorcycle	0.0000	0.5882	0.9817	0.4909	0.2909	**2.3517**
Carpooling	0.0430	0.1407	0.5479	0.5479	0.9550	**2.2345**
Motor-pooling	0.0227	0.0368	0.1636	0.1568	0.0727	**0.4526**
Car sharing	0.0000	0.0000	0.0000	0.0000	0.0000	**0.0000**
Total	**0.2909**	**1.7012**	**8.5610**	**5.9062**	**9.7031**	**26.1624**

In Table 3, the high value of the total CO_2 emissions of the commuters coming from the $5 \div 10$ km distance area is caused by their mobility preferences, which are mainly oriented toward the private cars, and by the number of students pertinent to this area.

Therefore, starting from the daily CO_2 emissions and using an energy factor, EF (toe/tCO_2), that links these emissions with the fossil-fuel energy consumption (conversion and Emission factors, Italy; report associated to SiReNa 20 (in Italian), http://www.energialombardia.eu/c/document_library/get_file?uuid=675ad6f1, 2019) (accessed on 18 September 2021) of car engines, it is now possible to determine the energy consumption C_{zm} per zone and mobility modality (toe), as reported in Table 4:

$$C_{zm} = E_{zm} * EF \tag{3}$$

These results represent the baseline scenario (Scenario 0) of the distribution of the mobility of the university commuter students. This scenario realized the amounts of CO_2 emissions and energy consumption shown in Tables 3 and 4, respectively. In the following, the actions taken by the University of Palermo in order to improve this impactful configuration are described. The new configuration represents Scenario 1.

Table 4. *SCENARIO 0*—daily energy consumption by zone and mobility modality and by vehicle occupation for all commuters, C_{zm} (toe).

Modalities of Mobility	CO_2 Emissions per Distance (D) of Origins from the Campus					Total (Tons of CO_2)
	$D \leq 3$ km	$3 < D \leq 5$ km	$5 < D \leq 10$ km	$10 < D \leq 20$ km	$D > 20$ km	
Walking	0.00000	0.00000	0.00000	0.00000	0.00000	**0.00000**
Biking	0.00000	0.00000	0.00000	0.00000	0.00000	**0.00000**
Public transportation	0.00342	0.01027	0.03846	0.01949	0.06199	**0.13362**
Car	0.66743	2.77650	20.42326	14.01596	24.91727	**62.80042**
Motorcycle	0.00000	1.75291	2.92553	1.46276	0.86682	**7.00802**
Carpooling	0.12807	0.41930	1.63284	1.63284	2.84590	**6.65893**
Motor-pooling	0.06772	0.10956	0.48759	0.46727	0.21671	**1.34884**
Car sharing	0.00000	0.00000	0.00000	0.00000	0.00000	**0.00000**
Total	**0.86663**	**5.06853**	**25.50767**	**17.59832**	**28.90869**	**77.94983**

2.2. *Implementing a Greener Mobility of the Commuter Students*

As it is possible to see in Table 2, although part of the trips is made by biking or walking, a significant component of the mobility is made by typically polluting private means, such as cars and motorcycles. Therefore, there is large room for improving the environmental performances of the mobility pattern. Among possible strategies, encouraging students to assume a more sustainable commuting behavior can pursue this target.

To achieve this goal, an effective way to facilitate the communication between the university governance and the commuter students may consist of the use of new information and communication technologies, in the belief that a proper modeling of the relationship between environment and subject is becoming increasingly important in the governance of new smart cities [68], where users represent the central points of the technological applications. In particular, tools based on smartphone apps seem to be the most effective choice today, as also reported in some recent works of the literature [69–71]. With this intent, a smartphone app based on an info-mobility Decision Support System has been expressly developed [72].

Such Decision Support System, named TrafficO2 (www.trafficO2.com) (accessed on 18 September 2021), has been a social innovation project conducted by the PUSH design lab from 2013 to 2016 and co-financed by the Italian Ministry of University and Research.

The project intends to decrease private traffic intensity and limit pollution, not through policies promoted by city administrations, but simply by involving social applications supported by smart technological devices (smartphones and/or tablets). TrafficO2, the smartphone app here introduced [72,73], is an info-mobility Decision Support System whose main aim is to push people especially commuter students toward more sustainable mobility behaviors. This change in transport habits is being encouraged via incentives proportionate to responsible choices. In detail, participants obtain "environmental points" as a reward for their sustainable mobility choices. Being a Decision Support System [74] each user is asked to log in and take a survey based on which they will receive a personalized improvement Scenario. Specifically, based on personal route and mobility modality, the app provides some alternative route options to which some parameters are associated (i.e., travel time, emitted and saved CO_2 and burnt calories), along with related O2 points (i.e., a virtual currency), and cumulative score. This makes it possible for the commuter to immediately know his/her achievable improvement, thus being more stimulated in attaining it. Furthermore, with the aim of encouraging the use of the app (hence, promoting sustainable behaviors), users can challenge one another by using the app to increase their O2 points and also play with the provided information. The TrafficO2 platform is thus a sort of a citizens' game [75] intended to encourage sustainable and environmentally friendly trips. Although the method is specifically designed to push people toward a soft mobility (i.e., walking and biking), the other transport modes between home and the university campus that are actually used are also considered, that is, public transportation, individual private transportation (cars and motorcycles) and shared mobility (car and motor sharing and carpooling).

The user's travel lengths and modalities (i.e., the way the user moves) are recorded and managed by using GPSs and accelerometers, sensors that are commonly present in smartphones and are able to detect the motion system with a high level of accuracy. A dedicated algorithm-based software that was trained by using a Fast Fourier Transform [76] was specifically designed for this purpose. Figure 3 illustrates screenshots of the software interface that appear to the users.

Although commuters are thought to be less sensitive to weather conditions than non-commuters [77], weather conditions are also taken into account by TrafficO2 by means of proper additional factors added to the baseline O2 points per km, especially on cloudy and rainy days.

In order to verify the feasibility of the TrafficO2 app, the method was firstly field-tested by inviting a small number of testers to install the mobile app and participate in the challenge [72]. Subsequently, by June 2015, the in-field testing was extended to a sample of 357 students, where the length of the daily one-way home–university campus trip was estimated through the use of a specific questionnaire and a GoogleMaps©TM (https://www.google.it/maps) (accessed on 18 September 2021) analysis of the routes used by each member of the sample. The app was expressly designed to encourage the transition to walking, cycling, public transport and vehicle sharing, without completely excluding trips by car or motorcycle.

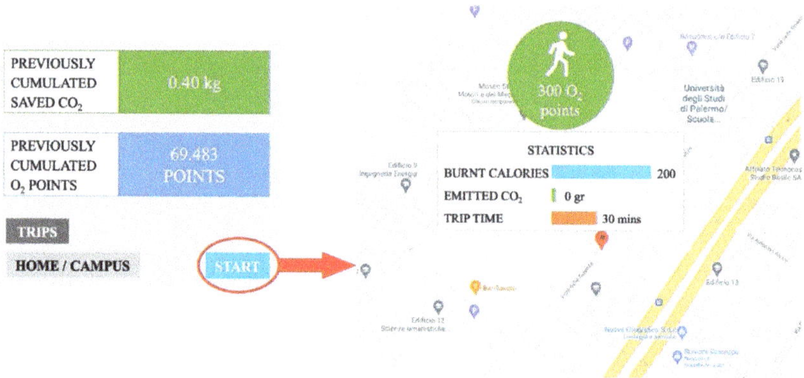

Figure 3. Mobile-phone screenshots of the app shown to the commuter users.

The proposed reward scheme was field-tested by using a sample of commuter students. The new mobility percentages, *MS'*, by distances and transportation modalities that emerged from testing the selected sample of students (Table 5) were attributed to the totality of the commuters gravitating around the campus in order to assess the whole energy and environmental benefits if they all chose to apply to the program.

Table 5. *SCENARIO 1*—share of commuters by zone and modality (MS'_{zm}) and related numbers (NC'_{zm}) per zone and per modality.

Modalities of Mobility	**Shares and Related Numbers of Commuters per Distance (*D*) of Origins from the Campus**									
	$D \le 3$ **km**		$3 < D \le 5$ **km**		$5 < D \le 10$ **km**		$10 < D \le 20$ **km**		$D > 20$ **km**	
	MS_{zm} (%)	NC_{zm}	MS_{zm} (%)	NC_{zm}	MS_{zm} (%)	NC_{zm}	MS_{zm} (%)	NC_{zm}	MS_{zm} (%)	NC_{zm}
Walking	67	5025	55	3575	0	0	0	0	0	0
Biking	12	900	20	1300	17	1148	0	0	0	0
Public transportation	10	750	13	845	32	2160	22	500	48	960
Car	0	0	0	0	6	405	21	473	13	260
Motorcycle	0	0	0	0	0	0	2	45	0	0
Carpooling	6	450	9	553	36	2430	42	954	37	730
Moto-pooling	5	375	4	228	9	608	12	279	3	50
Car sharing	0	0	0	0	0	0	0	0	0	0

The comparison of Table 5 with Table 2 indicates a significant change in the modes of students' travel to the campus as a result of the solicitations proposed by the app scheme. In addition, the aggregate percentage values, related to the modes of travel, indicate a considerable change in the performance of the mobility structure (see Figures 4 and 5), which tends to favor the less impactful methods.

This modified mobility implies a reduction in the amount of CO_2 released by commuters on their way from home to campus, assuming 200 working days in a year for students, as reported in Figure 6.

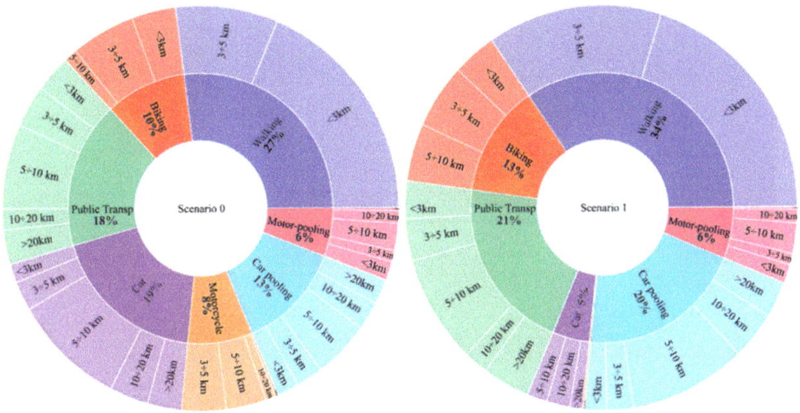

Figure 4. Percentages breakdown of the mobility means in the ex-ante (0) and improved ex-post (1) scenarios by origin distances, in reference to the total number (25,000) of commuters.

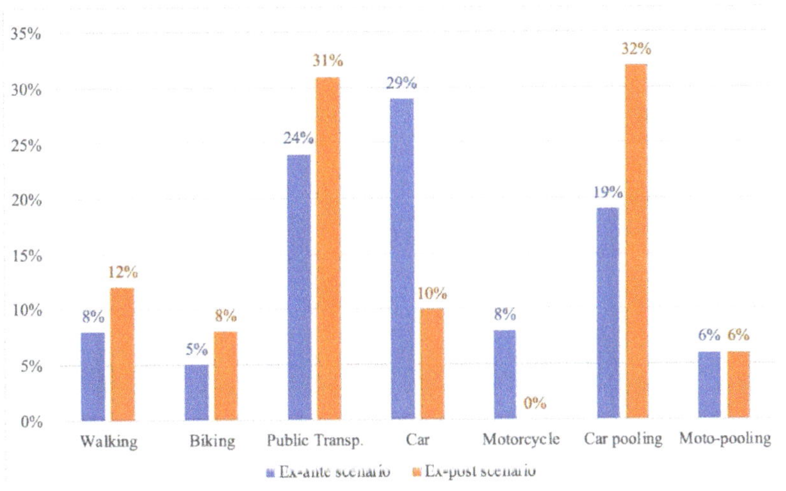

Figure 5. Aggregate percentages of kilometers covered by the mobility means in the actual ex-ante (0) and improved ex-post (1) scenarios, in reference to the total distance traveled by all commuters.

On the other hand, for the 25,000 students commuting to the campus from the periphery of Palermo (and its provincial territory), the pertinent energy required is equal to 15,591 and 6811 toe for the actual (ex-ante) and new improved (ex-post) scenarios, respectively. Such a significant enhancement, which consists in a reduction of up to 8780 toe, is highlighted in the graph shown in Figure 7. Data assumed for energy conversions through this study are 1 toe = 11,628 kWh for primary fuels (that is, 1 toe = 41.860 GJ) and 1 toe = 5347.59 kWh for electric energy (1 kWh = $0.187 * 10^{-3}$ toe).

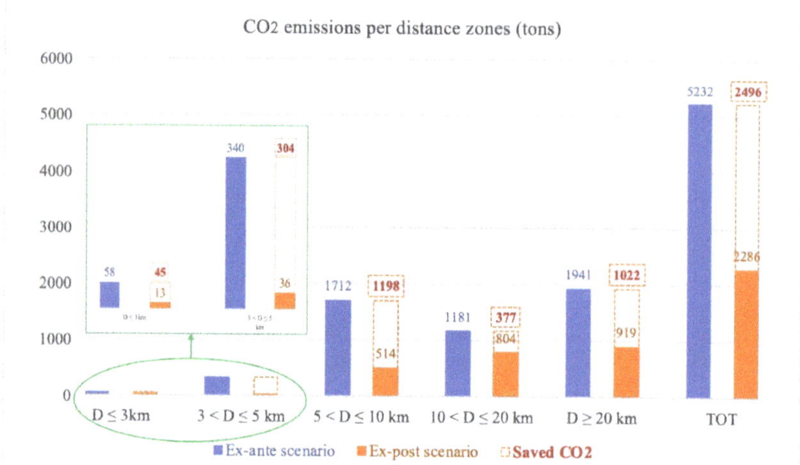

Figure 6. Yearly CO_2 (tons) releases and saved in the actual ex-ante (0) and improved ex-post (1) scenarios.

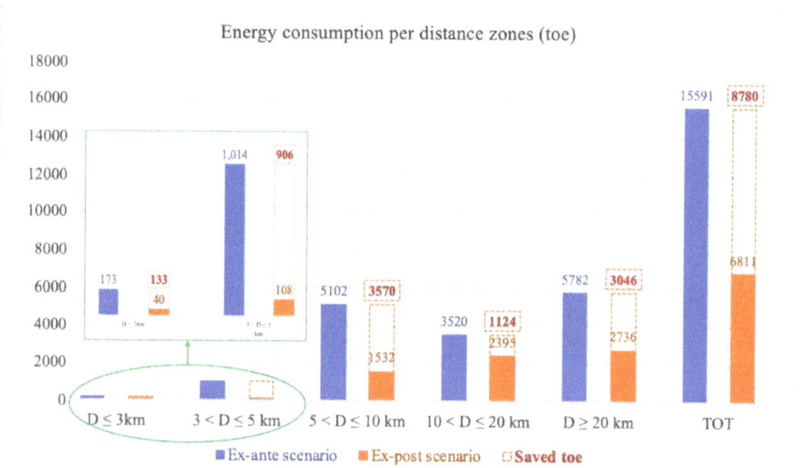

Figure 7. Yearly fossil fuels energy amounts (toe) involved in the actual ex-ante (0) and improved ex-post (1) scenarios.

The significant reduction in CO_2 emissions and energy use associated with the new hypothesized commuters' mobility configuration is certainly an important contribution that signals how a greener mobility (adopted by this category of students) could be effective for sustainability purposes.

The question now arises whether the universities (or any other Public Administrations that adopts similar incentive policies) may be entitled to receive tangible benefits due to the adoption of such more sustainable practices, for instance, by acquiring credits corresponding to the avoided carbon emissions and to the energy savings achieved (in this case, related to the new student-mobility configuration).

3. A Hypothesis of Acquisition of Certificates by the University

The following explores the potential of applying to a credits system for a university that adopts effective policies concerning the mobility modalities of its commuter students.

The Italian system, specifically designed for the access to the environmental market, the so-called "white certificates" or "Titoli di Efficienza Energetica" (TEE), was introduced in January 2017 [78] by a decree of the Italian Ministry of the Economic Development and further modified by a Ministry Decree released in May 2018 [79]. Finally, in May 2019, an operative guide was published [80] that introduced relevant changes concerning algorithms used for computing energy savings in the climatization of buildings.

The TEE scheme indicates the primary energy savings to be mandatorily achieved (after the implementation of energy efficiency actions) by the distributors of electric energy and natural gas with more than 50,000 customers. Entrusted entities may fulfill their energy-saving obligations by directly carrying out energy-efficiency interventions or by purchasing credits corresponding to the exceeding of their emission limits from another voluntary subject admitted to the TEE mechanism.

For each ton of oil equivalent (toe) of energy saving achieved through the adoption of energy-efficiency measures, a credit is recognized for a period (from three to ten years), depending on the type to which each project belongs. The targets indicated for Italy for the years 2017, 2018, 2019 and 2020 were 7.14, 8.32, 9.71 and 11.19 Mtoe, respectively.

Public administrations can also benefit from credits to be used for the refurbishment of highly energy-intensive public services, such as public lighting and urban mobility. The projects eligible to receive white certificates by the public administrations are those shown in Table 6 [53].

Table 6. Projects eligible for the efficiency transfer system in the public administrations.

Sectors	Allowable Projects
Industry	Plants of thermal energy; power quality systems; electric engines; energy recovery in the re-gasifying plants.
Networks, services and transportation	Energy efficiency of existing district heating and cooling; new fleets of transportation means fed by natural gas, liquefied natural gas, liquefied gas petroleum and hydrogen; efficiency of electric, gas and hydraulic networks; energy efficiency of data computing centers.
Civil	Installation of heating systems and warm-air generators; thermal insulation interventions; retrofit and realization of zero energy buildings.
Behavioral	Adoption of efficient systems for signaling and management; adoption of data analysis systems for single plants; adoption of action aimed at the utilization of low emission vehicles.

These projects are awarded white certificates if they generate additional energy savings, i.e., primary energy savings calculated as the difference between baseline consumption and post-operam energy consumption.

It is interesting to note that, among the sectors included in the TEE scheme, behavioral interventions are also covered, although it should be noted that a relevant sector from the point of view of the CO_2 emissions, such as transportation/mobility, it is not yet directly included among the actions eligible for the assignment of such credits.

However, it might be reasonable to propose to include—with minor changes to the structure of the scheme—sustainable mobility practices among the behavioral and virtuous actions that result in a reduction of the GHG emissions of the sector and, therefore, as candidate measures for the nomination of credits to be traded in the trading platforms.

From another perspective, it should be noted that the energy consumption and corresponding pollutant emission associated with commuter mobility pattern cannot be directly attributed to the campus area itself. However, the more environmentally sustainable and energy efficient habits adopted by campus users (mainly students) could be indirectly attributed to the university administration, due to the new low-carbon governance policies [81].

Hence, assigning to the University of Palermo the TEE certificates related to the environmental benefits, deriving from the choice of a more sustainable mobility pattern adopted by the commuter students, appears to be a sensible proposal. In fact, since this behavior would contribute to improve, at the same time, the air quality of a certain area of the city, the related energy savings could be included among the measures implemented by the university toward its sustainable low-carbon path.

The combination of the above-cited considerations—i.e., (1) the fact that the transportation sector has, to date, been scarcely considered in the TEE scheme and (2) the possibility that behavioral models could be promoted among the eligible actions for environmental and energy credits—suggests that special attention should be paid to commuter mobility if affected by new and greener sustainable behavioral models.

The application presented here showed how the use of ICT based technology allows us to restructure the commuters' mobility, resulting in an energy saving of 8780 toe/y. In exchange for approximately 128 €/toe, which represents the average of the TEE value in Italy, the University of Palermo might easily count on an interesting budget that could be used both to offer additional services to students and to implement further energy-saving policies, which, with a flywheel effect, could then produce other positive effects in terms of climatic impacts. This would place the universities (but also other institutions that decide to adhere to such policies) at the center of the scheme proposed by the European directives. In fact, the Clean Energy Package proposed a set of fundamental Standards aimed at achieving a climate-neutral economy by 2050, involving seven strategic areas, including energy efficiency and the use of energy from renewable sources, as well as eight European Directives, including the "Renewable Energy Directive (RED II)" 2018/2001/EU [82] and the "Electricity Market Directive (EMD)" 2019/944/EU [83].

4. Discussion

The proposal presented here starts from the consideration that a very important sector from the CO_2 emissions standpoint, such as mobility, is not yet fully included among the actions eligible for the acquisition of energy efficiency credits, while the white certificates scheme takes into account behavioral patterns. On the other hand, the European Parliament encourages citizens to participate in the European Union's energy efficiency process. The combination of these aspects leads to propose the sustainability of commuter students' mobility practices among the eligible actions for universities to obtain such credits.

However, a number of limitations emerge from the work presented here that should be appropriately highlighted in order to allow its application to other contexts and situations. First of all, the study is applied to a sample of students at the University of Palermo, while its results are extended to the entire audience of campus commuters. Although the sample is statistically representative of this audience, a study extended to all commuters would allow for more robust conclusions to be drawn from the results. In addition, considerations of the magnitude of GHGs emission savings (and energy consumption) from changing student mobility mode should be tested on other categories of commuters in order to estimate their true effectiveness.

On the other hand, it must be stressed that this proposal is very well contextualized in the current debate on sustainable development. In fact, this scheme seems to be very much in line with the desirable involvement of the citizens, as requested by the European Commission. Indeed, according to guidelines established by the European Parliament [84,85], the new concept of "community of renewable energy" is introduced. This means that citizens are encouraged to take part in the EU energy-efficiency process, paying cheaper energy bills and, much more importantly, self-consuming the energy produced by renewable energy plants.

In addition, these guidelines introduce and regulate a new energy system, no longer centralized or hierarchical, but distributed and collaborative: energy communities and self-consumption, in which citizens take an active role in the process of decarbonization of the energy system, no longer acting only as consumers but also as producers and managers of clean energy (prosumer), thus limiting barriers and promoting and fostering the development of renewable energies. These new legislative and technical tools, operating in the direction of an active involvement of citizens toward the decarbonization of the energy production and consumption sectors, are in line with the proposal made here.

Moreover, considering that the Italian system of the white certificates explicitly considers the role of citizens involvement and that the mobility sector does not appear to be fully exploited at the moment, it can be deduced that there is a favorable situation at the regulatory level (both European and Italian) for the promotion of policies aimed at enhancing the behavior of specific groups of users toward more sustainable choices, by rewarding, at the same time, the institutions and administrations that adopt such choices.

Of course, when universities access the economic benefits of acquiring these credits, they could transform part of these extra earnings into services for student. Some of these services could be benefits that have, in turn, a flywheel effect on students' propensity to make more sustainable mobility choices. Advantages include substantial reductions in university fees, awarding of formative university credits (CFU)—analogous to those students usually get from laboratory/field activities—and the provision of smartphones and/or tablets (by means of which further promoting the use of the mobility app game). This would likely induce a large amount of commuting students to adopt more sustainable behaviors.

Among the practical implications of this study is that, if institutions were extensively involved in the scheme proposed here and could enter the current energy trading and exchange markets, the process of facilitating countries' sustainability paths would receive a major boost forward.

However, it is clear that a change/revolution of the normative context of white certificates is highly desirable.

5. Conclusions

The field test, which involved a sample of students, showed a first feasibility of the proposal, which can be included among the practical results of the study.

The advantages for the University of Palermo in facilitating a more sustainable mobility of its students, which daily commute to and from the campus and the practical benefits for commuters applying to the campaign, through the rewards that the university provides them, are well evident.

Among the findings of the present analysis, it is noteworthy that the proposed student participation scheme has a strong educational value, as it involves young EU citizens who can acquire sustainability practices that will be part of their life background over the years.

The novelty of the proposal mainly relies on the possibility of directly engaging the educational institutions in the countries' path toward the environmental sustainability.

The study certainly opens to future works, aimed at testing its feasibility and effectiveness to different categories of commuters, in addition to university students. In this sense, an analogous application of the method to another class of commuters, for example, public employees that daily reach their working sites, would be highly recommended.

Although the proposed method for the acquisition of efficient credits by the universities cannot be directly included in the funding mechanisms currently operating, its implementation would require non-substantial changes to some of the current schemes (for example, the Italian so-called white certificates).

Certainly, such an implementation would be an effective way to involve institutions and local administrations in the path toward the greenhouse-gases-emission abatement and the decarbonization of the anthropogenic activities, with particular regard to those related to the mobility sector.

Author Contributions: Conceptualization, L.C., S.D.D., G.P., G.S., D.S. and G.R.; formal analysis, L.C., S.D.D., G.P., G.S., D.S. and G.R.; investigation, S.D.D. and D.S.; methodology, L.C., S.D.D., G.P., G.S., D.S. and G.R.; software, S.D.D. and D.S.; supervision, G.R.; visualization, L.C., S.D.D., G.P., G.S., D.S. and G.R.; writing—original draft, L.C., S.D.D., G.P., G.S., D.S. and G.R.; writing—review and editing, L.C., S.D.D., G.P., G.S., D.S. and G.R. All authors have read and agreed to the published version of the manuscript.

Funding: This research received no external funding.

Conflicts of Interest: The authors declare no conflict of interest.

References

1. Mobility and Transport. Available online: http://ec.europa.eu/transport (accessed on 18 September 2021).
2. Statistics Report on Energy Efficiency Indicators. Highlights. Available online: https://www.iea.org/reports/energy-efficiency-indicators (accessed on 18 September 2021).
3. Energia nel settore Trasporti 2005-2019. Quadro statistico di riferimento e monitoraggio target EU. *Energy in Transport Sector 2005—2019. Reference Statistical Framework and Monitoring of EU Targets*. Available online: https://www.gse.it/documenti_site/Documenti%20GSE/Rapporti%20statistici/Energia%20nel%20settore%20Trasporti%202005-2019.pdf (accessed on 18 September 2021). (In Italian)
4. Sarigiannis, D.A.; Kontoroupis, P.; Nikolaki, S.; Gotti, A.; Chapizanis, D.; Karakitsios, S. Benefits on public health from transport-related greenhouse gas mitigation policies in Southeastern European cities. *Sci. Total Environ.* **2017**, *579*, 1427–1438. [CrossRef]
5. Total Greenhouse Gas Emission Trends and Projections in Europe. Available online: https://www.eea.europa.eu/data-and-maps/indicators/greenhouse-gas-emission-trends-7/assessment (accessed on 18 September 2021).
6. Report Global Energy Review 2020. Available online: www.iea.org/reports/global-energy-review-2020 (accessed on 18 September 2021).
7. Filimonau, V.; Archer, D.; Bellamy, L.; Smith, N.; Wintrip, R. The carbon footprint of a UK University during the COVID-19 lockdown. *Sci. Total Environ.* **2021**, *756*, 143964. [CrossRef]
8. Italian Urgent Actions against COVID-19 Epidemic (Misure Urgenti in Materia di Salute, Sostegno al Lavoro e All'economia, Nonché di Politiche Sociali Connesse All'emergenza Epidemiologica da COVID-19). *Supplemento Ordinario alla "Gazzetta Ufficiale della Repubblica Italiana"*. n. 128, 19 May 2020—Serie Generale. Available online: https://def.finanze.it/DocTribFrontend/getAttoNormativoDetail.do?ACTION=getArticolo&id=%7B83672E3A-FEE0-4C97-9D4F-87790B110751%7D&codiceOrdinamento=200022200000000&articolo=Articolo%20222 (accessed on 18 September 2021).
9. Fenton, P.; Chimenti, G.; Kanda, W. The role of local government in governance and diffusion of Mobility-as-a-Service: Exploring the views of MaaS stakeholders in Stockholm. *J. Environ. Plan. Manag.* **2020**, *63*, 2554–2576. [CrossRef]
10. Peltomaa, J.; Tuominen, A. The orchestration of sustainable mobility service innovations: Understanding the manifold agency of car sharing operators. *J. Environ. Plan. Manag.* **2021**. [CrossRef]
11. Aburukba, R.; Al-Ali, A.R.; Riaz, A.H.; Al Nabulsi, A.; Khan, D.; Khan, S.; Amer, M. Fog Computing Approach for Shared Mobility in Smart Cities. *Energies* **2021**, *14*, 8174. [CrossRef]
12. Corriere, F.; Rizzo, G.; Guerrieri, M. Estimation of air pollutant emissions in "turbo" and in conventional roundabouts. *Appl. Mech. Mater.* **2013**, *394*, 597–604. [CrossRef]
13. Thaller, A.; Posch, A.; Dugan, A.; Steininger, K. How to design policy packages for sustainable transport: Balancing disruptiveness and implementability. *Transp. Res. D Transp. Environ.* **2021**, *91*, 102714. [CrossRef]
14. Melkonyan, A.; Koch, J.; Lohmar, F.; Kamath, V.; Munteanu, V.; Schmidt, J.A.; Bleischwitz, R. Integrated urban mobility policies in metropolitan areas: A system dynamics approach for the Rhine-Ruhr metropolitan region in Germany. *Sustain. Cities Soc.* **2020**, *61*, 102358. [CrossRef]
15. Nematchoua, M.K.; Deuse, C.; Cools, M.; Reiter, S. Evaluation of the potential of classic and electric bicycle commuting as an impetus for the transition toward environmentally sustainable cities: A case study of the university campuses in Liege, Belgium. *Renew. Sust. Energy Rev.* **2020**, *119*, 109544. [CrossRef]
16. Frank, L.D.; Pivo, G. Impacts of mixed use and density on utilization of three modes of travel: Single-occupant vehicle, transit, and walking. *Transp. Res. Record.* **1994**, *1466*, 44–52. Available online: http://worldcat.org/isbn/0309060729 (accessed on 18 September 2021).
17. Landis, B.W.; Vattikuti, V.R.; Brannick, M.T. Real-time human perceptions: Toward a bicycle level of service. *Transp. Res. Record.* **1997**, *1578*, 119–131. [CrossRef]
18. Cervero, R.; Duncan, M. Walking, Bicycling, and Urban Landscapes: Evidence from the San Francisco Bay Area. *Am. J. Public Health* **2003**, *93*, 1478–1483. [CrossRef] [PubMed]
19. Cervero, R.; Sarmiento, O.L.; Jacoby, E.; Gomez, L.F.; Neiman, A. Influences of built environments on walking and cycling: Lessons from Bogotá. *Int. J. Sustain. Transp.* **2009**, *3*, 203–226. [CrossRef]
20. Winters, M.; Brauer, M.; Setton, E.M.; Teschke, K. Built environment influences on healthy transportation choices: Bicycling versus driving. *J. Urban Health* **2010**, *87*, 969–993. [CrossRef] [PubMed]
21. Dill, J.; Voros, K. Factors affecting bicycling demand: Initial survey findings from the Portland, Oregon, Region. *Transp. Res. Record.* **2007**, *2031*, 9–17. [CrossRef]
22. Larsen, J.; El-Geneidy, A. Beyond the quarter mile: Re-examining travel distances by active transportation. *Can. J. Urban Res.* **2010**, *19*, 70–88. Available online: http://www.jstor.org/stable/26193275 (accessed on 18 September 2021).
23. Saelens, B.E.; Sallis, J.F.; Frank, L.D. Environmental correlates of walking and cycling: Findings from the transportation, urban design, and planning literatures. *Ann. Behav. Med.* **2003**, *25*, 80–91. [CrossRef]

24. Rybarczyk, G. Simulating bicycle wayfinding mechanisms in an urban environment. *Urban Plan. Transp. Res.* **2014**, *2*, 89–104. [CrossRef]
25. Lamíquiz, P.J.; López-Domínguez, J. Effects of built environment on walking at the neighborhood scale. A new role for street networks by modelling their configurational accessibility? *Transp. Res. A Policy Pract.* **2015**, *74*, 148–163. [CrossRef]
26. Corriere, F.; Peri, G.; Rizzo, G.; La Rocca, V. Environmental implications of traffic flow delays: A model for urban streets. *Appl. Mech. Mater.* **2013**, *260*, 1167–1172. [CrossRef]
27. Sardianou, E.; Nioza, E. Who are the eco-bicyclists? *Transport. Res. D Transp. Environ.* **2015**, *34*, 161–167. [CrossRef]
28. Badland, H.M.; Schofield, G.M.; Garrett, N. Travel behavior and objectively measured urban design variables: Associations for adults traveling to work. *Health Place* **2008**, *14*, 85–95. [CrossRef]
29. Zhao, P. The Impact of the Built Environment on Individual Workers' Commuting Behavior in Beijing. *Int. J. Sustain. Transp.* **2013**, *7*, 389–415. [CrossRef]
30. Turoń, K.; Kubik, A.; Chen, F. When, What and How to Teach about Electric Mobility? An Innovative Teaching Concept for All Stages of Education: Lessons from Poland. *Energies* **2021**, *14*, 6440. [CrossRef]
31. Jacoby, B. Adapting the institution to meet the needs of commuter students. In *Metropolitan Universities: An Emerging Model in American Higher Education*; Johnson, D.M., Bell, D.A., Eds.; University of North Texas Press: Denton, TX, USA, 1995; pp. 51–62.
32. Balsas, C.J.L. Sustainable transportation planning on college campuses. *Transp. Policy* **2003**, *10*, 35–49. [CrossRef]
33. Clark, M.R. Succeeding in the city: Challenges and best practices on urban commuter campuses. *About Campus Enrich. Stud. Learn. Exp.* **2006**, *11*, 2–8. [CrossRef]
34. Molina-García, J.; Castillo, I.; Sallis, J.F. Psychosocial and environmental correlates of active commuting for university students. *Prev. Med.* **2010**, *51*, 136–138. [CrossRef] [PubMed]
35. Wilkinson, S.; Badwan, K. Walk this way: The rhythmic mobilities of university students in Greater Manchester, UK. *Mobilities* **2021**, *16*, 373–387. [CrossRef]
36. Lee, M.C.; Orenstein, M.R.; Richardson, M.J. Systematic Review of Active Commuting to School and Children's Physical Activity and Weight. *J. Phys. Act. Health.* **2008**, *5*, 930–949. [CrossRef] [PubMed]
37. Sisson, S.B.; Tudor-Locke, C. Comparison of cyclists' and motorists' utilitarian physical activity at an urban university. *Prev. Med.* **2008**, *46*, 77–79. [CrossRef]
38. Whalen, K.E.; Páez, A.; Carrasco, J.A. Mode choice of university students commuting to school and the role of active travel. *J. Transp. Geogr.* **2013**, *31*, 132–142. [CrossRef]
39. Kerr, A.; Lennon, A.; Watson, B. The call of the road: Factors predicting students' car traveling intentions and behavior. *Transportation* **2010**, *37*, 1–13. [CrossRef]
40. Rybarczyk, G. Toward a spatial understanding of active transportation potential among a university population. *Int. J. Sustain. Transp.* **2018**, *12*, 625–636. [CrossRef]
41. Bopp, M.; Kaczynski, A.; Wittman, P. Active commuting patterns at a large, Midwestern college campus. *J. Am. Coll. Health* **2011**, *59*, 605–611. [CrossRef]
42. Shannon, T.; Giles-Corti, B.; Pikora, T.; Bulsara, M.; Shilton, T.; Bull, F. Active commuting in a university setting: Assessing commuting habits and potential for modal change. *Transp. Policy* **2006**, *13*, 240–253. [CrossRef]
43. Klöckner, C.A.; Friedrichsmeier, T. A multi-level approach to travel mode choice—How person characteristics and situation specific aspects determine car use in a student sample. *Transport. Res. F-Traf.* **2011**, *14*, 261–277. [CrossRef]
44. Delmelle, E.M.; Delmelle, E.C. Exploring spatio-temporal commuting patterns in a university environment. *Transp. Policy* **2012**, *21*, 1–9. [CrossRef]
45. Lundberg, B.; Weber, J. Non-motorized transport and university populations: An analysis of connectivity and network perceptions. *J. Transp. Geogr.* **2014**, *39*, 165–178. [CrossRef]
46. Moniruzzaman, M.; Farber, S. What drives sustainable student travel? Mode choice determinants in the Greater Toronto Area. *Int. J. Sustain. Transp.* **2018**, *12*, 367–379. [CrossRef]
47. Shields, R. The sustainability of international higher education: Student mobility and global climate change. *J. Clean. Prod.* **2019**, *217*, 594–602. [CrossRef]
48. Brand, C.; Dons, E.; Anaya-Boig, E.; Avila-Palencia, I.; Clark, A.; De Nazelle, A.; Gascon, M.; Gaupp-Berghausen, M.; Gerike, R.; Götschi, T.; et al. The climate change mitigation effects of daily active travel in cities. *Transp. Res. Part D Transp. Environ.* **2021**, *93*, 102764. [CrossRef]
49. Sobrino, N.; Arce, R. Understanding per-trip commuting CO_2 emissions: A case study of the Technical University of Madrid. *Transp. Res. Part D Transp. Environ.* **2021**, *96*, 102895. [CrossRef]
50. Fissi, S.; Romolini, A.; Gori, E.; Contri, M. The path toward a sustainable green university: The case of the University of Florence. *J. Clean. Prod.* **2021**, *279*, 123655. [CrossRef]
51. Filho, W.L.; Amaro, N.; Avila, L.V.; Brandli, L.; Damke, L.I.; Vasconcelos, C.R.P.; Hernandez-Diaz, P.M.; Frankenberger, F.; Fritzen, B.; Velazquez, L.; et al. Mapping sustainability initiatives in higher education institutions in Latin America. *J. Clean. Prod.* **2021**, *315*, 128093. [CrossRef]
52. Bautista-Puig, N.; Sanz-Casado, E. Sustainability practices in Spanish higher education institutions: An overview of status and implementation. *J. Clean. Prod.* **2021**, *295*, 126320. [CrossRef]

53. Inter-Ministerial Decree on New Rules for White Certificates (Nuove regole per i Certificati Bianchi). In *Gazzetta Ufficiale della Repubblica Italiana Serie Generale—n. 128*; Italian Ministry for the Economic Development, Ministerial Decree 21 May 2021. Available online: https://www.gazzettaufficiale.it/eli/id/2021/05/31/21A03391/sg (accessed on 18 September 2021).
54. Ribeiro, P.; Fonseca, F.; Meireles, T. Sustainable mobility patterns to university campuses: Evaluation and constraints. *Case Stud. Transp. Policy* **2020**, *8*, 639–647. [CrossRef]
55. Dell'Olio, L.; Cordera, R.; Ibeas, A.; Barreda, R.; Alonso, B.; Moura, J.L. A methodology based on parking policy to promote sustainable mobility in college campuses. *Transp. Policy* **2019**, *80*, 148–156. [CrossRef]
56. Website of the University of Palermo. Data on departments, degree courses and student enrollment at the University of Palermo. Available online: https://www.unipa.it (accessed on 18 February 2021).
57. Communication from the Commission to the European Parliament, the Council, the European Economic and Social Committee and the Committee of the Regions. A Policy Framework for Climate and Energy in the Period from 2020 to 2030. COM(2014) 15 Final. Brussels. 2014. Available online: https://eur-lex.europa.eu/legal-content/EN/TXT/?uri=COM:2014:15:FIN (accessed on 18 September 2021).
58. Energy Roadmap 2050 of the European Commission. Available online: https://ec.europa.eu/clima/policies/strategies/2050_en (accessed on 18 September 2021).
59. The UN Sustainable Development Goals. Available online: https://www.un.org/sustainabledevelopment (accessed on 18 February 2021).
60. Sustainable Development Goal 7: Ensure Access to Affordable, Reliable, Sustainable and Modern Energy for All. Available online: https://www.un.org/sustainabledevelopment/energy/ (accessed on 18 February 2021).
61. Sustainable Development Goal 11: Make Cities Inclusive, Safe, Resilient and Sustainable. Available online: https://www.un.org/sustainabledevelopment/cities (accessed on 18 February 2021).
62. Di Dio, S.; La Gennusa, M.; Peri, G.; Rizzo, G.; Vinci, I. Involving people in the building up of smart and sustainable cities: How to influence commuters' behaviors through a mobile app game. *Sustain. Cities Soc.* **2018**, *42*, 325–336. [CrossRef]
63. Studenti e Bacini Universitari. Istituto Nazionale di Statistica, Roma. ISBN 978-88-458-1909-4. Available online: https://www.istat.it/it/files/2016/11/Studenti-e-bacini-universitari.pdf (accessed on 18 September 2021). (In Italian)
64. Di Dio, S.; Massa, F.; Nucara, A.; Peri, G.; Rizzo, G.; Schillaci, D. Pursuing softer urban mobility behaviors through game-based apps. *Heliyon* **2020**, *6*, e03930. [CrossRef]
65. Statistics of IEA for CO_2 Emissions from Fuel Combustion. Available online: http://energyatlas.iea.org (accessed on 19 September 2021).
66. Ntziachristos, L.; Samaras, Z. *Copert III Programme Computer to Calculate Emissions from Road Transport*; Technical Report 49; European Environment Agency: Copenhagen, Denmark, 2000.
67. Ntziachristos, L.; Kouridis, C. EMEP Corinair Emissions Inventory Guidebook 2007, Group 7—Road Transport. Available online: https://www.eea.europa.eu/publications/EMEPCORINAIR5/page016.html (accessed on 19 February 2021).
68. Marino, C.; Nucara, A.; Peri, C.; Pietrafesa, M.; Pudano, A.; Rizzo, G. An MAS-based subjective model of indoor adaptive thermal comfort. *Sci. Technol. Built Environ.* **2015**, *21*, 114–125. [CrossRef]
69. Ben-Elia, E.; Erev, I.; Shiftan, Y. The combined effect of information and experience on drivers' route-choice behavior. *Transportation* **2008**, *35*, 165–177. [CrossRef]
70. Holton, M. Walking with technology: Understanding mobility-technology assemblages. *Mobilities* **2019**, *14*, 435–451. [CrossRef]
71. Attard, M.; Camilleri, M.P.J.; Muscat, A. The technology behind a shared demand responsive transport system for a university campus. *Res. Transp. Bus. Manag.* **2020**, *36*, 100463. [CrossRef]
72. Di Dio, S.; Lo Casto, B.; Micari, F.; Rizzo, G.; Vinci, I. Mobility, Data and Behavior: The TrafficO2 Case Study. In *Handbook of Research on Social, Economic, and Environmental Sustainability in the Development of Smart Cities*; Vesco, A., Ferrero, F., Eds.; IGI Global: Hershey, PA, USA, 2015; pp. 382–406. Available online: https://www.igi-global.com/chapter/mobility-data-and-behavior/130976 (accessed on 18 September 2021).
73. Guerrieri, M.; La Gennusa, M.; Peri, G.; Rizzo, G.; Scaccianoce, G. University campuses as small-scale models of cities: Quantitative assessment of a low carbon transition path. *Renew. Sustain. Energy* **2019**, *113*, 109263. [CrossRef]
74. Kwai Fun, R.; Wagner, C. Weblogging: A study of social computing and its impact on organizations. *Decis. Support Syst.* **2008**, *45*, 242–250. [CrossRef]
75. Hollander, Y.; Prahker, J.N. The applicability of non-cooperative game theory in transport analysis. *Transportation* **2006**, *33*, 481–496. [CrossRef]
76. Manzoni, V.; Manilo, D.; Kloeckl, K.; Ratti, C. *Transportation Mode Identication and Real-Time CO_2 Emission Estimation Using Smartphones, How CO_2 GO Works—Technical Report, Report of SENSEable City Lab*; Massachusetts Institute of Technology: Cambridge, MA, USA; Dipartimento di Elettronica e Informazione, Politecnico di Milano: Milan, Italy, 2010; Available online: http://senseable.mit.edu/co2go/images/co2go-technical-report.pdf (accessed on 18 July 2019).
77. Liu, C.; Susilo, Y.O.; Karlstrom, A. Investigating the impacts of weather variability on individual's daily activity–travel patterns: A comparison between commuters and non-commuters in Sweden. *Transport. Res. A Pol.* **2015**, *82*, 47–64. [CrossRef]

78. Determination of National Quantitative Objectives for Energy Saving to Be Achieved by Power and Gas Distribution Enterprises for the Period 2017–2020 (Determinazione Degli Obiettivi Quantitativi Nazionali di Risparmio Energetico che Devono Essere Perseguiti Dalle Imprese di Distribuzione Dell'energia Elettrica e il Gas per Gli Anni dal 2017 al 2020 e per L'approvazione Delle Nuove Linee Guida per la Preparazione, L'esecuzione e la Valutazione dei Progetti di Efficienza Energetica) (17A02375) (GU Serie Generale n.78 del 03-04-2017). Available online: https://www.gazzettaufficiale.it/gazzetta/serie_generale/caricaDettaglio?dataPubblicazioneGazzetta=2017-04-03&numeroGazzetta=78 (accessed on 19 October 2021). (In Italian)
79. Modification of the DM 11/01/2017 Concerning Determination of National Quantitative Objectives for Energy Saving to Be Achieved by Power and Gas Distribution Enterprises for the Period 2017–2020 (Modifica e Aggiornamento del Decreto 11 Gennaio 2017, Concernente la Determinazione Degli Obiettivi Quantitativi Nazionali di Risparmio Energetico che Devono Essere Perseguiti Dalle Imprese di Distribuzione Dell'energia Elettrica e il Gas per Gli Anni dal 2017 al 2020 e per L'approvazione Delle Nuove Linee Guida per la Preparazione, L'esecuzione e la Valutazione dei Progetti di Efficienza Energetica). (18A04609) (GU Serie Generale n.158 del 10-07-2018). Available online: https://www.gazzettaufficiale.it/eli/gu/2018/07/10/158/sg/pdf (accessed on 19 October 2021). (In Italian)
80. Directorial Decree Reporting Guidelines for the Release of White Certificates Deriving from No Energy Efficiency Projects (Guida Operativa per L'emissione dei Certificati Bianchi Non Derivanti da Progetti di Efficienza Energetica). Italian Ministry of Economical Development. Available online: https://www.mise.gov.it/images/stories/normativa/DM-Certificati-Bianchi_2017.pdf (accessed on 19 October 2021). (In Italian)
81. Energy Efficiency Credits (or White Certificates) Italy. Available online: https://www.gse.it/servizi-per-te/efficienza-energetica/certificati-bianchi (accessed on 18 September 2021). (In Italian)
82. Directive (EU) 2018/2001 of the European Parliament and of the Council of 11 December 2018 on the Promotion of the Use of Energy from Renewable Sources (Text with EEA Relevance). Available online: http://data.europa.eu/eli/dir/2018/2001/oj (accessed on 19 October 2021).
83. Directive (EU) 2019/944 of the European Parliament and of the Council of 5 June 2019 on Common Rules for the Internal Market for Electricity and Amending Directive 2012/27/EU (Text with EEA Relevance). Available online: http://data.europa.eu/eli/dir/2019/944/oj (accessed on 19 October 2021).
84. EU Emissions Trading System. Available online: https://ec.europa.eu/clima/policies/ets_en (accessed on 18 September 2021).
85. Directive 2008/1/EC of the European Parliament and of the Council of 15 January 2008 Concerning Integrated Pollution Prevention and Control (Codified Version) (Text with EEA Relevance). Available online: http://data.europa.eu/eli/dir/2008/1/oj (accessed on 19 October 2021).

International Journal of
Environmental Research and Public Health

MDPI

Article

The Impact of Green Credit on the Green Innovation Level of Heavy-Polluting Enterprises—Evidence from China

Zhifeng Zhang [1], Hongyan Duan [2], Shuangshuang Shan [3,*], Qingzhi Liu [4,*] and Wenhui Geng [1]

[1] School of Economics, Qingdao University, Qingdao 266071, China; sasha_china@hotmail.com (Z.Z.); wh.geng@outlook.com (W.G.)
[2] Department of Economics, The University of Sheffield, Sheffield S10 2TN, UK; hduan4@sheffield.ac.uk
[3] School of Foreign Language Education, Qingdao University, Qingdao 266071, China
[4] Department of Economics, Shandong University of Science and Technology, Taian 271019, China
* Correspondence: sss@qdu.edu.cn (S.S.); tajwk@126.com (Q.L.)

Abstract: This article uses the "Green Credit Guidelines" promulgated in 2012 as an example to construct a quasi-natural experiment and uses the double difference method to test the impact of the implementation of the "Green Credit Guidelines" on the green innovation activities of heavy-polluting enterprises. The study found that, in comparison to non-heavy polluting enterprises, the implementation of green credit policies inhibited the green innovation of all heavy-polluting enterprises. In the analysis of heterogeneity, this restraint effect did not differ significantly due to the nature of property rights and the company's size. The mechanism test showed that green credit policy limits the efficiency of business investment and increases the cost of financing business debt. Eliminating corporate credit financing, particularly long-term borrowing, negatively impacts the green innovation behavior of listed companies.

Keywords: green credit; heavy pollution enterprise; green innovation; investment efficiency; financing constraint; difference-in-difference model

Citation: Zhang, Z.; Duan, H.; Shan, S.; Liu, Q.; Geng, W. The Impact of Green Credit on the Green Innovation Level of Heavy-Polluting Enterprises—Evidence from China. *Int. J. Environ. Res. Public Health* **2022**, *19*, 650. https://doi.org/10.3390/ijerph19020650

Academic Editor: Roberto Alonso González Lezcano

Received: 9 December 2021
Accepted: 5 January 2022
Published: 6 January 2022

1. Introduction

Over the last few years, due to the impact of greenhouse gas, particularly carbon dioxide emissions, global warming and climate change issues have become increasingly severe, attracting the attention of many countries. Green technological innovation is considered to be an important means to achieve sustainable development. Technological change, financial liberalization and globalization have reinforced the boundaries among countries on technological capabilities and competitiveness [1]. Within the development of green management around the world, industry competition has become more complex and uncertain. The development of the majority of products and technologies is evolving towards a green structure. When planning commercial strategies, taking environmental impact into consideration has led to major changes in the social system and competition area [2,3]. As the main consumer of resources and energy, heavy-polluting enterprises are the main producers of environmental pollution [4]. Heavy-polluting industries represented by electricity and steel are pillar industries that drive economic development. However, they are also the main culprits of environmental problems [5]. Heavy-polluting companies should take active social responsibility and implement the concept of developing environmental protection. In the process of green transformation, green innovation should serve as a new perspective, product and management system for addressing environmental problems. The authors of [6,7] pointed out that research into environmental innovation is still in its infancy. Therefore, focusing on enterprises in heavy-polluting industries, the relationship between green credit policies and green technological innovation remains to be further investigated.

Through the guidance of green technology innovation policies, companies could improve resource utilization efficiency and achieve a win–win development of social energy conservation and emission reduction [8,9]. The government typically implements green technology innovation policies based on the following two elements: environmental monitoring and funding restrictions. Ref. [10] pioneered empirical research in this area and used manufacturing data in the United States to confirm that environmental regulation could, to some extent, promote companies' innovation. By limiting credit allocation and support to highly polluting and energy-consuming enterprises, more loan funds could be directed to environmentally friendly projects [11]. Theoretically, the Porter hypothesis suggests that a reasonable and strict environmental policy has a compensatory effect, prompting firms to internalize the pollution cost and improve innovation ability. However, green innovation is characterized by high inputs, high risks, long lead times and strong environmental externalities [12]. There is undoubtedly a need for reasonable and effective market intervention by the government. The government should take relevant policy measures to promote the green innovation. It is evident that the question of how to promote green transformation of enterprises through the promotion of technological innovation is an issue to be urgently explored.

Before the implementation of green credit in China, the International Finance Corporation (IFC) first proposed the concept of green credit in 2002, the "Equator Principles". The "Equator Principles" aims to evaluate the environmental and social risks in project financing. To reduce pollution emissions and support high-quality economic development, the Chinese government announced a series of green finance policies aimed at reducing environmental degradation. Green credit is one of the most important green financial instruments implemented by the government. Financial institutions are encouraged to direct capital to cleaner production [13]. The "Opinions on Implementing Environmental Protection Policies and Regulations to Prevent Credit Risks", issued in 2007, combined environmental regulation with credit regulation. This document made corporate environmental compliance one of the prerequisites for loan approval. However, due to the lack of clear implementation rules, the green credit policy is still in the theoretical stage. In 2012, the "Green Credit Guidelines" (GCP) were introduced, the first specific guidelines for financial institutions to carry out green credit. At present, some traditional heavy industries are still an important part of the national economy. Simply shutting down a large number of heavily polluting enterprises may lead to a shock in industrial development, unemployment and economic growth. Consequently, it is very important to find a way that would protect the environment and maintain stable economic development. In view of this, this article studies the impact of green credit on the level of green innovation of heavy-polluting enterprises.

The objective of this paper is to analyze the effectiveness of green credit policies. This article therefore draws up an econometric model. Variables include the level of green innovation, the effectiveness of investments, the level of debt financing and other factors. This study examines the impact of green credit policies on the level of green innovation of high-polluting companies. The marginal contributions of this article are as follows: First, concerning the effects of green credit policies, this article focuses on samples of highly polluting firms. This study will provide a practical basis for further investigation. Second, the green credit policy plays an important role in environmental oversight. Previous research on green credit policies has been subject to numerous omissions and shortcomings. However, this paper should not only look at the effects of green credit policies, but also discuss the mechanism of other possible factors which may work. Third, this paper enriches the research topics related to environmental regulation and pollution reduction. On the one hand, there is a lack of research on the level of green innovation in heavy polluters. On the other hand, this paper fully considers the problem of policy failure under the conditions of "strong government and weak society", and provides a research basis for the full implementation of pollution reduction policies.

2. Literature Review and Theoretical Hypothesis

2.1. Literature Review

In recent years, in the face of an increasingly severe ecological environment, the Chinese government has paid more attention to the use of financial products in environmental governance and introduced a series of policies in the field of green credit. The subject of this paper is the impact of the implementation of green credit policies on the green innovation capacity of heavily polluting enterprises. What the green credit policy is actually trying to achieve is an improvement in society's pollution reduction results. The improvement of the green innovation capacity of heavy polluters is only one path to achieving improved environmental performance of enterprises. As the indicators of the results of pollution reduction by enterprises have only been emphasized in recent years, the indicators are cumbersome. And the indicators are not of a uniform form. This has caused difficulties in the collation of data. This paper therefore focuses its attention on the impact of the implementation of green credit policies on the green innovation capacity of heavily polluting enterprises.

Current research on green credit policy is mainly divided into two main topics: theoretical analysis and effect assessment. More specifically, early in the study research, researchers were most interested in the need to implement green credit policies and the barriers to implementation. Ref. [14] elaborated systematically on green credit's connotation and strategic value. Guo [15] thoroughly analyzed the challenges of implementing green credit guidelines and proposed a series of practical suggestions. Furthermore, some studies have assessed the performance of commercial banks and financial institutions in the implementation of green credit principles through model building and empirical analysis [16].

With the deepening of the operation of the policy, researchers are gradually focusing on the quantitative evaluation of the application effect of the green credit policy. Furthermore, research on this subject can be discussed from both a macro and a micro perspective.

At the macroscopic impact level, scholars have conducted in-depth discussions on the impact of green credit on the overall environmental quality. The authors of [17] found that green credit can reduce environmental pollution through three intermediary channels: improving business performance, fostering business innovation, and promoting the modernization of industrial structures. Ref. [18] used the spatial Dubin model to analyze the impact of green credit on China's green economy and its transmission mechanism. They found that this policy can not only improve the local green economy, but also present Spatial spillover effects, which can promote the development of the green economy in surrounding areas to a certain extent. Based on China's provincial panel data, Zhang et al. [19] concluded that the green credit can reduce China's carbon emissions by encouraging modernization of industrial structures and technological innovation. Ref. [20] also confirmed that green credit has a major impact on promoting green and sustainable development in China. At the same time, environmental pollution is closely related to the industrial structure [21]. Some researchers have investigated the relationship between green credit and the industrial system of China. Ref. [22] demonstrated that green credit has a significant positive impact on the modernization of industrial structures as a whole, and Shao et al. [23] examined the dynamic development relationship between green credit and the rationalization of industrial structures in an innovative way. It turns out that there are three stages of degree of coupling from the bottom up. Implementing the green credit policy will help guide the rational allocation of resources and promote the development of the industry.

At the micro-impact level, most existing research is conducted around the two main bodies of companies and banks. For commercial banks, academics focus primarily on the impact of green credit implementation on bank performance. Ref. [24] used the systematic GMM regression method to test the relationship between green credit and the sustainable competitiveness of commercial banks. They noted that green credit policies could improve the performance of the bank's total assets. King and Levine [25] also indicated that green credit could indeed improve the bank's operational performance by encouraging the upgrading of the credit structure of commercial banks and reducing credit risk. However, some scholars' studies have reached different conclusions. Luo et al. [26] developed a comprehensive rating index for commercial bank capabilities using factor analysis. The study found that green credit has a significant impact on improving the overall competitive position of banks, but with the progressive implementation of policies, this promotional effect will tend to become weaker. Yin [27] estimated that green credit would weaken commercial banks' short-term financial performance, particularly for small and medium-sized commercial banks.

At the enterprise level, most scholars evaluate the policy effect of green credit from enterprises' investment and financing status. Liu et al. [28] concluded that green credit policy harms investment and the financial situation of high-pollution and energy-intensive companies. Lemmon and Roberts [29] also confirmed that the green credit policy could limit the bank's credit support to heavily polluting enterprises, which affects the financing activities of the enterprises to a certain extent. Li et al. [30] found that green credit will reduce the scale of debt financing of heavily polluting companies and increase costs by constructing a double differential model. Similarly, Peng et al. [31] have also found that green credit policies impact the extent to which high-polluting companies finance their debt. Zhang et al. [32] believed that green credit policies could promote short-term financing of "two highs" enterprises but negatively affect long-term funding and investment behavior. In addition, some scholars choose to focus on the impact of the implementation of green credit on the green behavior of enterprises. Research by [33] proves that green credit policies can help to increase investment in environmental protection by polluting companies. Furthermore, this promotion will vary depending on the nature and scale of the enterprise and the level of commercialization in the region. Zhang et al. [34] found that implementing Green Credit Guidelines helps businesses invest in renewable energy, and this promotion is heterogeneous. In addition, there is considerable academic interest in whether green credit influences business development performance. They found that green credit can increase the value of new energy businesses in a sustainable and long-term way [35]. Also, it will reduce the corporate performance of heavily polluting companies [36].

An analysis of many pieces of literature shows that research on the political impact of green credit is abundant at the macro-economic level. Furthermore, from a microeconomic perspective, the discussion on the effect of this policy on the performance of banks and investment and corporate finance is also very comprehensive. The fundamental objective of implementing the green credit policy is to encourage enterprises to proactively develop production and operation while respecting the environment. Green innovation is clearly an essential element of green transformation and company modernization. Unfortunately, at this point, little literature focuses on the specific effects of green credit policy on green innovation and its impact mechanism, and there are some differences in the conclusions drawn by existing studies. Ling et al. [37] used a difference-in-difference model to empirically analyze that green credit could negatively affect R&D investment and innovation output of enterprises when taking long-term debt as an intermediary, and this constraint has nothing to do with ownership rights and corporate scale. Caragnano [11] came to the same conclusion in their research. They believe that this policy reduces the scale of credit and increases the cost of credit for heavily polluting enterprises, leading to the intensification of credit constraints. However, the study of [38] noted that the green credit policy positively affects the technological innovation of high-polluting companies, and with increased commercialization, this promotional effect will be more meaningful. Hong et al. [39] are also of the opinion that Green Credit can promote innovation in green technologies across businesses. Furthermore, this influence will be heterogeneous depending on the type of ownership of the enterprise and the size. Liu et al. [40] proved that the implementation of green credit existed in the Porter effect by adopting PSM-DID. Hu et al. [41] also reached a similar conclusion. Guo et al. [42] found that green credit policies can effectively promote green technology innovation in one area, but there is no space spillover effect.

To sum up, the analysis of the micro effect of green credit in the existing literature is relatively limited, and there is a lack of relevant discussion on whether green credit can induce enterprise innovation transformation. At the same time, whether the implementation of this policy can promote enterprise green innovation has yet to be unified. In terms of research content, the above papers pay more attention to the direct impact of green credit policies on enterprises and banks, and neglect to fully sort out the policy mechanism. This article attempts to make up for these shortcomings. Concerning research samples, the scope of research in the existing literature is broader, and there is a lack of research on specific industries. This article uses highly polluting Chinese companies as a research sample to analyze the effects of policies at the industry level. In terms of empirical research, this article adopts the difference-in-difference method, which is appropriate for analyzing policies implemented in different regions and at different times.

2.2. Theoretical Hypothess

2.2.1. Green Credit Policy and Green Innovation Level

At present, there is no unified opinion in the academic circles on the impact of environmental supervision policies represented by the "Green Credit Guidelines" on the innovation capabilities of enterprises. Pigou proposed the "Pigou Tax" in 1932, establishing a precedent for environmental control. Subsequently, Coase criticized Pigou's method of correcting externalities. This is due to the fact that the "Pigou tax" restricts economic choices and stresses the important role of property rights and property rights transactions in environmental monitoring. According to using data on firms in major European countries, Rubashkina et al. [43] found that environmental regulation had an important role in facilitating their innovation. Hong et al. [39] states that there is an upward trend in the level of green innovation among firms, and an upward trend after the enactment of green credit. But what role does green credit policy play in this? Does it actively contribute to the promotion of green innovation capacity? As an environmental economic policy, the effect of green credit on enterprise technological innovation is mostly centered on the theoretical mechanisms of "Following cost "and "Porter hypothesis ". Following cost effect is reflected in the fact that environmental regulations will increase the production cost and pollution control cost of the enterprise. This produces a crowding-out effect on R&D investment activities and reduces the productivity of enterprises. The Porter hypothesis focuses on the innovation compensation effect. The Porter hypothesis as a reasonable environmental regulation has a positive effect on encouraging companies' innovation.

Whaller and Whitehead [44] argues that environmental regulatory policies limit the ability of firms to innovate technologically by increasing the cost of production and operation and limiting the flow of finance to less polluting innovation projects. Lenoard [45] argues that companies subject to stringent environmental regulations can lose domestic and international market share and face increased investment costs due to environmental regulations. Consequently, some companies will reorganize production and investment in areas where monitoring is weak, which does not have a good impact on the environment. Yuan and Xiang [46] used data from Chinese manufacturers to conclude that rising pollution control costs inhibited companies' innovation production. Kneller and Manderson [47] used environmental protection expenses to assess environmental regulations. They concluded that environmental law had not increased R&D investment in the UK manufacturing sector. The reason is that even though environmental regulation has increased investment in environmental R&D, it has been predatory. Shi et al. [48] estimated the impact of China's pilot carbon emissions trading policy on business innovation outcomes and concluded that this policy significantly undermined the innovation of regulated and non-regulated firms. Based on the above analysis, the following assumption is proposed:

Hypothesis 1 (H1). *Following the promulgation of the "Green Credit Guidelines" in relation to non-polluting companies, highly polluting companies' level of green innovation decreased considerably.*

2.2.2. The Moderating Effect of Enterprise Investment Efficiency

Figure 1 illustrates the mechanism of action of several variables in the theoretical model. The moderating effect is whether it will be affected by the moderator variable Z during the study of the influence of X on Y. There are obvious differences between industries with respect to the efficiency of investment by Chinese companies. This further implies that the impact of the level of green credit of enterprises on the innovation ability of enterprises may be unbalanced and insufficient due to differences in investment efficiency in industries and regions. Based on the different levels of investment, what is the impact of green credit on the green innovation capabilities of polluting companies? The effect of varying levels of investment efficiency of enterprises on green innovation capabilities is mainly reflected in the following two aspects.

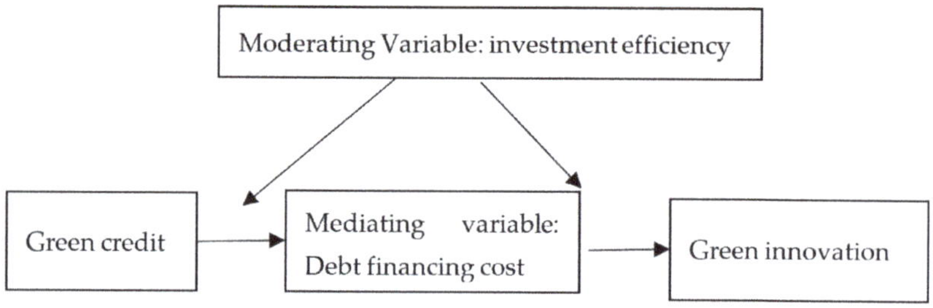

Figure 1. Types of variables in the theoretical model.

First of all, in the process of market-oriented reforms, the degree of local government intervention in enterprises within its jurisdiction also shows obvious differences across industries, which will also affect the innovation behavior of enterprises. An important feature in regions and industries with relatively high investment efficiency is that local governments have less improper and excessive intervention in enterprises within their jurisdiction. Moreover, local governments can also provide more convenient institutional infrastructure conditions for innovative financing of enterprises within their jurisdiction. For example, building enterprise information databases, setting up regional policy innovation guidance funds, implementing scientific and technological innovation guidance plans, and introducing preferential fiscal and tax policies for scientific and technological innovation, etc. All of this helps to increase opportunities for companies to obtain external loans, boosting entrepreneurial innovation [49]. Conversely, local governments have more stringent qualifications for obtaining green credits for highly polluting companies in areas where the optimization and reform of the market-oriented business environment is relatively slow. Therefore, the uncertainty of external policies is greater, and local governments will restrict the innovation decisions of companies more. As a result of the adverse effects of various government policies, the risk of business innovation will be higher. Banks are reluctant to lend funds to companies with high risks and uncertain returns, which will hinder business innovation [50].

Secondly, the allocation of credit resources also shows obvious differences between sectors and regions. Banks in various areas have "relaxing forces", and the distribution of credit resources will influence whether firms can obtain adequate credit financing support when carrying out investment activities [51]. Where the allocation of credit resources is more market-oriented, the autonomy of financial intermediaries such as banks is stronger. Banks are better equipped to gather and process business information, reducing the problem of information asymmetry between banks and businesses. To a certain extent, this contributes to a reduction in credit approval procedures and procedures for banks and other financial institutions. Consequently, it can effectively address the shortage of R&D funds and free up space for companies to improve investment efficiency [52]. Enhancing the effectiveness of investments further frees entrepreneurship from innovation and strengthens the enthusiasm for business innovation [34].

Hypothesis 2 (H2). *When firms' investment efficiency is weak, the inhibiting effect of green credit policy on firms' innovation capacity will be reinforced.*

2.2.3. Green Credit, Corporate Debt Financing Costs and Corporate Green Innovation Capabilities

Supply factors in financial markets influence corporate funding decisions [29,53]. The rapid expansion of industries with high pollution and high energy consumption leads to the continuous increase in the discharge of industrial waste water and waste gas, which intensifies the deterioration of the environment and brings negative externalities. In the production process, the company harmed the external environment without compensation, i.e., the external diseconomy of production was produced [54]. In economic theory, common approaches to negative externalities include taxation and explicit property rights. That is, by taxing the non-economic external enterprise exactly at the marginal cost of the external enterprise or by defining property rights according to the Coase theorem. Nevertheless, it is difficult for the former to estimate the cost of externalities in monetary terms. In the latter case, the transaction cost cannot be zero in practice [55]. Implementing green credit requires banks to consider compliance with environmental testing standards as a significant precondition for credit approval in credit activities. This increases the borrowing threshold of the companies with high pollution and high energy consumption and can essentially be considered as a macro-economic policy tool to promote environmental protection that uses economic levers to guide environmental protection, internalizing the costs of corporate environmental pollution [56]. Government and the financial sector share information about business environmental protection, which helps to understand the relationship between environmental protection and financial credit. Negative signals could be sent to the "two high" enterprises, affecting their production and operation decisions and resource allocation. At the same time, it can send signals to the capital market to strengthen the management and supervision of corporate environmental information disclosure, thereby reducing the willingness of external creditors to provide debt capital. Following the "Green Credit Guidelines" formal implementation, high-polluting companies will face increased public pressure and moral condemnation, and they may even face risks of environmental disputes, causing external creditors to divest or turn down loan extensions. As a result, the level of debt financing of highly polluting companies is declining [31]. As shown in Figure 1, green credit can initially affect the cost to finance corporate debt, and then affect the green innovation ability of high-polluting companies by affecting the cost of financing corporate debt. The cost of debt funding may be used as an intermediary variable. Based on the foregoing analysis, this paper suggests the following assumption:

Hypothesis 3 (H3). *Green credit policy may increase the debt financing cost of enterprises and then reduce the green technology innovation of enterprises.*

3. Data and Methods

3.1. Data and Variables

This article mainly selects the data of China's listed companies from 2010 to 2019. Based on the previous search objectives, this article selects the relevant data and tries to explain how policy works by analyzing mechanisms. In accordance with previous research objectives, this document selects relevant data. There are three data sources: First, the number of green invention patent applications mainly comes from the State Intellectual Property Office (http://pss-system.cnipa.gov.cn/sipopublicsearch/portal/uiIndex.shtml accessed on 9 December 2021). We specifically determine green patents based on the international patent classification in the "Green List of International Patent Classifications" issued by the World Intellectual Property Organization (WIPO) in 2010 (https://www.wipo.int/Classification/ipc/greeninventory/home accessed on 9 December 2021). Then, the financial data in the control variables, such as company size, asset-liability ratio, company life, ROA, proportion of tangible assets, cash holding rate, ownership concentration, earnings volatility, Tobin's Q, stock return rate, and whether to disclose social responsibility report, are mainly from the CSMAR database.

The variable explained in this paper is the level of green innovation, which is represented by the natural log of the number of green patent applications. Although the selection of patents to measure the level of technological innovation has a certain degree of one-sidedness, patent data is still the only observable variable in the measure of technological innovation. Therefore, based on the study of [57], the number of patent licenses is selected as a surrogate indicator of enterprise technological innovation.

The explanatory variable of this article is the green credit policy. As for the definition of heavy polluting enterprises, [58] used the research to compare the Guidelines on Industry Classification of Listed Companies issued by the China Securities Regulatory Commission (CSRC) with the Classified Management Directory of Listed Companies' Environmental Protection Verification Industry issued by the Ministry of Environmental Protection, so as to screen out samples of heavy polluting enterprises. It includes the mining industry, textile and garment fur industry, metal and nonmetal industry, petrochemical plastic industry, food and beverage industry, water, electricity and gas industry, biomedicine industry, paper making and printing industry, etc. By sampling highly polluting companies, we analyze the effect of green credit policy.

This paper selects investment efficiency as the moderator variable. Among them, the statistical method of the cost of debt financing is that of financial charges/total liabilities. The way of measuring investment efficiency is based on the measurement model described in [59]. This model has been widely used in the field of corporate finance as it allows the direct measurement of the investment efficiency of a given firm in a given year.

$$Inveffi_{it} = \beta_0 + \beta_1 Invest_{i,t-1} + \beta_2 Growth_{i,t-1} + \beta_3 Lev_{i,t-1} + \beta_4 Cash_{i,t-1} + \beta_5 Age_{i,t-1} + \sum Ind + \sum Year + \varepsilon_{it} \quad (1)$$

Where $Inveffi_{it}$ is the amount of capital investment, which is equal to (capital expenditure + M&A expenditure-income from selling long-term assets-depreciation)/total assets; $Growth_{i,t-1}$ is equal to the growth rate of operating income; $Lev_{i,t-1}$ is the asset-liability ratio; $Cash_{i,t-1}$ is equal to cash and cash equivalents/Total assets; $Age_{i,t-1}$ is the listing period, which is equal to the natural logarithm of the company's listing period. In addition, the model also controls the industry fixed effect Ind and the annual fixed effect Year. The residual of this formula is the investment efficiency. When the residual $\varepsilon_{it} > 0$, it indicates that the company has overinvested. When the residual $\varepsilon_{it} < 0$, it indicates that the enterprise has insufficient investment.

This paper takes debt financing cost as an intermediary variable, and the method of measuring debt financing cost is to divide the financial expenses of the enterprise by the total debt. In order to control the heterogeneous characteristics of the company, this article also uses the following control variables: company size, leverage level, company age, ROA, tangible asset ratio, cash holding ratio, equity concentration, whether to publish social responsibility reports and the degree of profit volatility, Tobin Q, stock yield. The specific variable definitions in the text are shown in Table 1.

In order to mitigate the influence of extreme values on empirical findings, this article winsorizes continuous variables that are less than 1% (or greater than 99%) of the quantile. To alleviate the endogenous problem, the control variables of the investment and financing equation (i.e., Equation (3)) in the regression analysis are all lagging one period (except for corporate age, equity concentration and corporate social responsibility). At the same time, the standard deviation of the test results is the adjustment of the cluster at the company level. Table 2 presents descriptive statistics of the main variables covered by the study.

Table 1. Variable description.

Variable	Statistic	Description
Green innovation level	lngp	Ln (1 + Number of green patent applications)
Group dummy variable	treated	Heavy polluting enterprise = 1; Non-heavy polluting enterprises = 0
Event dummy variable	post	The value for 2012 and later is 1. Otherwise, the value is 0
Investment efficiency	inveffi	Measured by Richardson's (2006) model
Debt financing cost	debt	Total financial expenses/liabilities
Company size	size	The natural log of total assets at year end
Leverage	lev	Asset-liability ratio
Company age	age	The number of years the company has been listed
Return on assets	roa	Net profit/Total average assets
Proportion of tangible assets	tar	(Owners' equity − Intangible Assets − Deferred Assets)/Total assets amount
Cash holding ratio	cash	Cash and cash equivalents ending balance/current liabilities
Ownership concentration	equity	Shareholding ratio of the company's largest shareholder
Social responsibility	public	Public social responsibility report = 1; Non-disclosure of social responsibility report = 0
Earning volatility	std	Standard deviation of return on assets in years t−3 to T
Tobin's Q	tq	(Market value of tradable shares + par value of non-tradable shares)/(Total Assets − net intangible assets − net goodwill)
Return on stock	ret	Annual return on individual shares

Table 2. Descriptive statistics.

Variable	Obs	Mean	Std. Dev.	Min	Max
lngp	12,378	0.2871725	0.7132743	0	6.590301
po	12,420	0.5273752	0.4992701	0	1
after	12,420	0.8	0.4000161	0	1
size	12,419	22.24249	1.331667	14.75859	28.63649
lev	12,419	0.4632725	0.6146905	0.0070799	29.69759
age	12,420	2.793565	0.397153	0.6931472	3.688879
roa	12,419	0.0506745	0.3824283	−28.94023	22.00289
tar	12,419	0.9304783	0.079834	0.317304	1
cash	12,419	0.1745579	0.1345231	0.0001508	0.9147874
equity	12,420	34.32527	15.02518	0.2863	89.9858
public	12,368	0.3036061	0.4598331	0	1
std	12,420	0.0949768	4.084318	0.0006314	453.1186
tq	12,048	2.164018	2.746482	0.683714	122.1895
ret	12,410	435.1414	39555.46	−353.706	4324004
inveffi	11,014	0.0412461	0.0512885	4.69×10^{-6}	0.4645226
debt	12,420	0.0111637	0.1502056	−2.454517	14.79254

3.2. Methods

The impact of green credit policy on the green technology innovation of heavily polluting companies is mainly achieved through political shocks. Specifically, first, the implementation of the green credit policy has reduced the ability of high-polluting companies to secure loans for green innovation. At the same time, high-polluting companies have spent more on reducing corporate pollution to cope with public monitoring of corporate environmental effects. To some degree, fewer funds are used to research companies' green patents [60,61].

A higher level of green credit will raise the threshold for companies to access green credit funds and reduce green technology innovation among companies. On the contrary, as the level of innovation in green technologies decreases, it will be harder for companies to obtain green credit funds from banks. In this way, there is a mutual causality between the explanatory variable and the explained variable. This will establish a correlation between the explanatory variable and the error term, resulting in endogenous problems and inconsistent parameter estimates [62]. The policy is exogenous, and the difference-in-difference method may effectively mitigate the endogenous problem. Additionally, the DID model can not only control unobservable individual heterogeneity between samples, but also maintain the influence of unobservable demographic factors that change over time. Therefore, a consistent estimate of policy effects could be obtained. The DID method has these excellent properties and has been extensively used in policy assessment.

On this basis, we use the "Green Credit Guidelines" incident released by the China Banking Regulation Commission on 24 February 2012, as a political shock. Before the publication of the "Green Credit Guidelines" in 2012, credit policies of banking financial institutions paid little attention to green development issues. After 2012, banking financial institutions are required to clarify the direction and focus areas of green credit support. This paper uses the DID model to evaluate green credit guidelines' impact on green technological innovation. The specific model is as follows:

$$Greeninnovation_{it} = \alpha + \beta treated_i \times post_t + \gamma X_{it} + \delta_i + \lambda_t + \varepsilon_{it} \quad (2)$$

Among them, $Greeninnovation_{it}$_it refers to the number of green invention patent applications of a company (divided by the number of invention patent applications), and represents the company's green innovation level. $treated_i$ is the group dummy variable, the treatment group company is 1, otherwise it is 0 (As companies in heavy polluting industries are directly affected by the green credit guidelines, they are treated as a treatment group and non-heavy polluting industries as a control group). $post_t$ is an event dummy variable, and the value is 1 in 2012 and later, otherwise the value is 0. $treated_i \times post_t$ are DID variables. X_{it} includes a series of enterprise-level control variables. β is the coefficient of the interaction term, which measures the impact of green credit standards on green technological innovation. At the same time, δ_i is an individual fixed effect, and λ_t is a time fixed effect to capture the influence of time-invariant enterprise-level factors and time-related factors.

In this paper, the impact of green credit on the technological innovation of heavily polluting enterprises is estimated by using the differential difference model of panel data. This paper further examines whether the moderating effect of investment efficiency exists. Therefore, based on model (2), investment efficiency is added as an intermediary variable.

$$Greeninnovation_{it} = \alpha + \beta_1(treaed_i \times post_t) + \beta_2(treated_i \times post_t \times Efficiency_{it}) + \gamma X_{it} + \delta_i + \lambda_t + \varepsilon_{it} \quad (3)$$

Moreover, the implementation of green credit policies may indirectly impact green innovation capacities by altering the debt financing costs of high-polluting companies. In other words, the cost of debt finance has a mediating effect on developing the green innovation capacity of heavy polluting enterprises inhibited by green credit. As shown in Figure 1, the mediating effect means that the influence relationship between dependent variable and independent variable is not a direct causal chain relationship (X→Y), but an indirect influence is generated through some intermediate variable M (X→M→Y). This paper draws on the stepwise regression method proposed by [63] by constructing the following recursive model to test the mechanism of debt financing costs affecting the level of green innovation of urban enterprises. Among them, β_1 in formula 4 measures the total effect of green credit policy on the company's green innovation capability. In formula 5, γ_1 measures the direct impact of green credit policies on the increase in debt financing costs of heavily polluting enterprises. And τ_2 measures the mediating effect of debt financing costs, that is, the degree of indirect influence of green credit on enterprises' level of green innovation of enterprises by changing the debt financing costs of heavily polluting enterprises.

$$Greeninnovation_{it} = \beta_0 + \beta_1 D_{it} + \beta_2 X_{it} + \delta_i + \lambda t + \varepsilon_{it} \tag{4}$$

$$Debt_{it} = \gamma_0 + \gamma_1 D_{it} + \gamma_2 X_{it} + \delta_i + \lambda t + \varepsilon_{it} \tag{5}$$

$$Greeninnovation_{it} = \tau_0 + \tau_1 D_{it} + \tau_2 Debt_{it} + \tau_3 X_{it} + \delta_i + \lambda t + \varepsilon_{it} \tag{6}$$

4. Results

4.1. Basic Regression

This article uses the DID method to measure the impact of green credit on the level of corporate green innovation. At the same time, in order to determine whether the fixed-effect model or the random-effect model should be used, this paper uses the LM test and the Hausman test. The test results show that the two-way fixed-effects model should be used. Table 3, from left to right, represents the results of Pooled panel regression, individual random effect, individual fixed effect and bidirectional fixed effect, respectively.

Table 3. Basic return.

	(1)	(2)	(3)	(4)
did	−0.188 ***	−0.028	−0.002	−0.070 ***
	[0.013]	[0.017]	[0.017]	[0.027]
size	0.203 ***	0.128 ***	0.079 ***	0.062 ***
	[0.010]	[0.016]	[0.017]	[0.017]
lev	−0.01	0.007	0.006	0.017
	[0.014]	[0.010]	[0.010]	[0.011]
age	−0.076 ***	0.068 **	0.173 ***	−0.113
	[0.016]	[0.032]	[0.044]	[0.082]
roa	−0.011	0.009	0.008	0.016
	[0.015]	[0.007]	[0.007]	[0.010]
tar	0.229 ***	0.213 **	0.155	0.147
	[0.069]	[0.099]	[0.100]	[0.100]
cash	0.325 ***	0.041	0.034	0.026
	[0.052]	[0.056]	[0.057]	[0.058]
equity	−0.004 ***	−0.001	0	0
	[0.001]	[0.001]	[0.001]	[0.001]
public	0.093 ***	0.047 **	0.022	0.015
	[0.015]	[0.023]	[0.026]	[0.026]
std	−0.008	0.008	0.008	0.007
	[0.010]	[0.015]	[0.014]	[0.013]
tq	0.015 ***	0.007 ***	0.004 **	0.003
	[0.003]	[0.003]	[0.002]	[0.002]
ret	0	0	0	0
	[0.000]	[0.000]	[0.000]	[0.000]
_cons	−4.149 ***	−2.936 ***	−2.102 ***	−0.888 **
	[0.233]	[0.375]	[0.385]	[0.441]
Year-fixed effect	Control	Control	Control	Control
Firm-fixed effect	Control	Control	Control	Control
N	12048	12048	12048	12048
R-squared	0.136	0.107	0.703	0.705

Notes: *** and ** indicate significant at the 1% and 5% levels, respectively.

Table 3 shows how green credit policies can limit companies' green technological innovation. The DID coefficient is −0.07 and passed the 1% significance test. After implementing the green credit policy, banks will raise the loan threshold to improve their green rating. This leads to higher financing costs for polluters. Compared with non-green patents, green technology patents have higher technical requirements and more investment, which may not be substantially increased in the short term, but will decline.

4.2. Robustness Test

This paper used two methods to verify the accuracy of the conclusions. The first method was parallel trend testing. The second method was the placebo test.

4.2.1. Parallel Trend Test

The assumption of parallel trend is the premise of using the time-varying DID model, requiring the lngp of the treatment group and the control group to have the same changing direction before implementing the green credit policy. Therefore, this paper adopts the time trend diagram of the treatment group and the control group to conduct a parallel trend test, as shown in Figure 2. Before the policy time point, the trend of the average growth trend was basically parallel, but after the implementation of the policy, the gap gradually widened, indicating that the green credit policy is effective. Therefore, by plotting the time trend graph for the treatment and control groups, a rough conclusion can be drawn that addresses the parallel trend assumption. Before the implementation of the Green Credit Policy, the trend of growth in the levels of green patents of polluting and non-polluting enterprises was more or less the same. After implementing the green credit policy, the growth of the green innovation capacity of heavy-polluting enterprises was relatively slow. It is pointed out that the innovation capacity of heavy polluting enterprises may be hampered by the green credit policy.

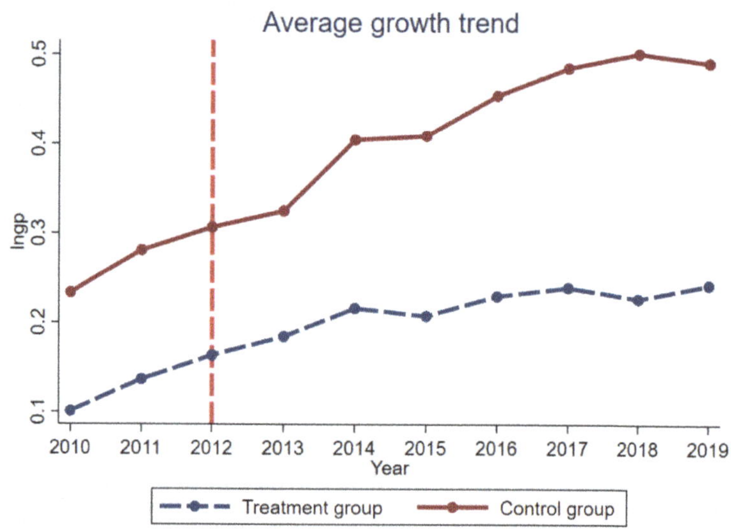

Figure 2. Parallel trend test.

4.2.2. Placebo Test

The basic idea behind the double-difference placebo test is to estimate the duration of the dummy treatment group or dummy policy. If the coefficient of the "pseudo-political fictitious variable" remains significant in the fictitious situation, this means that the result of the initial estimation is likely to be biased. Changes in the level of green innovation of heavy pollutant companies may have been influenced by other political or random factors. This paper randomly selected the interaction term 500 times to check whether the coefficient is significantly different from the baseline estimation result and draws the distribution diagram of the regression coefficient. As shown in Figure 3, randomized coefficients are expected to follow a normal distribution and thus pass the placebo test.

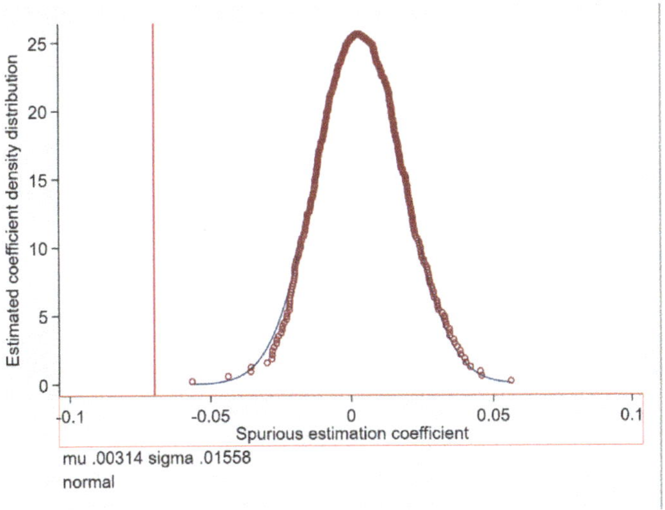

Figure 3. Placebo test.

4.3. Analysis of Heterogeneity

The nature and scope of company ownership may result in differences in the effectiveness of green credit policies. In general, compared to state-owned enterprises, non-state enterprises are less sensitive to environmental impacts in their day-to-day production and operations, and their consciousness of social responsibility is relatively weak. At the same time, enterprises of different sizes may have some differences in operational efficiency and financing channels. Therefore, differences in corporate ownership and size can lead to different characteristics of green innovation under the influence of green credit policies.

In order to explore the micro effects of green credit policies under different enterprise attributes, sample companies are divided into state-owned enterprises and non-state-owned enterprises according to different ownership attributes of enterprises. The sampled enterprises were divided into three quartiles based on differences in the size of the enterprise. The first third of the largest companies are defined as large companies, and the last two thirds are defined as small and medium-sized companies. The DID model is used to analyze the heterogeneous impact of green credit policies on green technological innovation. The empirical results are shown in the table below.

Table 4 shows that the heterogeneous impact of green credit policies on green innovation is mostly reflected in business property rights. Specifically, in the sub-sample regression of state-owned enterprises and non-state-owned enterprises, the coefficients of the interaction terms are −0.0599 and −0.0867, respectively, and the former does not pass the significance test. This shows that the inhibition effect of the green credit policy on the green innovation of heavily polluting enterprises is significant in the sample of non-state-owned enterprises, but not in the sample of state-owned enterprises. In the sub-sample regression of large enterprises and small and medium enterprises, the coefficients of the interaction terms are −0.167 and −0.0384, respectively, and neither of them has passed the significance test. This indicates that the policy inhibition effect of green credit on enterprises' green innovation will not be more different due to the size of enterprises.

Table 4. Heterogeneity analysis.

	(5)	(6)	(7)	(8)
	State-Owned	Non-State-Owned	Large Firms	Small Firms
did	−0.0599	−0.0867 **	−0.167	−0.0384
	(−1.32)	(−2.67)	(−1.94)	(−1.72)
size	0.0388	0.0842 ***	0.206 **	0.0580 ***
	−1.44	−3.62	−3.21	−3.47
lev	0.0763	0.0204	−0.0623	0.0104
	−1.1	−1.9	(−0.50)	−1
age	−0.237	−0.0262	−0.38	0.007
	(−0.78)	(−0.34)	(−1.25)	−0.11
roa	0.0628	0.0183	0.285	−0.0048
	−1.44	−1.45	−1.47	(−0.59)
tar	−0.0126	0.166	−0.133	0.0231
	(−0.05)	−1.42	(−0.38)	−0.28
cash	−0.14	0.0276	−0.0376	0.0418
	(−1.20)	−0.44	(−0.20)	−0.77
equity	−0.00117	−0.00098	−0.00066	-9.2×10^{-5}
	(−0.72)	(−0.86)	(−0.35)	(−0.10)
public	0.00318	0.0128	−0.0509	0.0445
	−0.09	−0.36	(−1.30)	−1.52
std	0.0384	−0.0003	0.0361	−0.03
	−1.63	(−0.07)	−1.61	(−1.84)
tq	−0.00073	0.00538 *	0.0372	0.00196
	(−0.17)	−2.03	−1.59	−1.28
ret	-7.35×10^{-8} ***	0.000000591 ***	0.000139	-3.62×10^{-8}
	(−11.23)	−22.11	−0.91	(−1.21)
_cons	0.218	−1.663 **	−3.052	−1.120 **
	−0.18	(−3.12)	(−1.77)	(−2.60)
Year-fixed effect	Control	Control	Control	Control
Firm-fixed effect	Control	Control	Control	Control
N	5483	6153	5094	6861
R-squared	0.1405	0.1356	0.1963	0.1357

Notes: ***, ** and * indicate significant at the 1%, 5% and 10% levels, respectively.

4.4. Mechanism Analysis

The results of Table 3 show that the implementation of green credit has hampered the ecological innovation capabilities of high-polluting companies. Concerning hypothesis 2, this article focuses on the moderating effect of investment efficiency and introduces the term interaction between investment efficiency and policy into the model. The moderating effect of investment efficiency is shown in the first column of Table 5. After introducing a regulated variable, the estimated coefficient of green credit policy is always significantly negative. The assessment of the coefficient of the adjustment variable shows that the coefficient of the interaction term between green credit policy and investment efficiency is significantly negative. The results show that the relationship between the implementation of green credit policies and the green innovation capabilities of heavily polluting companies will be negatively regulated by investment efficiency. Hypothesis 2 has been confirmed.

In order to further identify the internal mechanism of green credit policies, it is necessary to test the mediation effect of debt financing costs. According to the stepwise regression method, the models 4~6 are regressed. It can be seen from Table 5 that the coefficients of β_1,τ_1 and τ_2 are all significant, so the intermediary variables are path dependent. Specifically, implementing green credit policies will lead to increased corporate debt costs. According to the procedure of the intermediary effect test, the intermediary effect of debt financing costs is −0.144. Green credit policy indirectly inhibits the level of green innovation capacity of firms by increasing the debt financing costs of highly polluting firms. At the same time, the estimated coefficient of the green credit policy is significantly negative under different models, which means that part of the intermediary effect of debt financing costs is significant. The above results indicate that the implementation of the green credit policy will increase the debt financing cost of heavily polluting companies, thereby inhibiting the development of the level of green innovation for heavily polluting companies. Hypothesis 3 has been confirmed.

Table 5. Mechanism analysis.

	(9)	(10)	(11)	(12)
	Regulating Effect	Mediating Effect		
did	−0.206 ***	−0.188 ***	0.00237 *	−0.188 ***
	(−13.58)	(−14.71)	(−2.26)	(−14.69)
did_inveffi	0.321			
	−1.83			
debt				−0.144 **
				(−3.49)
size	0.224 ***	0.203 ***	0.00125	0.204 ***
	−18.79	−20.42	−1.89	−20.44
lev	−0.115 **	−0.01	0.0244 ***	−0.00651
	(−2.72)	(−0.69)	−3.33	(−0.46)
age	−0.114 ***	−0.0757 ***	0.00196	−0.0754 ***
	(−6.02)	(−4.77)	−1.19	(−4.75)
roa	−0.436 ***	−0.0109	0.00913	−0.00963
	(−5.62)	(−0.75)	−1.09	(−0.68)
tar	0.320 ***	0.229 ***	0.00712	0.230 ***
	−4.2	−3.33	−1.16	−3.34
cash	0.452 ***	0.325 ***	−0.176 ***	0.300 ***
	−6.14	−6.23	(−14.87)	−5.43
equity	−0.00347 ***	−0.00359 ***	−0.0000696 *	−0.00360 ***
	(−6.30)	(−7.07)	(−2.22)	(−7.09)
public	0.0844 ***	0.0929 ***	−0.00258 *	0.0925 ***
	−5.31	−6.12	(−2.20)	−6.09
std	−0.337 ***	−0.00774	−0.00256	−0.00811
	(−4.88)	(−0.76)	(−0.67)	(−0.81)
tq	0.0257 ***	0.0154 ***	−0.000323	0.0154 ***
	−7.11	−5.19	(−1.14)	−5.2
ret	1.62×10^{-8}	8.47×10^{-9}	1.36×10^{-9}	8.67×10^{-9}
	−0.89	−0.39	−1.23	−0.4
_cons	−4.543 ***	−4.149 ***	−0.00839	−4.151 ***
	(−16.61)	(−17.82)	(−0.48)	(−17.83)
Year-fixed effect	Control	Control	Control	Control
Firm-fixed effect	Control	Control	Control	Control
N	10770	12048	12048	12048
R-squared	0.1405	0.1356	0.1963	0.1357

Notes: ***, ** and * indicate significant at the 1%, 5% and 10% levels, respectively.

After implementing green credit, financial institutions reduced the long-term debt of polluting companies to avoid risks. This will impede investment in R and D and the generation of business innovation. The implementation of green credit will harm the company's green innovation. Mechanism analysis found that the credit constraints caused by the reduction of credit scale and the increase of credit costs are the main mechanism of action [11].

5. Discussion

This study makes a significant contribution to exploring the relationship between green credit policies and the green innovation capacity of highly polluting firms. Based on the implementation of green credit policies in China, this paper uses a difference-in-difference approach to identify policy impacts. This paper finds that the implementation of green credit policies inhibits the ability of heavily polluting firms to innovate green. This paper adopts a similar research methodology to [39], but the findings are quite different. Hong et al. [39] believes that the implementation of the green credit policy has improved the company's green innovation capabilities. The research sample used in this article is not the same as that of the above research. This article focuses on heavy-polluting companies. The reason is that the current environmental pollution is mainly affected by polluting emissions from heavily polluting companies. However, this article does not consider that the green credit policy has no positive effect on heavily polluting companies. This article believes that the credit restraint effect and information transmission effect caused by policies reduce the credit resources and commercial credit available to enterprises, leading to a decline in the level of technological innovation. Moreover, this paper argues that the decline of green innovation may be triggered by the fact that it takes some time for the financial steering role of green credit and the resource allocation role of R&D investment to manifest. In the meantime, a study by [16] explains this point in a different light. It argues that switching social capital from polluting industries to non-polluting industries can facilitate green innovation in non-polluting industries, which in turn can lead to environmental improvements. That might be another explanation of the conclusions of that document.

In this paper, investment efficiency is considered the moderating variable and the cost of debt financing is considered the mediating variable in the analysis of the mechanism. Some existing studies concentrate on the unique impact of green credit policies. For example, Li et al. [64] argued that implementing green credit policies reduced the cost of debt financing to highly polluting companies. Zhang et al. [32] found that implementing green credit guidelines helps companies invest in renewable energy. These articles do not analyze the interactive effects that other influencing factors may have. This article integrates the impact of investment efficiency and debt financing costs into the mechanism analysis of this article, trying to reveal the mechanism of green credit inhibiting technological innovation of polluting enterprises. The results of this article show that investment efficiency has not played a moderating role. Wang et al. [65] pointed out that green credit can improve the investment efficiency of enterprises. However, the research results of this article do not confirm that the improvement of investment efficiency will affect the effect of green credit policy on the level of green technology innovation. Moreover, the results show that an increase in the cost of debt financing can make policy implementation more effective. The results of this study are the same as those obtained by [56]. Both articles argue that the implementation of green credit policies will lead to an increase in the cost of debt financing and thus less funding for green innovation by heavy polluters.

In the meantime, this article breaks down the research sample into small and medium-sized enterprises (SMEs) and large enterprises. This article argues that the disincentive effect of green credit on corporate green innovation does not differ by company size. This differs from the conclusions reached by [66]. Singh et al. [66] uses environmental performance as the explained variable, and the research shows that the effects of green policies will vary depending on the size of the company. This paper argues that company size is not a critical factor in determining whether green policies are effective. At the same time, the research results of this article conclude that green credit is significant in the sample of non-state-owned enterprises, but not in the sample of state-owned enterprises. This is the same as the conclusion of [67], who believes that compared with private enterprises, state-owned enterprises have more financing channels. Therefore, the restrictions of green credit policies will have a greater impact on private enterprises.

There are several limitations to this study. Firstly, since the enactment of the green credit policy, it has been more difficult for the heavily polluting enterprises to access social capital. Therefore, it is worth considering whether this social capital has gone into non-heavily polluting enterprises and improved environmental benefits. This is a direction that may require further consideration going forward. Then, the ability of companies to innovate in green is only one way for them to reduce their pollution levels. Innovation is not the ultimate goal. Reducing pollution is a desired result of green credit policies. Future research will focus on indicators that represent the level of pollution reduction of high-polluting enterprises. However, due to the complexity of the current corporate pollution reduction indicators, there is no uniformity. As a result, data collection is more difficult.

6. Conclusions

Based on the panel data of China's A-share non-financial listed companies from 2010 to 2019, this paper constructs a DID model to study the impact of green credit guidelines on the green innovation capabilities of heavily polluting companies. With respect to the impact of environmental regulation on business technological innovation, Porter's weak hypothesis remains controversial. This study uses Chinese listed companies as a sample to empirically test the inhibitory effect of green credit standards on companies' green innovation capabilities, which are manifested in three aspects: (1) Under the green credit policy, it is difficult for heavily polluting enterprises to obtain more credit support and better loan interest rates for a short time, leading to difficulty for enterprises to have enough funds to research green innovative products and technologies, (2) The implementation of green credit policy leads to the restriction of green credit from commercial banks for heavily polluting enterprises, which stimulates enterprises to increase commercial credit instead of debt financing. However, due to the differences in the ability of different heavy polluting enterprises to obtain commercial credit, many heavy polluting enterprises find it difficult to obtain enough funds to supplement the credit gap of commercial banks [68], (3) Pilot policies are a gradual process, and green projects are indeed characterized by long cycles, high risks and high evaluation costs. There is a gradual change in the attitude and evaluation of financial institutions towards green projects. The support for green projects is obviously supported by the amount of financial resources, but there is no preferential financing cost [69].

Author Contributions: Conceptualization, H.D. and Z.Z.; methodology, H.D. and Q.L.; software, Z.Z.; validation, S.S., W.G.; formal analysis, H.D.; investigation, Z.Z.; resources, W.G.; data curation, Q.L.; writing—original draft preparation, H.D.; writing—review and editing, Z.Z.; visualization, H.D.; supervision, Z.Z.; project administration, Z.Z. All authors have read and agreed to the published version of the manuscript.

Funding: This research was funded by Cooperation and Innovation International Project Fund (2021-HSZ029).

Institutional Review Board Statement: Not applicable.

Informed Consent Statement: Not applicable.

Data Availability Statement: Not applicable.

Conflicts of Interest: The authors declare no conflict of interest.

References

1. Leichenko, R.; O'Brien, K. *Environmental Change and Globalization: Double Exposures*; Oxford University Press: Oxford, UK, 2018.
2. Schiederig, T.; Tietze, F.; Herstatt, C. Green innovation in technology and innovation management—An exploratory literature review. *Rd Manag.* **2012**, *42*, 180–192. [CrossRef]
3. Azzone, G.; Bertelè, U.; Noci, G. At last we are creating environmental strategies which work. *Long Range Plan.* **1997**, *30*, 478–571. [CrossRef]
4. Wu, H.G.; Wang, S.H. Do bond market participants pay attention to corporate environmental information?—Empirical evidence from China's heavily polluting listed companies. *Account. Res.* **2016**, *9*, 68–74.
5. Wang, K.; Zhang, X. The effect of media coverage on disciplining firms' pollution behaviors: Evidence from Chinese heavy polluting listed companies. *J. Clean. Prod.* **2021**, *280*, 123035. [CrossRef]
6. Rennings, K. Redefining innovation—Eco-innovation research and the contribution from ecological economics. *Ecol. Econ.* **2000**, *32*, 319–332. [CrossRef]
7. Andersen, D.C. Do credit constraints favor dirty production? Theory and plant-level evidence. *J. Environ. Econ. Manag.* **2017**, *84*, 189–208. [CrossRef]
8. Porter, M.E.; Van der linde, C. Toward a New Conception of the Environment-Competitiveness Relationship. *J. Econ. Perspect.* **1995**, *9*, 97–118. [CrossRef]
9. Li, Z.; Liao, G.; Albitar, K. Does corporate environmental responsibility engagement affect firm value? The mediating role of corporate innovation. *Bus. Strategy Environ.* **2020**, *29*, 1045–1055. [CrossRef]
10. Palmer, K.; Oates, W.E.; Portney, P.R. Tightening Environmental Standards: The Benefit-Cost or the No-Cost Paradigm? *J. Econ. Perspect.* **1995**, *9*, 119–132. [CrossRef]
11. Caragnano, A.; Mariani, M.; Pizzutilo, F.; Zito, M. Is it worth reducing GHG emissions? Exploring the effect on the cost of debt financing. *J. Environ. Manag.* **2020**, *270*, 110860. [CrossRef]
12. Ling, S.; Han, G.; An, D.; Hunter, W.C.; Li, H. The impact of green credit policy on corporate green innovation. *Stud. Sci. Sci.* **2021**, *18*, 1–23.
13. He, L.; Liu, R.; Zhong, Z.; Wang, D.; Xia, Y. Can green financial development promote renewable energy investment efficiency? A consideration of bank credit. *Renew. Energy* **2019**, *143*, 974–984. [CrossRef]
14. He, D.; Zhang, X. Thoughts on several issues in the promotion of green credit by Chinese commercial banks. *Shanghai Financ.* **2007**, *12*, 4–9.

15. Guo, P. Financial policy innovation for social change: A case study of China's green credit policy. *Int. Rev. Sociol.* **2014**, *24*, 69–76. [CrossRef]
16. Xu, L. On the evaluation of performance system incorporating "green credit" policies in China's financial industry. *J. Financ. Risk Manag.* **2013**, *2*, 33–37. [CrossRef]
17. Zhang, K.; Li, Y.; Qi, Y.; Shao, S. Can green credit policy improve environmental quality? Evidence from China. *J. Environ. Manag.* **2021**, *298*, 113445. [CrossRef] [PubMed]
18. Lei, X.; Wang, Y.; Zhao, D.; Chen, Q. The local-neighborhood effect of green credit on green economy: A spatial econometric investigation. Environ. *Sci. Pollut. Res.* **2021**, *28*, 65776–65790. [CrossRef]
19. Zhang, S.; Wu, Z.; Wang, Y.; Hao, Y. Fostering green development with green finance: An empirical study on the environmental effect of green credit policy in China. *J. Environ. Manag.* **2021**, *296*, 113159. [CrossRef]
20. Wang, M.; Liao, G.; Li, Y. The relationship between environmental regulation, pollution and corporate environmental responsibility. *Int. J. Environ. Res. Public Health* **2021**, *18*, 8018. [CrossRef] [PubMed]
21. Oosterhaven, J.; Broersma, L. Sector structure and cluster economies: A decomposition of regional labour productivity. *Reg. Stud.* **2007**, *41*, 639–659. [CrossRef]
22. Xu, S.; Zhao, X.; Yao, S. Analysis of the effect of green credit on the upgrading of industrial structure. *J. Shanghai Univ. Financ. Econ.* **2018**, *20*, 59–72.
23. Shao, C.; Wei, J.; Liu, C. Empirical analysis of the influence of green credit on the industrial structure: A case study of China. *Sustainability* **2021**, *13*, 5997. [CrossRef]
24. He, L.; Wu, C.; Zhong, Z.; Zhu, J. Green credit, internal and external policies, and commercial bank competitiveness: Based on an empirical study of 9 listed commercial banks. *Financ. Econ. Res.* **2018**, *33*, 91–103.
25. King, R.G.; Levine, R. Finance and growth: Schumpeter might be right. *Q. J. Econ.* **1993**, *108*, 717–737. [CrossRef]
26. Luo, S.; Yu, S.; Zhou, G. Does green credit improve the core competence of commercial banks? Based on quasi-natural experiments in China. *Energy Econ.* **2021**, *100*, 105335. [CrossRef]
27. Yin, X. Research on the impact of green credit on the financial performance of commercial banks. *Financ. Mark.* **2021**, *6*, 71. [CrossRef]
28. Liu, J.-Y.; Xia, Y.; Fan, Y.; Lin, S.-M.; Wu, J. Assessment of a green credit policy aimed at energy-intensive industries in China based on a financial CGE model. *J. Clean. Prod.* **2017**, *163*, 293–302. [CrossRef]
29. Lemmon, M.; Roberts, M.R. The response of corporate financing and investment to changes in the supply of credit. *J. Financ. Quant. Anal.* **2010**, *45*, 555–587. [CrossRef]
30. Li, W.; Cui, G.; Zheng, M. Does green credit policy affect corporate debt financing? Evidence from China. *Environ. Sci. Pollut. Res.* **2021**, 1–10. [CrossRef] [PubMed]
31. Peng, B.; Yan, W.; Elahi, E.; Wan, A. Does the green credit policy affect the scale of corporate debt financing? Evidence from listed companies in heavy pollution industries in China. *Environ. Sci. Pollut. Res.* **2021**, *29*, 755–767. [CrossRef]
32. Zhang, K.; Wang, Y.; Huang, Z. Do the green credit guidelines affect renewable energy investment? Empirical research from China. *Sustainability* **2021**, *13*, 9331. [CrossRef]
33. Yang, Z.; Fang, H. Research on green productivity of chinese real estate companies—Based on SBM-DEA and TOBIT models. *Sustainability* **2020**, *12*, 3122. [CrossRef]
34. Zhang, M.; Xu, H.; Feng, T. Business environment, relational lending and technological innovation of small and medium-sized enterprises. *J. Shanxi Univ. Financ. Econ.* **2019**, *41*, 35–49.
35. Lai, X.; Yue, S.; Chen, H. Can green credit increase firm value? Evidence from Chinese listed new energy companies. *Environ. Sci. Pollut. Res.* **2021**, 1–19. [CrossRef]
36. Yao, S.; Pan, Y.; Sensoy, A.; Uddin, G.S.; Cheng, F. Green credit policy and firm performance: What we learn from China. *Energy Econ.* **2021**, *101*, 105415. [CrossRef]
37. Ling, S.; Han, G.; An, D.; Hunter, W.C.; Li, H. The impact of green credit policy on technological innovation of firms in pollution-intensive industries: Evidence from China. *Sustainability* **2020**, *12*, 4493. [CrossRef]
38. Hao, F.; Xie, Y.; Liu, X. The impact of green credit guidelines on the technological innovation of heavily polluting enterprises: A quasi-natural experiment from China. *Math. Probl. Eng.* **2020**, *2020*, 8670368. [CrossRef]
39. Hong, M.; Li, Z.; Drakeford, B. Do the green credit guidelines affect corporate green technology innovation? Empirical research from China. Int. J. Environ. Res. *Public Health* **2021**, *18*, 1682.
40. Liu, S.; Xu, R.; Chen, X. Does green credit affect the green innovation performance of high-polluting and energy-intensive enterprises? Evidence from a quasi-natural experiment. *Environ. Sci. Pollut. Res.* **2021**, *28*, 65265–65277. [CrossRef]
41. Hu, G.; Wang, X.; Wang, Y. Can the green credit policy stimulate green innovation in heavily polluting enterprises? Evidence from a quasi-natural experiment in China. *Energy Econ.* **2021**, *98*, 105134. [CrossRef]
42. Guo, Q.; Zhou, M.; Liu, N.; Wang, Y. Spatial effects of environmental regulation and green credits on green technology innovation under low-carbon economy background conditions. *Int. J. Environ. Res. Public Health* **2019**, *16*, 3027. [CrossRef] [PubMed]
43. Rubashkina, Y.; Galeotti, M.; Verdolini, E. Environmental regulation and competitiveness: Empirical evidence on the Porter Hypothesis from European manufacturing sectors. *Energy Policy* **2015**, *83*, 288–300. [CrossRef]
44. Whaller, N.; Whitehead, B. It's not easy being green. *Harv. Bus. Rev.* **1994**, *72*, 46–52.

45. Leonard, H.J. *Pollution and the Struggle for the World Product: Multinational Corporations, Environment, and International Comparative Advantage*; Cambridge University Press: Cambridge, UK, 2006.
46. Yuan, B.; Xiang, Q. Environmental regulation, industrial innovation and green development of Chinese manufacturing: Based on an extended CDM model. *J. Clean Prod.* **2018**, *176*, 895–908. [CrossRef]
47. Kneller, R.; Manderson, E. Environmental regulations and innovation activity in UK manufacturing industries. *Resour. Energy Econ.* **2012**, *34*, 211–235. [CrossRef]
48. Shi, B.; Feng, C.; Qiu, M.; Ekeland, A. Innovation suppression and migration effect: The unintentional consequences of environmental regulation. *China Econ. Rev.* **2018**, *49*, 1–23. [CrossRef]
49. Feng, T.; Zhang, M. Business environment, financial development and enterprise technological innovation. *Technol. Prog. Countermeas.* **2020**, *37*, 147–153.
50. Zadeh, M.H.; Magnan, M.; Cormier, D.; Hammami, A. Environmental and social transparency and investment efficiency: The mediating effect of analysts' monitoring. *J. Clean. Prod.* **2021**, *322*, 128991. [CrossRef]
51. Chava, S.; Oettl, A.; Subramanian, A.; Subramanian, K.V. Banking deregulation and innovation. *J. Financ. Econ.* **2013**, *109*, 759–774. [CrossRef]
52. Arrow, K.J.; Hurwicz, L. Competitive stability under weak gross substitutability: Nonlinear price adjustment and adaptive expectations. *Int. Econ. Rev.* **1962**, *3*, 233–255. [CrossRef]
53. Faulkender, M.; Petersen, M.A. Does the source of capital affect capital structure? *Rev. Financ. Stud.* **2006**, *19*, 45–79. [CrossRef]
54. Randall, A. Market solutions to externality problems: Theory and practice. *Am. J. Agric. Econ.* **1972**, *54*, 175–183. [CrossRef]
55. Meade, J.E. *The Theory of Economic Externalities: The Control of Environmental Pollution and Similar Social Costs*; Brill Book Archive: Leiden, The Netherlands, 1973; Volume 2.
56. Dong, Q. The impact of technological finance on the total factor productivity of city commercial banks—Based on the perspective of moderating effect and mediating effect. *Financ. Theory Pract.* **2018**, *9*, 38–44.
57. Qi, S.; Lin, S.; Cui, J. Can the environmental rights trading market induce green innovation?—Evidence based on green patent data of Chinese listed companies. *Econ. Res.* **2018**, *53*, 129–143.
58. Shen, H.; Ma, Z. Regional economic development pressure, corporate environmental performance and debt financing. *Financ. Res.* **2014**, *2*, 153–166.
59. Richardson, S. Over-investment of free cash flow. *Rev. Account. Stud.* **2006**, *11*, 159–189. [CrossRef]
60. Yang, X.; Yao, Y. Environmental compliance and firm performance: Evidence from China. *Oxf. Bull. Econ. Stat.* **2012**, *74*, 397–424. [CrossRef]
61. Hamamoto, M. Environmental regulation and the productivity of Japanese manufacturing industries. *Resour. Energy Econ.* **2006**, *28*, 299–312. [CrossRef]
62. Antonakis, J.; Bendahan, S.; Jacquart, P.; Lalive, R. On making causal claims: A review and recommendations. *Leadersh. Q.* **2010**, *21*, 1086–1120. [CrossRef]
63. Baron, R.M.; Kemmy, D.A. The moderator mediator variable distinction in social psychological research. *J. Pers. Soc. Psychol.* **1986**, *51*, 1173–1182. [CrossRef]
64. Li, C.; Lu, N.; Li, D.; Wang, X. Corporate green innovation: Government regulation, information disclosure and investment strategy evolution. *Stud. Sci. Sci.* **2021**, *39*, 180–192.
65. Wang, Y.L.; Lei, X.D.; Long, R.Y. Can green credit policy promote the corporate investment efficiency? *China Popul. Resour. Environ.* **2021**, *31*, 123–133.
66. Singh, S.K.; Del Giudice, M.; Chierici, R.; Graziano, D. Green innovation and environmental performance: The role of green transformational leadership and green human resource management. *Technol. Forecast. Soc. Chang.* **2020**, *150*, 119762. [CrossRef]
67. Yu, B. How Green Credit Policy Affects Technological Innovation of Heavy-polluting Enterprises? *Econ. Manag.* **2021**, *11*, 35–51.
68. Chen, X.; Shi, Y.; Song, X. Green credit constraints, commercial credit and corporate environmental governance. *Int. Financ. Stud.* **2019**, *12*, 13–22.
69. Li, R.; Liu, L. Green finance and green innovation of enterprises. *J. Wuhan Univ. Philos. Soc. Sci.* **2021**, *74*, 126–140.

buildings

MDPI

Article

Understanding Occupants' Thermal Sensitivity According to Solar Radiation in an Office Building with Glass Curtain Wall Structure

Sung-Kyung Kim, Ji-Hye Ryu *, Hyun-Cheol Seo and Won-Hwa Hong

School of Architectural Civil, Environmental and Energy Engineering, Kyungpook National University, Daegu 41566, Korea; kimsg1321@gmail.com (S.-K.K.); notsools@gmail.com (H.-C.S.); hongwh@knu.ac.kr (W.-H.H.)
* Correspondence: ryou0407@knu.ac.kr

Abstract: The thermal comfort of occupants in the increasing number of modern buildings with glass curtain wall structures is of significant research interest. As the thermal sensitivity of building occupants varies with building features, situational factors, and the human body's thermal balance, it is necessary to derive the comfort temperature based on field research, which was conducted in this study in a South Korean office building with a glass curtain wall structure. The influence of solar radiation on the indoor thermal environment and thermal comfort obtained by measurements and occupant questionnaires was analyzed using cumulative graphs and a sensitivity analysis. The observed changes in operative temperature over time confirmed that occupant comfort was significantly affected by the radiant temperature. Based on this result, two groups (Group A near the windows and Group B near the interior corridor) were defined for analysis. Owing to the influx of solar radiation, Group A was more sensitive to changes in the thermal environment (0.67/°C) than Group B (0.49/°C), and the derived comfort temperature for each group differed from the set temperature by approximately ±2 °C. Thus, it was confirmed that the solar radiation introduced through a glass curtain wall building has a direct impact on the indoor thermal environment and occupant comfort according to location.

Keywords: glass curtain wall structure; solar radiation; office building; thermal environment; thermal comfort; operative temperature; thermal sensitivity

Citation: Kim, S.-K.; Ryu, J.-H.; Seo, H.-C.; Hong, W.-H. Understanding Occupants' Thermal Sensitivity According to Solar Radiation in an Office Building with Glass Curtain Wall Structure. *Buildings* **2022**, *12*, 58. https://doi.org/10.3390/buildings12010058

Academic Editors: Roberto Alonso González Lezcano, Francesco Nocera and Rosa Giuseppina Caponetto

Received: 2 December 2021
Accepted: 5 January 2022
Published: 7 January 2022

1. Introduction

With the rise of the modern construction industry, comfort, beauty, and constant balance have been sought in the field of architecture. In this regard, transparent envelopes (e.g., glazed facades, glass curtain walls, glass domes, and skylight windows) have been applied to many large public buildings [1–3]. The indoor thermal environments of such structures, including the indoor air temperature, are significantly affected by solar radiation either directly or indirectly depending on the external characteristics of the structure. Thus, the thermal comfort of building occupants will be affected by variations in solar radiation throughout the building. In a previous study related to solar radiation, the radiant temperature was identified as the main cause of a non-uniform indoor thermal environment [4]. Furthermore, the radiant temperature may act as an important parameter in the thermal exchange between the human body and the surrounding environment [5]. This exchange eventually affects the indoor air temperature and the thermal comfort of the occupants [1–3,6–10]. In other words, high solar radiation in summer has a negative impact on the thermal comfort of building occupants [11–14]. In addition, the increased heat provided by solar radiation requires more energy to power cooling devices [14]. As occupants near high-temperature areas may feel more discomfort, it is important to seek methods to maintain overall thermal comfort throughout transparent envelope buildings [1].

Thermal comfort is affected by situations beyond the human body's heat balance physics, such as climate setting, social conditions, economic considerations, other situational factors, and particularly the building exterior. Nielsen [15] exposed six subjects to an artificial "sun" and proved that solar radiation has an important influence on the physiological condition of the human body. A number of studies have also mentioned that solar radiation affects indoor thermal sensation [16–18]. However, previous studies currently consider only basic factors (temperature and humidity) when studying the thermal comfort of occupants, and most of them do not consider solar radiation [1]. This cannot take into account the effects of intense solar radiation and hot weather on indoor radiation temperatures in summer. In addition, there is a limit to analyzing high-rise buildings of transparent sheath structure with previous studies because there may be differences in radiation temperature and indoor air temperature [1]. Therefore, it is necessary to determine how much solar radiation affects indoor thermal environment and occupant comfort [1]. As transparent envelopes are widely used in modern buildings [19–21], research on the thermal comfort related to the solar radiation permitted through such envelopes is clearly required.

Office space is the representative use of buildings with transparent envelopes. In offices, heating, ventilation, and air-conditioning (HVAC) systems cannot be controlled in individual units, and physical control (such as that provided by discrete temperature control systems, windows, and blinds) is limited. This limited control of the indoor thermal environment affects the building performance and the thermal comfort of its occupants. As a result, it is difficult to ensure occupant comfort in public buildings or large office buildings with transparent envelopes. Yet thermal comfort plays an important role in the satisfaction of office occupants with their environment, as manifested in work productivity, and other work performance metrics [22–24]. Indeed, the thermal environment of an office has been found to be correlated with work efficiency in addition to the comfort, health, and safety of building occupants [25–27]. Mak et al. [28] mentioned that among the aspects of indoor thermal environment, temperature has the largest impact on the productivity of office building occupants. Maula et al. [29] showed that inappropriate temperature adversely affects the mood, motivation, and concentration of building occupants. It has also been observed that work productivity decreases when the indoor air temperature increases from a medium level (e.g., 21 to 25 °C) to a high level (e.g., 26 °C or higher) [30,31]. Notably, any estimate of thermal comfort is affected by the temperature in the immediate vicinity of the human body [1]. Therefore, it is necessary to conduct research on the aspects of the indoor thermal environment that have the largest impact on thermal comfort and work productivity in offices [25,32].

When this is integrated, there is a lack of research on thermal comfort associated with solar radiation in modern buildings. Therefore, the thermal comfort of modern buildings (curtain walls) lacking prior research is studied. In particular, since the curtain wall structure is highly influenced by solar radiation, an analysis was conducted in consideration of this. Unlike previous studies, this study studied the correlation between solar radiation and comfort introduced into the curtain wall structure. A previous study of office thermal environments [33] found that different occupants in the same space often have different thermal preferences. Additionally, the non-uniform indoor thermal environment directly affects the heat released from the human body [5]. Thus, the typical thermal environment of an office building, which depends on the characteristics of the building and space within, cannot guarantee the comfort of all building occupants. The building envelope structure, building type, indoor thermal environment control, and occupant characteristics are all important information when conducting research to improve building energy use and occupant comfort [33]. Indeed, identifying such information addresses the limitations of previous research on the thermal comfort of occupants in buildings [2,34]. Huizenga et al. [35] evaluated the window performance for a human's thermal comfort in various windows systems (solar heat gain coefficient, U-value, solar transmissivity, window region and frame, etc.). They concluded that this new high-performance window can gain solar heat and reduce cooling cost during the summer season and relieve thermal discomfort. Moreover, simulation studies have shown that solar radiation [36] and thermal characteristics [37] of windows could have a substantial effect on occupants' thermal comfort [38]. Therefore, an analysis of the thermal environment according to occupant location in an office is required to inform research on occupant comfort in transparent envelope buildings.

In this study, a field experiment was therefore performed in an actual office building with a transparent envelope consisting of curtain walls instead of a laboratory (chamber) to reliably reflect the actual indoor thermal environment of an office and inform an analysis of the thermal comfort of its occupants. Unlike previous studies, the changes in indoor air temperature and radiant temperature over time were examined to investigate the influence of solar radiation on occupant comfort. The thermal comfort of the occupants who responded to changes in the indoor thermal environment was thus analyzed according to their location relative to the curtain wall. Different comfort temperatures were then derived and analyzed based on the thermal sensitivity of the occupants according to location.

By identifying thermal comfort levels in the non-uniform indoor thermal environment of a building with a transparent envelope, the results of this study contribute to the preparation of efficient measures for individual thermal control to improve the overall thermal comfort of office occupants.

2. Methods

Objective physical data and subjective personal data were collected for analysis in this study using field experiments [39–42]. The physical factors of the indoor thermal environment are the objective data measured using equipment, whereas the personal factors are the subjective data obtained through a questionnaire survey. The factors that affect the thermal comfort of indoor occupants include: (1) environmental factors, such as the air temperature, relative humidity, wind speed, and radiant temperature, and (2) individual factors, such as clothing and activities [43]. Therefore, in this study, the environmental factors related to occupant comfort were set as objective physical factors based on previous studies. These consisted of the temperature and humidity [44,45], which are the basic descriptors of the indoor environment. As office characteristics in summer [46] were the subject of this study, the average clothing insulation (clo) level and the metabolic rate (met) were calculated to be 0.5 and 1.2, respectively. The subjective data were collected from office occupants using a questionnaire. Prior consent was acquired from the participants for all processes, including data survey, sharing, storage, and requirements.

2.1. Field Data Collection

Laboratory chamber research relies upon an artificial environment and provides a limited ability to simulate and measure factors such as solar radiation and wind speed [2,47]. This study accordingly targeted a transparent envelope building to conduct field research on the correlation between solar radiation and thermal comfort [2] using equipment in an actual office space. The target building was an office building at K University in Daegu, South Korea, with a curtain wall structure through which a large quantity of heat is introduced by solar radiation (Table 1). Notably, Daegu exhibits slightly higher temperature than the surrounding areas because its basin topography inhibits the release of heat. In addition, the target building experiences a large influx of solar radiation because school buildings up to four stories in height are distributed around it. The target building has transparent curtain walls on its north and east faces that consist of highly air-tight, low-e double glazing with insulation film. U-value is 1.690 W/m^{2}K, and solar heat gain coefficient (SHGC) is 0.486. The experimental space was located in the northeast corner of the ninth floor of the office building and had an area of approximately 133 m^2 (15.78 m × 8.46 m). The indoor air temperature was set to 26 °C based on domestic regulations related to indoor air temperature in summer [48]. Three system air conditioners and eight energy recovery ventilation systems (ERVs) with 0.5 m × 0.5 m square vents were installed in the ceiling of the experimental space. These cooling and ventilation systems were controlled by the central HVAC system.

Table 1. Overview of the target building.

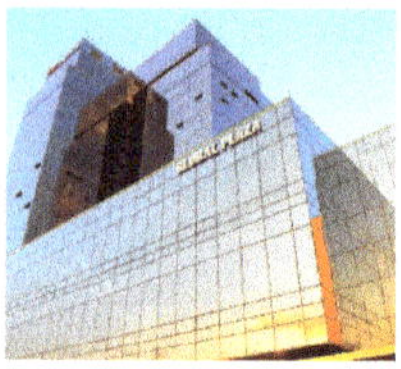

Category	Content
Location	Sangyeok-dong, Buk-gu, Daegu
Scale	One basement floor and 17 floors above the ground
Facility	Building G of K University
Total floor area	37,277 m^2
Experimental area	133 m^2
Facility use	Office space
Cooling method	Central HVAC system (central cooling system)
Building features	24 mm low-e double glass
U-value	1.690 W/m^2K
SHGC	0.486

The experiments were performed from 09:00 to 18:00, except during lunch time from 11:30 to 13:00, every day in July when the average outdoor air temperature was higher than 30 °C. During the experimental period, the average outdoor temperature was 32.4 °C, the maximum temperature was 35.5 °C, and the standard deviation was 2.2. The indoor air temperature, relative humidity, wind speed, and radiant temperature were recorded every 15 min using the equipment detailed in Table 2. These instruments were located at 40 equipment points arranged in a 2 m × 2 m grid 1.2 m above the floor, as shown in Figure 1 (additional measurements were performed under the air conditioner vents to consider their influence). Figure 1 also shows the locations of the questionnaire respondents (subject points).

Table 2. Test range and precision of the measurement instruments.

Model	Environmental Parameters Measured	Test Range	Precision	Resolution
TESTO 480	Air temperature (T_A, °C) Radiant temperature (T_r, °C)	0–50 °C 0–120 °C	±0.1 °C −40 to 1000 °C	0.1 °C -
Data logger	Air temperature (T_A, °C)	0–50 °C		-

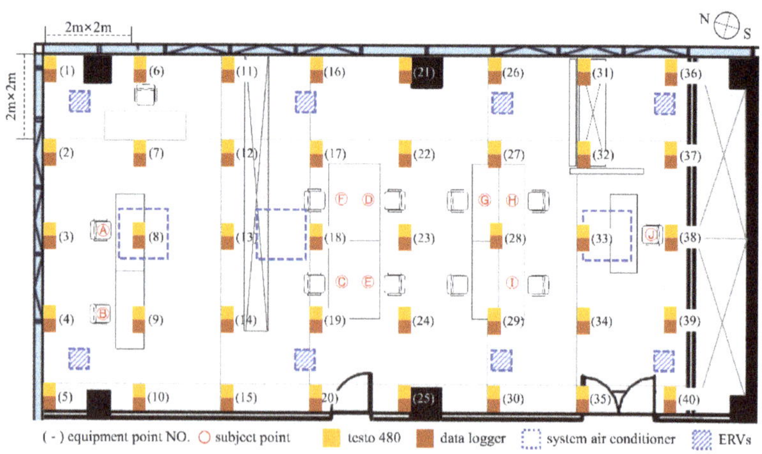

Figure 1. Locations of measurement instruments and questionnaire respondents.

2.2. Subjects and Thermal Comfort Questionnaire

The heat dissipation rate of a subject's body is proportional to the amount of activity they undertake, and varies depending on their, clothing, metabolic rate, and body surface area. The standard deviations (σ) of the amount of clothing and the metabolic rate of the subjects who participated in this study were found to be between approximately 10–20%, thereby minimizing their influence on the experiment results [49]. The subjects were all in their twenties and thirties, and a total of 40 office occupants (17 male and 23 female) in the study area were randomly selected to complete the questionnaire. All subjects were healthy and took no medication. They were requested to avoid alcohol, smoking, and intense physical activities at least 12 h before the experiments [2]. Table 3 shows the personal characteristics of the subjects, as obtained through the questionnaire.

Table 3. Personal characteristics of the experimental subjects.

Subjects	Age		Height (cm)	
	Mean	σ	Mean	σ
Male (N:17)	26.4	1.5	175	6.5
Female (N:23)	25.6	1.8	166.3	6.2

σ is standard deviation.

The subjects entered the experimental space 30 min before the start of the experiment to ensure time for adaptation to the thermal environment. Each subject then completed a questionnaire to identify their comfort sensation vote (CSV) and thermal sensation vote (TSV) [50] every 15 min starting at the beginning of the experiment; the questionnaire response interval was same as the objective data measurement interval.

The two questionnaire items were ranked on a seven-point scale based on the seven-level sensory scale of the ASHRAE Standard and ISO 10551 [44,51,52], as shown in Figure 2. For TSV, a ranking of 1 indicates feeling cold, 4 indicates feeling neutral, and 7 indicates feeling hot; for CSV, a ranking of 1 indicates feeling very uncomfortable, 4 indicates feeling neutral, and 7 indicates feeling very comfortable.

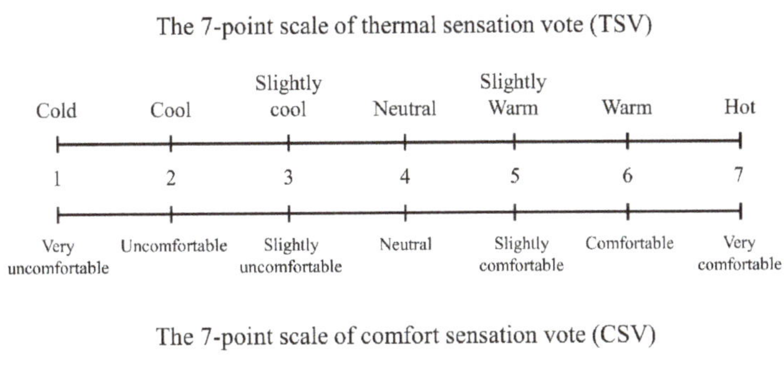

Figure 2. Questionnaire items and rating scale used in this study: (**top**) the seven-point scale for the thermal sensation vote (TSV) and (**bottom**) the seven-point scale for the comfort sensation vote (CSV).

3. Results and Discussion

Table 4 is the average hourly data for solar radiation in the experimental area (Daegu) at the time of the experiment. At 14:00 of the day, the highest solar radiation was 2.97 MJ/m^2, and at 18:00, the lowest solar radiation was 1.03 MJ/m^2.

Table 4. Mean solar radiation data per hour in the experimental area.

(MJ/m^2)	Time									
	9:00	10:00	11:00	12:00	13:00	14:00	15:00	16:00	17:00	18:00
Solar radiation	1.56	1.62	2.28	2.58	2.70	2.97	2.78	2.00	1.5	1.03

Table 5 summarizes the physical and subjective data measured in this study. The average of T_A was 25.7 °C, but the average of T_r was 26.7 °C. The average of TSV was slightly warm, and the average of CSV was derived as neutral.

Table 5. Summary of physical and subjective data.

Data	Physical		Subjective	
	T_A (°C)	T_r (°C)	TSV	CSV
Max	30.5	35.5	-	-
mean	25.7	26.7	5	4
σ	1.5	2.7	1.5	1.3

σ is standard deviation.

3.1. Occupant Thermal Comfort according to the Difference between Indoor Air Temperature and Radiant Temperature

Figure 3 shows the changes in indoor air temperature (T_A) and radiant temperature (T_r) over time. Both T_A and T_r were high near the windows in the north and in the afternoon. During the experiment, T_A ranged from a minimum of 23.15 °C at 10:00 to a maximum of 28.93 °C at 17:00, while T_r ranged from a minimum of 23.25 °C at 10:00 to a maximum of 33.35 °C at 17:00. Though the minima and maxima of both temperatures each occurred at the same time of day, T_A increased from north to south whereas T_r increased from northwest to southeast.

The distribution of T_r showed notable characteristics that were not observed in that of T_A; T_r increased in the central part of the indoor space over time and was exceptionally high in the southeast direction. These differences resulted from the presence of furniture (a partition) installed in the office space, suggesting that the radiant temperature was exceptionally high because the heat could not be dissipated in the air.

Figure 4a,b show the TSV and CSV responses of the subjects, respectively, according to T_A. The blue area indicates that the indoor air temperature is the same as the radiant temperature, whereas the red area indicates that these temperatures are different. In Figure 4a, when T_A = 28 °C (ii), the responses exhibit similar distributions regardless of T_r, with the largest percentage of responses (~35%) indicating the slightly warm TSV (5) when T_r = 28 °C (blue), whereas when T_r = 30 °C (red), the largest percentage of responses (~43%) indicated the neutral TSV (4). However, when T_A = 26 °C (i), a wider distribution of responses can be observed for T_r = 28 °C (red) than for T_r = 26 °C (blue), with ~44% indicating the neutral TSV (4) and 20% each indicating the cold (1) cool (2), and slightly warm (5) TSVs in the former case. Thus, the distribution of TSV responses was wider when T_r was not the same as T_A. Therefore, TSV results responded the most to the neutral when the indoor temperature was 26 degrees (i). In addition, when the indoor temperature was 28 degrees (ii), the response was highest to neutral and slimly warm.

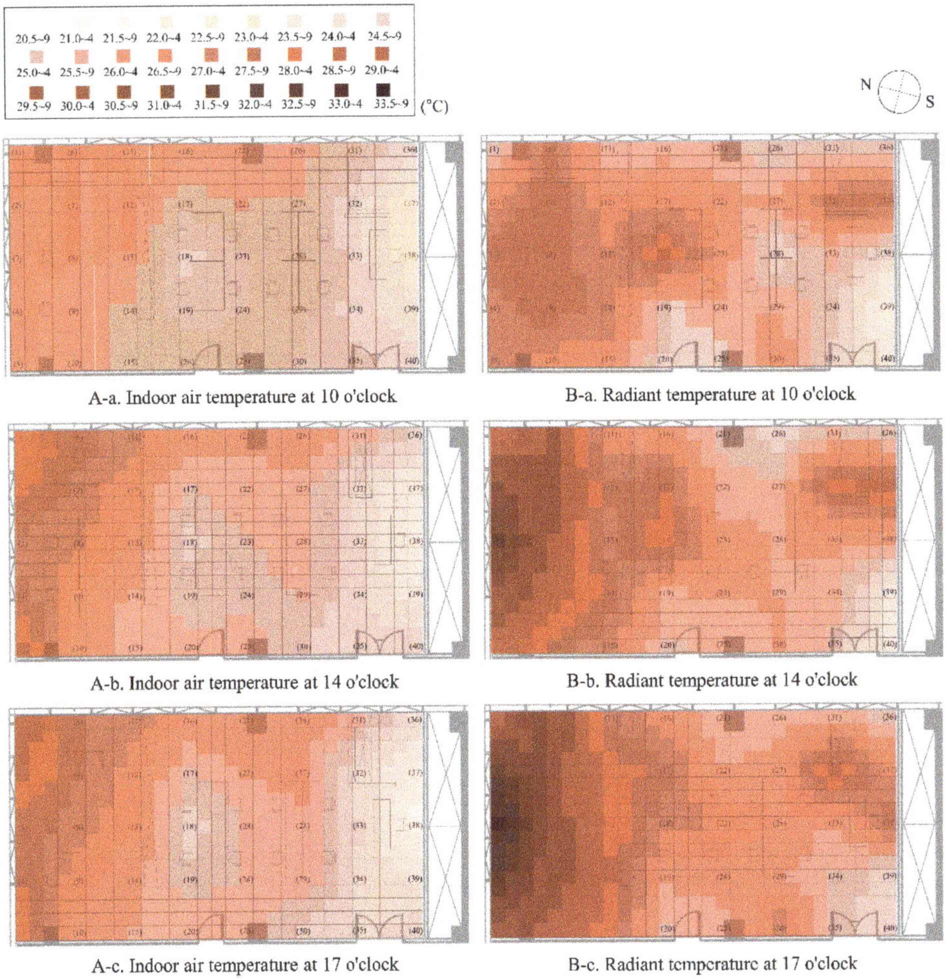

Figure 3. Changes in indoor air temperature T_A (**A**) and radiant temperature T_r (**B**) at 10:00 (**a**), 14:00 (**b**) and 17:00 (**c**).

In Figure 4b, when T_A = 26 °C (i), the largest percentage of responses indicated the neutral CSV (4) whether T_r = 26 or 28 °C. However, when T_r = 26 °C (blue), more responses were distributed to the two uncomfortable CSVs (2 and 3), whereas when T_r = 28 °C (red), more responses were distributed to the two comfortable CSVs (5 and 6). When T_A = 28 °C (ii), the same percentage of responses (28%) indicated the comfortable CSV (6) for T_r = 28 and 30 °C. However, 43% of responses indicated the neutral CSV (4) when T_r = 30 °C (red), whereas only ~20% of responses indicated the neutral CSV (4) when T_r = 28 °C, with 28% indicating the slightly uncomfortable CSV (3). Thus, the distribution of CSV responses was wider when T_r = T_A. Therefore, most of the occupants responded to the neutral when the indoor temperature was 26 degrees (i). In addition, when the indoor temperature was 28 °C (ii), the response was high to neutral and comfortable.

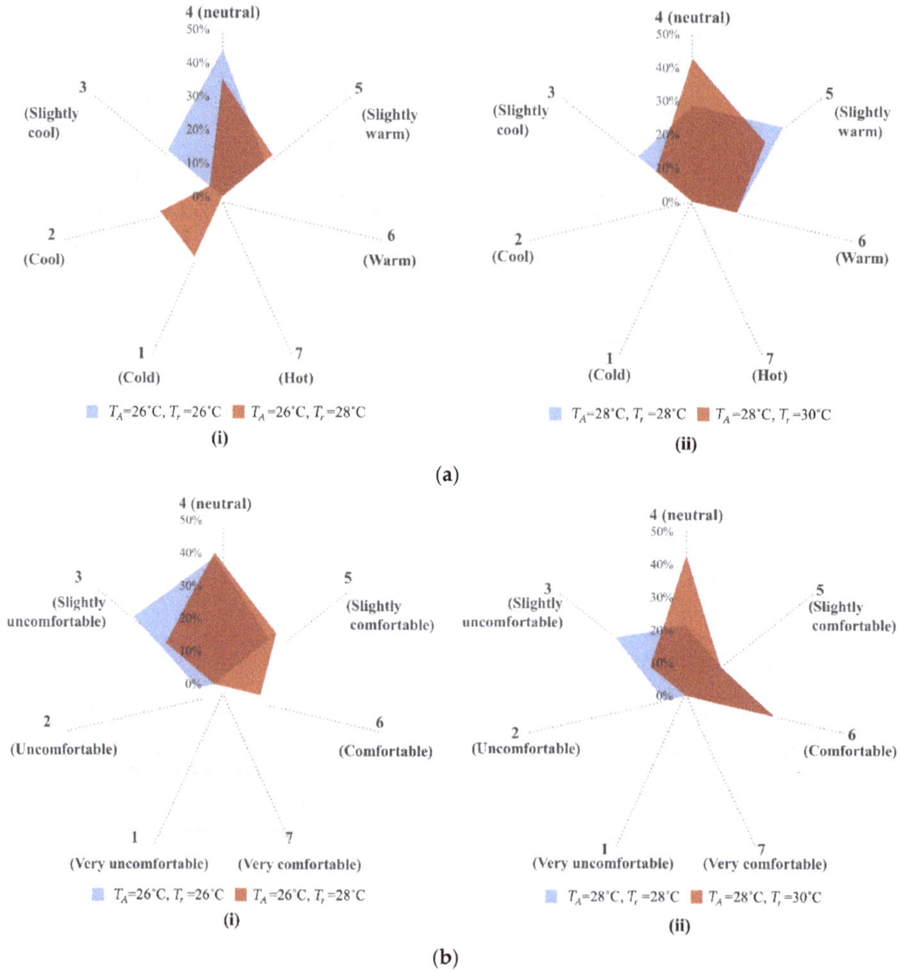

Figure 4. Thermal comfort response results according to the difference between the T_A and T_r: (**a**) TSV for (**i**) T_A = 26 °C and (**ii**) T_A = 28 °C, and (**b**) CSV for (**i**) T_A = 26 °C and (**ii**) T_A = 28 °C.

The analysis results presented in Figure 4 indicate a clear difference between the TSV and CSV results. In addition, considerably different thermal comfort results were observed according to the indoor air temperature and radiant temperature. In particular, when the indoor air temperature was different from the radiant temperature, the TSVs of the occupants were distributed among several different and often opposing scores. In other words the blue areas in Figure 4 indicate an even distribution across the five vertices, whereas the red areas indicate an uneven distribution with a high response at a few specific vertices. It was also found that the comfort of the occupants varied depending on both the radiant temperature and the indoor air temperature. This confirms the influence of the building characteristics (curtain walls); it appears that the radiant temperature showed significant changes under the influence of the solar radiation introduced through the curtain walls, which also had a significant influence on thermal comfort. Thus, a simple comparison between the indoor air temperature and radiant temperature is only of limited utility when analyzing the thermal comfort of office occupants. To provide a more detailed analysis, thermal comfort was estimated in Section 3.2 based on the accumulated mean thermal sensation vote (mTSV) according to the temperature change.

3.2. Thermal Sensation Changes and Comfort Temperature over Time

The changes in thermal sensations of the subjects were analyzed using the TSV reported at each location. In previous studies, TSV has been used as a representative index for general thermal comfort evaluation [53]. The changes in TSV over time are shown in Figure 5, in which the greater the value, the larger the change. The average change in TSV at all ten subject locations was 0.55, with an average maximum of 1.80 and an average minimum of 0, indicating that there were subjects who experienced no thermal change. A σ of 0.45 was calculated for all data. At 10:00, 14:00, and 17:00, the average change in TSV was 1.22, 1.12, and 1.23, respectively, at point A; 0.58, 1.08, and 0.71, respectively, at point B; 0.02, 0.35, and 0.40, respectively, at point C; 0.90, 1.80, and 1.05, respectively, at point D; 0.13, 0.17, and 0.32, respectively, at point E; 0.34, 0.69, and 0.50, respectively, at point F; 0.31, 0.61, and 0.67, respectively, at point G; 0.52, 0.92, and 0.25, respectively, at point H; 0.00, 0.06, and 0.05, respectively, at point I; and 0.21, 0.20, and 0.11, respectively, at point J. Thus, the changes in TSV at point D were the largest, followed by those at A, B, H, G, F, C, E, J, and I.

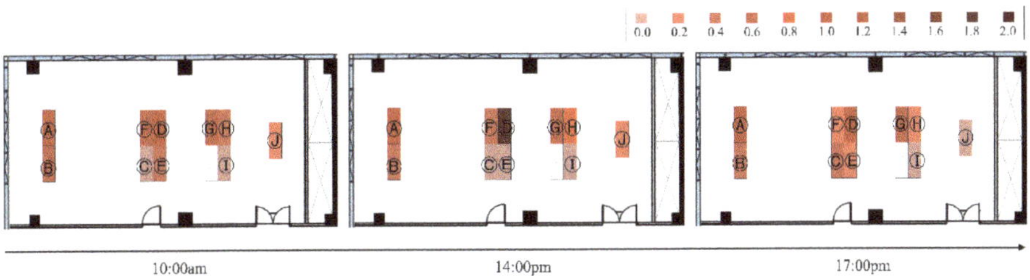

Figure 5. Changes in the thermal sensations of the subjects.

The changes in TSV at each point were divided into two groups according to their proximity to the windows. Points A, B, D, F, G, and H, which showed changes exceeding the average, were combined together in Group A (Male 50: Female 50); all of these points were close to the windows, where they received high solar radiation. Points C, E, I, and J, which showed changes smaller than the average, were combined together in Group B (Male 15: Female 75); all of these points were relatively far from the windows and closer to the interior corridor. The average and σ of the change in the TSV of Group A were 0.81 and 0.13, respectively, whereas those of Group B were 0.17 and 0.07, respectively, confirming a significant difference between the thermal comfort experienced by the two groups over the course of the day.

The overall σ of the changes in TSV was 1.31. The mTSV was calculated to quantify the change in TSV over the course of the day, with a positive value indicating a change to a warmer sensation, zero indicating no change, and a negative value indicating a change to a cooler sensation. For Group A, mTSV was 5 (slightly warmer) and the corresponding σ was 1.25. For Group B, mTSV was 3 (slightly cooler) and the corresponding σ was 1.19.

The mTSV results of each group were analyzed using a Probit regression analysis to estimate their respective levels of thermal comfort [54]; the results are shown in Figure 6. In Figure 6a, the highest curve represents the warm TSV (6) and the lowest curve represents the cold TSV (1). As the temperature increases from 23 to 28 °C, the curves representing the warm (6) and slightly warm (5) TSVs increase faster than the others. In Figure 6b, Group B only reported only five TSVs from cold (1) to slightly warm (5); the highest curve represents the slightly warm TSV (5) and the lowest curve represents the cold TSV (1). As the temperature increases from 22 to 26 °C, the curve representing the slightly warm TSV (5) increases faster than the others.

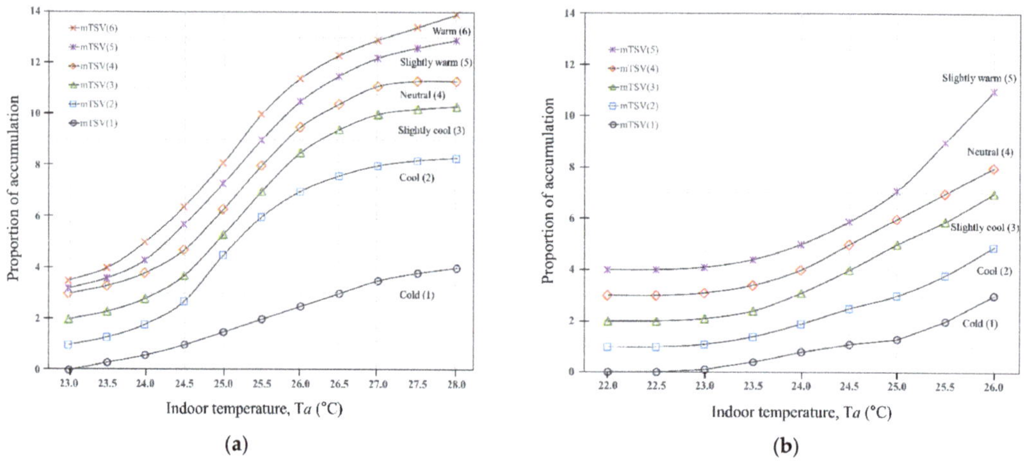

Figure 6. Proportions of mTSV: (**a**) Group A (window); (**b**) Group B (corridor).

For both groups, the lowest curve represents the cold TSV (1), but a generally warmer thermal sensation scale is shown in Figure 6a than in Figure 6b because the highest curve in the former represents the warm TSV (6) whereas that in the latter represents the slightly warm TSV (5). In addition, the proportion of cold TSV (1) decreases with increasing indoor air temperature in Figure 6a but increases with increasing indoor air temperature in in Figure 6b. The comprehensive analysis results thus confirm that Group A felt warmer than Group B, indicating that the vicinity of Group A to the windows resulted in a higher temperature in the same office space. Based on these results, it can be determined that a clear difference in comfort temperature exists between the two groups and thus in the thermal environments of their respective spaces.

The comfort temperature results for each group, derived by regression analysis of the neutral score in Figure 6a,b, are shown in Table 6. The comfort temperature was derived from the T_{op} and the mean of TSV. It was found to be at a significant level through the derived R^2 and p values. The average comfort temperature for all groups was found to be 26.6 °C. Goto et al. [55], who used the same indoor set temperature as this study (26 °C), stated that the comfort temperature preferred in office buildings was approximately 26 °C. Furthermore, Madhavi et al. [56] identified 27.1 °C as the comfort temperature, which is also similar to the average comfort temperature obtained in this study.

Table 6. Regression analysis of comfort temperature according to group.

Group	Regression Equation	R^2	p Value	Comfort Temperature
Group A	y = 0.402x − 9.968	0.515	0.000	24.7 °C
Group B	y = 0.307x − 8.735	0.378	0.001	28.4 °C

The comfort temperature for Group A was found to be 24.7 °C for whereas that for Group B was 28.4 °C. Thus, the respondents in Group A felt comfortable at a temperature approximately 2 °C lower than the current indoor set temperature of 26 °C, whereas those in Group B felt comfortable at a temperature approximately 2 °C higher than the set temperature. Consequently, the comfort temperatures in different spaces differed by approximately 3.7 °C, indicating that the comfort temperature is clearly dependent on the occupant location, even in the same space.

Tanabe et al. [57] performed experiments in six different office buildings, finding that the occupant thermal satisfaction level was 75% at an indoor air temperature of 25 °C, but dropped to 40% at 28 °C. However, a comfort temperature of 28.4 °C was obtained for

Group B in this study. Thus, despite a consistent temperature of 28°C, the analysis results were different depending on the presence of solar radiation and occupancy environment.

3.3. Analysis of Sensitivity to the Mean Thermal Sensation and Indoor Operative Temperature

Figure 7 shows the sensitivity analysis of the mean thermal sensation (MTS) to the indoor operative temperature (T_{op}) for Groups A and B, in which a strong positive correlation can be observed between MTS and T_{op} [39]. In the figure, the size of the bubble is proportional to the number of responses to the temperature change in the TSV results, and the slope of the regression equation thus represents the thermal sensitivity of the group to changes in T_{op}. A low sensitivity indicates that the temperature change is not felt, whereas a high sensitivity indicates that the temperature change is directly felt. The overall average sensitivity was found to be 0.58/°C. The slope for Group A (0.67/°C) is higher than that for Group B (0.49/°C), indicating that Group A was more sensitive to changes in the indoor air temperature, and that Group B could accept a higher temperature. Therefore, Group B can set the temperature higher than 26 °C. Group B feels that they are comfortable with the temperature higher than average. This control can save cooling energy and at the same time, can keep the comfort of occupants having the characteristics of Group B. This will be a positive control.

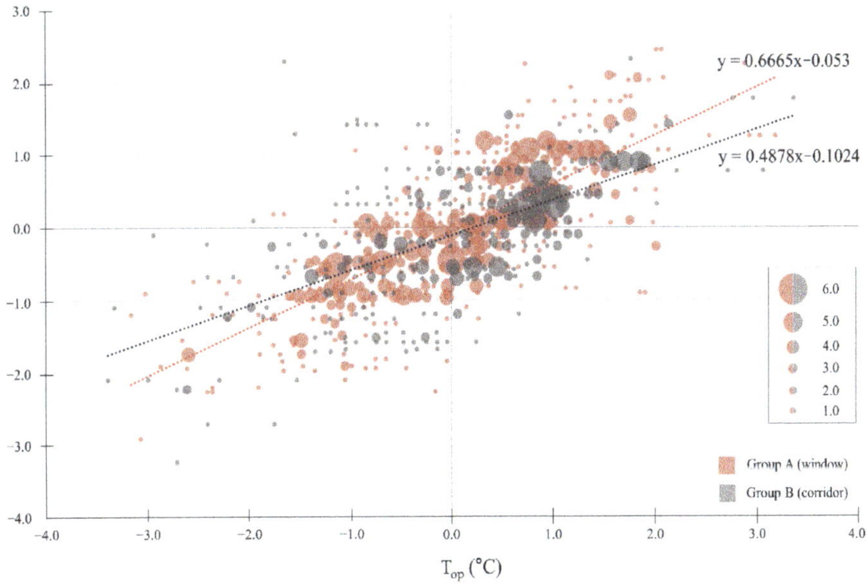

Figure 7. Regression analysis of mean thermal sensation (MTS) and indoor operative temperature (T_{op}).

Group B was likely less sensitive than Group A because the increase in solar radiation admitted through the curtain wall over the course of the day primarily affected Group A. In addition, the amount of change in MTS with temperature confirmed that Group A could not adapt to the temperature change and reacted more sensitively because the large temperature change in the area near the windows owing to the influx of solar radiation. Therefore, a temperature lower than the setting temperature is needed to Group A. Going further, temperature control by hour for reacting to the influence of solar radiation is needed. Thus, the results of this study indicate that sensitivity differs significantly according to the indoor thermal environment at the occupant location in an office space.

A previous study on thermal comfort in various building types [58] found that the universally adopted sensitivity (Griffiths constant) was close to 0.5/°C by Michael Humphreys. This value is not significantly different from the sensitivity results derived in this study; it is particularly similar to the sensitivity result obtained for Group B (0.49/°C). Furthermore, the comfort temperature (28.7 °C in [59] compared to 28.4 °C for Group B in this study) of the occupants with low sensitivity (0.255/°C in [59] compared to 0.49/°C for Group B in this study) was found to be relatively high. These occupants can clearly accept higher temperatures in summer.

Indeed, this study showed similar estimates for sensitivity as previous studies. Rupp et al. [58] estimated that the thermal sensitivity of office buildings in a subtropical climate, which is similar to the climate of Korea, was 0.568/°C. They also derived a sensitivity of approximately 0.440/°C in air-conditioned offices. These circumstances are comparable to those obtained through field research in summer in this study, but the derived results are different. Additional data are therefore required to confirm the validity of these results. Rupp et al. [58] mentioned that it remained necessary to avoid reliance on universal thermal sensitivity results by conducting further research because thermal sensitivity is not constant. They also emphasized the necessity of deriving the comfort temperature based on field research data. The field research conducted in this study was accordingly used to derive the comfort temperatures. However, research including more variables remains required to compensate for the limitations of such field research at present.

Thermal comfort is significantly affected by the exterior, type, and geographical location of a building along with situational factors and the human body's thermal balance [39]. In this study, field measurements were performed, and subjective sensations collected in an office space experiencing a large influx of solar radiation in a building with a transparent envelope. The analysis confirmed that the solar radiation introduced into an indoor space has a direct impact on the indoor air temperature and the thermal comfort of the occupants. Similarly, Moon [15] conducted research on the relationship between solar radiation and indoor thermal comfort and emphasized that solar radiation must be considered during the design of HVAC systems, as solar radiation increases body temperature [11,17]. Since numerical data describing the influx of solar radiation were insufficient in this study, it remains necessary to collect additional relevant data. The inclusion of such data should be further discussed in future research to obtain definitive results describing thermal comfort in buildings. Thus, in future work, solar radiation data will be measured, and revised regression coefficients will be estimated using all relevant data.

4. Conclusions

In this study, the influence of solar radiation on the indoor thermal environment and thermal comfort of occupants in an office building with a transparent envelope was analyzed using measurements and questionnaire responses. The analysis results showed that there was a clear difference between the indoor air temperature and radiant temperature owing to the transparent envelope of the building. The comfort of occupants in a group subjected to the significant influence of solar radiation (Group A) was compared with that of a group less affected by solar radiation (Group B), confirming the effect of solar radiation. The overall average sensitivity of the questionnaire respondents was 0.58/°C, and the average comfort temperature was found to be 26.6 °C. The sensitivity of Group A was 0.67/°C—higher than the average sensitivity—whereas that of Group B was 0.49/°C—lower than the average sensitivity. The comfort temperature of Group A was 24.7 °C—approximately 2 °C lower than the set temperature (26 °C)—whereas that of Group B was 28.4 °C—approximately 2 °C higher than the set temperature. In the analysis results, the two groups exhibited prominent differences in comfort according to the influence of solar radiation in a single office space. This indicates that solar radiation affects the indoor operative temperature, which is directly related to the thermal comfort of the occupants.

The derived comfort temperatures differed from the set temperature by approximately ±2 °C depending on the occupant location in the office. In particular, it was found that the solar radiation introduced through the transparent envelope eventually had a direct impact on the indoor thermal environment of the office and the comfort of its occupants. As a result, the simple form of temperature control typically applied through the central HVAC system in an office building can create a thermal imbalance among occupants. Therefore, the results of this study could be used to account for the effects of solar radiation through transparent envelopes when investigating individualized measures to properly control the indoor thermal environment and thereby maintain the thermal comfort of occupants. Additional research on the relationship between the thermal comfort of occupants and solar radiation remains to be conducted by collecting numerical data describing the solar radiation inside building spaces.

Author Contributions: Conceptualization, S.-K.K. and J.-H.R.; methodology, S.-K.K. and J.-H.R.; formal analysis, S.-K.K.; investigation, S.-K.K.; writing—original draft preparation, S.-K.K. and J.-H.R.; writing—review and editing, H.-C.S. and W.-H.H. All authors have read and agreed to the published version of the manuscript.

Funding: This work was supported by a National Research Foundation of Korea (NRF) grant funded from the Korean government (MSIP, South Korea) (No.2020R1C1C1007127).

Institutional Review Board Statement: The study was conducted according to the guidelines of the Declaration of Helsinki. Nonetheless, ethical review and approval were waived for this study, due to the characteristics of the study: no medical experiments were performed on human; Subjects were informed of the objectives of the study and expressed their consent by self-enrolling in the survey; occupants' data was collected under written given consent; data was anonymised.

Informed Consent Statement: Informed consent was obtained from all subjects involved in the study.

Data Availability Statement: The data presented in this study are available on request from authors.

Acknowledgments: This research was supported by Basic Science Research Program through the National Research Foundation of Korea (NRF) funded by the Ministry of Education (NRF-2019R1A6A3A01096814). This work was supported by NRF (National Research Foundation of Korea) Grant funded by the Korean Government (NRF-2019-Global Ph.D. Fellowship Program).

Conflicts of Interest: The authors declared no potential conflict of interest with respect to the research, authorship, and/or publication of this article.

References

1. Dong, Q.; Li, S.; Han, C. Numerical and experimental study of the effect of solar radiation on thermal comfort in a radiant heating system. *J. Build. Eng.* **2020**, *32*, 101497. [CrossRef]
2. Zhang, H.; Yang, R.; You, S.; Zheng, W.; Zheng, X.; Ye, T. The CPMV index for evaluating indoor thermal comfort in buildings with solar radiation. *Build. Environ.* **2018**, *134*, 1–9. [CrossRef]
3. Zhang, T.; Chen, Q. Novel air distribution systems for commercial aircraft cabins. *Build. Environ.* **2007**, *42*, 1675–1684. [CrossRef]
4. Song, C.; Duan, G.; Wang, D.; Liu, Y.; Du, H.; Chen, G. Study on the influence of air velocity on human thermal comfort under non-uniform thermal environment. *Build. Environ.* **2021**, *196*, 107808. [CrossRef]
5. Atmaca, I.; Kaynakli, O.; Yigit, A. Effects of radiant temperature on thermal comfort. *Build. Environ.* **2007**, *42*, 3210–3220. [CrossRef]
6. Al-Masrani, S.M.; Al-Obaidi, K.M.; Zalin, N.A.; Isma, M.I.A. Design optimisation of solar shading systems for tropical office buildings: Challenges and future trends. *Sol. Energy* **2018**, *170*, 849–872. [CrossRef]
7. Cheng, C.L.; Chen, C.L.; Chou, C.P.; Chan, C.Y. A mini-scale modeling approach to natural daylight utilization in building design. *Build. Environ.* **2007**, *42*, 372–384. [CrossRef]
8. Karlsen, L.; Heiselberg, P.; Bryn, I.; Johra, H. Verification of simple illuminance based measures for indication of discomfort glare from windows. *Build. Environ.* **2015**, *92*, 615–626. [CrossRef]
9. Baker, N.; Steemers, K. *Daylight Design of Buildings: A Handbook for Architects and Engineers*; Routledge: London, UK, 2014.
10. Munaaim, M.A.C.; Al-Obaidi, K.M.; Ismail, M.R.; Rahman, A.M.A. A review study on the application of the fibre optic daylighting system in Malaysian buildings. *Int. J. Sustain. Build. Technol. Urban Dev.* **2014**, *5*, 146–158. [CrossRef]
11. Yang, R.; Zhang, H.; You, S.; Zheng, W.; Zheng, X.; Ye, T. Study on the thermal comfort index of solar radiation conditions in winter. *Build. Environ.* **2020**, *167*, 106456. [CrossRef]
12. O'Brien, W.; Kapsis, K.; Athienitis, A.K. Manually-operated window shade patterns in office buildings: A critical review. *Build. Environ.* **2013**, *60*, 319–338. [CrossRef]
13. Al-Obaidi, K.M.; Ismail, M.A.; Rahman, A.M.A. Effective use of hybrid turbine ventilator to improve thermal performance in Malaysian tropical houses. *Build. Serv. Eng. Res. Technol.* **2016**, *37*, 755–768. [CrossRef]

14. Wu, J.; Li, X.; Lin, Y.; Yan, Y.; Tu, J. A PMV-based HVAC control strategy for office rooms subjected to solar radiation. *Build. Environ.* **2020**, *177*, 106863. [CrossRef]
15. Moon, J.H.; Lee, J.W.; Jeong, C.H.; Lee, S.H. Thermal comfort analysis in a passenger compartment considering the solar radiation effect. *Int. J. Therm. Sci.* **2016**, *107*, 77–88. [CrossRef]
16. Roller, W.L.; Goldman, R.F. Prediction of solar heat load on man. *J. Appl. Physiol.* **1968**, *24*, 717–721. [CrossRef]
17. Nielsen, B. Solar heat load: Heat balance during exercise in clothed subjects. *Eur. J. Appl. Physiol.* **1990**, *60*, 452–456. [CrossRef] [PubMed]
18. Hodder, S.G.; Parsons, K. The effects of solar radiation on thermal comfort. *Int. J. Biometeorol.* **2007**, *51*, 233–250. [CrossRef]
19. Zhu, W.S. The application of glass materials in building design. *Adv. Mater. Res.* **2013**, *706–708*, 516–519. [CrossRef]
20. Collin, S.; Jackson, K.A. Effects of the network environment on the vibrational modes of glass building blocks. *Strahlentherapie* **1964**, *123*, 463–496.
21. Nikitin, Y.; Murgul, V.; Vatin, N.; Pukhkal, V. Uses of glass in architecture: Heat losses of buildings based on translucent structures. *Appl. Mech. Mater.* **2014**, *680*, 481–485. [CrossRef]
22. al Horr, Y.; Arif, M.; Kaushik, A.; Mazroei, A.; Katafygiotou, M.; Elsarrag, E. Occupant productivity and office indoor environment quality: A review of the literature. *Build. Environ.* **2016**, *105*, 369–389. [CrossRef]
23. Lan, L.; Wargocki, P.; Lian, Z. Quantitative measurement of productivity loss due to thermal discomfort. *Energy Build.* **2011**, *43*, 1057–1062. [CrossRef]
24. Humphreys, M.A. Quantifying occupant comfort: Are combined indices of the indoor environment practicable? *Build. Res. Inform.* **2005**, *33*, 317–325. [CrossRef]
25. Jazizadeh, F.; Ghahramani, A.; Becerik-Gerber, B.; Kichkaylo, T. Personalized thermal comfort-driven control in HVAC-Operated office buildings. In Proceedings of the 2013 ASCE International Workshop on Computing in Civil Engineering, Los Angeles, CA, USA, 23–25 June 2013.
26. Tarantini, M.; Pernigotto, G.; Gasparella, A. A co-citation analysis on thermal comfort and productivity aspects in production and office buildings. *Buildings* **2017**, *7*, 36. [CrossRef]
27. Mofidi, F.; Akbari, H. An integrated model for position-based productivity and energy costs optimization in offices. *Energy Build.* **2019**, *183*, 559–580. [CrossRef]
28. Mak, C.M.; Lui, Y.P. The effect of sound on office productivity. *Build. Serv. Eng. Res. Technol.* **2011**, *33*, 339–345. [CrossRef]
29. Maula, H.; Hongisto, V.; Östman, L.; Haapakangas, A.; Koskela, H.; Hyönä, J. The effect of slightly warm temperature on work performance and comfort in open-plan offices—A laboratory study. *Indoor Air* **2015**, *26*, 286–297. [CrossRef] [PubMed]
30. Hygge, S.; Knez, I. Effects of noise, heat and indoor lighting on cognitive performance and self-reported affect. *J. Environ. Psychol.* **2001**, *21*, 291–299. [CrossRef]
31. Lan, L.; Wargocki, P.; Wyon, D.P.; Lian, Z. Effects of thermal discomfort in an office on perceived air quality, SBS symptoms, physiological responses, and human performance. *Indoor Air* **2011**, *21*, 376–390. [CrossRef] [PubMed]
32. Gunay, H.B.; Shen, W.; Newsham, G.; Ashouri, A. Modelling and analysis of unsolicited temperature setpoint change requests in office buildings. *Build. Environ.* **2018**, *133*, 203–212. [CrossRef]
33. Shahzad, S.; Calautit, J.K.; Hughes, B.R.; Satish, B.K.; Rijal, H.B. Patterns of thermal preference and Visual Thermal Landscaping model in the workplace. *Appl. Energy* **2019**, *255*, 113674. [CrossRef]
34. Gennusa, M.L.; Nucara, A.; Pietrafesa, M.; Rizzo, G. A model for managing and evaluating solar radiation for indoor thermal comfort. *Sol. Energy* **2007**, *81*, 594–606. [CrossRef]
35. Huizenga, C.; Zhang, H.; Mattelaer, P.; Yu, T.; Arens, E.; Lyons, P. *Window Performance for Human Thermal Comfort*; Report to the National Fenestration Rating Council; Center for the Built Environment: Berkeley, CA, USA, 2006.
36. Lyons, P.; Arates, D.; Huizenga, C. Window performance for human thermal comfort. *ASHRAE Trans.* **1999**, *73*, 400–420.
37. Stegou-Sagia, A.; Antonopoulos, K.; Angelopoulou, C.; Kotsiovelos, G. The impact of glazing on energy consumption and comfort. *Energy Convers. Manag.* **2007**, *48*, 2844–2852. [CrossRef]
38. Bessoudo, M.; Tzempelikos, A.; Athienitis, A.K.; Zmeureanu, R. Indoor thermal environmental conditions near glazed facades with shading devices—Part I: Experiments and building thermal model. *Build. Environ.* **2010**, *45*, 2506–2516. [CrossRef]
39. Fang, Z.; Zhang, S.; Cheng, Y.; Fong, A. Field study on adaptive thermal comfort in typical air conditioned classrooms. *Build. Environ.* **2018**, *133*, 73–82. [CrossRef]
40. Abowitz, D.A.; Toole, T.M. Mixed method research: Fundamental issues of design, validity, and reliability in construction research. *J. Constr. Eng. Manag.* **2009**, *136*. [CrossRef]
41. Creswell, J.W.; Clark, V.L.P. *Designing and Conducting Mixed Methods Research*; SAGE Publications, USA, Inc.: Thousand Oaks, CA, USA, 2007; ISBN 978-1412975179-13.
42. Zou, P.X.; Xu, X.; Sanjayan, J.; Wang, J. A mixed methods design for building occupants' energy behavior research. *Energy Build.* **2018**, *166*, 239–249. [CrossRef]
43. Sarhadi, F.; Rad, V.B. The structural model for thermal comfort based on perceptions individuals in open urban spaces. *Energy Build.* **2020**, *185*, 107260. [CrossRef]
44. Gunnarsen, L.; Fanger, P.O.; Fanger, P.O. Adaptation to indoor air pollution. *Environ. Int.* **1992**, *18*, 43–54. [CrossRef]
45. Nguyen, A.T.; Singh, M.K.; Reiter, S. An adaptive thermal comfort model for hot humid South-East Asia. *Build. Environ.* **2012**, *56*, 291–300. [CrossRef]

46. Chapter 9: Thermal Comfort. In *ASHRAE Handbook Fundamentals;* American Society of Heating, Refrigerating and Air-Conditioning Engineers, USA, Inc.: Atlanta, GA, USA, 2009; pp. 1–9.
47. Trebilcock, M.; Soto-Muñoz, J.; Piggot-Navarrete, J. Evaluation of thermal comfort standards in office buildings of Chile: Thermal sensation and preference assessment. *Build. Environ.* **2020**, *183*, 107158. [CrossRef]
48. Ministry of Trade, Industry and Energy (MOTIE). *Regulation on Promotion of Rationalization of Energy Use by Public Institutions;* Ministry of Trade, Industry and Energy: Sejong, Korea, 2018.
49. Wu, Q.; Liu, J.; Zhang, L.; Zhang, J.; Jiang, L. Study on thermal sensation and thermal comfort in environment with moderate temperature ramps. *Build. Environ.* **2020**, *171*, 106640. [CrossRef]
50. Xiong, Y.; Liu, J.; Kim, J. Understanding differences in thermal comfort between urban and rural residents in hot summer and cold winter climate. *Build. Environ.* **2019**, *165*, 106393. [CrossRef]
51. Zhang, Y.; Zhao, R. Overall thermal sensation, acceptability and comfort. *Build. Environ.* **2008**, *43*, 44–50. [CrossRef]
52. International Standard ISO 10551: 2009. *Ergonomics of the Physical Environment-Subjective Judgement Scales for Assessing Physical Environment;* International Organization for Standardization (ISO):: Geneva, Switzerland, 2009; p. 5.
53. Luo, M.; Cao, B.; Damiens, J.; Lin, B.; Zhu, Y. Evaluating thermal comfort in mixed-mode buildings: A field study in a subtropical climate. *Build. Environ.* **2015**, *88*, 46–54. [CrossRef]
54. Khalid, W.; Zaki, S.A.; Rijal, H.B.; Yakub, F. Investigation of comfort temperature and thermal adaptation for patients and visitors in Malaysian hospitals. *Energy Build.* **2019**, *183*, 484–499. [CrossRef]
55. Goto, T.; Mitamura, T.; Yoshino, H.; Tamura, A.; Inomata, E. Long-term field survey on thermal adaptation in office buildings in Japan. *Building Environ.* **2007**, *42*, 3944–3954. [CrossRef]
56. Indraganti, M.; Ooka, R.; Rijal, H.B. Thermal comfort in offices in summer: Findings from a field study under the 'setsu-den'conditions in Tokyo. *Build. Environ.* **2013**, *61*, 114–132. [CrossRef]
57. Tanabe, S.; Iwahashi, Y.; Tsushima, S. Thermal comfort and productivity in offices under mandatory electricity savings after great East Japan earthquake. In Proceedings of the 7th Windsor Conference: The Changing Context of Comfort in an Unpredictable World Cumberland Lodge, Windsor, UK, 12–15 April 2012.
58. Rupp, R.F.; Kim, J.; Ghisi, E.; de Dear, R.J. Thermal sensitivity of occupants in different building typologies: The Griffiths Constant is a Variable. *Energy Build.* **2019**, *200*, 11–20. [CrossRef]
59. Liu, Y.; Dong, Y.; Song, C.; Wang, Y.; Liu, L.; Liu, J. A tracked field study of thermal adaptation during a short-term migration between cold and hot-summer and warm-winter areas of China. *Build. Environ.* **2017**, *124*, 90–103. [CrossRef]

International Journal of
Environmental Research and Public Health

MDPI

Article

The Impact of Family Socioeconomic Status on Elderly Health in China: Based on the Frailty Index

Wenjian Zhou [1], Jianming Hou [2,*], Meng Sun [2] and Chang Wang [3]

1 Northeast Asian Studies College, Jilin University, Changchun 130012, China; zhouwj20@mails.jlu.edu.cn
2 Center for Northeast Asian Studies, Jilin University, Changchun 130012, China; sunmeng_meng@jlu.edu.cn
3 School of Physical Education, Northeast Normal University, Changchun 130024, China; wangc358@nenu.edu.cn
* Correspondence: houjianming@jlu.edu.cn

Abstract: China is about to enter a moderate aging society. In the process of social and economic development, the family socioeconomic status and health status of the elderly have also changed significantly. Learning the impact of family socioeconomic status on elderly health can help them improve family socioeconomic status and better achieve healthy and active aging. Using the data of the Chinese Longitudinal Healthy Longevity Survey in 2018, this study firstly analyzed the impact of family socioeconomic status on elderly health using the multivariate linear regression model and quantile regression model, the heterogeneity of different elderly groups using subsample regression, and the mediation effects of three conditions associated with the family socioeconomic status of the elderly. The results show that family socioeconomic status has a negative effect on the frailty index, that is, it has a positive impact on elderly health. Family socioeconomic status has a higher positive impact on the health status of the middle and lower age elderly and rural elderly. Overall living status and leisure and recreation status both have mediation effects, while health-care status has no mediation effect.

Keywords: family socioeconomic status; elderly health; frailty index; mediation effect

Citation: Zhou, W.; Hou, J.; Sun, M.; Wang, C. The Impact of Family Socioeconomic Status on Elderly Health in China: Based on the Frailty Index. *Int. J. Environ. Res. Public Health* **2022**, *19*, 968. https://doi.org/10.3390/ijerph19020968

Academic Editors: Roberto Alonso González Lezcano, Francesco Nocera and Rosa Giuseppina Caponetto

Received: 8 December 2021
Accepted: 13 January 2022
Published: 15 January 2022

1. Introduction

According to the seventh national census of China, the number of people aged 60 and above in 2020 was 260 million accounting for 18.7% of the total population, and the number of people aged 65 and above was 190 million accounting for 13.5% of the total population [1]. Although China is still in the mild aging stage, it is about to enter a moderate aging society. The scale and proportion of the elderly population will continue to expand. The increasingly serious problem of the aging population not only brings great pressure to the country but also poses various threats to the health and security of the elderly.

With the increase of age, the physiological health of the elderly population is declining, and the mental health issue has become more prominent in recent years. The physical and mental health problems of the elderly bring a series of challenges to the construction of China's public health system, the construction of an age-friendly society, and the formulation of health standards for the elderly. In particular, China still has a typical dual economic structure at present. The health levels of the elderly population in urban and rural areas differ greatly, and they also face different health risks. At the same time, the socioeconomic status of the elderly begins to decline after a significant shift in their social roles, which often affects their overall living status, leisure and recreation status, health-care status, etc. Quality of life has an intuitive impact on the health status of the elderly. Leisure and recreational activities not only relieve the stress and tension in life, but also help to enhance social interaction among the elderly, maintain the stability of human body functions, and improve the psychological state. Health-care services, as a means of protection when health is at risk, play a last resort role in the health of the elderly.

The Outline of Healthy China 2030 Plan proposed to promote healthy aging and ensure the health of the elderly [2]. The fifth plenary session of the 19th CPC Central Committee approved the CPC Central Committee's Proposals on Formulating the 14th Five-Year Plan for National Economic and Social Development and the Long-Term Goals of 2035, which proposed to comprehensively promote the construction of a healthy China, give priority to the development of the people's health, implement the national strategy of actively responding to population aging, and actively develop human resources for the elderly [3]. The implementation of active aging and the development of human resources for the elderly can delay the decline of their socioeconomic status and promote active aging and healthy aging.

In a marriage-based family, the husband and wife are closely interdependent in life and economy. They support each other and share their weal and woe. Both parties determine the socioeconomic status of the entire family, which in turn has a very important impact on both parties. However, existing studies (reviewed in Section 2) have mostly analyzed the effects of older adults' socioeconomic status on their self-rated health, physical health, and mental health but less on their overall health status from the perspective of family socioeconomic status. Based on the above research backgrounds, it is of great theoretical and practical significance to analyze the impact, heterogeneity, and different mechanisms of the family socioeconomic status of the elderly on their comprehensive health status. Theoretically, it makes up for the shortage of research between family socioeconomic status and elderly health from a comprehensive perspective. Realistically, it calls for more attention to help the elderly improve their family socioeconomic status and comprehensive health status from different dimensions and reduce the inequalities within them, and provides a reference basis for the formulation of public health policy for the elderly, so that they can enjoy happy and healthy lives and successfully achieve healthy and active aging.

2. Literature Review

The health production theory suggests that people's optimal decisions about their health needs are influenced by a variety of factors, including health insurance, lifestyle, education, income status, and living environment [4]. The health causation theory holds that health is also influenced by social structural factors, and socioeconomic status of an individual affects their health status. The higher the socioeconomic status, the better the health status [5]. The social stratification theory assumes that the differences between social groups are universal. People have both natural and social differences. Natural differences are formed by the physical differences of people, whereas social differences are formed by people due to social factors, such as political, economic, cultural, and interaction relationships. It is based on certain criteria for distinguishing people's positions in social activities and social relations, and the common stratification criteria are economic income, occupation, education level, power, etc. [6]. The existence of social stratification structure leads to the inequality of socioeconomic status and family socioeconomic status.

Socioeconomic status based on the social stratification theory is the social class or position in which an individual or group is located and is a comprehensive reflection of education level, occupational rank, income level, etc. Inequality in socioeconomic status can lead to inequality in one's own health. Several scholars have revealed this phenomenon through their studies. Winkleby found that socioeconomic status plays a determinant role in almost all diseases and all stages of life [7]. He found that the household income of older adults has a positive effect on their life satisfaction and physical health status and occupational status only has a positive effect on their physical health status, but education has no effect on their life satisfaction and physical health status [8]. Zhang et al. concluded that elderly people with low socioeconomic status, poor income level, low education level, and manual labor-oriented jobs or no job mostly have severely underutilized health services or no health-care coverage at all, leading to the worsening of their own health status [9]. Kuo et al. examined the impact of socioeconomic status on colorectal cancer risk, staging, and survival under the National Health Insurance system in Taiwan [10].

However, these studies mainly analyze the different dimensions of socioeconomic status and lack a comprehensive consideration of socioeconomic status. Some scholars use the socioeconomic status index to study its impact and mechanism on the health of the elderly. Cristine et al. suggested that people with lower socioeconomic status are more likely to be in an unfavorable environment and have negative emotions and potential stress, which in turn have a negative impact on their health [11]. Xue et al. suggested that socioeconomic status affects the physical and mental health of older adults through mediating variables, such as sleep quality, dietary patterns, physical activities, and social participation [12]. Liu et al. found that socioeconomic status positively influences the health of older adults through food access, physical activities, recreational activities, and improving their overall well-being [13]. Wang et al. extended the study of the influence mechanism from a social capital perspective and found that high socioeconomic status groups increase their health advantage through a high frequency of social interactions with friends; low socioeconomic status groups mitigate the health disadvantage caused by low status through social trust [14]. However, these studies do not consider the impact of socioeconomic status from a family perspective.

Family socioeconomic status is a comprehensive reflection of the individual socioeconomic status of family members, and it is the social class or status of family members based on the family cooperation model. Unequal family socioeconomic status can negatively affect education, occupational status, and the health of children. Javier found that the lower the family socioeconomic status of elementary school students, the lower their scores in basic competencies [15]. Meng et al. investigated the family socioeconomic status in China and found that the socioeconomic status of students' families has important effects and constraints on the students' preferences with regard to the different types of higher education schools and majors [6]. Zhu et al. argued that the influence of family status on the youth's attainment of initial position is changing in a wave-like fashion [16]. Cheng et al. found that the family socioeconomic status of secondary school students is significantly and positively related to overall psychological quality and its dimensions [17]. Unequal family socioeconomic status can also lead to inequality in individual's health. However, only a few studies have focused on this aspect. Huang et al. concluded that a higher family socioeconomic status has a significant contribution to their own health in China [18]. Cao et al. thought consistently higher early family socioeconomic status and upward socioeconomic status mobility will lead to a higher incidence of good health in old age, while continuous lower early family socioeconomic status is the opposite, that is, the impact of early family environment on the elderly health is cumulative [19]. Ghasemi et al. found that subjective perception of family socioeconomic status can explain differences in health-related quality of life of low-income people in Iran [20]. Booysen et al. also found that family structure and family socioeconomic status both have an influence on public health [21]. However, these studies do not clarify how family socioeconomic status affects the comprehensive health status of the elderly.

Based on the above literature analyses, we think that many studies have been conducted on both socioeconomic status and family socioeconomic status, but the existing studies mainly focus on the influence of individual socioeconomic status on the health status in different dimensions of themselves, more on the intergenerational influence of family socioeconomic status on children and less on the impact and mechanism of family socioeconomic status on comprehensive health status. We know that when the socioeconomic status of a family is higher in real life, its members usually enjoy better living conditions, abundant leisure and entertainment activities, and high-quality medical and health services, which will have a positive effect on their health. Therefore, based on the above theories, this study creatively analyzes the impact and mechanism of family socioeconomic status on frailty index. In the present study, the total family income, the comprehensive years of education, and the comprehensive occupational rank before retirement of elderly couples were synthesized into the family socioeconomic status index. The frailty index was used as a measure of the comprehensive health status of the elderly. The impact of family socioeconomic status on elderly health was first analyzed, followed by the differences in the impact of family socioeconomic status on the health status of different elderly groups as well as the possible mechanisms of the impact. Figure 1 shows the specific theoretical analysis framework.

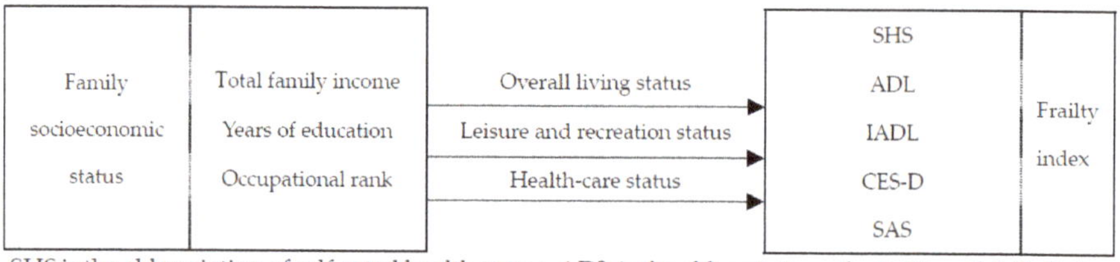

SHS is the abbreviation of self-rated health status. ADL is the abbreviation of activities of daily living. IADL is the abbreviation of instrumental activities of daily living. CES-D is the abbreviation of the center for epidemiological studies—depression. SAS is the abbreviation of the self-rated anxiety scale.

Figure 1. Framework diagram of theoretical analysis.

3. Study Design

3.1. Data

The data used in this study were obtained from the Chinese Longitudinal Healthy Longevity Survey in 2018 (CLHLS was downloaded from https://opendata.pku.edu.cn/dataverse/pku (accessed on 1 November 2021)), which is a national-wide and longitudinal survey of the elderly organized by the Center for Healthy Aging and Development Research/National Development Research Institute of Peking University. The detailed information about the survey design has been reported in previous research [22–24]. The samples were collected from 23 provinces of China, and the total number of valid samples was 15,874. The contents of the surviving respondents' questionnaires included the basic conditions, socioeconomic conditions, and various health conditions of the elderly, which cover all aspects of the elderly and meet the needs of the study. In the present study, elderly people aged 60 and above were included, and 7599 samples were obtained after deleting those samples with missing or invalid variable values.

3.2. Variable Descriptions

3.2.1. Explained Variable

The explained variable is the comprehensive health status of the elderly, and the frailty index is used as a measurement method. The frailty index, or cumulative health deficit index, refers to the proportion of health deficit indicators among all measures of health for an individual and can be understood as an accumulation of health deficits. Health deficits can be measured somatically, functionally, and psychologically [25]. The number of variables used to construct the index is not standardized, usually ranging from 30 to 70 and taking values between 0 and 1 [26]. Drawing on previous research results and combining data availability and research objectives, this study selected 32 indicators measuring health status to construct the frailty index, covering self-rated health status (SHS), activities of daily living (ADL), instrumental activities of daily living (IADL), the center for epidemiological studies–depression (CES-D), and the self-rated anxiety scale (SAS). The SHS was assigned in the following manner: 0, "very good"; 0.25, "good"; 0.5, "general"; 0.75, "bad"; and 1, "very bad". The ADL are reflected by the elderly's problems in bathing, dressing, toileting, indoor transferring, control of urination and defecation, and feeding (six aspects). For each aspect, if the elderly does not need assistance, a value of 0 was assigned; if the elderly needs one part assistance, a value of 0.5 was assigned; and if the elderly needs more than one part assistance, a value of 1 was assigned. The IADL are reflected by the questions of whether the elderly can go outside to visit neighbors, go shopping, make food, wash clothes, walk 1 km continuously, carry a 5 kg weight, crouch and stand three times continuously, and take public transportation by themselves (eight aspects). For each aspect, if the elderly can do so, a value of 0 was assigned; if the elderly encounters little difficulty, a value of 0.5 was assigned; if the elderly is unable to do so, a value of 1 was assigned. The CES-D consists of 10 questions, with regard to whether the older person is bothered by some small things, has difficulty in concentrating, feels sad or depressed, struggles to do things, has hope for the future, feels nervous or afraid, is as happy as when he or she was young, feels lonely, and feels unable to continue life as well as his or her sleep quality. For the seven questions reflecting negative emotions, the assigned values were as follows: 0, "never"; 0.25, "seldom"; 0.5, "sometimes"; 0.75, "often"; and 1, "always". For the three questions reflecting positive emotions with regard to whether the elderly has hope for the future and is as happy as when he or she was young as well as his or her sleep quality, they were assigned with the opposite values. The SAS is composed of seven questions with regard to whether the elderly feels uneasy, worried and annoyed, cannot stop or control worry, is worried too much about all kinds of things, is very nervous and finds it difficult to relax, is so anxious that he or she cannot sit still, easily gets annoyed or irritated, and feels as if something terrible is going to happen. We assigned the values according to the frequency of each problem: 0, "never"; 0.33, "for several days"; 0.67, "more than half of days"; and 1, "almost every day". Finally, the scores of the 32 indicators were summed and then divided by the theoretical maximum score of 32 to obtain the frailty index of each elderly person.

3.2.2. Explanatory Variable

The explanatory variable is the family socioeconomic status of the elderly, which consists of three dimensions: total family income, comprehensive years of education, and comprehensive occupational rank before retirement of the elderly couple (for the currently spouseless elderly, this study used their own years of education and occupational rank before retirement). The total family income is the total income of the whole family in the last year, which was processed logarithmically in this study. The range of years of education is 0–22 years, and those samples with 22 years or more of education were treated as 22 years. For the occupational level before retirement, in accordance with the study of Xue and Ge, the present study defined "professional, technical, governmental, institutional, managerial, and military personnel" as senior practitioners assigned with a value of 3; "commercial, service, and industrial workers" as intermediate practitioners with a value of 2; and the other options as general practitioners with a value of 1 [12]. For the years of education and occupational rank, previous studies have only considered the elderly individuals. Therefore, in the present study, the spouses of the elderly were also taken into consideration. We calculated the comprehensive years of education and occupational rank before retirement of the elderly couples in accordance with Zhu and Li's study, which enables to evaluate the advantages and disadvantages of the different types of family status more accurately using an approach based on the Pythagorean theorem [16,27]. Finally, the present study used the entropy weight method to synthesize the total family income, the comprehensive years of education, and the comprehensive occupational rank before retirement of elderly couples into a family socioeconomic status index. The entropy weight method is currently the main method of objective assignment method, which aims to assign weights to each evaluation index based on the degree of difference between its values and construct a composite index.

3.2.3. Control Variables

Based on the survey data and existing studies, this study selected the basic personal information and social security status of the elderly as control variables. The control variables included gender, age, marital status, residential area, co-residence mode, number of surviving children, whether or not he or she has retirement pension/public old-age insurance/private or commercial old-age insurance, and whether or not he or she has medical insurance [8,9,12–14]. In this study, we classified marital status into without spouse and with spouse, and residential area into urban and rural areas. The co-residence mode included living alone, living with family members, and living in an institution, which are generated into two dummy variables: whether or not living with family members and whether or not living in an institution.

3.2.4. Mediating Variables

The mediating variables were the overall living status, leisure and recreation status, and health-care status of the elderly. In the current study, two dichotomous variables, "is all of the financial support sufficient to pay for daily expenses" and "self-reported quality of life ("very bad", "bad", and "general" were merged into "bad", and "good" and "very good" were merged into "good")," were selected to construct the overall living status. If the financial support is sufficient and the quality of life is good, the overall living status is "good"; otherwise, it is "bad". The two dichotomous variables, "whether he or she exercises or not now" and "whether he or she has traveled in the past 2 years", were selected to construct the leisure and recreation status. If they exercise regularly and have traveled, the leisure and recreation status is good; otherwise, it is "bad". The two dichotomous variables, "whether he or she can get adequate medical service at present" and "whether he or she has regular physical examination once a year", were selected to construct the health-care status. If they can get adequate medical service at present and have regular physical examination once a year, the health-care status is good; otherwise, it is "bad". Table 1 shows the variables and data statistics.

Table 1. Variables and data statistics.

Continuous Variables	**Mean**	**Standard Deviation**	**Min**	**Max**
Health status	0.211	0.144	0	1
Family socioeconomic status	0.189	0.197	0	1
Age	83.872	11.488	60	117
Number of surviving children	3.437	1.786	0	11
Categorial Variables	**Categories**	***n***	**Percentages (%)**	**Average Frailty Index**
Gender	Female	4228	55.6	0.236
	Male	3371	44.4	0.181
Marital status	Without spouse	4519	59.5	0.252
	With spouse	3080	40.5	0.152
Residential area	Rural	3266	43.0	0.205
	Urban	4333	57.0	0.216
Living with family members	No	1623	21.4	0.214
	Yes	5976	78.6	0.210
Living in an institution	No	7326	96.4	0.207
	Yes	273	3.6	0.320
Old-age insurance	Do not have	3807	50.1	0.219
	Have	3792	49.9	0.203
Medical insurance	Do not have	1049	13.8	0.235
	Have	6550	86.2	0.207
Overall living status	Bad	2645	34.8	0.250
	Good	4954	65.2	0.191
Leisure and recreation status	Bad	7011	92.3	0.220
	Good	588	7.7	0.112
Health-care status	Bad	2438	32.1	0.261
	Good	5161	67.9	0.188

3.3. Models

3.3.1. Multiple Linear Regression Model

In the current study, we used the frailty index of the elderly as the explained variable and the family socioeconomic status index as the explanatory variable and added various control variables to establish a multiple linear regression model to analyze the influence of family socioeconomic status on the health of the elderly.

$$Y_i = \alpha + \beta_0 X_i + \sum_j \beta_j Z_{ij} \tag{1}$$

In Equation (1), Y_i is the frailty index of the ith elderly person, and α is a constant term. X_i is the explanatory variable, which indicates the family socioeconomic status index of the ith elderly person, and β_0 is its coefficient. Z_{ij} is the jth control variable of the ith elderly person, and β_j is the coefficient of each control variable.

3.3.2. Quantile Regression Model

Because of the high heterogeneity of the health status of older adults, the same family socioeconomic status may have different effects on older adults with different frailty status. Therefore, we also used the quantile regression model to analyze the effects of family socioeconomic status on frailty indices at different quartiles to verify whether the findings of the multiple linear regression model are still supported.

$$Q_{i\theta}(Y_i) = \alpha + \beta_{0\theta} X_i + \sum \beta_{j\theta} Z_{ij} \tag{2}$$

In Equation (2), $Q_{i\theta}(Y_i)$ denotes the conditional quantile of the frailty index for a given distribution of explanatory and control variables, where θ denotes the quantiles, and 10%, 25%, 50%, 75%, and 90% are selected in turn. The remaining variables and parameters are explained as in the multiple linear regression model above.

3.3.3. Mediating Effect Model

The mediating variables are the overall living status, leisure and recreation status, and health-care status of the elderly, all of which are dichotomous variables. When the mediating variable is a categorical variable, the mediation effect analysis needs to be conducted by calculating a confidence interval through a two-step regression method. The procedure for testing the mediating effect is as follows:

$$M = aX + \varepsilon_2 \tag{3}$$

$$Y = c'X + bM + \varepsilon_3 \tag{4}$$

where Y denotes the explained variable, X denotes the explanatory variable, and M denotes the mediating variable. Equation (3) represents the regression of the mediating variable on the explanatory variable, and logistic regression is used. Equation (4) represents the regression of the explained variable on both the explanatory and mediating variables, and linear regression is used. In the present study, we first used the Stata 15.0 software to obtain the estimated values of regression coefficients and robust standard errors of a and b. Then, we used the Medci command in the package of RMediation (downloaded from https://cloud.r-project.org/bin/windows/contrib/3.5/RMediation_1.1.4.zip (accessed on 5 November 2021)) of R 3.5.1 software (R Foundation for Statistical Computing, Vienna, Austria) to conduct the coefficient product distribution test to obtain the confidence interval of the mediating effect [28]. Moreover, if this confidence interval does not contain 0, it indicates the existence of the mediating effect [29].

4. Results

4.1. The Effect of Family Socioeconomic Status on Elderly Health

A multiple linear regression model was established as a benchmark model to analyze the effect of family socioeconomic status on elderly health. From Model 1 in Table 2, it can be seen that the family socioeconomic status of the elderly has a significantly negative effect on the frailty index at the 1% level, and for every 1 unit increase in the family socioeconomic status, the frailty index decreases by 0.050 units. We performed a multicollinearity test which indicated that the problem of multicollinearity was excluded in the multiple linear regression model.

Table 2. Regression results of the impact of family socioeconomic status on elderly health.

Variables	Model 1 OLS	Model 2 Q10	Model 3 Q25	Model 4 Q50	Model 5 Q75	Model 6 Q90
Explanatory variable						
Family socioeconomic status	−0.05 *** (0.009)	−0.041 *** (0.008)	−0.058 *** (0.007)	−0.058 *** (0.009)	−0.055 *** (0.012)	−0.067 *** (0.017)
Control variables						
Gender (Female)	−0.030 *** (0.003)	−0.017 *** (0.003)	−0.023 *** (0.003)	−0.028 *** (0.003)	−0.032 *** (0.004)	−0.039 *** (0.005)
Age	0.006 *** (0.000)	0.003 *** (0.000)	0.004 *** (0.000)	0.00 6*** (0.000)	0.007*** (0.000)	0.008 *** (0.000)
Marital status (Without spouse)	−0.012 *** (0.004)	0.001 (0.003)	−0.004 (0.004)	−0.015 *** (0.004)	−0.021 *** (0.006)	−0.022 *** (0.008)
Residential area (Rural)	0.007 ** (0.003)	0.002 (0.003)	0.006 * (0.003)	0.004 (0.003)	0.007 (0.004)	0.013 ** (0.006)
Living with family members (No)	0.031 *** (0.004)	0.012 *** (0.003)	0.018 ** (0.004)	0.031 *** (0.005)	0.037 *** (0.006)	0.040 *** (0.009)
Living in an institution (No)	0.106 *** (0.010)	0.044 *** (0.011)	0.058 *** (0.010)	0.100 *** (0.019)	0.145 *** (0.018)	0.173 *** (0.027)
Number of surviving children	−0.002 ** (0.001)	−0.002 ** (0.001)	−0.002 ** (0.001)	−0.003 *** (0.001)	−0.002 (0.001)	0.001 (0.002)
Old-age insurance (Do not have)	−0.001 (0.003)	−0.002 (0.003)	0.000 (0.003)	−0.003 (0.003)	−0.005 (0.005)	0.004 (0.006)
Medical insurance (Do not have)	−0.012 *** (0.004)	−0.002 (0.003)	−0.006 (0.004)	−0.014 ** (0.006)	−0.013 ** (0.006)	−0.013 (0.010)
Constant	−0.260 *** (0.014)	−0.148 *** (0.017)	−0.192 *** (0.013)	−0.264 *** (0.014)	−0.317 *** (0.022)	−0.290 *** (0.027)
R^2/Pseudo R^2	0.310	0.081	0.126	0.196	0.234	0.207

The robust standard errors are in parentheses in Model 1, and the statistic for measuring goodness-of-fit is R^2. The bootstrap standard errors are in parentheses in Models 2–6, with a sample size of 100, and the statistic for measuring goodness-of-fit is Pseudo R^2. * $p < 0.1$, ** $p < 0.05$, *** $p < 0.01$.

Because of the high heterogeneity of the health status of older adults, the same family socioeconomic status may have different effects on older adults with different frailty status. Then we also developed quantile regression models to analyze the effects of family socioeconomic status on the elderly health in different quantiles. Models 2–6 in Table 2 show that the effects of family socioeconomic status of older adults on the frailty index remain significantly negative at the 1% level, and the coefficients of the effects are, respectively, −0.041, −0.058, −0.058, −0.055, −0.067.

The results of the multivariate linear regression model and quantile regression models suggest that improving family socioeconomic status can reduce the frailty index and promote the health of the elderly.

4.2. Robustness Test

In the current study, the economic status compared with local people, the average years of education, and the average occupational level before retirement of elderly couples are integrated into the replaced family socioeconomic status index using the entropy weight method to conduct a robustness test. Models 7–12 in Table 3 show that the effects of replaced family socioeconomic status of older adults on the frailty index remain significantly negative at the 1% level, and the coefficients of the effects are, respectively, −0.070, −0.050, −0.071, −0.075, −0.081, −0.100. These results also demonstrate that the increase of family socioeconomic status can decrease the frailty index and promote the elderly health, indicating that the empirical results obtained above are reliable.

Table 3. Regression results after replacing the explanatory variable.

Variables	Model 7	Model 8	Model 9	Model 10	Model 11	Model 12
	OLS	Q10	Q25	Q50	Q75	Q90
Replaced family socioeconomic status	−0.070 ***	−0.050 ***	−0.071 ***	−0.075 ***	−0.081 ***	−0.100 ***
	(0.011)	(0.009)	(0.008)	(0.011)	(0.015)	(0.024)
Constant	−0.258 ***	−0.147 ***	−0.192 ***	−0.261 ***	−0.310 ***	−0.284 ***
	(0.014)	(0.015)	(0.014)	(0.016)	(0.021)	(0.024)
R^2/Pseudo R^2	0.311	0.082	0.127	0.197	0.235	0.209

The robust standard errors are in parentheses in Model 7, and the statistic for measuring goodness-of-fit is R^2. The bootstrap standard errors are in parentheses in Models 8–12, with a sample size of 100, and the statistic for measuring goodness-of-fit is Pseudo R^2. *** $p < 0.01$. The control variables in each model have been controlled.

4.3. Heterogeneity Analysis

The above analysis found that both residential area and age have significant influence on the health of the elderly. Therefore, we used the multiple linear regression model to continue to analyze the different effects of family socioeconomic status on the health of the elderly in different residential areas and at different ages.

Table 4 shows that the impacts of the family socioeconomic status of the urban and rural elderly on the frailty index are −0.043 and −0.088, both significant at the 1% level. However, the impact in urban areas is lower than rural areas.

Table 4. Results of multiple linear regression (with explanatory variable) by residential area.

Variables	Model 13		Model 14	
	Urban		Rural	
	Coefficient	Standard Deviation	Coefficient	Standard Deviation
Family socioeconomic status	−0.043 ***	0.011	−0.088 ***	0.018
Constant	−0.282 ***	0.019	−0.215 ***	0.021
n	4333		3266	
F value	228.130 ***		163.550 ***	
R^2	0.313		0.309	

*** $p < 0.01$. The control variables in each model have been controlled.

Table 5 shows that the effects of family socioeconomic status on the frailty index for the elderly aged 60–69 and 70–79 years (lower and middle age) are −0.043 and −0.088, both significant at the 1% level, whereas the effect of family socioeconomic status on the frailty index is no longer significant for the elderly aged 80 years and above (higher age).

Table 5. Results of multiple linear regression (with explanatory variable) by age.

Variables	Model 15		Model 16		Model 17	
	60–69 Years Old		70–79 Years Old		80 Years Old and Above	
	Coefficient	Standard Deviation	Coefficient	Standard Deviation	Coefficient	Standard Deviation
Family socioeconomic status	−0.086 ***	0.018	−0.094 ***	0.014	−0.009	0.014
Constant	0.046	0.115	−0.124 **	0.058	−0.423 ***	0.028
n	976		1977		4646	
F Value	10.910 ***		12.880 ***		144.100 ***	
R^2	0.116		0.080		0.220	

** $p < 0.05$, *** $p < 0.01$. The control variables in each model have been controlled.

4.4. Mediating Effect Analysis

The level of family socioeconomic status generally directly affects the overall living status, leisure and recreation status, and health-care status of the elderly. Therefore, those were selected as mediating variables to analyze their mediation effects in the influence of family socioeconomic status on elderly health. Table 6 shows the results after adding each mediating variable to the baseline linear regression model. From the comparison with Model 1, it can be seen that the absolute values of the impact coefficients of family socioeconomic status in Models 18–20 are becoming smaller and still significant at the 1% level, and that the impact coefficients of each mediating variable are significantly negative at the 1% level, which initially indicates the existence of mediation effects for each of the above mediating variables.

Table 6. Results of multiple linear regression adding mediating variables.

Variables	Model 18		Model 19		Model 20	
	Coefficient	Standard Deviation	Coefficient	Standard Deviation	Coefficient	Standard Deviation
	Explanatory variable					
Family socioeconomic status	−0.030 ***	0.009	−0.035 ***	0.009	−0.049 ***	0.009
	Mediating variables					
Overall living status	−0.071 ***	0.003				
Leisure and recreation status			−0.054 ***	0.004		
Health-care status					−0.032 ***	0.003
Constant	−0.243 ***	0.013	−0.243 ***	0.014	−0.217 ***	0.014
F value	392.380 ***		348.410 ***		332.720 ***	
R^2	0.363		0.319		0.319	

*** $p < 0.01$. The control variables in each model have been controlled.

We further tested the mediation effect by calculating the confidence interval through a two-step regression method. The results in Table 7 show that the 95% confidence intervals of the estimated mediation effects for the overall living status and leisure and recreation status are, respectively, [−0.116, −0.074] and [−0.184, −0.127]; they do not contain 0, indicating the existence of mediating effects in the impact of family socioeconomic status on elderly health. Moreover, the 95% confidence interval of the estimated mediation effect for the health-care status is [−0.014, 0.004] and contains 0, indicating the absence of the mediation effect.

Table 7. Estimated results of mediating effects.

Mediating Variables	Mediating Effect	Standard Deviation	95% Confidence Interval	Yes/No
Overall living status	−0.095	0.013	[−0.116, −0.074]	Yes
Leisure and recreation status	−0.155	0.017	[−0.184, −0.127]	Yes
Health-care status	−0.005	0.006	[−0.014, 0.004]	No

We set rho as 0, alpha as 0.1, and type as "mc" in the R software.

5. Discussion

In the current study, based on the CLHLS in 2018, the total family income, the comprehensive years of education, and the comprehensive occupational rank before retirement of the elderly couples were synthesized into a family socioeconomic status index that was used as the explanatory variable using the entropy weight method, and the frailty index was used as a measurement of the comprehensive health status of the elderly. First, we established the multiple linear regression model and quantile regression models to analyze the effects of family socioeconomic status on the health status of the elderly and conducted a robustness test using the replaced explanatory variable. Then, the heterogeneity of the effect of family socioeconomic status on the health status of the elderly among different residential areas and at different ages was analyzed. Finally, the overall living status, leisure and recreation status, and health-care status of older adults were used as mediating variables to analyze their mediation effects in the influence of family socioeconomic status on elderly health.

Family socioeconomic status has a positive impact on the health status of the elderly. This result is same to those of other researchers [18,20,21,30]. Family socioeconomic status reflects the individual's ability to obtain material and social resources [31]. Higher family socioeconomic status usually means higher total family income, education, and occupational rank [18]. Older adults with higher total family income tend to have better living conditions, participate in more leisure and entertainment activities to meet higher-lever needs, and purchase better health-care services to increase investment in health. Elderly families with higher years of education have acquired higher health awareness and literacy during their continuous learning and developed healthier living habits; they are more aware of various health risk factors and therefore more aware of their prevention, and are able to respond more quickly and effectively when they encounter diseases. Older households with higher occupational rank tend to have a higher proportion of pensions and have higher pensions; in addition, higher occupational rank tends to be accompanied by more available access to health-care services. Thus, higher family income, education, and occupational rank generally result in better health outcomes for older adults. Family socioeconomic status is a comprehensive reflection of the individual socioeconomic status of elderly couples, and it is the social class or status of elderly couples based on the family cooperation model. Therefore, the increase of family socioeconomic status can decrease the frailty index and promote the elderly health.

Due to the typical dual economic structure of urban and rural areas in China, the family socioeconomic status of the urban elderly is relatively higher (the average family socioeconomic status indices of the urban and rural elderly in the present study are, respectively, 0.237 and 0.126). Additionally, public health and medical resources in urban areas are more abundant and the allocation is more reasonable, while these conditions in rural areas are relatively poor. Under the influence of the law of diminishing marginal utility of the health production function [4,18], the family socioeconomic status of the urban elderly has lower influence on the frailty index. Some scholars also hold the analogous view [13,18]. In other words, when the family socioeconomic status changes by an equal amount, it has a higher impact on the health of the rural elderly.

Family socioeconomic status has a significantly positive influence on the health status of middle and lower age elderly, but not on higher age elderly, which is similar to the conclusion of other related studies [32,33]. When older adults reach the higher age, their physical functions continue to decline, and their health status becomes increasingly dependent on the individual and less influenced by other factors, including the family socioeconomic status, whereupon the effect of family socioeconomic status on the health of the higher age elderly is no longer significant.

A review study by Huang showed that there are four mediating pathways between socioeconomic status and health: material factors, lifestyle factors, psychosocial factors, and neighborhood [34]. Unlike that, we think that overall living status and leisure and recreation status have mediation effects in the influence of family socioeconomic status on the health status of the elderly, whereas health-care status has no mediation effect, which is different from the conclusion of other studies as well [12–14,35,36]. When older adults have a higher family socioeconomic status, on the one hand, their sources of living are often more abundant and their quality of life is usually higher, and thus their overall living status is better. They will pay more attention to direct investment in health. On the other hand, their health awareness tends to be higher, and it is more likely to increase the physical resistance through exercise and to relax by participating in various leisure and recreational activities. Therefore, overall living status and leisure and recreation status have mediation effects in the influence of family socioeconomic status on elderly health. With the expansion of medical insurance coverage and regular physical examination in China, not subject to the family socioeconomic status, more and more elderly people are able to be hospitalized in time when they fall ill and participate in annual routine medical checkups. As the basic public health services become more equalized, health-care status has no mediation effect in the effect of family socioeconomic status on elderly health.

There were several limitations to this research. First, the study only used the 2018 cross-sectional data, so we did not reveal the dynamic impact of family socioeconomic status on elderly health. Second, limited by the variables in CLHLS data, only 32 indicators were used to construct the frailty index. If more indicators can be obtained, the measurement of frailty index will be more accurate. Third, total family income and primary occupation rank before retirement of the elderly might be related to their health status, so there might be a reverse causality between family socioeconomic status and frailty index to some extent.

6. Conclusions

The main findings of this study are as follows:

1. This study explores the relationship between family socioeconomic status and the health status of the elderly in China from a comprehensive perspective. The improvement of the family socioeconomic status of the elderly will lower their frailty index, thereby promoting the improvement of their health.
2. The influence of family socioeconomic status on elderly health shows obvious urban–rural differences. Compared with the urban elderly, the family socioeconomic status of the rural elderly has a higher impact on the health of the elderly. As the public health and medical resources in urban areas are more abundant and the allocation is more reasonable, while these conditions in rural areas are relatively poor, the effect of promoting the health of the rural elderly by improving their family socioeconomic status is more significant.
3. The impacts of family socioeconomic status on the health of the elderly in different age groups are different. Family socioeconomic status has a significantly positive influence on the health status of middle and lower age elderly, but not on higher age elderly. As the elderly age, their physical functions continue to decline and their psychological status becomes more stable, and their health status becomes increasingly dependent on the individual and less influenced by other factors, including the family socioeconomic status.
4. Overall living status and leisure and recreation status have mediation effects in the influence of family socioeconomic status on the health status of the elderly, whereas health-care status has no mediation effect. Family socioeconomic status is to some extent the decisive factor of overall living status and leisure and recreation status. With the continuous equalization of China's medical and health services, the mediating role of health-care status in the impact has become weaker.

Based on the above research, we propose the following countermeasures:

1. Improve the old-age insurance system. Expand the coverage of old-age insurance and improve pension benefits. At the same time, increase the transfer payment to the elderly and strengthen the economic security ability for them to improve their living conditions.
2. Promote healthy aging of the elderly. Enlarge the enrollment scale of universities for the elderly and enrich the teaching contents. In particular, health education for the elderly should be strengthened to improve their health awareness and health literacy.
3. Accelerate the implementation of the delayed retirement policy and gradually postpone the retirement age of the elderly. At the same time, accelerate the development of human resources of the elderly to delay the decline of their occupational rank.
4. Improve the medical insurance system. Expand the coverage of medical insurance and increase the reimbursement ratio of medical expenses. At the same time, improve the level of health-care technology and improve the health-care status of the elderly.

5. Promote active aging of the elderly. On the one hand, the government and society should provide more leisure and recreational activities, places, and facilities; on the other hand, the elderly should be encouraged to participate in more recreational activities and other social activities.
6. Pay more attention to the key elderly populations. For example, public health policies should be strengthened for the rural elderly and the higher age elderly.

Author Contributions: Conceptualization, W.Z. and J.H.; methodology, M.S.; software, M.S.; validation, W.Z., J.H., M.S. and C.W.; formal analysis, W.Z.; writing—original draft preparation, W.Z.; writing—review and editing, J.H.; project administration, C.W. All authors have read and agreed to the published version of the manuscript.

Funding: This research received no external funding.

Acknowledgments: Data used for this research were provided by the study entitled "Chinese Longitudinal Longevity Survey" (CLHLS) managed by the Center for Healthy Aging and Development Studies, Peking University.

Conflicts of Interest: The authors declare no conflict of interest.

References

1. National Bureau of Statistics of China. The 7th Population Census Bulletin. Available online: http://www.stats.gov.cn/tjsj/tjgb/rkpcgb/qgrkpcgb/202106/t20210628_1818824.html (accessed on 1 December 2021).
2. The CPC Central Committee; State Council of China. The CPC Central Committee and the State Council Issue Healthy China 2030 Plan Outline. Available online: http://www.gov.cn/xinwen/2016-10/25/content_5124174.htm (accessed on 1 December 2021).
3. The CPC Central Committee. Proposal of the Central Committee of the Communist Party of China on Formulating the 14th Five-Year Plan for National Economic and Social Development and the Long-Term Goals for 2035. Available online: http://www.gov.cn/zhengce/2020-11/03/content_5556991.htm (accessed on 1 December 2021).
4. Grossman, M. Concept of Health Capital and Demand for Health. *J. Political Econ.* **1972**, *80*, 223–255. [CrossRef]
5. Su, Q.; Li, H. The Impact of Residents' Socioeconomic Status on Objective Health—An Empirical Analysis Based on the Panel Data of CHNS 1989–2015. *J. Fujian Agric. For. Univ. Philos. Soc. Sci.* **2021**, *4*, 60–69.
6. Meng, D.; Li, Z.; Zhou, S.; Zhu, X.; Su, L. A Study on the Correlation between Students' Family Socioeconomic Status and Types of Institutions of Higher Learning and Major Selection (PART I). *J. Yuzhou Univ. Soc. Sci. Ed.* **1996**, *3*, 64–75.
7. Winkleby, M.A.; Jatulis, D.E.; Fortmann, P. Socioeconomic Status and Health-How Education, Income, and Occupation Contribute to Risk-Factors for Cardiovascular-Disease. *Am. J. Public Health* **1992**, *6*, 816–820. [CrossRef] [PubMed]
8. Zhaiping, H. Socioeconomic Status and Social Support Network of the Rural Elderly and Their Physical and Mental Health. *Soc. Sci. China* **2002**, *3*, 135–148, 207.
9. Zhang, T.; Wang, C.; Yang, H.; Lin, H.; Zhang, T.; Wang, H.; Gong, G.; Zhang, X. Socioeconomic Status and Health Status of the Elderly. *Chin. Prim. Health Care* **2002**, *9*, 9–11.
10. Kuo, W.Y.; Hsu, H.S.; Kung, P.T.; Tsai, W.C. Impact of Socioeconomic Status on Cancer Incidence Risk, Cancer Staging, and Survival of Patients with Colorectal Cancer under Universal Health Insurance Coverage in Taiwan. *Int. J. Environ. Res. Public Health* **2021**, *18*, 12164. [CrossRef]
11. Schetter, C.D.; Schafer, P.; Lanzi, R.G.; Clark-Kauffman, E.; Raju, T.N.K.; Hillemeier, M.M. Shedding Light on the Mechanisms Underlying Health Disparities through Community Participatory Methods: The Stress Pathway. *Perspect. Psychol. Sci.* **2013**, *8*, 613–633. [CrossRef]
12. Xue, X.D.; Ge, K.X. The Effect of Socioeconomic Status on the Health of the Elderly in China: Evidence from the Chinese Longitudinal Healthy Longevity Survey. *Popul. Dev.* **2017**, *2*, 61–69.
13. Liu, C.P.; Wang, L.J. A Study of the Impact of Socio-Economic Status on the Health of the Elderly. *Chin. J. Popul. Sci.* **2017**, *5*, 40–50, 127.
14. Wang, F.; Ma, Y. Socioeconomic Status, Social Capital and Health Inequality. *J. Huazhong Univ. Sci. Technol. Soc. Sci. Ed.* **2020**, *6*, 59–66.
15. Gil-Flores, J. Measuring Primary School Students' Family Socioeconomic Status. *Rev. Educ.* **2013**, *362*, 298–322.
16. Zhu, Y.; Zhang, S. The Relative Influence of Education and Family Status on Youth's Initial Occupational Status: A Trend Analysis between 1977 and 2014. *Fudan Educ. Forum* **2020**, *6*, 79–86.
17. Cheng, G.; Liu, J.; Lin, N.; Huang, J.; Wang, X. The Relationship between Family Socioeconomic Status and Mental Health of Middle School Students: The Mediating Role of Psychological Quality. *J. Southwest Univ. Soc. Sci. Ed.* **2019**, *1*, 105–112.
18. Huang, Q.; Li, K.; Xiong, D. Family Socio Economic Status and Resident Health Research Based on Dual Perspectives of Lifestyle and Social Support. *J. Yunnan Univ. Finance Econ.* **2020**, *7*, 66–80.
19. Cao, G.; Du, B. Study on the Role of Early Family Socioeconomic Status and Parental Style on Health in Old Age. *Northwest Popul. J.* **2020**, *2*, 79–89.

20. Ghasemi, S.R.; Zangeneh, A.; Rajabi-Gilan, N.; Reshadat, S.; Saeidi, S.; Ziapour, A. Health-Related Quality of Life in Informal Settlements in Kermanshah, Islamic Republic of Iran: Role of Poverty and Perception of Family Socioeconomic Status. *East. Mediterr. Health J.* **2019**, *25*, 775–783. [CrossRef] [PubMed]
21. Booysen, F.; Botha, F.; Wouters, E. Conceptual Causal Models of Socioeconomic Status, Family Structure, Family Functioning and Their Role in Public Health. *BMC Public Health* **2021**, *21*, 191. [CrossRef] [PubMed]
22. Yang, Y.; Meng, Y. Is China Moving toward Healthy Aging? A Tracking Study Based on 5 Phases of CLHLS Data. *Int. J. Environ. Res. Public Health* **2020**, *17*, 4343. [CrossRef]
23. Ye, L.; Luo, J.; Shia, B.; Fang, Y. Multidimensional Health Groups and Healthcare Utilization Among Elderly Chinese: Based on the 2014 CLHLS Dataset. *Int. J. Environ. Res. Public Health* **2019**, *16*, 3884. [CrossRef]
24. Gu, L.; Cheng, Y.; Phillips, D.R.; Rosenberg, M. Understanding the Wellbeing of the Oldest-Old in China: A Study of Socio-Economic and Geographical Variations Based on CLHLS Data. *Int. J. Environ. Res. Public Health* **2019**, *16*, 601. [CrossRef] [PubMed]
25. Hwang, A.-C.; Lee, W.-J.; Huang, N.; Chen, L.-Y.; Peng, L.-N.; Lin, M.-H.; Chou, Y.-J.; Chen, L.-K. Longitudinal Changes of Frailty in 8 Years: Comparisons between Physical Frailty and Frailty Index. *BMC Geriatrics* **2021**, *21*, 726. [CrossRef]
26. Zeng, X. Comprehensive Index of Elderly Health Research Progress of Frailty Index. *Chin. J. Gerontol.* **2010**, *21*, 3220–3223.
27. Li, Y. Integration Journey: The Social Mobility Trajectory of Ethnic Minority Groups in Britain. *Soc. Incl.* **2018**, *6*, 270–281. [CrossRef]
28. Tofighi, D.; Mackinnon, D. RMediation: An R Package for Mediation Analysis Confidence Intervals. *Behav. Res. Methods* **2011**, *43*, 692–700. [CrossRef] [PubMed]
29. Fang, J.; Wen, Z.; Zhang, M. Mediation Analysis of Categorical Variables. *Psychol. Sci.* **2017**, *2*, 471–477.
30. Kong, F.; Xu, L.; Kong, M.; Li, S.; Zhou, C.; Zhang, J.; Ai, B. Association between Socioeconomic Status, Physical Health and Need for Long-Term Care among the Chinese Elderly. *Int. J. Environ. Res. Public Health* **2019**, *16*, 2124. [CrossRef]
31. Bian, F.; Wu, D. The Impact of Family Socioeconomic Status on Prosocial Behavior: A Survey of College Students in China. *Curr. Psychol.* **2021**. [CrossRef]
32. Yang, Y.; Sun, L.; Zhang, H.; Silin, H.; Xiao, Z. Allosatic Load and Its Relationship with Socioeconomic Health Disparities. *Adv. Psychol. Sci.* **2018**, *26*, 1475–1487. [CrossRef]
33. Crimmins, E.; Kim, J.; Seeman, T. Poverty and Biological Risk: The Earlier "Aging" of the Poor. *J. Gerontol. A Biol. Sci. Med. Sci.* **2009**, *64*, 286–292. [CrossRef]
34. Jieping, H. A System Review of Mechanism of SES to Health. *J. Beijing Inst. Technol. Soc. Sci. Ed.* **2014**, *6*, 52–60.
35. Xue, Y.; Lu, J.; Zheng, J.; Zhang, J.; Lin, H.; Qin, Z.; Zhang, C. The Relationship between Socioeconomic Status and Depression among the Older Adults: The Mediating Role of Health Promoting Lifestyle. *J. Affect. Disord.* **2021**, *285*, 22–28. [CrossRef] [PubMed]
36. Yang, Y.; Wang, S.; Chen, L.; Luo, M.; Xue, L.; Cui, D.; Mao, Z. Socioeconomic Status, Social Capital, Health Risk Behaviors, and Health-Related Quality of Life among Chinese Older Adults. *Health Qual. Life Outcomes* **2020**, *18*, 291. [CrossRef] [PubMed]

buildings

MDPI

Article

A Comparison of Energy Consumption in American Homes by Climate Region

Luciana Debs [1,*] and Jamie Metzinger [2]

[1] School of Construction Management Technology, Purdue University, West Lafayette, IN 47907, USA
[2] Department of Built Environment, Indiana State University, Terre Haute, IN 47809, USA; jamie.metzinger@indstate.edu
* Correspondence: ldecresc@purdue.edu

Abstract: The present research analyzes the impact of nine factors related to household demographics, building equipment, and building characteristics towards a home's total energy consumption while controlling for climate. To do this, we have surveyed single-family owned houses from the 2015 Residential Energy Consumption Survey (RECS) dataset and controlled the analysis by Building America climate zones. Our findings are based on descriptive statistics and multiple regression models, and show that for a median-sized home in three of the five climate zones, heating equipment is still the main contributor to a household's total energy consumed, followed by home size. Social-economic factors and building age were found relevant for some regions, but often contributed less than size and heating equipment towards total energy consumption. Water heater and education were not found to be statistically relevant in any of the regions. Finally, solar power was only found to be a significant factor in one of the regions, positively contributing to a home's total energy consumed. These findings are helpful for policymakers to evaluate the specificities of climate regions in their jurisdiction, especially guiding homeowners towards more energy-efficient heating equipment and home configurations, such as reduced size.

Keywords: RECS; energy consumption; residential construction; multiple regression analysis; Building America climate zones

Citation: Debs, L.; Metzinger, J. A Comparison of Energy Consumption in American Homes by Climate Region. *Buildings* **2022**, *12*, 82. https://doi.org/10.3390/buildings12010082

Academic Editors: Roberto Alonso González Lezcano, Francesco Nocera and Rosa Giuseppina Caponetto

Received: 19 November 2021
Accepted: 13 January 2022
Published: 16 January 2022

1. Introduction

In 2020, energy consumption in buildings, that is commercial and residential usage combined, accounted for approximately 40% of the total energy consumed in the United States [1]. Despite many Americans having to work and study from home due to workplace restrictions and local lockdowns because of the COVID-19 pandemic, total residential energy consumption including energy system losses presented a 4% reduction compared to that of 2019. Part of this result can be linked to warmer weather during winter, which helped to reduce the use of heating in homes [2]. While this information is positive, the increased time spent at home stresses the importance of understanding energy consumption patterns in American homes to further improve their efficiency and to provide guidance for policymakers on the matter. Additionally, topics related to energy consumption patterns are increasingly important to students and professionals of the built environment given the United Nations Sustainable Development Goal 7—affordable and clean energy [3].

It is well known that energy consumption in homes is mainly affected by physical characteristics of the home, household characteristics and behavior, home appliances, and exterior factors, including energy market and climate [4]. Physical characteristics of the home include building materials, home configuration, and size, among others. Household factors include behavioral factors, such as their level of environmental consciousness and also intrinsic characteristics, such as education, income, number of members. Home appliances include the different appliances and equipment in the home, given that some are more efficient than others. Exterior factors include primarily location and climate characteristics. It is well known that changes in weather can have a significant impact on the energy consumption of traditional homes [5].

Although isolated factors have been widely studied, few published research studies have explored the interaction of factors related to energy consumption in homes. Hirst et al. [6] have provided an interesting analysis of the contribution of several factors to a home's energy consumption, though the study is now decades old. Other recent studies also based on previous versions of the Residential Energy Consumption Survey (RECS) have provided a baseline on the effects of household and physical characteristics of homes, but they did not separate their analysis by climate zones. Furthermore, while they have provided interesting results, some of them did not control for housing type [4,7,8], or, when housing type was controlled for, researchers evaluated only electricity consumption [9]. A more nuanced analysis of total energy consumption by region and controlling for the most frequent home type in the United States—the single-family home—can provide targeted information to guide specific energy-related built environment policies and improvement efforts.

To this end, we propose reviewing the most recently published microdata of the Residential Energy Consumption Survey (RECS), which was collected during 2015, and comparing the results per climate zone. Regression models were developed per Building America climate zones [10] and include factors related to physical characteristics of the home, household characteristics, and appliances and equipment used in the homes. Providing analysis per climate type allows for a more nuanced view of the factors' contributions to the overall energy consumption in a home, while still being able to match with geographical regions. Therefore, the significance and originality of the present study lie in the combination of (1) its focus on the most common housing typology in the United States (the single-family, detached home), (2) the use of an updated and large dataset to analyze the contribution of factors that are known to influence a household's energy consumption, and (3) the analysis the results by climate region.

2. Background Literature

The analysis of factors influencing energy consumption in buildings is a complex matter [8]. This is mainly because of the number of different factors and their potential interactions influencing energy consumption, which make interpretation of results difficult. In fact, Jones et al. [11] have surveyed academic papers to find 62 factors that may affect energy consumption in homes. However, of those 62, only 20 factors were consistently found to positively influence energy consumption. Despite that, many researchers have worked to improve our understanding of residential energy consumption. Even though there are several factors to be included in the analysis, they can generally be summarized into four main categories: physical characteristics of the home, household characteristics and behavior, home appliances, and exterior factors. These categories are adapted from Estiri [4] and we have combined energy market and climate into exterior factors.

Perhaps the most evident factor that influences energy is climate [12]. This includes temperature and humidity, in addition to solar radiation, wind, and rain [13]. Many studies use heating degree days (HDD) and cooling degree days (CDD) to verify the impact of temperature on energy consumption, such as those conducted by Hojjati and Wade [14], Sanquist et al. [9], and Iraganaboina and Eluru [7].

Home appliances and equipment also have an impact on a home's energy consumption pattern. Iraganaboina and Eluru [7] have found that homes with more appliances are prone to higher energy consumption. Additionally, previous research debated the impact of Energy Star appliances on a home's energy consumption and identified significant results only for Energy Start refrigerators [15]. Energy Star is a governmental program that aids consumers to identify more energy-efficient appliances and equipment in the United States [16].

Furthermore, home heating and cooling equipment is known to have the largest impact on energy consumption in a home [17], followed usually by water heating equipment [18].

It is also well known that equipment and fuel choices impact total energy used in a home [17,18].

In terms of renewable energy generated on-site, Iraganaboina and Eluru [7] have found that homes with solar power were likely to have higher electricity use. To this result, Iraganaboina and Eluru [7] provide an interesting explanation based on the use of solar power to offset electricity costs, but have not explored the issue further.

Other factors affecting residential energy consumption include the building's physical characteristics, such as type, year of construction, and size. Energy consumption is usually higher for single-family homes, mostly due to their larger size [14]. Other research has found building size to have an impact on energy consumption. For example, home size was found to impact energy consumption, which can be linked to its effect on a building's heating and cooling loads [19]. However, previous research has found this effect to also vary per fuel, with constant increases for gas and decreases for electricity, which can be related to the choice of heating fuel [7]. The effect of size is difficult to measure because it is often correlated with other factors such as family size, room number, and housing type [4]. It is also well known that the average home size has increased in the United States, with an estimated increase of 27.9% between 1980 and 2005 [14]. However, preliminary data from the United States Census indicate a very small decrease in median size for newly sold homes from an all-time high of 2526 square feet (234.67 square meters) in 2014 to 2333 square feet (216.74 square meters) in 2020 [20].

Building age has also been identified by previous research as having a significant effect on a home's energy consumption [12,21–23]. However, a study on the European Union has found that the impact of building age is not linearly related to energy consumption. In that study, older homes (built before 1921) were found to be more energy efficient than the average of all homes, and homes built between 1947 and 1979 were found to be the worst performers [20]. In the United States, Kavousian et al. [19] also verified a reduced energy consumption for homes built before 1975 if compared to homes built between 1993 and 2003, while analyzing close to one thousand American households. They ponder that this could be due to newer homes having appliances that consume more energy, such as air-conditioners [19], which is also suggested by other researchers [12].

Education and income level have been found to impact energy usage. Salari and Javid [23] found that a head of household with a higher education degree is effectively associated with lower energy usage. In a recent study, Debs et al. [24] indicated that energy consumption was significantly influenced by the respondents' highest educational degree, though the same was not found significant when assessing its influence on the total number of energy star appliances in a home.

Higher income may be associated with having more technology and electronics usage, but it does not contribute to a considerable or statistically significant increase in energy consumption [9,24,25]. In fact, previous research associated higher income with being able to afford more energy-efficient equipment [26]. However, recent research conducted in the United Kingdom indicated that an increase in wealth correlated with higher energy consumption, especially for energy-poorer households [27].

Finally, it is generally accepted that a larger household will use more energy [9,28]. Additionally, individual factors also play a part in energy usage. For example, previous research suggests that gender influences energy consumption, with men using less energy than women [28]. However, recent findings challenge biological differences related to energy consumption and suggest that social gender roles may help explain these differences [29]. Moreover, retirees and those that work from home tend to use more energy than those that work outside of the home [28]; age positively affects energy consumption [30] and those living in the city may utilize services not available to those in rural areas, such as laundry and cooking outside of the house [9].

Residential Energy Consumption Survey (RECS) Overview

The Residential Energy Consumption Survey (RECS) is managed by the United States Energy Information Administration (US EIA) and collects data about the energy consumption of homes across the United States periodically since 1979. It collects not only information about household characteristics, but also behavior, home appliances, climate, and physical characteristics of the house. It includes different types of homes, such as mobile homes, single-family detached and attached homes, as well as apartments in multi-family buildings. The latest iteration of the RECS, here called RECS 2015, evaluates data collected between August 2015 and April 2016 [31].

RECS 2015 surveys, methodology information, microdata, and codebook are publicly available online [32]. For the 2015 survey, "multi-stage area probability random sampling" [31] (p. 8) was used, resulting in 5686 households surveyed. Data collection used a combination of methods, including online and mail surveys, as well as interview procedures. This means the data is based on interviewees' willingness to participate and give accurate answers. And, in addition to contacting households, RECS also obtained energy information from energy suppliers. It is also important to note that for several questions in RECS, invalid or missing data were imputed using statistical modeling. Data imputation was used for approximately two-thirds of the surveyed homes in RECS 2015 [30].

Several previous researchers have used RECS datasets to explore several energy-related topics. Among those, are the studies by Hojjati and Wade [14], who analyzed RECS data from 1980 to 2005; Sanquist et al. [9], who used the 2001 and 2005 iterations to evaluate electricity consumption; Steemers and Yun [12], who evaluated 2001 RECS data for heating and cooling energy consumptions; Estiri [4], who used the 2009 RECS data to evaluated factors contributing to the energy consumption of American homes; and, more recently, work by Karatasou and Santamouris [8] and by Iraganaboina and Eluru [7] used the 2015 RECS dataset. Karatasou and Santamouris [8] focused on the impact of socio-economic variables on energy consumption, and Iraganaboina and Eluru [7] provided a broad analysis of household composition, size, and characteristics, as well as the type of fuels consumed by residences in the United States.

3. Materials and Methods

The present study uses descriptive statistics and inferential statistics to evaluate how certain factors contribute to the energy consumption in a home. The factors selected for analysis were briefly discussed in the background literature of the present paper and relate to physical characteristics of the home (home size and year built), household composition (education, income, and the number of household members), and home equipment (space heating type, air conditioning type, water heater type and use of on-site generation of solar power).

Our analysis is also delimited to single-family owned homes, given that most homeowners are responsible for their home and appliances maintenance and energy costs. Single-family detached homes were chosen because they account for approximately 63.91% of the housing stock in the United States in 2019 [33], and their consumption characteristics can significantly differ from other types of housing [4,34,35]. This resulted in a sample size of n = 3288 homes from the 2015 RECS dataset. Furthermore, as mentioned previously, the RECS survey includes data imputed using statistical modeling and this imputed data was the one utilized in the present study.

First, descriptive statistics are presented. These include frequency of categorial factors' levels per climate zone and median, mean and standard deviation for home size, and the number of household members. Additionally, descriptive statistics of fuel type of heating and cooling equipment and water heating equipment are included. The goal of the descriptive analysis results is to give an overview of the data to be further analyzed by the inferential statistics.

Then, for inferential statistics, we started by performing an analysis of variance (ANOVA) to evaluate differences in total BTU consumed per climate region, followed by five regression models—one for each Building America climate zone. This removes the need to include heat and cooling degree days as factors, but still controls for climate variation. This also allows results to be grouped geographically, which can help with policy decisions. RECS 2015 includes information about a home's climate using both Building America climate zones and the International Energy Conservation Code (IECC) Climate Code. The choice to use Building America climate zones was made to reach a balance between a reasonable number of models to compare (five), in comparison to eleven if using the IECC zones. Building America climate zones were elaborated by Department of Energy (DOE) researchers and are based on simplifying the IECC climate zones [10].

Total energy consumption in this paper will be measured in BTU and accounts for energy used in a home from gas, electricity, propane, and fuel oil (or kerosene) sources. It does not include wood as a fuel source. Factors included in the multiple regression model are based on previous research and consider physical characteristics of the home, household characteristics, and home equipment. Figure 1 illustrates the conceptual framework of the proposed model.

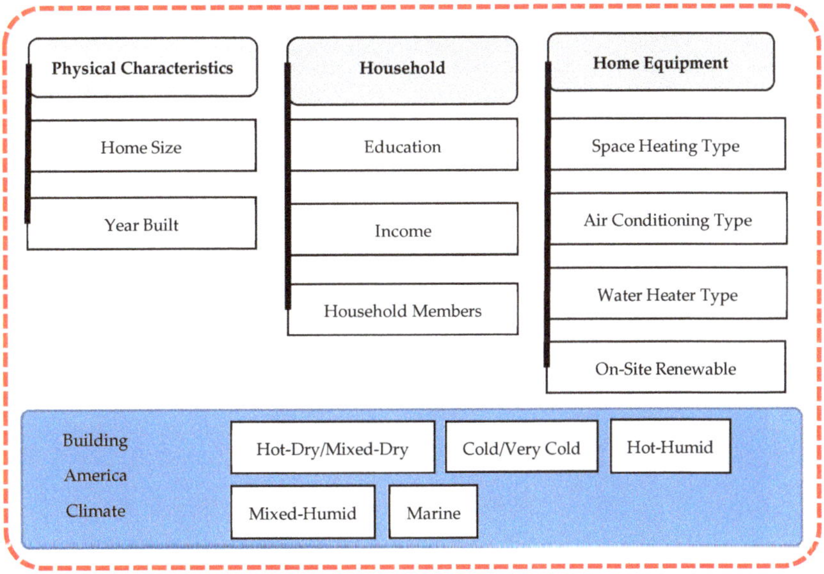

Figure 1. Proposed conceptual framework.

We also note that data from RECS for income and year built is presented as categorical. For income, data is collected in brackets of approximately \$20,000 to \$139,999, the following bracket includes incomes of \$140,000 or more. For the year built, data is presented in decades except for the first (for homes built before 1950) and the last bracket (for homes built 2010 to 2015). Because of the ordinal nature and reasonable spacing of most brackets of the categories in income and year built, both variables were treated as continuous in the regression model. This also simplifies the interpretation of the regression results [36]. Other variables in the model considered as continuous were the size of the home and the number of family members. All other variables are categorical and include education, type of heating equipment, type of air-conditioning equipment, type of water heating equipment, and on-site power generation from solar. Our working model for each Building America climate zone is represented by Equation (1):

$$Y_{TOTALBTU} = Intercept + \beta_{1\text{-}SIZE} + \beta_{2\text{-}YEAR} + \beta_{3\text{-}EDUCATION} + \beta_{4\text{-}INCOME} + \beta_{5\text{-}MEMBERS} + \beta_{6\text{-}HEATTYPE} + \beta_{7\text{-}ACTYPE} + \beta_{8\text{-}WATERTYPE} + \beta_{9\text{-}SOLAR} \quad (1)$$

where:

TOTALBTU = total energy consumption in thousand BTU (does not include wood),
SIZE = total heated square footage of home (continuous variable),
YEAR = year range a home was built (categorical, treated as a continuous variable),
EDUCATION = highest degree of education of respondent (categorical variable),
INCOME = household income (range) in 2014 (categorical, treated as a continuous variable),
MEMBERS = number of household members (discrete, treated as a continuous variable),
HEATTYPE = type of primary space heating equipment used in the home (categorical variable),
ACTYPE = type of primary air conditioning equipment used in the home (categorical variable),
WATERTYPE = type of primary water heater type used in the home (categorical variable),
SOLAR = existence of on-site solar energy generation (categorical variable).

Though appliances are found to influence a home's energy consumption [15], information about them was not included in the model because certain appliances did not apply to all respondents. Additionally, respondents could refuse to answer or indicate they "do not know" the answer to the question, making interpretation of responses too complicated and outside of the scope of the present research.

Regression models were evaluated using an automated backward stepwise approach in R Studio. The resulting model was additionally manually reviewed by researchers to remove any non-significant factors ($\alpha = 0.05$) also using a backward, stepwise approach.

4. Results

This section presents our results for the study. First, we present descriptive statistics related to the main factors utilized in the analysis. Following this, we present the results of our multiple regression analysis.

4.1. Descriptive Statistics

In this section, descriptive statistics focus on the factors included in our proposed conceptual framework, as well as fuel type for heating and cooling equipment and water heater fuel type. It considers only the data for our delimited sample of single-family, detached, and owned homes in the United States while providing estimates per Building America climate regions.

Climate. The distribution of homes per climate zone can be seen in Figure 2. Climate distribution for the sample indicated it included more homes built in the Cold/Very Cold climate zone (n = 37.41%), followed by Mixed-Humid (n = 25.85%), Hot-Humid (n = 17.61%), Hot-Dry/Mixed-Dry (n = 11.10%) and Marine (n = 8.03%). This distribution is expected, given the surface area coverage of each of the respective Building America climate regions analyzed.

Physical characteristics. The median house size in the sample was 2400 square feet with a standard deviation of 1284.5 square feet (119.33 square meters) (Table 1). Median size also varied by region, with Cold/Very Cold climate homes being larger and hot-humid homes being usually smaller. However, the standard deviation (SD) was considerably high (larger than 1000 square feet/92.9 square meters) for all regions.

Additionally, Figure 3 shows the relationship between home square footage and total energy consumption. Different colors and different shapes illustrate the data for each climate zone, as well as linear trendlines for each region. The graph shows that most houses are within 1000 square feet (92.9 square meters) and 4000 square feet (371.6 square meters), and the energy consumption is within 50 million and 125 million BTU (52.72 and 131.88 GJ). The spread of the data is larger for home size than for total energy consumption, but there are a few outliers.

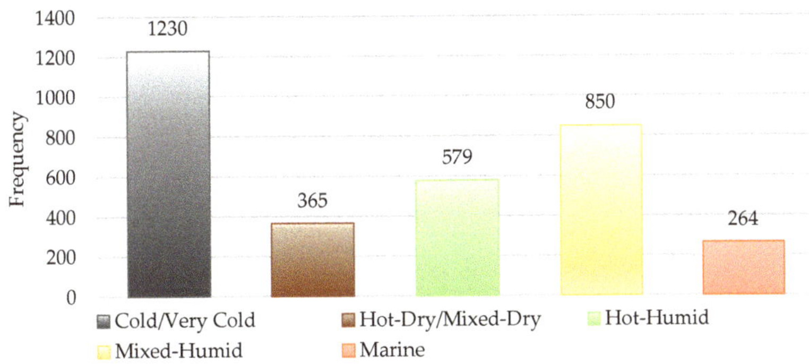

Figure 2. Distribution of homes per Building America climate zone (total n = 3288).

Table 1. Total square footage (sqft) and square meters (m^2) of home per climate zones (total n = 3288).

Climate Zone	Frequency	Median		Mean		SD	
		sqft	m^2	sqft	m^2	sqft	m^2
Cold/Very Cold	1230	2700	251	2889.64	268.46	1243.78	115.55
Hot-Dry/Mixed-Dry	365	2116	197	2402.85	223.23	1188.03	110.37
Hot-Humid	579	1904	177	2230.93	207.26	1130.66	105.04
Mixed-Humid	850	2519	234	2802.66	260.38	1408.21	130.83
Marine	264	1949	181	2245.54	208.62	1117.38	103.81
Total	3288	2400	223	2645.40	245.77	1284.51	119.33

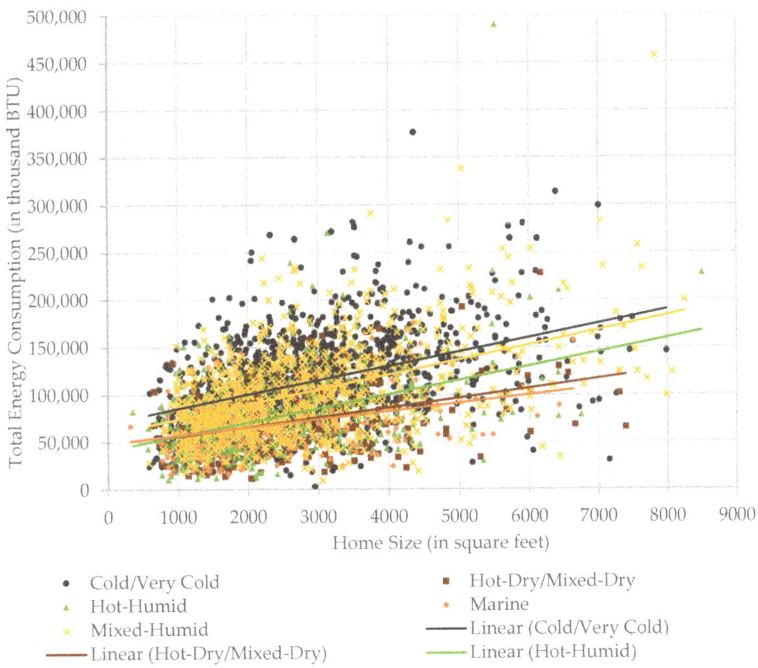

Figure 3. Box plot for the total square footage of homes per climate region.

The distribution of building age was fairly stable, with more homes being built between 2000 and 2009 (n = 16.8%) and before 1950 (n = 15.5%). The decades in between these two categories comprise between 10.2% (from 1960 to 1969) and 14.8% (between 1970 and 1979); homes built between 2010 and 2015 comprised the smallest percentage (n = 3.7%). Specific information for building age per climate region can be seen in Figure 4.

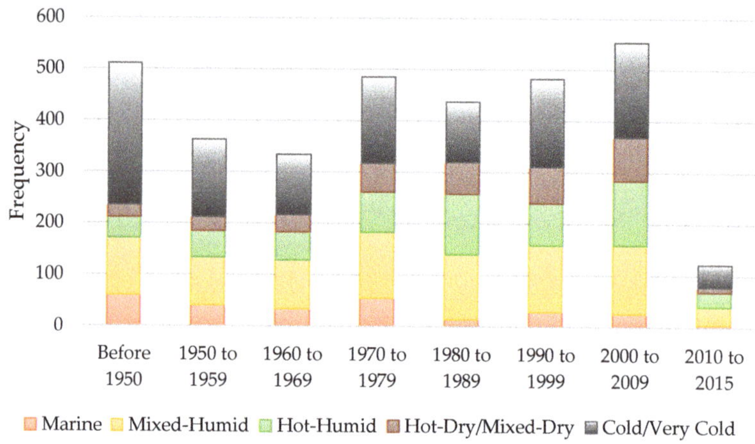

Figure 4. Year the home was built per Building America climate zone (total n = 3288).

Household characteristics. In terms of household education, about 32.8% of respondents indicated they had a college or an associate's degree, followed by an almost equal distribution of respondents with a high-school diploma or GED (n = 22.3%) and bachelor's degree (n = 22.1%); 17.8% of respondents had some sort of graduate degree, and only 5% had less than a high-school diploma or GED. This distribution seems to be similar for every region, as can be seen in Figure 5. We note that this question only asked for the respondent's highest educational degree and does not include information about the educational degrees of all household members.

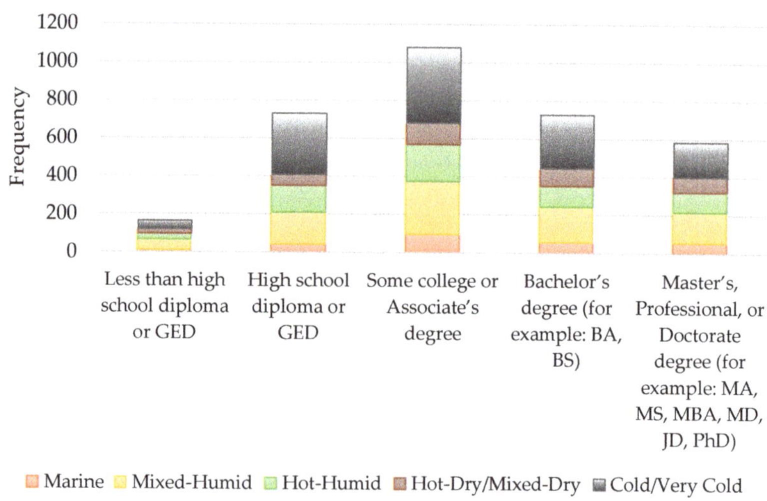

Figure 5. Household respondents' highest earned degree per climate zone (total n = 3288).

When asked about the income of the previous year (2014), the median answer indicated an income between $20,000 and $39,999 for their annual gross household income, with 18.8% of respondents indicating to fit that income bracket. Income seems to vary per region and Figure 6 shows the breakdown per income bracket for each Building America climate region. Hot-Dry/Mixed-Dry and Marine regions seem to have a more balanced sample across brackets than other regions.

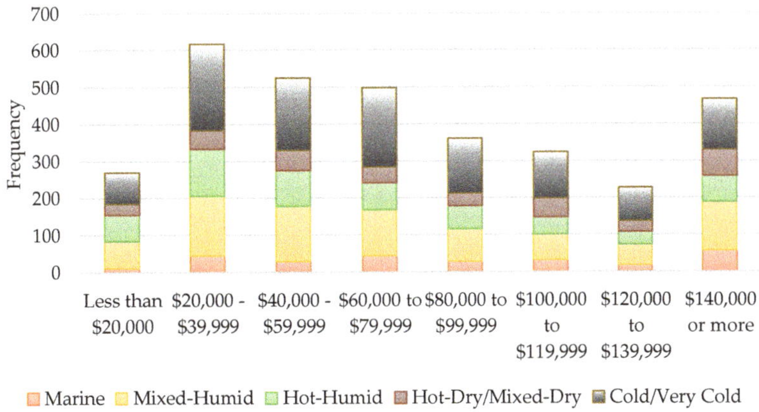

Figure 6. 2014 annual household income brackets per climate zone (total n = 3288).

In general, each household contained a minimum of one and a maximum of 11 members, with a mean of 2.69 people per household and a standard deviation of 1.396. In the case of household members, the median was 2 people per household for all regions. The mean number of people varied from a low of 2.60 in the Hot-Humid region to a high of 2.79 in the Hot-Dry/Mixed-Dry region. Figure 7 shows a box plot representation for the number of household members in each surveyed climate region and indicates a higher variability in the Marine, Mixed-Humid, and Hot-Dry/Mixed Dry regions, in which most homes house two to four people than Hot-Humid and Cold/Very Cold regions, in which most homes have two to three people only.

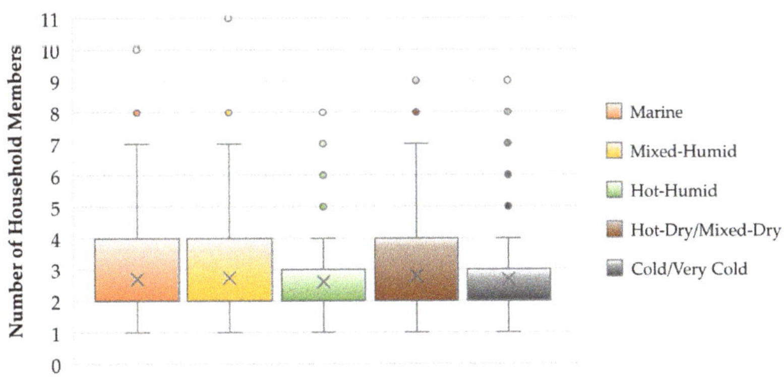

Figure 7. Box plot for the number of household members per climate region.

Equipment. In general, most of the surveyed homes utilized a central furnace as their main heating equipment (n = 65.9%), followed by heat pump (n = 14.8%). The remainder of the homes used other sources of heat (n = 17%) or heating was not applicable (n = 2.3%). When further analyzing equipment type per region, a central furnace is still the main type of equipment used, however, we can see heat pumps are proportionally more common in Hot-Humid, Mixed-Humid and Marine, than Cold/Very Cold and Hot-Dry/Mixed-Dry climates (see Figure 8).

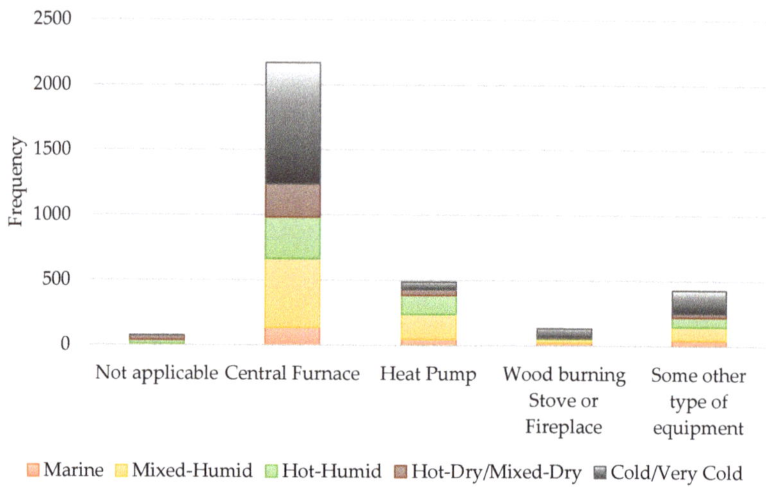

Figure 8. Type of main space heating equipment per climate zone (total n = 3288).

For main heating equipment fuel, most homes used natural gas from underground pipes (n = 54.6%), followed by electricity (n = 27.6%). Other fuels accounted for 15.5% of surveyed homes. For 2.3% of homes, heating fuel was not applicable. In all climate regions, electricity and piped natural gas were found to be the most prevalent fuels for main heating equipment in homes, but fuel oil/kerosene was found in almost as many homes as electricity for homes in the Cold/Very Cold climate. The breakdown can be seen in Table 2.

Table 2. Fuel used on main heating equipment per climate zones (total n = 3288).

Fuel Type	Frequency of Homes per Climate Zone				
	Cold/Very Cold	Hot-Dry/Mixed-Dry	Hot-Humid	Mixed-Humid	Marine
Not Applicable	1	32	30	1	10
Natural gas (piped)	808	243	192	425	128
Electricity	132	76	332	278	89
Fuel oil/kerosene	114	0	1	56	3
Propane (bottled gas)	93	9	15	62	10
Wood	76	5	9	28	24
Some other fuel	6	0	0	0	0
Total	1230	365	579	850	264

For air conditioning, most homes used a central air conditioning system (n = 69%), followed by individual window or wall, or portable units (n = 14.2%), and both a centralized system and individual units (n = 5.6%); for 11.6% of homes, air conditioning type was not applicable. When further analyzing per climate zone (Figure 9), we note a similar prevalence of central air-conditioning systems in all regions, except Marine. In the Marine climate zone, central air conditioning systems (n = 102) are almost as prevalent as not having air conditioning (n = 106).

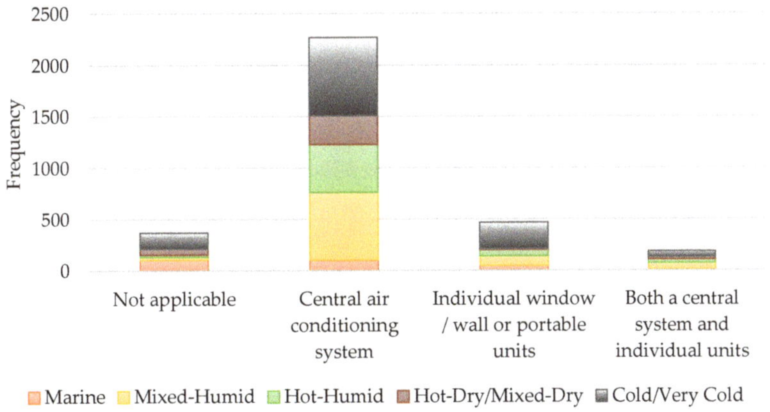

Figure 9. Type of main air conditioning equipment per climate zone (total n = 3288).

For water heaters, almost half of the homes used a medium storage-tank water heater (n = 48.7%), followed by water heaters with large storage tanks of 50 gallons (189.27 liters) or more (n = 38.2%). Small storage tank water heaters accounted for only 9.2% of the surveyed homes, and only 4% of homes had a tankless or on-demand water heater. This is similar to what is found in all regions, as can be seen in Figure 10. The two main fuel types used in water heaters were natural gas from underground pipes (n = 50.7%) and electricity (n = 41.2%), accounting for the vast majority of surveyed homes. When further analyzing per climate zone, results indicate that in all regions electricity and natural gas are the most prevalent fuel for water heating equipment. However, in Hot-Dry/Mixed-Dry regions, natural gas (n = 74.8%) is much more frequently used than electricity (n = 19.2%); this is similar for Cold/Very Cold regions, though with slightly lesser difference (natural gas n = 57.5% and electricity n = 30.9%). Only in Hot-Humid climate zones do homes seem to use electricity (n = 62.9%) for heating water more frequently than natural gas (n = 33.9%).

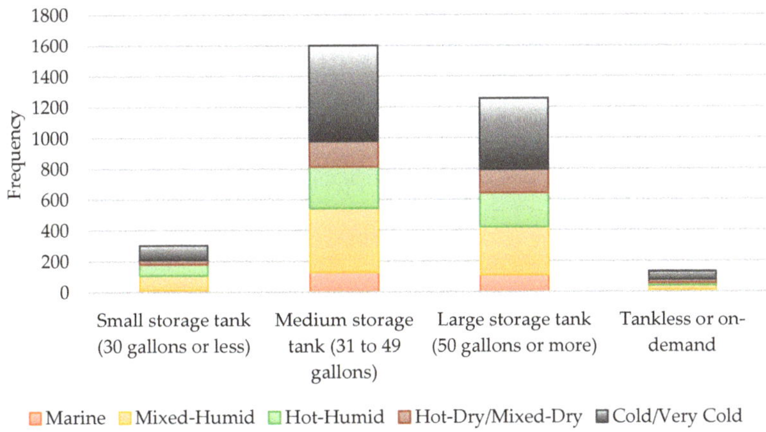

Figure 10. Type of water heating equipment per climate zone (total n = 3288).

Finally, when assessing the existence of on-site solar energy generation, we found that very few homes from the sample have this feature. For all climate zones, only 78 homes had on-site electricity generation from solar. Of those 78 homes, the region with most homes with solar power generation on-site was Hot-Dry/Mixed-Dry region (n = 30), followed by Cold/Very Cold (n = 15), Mixed-Humid (n = 13), Marine (n = 12) and Hot-Humid (n = 8).

4.2. Multiple Regression Analysis Results

First, a log transformation for total BTU was performed to improve the fit of residuals for every region. We note that for the Cold/Very Cold climate zone a quadratic transformation would yield a better model fit, but to standardize the procedures across the climate zones, a log transformation for total BTU was used in that region as well.

Second, a one-way ANOVA was run to evaluate differences in energy consumption between regions. The results indicate that we can reject the null hypothesis that all regions consume energy equally ($F = 168.315$, p-value < 0.001). Additionally, a box plot of LogBTU per climate region is presented in Figure 11 to help visualize results. A Tukey comparison between regions indicates that the five regions can be grouped into three main groups of total energy consumption—(1) Cold/Very Cold, (2) Mixed-Humid, and (3) remaining regions (Hot-Dry/Mixed-Dry, Hot-Humid, and Marine). We note that even though homes of some of the regions might have similar total energy consumption, we cannot assess if the distribution of that consumption—meaning how energy is spent in the home—is similar.

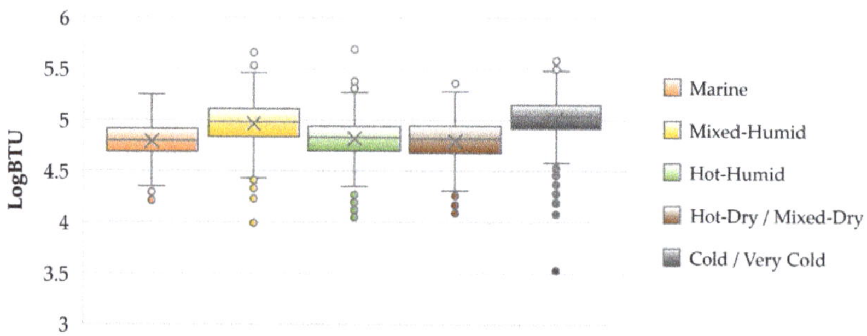

Figure 11. Box plot for LogBTU per climate region.

Five multiple regression models were then run for the present study—one for each Building America climate region. Equation (1), included in Section 3 (Methodology) represented the initial regression model. Final models vary per region, and Table 3 summarizes the parameter estimates in each of the factors. For factors treated as categorical, parameter estimates are included per level, if the factor was found significant at the 0.05 level. Size, year built, income, and the number of family members were treated as continuous variables. We note that the model did not present a significant result for education or type of water heater in any of the regions, therefore these factors were removed from Table 3 and Equation (2), which represents the revised model equation, which can still differ per climate region:

$$Y_{LOG\_TOTALBTU} = Intercept + \beta_{1\text{-}SIZE} + \beta_{2\text{-}YEAR} + \beta_{4\text{-}INCOME} + \beta_{5\text{-}MEMBERS} + \beta_{6\text{-}HEATTYPE} + \beta_{7\text{-}ACTYPE} + \beta_{9\text{-}SOLAR}. \quad (2)$$

The goodness of fit can be evaluated by the adjusted R-square value for each resulting model and varied from 0.2953 (Hot-Dry/Mixed-Dry region) to 0.4459 (Mixed-Humid region). We also note that even though a wood-burning fireplace or stove is included as a level of type of heating equipment, the wood consumption is not included in a home's total BTU usage in RECS and this information needs to be considered when analyzing homes that use this type of fuel.

Table 3. Parameter estimates and summary results of regression per region.

Factors	Climate				
	Cold/Very Cold	Hot-Dry/Mixed-Dry	Hot-Humid	Marine	Mixed-Humid
Estimate	9.066	9.991	10.36	9.899	9.843
Size [1]	0.0106	0.01052	0.01497	0.01108	0.00868
Year Built [2]	−0.0293	NS	−0.0485	NS	−0.02724
Income [3]	0.03301	0.02964	0.04807	NS	0.06760
Number Family Members	0.04976	0.06029	0.1021	0.05041	0.05165
Type of Heating Equipment					
Not applicable	Baseline	Baseline	Baseline	Baseline	Baseline
Central Furnace	1.978	0.4007	0.2794	0.7212	1.040
Heat Pump	1.547	0.1440	0.07365	0.6331	0.6779
Wood burning fireplace or stove	1.422	0.0278	−0.1966	0.3597	0.3683
Some other equipment	1.912	0.4322	0.1649	0.7275	0.9837
Type of Air-Conditioning			NS		
Not applicable	Baseline	Baseline		Baseline	Baseline
Central system	0.1152	0.2006		0.1617	0.1048
Individual unit(s)	0.0990	0.08995		0.1237	0.0457
Central & individual unit(s)	0.1442	0.06971		0.4219	0.1993
Solar Energy	NS	NS	NS		NS
Has solar				0.2367	
No solar				Baseline	
Adjusted R	0.3359	0.2953	0.3461	0.3102	0.4459
p-Value	<0.0001	<0.0001	<0.0001	<0.0001	<0.0001

Notes: Not Significant (NS). [1] in hundred square feet. [2] in decades for homes built after 1950. All homes before 1950 are combined. [3] in $20,000 increments until more than $140,000 per year. Categorical levels are italicized.

Cold and Very Cold Climate. This zone covers a large area of the United States. For this region, the reduced model contained all the revised Equation (2) variables, except for solar energy. The variable that had the largest single-increment impact on the total BTU consumed by a household was type of heating equipment. This was compared to a baseline of "not applicable" heating equipment, which was only found in one home of this region. For the homes that had applicable heating equipment, a central furnace and some other equipment were found to very similarly contribute to the energy consumption of the home, while heat pumps consumed less. Furthermore, in this climate newer homes were found to significantly consume less energy, though the amount reduced per decade younger is small ($\beta_2 = -0.0293$). Contributions of the number of household members and income were found to also have small, though statistically significant increments. Based on the findings, the researchers evaluated Spearman correlations between the four variables treated as continuous, namely, year built, number of household members, income, and home size as seen in Table 4. All correlations were significant at the $\alpha = 0.01$ level. However, we note that all correlations were weak ($0.1 < \rho < 0.4$), or very weak, in the case of the number of household members and year built ($\rho = 0.096$). The associations between income and number of household members ($\rho = 0.337$) and income and home size ($\rho = 0.352$), despite weak, were higher than the other correlations coefficients. We also note that, even though a small parameter estimate was found for the contribution of total square footage ($\beta_1 = 0.0106$), the median home size in this region is 2700 square feet (251 square meters), making size the second largest contributor to total energy consumption for a median-sized home in Cold and Very Cold Climate, after heating equipment.

Table 4. Correlation analysis—Cold/Very Cold Climate (Spearman's ρ).

	Year Built	Number of Household Members	Income	Home Size
Year Built	1.00			
Number of Household Members	0.096 **	1.00		
Income	0.257 **	0.337 **	1.00	
Home Size	0.156 **	0.180 **	0.352 **	1.00

Notes: ** Correlation is significant at the 0.01 level.

Hot-Dry and Mixed-Dry Climate. This climate is found mainly in the southwest of the United States. For this region, the reduced model contained all the revised Equation (2) variables, except for solar energy and year built. And, similarly to the Very Cold and Cold climate zones, the variable that had the largest single-increment impact on the total BTU consumed by a household was the type of heating equipment, again compared to a baseline of "not applicable" heating equipment, which was found in 32 homes of this region. For the homes that had applicable heating equipment, a central furnace and some other equipment were found to very similarly contribute to the energy consumption of the home, while heat pumps were found to consume the least energy of the distinct types of heating equipment. Contributions of income were found to be small, compared to the number of family members. Our Spearman correlation analysis between the variables treated as continuous showed significance for all correlations, with the exceptions of the number of household members and year home was built, and income and year built, as seen in Table 5. Even when correlation was determined to be significant, all were considered weak. Interestingly, here the largest correlation coefficient was for the association between home size and year built ($\rho = 0.373$). In this region, the median size of homes is also considerably less than those in Cold and Very Cold climate ($\tilde{x} = 2116$). Considering the contribution of total square footage ($\beta_1 = 0.01052$), size was found to be the largest contributor to total energy consumption for a median-sized home (2116 square feet/197 square meters) that did not use a central furnace or some other type of heating equipment in the Hot-Dry and Mixed-Dry climate. For homes with a central furnace—the most frequent type of heating equipment in this region—or some other heating equipment, heating equipment was the largest contributor to energy usage in this climate, followed by home size. Finally, central air conditioning systems in this region have a higher contribution to the total energy consumed in the home, compared to other types of air conditioning systems for this factor. In fact, central air conditioning in Hot-Dry and Mixed-Dry climate are an important factor in the total energy consumed in these homes, given that it is the most frequent type of air-conditioning system used in this climate (see Figure 7).

Table 5. Correlation analysis—Hot-Dry and Mixed-Dry Climate (Spearman's ρ).

	Year Built	Number Household Members	Income	Home Size
Year Built	1.00			
Number of Household Members	0.092	1.00		
Income	0.071	0.231 **	1.00	
Home Size	0.373 **	0.159 **	0.294 **	1.00

Notes: ** Correlation is significant at the 0.01 level.

Hot-Humid Climate. This climate is found in the southeast of the United States. For this region, the reduced model contained all the revised Equation (2) variables, except for solar energy and air conditioning. Newer homes in this climate tend to consume less energy ($\beta_2 = -0.0485$). Similarly to the previously analyzed climate zones, the variable that had the largest single-increment impact on the total BTU consumed by a household was type of heating equipment. Thirty homes had "not applicable" heating equipment in this region. For the homes that had applicable heating equipment, central furnaces consumed more energy, followed by some other equipment, and then heat pumps. Homes with a fireplace or wood-burning stove were found to contribute negatively to the increment of energy consumed. The authors note that wood was not included in the total energy estimate used in the models. Only 11 houses using one of these equipment types were found in this climate zone. In this climate region, all but one of the Spearman correlations analyzed were found to be significant, as presented in Table 6. All significant correlations were found to be weak, with the associations between income and year built ($\rho = 0.349$), home size and year built ($\rho = 0.324$), and income and home size ($\rho = 0.378$) presenting the largest coefficient values. In this region, the median size of homes is 1904 square feet (177 square meters). Therefore, considering the contribution of total square footage ($\beta_1 = 0.01497$), size is the largest contributor to total energy consumption for a median-sized home in this climate, ahead of heating equipment, including central furnace, which is still the most frequent heating equipment used in homes in this climate zone.

Table 6. Correlation analysis—Hot-Humid Climate (Spearman's ρ).

	Year Built	Number Household Members	Income	Home Size
Year Built	1.00			
Number of Household Members	0.245 **	1.00		
Income	0.349 **	0.209 **	1.00	
Home Size	0.324 **	0.049	0.378 **	1.00

Notes: ** Correlation is significant at the 0.01 level.

Marine Climate. This climate is found along the west coast of the United States. For this region, the reduced model contained all Equation (2) variables, except for year built and income. This climate was the only one in which solar energy generation on-site was significant, however, it was found to have a positive contribution to the total energy consumption of the home. Similarly to the previously analyzed climate zones, the variable that had the largest single-increment impact on the total BTU consumed by a household was type of heating equipment. Heating equipment was "not applicable" for only 10 homes in this region. For the homes that had applicable heating equipment, a central furnace and some other equipment consumed more energy, followed by heat pumps. The number of family members had a small contribution to the total energy consumed in homes ($\beta_5 = 0.05041$). The Spearman correlation analysis for this region indicated significance in only three associations (see Table 7): between income and the number of household members, between size and year built, and size and income. Of those, the largest correlation coefficient was found between income and number of household members ($\rho = 0.334$). In this region, the median size of homes is very similar to what was found in the Hot-Humid region and is equal to 1949 square feet (181 square meters). Interestingly, in this case, size was not found to be one of the largest contributors to energy use in a median-sized home, contributing less than most heating equipment, solar power, and at least one of the cooling equipment options.

Table 7. Correlation analysis—Marine Climate (Spearman's ρ).

	Year Built	Number Household Members	Income	Home Size
Year Built	1.00			
Number of Household Members	0.092	1.00		
Income	0.024	0.334 **	1.00	
Home Size	0.183 **	0.065	0.188 **	1.00

Notes: ** Correlation is significant at the 0.01 level.

Mixed-Humid Climate. This climate is found in the lower half-east of the United States, in between the Hot-Humid and Cold/Very Cold and Hot-Humid climates. For this region, the reduced model contained all the original variables, except for solar energy. Year built was the only variable to negatively contribute to the total energy consumption in homes. Similarly to other climate zones, the variable that had the largest single-increment impact on the total BTU consumed by a household was type of heating equipment. Heating equipment was "not applicable" for only one home in this. For the homes that had applicable heating equipment, a central furnace and some other equipment were found to very similarly contribute to the energy consumption of the home, while heat pumps consumed less. Contributions of income and the number of family members were found to be fairly similar. Similar to the Cold and Very Cold climate region, the Spearman correlation analysis for this climate region showed significance at the $\alpha = 0.01$ level for all relations shown in Table 8. However, differently than all other regions, the relationship between income and home size in the Mixed-Humid climate was found to be moderate ($\rho = 0.457$), followed by a weak correlation between income and number of household members ($\rho = 0.368$). Additionally, for this region, individual window/wall or portable units contributed less than central air conditioning systems, which in turn contributed less than both a central and individual unit to the total BTU consumed in a home. In this region, the median size of homes is 2519 square feet (234 square meters), which is second only to the median home size in Cold and Very Cold climate region. Considering the contribution of total square footage ($\beta_1 = 0.00868$), similarly to Cold and Very Cold climate region, size is the second largest contributor to total energy consumption for a median-sized home in the Hot-Dry and Mixed-Dry climate.

Table 8. Correlation analysis—Mixed-Humid Climate (Spearman's ρ).

	Year Built	Number Household Members	Income	Home Size
Year Built	1.00			
Number of Household Members	0.192 **	1.00		
Income	0.227 **	0.368 **	1.00	
Home Size	0.207 **	0.160 **	0.457 **	1.00

Notes: ** Correlation is significant at the 0.01 level.

5. Discussion

Even though energy consumption patterns can be affected by several different factors, resulting in a complex analysis [8], the ability to analyze data per Building America climate regions has provided some interesting discussion topics. For example, the use of solar power did not appear to be a significant factor in four of the five analyzed regions. This factor was only found to be relevant in the marine region, though only 12 of the 264 homes surveyed in this climate had this feature. When the existence of solar power was a relevant factor, it was found to positively contribute to a household's energy consumption—a finding that can be related to Iraganaboina and Eluru [7] who analyzed the same dataset while controlling it per fuel type and used all types of housing units and found that energy consumption in homes that had solar power tended to be higher than homes without solar power. This finding might be due to the marine region including a portion of the state of California, whose residential solar power market is considered more mature than other states [37] and retail energy costs are among the higher in the United States [38]. However, we note that RECS data is not separated by state, but only by census division, therefore this should be further researched. Furthermore, included in the analyzed marine climate region are some of the largest technology-focused metropolitan areas in the United States, including San Francisco, San Jose, and Seattle [39]. This is relevant when considering that previous research [40] suggests that residential solar power generation is linked to behavioral factors. Specifically, consumers that are more innovation-driven and have stronger pro-environment beliefs are more likely to be interested in residential solar photovoltaic panels [40]. Future research on building, household, and home equipment characteristics specific to homes with on-site solar power generation could help clarify this matter.

Additionally, we verified that size was a large contributor to the total energy consumed in a home in most regions. For three of five regions, it was found to frequently be the second largest contributing factor to total energy consumption for median-sized homes. In those regions, heating equipment was the largest contributor to total energy consumption, which concurs with the United States Energy Information Administration [41] information on different contributors to a home's end-use energy consumption. In one region—Hot-Humid climate—size was seen as the largest contributor, and this is probably due to the reduction in the use of heating. Other studies have also assessed the contribution of home size (sometimes total home square foot, such as Estiri [4], and Iraganaboina and Eluru [7]; and other times only heated square footage, such as Karatasou and Santamouris [8]) and indicated that a larger home size positively contributes to total energy consumption in a home.

Our findings also concur with previous research, in that weather and the home's physical characteristics (and equipment) contribute more to its total energy consumption than household characteristics [4,19]. However, previous researchers [4,12] also warn about interactions between households' and buildings' characteristics. In our case, we only assessed correlations between year built, size, income, and the number of family members, which in most regions resulted in significant, but weak correlations. Moderate and significant correlation between income and home size was only found for the Mixed-Humid climate. This shows the need for more in-depth, regional analysis to guide local policymaking; and it suggests the need to further educate people on energy-efficient home options, as also suggested by Estiri [4] especially for homes in the Mixed-Humid climate.

Finally, education and water heaters were not found to be significant factors in the analysis for any of the regions. This is interesting and contradicts recent findings related to the influence of education in a home's energy consumption by Debs et al. [24] on the same dataset (though analysis was not controlled by climate zone) as well as Salari and Javid [22], who used a combination of United States EIA data for energy consumption and American Community Survey (ACS) for demographic data and have analyzed the results at the state level. Our findings seem to be more aligned with an indirect effect of household socio-economic characteristics on total energy consumption, as proposed by Karatasour and Santamouris [8]. However, we caution interpretation of this factor, given that RECS does not ask about the educational level of all household members, but just the highest education completed by the respondent of the survey, therefore the influence of education as measured in this dataset may be incomplete.

6. Conclusions

The present study has analyzed factors influencing the total energy consumption in single-family homes in the United States using data from the 2015 RECS and controlling by Building America climate zones. We have originally analyzed the impact of nine factors: total home size, year built, respondent's education, annual household gross income, number of household members, type of heating equipment, type of air conditioning equipment, type of water heater equipment, and the existence of on-site solar power generation. Our results indicate that education and water heater type are not significantly associated with total energy consumed in a home in any of the studied climate regions. In most regions, heating equipment type was the largest contributor to the total energy consumed in a median-sized home, followed by home size.

In the Hot-Humid zone, size was the largest contributor to the total energy consumed in a median-sized home. Additionally, in the Mixed-Humid climate, income and total square footage were positively and moderately correlated. These findings, and the fact that home size is a large contributor to the total energy consumption in a median-sized home in most climate regions suggest that policies and programs aiming to educate households into more energy-efficient options for home configurations could help reduce total energy consumption in at least one climate region. Additionally, the findings can be helpful to encourage conversations among built-environment professionals and how they can guide clients into choosing more energy-efficient home equipment and space configurations.

Furthermore, the direct effect of social-economic factors, such as income and number of household members was small, but other researchers indicate the indirect influence of those factors. Interestingly also, on-site solar power generation was not found to be significant in most regions, and when it was, it was positively associated with total energy consumption. This information is relevant because many states have incentives for the use of on-site solar power in homes, such as Arizona, California, and New York. Even though on-site solar power in homes is helpful to reduce the impact of grid dependency, it cannot be seen as a strategy to reduce total energy consumption because many of the homes are usually still connected to the electrical grid.

Further research could explore a similar analysis using other housing configurations, as well as for rental units to explore factors that can be considered significant to a home's energy consumption and, therefore, help guide policy and incentives. Other suggestions for further exploration are (1) to continue to study the relationship between households' socioeconomic status and a home's physical characteristics and equipment choice, (2) to perform a historical investigation of trends to further understand the evolution of home physical characteristics, appliances and equipment use and its impact in energy consumption, (3) to compare building, household and equipment characteristics of homes with on-site solar power generation in different climate regions, and (4) to compare the models developed in the present research with actual data from buildings in each of the climate regions, taking into account typical envelope features, such as building orientation, window areas, and materials' thermal transmittances, among others.

Author Contributions: Conceptualization, L.D. and J.M.; formal analysis, L.D.; investigation, L.D. and J.M.; methodology, L.D. and J.M.; visualization, L.D.; writing—original draft, L.D. and J.M.; writing—review & editing, L.D. and J.M. All authors have read and agreed to the published version of the manuscript.

Funding: This research received no external funding.

Institutional Review Board Statement: Not applicable.

Informed Consent Statement: Not applicable.

Data Availability Statement: Publicly available datasets were analyzed in this study. The data can be found inn United States Energy Information Administration, 2015 Residential Energy Consumption Survey (RECS) microdata webpage here: https://www.eia.gov/consumption/residential/data/2015/index.php?view=microdata (accessed on 1 July 2021).

Conflicts of Interest: The authors declare no conflict of interest.

References

1. US EIA. Energy Consumption by Sector. In *Monthly Energy Review*; July 2021. Available online: https://www.eia.gov/totalenergy/data/monthly/pdf/sec2.pdf (accessed on 20 August 2021).

2. US EIA. Despite More People Staying at Home, U.S. Residential Use Fell 4% in 2020. May 2021. Available online: https://www.eia.gov/todayinenergy/detail.php?id=47976 (accessed on 20 August 2021).
3. United Nations. Transforming Our World: The 2030 Agenda for Sustainable Development. 2015. Available online: https://sdgs.un.org/publications/transforming-our-world-2030-agenda-sustainable-development-17981 (accessed on 6 October 2021).
4. Estiri, H. Building and household X-factors and energy consumption at the residential sector: A structural equation analysis of the effects of household and building characteristics on the annual energy consumption of US residential buildings. *Energy Econ.* **2014**, *43*, 178–184. [CrossRef]
5. Fikru, M.G.; Gautier, L. The impact of weather variation on energy consumption in residential houses. *Appl. Energy* **2015**, *144*, 19–30. [CrossRef]
6. Hirst, E.; Goeltz, R.; Carney, J. Residential energy use: Analysis of disaggregate data. *Energy Econ.* **1982**, *4*, 74–82. [CrossRef]
7. Iraganaboina, N.C.; Eluru, N. An examination of factors affecting residential energy consumption using a multiple discrete continuous approach. *Energy Build.* **2021**, *240*, 110934. [CrossRef]
8. Karatasou, S.; Santamouris, M. Socio-economic status and residential energy consumption: A latent variable approach. *Energy Build.* **2019**, *198*, 100–105. [CrossRef]
9. Sanquist, T.F.; Orr, H.; Shi, B.; Bittner, A.C. Lifestyle factors in U.S. residential electricity consumption. *Energy Policy* **2012**, *42*, 354–364. [CrossRef]
10. Baechler, M.; Gilbride, T.L.; Cole, P.C.; Hefty, M.G.; Ruiz, K. *High-Performance Home Technologies: Guide to Determining Climate Regions by County*; Building America Best Practices Series; Pacific Northwest National Laboratory, U. S. Department of Energy (DOE)—Building Technologies Office, 2015; Volume 7.3. Available online: https://www.energy.gov/sites/prod/files/2015/10/f27/ba_climate_region_guide_7.3.pdf (accessed on 18 November 2021).
11. Jones, R.V.; Fuertes, A.; Lomas, K.J. The socio-economic, dwelling and appliance related factors affecting electricity consumption in domestic buildings. *Renew. Sustain. Energy Rev.* **2015**, *43*, 901–917. [CrossRef]
12. Steemers, K.; Yun, G.Y. Household energy consumption: A study of the role of occupants. *Build. Res. Inf.* **2009**, *37*, 625–637. [CrossRef]
13. Delzendeh, E.; Wu, S.; Lee, A.; Zhou, Y. The impact of occupants' behaviours on building energy analysis: A research review. *Renew. Sustain. Energy Rev.* **2017**, *80*, 1061–1071. [CrossRef]
14. Hojjati, B.; Wade, S.H. US household energy consumption and intensity trends: A decomposition approach. *Energy Policy* **2012**, *48*, 304–314. [CrossRef]
15. Ohler, A.M.; Loomis, D.G.; Ilves, K. A study of electricity savings from energy star appliances using household survey data. *Energy Policy* **2020**, *144*, 111607. [CrossRef]
16. US Environmental Protection Agency (EPA). About Energy Star—2020. Available online: https://www.energystar.gov/sites/default/files/asset/document/2021%20About%20ENERGY%20STAR%20Overview%204.12.21%20v1.pdf (accessed on 6 October 2021).
17. Shah, V.P.; Debella, D.C.; Ries, R.J. Life cycle assessment of residential heating and cooling systems in four regions in the United States. *Energy Build.* **2008**, *40*, 503–513. [CrossRef]
18. Maguire, J.; Fang, X.; Wilson, E. *Comparison of Advanced Residential Water Heating Technologies in the United States (No. NREL/TP-5500-55475)*; National Renewable Energy Lab (NREL): Golden, CO, USA, 2013.
19. Kavousian, A.; Rajagopal, R.; Fischer, M. Determinants of residential electricity consumption: Using smart meter data to examine the effect of climate, building characteristics, appliance stock, and occupants' behavior. *Energy* **2013**, *55*, 184–194. [CrossRef]
20. U.S Census. New Single-Family Homes in 2020. Available online: https://www.census.gov/construction/chars/xls/squarefeet_cust.xls (accessed on 3 September 2021).
21. Aksoezen, M.; Daniel, M.; Hassler, U.; Kohler, N. Building age as an indicator for energy consumption. *Energy Build.* **2015**, *87*, 74–86. [CrossRef]
22. Salari, M.; Javid, R.J. Residential energy demand in the United States: Analysis using static and dynamic approaches. *Energy Policy* **2016**, *98*, 637–649. [CrossRef]
23. Salari, M.; Javid, R.J. Modeling household energy expenditure in the United States. *Renew. Sustain. Energy Rev.* **2017**, *69*, 822–832. [CrossRef]
24. Debs, L.; Kota, B.R.; Metzinger, J. Recent Energy Consumption Trends in American Homes. In Proceedings of the Associated Schools of Construction 57th Annual International Conference (Virtual), California State University, Chico, CA, USA, 5–9 April 2021.
25. Juarex, D.A.; Walke, A.D. Residential electricity consumption in Seattle. *Energy Econ.* **2012**, *34*, 1693–1699.
26. Bhattacharjee, S.; Reichard, G. Socio-economic factors affecting individual household energy consumption: A systematic review. In Proceedings of the ASME 2011 5th International Conference on Energy Sustainability, Washington, DC, USA, 7–10 August 2011.
27. Bao, H.X.; Li, S.H. Housing wealth and residential energy consumption. *Energy Policy* **2020**, *143*, 111581. [CrossRef]
28. Fong, W.K.; Matsumoto, H.; Lun, Y.F.; Kimura, R. Influences of Indirect Lifestyle aspects and climate on household energy consumption. *J. Asian Archit. Build. Eng.* **2018**, *6*, 395–402. [CrossRef]
29. Grünewald, P.; Diakonova, M. Societal differences, activities, and performance: Examining the role of gender in electricity demand in the United Kingdom. *Energy Res. Soc. Sci.* **2020**, *69*, 101719. [CrossRef]
30. Estiri, H.; Zagheni, E. Age matters: Ageing and household energy demand in the United States. *Energy Res. Soc. Sci.* **2019**, *55*, 62–70. [CrossRef]

31. US EIA. 2015 RECS Household Characteristics Technical Documentation Summary (Webpage). Available online: https://www.eia.gov/consumption/residential/reports/2015/methodology/index.php (accessed on 13 July 2021).
32. US EIA. 2015 RECS Survey Data. Microdata. Available online: https://www.eia.gov/consumption/residential/data/2015/index.php?view=microdata (accessed on 18 November 2021).
33. US Census Bureau. American Housing Survey 2019 [Summary Tables]. 2020. Available online: https://www.census.gov/programs-surveys/ahs/data.html (accessed on 15 July 2021).
34. Estiri, H.; Gabriel, R.; Howard, E.; Wang, L. *Different Regions, Differences in Energy Consumption: Do Regions Account for the Variability in Household Energy Consumption*; Working Paper, 134; Center for Statistics and the Social Sciences University of Washington: Seattle, WA, USA, 2013. Available online: https://csss.uw.edu/files/working-papers/2013/wp134.pdf (accessed on 23 September 2021).
35. Kaza, N. Understanding the spectrum of residential energy consumption: A quantile regression approach. *Energy Policy* **2010**, *38*, 6574–6585. [CrossRef]
36. Pasta, D.J. Learning when to be discrete: Continuous vs. categorical predictors. In Proceedings of the SAS Global Forum, Washington, DC, USA, 22–25 March 2009. Available online: https://support.sas.com/resources/papers/proceedings09/248-2009.pdf (accessed on 29 December 2021).
37. Bao, Q.; Sinitskaya, E.; Gomez, K.J.; MacDonald, E.F.; Yang, M.C. A human-centered design approach to evaluating factors in residential solar PV adoption: A survey of homeowners in California and Massachusetts. *Renew. Energy* **2020**, *151*, 503–513. [CrossRef]
38. US EIA. State Electricity Profiles (Data for 2020). November 2021. Available online: https://www.eia.gov/electricity/state/ (accessed on 29 December 2021).
39. Atkinson, R.; Muro, M.; Whiton, J. *The Case for Growth Centers*; Brookings Institution: Washington, DC, USA, 2019. Available online: https://pubs.aeaweb.org/doi/pdfplus/10.1257/jep.34.3.99 (accessed on 29 December 2021).
40. Wolske, K.S.; Stern, P.C.; Dietz, T. Explaining interest in adopting residential solar photovoltaic systems in the United States: Toward an integration of behavioral theories. *Energy Res. Soc. Sci.* **2017**, *25*, 134–151. [CrossRef]
41. US EIA. Use of Energy Explained. Energy Use in Homes. June 2021. Available online: https://www.eia.gov/energyexplained/use-of-energy/homes.php (accessed on 6 October 2021).

International Journal of
Environmental Research and Public Health

MDPI

Review

Sustainability of Heating, Ventilation and Air-Conditioning (HVAC) Systems in Buildings—An Overview

Nilofar Asim [1,*], Marzieh Badiei [2], Masita Mohammad [1], Halim Razali [1], Armin Rajabi [3], Lim Chin Haw [1] and Mariyam Jameelah Ghazali [3,*]

1 Solar Energy Research Institute, Universiti Kebangsaan Malaysia, Bangi 43600, Malaysia; masita@ukm.edu.my (M.M.); drhalimrazali@ukm.edu.my (H.R.); chinhaw.lim@ukm.edu.my (L.C.H.)
2 Independent Researcher, Razavi 16, Mashhad 91777-35843, Iran; gbadiei317@gmail.com
3 Department of Mechanical and Manufacturing Engineering, Faculty of Engineering and Built Environment, Universiti Kebangsaan Malaysia, Bangi 43600, Malaysia; arminukm50@siswa.ukm.edu.my
* Correspondence: nilofarasim@ukm.edu.my (N.A.); mariyam@ukm.edu.my (M.J.G.)

Citation: Asim, N.; Badiei, M.; Mohammad, M.; Razali, H.; Rajabi, A.; Chin Haw, L.; Jameelah Ghazali, M. Sustainability of Heating, Ventilation and Air-Conditioning (HVAC) Systems in Buildings—An Overview. *Int. J. Environ. Res. Public Health* **2022**, *19*, 1016. https://doi.org/10.3390/ijerph19021016

Academic Editors: Roberto Alonso González Lezcano, Francesco Nocera and Rosa Giuseppina Caponetto

Received: 1 December 2021
Accepted: 13 January 2022
Published: 17 January 2022

Abstract: Increasing demand on heating, ventilation, and air-conditioning (HVAC) systems and their importance, as the respiratory system of buildings, in developing and spreading various microbial contaminations and diseases with their huge global energy consumption share have forced researchers, industries, and policymakers to focus on improving the sustainability of HVAC systems. Understanding and considering various parameters related to the sustainability of new and existing HVAC systems as the respiratory system of buildings are vital to providing healthy, energy-efficient, and economical options for various building types. However, the greatest opportunities for improving the sustainability of HVAC systems exist at the design stage of new facilities and the retrofitting of existing equipment. Considering the high available percentage of existing HVAC systems globally reveals the importance of their retrofitting. The attempt has been made to gather all important parameters that affect decision-making to select the optimum HVAC system development considerations among the various opportunities that are available for sustainability improvement.

Keywords: HVAC systems; sustainability; energy efficient; indoor air quality; water recovery; retrofitting

1. Introduction

Population growth, modern technologies, and lifestyles are among the reasons for the necessity of heating, ventilation, and air conditioning (HVAC) systems in various types of buildings. Meanwhile, HVAC systems have an important role in the comfort and safety of indoor air quality (IAQ). However, these systems account for 40–60% of energy usage in buildings [1] or 15% of the world's total energy consumption (Rafique 2018). These facts illustrate the importance of considering HVAC sustainability development by researchers, industries, and policymakers. Furthermore, sustainability considerations and innovations in HVAC systems are necessary to provide a remarkable, healthy, productive, and sustainable built environment for occupants while reducing energy consumption and costs [2].

For the sustainable development of all three pillars, namely, economic, environmental, and social, reaching the immediate and long-term benefits of people, the planet, and prosperity must be carefully considered [3].

Various affecting parameters must be considered to improve the sustainability of HVAC systems. A remarkable understanding of human-in-the-loop HVAC systems could facilitate and improve the achievement of sustainability (Figure 1) [4]. Considering all the related parameters will help minimize energy usage without compromising occupant thermal comfort.

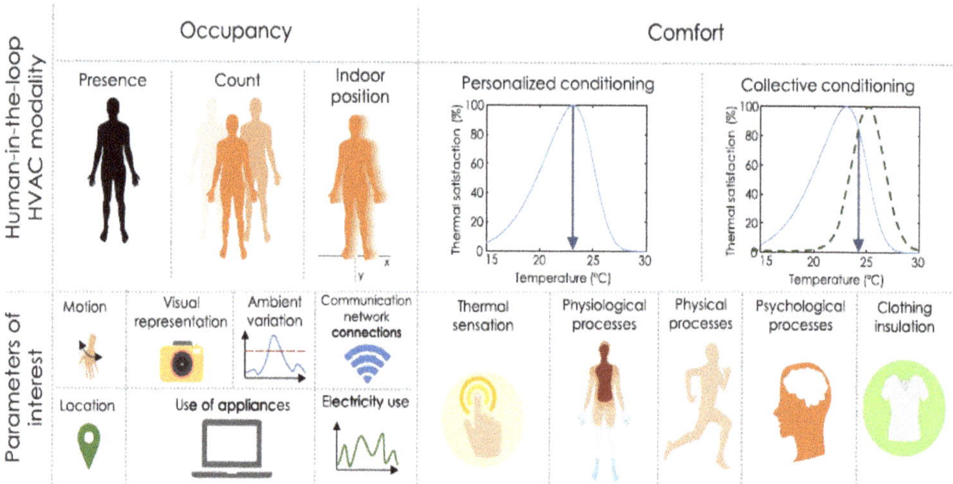

Figure 1. Human-in-the-loop HVAC modalities of occupancy and comfort along with their parameters of interest [4].

The assessment of measurement and modeling techniques and their performance are important in planning to achieve sustainable HVAC systems considering occupancy, comfort, and building type [4].

Despite the availability of various methods that can be used in building design and retrofitting to improve the HVAC system performance [5,6], this paper only studies the parameters that directly deal with HVAC sustainability improvement. However, many of these parameters, such as energy, environment, and water recovery, overlap with one another.

2. Energy

The high energy share of HVAC systems in buildings, which increase greenhouse gas emissions and costs, motivates researchers to study the various parameters related to reducing energy consumption and finding sustainable solutions for HVAC systems [7,8]. Many studies have been conducted to develop advanced design and control strategies to optimize energy, thermal, and environmental performance and to make these strategies cost-effective for HVAC systems [2,9–11].

Renewable energies could improve the sustainability of HVAC systems directly or indirectly. Considering the climate and geographical conditions, the use of various heating and cooling technologies that utilize renewable energy sources in HVAC systems in the building are very important options in improving sustainability.

Desiccant heating, cooling, and ventilation [12–15]; evaporative passive cooling [16,17]; solar heating and cooling systems [18,19]; geothermal heating and cooling systems [20]; and biomass heating and cooling technologies [21,22] are examples of renewable technologies that are used in HVAC systems in buildings.

Various HVAC system designs that utilize renewable energy sources have been developed and explored [23,24]. Ma et al. [2] studied the HVAC systems in solar-powered decathlon houses developed in the USA. They found that most of them used heat pumps for space heating and cooling. After 2005, more than half of houses utilized energy/heat recovery ventilators for improving the HVAC performance. Meanwhile, various other technologies such as phase change materials, night-time radiative cooling, evaporative cooling, and desiccant dehumidification are employed for electrical energy saving in HVAC systems.

Modified and improved designs for various components in HVAC systems, such as dampers dampers [25,26], filters [27,28], humidifier, dehumidifier [29,30], heating and cooling coils [31], and ducts and fans [27,32], can reduce the energy consumption of such systems while optimizing their performance [13].

Waste heat and energy recovery are important for reducing energy usage in HVAC systems [33–36].

Air-to-air heat exchangers [37] and heat pipe heat exchangers (HPHE) with different forms and designs can be used as heat recovery equipment for the air quality improvement in HVAC systems [33,38–45]. A study showed that the use of a U-shaped HPHE in a hospital could reach 7.64% higher effectiveness or heat recovery of up to 608.45 W [44].

Shahsavar et al. [36] developed an air handling unit design equipped with primary and secondary heat recovery units and could increase the efficiency by 43.75%.

The use of liquid-to-air membrane energy exchangers [46,47], porous metal foam heat exchangers [48], nanofluid as heat transfer fluid [49], phase change material as heat transfer media [50–53], membrane heat exchanger [54–56], and polymer heat exchangers [57,58] affect the energy consumption and recovery and sustainability of HVAC systems positively.

The integration of various energy sources instead of one energy source using multicarrier/multiconverters to cover energy loads is another effective method for reducing energy and cost in HVAC systems. Fabrizio et al. [59] reviewed various integrated designs for HVAC and hot water production systems in buildings based on their advantages and disadvantages and presented their efficiencies for energy recovery. They found that for obtaining optimal results for multienergy systems, the appropriate manufacture data for system design and performance calculation is needed.

The application of ultrasonic energy in HVAC systems for process enhancement or system efficiency improvement, such as air humidification/dehumidification, desiccant regeneration, air purification, heat exchanger, defrosting, and evaporator, has been explored by many researchers [60–64].

Improving the ventilation components in HVAC systems plays an important role in optimizing energy efficiency and improving IAQ [65–67]. However, researchers have developed many energy-efficient ventilation methods, such as natural and hybrid ventilation strategies for buildings. Their studies also showed that occupants' behavior affects energy consumption. The study showed that ventilation was interrelated with various factors, such as indoor and outdoor conditions, building characteristics and application, and occupants' behavior [65]. Thus, many factors must be considered in designing sustainable ventilation systems.

The effective management of mixed-mode (MM) buildings, which utilize natural and mechanical ventilation systems (hybrid), reduces the energy consumption of HVAC systems in a building; however, the reduction percentage depends on the climate, building type, and evaluation assumptions [68].

The use of various prediction models to estimate energy consumption based on various parameters in building and HVAC system designs could help us to determine the optimum parameters for reducing energy consumption [69–71]. Meanwhile, new integrated designs that implant programmed control systems are very efficient in developing energy-efficient HVAC systems in buildings [33,72,73]. Smart technologies could be predictive/responsive/adaptive against weather, users, grids, and other variables. The use of these smart technologies in buildings and HVAC systems could reduce energy and cost remarkably [7,73] (Figure 2). Figure 3 presents the managing level of adaptive–predictive control strategies in the smart building through a cloud platform. Cloud technology provides additional benefits and functions to the system, and the local controller could still manage the control in case of disconnection.

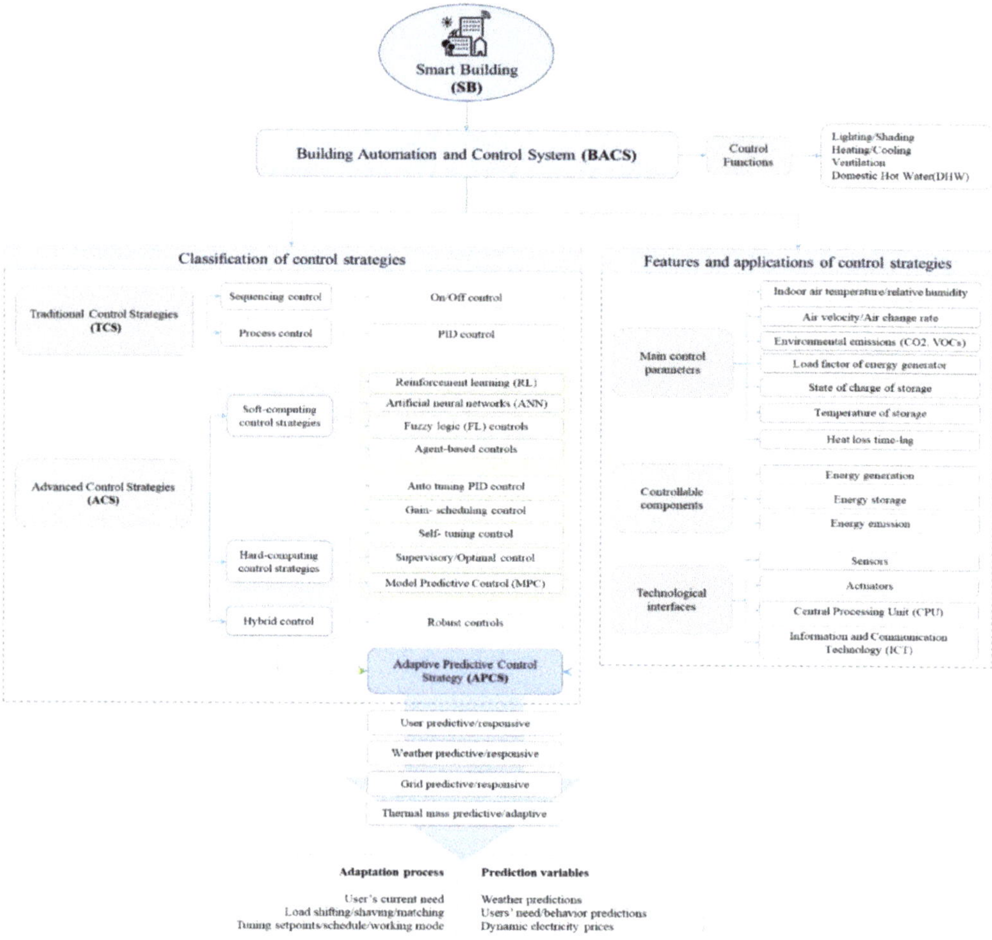

Figure 2. Features, applications, and functions of building automation and control system (BACS) in buildings and HVAC systems [7].

The progress in artificial intelligence provides a lot of opportunities for developing a smart built environment (SBE) and smart energy consumption. Figure 4 presents the energy flow charts between the supply side of smart energy system (SES) categories and the demand side in the SBE [74]. In the SBE, the use of nonrenewable energy sources reduced greenhouse gas emissions and cost considering the provision of a more sustainable built environment. Su [74] presented some methodologies, system optimizations, and holistic designs for developing SESs and discussed future challenges that require attention. Based on the presented macroscopic view, the fraction of energy can be optimized when the control of the transient fraction of power is adjusted properly. The optimization of the transient fraction of power from different energy forms needs to be considered based on the trade form between the supply side of SESs and the demand side of the SBE.

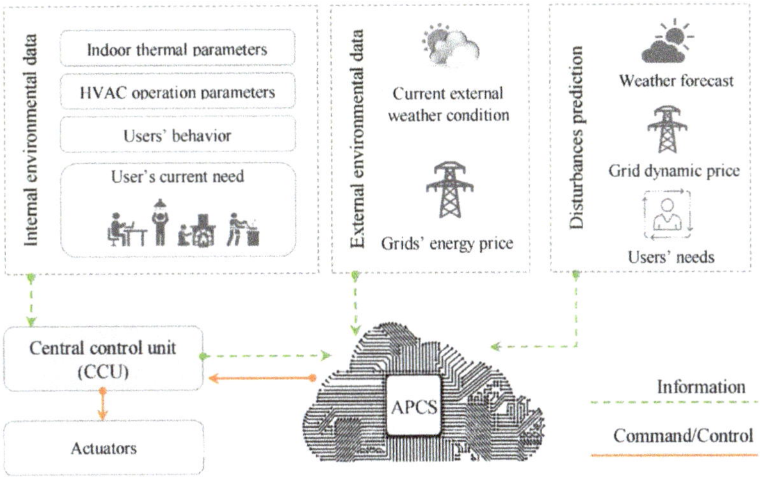

Figure 3. Application of adaptive–predictive control strategies (APCS) as a supervisory control system through a cloud platform [7].

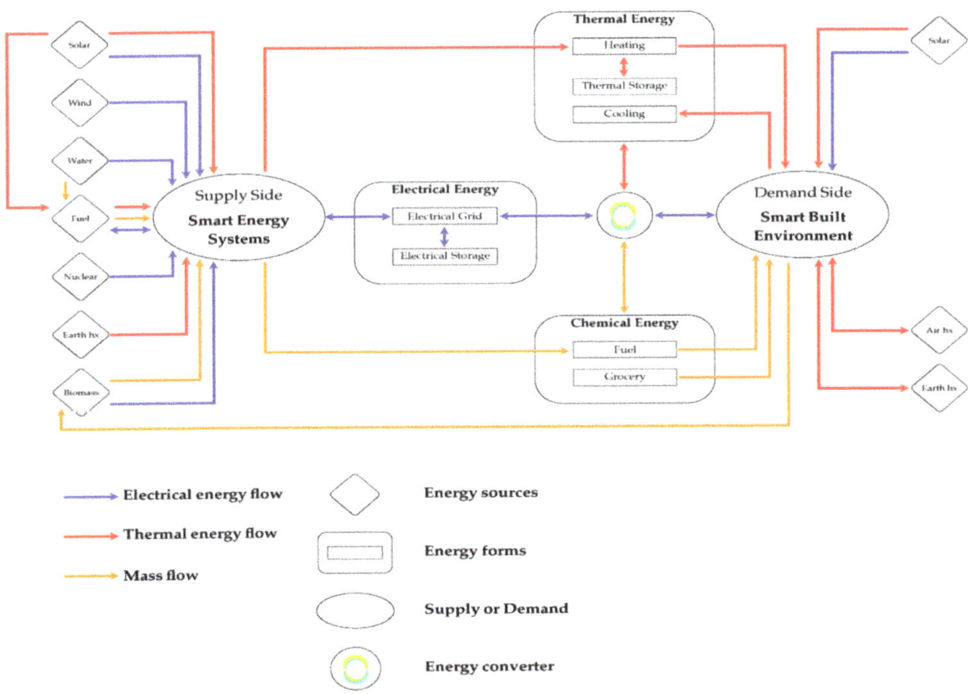

Figure 4. Energy flow charts between the supply side SESs and the demand side SBE [74] (Su 2020).

The use of various decision-making methods, such as multicriteria decision-making (MCDM) methods, could help researchers to find the optimum design for different building types and operation conditions [75,76].

Despite the availability of various modeling techniques developed for improving the control strategy of HVAC systems, finding the optimum model depends on various parameters; moreover, decision makers must be informed about the role, application, advantages, disadvantages, and outcomes of different modeling techniques to find the best option for their application [66,75,77].

Shi et al. [70] investigated a well-validated building simulation model to compare the performance of 12 existing HVAC system strategies in decreasing energy usage, peak demand, and energy cost for decision making in the real world.

3. Environment and Society (Thermal Comfort and IAQ)

Spending more than 80% of peoples' time indoors reveals the importance of IAQ on the health and comfort of occupants [78]. Studies have shown that low IAQ decreases the work performance of occupants [79–81].

IAQ in buildings, such as temperature, humidity, airflow, and cleanliness, is directly related to HVAC systems and is considered the respiratory system of buildings [82]. However, improperly designed or operated HVAC systems could contain and develop various microbial contaminations and cause serious health issues for occupants. Recently, various outbreaks of severe epidemic diseases, such as COVID-19, SARS, MERS, and H7N9, and the importance of controlling the spread of various microbial contaminations in HVAC systems, have become critical subjects to consider in the sustainability development of such systems. The microbial contaminations could have been generated in different ways, such as by people (talking/sneezing), pets, carpets, and toilets (Figure 5). These viruses could survive and grow in various HVAC components, such as air ducts, filters, heat exchangers, and fan coils because of their suitable environmental conditions for microbial contaminations [82].

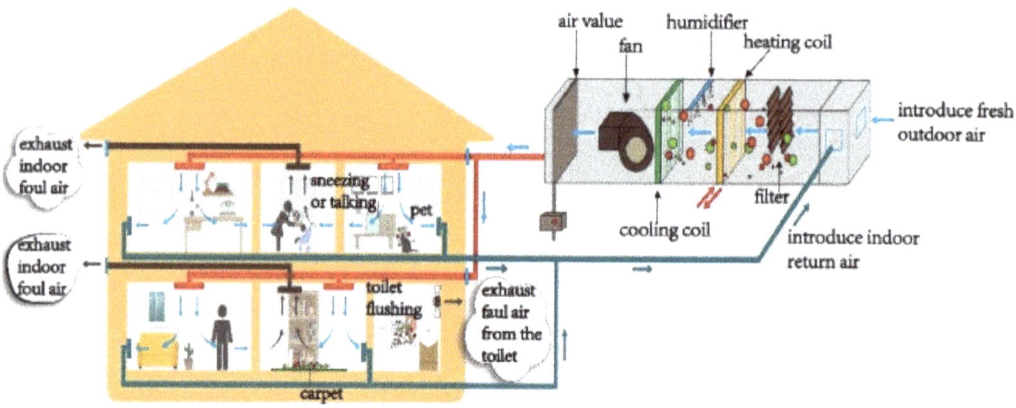

Figure 5. Schematic of microbial contamination in a HVAC system of residential buildings [82].

These microbial contaminations diffuse and spread indoors in the form of aerosols or accumulated dust (i.e., suspended particulate matter) with supply airflow and affect the occupants' health [83]. Microbial contamination with a particle size smaller than 10 μm could be inhaled into the lungs and might cause various respiratory diseases [82]. Therefore, microbial contamination control in HVAC systems is vital for human health and IAQ. Some researchers have used the dehumidifier condensed water to measure volatile organic contaminants and nanoparticles in indoor air [84–86].

Liu et al. [82] reviewed various microbial contamination characteristics, and growth, reproduction, and transmission mechanisms caused by HVAC systems to determine effective control methods. They found that filters, heat exchangers (e.g., cooling coil and evaporative condenser), and ventilation ducts are the common components of microbial contamination because their environmental conditions are suitable for their survival and growth.

To prevent microbial contamination in HVAC systems, the control of pollution sources, the regulation of air parameters, and the operation of HVAC systems must be considered completely [82].

Sukarno et al. [33] developed an HVAC system design by adding a heat pipe heat exchanger to remove contaminated air in the airborne infection isolation room in a hospital.

Santos et al. [87] studied various strategies to minimize the risk of COVID-19 infection within the indoor environment through an HVAC system design. They concluded that UV-C lamps, pressure control, air renewal and filtration, restroom actions, and humidity control are effective strategies for minimizing the transmission of airborne infections within the built environment (Figure 6).

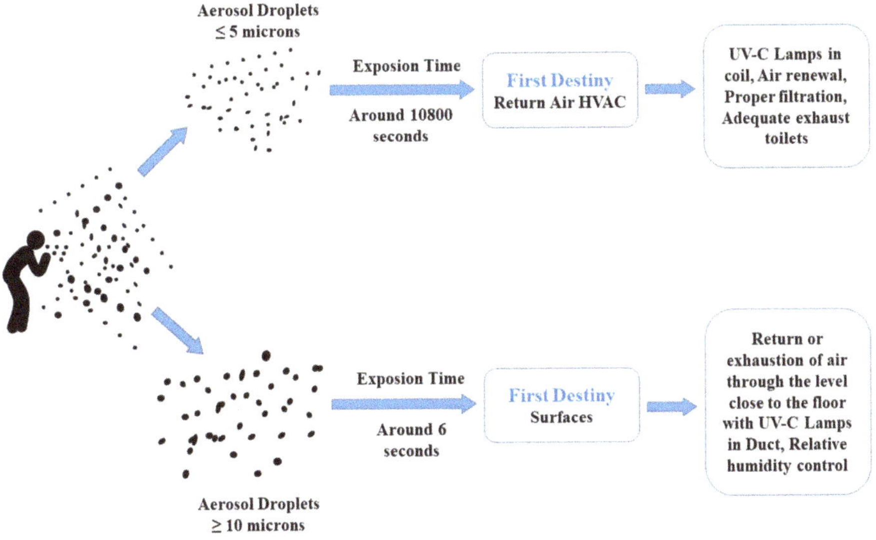

Figure 6. Contagion sources vs. strategies to prevent contagion. Reproduced with permission from [87].

Air filtration and purification technologies could modify the IAQ of buildings effectively [88]. However, the influence of various parameters on the performance of these technologies must be considered [89].

Photocatalysis, plasma, UV, microwave sterilization, and physical adsorption are among the common air purification technologies that are combined with HVAC systems to control indoor microbial contaminations [82,90]. However, finding an optimum microbial contamination removal technology needs the consideration of various parameters in HVAC systems. Table 1 presents the comparison of various purification and filtration technologies used in buildings.

Table 1. Comparison of different purification and filtration technologies in building environments [82,91].

Technologies	Target	Advantages	Disadvantages	Efficiency
Fiber filtration	Particles, microorganisms	Low cost, convenient installation	Resistance related to the purification efficiency, mid- and high efficiency of high-resistance filters	Can achieve 99.99%
Electrostatic dust removal	Particles, microorganisms	High efficiency and wide range of particle size, small pressure loss	High investment, efficiency decline after dust discharge, easy to breakdown electric field	50% (some only 20%)

Table 1. *Cont.*

Technologies	Target	Advantages	Disadvantages	Efficiency
Ultraviolet sterilization	Microorganisms	High efficiency, safe and convenient, short reactive time, no residual toxicity, no pollution, low resistance, low cost	Poor dynamic sterilization effect, short service life, UV lamp should be close to the irradiated material, can be influenced by environmental factors, and suspended particles greatly produce secondary pollution	82.90%
Activated carbon adsorption	Nearly all pollutants except biological ones	Wild sources, wide pollutant purifying range, does not easily cause secondary pollution	Saturated regeneration problems, high resistance, poor mineral processing	
Plasma	All indoor pollutants	Wide range of pollutants	Cannot completely degrade pollutants, high energy consumption, and production of by-products (ozone and nitrogen oxides)	66.70%; Cold plasma air filter: 85–98%
Negative ions	Particles, microorganisms	Accelerate metabolism, strengthen cell function, effective to some disease	Produce ozone, cause secondary pollution, dust deposition damages walls	73.40%
Photocatalysis	TVOC, microorganisms, and other inorganic gaseous pollutants	Wide range of purification, mild reaction conditions, no adsorption saturation phenomenon, long service life	Compared with the activated carbon adsorption technology, purification process is slower, easily causes secondary pollution if response is not completed, unable to remove particulate pollutants	75% (some may only 30% or even negative)
Trombe wall	Effective particles (diameter) >10 μm and <0.01 μm	60-year service life	Useless for 0.1–1 μm	99.4% for PM10
Biofilter	Mixture of VOCs	Effective odor control method		Dynamic botanical air filtration system: >33% for toluene and 90% for formaldehyde; integrated biofiltration system: 99%
Microwave sterilization	Bacterial and fungal aerosols	Heating uniformity, rapid sterilization, and no residue combination of thermal and nonthermal effects; under atmospheric pressure, microwaves can induce argon plasma disinfection	Radiation is harmful to human health	30–40% of bacterial and fungal aerosols in the environment can survive for 1.7 min under microwave high-power radiation

To improve the performance of purification techniques, a combination of strategies, such as plasma combined with photocatalysis and plasma with activated carbon, could be adopted [82].

Paying attention to healthy ventilation is vital when improving the thermal comfort of a building using HVAC systems.

4. Water Recovery

As a most treasured resource in the world, the investigation of water sustainability in buildings and HVAC systems is crucial. HVAC systems are considered air–water harvesting systems that liquefy the water vapor available in the air as they condensate; they are also a potential water source [92]. The recovery of condensate has more value, especially in a hot and dry climate which has water scarcity.

The amount of condensate depends on relative humidity (RH), temperature, air speed, and HVAC system type [93–95].

Unfortunately, in most cases, the condensate is removed and disposed in sanitary drain [94].

Meanwhile, untreated condensate can be the origin of aerosols, which are responsible for microbial contamination in HVAC systems [96]. Water recovery from HVAC systems is also an important issue for water sustainability and building energy recovery, as well as a healthy environment.

Algarni et al. [94] reviewed various condensate recovery systems in HVAC systems, the potential application of the collected water, and the quality characteristics of the condensate water (Figure 7). They found that planning for a condensate recovery system at the design stage of a building efficiently increased the ease and performance of collecting, storing, and reusing the condensate in the buildings.

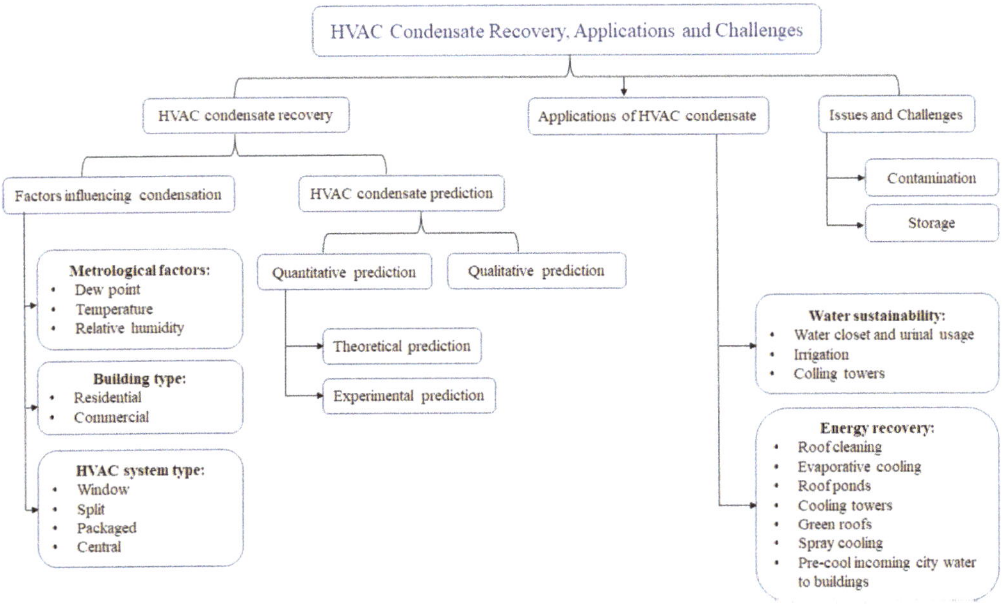

Figure 7. Overview of HVAC condensate recovery, applications, and challenges. Reprinted with permission from [94].

Although many researchers have studied the usage of condensate as potable water because of its high quality (i.e., low mineral and chemical content), the use of proper disinfection methods, such as UV, chlorine, and ozone disinfection, is required to eliminate the potential hazard of microbial contamination [96].

Despite the availability of various studies on the water recovery of HVAC systems, many subjects still need more attention. The application of condensate in evaporative cooling, spray cooling, roof ponds, and green roofs are among the interesting areas that require further research. The separate condensate piping in the plumbing and drainage system in the design stage of HVAC systems could bring more value. More attention to the storage and contamination of condensate based on its end usage plan and optimized water recovery systems as a part of HVAC systems is required [94,97].

Researchers have developed various designs for water and energy recovery from HVAC systems [35,98–102]. Cattani et al. [103] developed an integrated system of HVAC for water production. They also simulated a one-year period of water saving for this integrated system to evaluate its effectiveness. The life cycle assessment showed that rainwater and condensate recovery are sustainable options for meeting the water demands in urban buildings [104,105].

Meanwhile, the development of new designs, such as tri-generation systems [106,107] for combined systems could provide many advantages for building sustainability.

Yoon et al. [108] used the condensate for water spraying in a portable air conditioner to increase the coefficient of performance (COP) by 16%.

Tan et al. [109] explored the increase of condensate recovery by coupling a heat pump and membrane distillation (MD). They found that the coupling of MD with the thermoelectric cooler reduced the energy consumption because of the cooling provided by the MD. Meanwhile, the condensate increased because of the improvement in the thermoelectric efficiency.

5. Retrofitting of Existing HVAC Systems (Modification of Old HVAC Systems)

The fact that more than 25% of existing buildings in Europe are more than 70 years old [110,111], 60% of residential building in the US are more than 30 years old [112], and a high percentage of developing countries are currently using low sustainability concepts suggests the importance of considering their retrofitting [113,114]. Retrofitting of existing buildings could decrease the global energy consumption and environmental impact remarkably [6].

Considering the high energy consumption of HVAC systems in buildings, their low sustainability reveals the vital attention required for their modification. This retrofitting could reduce the environmental impacts of the built environment. However, optimum decision making that considers various important parameters, such as energy modeling and assessment, retrofit designs, cost, and risk assessment, is crucial [115,116].

Toosi et al. [113] reviewed the life cycle sustainability assessment of studies conducted for building energy retrofitting to determine the life cycle environmental impacts, economic aspects, and the social dimensions of a product, service, or process. They found that the lack of life cycle inventory databases was the main barrier in the life cycle sustainability assessment. Meanwhile, considering other parameters such as future energy mixes, user behavior impacts, macroeconomic parameters, and so on, is important for sustainability assessments.

The recommended steps for the energy retrofitting of a building [112] are listed as follows:

1. Measurement of HVAC system performance.
2. Identification of potential retrofit alternatives, such as smart controlling systems, upgrading mechanical systems, energy and water recovery, and utilization of renewable energy sources.
3. Establishment of the relation between the investment of retrofitting and the sustainability performance.

Formulation of an optimization model for retrofit investments allocation.

Modification in HVAC systems as a cost-saving opportunity has an important effect on the environmental sustainability of buildings [117]. Monitoring and controlling the HVAC systems is crucial in managing and optimizing the sustainability of HVAC systems. Energy-efficient building designs, considering the important effects of building reflection and insulation on the HVAC system's performance, and the energy retrofitting of the building's design, are more effective and easier than upgrading the HVAC systems [117].

According to Patel et al. [117], some useful modification for existing HVAC systems include:

Utilizing energy monitoring and control systems (smart systems): the use of smart monitoring and control technologies in HVAC systems could decrease the energy usage of HVAC systems remarkably [67].

Discharge air temperature management: by setting higher discharge air temperatures, the energy for subsequent reheating of cooled make-up air could be reduced and energy could be saved.

Variable-air-volume systems: the optimization of air flow into the building, based on its requirements, by adjusting the air flow within the HVAC ductwork could reduce load and save energy.

Duct leakage repair: duct leakage is responsible for significant energy waste in HVAC systems. Repairing duct leakage could improve energy usage by 30%.

Adjustable speed drives: adjustable speed drives could be used in variable volume air handlers, recirculation fans, chiller pumps, and water pumps to reduce energy consumption.

Heat recovery systems: various heat recovery systems could be used in HVAC systems to reduce energy consumption [67].

Improvement of chiller: various concepts, such as decreasing the temperature of the condenser water and installing separate high-temperature chillers for process cooling, could improve energy efficiency.

Fan modification: selecting the appropriate size and shape of the sheaves of a fan could optimize its efficiency and air flow and decrease energy consumption.

Exhaust fans improvement: changing traditional centrifugal exhaust fans with mixed flow impeller exhaust fans could increase efficiency by 25%. They are also cheaper to install and maintain.

Cooling water recovery: recycling secondary treated cooling water in chiller systems could improve the sustainability of systems.

Solar air heating: in cold climates, the use of solar heating systems, such as a solar wall, not only reduces energy consumption but also provides clean fresh air and reduce emissions.

Filter's modification: utilizing improved filters or filter slots to avoid pressure drops could improve the energy usage in HVAC systems.

Meanwhile, the importance of HVAC system maintenance in terms of energy consumption must not be ignored [117].

6. Discussion and Conclusions

Recent pandemic diseases, such as COVID-19, SARS, H7N9, and MERS, and the fact that people spend more than 80% of their time inside buildings show the importance of designing sustainable HVAC systems. Moreover, HVAC systems are the respiratory system of a building, and the potential risk to develop various microbial contaminations that threaten occupant health and work performance shows the urgency to improve its sustainability and performance.

Meanwhile, the high percentage of existing unsustainable HVAC systems globally shows the vital need for their retrofitting to mitigate environmental, energy, and economical issues. However, controlling and maintaining modified HVAC systems for their sustainability needs careful attention.

However, the optimum design and retrofitting plan of the HVAC system depends on the building types, climatic conditions, and effective parameters for the requested sustainability. Moreover, the decision makers could use decision-making methods to develop optimum plans that consider the various advantages and disadvantages and the potential risk of each option [75,118,119]. Some important recommendations for the better optimization of HVAC systems in buildings are listed as follows:

- Improvement and retrofitting of the building design are very effective for improving the performance of HVAC systems.
- All decision-making parameters for the planning of sustainable HVAC systems, such as occupancy, comfort, health, building type, and cost must be extensively studied.
- Important parameters must be considered in using renewable technologies in HVAC systems to achieve sustainability.
- The use of developed and advanced designs and control strategies in the HVAC systems could increase their sustainability remarkably.

- Improving IAQ and occupants' health by focusing on ventilation systems and microbial contamination prevention in HVAC systems.
- Water and energy recovery in HVAC systems are crucial parameters for improving sustainability.
- The retrofitting of the existing HVAC system is a vital action in the current situation.
- Optimum plans need to take into account all the advantages and disadvantages of various options while considering the available facilities, conditions, risks, and cost.

Funding: This study was partially supported by the Universiti Kebangsaan Malaysia's grants (DPK-2019-001 and GP-K019259).

Informed Consent Statement: Not applicable.

Conflicts of Interest: The authors declare no conflict of interest.

References

1. Pérez-Lombard, L.; Ortiz, J.; Pout, C. A review on buildings energy consumption information. *Energy Build.* **2008**, *40*, 394–398. [CrossRef]
2. Ma, Z.; Ren, H.; Lin, W. A review of heating, ventilation and air conditioning technologies and innovations used in solar-powered net zero energy Solar Decathlon houses. *J. Clean. Prod.* **2019**, *240*, 118158. [CrossRef]
3. Muralikrishna, I.V.; Manickam, V. Chapter Two—Sustainable Development. In *Environmental Management*; Butterworth-Heinemann: Oxford, UK, 2017; pp. 5–21.
4. Jung, W.; Jazizadeh, F. Human-in-the-loop HVAC operations: A quantitative review on occupancy, comfort, and energy-efficiency dimensions. *Appl. Energy* **2019**, *239*, 1471–1508. [CrossRef]
5. Touchaei, A.G.; Hosseini, M.; Akbari, H. Energy savings potentials of commercial buildings by urban heat island reduction strategies in Montreal (Canada). *Energy Build.* **2016**, *110*, 41–48. [CrossRef]
6. Ma, Z.; Cooper, P.; Daly, D.; Ledo, L. Existing building retrofits: Methodology and state-of-the-art. *Energy Build.* **2012**, *55*, 889–902. [CrossRef]
7. Gholamzadehmir, M.; Del Pero, C.; Buffa, S.; Fedrizzi, R.; Aste, N. Adaptive-predictive control strategy for HVAC systems in smart buildings—A review. *Sustain. Cities Soc.* **2020**, *63*, 102480. [CrossRef]
8. Dezfouli, M.M.S.; Moghimi, S.; Azizpour, F.; Mat, S.; Sopian, K. Feasibility of saving energy by using VSD in HVAC system, a case study of large scale hospital in Malaysia. *WSEAS Trans. Environ. Dev.* **2014**, *10*, 15–25.
9. Huang, P.; Huang, G.; Wang, Y. HVAC system design under peak load prediction uncertainty using multiple-criterion decision making technique. *Energy Build.* **2015**, *91*, 26–36. [CrossRef]
10. Huang, S.; Ma, Z.; Wang, F. A multi-objective design optimization strategy for vertical ground heat exchangers. *Energy Build.* **2015**, *87*, 233–242. [CrossRef]
11. Pérez-Lombard, L.; Ortiz, J.; Coronel, J.F.; Maestre, I.R. A review of HVAC systems requirements in building energy regulations. *Energy Build.* **2011**, *43*, 255–268. [CrossRef]
12. Asim, N.; Amin, M.H.; Alghoul, M.; Badiei, M.; Mohammad, M.; Gasaymeh, S.S.; Amin, N.; Sopian, K. Key factors of desiccant-based cooling systems: Materials. *Appl. Therm. Eng.* **2019**, *159*, 113946. [CrossRef]
13. Rafique, M.M.; Rehman, S. Renewable and Sustainable Air Conditioning. In *Sustainable Air Conditioning Systems*; Books on Demand: Norderstedt, Germany, 2018.
14. Enteria, N.; Awbi, H.; Yoshino, H. Advancement of the Desiccant Heating, Ventilating, and Air-Conditioning (DHVAC) Systems. In *Desiccant Heating, Ventilating, and Air-Conditioning Systems*; Springer: Singapore, 2017; pp. 1–9.
15. Pottathara, Y.B.; Tiyyagura, H.R.; Ahmad, Z.; Sadasivuni, K.K. Graphene Based Aerogels: Fundamentals and Applications as Supercapacitors. *J. Energy Storage* **2020**, *30*, 101549. [CrossRef]
16. Emdadi, Z.; Maleki, A.; Azizi, M.; Asim, N. Evaporative Passive Cooling Designs for Buildings. *Strat. Plan. Energy Environ.* **2019**, *38*, 63–80. [CrossRef]
17. Emdadi, Z.; Maleki, A.; Mohammad, M.; Asim, N.; Azizi, M. Coupled Evaporative and Desiccant Cooling Systems for Tropical Climate. *Int. J. Environ. Sci.* **2017**, *2*, 262–278.
18. Sarbu, I.; Sebarchievici, C. *Solar Heating and Cooling Systems: Fundamentals, Experiments and Applications*; Elsevier: Amsterdam, The Netherlands, 2017.
19. Wang, R.; Xu, Z.; Ge, T. Introduction to solar heating and cooling systems. In *Advances in Solar Heating and Cooling*; Woodhead Publishing: Sawston, UK, 2016; pp. 3–12. [CrossRef]
20. Soltani, M.; Kashkooli, F.M.; Dehghani-Sanij, A.; Kazemi, A.; Bordbar, N.; Farshchi, M.; Elmi, M.; Gharali, K.; Dusseault, M.B. A comprehensive study of geothermal heating and cooling systems. *Sustain. Cities Soc.* **2019**, *44*, 793–818. [CrossRef]
21. Wegener, M.; Malmquist, A.; Isalgue, A.; Martin, A. Biomass-fired combined cooling, heating and power for small scale applications—A review. *Renew. Sustain. Energy Rev.* **2018**, *96*, 392–410. [CrossRef]

22. Wang, Z.X.; Li, H.Y.; Zhang, X.F.; Wang, L.W.; Du, S.; Fang, C. Performance Analysis on a Novel Micro-Scale Combined Cooling, Heating and Power (Cchp) System for Domestic Utilization Driven by Biomass Energy. *Renew. Energy* **2018**, *96*, 392–410. [CrossRef]
23. Khalid, F.; Dincer, I.; Rosen, M. Development and analysis of sustainable energy systems for building HVAC applications. *Appl. Therm. Eng.* **2015**, *87*, 389–401. [CrossRef]
24. Lucentini, M.; Naso, V.; Borreca, M. Parametric Performance Analysis of Renewable Energy Sources HVAC Systems for Buildings. *Energy Procedia* **2014**, *45*, 415–423. [CrossRef]
25. Nassif, N. Performance analysis of supply and return fans for HVAC systems under different operating strategies of economizer dampers. *Energy Build.* **2010**, *42*, 1026–1037. [CrossRef]
26. Kialashaki, Y. Energy and economic analysis of model-based air dampers strategies on a VAV system. *Int. J. Environ. Sci. Technol.* **2018**, *16*, 4687–4696. [CrossRef]
27. Alavy, M.; Li, T.; Siegel, J.A. Energy use in residential buildings: Analyses of high-efficiency filters and HVAC fans. *Energy Build.* **2020**, *209*, 109697. [CrossRef]
28. Grainge, Z. HVAC efficiency: Can filter selection reduce HVAC energy costs? *Filtr. Sep.* **2007**, *44*, 20–22. [CrossRef]
29. Shamim, J.A.; Hsu, W.-L.; Paul, S.; Yu, L.; Daiguji, H. A review of solid desiccant dehumidifiers: Current status and near-term development goals in the context of net zero energy buildings. *Renew. Sustain. Energy Rev.* **2021**, *137*, 110456. [CrossRef]
30. Chua, K.; Chou, S.; Islam, M. Integrating Composite Desiccant and Membrane Dehumidifier to Enhance Building Energy Efficiency. *Energy Procedia* **2017**, *143*, 186–191. [CrossRef]
31. Wang, Y.W.; Cai, W.J.; Soh, Y.C.; Li, S.J.; Lu, L.; Xie, L. A simplified modeling of cooling coils for control and optimization of HVAC systems. *Energy Convers. Manag.* **2004**, *45*, 2915–2930. [CrossRef]
32. Yildiz, A.; Ersöz, M.A. The effect of wind speed on the economical optimum insulation thickness for HVAC duct applications. *Renew. Sustain. Energy Rev.* **2016**, *55*, 1289–1300. [CrossRef]
33. Sukarno, R.; Putra, N.; Hakim, I.I.; Rachman, F.F.; Mahlia, T.M.I. Utilizing heat pipe heat exchanger to reduce the energy consumption of airborne infection isolation hospital room HVAC system. *J. Build. Eng.* **2021**, *35*, 102116. [CrossRef]
34. Koç, A.; Yağlı, H.; Bilgic, H.H.; Koç, Y.; Özdemir, A. Performance analysis of a novel organic fluid filled regenerative heat exchanger used heat recovery ventilation (OHeX-HRV) system. *Sustain. Energy Technol. Assess.* **2020**, *41*, 100787. [CrossRef]
35. Eades, W.G. Energy and water recovery using air-handling unit condensate from laboratory HVAC systems. *Sustain. Cities Soc.* **2018**, *42*, 162–175. [CrossRef]
36. Goldanlou, A.S.; Kalbasi, R.; Afrand, M. Energy usage reduction in an air handling unit by incorporating two heat recovery units. *J. Build. Eng.* **2020**, *32*, 101545. [CrossRef]
37. Liu, W.; Kalbasi, R.; Afrand, M. Solutions for enhancement of energy and exergy efficiencies in air handling units. *J. Clean. Prod.* **2020**, *257*, 120565. [CrossRef]
38. Abd El-Baky, M.A.A. Heat pipe heat exchanger for heat recovery in air conditioning. *Appl. Therm. Eng.* **2007**, *27*, 795–801. [CrossRef]
39. Mardiana-Idayu, A.; Riffat, S. Review on heat recovery technologies for building applications. *Renew. Sustain. Energy Rev.* **2012**, *16*, 1241–1255. [CrossRef]
40. Putra, N.; Winarta, S.M.A. Experimental Study of Heat Pipe Heat Exchanger Multi Fin for Energy Efficiency Effort in Operating Room Air System. *Int. J. Technol.* **2018**, *9*, 291–319.
41. Ahmadzadehtalatapeh, M.; Yau, Y. The application of heat pipe heat exchangers to improve the air quality and reduce the energy consumption of the air conditioning system in a hospital ward—A full year model simulation. *Energy Build.* **2011**, *43*, 2344–2355. [CrossRef]
42. Cuce, P.M.; Riffat, S. A comprehensive review of heat recovery systems for building applications. *Renew. Sustain. Energy Rev.* **2015**, *47*, 665–682. [CrossRef]
43. Fikri, B.; Sofia, E.; Putra, N. Experimental analysis of a multistage direct-indirect evaporative cooler using a straight heat pipe. *Appl. Therm. Eng.* **2020**, *171*, 115133. [CrossRef]
44. Kusumah, A.S.; Hakim, I.I.; Sukarno, R.; Rachman, F.F.; Putra, N. The Application of U-shape Heat Pipe Heat Exchanger to Reduce Relative Humidity for Energy Conservation in Heating, Ventilation, and Air Conditioning (HVAC) Systems. *Int. J. Technol.* **2019**, *10*, 291–319.
45. Martínez, F.J.R.; Plasencia, M.A.Á.-G.; Gómez, E.V.; Díez, F.V.; Martín, R.H. Design and experimental study of a mixed energy recovery system, heat pipes and indirect evaporative equipment for air conditioning. *Energy Build.* **2003**, *35*, 1021–1030. [CrossRef]
46. Abdel-Salam, M.R.; Fauchoux, M.; Ge, G.; Besant, R.W.; Simonson, C.J. Expected energy and economic benefits, and environmental impacts for liquid-to-air membrane energy exchangers (LAMEEs) in HVAC systems: A review. *Appl. Energy* **2014**, *127*, 202–218. [CrossRef]
47. Abdel-Salam, M.R.; Besant, R.W.; Simonson, C.J. Performance Testing of 2-Fluid and 3-Fluid Liquid-to-Air Membrane Energy Exchangers for Hvac Applications in Cold–Dry Climates. *Int. J. Heat Mass Transfer.* **2016**, *106*, 558–569. [CrossRef]
48. Kuruneru, S.T.W.; Vafai, K.; Sauret, E.; Gu, Y. Application of porous metal foam heat exchangers and the implications of particulate fouling for energy-intensive industries. *Chem. Eng. Sci.* **2020**, *228*, 115968. [CrossRef]
49. Awais, M.; Ullah, N.; Ahmad, J.; Sikandar, F.; Ehsan, M.M.; Salehin, S.; Bhuiyan, A.A. Heat transfer and pressure drop performance of Nanofluid: A state-of- the-art review. *Int. J. Thermofluids* **2021**, *9*, 100065. [CrossRef]

50. Shao, J.; Darkwa, J.; Kokogiannakis, G. Review of phase change emulsions (PCMEs) and their applications in HVAC systems. *Energy Build.* **2015**, *94*, 200–217. [CrossRef]
51. Abu-Hamdeh, N.H.; Melaibari, A.A.; Alquthami, T.S.; Khoshaim, A.; Oztop, H.F.; Karimipour, A. Efficacy of incorporating PCM into the building envelope on the energy saving and AHU power usage in winter. *Sustain. Energy Technol. Assess.* **2021**, *43*, 100969. [CrossRef]
52. Sun, W.; Zhang, Y.; Ling, Z.; Fang, X.; Zhang, Z. Experimental investigation on the thermal performance of double-layer PCM radiant floor system containing two types of inorganic composite PCMs. *Energy Build.* **2020**, *211*, 109806. [CrossRef]
53. Nariman, A.; Kalbasi, R.; Rostami, S. Sensitivity of AHU power consumption to PCM implementation in the wall-considering the solar radiation. *J. Therm. Anal.* **2021**, *143*, 2789–2800. [CrossRef]
54. Nasif, M.; Al-Waked, R.; Morrison, G.; Behnia, M. Membrane heat exchanger in HVAC energy recovery systems, systems energy analysis. *Energy Build.* **2010**, *42*, 1833–1840. [CrossRef]
55. Rasouli, M.; Akbari, S.; Simonson, C.J.; Besant, R.W. Energetic, economic and environmental analysis of a health-care facility HVAC system equipped with a run-around membrane energy exchanger. *Energy Build.* **2014**, *69*, 112–121. [CrossRef]
56. Albdoor, A.K.; Ma, Z.; Cooper, P.; Al-Ghazzawi, F.; Liu, J.; Richardson, C.; Wagner, P. Air-to-air enthalpy exchangers: Membrane modification using metal-organic frameworks, characterisation and performance assessment. *J. Clean. Prod.* **2021**, *293*, 126157. [CrossRef]
57. T'Joen, C.; Park, Y.; Wang, Q.; Sommers, A.; Han, X.; Jacobi, A. A review on polymer heat exchangers for HVAC&R applications. *Int. J. Refrig.* **2009**, *32*, 763–779. [CrossRef]
58. Jabbour, J.; Russeil, S.; Mobtil, M.; Bougeard, D.; Lacrampe, M.-F.; Krawczak, P. High performance finned-tube heat exchangers based on filled polymer. *Appl. Therm. Eng.* **2019**, *155*, 620–630. [CrossRef]
59. Fabrizio, E.; Seguro, F.; Filippi, M. Integrated HVAC and DHW production systems for Zero Energy Buildings. *Renew. Sustain. Energy Rev.* **2014**, *40*, 515–541. [CrossRef]
60. Yao, Y. Research and applications of ultrasound in HVAC field: A review. *Renew. Sustain. Energy Rev.* **2016**, *58*, 52–68. [CrossRef]
61. Ruiz, J.; Martínez, P.; Martín, Í.; Lucas, M. Numerical Characterization of an Ultrasonic Mist Generator as an Evaporative Cooler. *Energies* **2020**, *13*, 2971. [CrossRef]
62. Martínez, P.; Ruiz, J.; Martín, Í.; Lucas, M. Experimental study of an ultrasonic mist generator as an evaporative cooler. *Appl. Therm. Eng.* **2020**, *181*, 116057. [CrossRef]
63. Arun, B.S.; Mariappan, V.; Maisotsenko, V. Experimental study on combined low temperature regeneration of liquid desiccant and evaporative cooling by ultrasonic atomization. *Int. J. Refrig.* **2020**, *112*, 100–109. [CrossRef]
64. Song, J.; Tian, W.; Xu, X.; Wang, Y.; Li, Z. Thermal performance of a novel ultrasonic evaporator based on machine learning algorithms. *Appl. Therm. Eng.* **2019**, *148*, 438–446. [CrossRef]
65. Chenari, B.; Carrilho, J.D.; da Silva, M.G. Towards sustainable, energy-efficient and healthy ventilation strategies in buildings: A review. *Renew. Sustain. Energy Rev.* **2016**, *59*, 1426–1447. [CrossRef]
66. Ma, N.; Aviv, D.; Guo, H.; Braham, W.W. Measuring the right factors: A review of variables and models for thermal comfort and indoor air quality. *Renew. Sustain. Energy Rev.* **2021**, *135*, 110436. [CrossRef]
67. Curto, D.; Franzitta, V.; Longo, S.; Montana, F.; Sanseverino, E.R. Investigating energy saving potential in a big shopping center through ventilation control. *Sustain. Cities Soc.* **2019**, *49*, 101525. [CrossRef]
68. Gomis, L.L.; Fiorentini, M.; Daly, D. Potential and practical management of hybrid ventilation in buildings. *Energy Build.* **2021**, *231*, 110597. [CrossRef]
69. Kim, D.D.; Suh, H.S. Heating and cooling energy consumption prediction model for high-rise apartment buildings considering design parameters. *Energy Sustain. Dev.* **2021**, *61*, 1–14. [CrossRef]
70. Shi, H.; Chen, Q. Building energy management decision-making in the real world: A comparative study of HVAC cooling strategies. *J. Build. Eng.* **2020**, *33*, 101869. [CrossRef]
71. Seo, J.; Ooka, R.; Kim, J.T.; Nam, Y. Optimization of the HVAC system design to minimize primary energy demand. *Energy Build.* **2014**, *76*, 102–108. [CrossRef]
72. Pang, Z.; Chen, Y.; Zhang, J.; O'Neill, Z.; Cheng, H.; Dong, B. Nationwide HVAC energy-saving potential quantification for office buildings with occupant-centric controls in various climates. *Appl. Energy* **2020**, *279*, 115727. [CrossRef]
73. Stopps, H.; Huchuk, B.; Touchie, M.F.; O'Brien, W. Is anyone home? A critical review of occupant-centric smart HVAC controls implementations in residential buildings. *Build. Environ.* **2021**, *187*, 107369. [CrossRef]
74. Su, Y. Smart energy for smart built environment: A review for combined objectives of affordable sustainable green. *Sustain. Cities Soc.* **2020**, *53*, 101954. [CrossRef]
75. Bac, U.; Alaloosi, K.A.M.S.; Turhan, C. A comprehensive evaluation of the most suitable HVAC system for an industrial building by using a hybrid building energy simulation and multi criteria decision making framework. *J. Build. Eng.* **2021**, *37*, 102153. [CrossRef]
76. Porowski, M. Energy optimization of HVAC system from a holistic perspective: Operating theater application. *Energy Convers. Manag.* **2019**, *182*, 461–496. [CrossRef]
77. Afroz, Z.; Shafiullah, G.; Urmee, T.; Higgins, G. Modeling techniques used in building HVAC control systems: A review. *Renew. Sustain. Energy Rev.* **2018**, *83*, 64–84. [CrossRef]

78. Steinemann, A.; Wargocki, P.; Rismanchi, B. Ten questions concerning green buildings and indoor air quality. *Build. Environ.* **2017**, *112*, 351–358. [CrossRef]
79. EPA. *Indoor Air Quality and Student Performance*; United States Environmental Protection Agency, Indoor Environments Division Office of Radiation and Indoor Air: Washington, DC, USA, 2000.
80. Al Horr, Y.; Arif, M.; Katafygiotou, M.; Mazroei, A.; Kaushik, A.; Elsarrag, E. Impact of indoor environmental quality on occupant well-being and comfort: A review of the literature. *Int. J. Sustain. Built Environ.* **2016**, *5*, 1–11. [CrossRef]
81. Che-Ani, A.I.; Tawil, N.M.; Musa, A.R.; Yahaya, H.; Tahir, M.M. The Architecture Studio of Universiti Kebangsaan Malaysia (UKM): Has the Indoor Environmental Quality Standard Been Achieved? *Asian Soc. Sci.* **2012**, *8*, 174. [CrossRef]
82. Liu, Z.; Ma, S.; Cao, G.; Meng, C.; He, B.-J. Distribution characteristics, growth, reproduction and transmission modes and control strategies for microbial contamination in HVAC systems: A literature review. *Energy Build.* **2018**, *177*, 77–95. [CrossRef]
83. Abdulaali, H.S.; Usman, I.M.S.; Hanafiah, M.M.; Abdulhasan, M.J.; Hamzah, M.T.; Nazal, A.A. Impact of poor indoor environmental quality (Ieq) to inhabitants health, wellbeing and satisfaction. *Int. J. Adv. Sci. Technol.* **2020**, *29*, 1284–1296.
84. Roll, I.B.; Halden, R.U.; Pycke, B.F. Indoor air condensate as a novel matrix for monitoring inhalable organic contaminants. *J. Hazard. Mater.* **2015**, *288*, 89–96. [CrossRef]
85. Cobo-Golpe, M.; Ramil, M.; Cela, R.; Rodríguez, I. Portable dehumidifiers condensed water: A novel matrix for the screening of semi-volatile compounds in indoor air. *Chemosphere* **2020**, *251*, 126346. [CrossRef] [PubMed]
86. Silva, L.F.O.; Pinto, D.; Enders, M.S.P.; Hower, J.C.; Flores, E.M.M.; Müller, E.I.; Dotto, G.L. Portable dehumidifiers as an original matrix for the study of inhalable nanoparticles in school. *Chemosphere* **2021**, *262*, 127295. [CrossRef] [PubMed]
87. Santos, A.F.; Gaspar, P.D.; Hamandosh, A.; de Aguiar, E.B.; Filho, A.C.G.; de Souza, H.J.L. Best Practices on HVAC Design to Minimize the Risk of COVID-19 Infection within Indoor Environments. *Braz. Arch. Biol. Technol.* **2020**, *63*, e20200335. [CrossRef]
88. Abdulaali, H.S.; Hanafiah, M.M.; Usman, I.M.; Nizam, N.U.M.; Abdulhasan, M.J. A review on green hotel rating tools, indoor environmental quality (Ieq) and human comfort. *Int. J. Adv. Sci. Technol.* **2020**, *29*, 128–157.
89. Li, T.; Siegel, J.A. Assessing the Impact of Filtration Systems in Indoor Environments with Effectiveness. *Build. Environ.* **2021**, *187*, 107389. [CrossRef]
90. Nath, R.K.; Zain, M.; Jamil, M. An environment-friendly solution for indoor air purification by using renewable photocatalysts in concrete: A review. *Renew. Sustain. Energy Rev.* **2016**, *62*, 1184–1194. [CrossRef]
91. Liu, G.; Xiao, M.; Zhang, X.; Gál, C.; Chen, X.; Liu, L.; Pan, S.; Wu, J.; Tang, L.; Clements-Croome, D. A review of air filtration technologies for sustainable and healthy building ventilation. *Sustain. Cities Soc.* **2017**, *32*, 375–396. [CrossRef]
92. Tu, Y.; Wang, R.; Zhang, Y.; Wang, J. Progress and Expectation of Atmospheric Water Harvesting. *Joule* **2018**, *2*, 1452–1475. [CrossRef]
93. Ahmed, H.M. The Amount of Fresh Water Wasted as by Product of Air Conditioning Systems: Case Study in the Kingdom of Bahrain. In Proceedings of the 2019 International Conference on Fourth Industrial Revolution (ICFIR), Manama, Bahrain, 19–21 February 2019; pp. 1–4.
94. Algarni, S.; Saleel, C.; Mujeebu, M.A. Air-conditioning condensate recovery and applications—Current developments and challenges ahead. *Sustain. Cities Soc.* **2018**, *37*, 263–274. [CrossRef]
95. Habeebullah, B.A. Potential use of evaporator coils for water extraction in hot and humid areas. *Desalination* **2009**, *237*, 330–345. [CrossRef]
96. Hermes, J. Air Conditioning Condensate Recovery. 2021. Available online: https://www.environmentalleader.com/2013/01/air-conditioning-condensate-recovery (accessed on 1 December 2021).
97. Scalize, P.S.; Soares, S.S.; Alves, A.C.F.; Marques, T.A.; Mesquita, G.G.M.; Ballaminut, N.; Albuquerque, A.C.J. Use of condensed water from air conditioning systems. *Open Eng.* **2018**, *8*, 284–292. [CrossRef]
98. Magrini, A.; Cartesegna, M.; Magnani, L.; Cattani, L. Production of Water from the Air: The Environmental Sustainability of Air-conditioning Systems through a More Intelligent Use of Resources. The Advantages of an Integrated System. *Energy Procedia* **2015**, *78*, 1153–1158. [CrossRef]
99. Magrini, A.; Cattani, L.; Cartesegna, M.; Magnani, L. Water Production from Air Conditioning Systems: Some Evaluations about a Sustainable use of Resources. *Sustainability* **2017**, *9*, 1309. [CrossRef]
100. Tu, R.; Hwang, Y. Performance analyses of a new system for water harvesting from moist air that combines multi-stage desiccant wheels and vapor compression cycles. *Energy Convers. Manag.* **2019**, *198*, 111811. [CrossRef]
101. Magrini, A.; Cattani, L.; Cartesegna, M.; Magnani, L. Integrated Systems for Air Conditioning and Production of Drinking Water—Preliminary Considerations. *Energy Procedia* **2015**, *75*, 1659–1665. [CrossRef]
102. Cuviella-Suárez, C.; Colmenar-Santos, A.; Borge-Diez, D.; López-Rey, Á. Reduction of water and energy consumption in the sanitary ware industry by an absorption machine operated with recovered heat. *J. Clean. Prod.* **2021**, *292*, 126049. [CrossRef]
103. Cattani, L.; Magrini, A.; Cattani, P. Water Extraction from Air by Refrigeration—Experimental Results from an Integrated System Application. *Appl. Sci.* **2018**, *8*, 2262. [CrossRef]
104. Ghimire, S.R.; Johnston, J.M.; Garland, J.; Edelen, A.; Ma, X.C.; Jahne, M. Life cycle assessment of a rainwater harvesting system compared with an AC condensate harvesting system. *Resour. Conserv. Recycl.* **2019**, *146*, 536–548. [CrossRef]
105. Arden, S.; Morelli, B.; Cashman, S.; Ma, X.; Jahne, M.; Garland, J. Onsite Non-potable Reuse for Large Buildings: Environmental and Economic Suitability as a Function of Building Characteristics and Location. *Water Res.* **2020**, *191*, 116635. [CrossRef]

106. Gurubalan, A.; Maiya, M.; Geoghegan, P.J. Tri-generation of air conditioning, refrigeration and potable water by a novel absorption refrigeration system equipped with membrane dehumidifier. *Appl. Therm. Eng.* **2020**, *181*, 115861. [CrossRef]
107. Akgül, A.; Seçkiner, S.U. Optimization of biomass to bioenergy supply chain with tri-generation and district heating and cooling network systems. *Comput. Ind. Eng.* **2019**, *137*, 106017. [CrossRef]
108. Yoon, I.J.; Son, C.H.; Moon, C.G.; Kong, J.Y. Performance characteristics of portable air conditioner with condensate-water spray. *IOP Conf. Series: Mater. Sci. Eng.* **2019**, *675*, 12043. [CrossRef]
109. Tan, Y.Z.; Han, L.; Chew, N.G.P.; Chow, W.H.; Wang, R.; Chew, J.W. Membrane distillation hybridized with a thermoelectric heat pump for energy-efficient water treatment and space cooling. *Appl. Energy* **2018**, *231*, 1079–1088. [CrossRef]
110. Vilches, A.; Garcia-Martinez, A.; Sanchez-Montañes, B. Life cycle assessment (LCA) of building refurbishment: A literature review. *Energy Build.* **2017**, *135*, 286–301. [CrossRef]
111. Lavagna, M.; Baldassarri, C.; Campioli, A.; Giorgi, S.; Valle, A.D.; Castellani, V.; Sala, S. Benchmarks for environmental impact of housing in Europe: Definition of archetypes and LCA of the residential building stock. *Build. Environ.* **2018**, *145*, 260–275. [CrossRef]
112. Jafari, A.; Valentin, V. An Investment Allocation Approach for Building Energy Retrofits. In *Construction Research Congress*; ASCE: Reston, VA, USA, 2016; pp. 1061–1070. [CrossRef]
113. Toosi, H.A.; Lavagna, M.; Leonforte, F.; Del Pero, C.; Aste, N. Life Cycle Sustainability Assessment in Building Energy Retrofitting; A Review. *Sustain. Cities Soc.* **2020**, *60*, 102248. [CrossRef]
114. Ardente, F.; Beccali, M.; Cellura, M.; Mistretta, M. Energy and environmental benefits in public buildings as a result of retrofit actions. *Renew. Sustain. Energy Rev.* **2011**, *15*, 460–470. [CrossRef]
115. Ruggeri, A.; Gabrielli, L.; Scarpa, M. Energy Retrofit in European Building Portfolios: A Review of Five Key Aspects. *Sustainability* **2020**, *12*, 7465. [CrossRef]
116. Jafari, A.; Valentin, V. An optimization framework for building energy retrofits decision-making. *Build. Environ.* **2017**, *115*, 118–129. [CrossRef]
117. Patel, P. Energy saving by modification in hvac as a cost saving opportunity for industries. *Int. J. Pharm. Sci. Res.* **2013**, *4*, 3347–3356.
118. Feng, W.; Wei, Z.; Sun, G.; Zhou, Y.; Zang, H.; Chen, S. A conditional value-at-risk-based dispatch approach for the energy management of smart buildings with HVAC systems. *Electr. Power Syst. Res.* **2020**, *188*, 106535. [CrossRef]
119. Shi, W.; Jin, X.; Wang, Y. Evaluation of energy saving potential of HVAC system by operation data with uncertainties. *Energy Build.* **2019**, *204*, 109513. [CrossRef]

International Journal of
Environmental Research and Public Health

MDPI

Article

The Impact of Air Pollution Perception on Urban Settlement Intentions of Young Talent in China

Lianying Yao [1,2], Xuewen Li [3,*], Rongrong Zheng [4] and Yiye Zhang [4]

1 School of Economics, Zhejiang University of Technology, Hangzhou 310014, China; yaolianying@zju.edu.cn
2 Global Institute for Zhejiang Merchants Development, Zhejiang University of Technology, Hangzhou 310014, China
3 School of Public Affairs, Zhejiang University, Hangzhou 310058, China
4 School of Public Administration, Zhejiang University of Finance and Economics, Hangzhou 310018, China; 15068553536@163.com (R.Z.); zhangyiye@zufe.edu.cn (Y.Z.)
* Correspondence: lixuewen@zju.edu.cn

Abstract: In recent years, with the public paying more and more attention to the problem of air pollution, the impact of air quality on migration has gradually become a growing concern. However, in the current context of cities' efforts to "attract talent" in China, research on the impact of air pollution on the flow or dwelling willingness of young talent is relatively limited. Based on the theory of planned behavior and from the perspective of subjective perception, this paper uses a regulated model to explore the impact mechanism of air pollution perception on young talent urban settlement intentions. Taking Hangzhou as a case, this study surveyed 987 individuals who were classified as young talent to explore the impact of air pollution perception on urban settlement intentions in China. The research shows that air pollution perception has a significant impact on young talent urban settlement intentions, and this impact is achieved through the intermediary effect of residential satisfaction. Place attachment of young talent to cities cannot significantly regulate the impact of air pollution perception on residential satisfaction, but it can significantly regulate the relationship between residential satisfaction and urban settlement intentions. That is to say, although place attachment cannot reduce the decline in residential satisfaction brought by air pollution perception, it can weaken the negative impact of air pollution perception on dwelling willingness through a decline in residential satisfaction. This paper contributes to a deeper understanding of the relationship between air quality and young talent settlement intentions.

Keywords: air pollution perception; young talent; urban settlement intentions; residential satisfaction; place attachment

Citation: Yao, L.; Li, X.; Zheng, R.; Zhang, Y. The Impact of Air Pollution Perception on Urban Settlement Intentions of Young Talent in China. *Int. J. Environ. Res. Public Health* **2022**, *19*, 1080. https://doi.org/10.3390/ijerph19031080

Academic Editors: Roberto Alonso González Lezcano, Francesco Nocera and Rosa Giuseppina Caponetto

Received: 29 November 2021
Accepted: 13 January 2022
Published: 19 January 2022

1. Introduction

In recent years, with the sustained and stable development of China's economy and society, the attraction of China's living environment to international immigrants has continued to increase. In 2020, the number of foreign persons living in the mainland reached 850,000, which rose from 600,000 in 2010, an increase of 42% (China National Bureau of Statistics, 2021). At the same time, along with a series of policies aimed at encouraging reasonable population migration, various traditional barriers that restrict population mobility have been broken down. Meanwhile, intensive regional competition has made attracting and retaining young talent an important approach to obtaining development advantages. The urban settlement of young talent has been an important issue in China. For example, in recent years, large- and medium-sized cities, such as Hangzhou, Nanjing, Wuhan, Zhengzhou, Chengdu, and Xi'an, have introduced "New Deals" for young talent, beginning a "talent grabbing" war. Retaining young talent for long-term residencies and, thus, developing cities has become a common concern for city administration and demographic researchers. Yet, young talent endures unstable career developments and a lack of social integration, owing to their short stays in new cities. This results in their increased willingness to move among cities, which makes urban settlement challenging [1]. The theory of planned behavior (TPB) suggests that psychological factors (such as attitude, subjective norms, and perceptual behavioral control) indirectly influence individual behavior through behavioral intentions [2]. Based on the TPB, scholars such as Weng and McElroy, proposed the concept of talent urban settlement intentions [3]; that is, the willingness of talent to work and live in a city for a long time. From this concept we can regard "settlement intentions" as a kind of attitude and behavior tendency, which reflects a comprehensive evaluation of talent from various aspects of a city and is a good indicator of a city's ability to retain talent. A comprehensive analysis of the influencing factors of the willingness of talent to settle down can help city administration understand what such talent need from the city and thus enact targeted and efficient public policies and provide public goods.

Various studies have been conducted on urban settlement intentions and their influencing factors on population migration between countries, cities, and urban–rural areas. Related studies show that economic factors (e.g., income level and cost of living) [4], personal factors (e.g., education, occupation, and mobility distance) [5,6], amenities (e.g., entertainment and recreational facilities, cultural facilities, consumer shopping, green parks, and public cultural activities) [7], policy (e.g., household registration and subsidies) [8,9], and social factors (e.g., family and friends' connections, traditional attitudes, and cultural inclusion) [10] are all important influencing factors in urban settlement intentions. In addition, when examining the influencing factors of overseas immigration, Poprawe believes that political corruption can easily lead people to emigrate abroad [11]; Bertoli and Moraga found that the migration situation between the two countries is affected, not only by various factors between the two countries, but also by the policies of a third country [12].

In recent years, as environmental hazards, e.g., air pollution, have become increasingly serious, more individuals consider air quality an important factor when choosing a place of residence (for physical and mental health purposes). A survey conducted by New Fortune magazine in 2013 found that the environment had become one of the important factors to promote to Chinese residents to consider international migration [13]. Based on city level data, Qin and Zhu's research confirmed that, during a period of increasing air pollution, people retrieve "immigrants" through the Internet more frequently [14]. Kohlhuber et al. found that highly educated people are more concerned about air quality [15]. Jacquemin et al. further found that educational attainment was highly correlated with the level of perceived annoyance [16]; particularly, respondents with a graduate degree or higher were found to be the most sensitive to poor air quality. These findings suggest that young talent are more sensitive and concerned about air pollution, and that this may consequently influence their choice of cities when seeking long-term employment. However, existing studies related to population migration settlement have often neglected the topic of air quality [17]. Further, the impact mechanism of air pollution perception on urban settlement intentions has not been examined, although perception is considered important for initiating actions. With increasing concerns about air pollution, it is necessary to introduce air quality factors into analyses, focusing on their impact on the urban settlement intentions of young talent in China.

This paper is devoted to studying the impact of air pollution perception on the willingness of young talent to settle down in Chinese cities, based on the perspective of the inter-city talent competition using young talent as the research subjects. This study further shows how, and under what circumstances, air pollution perceptions affect the willingness of young talent to settle down in cities. Specifically, this study proposes urban residential satisfaction as a mediating variable and empirically tests its mediating role. It also suggests and tests the moderating role of place attachment in the relationship between air pollution perception and urban settlement intentions. The study systematically investigates the impact mechanisms and boundary conditions of air pollution perception on urban settlement intentions. It further provides theoretical references for city administration to improve the urban talent environment, urban talent attraction, and their retention. The study is structured as follows. Section 2 reviews existing studies and proposes hypotheses for testing. Section 3 introduces the research method and design used in this study. Section 4 presents the empirical results and conducts an in-depth discussion to interpret the results. Section 5 concludes this study by determining future studies.

2. Literature Review and Hypotheses Formulation

2.1. Impact of Air Pollution Perception on the Urban Settlement Intentions of Young Talent

By referring to perceived quality research, based on the consumer perspective [18], air pollution perception is defined as people's opinion formed by the air pollution conditions around them and considers the processes by which the opinion is modified. Although there is no research that directly examines the impact of air pollution perception on the willingness of young talent to settle in cities, many scholars have conducted exploratory studies about the relationship between subjective and objective environmental quality and the migration and settlement of a population. Chen et al. analyzed the impact of air pollution on population migration in China from 1996 to 2010 [19] and found that, within the study period, air pollution reduced the in-migration of mobile populations by 50% in a county, ultimately reducing the total population by 5% through net out-migration. However, as Gronroos et al. [20] stated, customer satisfaction regarding a service stems from comparing the customer's perception of a service and their expectations from the service. Accordingly, air pollution perception is a direct reflection of objective air quality, a complement of, and development in, objective air quality, and is a more direct influencing factor in decision-making. Air pollution perception may influence the willingness of young talent to settle down in cities in three ways. Concerns about their own and their family's health may influence the willingness of young talent to settle down in cities. Air pollution can cause respiratory diseases, physiological dysfunctions, and irritate mucosal tissues, such as the eyes and nose, resulting in illnesses or the recurrence of old illnesses in people with a history of respiratory diseases [21]. Continuing to live in a polluted environment may place residents at an increased risk of contracting heart disease and lung cancer [22]. Sun et al. [17] analyzed data from a 2014 survey conducted by the National Health and Family Planning Commission in eight cities, including Beijing, Xiamen, and Shenzhen, and found that, as the concentration of PM2.5 increased, people's health-related expectations decreased significantly. Consequently, young talent may choose to leave such cities. The willingness of young talent to settle in cities may also be influenced by air pollution surpassing all other environmental issues and increasingly affecting residents' trust in the government, becoming a political, societal, and living condition issue [23]. Wang and Han [24] found that air pollution perception significantly affects the public's evaluation of the government's performance. They also found that poor air perception may cause young talent to lose trust in local governments, thus losing interest in settling down in a city. Moreover, additional living expenses for young talent caused by air pollution perception may also influence their willingness to settle down. Further, they are required to pay for the explicit costs of protective equipment, such as air purifiers, and shoulder various hidden costs, such as reduced labor efficiency [25] and increased workdays owing to air pollution. For example, studies show that a 1% increase in suspended particulate matter in the air is associated with a significant increase of 0.44% in the number of workdays lost [26]. The combination of these costs is not negligible and constitutes a "push" factor in migrating from cities.

Therefore, to further explore the relationship between air pollution perception and the settlement intentions of young talent, this study proposes the following hypothesis based on the abovementioned analysis:

Hypothesis 1 (H1). *Air pollution perception has a significant negative effect on the urban settlement intentions of young talent.*

2.2. The Mediating Role of Residential Satisfaction between Air Pollution Perception and the Urban Settlement Intentions of Young Talent

2.2.1. Air Pollution Perception and Urban Residential Satisfaction

Satisfaction occurs when people's inner desires and all their subjective feelings are in tune with each other. It is reflected in a person's psychological state, when one is extremely pleased and comfortable [27]. Scholars, such as You and Chen [28], defined urban residential satisfaction as the public's satisfaction assessment, based on the accumulation of all environmental feelings. An empirical study on the elderly found that subjective evaluations, that is, perceived factors, explained the degree of variation in residential satisfaction much more effectively than objective environmental variables [29]. Objectively measured air quality ultimately affects residential satisfaction by influencing the subjective perceptions of young talent. Air pollution directly triggers sensory discomfort, which consequently causes negative emotions. Moreover, studies show that, although individuals have many behavioral beliefs, only a relatively small number of these are accessible at any given time and in any given context. These obtainable beliefs, also referred to as salient beliefs, are the cognitive and emotional bases for behavioral attitudes, subjective norms, and perceptual behavioral control [30]. Young talent is more concerned about air quality and have higher expectations regarding this issue [31]. Therefore, for young talent, air pollution perception becomes a salient belief that profoundly influences residential satisfaction. If their perception of air quality differs from their preferred conditions, it causes a negative assessment of their satisfaction with urban living. Therefore, perceived air pollution is a subjective perception and an important aspect of the urban environment from the point of view of young talent and is likely to significantly influence residential satisfaction.

Accordingly, the study hypothesizes the following:

Hypothesis 2a (H2a). *Air pollution perception has a significant negative impact on the urban residential satisfaction of young talent.*

2.2.2. Residential Satisfaction and the Urban Settlement Intention of Young Talent

People tend to follow practices that satisfy them. In other words, satisfaction drives loyalty. Cardozo [32] suggested that customers are more likely to purchase a product again (or other goods) if they are satisfied with a merchant's production. Similarly, if young talent has high-level residential satisfaction in a city, they are more likely to continue living there. In other words, residential satisfaction generates a willingness to settle down in cities. Weng et al. [33] proposed the concept of regional commitment in his study on talent agglomeration, arguing that, if the regional environment matches the growth and living needs of talent, that is, if they experience good residential satisfaction, it can generate regional commitment between the talent and the city. This will, in turn, result in the desire to actively work to promote regional development. Therefore, residential satisfaction evaluates the degree to which the needs of young talent are met. According to customer loyalty and regional commitment theories, high-level urban residential satisfaction can make young talent emotionally "loyal" to a city, promote strong regional commitments, and make them willing to invest more in regional development. Liang [34] found that satisfaction with urban life has a significant impact on the willingness of a migrant population to settle down, especially those who are "relatively satisfied" and "very satisfied". Yao [35] conducted a large-scale questionnaire survey of foreign residents in Shanghai and found that the higher the satisfaction of foreign migrants with the city and community, the greater the likelihood of their long-term residence in Shanghai.

Accordingly, this study hypothesizes the following:

Hypothesis 2b (H2b). *Residential satisfaction has a significant positive impact on the urban settlement intentions of young talent.*

2.2.3. Residential Satisfaction Plays an Intermediary Role in the Impact of Air Pollution Perception on the Urban Settlement Intentions of Young Talent

Residential satisfaction reflects whether residents' various expectations and needs from a city are met, resulting in a pleasant and positive state of mind [36]. It essentially reflects the comparison of people's perceptions with their expectations in the context of various urban residence-related factors and satisfaction arises when perceptions meet expectations [37]. Young talent is a group of urban residents who are significantly concerned with environmental issues and the impact of air quality factors on health [31]. If their perception of air quality is not satisfactory, they will feel dissatisfied and choose to relocate to a better environment. Previous research further shows that residential satisfaction is a positive psychological mechanism that can explain proactive psychological processes, such as urban settlement intentions. Further, it links the perceived environment with the intentions of long-term residence [38]. Therefore, this study argues that, for young talent, residential satisfaction may be a psychological mechanism that can effectively convey perceived environmental quality as a livability characteristic; that is, the perception by young talent of air pollution is influenced by the psychological mechanisms of residential satisfaction. This further impacts their willingness to stay in a new city.

This study therefore combines the Hypotheses H2a and H2b and proposes the following hypothesis:

Hypothesis 2 (H2). *Residential satisfaction plays an intermediary role in the relationship between air pollution perceptions and the urban settlement intentions of young talent.*

In other words, air pollution perceptions influence the urban settlement intentions of young talent through residential satisfaction.

2.2.4. The Moderating Role of Place Attachment in the Relationship between Residential Satisfaction and Urban Settlement Intentions

Place attachment is a concept in psychology that characterizes the emotional bond and psychological identity between an individual and a specific environment. It refers to an individual's emotional response to their interaction with the environment and reflects a deep emotional connection to the place. Cultural and social characteristics modify this human–place relationship [39]. Psychological attachments to a place, or place attachment, occurs when individuals assign specific values to places in human–place interactions and form a positive emotional tie [40,41]. Place attachment may arise from cognition (i.e., the more you know about a place, the more you love it), well-known or reciprocal social networks, or a special emotional connection [42]. Casen et al. [43] suggest that people's attitudes and behaviors toward a particular place are significantly influenced by the emotions, meanings, and values that they assign to that place. Young talent, after working and living in a city, become inextricably linked to the city in various ways. A positive link generates positive emotions and is assigned special values, thus developing place attachment. Greater place attachment means that they have special emotional and social ties to a city and a deeper sense of identity and belonging. Therefore, they are likely to give better satisfaction ratings, even when they perceive air quality as being poor.

Therefore, this paper hypothesizes the following:

Hypothesis 3a (H3a). *Place attachment inversely regulates the relationship between air pollution perception and urban settlement intentions.*

In other words, relative to weaker place attachment, stronger place attachment will weaken the impact of poor air pollution perceptions on residential satisfaction.

Further, place attachment may not only affect the relationship between perceived air pollution and attitude, but it may also influence the relationship between attitude and behavioral intentions. Although there is still no research in this area, studies in other fields have found similar findings. Scholars studying the loyalty of tourists to tourist destinations show that place attachment significantly influences the relationship between tourist perceptions of a destination and satisfaction with tourism, as well as loyalty [44]. Li and Zhou [45] found that place attachment, as a moderating variable, significantly reinforced positive behavior among tourists, such as protecting tourist attraction sites. Therefore, in conjunction with the analysis above, it can be hypothesized that this moderating factor may exist between residential satisfaction and the urban settlement intentions of young talent. The inclination of young talent to leave a city owing to lower residential satisfaction arising from what they perceive to be poor air quality may be weakened when there is good place attachment. Therefore, this study suggests that place attachment may have a moderating effect on the relationship between residential satisfaction and the willingness to settle down. Accordingly, this study proposes the following hypothesis:

Hypothesis 3b (H3b). *Place attachment plays a moderating role in the relationship between residential satisfaction and the urban settlement intentions of young talent and enhances the positive impact of residential satisfaction on the willingness to settle down.*

Based on the above analysis, this study argues that place attachment between young talent and a city creates a deep emotional connection and a special value ascription between them and the environment. This consequently changes their satisfaction assessment of the air quality of the living environment and the resulting urban settlement intentions.

Combining H3a and H3b, this study proposes the following hypothesis:

Hypothesis 3 (H3). *Place attachment plays a moderating role among the relationship of air pollution perception, residential satisfaction, and urban settlement intentions; despite a greater place attachment, young talent may still suffer lower residential satisfaction owing to poor air quality. However, the moderating role of place attachment weakens the impact of residential satisfaction on their urban settlement intentions.*

The proposed hypotheses can be further summarized, as in Figure 1.

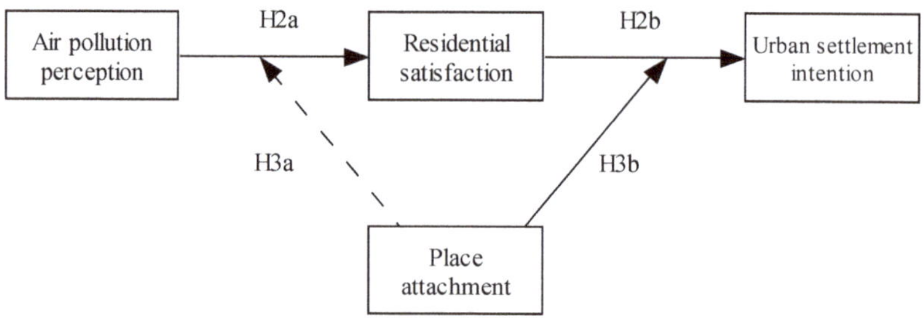

Figure 1. The conceptual model.

3. Materials and Methods

3.1. Data Collection

This study took Hangzhou as the research area. Hangzhou is the capital city of Zhejiang Province, located in the south of China. The city covers a total area of 16,850 square kilometers and the local GDP is 1.61 trillion CNY (Chinese Yuan, namely 0.23 trillion US dollars) with a residential population of 11.936 million in 2020 (Hangzhou Municipal Bureau of Statistics, 2021, the data mentioned below in this paragraph area also from this). Hangzhou is devoted to developing a digital economy and achieving high-quality development, which needs a large amount of young talent. By the end of 2020, Hangzhou's talent pool expanded to 2.945 million people with an annual increase of 5.2%. The net inflow rate of talent and overseas talent ranked at the top in China, and, for 10 consecutive years, Hangzhou has been rated as being among the "Ten Most Attractive Chinese Cities for Foreigners" (Hangzhou Municipal Bureau of Statistics, 2021). Hangzhou is becoming one of the most dynamic cities in China and is therefore suitable for investigating the young talent settlement intentions and the influence of air pollution perceptions [46].

According to the World Health Organization, People aged 14 to 44 are classified as young people. So, in this study, "young talent" refer to those who have a Junior college degree or above and are under the age of 44. This study uses data gathered from a questionnaire survey conducted by the research team, from April to June 2018, at the Hangzhou Future Sci-Tech City, the Hangzhou Economic and Technological Development Zone, Hangzhou High-Tech Zone (Binjiang), and key office buildings in central urban districts, where the inflow of young talent to Hangzhou is more concentrated. The target population of the questionnaire survey was young talent working in Hangzhou. The survey adopted a stratified random sampling method. With support from relevant government departments, survey respondents were randomly selected from a list of enterprises and their employees. A total of 1200 questionnaires were distributed with 300 for each abovementioned region. Overall, 1089 responses were collected, and, of these, 102 were excluded due to incomplete or invalid data. The final valid number of questionnaire responses was 987. Table 1 provides basic information about the survey respondents. A total of 807 (81.8% of the total sample) had a bachelor's degree or above. This included 49 (5%) with a doctoral degree and 176 (17.8%) with a master's degree. Further, 702 (71.1%) had an annual income of CNY 80,000 or more and 761 (77.1%) were under 35 years old. Based on age, educational attainment, and income level, the survey sample mainly consisted of young people with high educational attainments.

Table 1. Sample of the respondents.

Statistical Indicators	Ratio
Gender	
Male	55.5%
Female	44.5%
Age (years)	
Below 22	2.3%
Between 22 and 27	32.1%
Between 27 and 35	42.7%
Above 35	22.9%
Education	
Junior college	18.2%
Bachelor	59.0%
Master	17.8%
Ph.D.	5.0%
Hometown	
Hangzhou	19.8%
Outside Hangzhou but within Zhejiang	34.2%
Outside Zhejiang or China	46.0%
City of final graduation	
Zhejiang	48.6%
Outside Zhejiang	51.4%
Annual income (CNY)	
Below 80,000	28.9%
Between 80,000 and 150,000	38.2%
Between 150,000 and 250,000	18.2%
Between 250,000 and 350,000	7.6%
Above 350,000	7.1%

3.2. Measurement

The questionnaire's measurement scales were based on those used by previous related studies. A small-scale pre-survey and analysis were conducted before the large-scale survey. During this process, the research team communicated with the respondents comprehensively and used their input to improve the questionnaire in terms of reliability, validity, readability, and semantic accuracy to avoid any possible ambiguities arising from terminology. Chinese was used as the common language and due attention was also paid to minimize information loss during translation in paper writing [47]. The questionnaire items used a five-point Likert scale, and each respondent answered based on their judgment. In the questionnaire, an answer of 0 corresponded to "no such problem", 1 to "average", 2 to "not serious", 3 to "not very serious", 4 to "quite serious", and 5 to "very serious".

Based on Li [48] and Wang and Han [24], this study measured air pollution perception using three items, "the severity of PM2.5 in Hangzhou", "the air in Hangzhou is gray", and "the air is smelly in Hangzhou". To evaluate place attachment, this study referenced the studies by Kyle et al. [49] and Williams and Vaske [50]. Seven items are used to measure place attachment, "I like the cultural heritage of Hangzhou", "the landscape of Hangzhou gives me a sense of belonging", "Hangzhou possesses all kinds of living facilities that I want", "I have a good time with my colleagues (neighbors) in Hangzhou", "the help provided by the people around me makes me feel very warm", "I often feel respected in my life", and "I am willing to make efforts to make Hangzhou become better". To evaluate urban settlement intentions, the scale, based on the settlement intention scale developed by Hu and Weng [51] was adjusted so that it included four questionnaire items: "I am willing to stay and live in Hangzhou for a long time", "I have not considered the idea of settling in other similar cities", "if I were to choose again, I would still choose to work and live in Hangzhou", and "if I have the opportunity, I would recommend my relatives and friends from other places to live in Hangzhou". Satisfaction of living in a city was evaluated using three items, "I am happy to be able to work and live in this area", "I am satisfied with the living environment in the city", and "I often feel spiritually happy living here". Simultaneously, drawing on the results from existing research, this study selected seven control variables: gender, age, education, time spent in Hangzhou, income, development expectations, and family and friends in Hangzhou. Among them, gender and education were dummy variables. Variable "1" represented male in the gender variable and having at least one family member or friend in Hangzhou in the family and friends variable. Regarding the education variable, an educational attainment of junior college was considered a reference point. Other variables, such as age, time spent in Hangzhou, income, and career development expectations, were considered as continuous variables.

4. Results

4.1. Reliability and Validity Tests of the Questionnaire

This study used Cronbach's alpha coefficient to test the reliability of the measurement's variables to ensure the reliability and validity of the questionnaire. The results showed that the reliability of the four scales of place attachment, residential satisfaction, air pollution perception, and urban settlement intentions were 0.868, 0.974, 0.912, and 0.934, respectively. All four results were greater than 0.7 and, thus, had good reliability [52]. Further, according to the method suggested by Fornell et al. [53], this study used AMOS 24.0 (software to analyze structural equation modeling) to conduct a confirmatory factor analysis (CFA) on the four main variables to calculate the square root of the average variance extracted (AVE) value of each variable. The discriminant validity of each variable was tested by comparing the square root of the AVE value of each variable with the correlation coefficient between the latent variables, as shown in Table 2. The square root of the AVE value of all the variables was greater than the correlation coefficients. This indicated a good discriminant validity among the variables.

In addition, this study conducted a structural validity test on the four variables. The results showed that all the factor loading values in the four-factor model (model fit indices: $X^2/\text{df} = 4.684$, RMSEA = 0.078, IFI = 0.925, CFI = 0.918) (X^2 denotes chi-square test, which can assess overall fit and the discrepancy between the sample and fitted covariance matrices. df denotes model degrees of freedom. The chi-square value and model degrees of freedom can be used to calculate a p-value. Model is good fit if p-value > 0.05. RMSEA is an abbreviation for Root mean Square Error of Approximation. It is a parsimony-adjusted index, which is good fit if RMSEA < 0.08. IFI is an abbreviation for incremental fit index with values greater than approximately 0.90. CFI is an abbreviation for comparative fit index, which is good fit if CFI ≥ 0.90) were significantly higher than the general recommendation of 0.4, indicating that the measurement items of each variable could be better aggregated and effectively reflect the same construct. The results also showed that the four-factor model substantially fit indicators better than the other factor models. In summary, the tests described above indicate that the data of this questionnaire have high reliability and validity.

Table 2. Reliability and validity tests.

Variable	Mean	S.D.	1	2	3	4
Air pollution perception	2.562	1.009	**0.690**			
Place attachment	3.773	0.625	0.616 ***	**0.800**		
Residential satisfaction	3.821	0.759	0.218 ***	0.284 ***	**0.075**	
Urban settlement intention	3.800	0.721	0.451 ***	0.437 ***	0.511 ***	**0.780**

Note: The numbers in bold form a diagonal, and the diagonal line demonstrates the square root of the average variance extracted (AVE) value, and below the diagonal is the correlation coefficient of each variable. *** $p < 0.01$ with two-tailed test.

4.2. Testing the Main Effect

Models 1 and 2 in Table 3 show that, after controlling the relevant variables, the independent variable of air pollution perception significantly impacts the dependent variable of urban settlement intentions. The R^2 changes significantly, supporting H1 (β = −0.077, $p < 0.01$). Particularly, it is worth pointing out that, among the control variables, family and friends in Hangzhou and career development expectations have a significant impact on urban settlement intentions. In other words, migrant talent with family and friends in Hangzhou are more willing to settle in Hangzhou permanently. Additionally, development expectations are also a key influencing variable of urban settlement intentions. Development expectations depend on one's judgment of future employment and development prospects; the better the expectation, the greater the cost of "giving up." In 2019, the added value of Hangzhou's core digital economy industry was CNY 379.5 billion, which increased by 15.1% compared with 2018. Contrastingly, the growth was 14.6% for the e-commerce industry, 13.6% for the Internet-of-Things industry, and 15.7% for the software and information service industry. Such growths resulted from the rapid development of high-tech industries, which provide a career platform for young talent and raises their development expectations. These improvements made Hangzhou one of the top cities in China, in terms of young talent inflow.

4.3. Testing the Mediating Effects

Models 3–6 tested the mediating effects of air pollution perception on residential satisfaction and further influence on the urban settlement intentions of young talent. Firstly, according to the results of Models 3 and 4 in Table 3, the control variables, such as age and career development expectations, had a significant influence on residential satisfaction and remained robust both in Models 3 and 4. After the inclusion of the key independent variables air pollution perception in Model 4, its effect on residential satisfaction was significant (β = −0.167, $p < 0.001$), with R^2 changing to 0.024, further enhancing the model's explanatory power. Therefore, Hypothesis H2a was supported. Further, intermediary variables were included in Model 5. The results showed that residential satisfaction had a significant influence on the urban settlement intentions of young talent (β = 0.530, $p < 0.001$). The model's explanatory power increased by 23.3%, based on the amount of change in R^2; thus, supporting Hypothesis H2b. In addition, this study further examined the effect of perceived air quality and residential satisfaction on settlement intentions. Model 6 incorporated both the independent variable of air pollution perception and the mediating variable of residential satisfaction. The empirical results showed that residential satisfaction had a significant influence on settlement intentions (β = 0.532, $p < 0.001$), while the influence of air pollution perception became insignificant (β = −0.012, $p > 0.05$). After adding both the mediating and independent variables, the independent variable in the model became insignificant. Contrastingly, the mediating variable remained significant, according to the evaluation method of Baron and Kenny [54]. This indicates that residential satisfaction plays a mediating role between air pollution perception and urban settlement intentions altogether, thus verifying Hypothesis H2.

To further test the mediating effects, this study conducted a bootstrap test using the PROCESS macro for SPSS/SAS developed by Hayes [55], and repeated the sample 5000 times. The results showed that the indirect effect of air pollution perception on urban settlement intentions through residential satisfaction was 0.0886, with a 95% confidence interval of [0.055, 0.124] and $p < 0.001$. According to the criteria proposed by Preacher and Hayes [56] for testing mediating effects, if the confidence interval of the indirect effect does not include 0, then the indirect effect reaches a significant level. The empirical results show that the exclusion of a value of 0 also confirmed Hypothesis H2.

Table 3. Testing main effect and mediating effects of residential satisfaction.

Variable	Urban Settlement Intention		Residential Satisfaction		Urban Settlement Intention	
	Model 1	Model 2	Model 3	Model 4	Model 5	Model 6
Key variable						
Air pollution perception		−0.077 ** (0.031)		−0.167 *** (0.031)		−0.012 (0.027)
Mediating variable						
Residential satisfaction					0.530 *** (0.027)	0.532 *** (0.027)
Control variable						
Gender	−0.137 ** (0.061)	−0.139 ** (0.061)	−0.166 (0.062)	−0.169 ** (0.061)	−0.049 (0.052)	−0.049 (0.052)
Age	0.091 * (0.050)	0.090 ** (0.050)	0.084 * (0.050)	0.082 * (0.050)	0.046 (0.042)	0.045 (0.038)
Edu1	−0.137 * (0.179)	−0.143 * (0.079)	−0.001 (0.080)	−0.013 (0.079)	−0.137 ** (0.066)	−0.136 (0.067)
Edu2	−0.112 (0.103)	−0.116 (0.103)	−0.021 (0.104)	−0.029 (0.103)	−0.101 (0.087)	0.100 (0.087)
Edu3	0.047 (0.160)	0.041 (0.160)	0.090 (0.162)	0.079 (0.060)	−0.001 (0.035)	0.001 (0.135)
Time spent in Hangzhou	0.033 (0.035)	0.030 ** (0.035)	0.006 (0.035)	0.013 (0.035)	0.037 ** (0.029)	0.037 ** (0.029)
Annual income	0.029 (0.031)	0.032 (0.031)	0.034 (0.032)	0.041 (0.031)	0.011 (0.026)	0.010 (0.026)
Career development expectations	0.465 *** (0.032)	0.433 *** (0.034)	0.432 *** (0.032)	0.363 *** (0.034)	0.236 *** (0.029)	0.240 *** (0.031)
Family and friends	0.433 ** (0.090)	0.430 *** (0.085)	0.136 ** (0.043)	0.113 ** (0.087)	0.237 ** (0.079)	0.337 ** (0.093)
Constant	−1.808 *** (0.170)	−1.696 *** (0.175)	−1.875 *** (0.172)	−1.632 *** (0.176)	−0.815 ** (0.152)	−0.828 (0.155)
R^2	0.188	0.193	0.166	0.190	0.421	0.422
Adjusted R^2	0.181	0.185	0.159	0.183	0.416	0.414
ΔR^2	–	0.05 ***	–	0.024 ***	0.233 ***	0.001 ***
F	28.274 ***	25.948 ***	24.387 ***	25.485 ***	359.169 ***	10.200 *
VIF	1.880	1.879	1.879	1.880	1.879	1.880

Note: Standard errors in parentheses; * $p < 0.10$, ** $p < 0.05$, *** $p < 0.01$ with two-tailed test; all the regression coefficients were non-standardized. VIF, Variance Inflation Factor.

4.4. Testing the Moderating Effects

Hypothesis H3a proposes that place attachment has a positive moderating effect on the relationship between air pollution perception and residential satisfaction. In other words, greater place attachment can weaken the effect of air pollution perception on residential satisfaction and offset the decrease in residential satisfaction caused by poor air quality. To test this hypothesis, residential satisfaction was set as the dependent variable per the three-step test method of moderated hierarchical regression analyses. Hierarchical regression was established to sequentially incorporate the control variable, standardized independent variable, moderating variable, the product of the moderating variable, and independent variable into the equation, as shown in Models 7 and 8 in Table 4. The interaction term insignificantly influenced residential satisfaction (β = 0.004, $p > 0.05$). Therefore, Hypothesis H3a was not verified. Further, this study used the same approach to test the moderating role of place attachment between residential satisfaction and urban settlement intentions. Models 9 and 10 showed the empirical results, where the product term had a significant influence on settlement intentions, with β = 0.024 ($p < 0.01$) and $\Delta R^2 = 0.132$ ($p < 0.05$). Therefore, Hypothesis H3b was verified; in other words, the relationship between residential satisfaction and urban settlement intentions is significantly stronger when place attachment is stronger.

Table 4. Testing the moderating effects of place attachment.

Variable	Residential Satisfaction		Urban Settlement Intention	
	Model 7	Model 8	Model 9	Model 10
Key variable	−0.078 ** (0.033)	−0.077 ** (0.033)		
Air pollution perception	−0.078 ** (0.033)	−0.077 ** (0.033)		
Moderating variable				
Place attachment	0.271 *** (0.040)	0.273 *** (0.042)	0.114 *** (0.023)	0.123 *** (0.024)
Mediating variable				
Residential satisfaction			0.357 *** (0.020)	0.361 *** (0.020)
Interaction		0.004 (0.025)		0.024 ** (0.013)
Control variable				
Gender	−0.148 ** (0.059)	−0.113 ** (0.045)	−0.032 (0.037)	−0.033 (0.037)
Age	0.050 (0.049)	0.038 (0.037)	0.021 (0.030)	0.020 (0.033)
Edu1	−0.048 (0.077)	0.036 (0.059)	0.116 ** (0.047)	0.117 ** (0.047)
Edu2	−0.062 (0.101)	0.047 (0.076)	0.041 (0.097)	0.092 * (0.062)
Edu3	0.014 (0.040)	0.013 (0.119)	0.089 (0.062)	0.045 (0.097)
Time spent in Hangzhou	0.003 (0.034)	0.002 (0.026)	0.029 * (0.021)	0.028 * (0.021)
Annual income	0.051 * (0.031)	0.039 * (0.023)	0.014 (0.019)	0.014 (0.019)
Career development expectations	0.214 *** (0.040)	0.213 *** (0.040)	0.103 *** (0.025)	0.100 *** (0.025)
Family and friends	0.211 ** (0.097)	0.330 ** (0.091)	0.235 ** (0.089)	0.326 ** (0.063)
Constant	0.949 (0.198)	−0.950 *** (0.199)	3.513 *** (0.124)	3.516 *** (0.123)
R^2	0.227	0.227	0.306	0.438
Adjusted R^2	0.219	0.219	0.301	0.431
ΔR^2	0.061	0.00	0.118	0.132
F	28.717 ***	26.082	75.341 ***	68.948 ***
VIF	1.981	2.227	1.885	1.888

Note: Standard errors in parentheses; * $p < 0.10$, ** $p < 0.05$, *** $p < 0.01$ with two-tailed test; all the regression coefficients were non-standardized.

To visualize the moderating role played by place attachment in the relationship between residential satisfaction and settlement intentions, this study plotted the moderating relationship based on the method recommended by Aiken and West [57]. Each chosen variable had one standard deviation above and below the mean. Further, the moderating relationship is plotted in Figure 2, and shows the difference in the relationship between residential satisfaction and settlement intentions when young talent has different levels of place attachment to the city. With greater place attachment, a slight change in residential satisfaction promotes an increase in urban settlement intentions. Conversely, a weaker place attachment weakens the positive impact of residential satisfaction on urban settlement intentions.

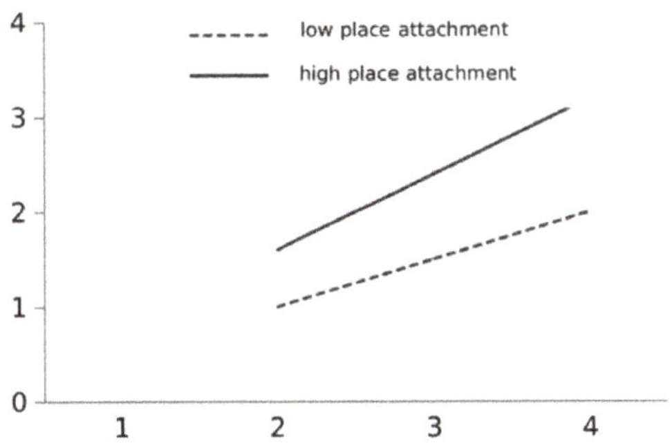

Figure 2. The regulatory role of place attachment on the relationship between residential satisfaction and urban settlement intention.

Moreover, this study uses the PROCESS plug-in for SPSS/SAS developed by Hayes to further test the adjusted mediating effect by repeating the sample 5000 times using the bootstrap method. The empirical results show that the mediating effect of residential satisfaction between air pollution perceptions and urban settlement intentions differs significantly at different levels of place attachment. Air pollution perceptions had a stronger indirect negative effect on urban settlement intentions at lower levels of place attachment ($\beta = -0.071$, $p < 0.001$), whereas at higher levels of place attachment, it had a weaker negative effect on settlement intentions ($\beta = -0.038$, $p < 0.001$), ($\Delta\beta = -0.033$, $p < 0\ 05$), with a 95% confidence interval of [−0.021, −0.001], which does not include 0. Therefore, Hypothesis H3 was also empirically supported. With a greater level of place attachment, young talent may still experience residential dissatisfaction due to poor air quality. However, the impact of residential dissatisfaction on urban settlement intentions is weakened by greater place attachment.

5. Discussion

Based on data obtained from 987 questionnaires collected from a sample group of young talent in Hangzhou, this study explored the influence of perceived air quality on urban settlement intentions. Hypotheses 1, 2, 2a, 2b, 3 and 3b were supported, whereas Hypothesis 3a was rejected. The findings of this study are as follows. First, air pollution perceptions significantly influence the urban settlement intentions of young talent; the poorer their air pollution perception, the weaker the urban settlement intentions. Second, residential satisfaction significantly mediates the relationship between air pollution perception and urban settlement intentions. In other words, a poorer air quality perception reduces residential satisfaction among young talent, thus weakening their urban settlement intentions. In conclusion, place attachment has a significant moderating effect on the relationship between residential satisfaction and settlement intentions. However, it insignificantly affects the relationship between air pollution perception and residential satisfaction. Compared with a weaker level of place attachment, a greater level of place attachment does not change the dissatisfaction associated with poorer perceived air quality. Instead, it can weaken the effect that this dissatisfaction has on settlement intentions.

Given the current situation of talent competition among various cities, this study focuses on the urban settlement intentions of young talent at an earlier stage. For the first time, it introduces the perceived air quality factor into the analysis of the influencing factors of the urban settlement intentions of young talent. This study examined the influence mechanism of air pollution perception on the urban settlement intentions of young talent. This study also verified the applicability of the demographic characteristics, economic development, and socio-cultural factors proposed by Woon et al. [4], which influence population migration, on young talent. The idea that young and highly educated people are more concerned about air pollution, as suggested by Jacquemin et al. [16], was expanded and confirmed, further corroborating the idea that young talent also choose to "vote with their feet" in the face of environmental pollution, as demonstrated by Banzhaf and Walsh [58]. In addition, unlike in previous studies, which used objective indicators to examine the impact of specific air pollutants on population migration and settlement, this study explored the psychological mechanism of the impact of air quality on the settlement intentions of young talent, starting from the concept of perceived air quality and with the help of factors, such as residential satisfaction and place attachment. This line of exploration is a useful supplement to studies on the impact of objective air quality on the spatial mobility of labor forces. Furthermore, based on the TPB, this study explored, for the first time, the influence mechanism of the relationship between perceived air quality and the settlement intentions of young talent. It was found that residential satisfaction mediates the relationship altogether, thus uncovering the transmission mechanism from better and worse perceived air quality to the strength of urban settlement intentions. The study demonstrated that air pollution perception significantly influences the satisfaction of young talent with urban living, affecting their settlement intentions. Urban air quality should also become an important aspect of the urban talent environment and be incorporated in the government's public service provisions; thus, the study provides a reference for subsequent studies related to talent environment construction and evaluation. Fourth, this study tested the moderating role of place attachment, an important concept in geography that refers to the emotional interaction between people and specific places, in the relationship among the independent (air pollution perception), mediating (residential satisfaction), and dependent (settlement intention) variables. The findings of this study expand Li and Zhou's research [45] on the moderating role of place attachment. Additionally, based on the results of the empirical analysis, it was verified that, in terms of human–place interaction, place attachment does not have a moderating effect on the relationship between air pollution perception and residential satisfaction. Place attachment, however, has a moderating effect on the impact of residential satisfaction on settlement intentions. Therefore, this study explained, in more detail, the influence mechanism of air pollution perception on the urban settlement intentions of young talent.

6. Conclusions

This study empirically examined the significant influence of air pollution perception on the urban settlement intentions of young talent and explained its influence mechanism. In the context of fierce competition for talent across various cities, this study's findings serve as an important reference for cities to construct an advantageous ecological environment for their talent and enhance the city's competitiveness for young talent. First, various cities are currently attracting talent through different policies, such as relaxing household registration restrictions and providing subsidies. However, the influence of environmental factors, such as air pollution on young talent, should not be ignored. Air pollution management should be enhanced through the strategic construction of an urban talent environment to promote high-quality development. Air quality should further be improved continuously through measures such as adjusting industrial structures and strengthening pollution control and dust management in key industries. Second, as improving air pollution control involves complex factors, such as industrial transformation and upgrades and synergy between multiple locations, it must be a long-term process. Greater place attachment can offset the reduction of urban settlement intentions caused by low residential satisfaction due to air pollution. Based on relevant sources, city managers can enhance place attachment to their respective cities by strengthening and improving publicity, creating a compassionate and welcoming image, building community exchange platforms to facilitate social integration, creating opportunities to attract young talent to participate in urban governance, and increasing the understanding and identity of young talent within the city. In conclusion, guided by the various housing needs of young talent, it is necessary to improve the supply of various public goods in the city, enhance urban governance, and implement multiple measures to improve residential satisfaction in the city.

This study, however, has some limitations. First, the survey data were obtained from Hangzhou. Although the inflow of young talent to Hangzhou in recent years has been among the highest in China and the survey sample shows that the sources of talent are also distributed across the country, the survey is inevitably influenced by the geographical characteristics of Hangzhou. Surveys and studies with greater coverage are yet to be conducted to verify whether the research findings can be generalized to the national level. Second, while semi-structured interviews were conducted with young talent, the formal survey was conducted in a relatively short period, making it difficult to properly reflect the dynamic interactions among variables, such as air pollution perception, residential satisfaction, place attachment, and settlement intentions. Follow-up studies can adopt a longitudinal tracking approach to conduct an extensive analysis of the relationship among these variables. This approach would improve the persuasiveness of the research findings. In conclusion, regarding the influence mechanism of air pollution perception on urban settlement intention, whether other variables can be included in the research model should be further explored in future studies.

Author Contributions: The individual contribution and responsibilities of the authors are listed as follows: L.Y. proposed and designed the research, and proofread the manuscript; X.L. collected the data and completed empirical analysis; R.Z. conducted literature review and discussions; Y.Z. helped collect the data and edit the final manuscript. All authors have read and agreed to the published version of the manuscript.

Funding: This research was jointly funded by The Key Projects of Soft Science in Zhejiang Province of China (grant numbers 2020C35061 and 2022C25028) and National Natural Science Foundation of China (grant number 72074192). This research was also supported by the Urban Emergency Management Research Innovation Team of Zhejiang University of Finance & Economics.

Institutional Review Board Statement: Not applicable. Our study was based on data from the questionnaire that the respondents were willing to answer and the questions in the questionnaire did not involve ethical issue.

Informed Consent Statement: Informed consent was obtained from all subjects involved in the study.

Data Availability Statement: Data will be made available upon request.

Acknowledgments: The authors would like to thank the respondents who provided helps for the pilot study, interview, and formal survey.

Conflicts of Interest: The authors declare no conflict of interest.

References

1. Zhang, W.H.; Luan, B.; Cai, S.S. A comparative study of willingness to stay in a city between new white collor workers and new generation of rural migrant workers. *Fujian Trib. Humanit. Soc. Sci.* **2018**, *8*, 140–147. (In Chinese)
2. Ajzen, I. The theory of planned behavior. *Organ. Behav. Hum. Decis. Processes* **1991**, *50*, 179–211. [CrossRef]
3. Weng, Q.X.; McElroy, J.C. HR environment and regional attraction: An empirical study of industrial clusters. *Aust. J. Manag.* **2010**, *35*, 81–95.
4. Woon, Y.F. Labor migration in the 1990s: Home ward orientation of migrants in the Pearl River delta region and its implications for interior China. *Mod. China* **1999**, *25*, 475–512. [CrossRef]
5. Fu, X.Q. A Study on the differences in residence intentions between the new and old generations of floating population: Taking Beijing, Shanghai, and Guangzhou as examples. *World Surv. Res.* **2017**, *7*, 28–32. (In Chinese) [CrossRef]
6. Yang, Q.; Li, P.J. The family development ability of the new generation of migrant workers and the willingness to stay in the city: An empirical study based on the data of the 2014 "Migrant Population Dynamics Monitoring Survey". *China Youth Study* **2017**, *10*, 50–56. (In Chinese) [CrossRef]
7. Chen, J.; Liu, Z.J.; Chen, M.; Ye, X.G. An empirical study on the impact of perception of the talent environment on the flow willingness to overseas High-level talents: Taking Guangdong Province as an example. *Sci. Technol. Manag. Res.* **2018**, *1*, 163–169. (In Chinese) [CrossRef]
8. Zhao, Y.H. Causes and consequences of return migration: Recent evidence from China. *J. Comp. Econ.* **2002**, *30*, 376–394. [CrossRef]
9. Wang, W.W.; Fan, C.C. Success or failure: Selectivity and reasons of return migration in Sichuan and Anhui, China. *Environ. Plan.* **2006**, *38*, 939–958. [CrossRef]
10. Zeng, X.H.; Qin, W. Analysis on the influencing factors of migrant workers' tendency to stay in the city. *Popul. Econ.* **2003**, *3*, 50–54. (In Chinese)
11. Poprawe, M. On the Relationship Between Corruption and Migration: Empirical Evidence from a Gravity Model of Migration. *Public Choice* **2015**, *3*, 337–354. [CrossRef]
12. Bertoli, S.; Moraga, F.H. Multilateral Resistance to Migration. *J. Dev. Econ.* **2013**, *2*, 79–100. [CrossRef]
13. Qin, Y.; Zhu, H. Run Away? Air Pollution and Emigration Interests in China. *J. Popul. Econ.* **2018**, *31*, 235–266. [CrossRef]
14. Wang, H.Y.; Liu, G.F. *China International Migration Report*; Social Science Literature Press: Beijing, China, 2015. (In Chinese)
15. Kohlhuber, M.; Mielck, A.; Weiland, S.K.; Bolte, G. Social inequality in perceived environmental exposures in relation to housing conditions in Germany. *Environ. Res.* **2006**, *101*, 246–255. [CrossRef] [PubMed]
16. Jacquemin, B.; Sunyer, J.; Forsberg, B.; Götschi, T.; Bayer-Oglesby, L.; Ackermann-Liebrich, U.; Marco, R.D.; Heinrich, J.; Jarvis, D.; Torén, K. Annoyance due to air pollution in Europe. *Int. J. Epidemiol.* **2007**, *36*, 809–820. [CrossRef]
17. Sun, W.Z.; Zhang, X.N.; Zheng, S.Q. Air pollution and spatial mobility of labor force: Study on the migrants' job location choice. *Econ. Res. J.* **2019**, *11*, 102–115. (In Chinese)
18. Mitran, D.; Golder, P.N. How does objective quality affect perceived quality? Short-term effects, long-term effects, and as asymmetries. *Mark. Sci.* **2006**, *25*, 230–247. [CrossRef]
19. Chen, S.; Oliva, P.; Zhang, P. The Effect of Air Pollution on Migration: Evidence from China. 2017. Available online: https://www.nber.org/system/files/working_papers/w24036/w24036.pdf (accessed on 10 September 2021).
20. Gronroos, C. An applied service theory. *J. Mark.* **1982**, *7*, 46–56.

21. Katsouyanni, K.; Grypairs, A.; Samoli, E. Short-term effects of air pollution on health. *Encycl. Environ. Health* **2011**, *4*, 51–60. [CrossRef]
22. Schwartz, J. Long-term effects of particulate air pollution on human health. *Encycl. Environ. Health* **2011**, *12*, 520–527. [CrossRef]
23. Wang, X.Y.; He, X.B. Research on the influence mechanism of air pollution on the trust of urban resident government. *Chin. J. Popul. Sci.* **2017**, *4*, 97–107. (In Chinese)
24. Wang, Y.J.; Han, D.L. Air quality, environmental pollution perception and local government environmental governance evaluation. *China Soft Sci.* **2019**, *8*, 41–50. (In Chinese) [CrossRef]
25. Jones, B.A.; Fleck, J. Shrinking Lakes, air pollution, and human health: Evidence from California's Salton Sea. *Sci. Total Environ.* **2020**, *1*, 136–148. [CrossRef] [PubMed]
26. Sherefkin, R. Ford Blames Its Suppliers for Quality Problems, Demands Improvement. 2002. Available online: https://www.autoweek.com/news/a2108396/ford-blames-its-suppliers-quality-problems-demands-improvement/ (accessed on 8 September 2021).
27. Zhang, Y.G.; Wong, I.K.; Cheng, J.J.; Yu, X.Y.; Chen, X. The influence of multidimensional deconstruction of stressors on enhancing urban residents' well-being: From the perspective of rural tourism and leisure involvement. *Geogr. Res.* **2019**, *38*, 971–987. (In Chinese)
28. You, J.X.; Chen, Q. Urban management pattern oriented by public satisfaction. *J. Public Manag.* **2004**, *1*, 51–57. (In Chinese)
29. Rojo-Pere, F.; Fernandez-Mayoralas, F.G.; Pozo-Rivera, E.; Rojo-Abuin, J.M. Ageing in place: Predictors of the residential satisfaction of elderly. *Soc. Indic. Res.* **2001**, *54*, 173–208. [CrossRef]
30. Fishbein, M.; Ajzen, I. *Belief, Attitude, Intention, and Behavior: An Introduction to Theory and Research*; Addison-Wesley: Reading, MA, USA, 1975.
31. Fischer, G.W.; Morgan, M.G. What risks are people concerned about. *Risk Anal.* **1991**, *11*, 303–314. [CrossRef]
32. Cardozo, R. An experimental study of customer effort, expectation and satisfaction. *J. Mark. Res.* **1965**, *2*, 244–249. [CrossRef]
33. Weng, Q.X.; Yang, S.C.; Cao, W.L. The influence of regional environment on talent commitment and rooting willingness. *Sci. Res. Manag.* **2014**, *35*, 154–160. (In Chinese)
34. Liang, S.K. An analysis of influencing factors of settling willingness of floating population. *Popul. Soc.* **2016**, *2*, 63–74. (In Chinese)
35. Yao, L.Y. Influencing factors of young talents' urban dwelling willingness. *Contemp. Young Res.* **2019**, *5*, 51–60. (In Chinese)
36. He, Z.J.; Wang, Y.; Li, Y. Analysis on the perception dimensions of residential satisfaction in new-type rural communities. *Henan Soc. Sci.* **2018**, *26*, 82–88. (In Chinese)
37. Amerigo, M.; Aragones, J.I. A theoretical and methodological approach to the study of residential satisfaction. *J. Environ. Psychol.* **1997**, *17*, 83–90. [CrossRef]
38. Spear, A. Residential satisfaction as an intervening variable in residential mobility. *Demography* **1974**, *11*, 173–188. [CrossRef] [PubMed]
39. Steel, E.F. *The Sense of Place*; CBI Publishing: Boston, MA, USA, 1981.
40. Williams, D.R.; Patterson, M.; Roggen, J.W.; Watson, A.E. Beyond the commodity metaphor: Examining emotional and symbolic attachment to place. *Leis. Sci.* **1992**, *14*, 29–46. [CrossRef]
41. Raymond, C.M.; Brown, G.; Robinson, G.M. The influence of place attachment and moral and normative concerns on the conservation of native vegetation: A test of two behavioral models. *J. Environ. Psychol.* **2011**, *31*, 323–335. [CrossRef]
42. Wang, X.; Aoki, N.; Xu, S.B. Reflection on displacement in the context of inner-city redevelopment from the perspective of place attachment: A case study of the demolition project of Xigunan, Tianjin. *Hum. Geogr.* **2019**, *5*, 44–52. (In Chinese)
43. Cassn, W. Emotion and rationality: The characterization and evaluation of opposition to renewable energy projects. *Emot. Space Soc.* **2009**, *2*, 62–69. [CrossRef]
44. Yuksel, A.; Yuksel, F.; Billim, Y. Destination attachment: Effects on customer satisfaction and cognitive, affective and conative loyalty. *Tour. Manag.* **2010**, *31*, 274–284. [CrossRef]
45. Li, Q.C.; Zhou, L.Q. The impact of perceived outcome efficacy on tourists' decision to adopt environmental behaviors. *J. Zhejiang Univ. Sci. Ed.* **2015**, *42*, 460–464. (In Chinese) [CrossRef]
46. Yao, Y.L. Migration experience and social integration: An analysis of the influencing factors of foreign floating population's residence willingness in Shanghai. *Fujian Trib. Humanit. Soc. Sci.* **2019**, *9*, 95–103. (In Chinese)
47. Peng, Y.; Gu, X.; Zhu, X.; Zhang, F.; Song, Y. Recovery evaluation of villages reconstructed with concentrated rural settlement after the Wenchuan earthquake. *Nat. Hazards* **2020**, *104*, 139–166. [CrossRef]
48. Li, J. Research on the Relationship between Perceived Air Quality and Public Satisfaction and Environmental Behavior Willingness. Master's Thesis, China Jiliang College, Hangzhou, China, 2016. (In Chinese)
49. Kyle, G.T.; Mowen, A.J.; Tarrant, M. Linking place preferences with place meaning: An examination of the relationship between place motivation and place attachment. *J. Environ. Psychol.* **2004**, *24*, 439–454. [CrossRef]
50. Williams, D.R.; Vaske, J.J. The measurement of place attachment: Validity and generalize ability of a psychometric approach. *For. Sci.* **2003**, *49*, 830–840.
51. Hu, B.; Weng, Q.X. The influence of industrial clusters' character on the staying will: An empirical research on four industrial clusters in China. *Ind. Eng. Manag.* **2008**, *5*, 113–119. (In Chinese) [CrossRef]
52. Peng, Y.; Zhu, X.; Zhang, F.; Huang, L.; Xue, J.; Xu, Y. Farmers' risk perception of concentrated rural settlement development after the 5.12 Sichuan Earthquake. *Habitat Int.* **2018**, *71*, 169–176. [CrossRef]

53. Fornell, C.; Larckerd, F. Evaluating structural equation models with unobservable variables and measurement error. *J. Mark. Res.* **1981**, *66*, 39–50. [CrossRef]
54. Baron, R.M.; Kenny, D.A. The moderator-mediator variable distinction in social psychological research: Conceptual strategic and statistical considerations. *J. Personal. Soc. Psychol.* **1986**, *51*, 1173–1182. [CrossRef]
55. Hayes, A.F. *An Introduction to Mediation, Moderation, and Conditional Process Analysis*; Guilford Press: New York, NY, USA, 2013.
56. Preacher, K.J.; Hayes, A.F. Asymptotic and resampling strategies for assessing and comparing indirect effects in multiple mediator model. *Behav. Res. Methods* **2008**, *40*, 879–891. [CrossRef]
57. Aiken, L.S.; West, S.G. Multiple regression: Testing and interpreting interactions. *J. Oper. Res. Soc.* **1994**, *45*, 119–120.
58. Banzhaf, H.S.; Walsh, R.P. Do people vote with their feet? An empirical test of Tiebout. *Am. Econ. Rev.* **2008**, *98*, 843–863. [CrossRef]

International Journal of
Environmental Research and Public Health

MDPI

Article

A Blessing or a Curse? Exploring the Impact of Environmental Regulation on China's Regional Green Development from the Perspective of Governance Transformation

Xianpu Xu *, Xiawan Li and Lin Zheng

School of Business, Xiangtan University, Xiangtan 411105, China; lxwxtu20@163.com (X.L.); zlxtu517@126.com (L.Z.)
* Correspondence: xuxianpu@xtu.edu.cn

Abstract: China's rapid economic growth has caused serious problems, such as environmental pollution and resource exhaustion. Only by improving the green total factor productivity (GTFP) can China's economic development get out of the dual dilemmas of environmental degradation and resources exhaustion. Although environmental regulation helps to improve China's productivity, its impact on GTFP is still controversial and deserves careful investigation. In this context, this study adopts the global Malmquist-Luenberger productivity index to measure the GTFP change of China's 30 provinces over the period of 2003 to 2017 and then it uses the fixed-effect dynamic panel model to investigate the impact of environmental regulation on GTFP from the perspective of governance transformation. The results show that: (1) there is a nonlinear U-shaped relationship between environmental regulation and GTFP, indicating that the Porter hypothesis is verified in China. More notably, the values of environmental regulation are still located on the left side of the U-shaped curve at present, which means that the promotional effect of environmental regulation on GTFP has not been realized fully. (2) The U-shaped relationship shows significant regional heterogeneity. The western region demonstrates the highest level of significance, followed by the eastern region. However, the U-shaped relationship is insignificant in the central region. (3) Governance transformation can not only significantly improve GTFP but it can also accelerate the realization of the Porter hypothesis by inspiring the innovative enthusiasm of enterprises, which means that governance transformation can contribute to the achievement of the improved effects of environmental regulation on GTFP. (4) R&D investment can significantly improve GTFP, where the impacts of trade openness and factor endowment were significantly negative and the influence of foreign direct investment was not significant. These conclusions provide a good reference point for optimizing the relationship between the government and the market, as well as promoting regional green and high-quality development in China.

Keywords: green total factor productivity; environmental regulation; governance transformation; the U-shaped relationship; global Malmquist-Luenberger index

Citation: Xu, X.; Li, X.; Zheng, L. A Blessing or a Curse? Exploring the Impact of Environmental Regulation on China's Regional Green Development from the Perspective of Governance Transformation. *Int. J. Environ. Res. Public Health* **2022**, *19*, 1312. https://doi.org/10.3390/ijerph19031312

Academic Editors: Roberto Alonso González Lezcano, Francesco Nocera and Rosa Giuseppina Caponetto

Received: 27 December 2021
Accepted: 21 January 2022
Published: 25 January 2022

1. Introduction

Since the reform and expansion in 1978, China has achieved remarkable economic growth achievements which benefited greatly from the large scale of the government's leading investment and factor input [1–3]. However, extensive economic development, at the cost of high energy consumption and high emissions, has caused severe problems of resource exhaustion and environmental pollution, which have seriously affected the sustainable growth of China's economy, as shown in Figure 1. Currently, as the world's second-largest economy, China is facing the dual pressure of economic development and environmental protection. Meanwhile, China's economy has entered a "new normal" period, shifting from high-speed growth to high-quality development and total factor productivity (hereafter, TFP) has become the core indicator to measure the degree of high-quality economic development [4,5]. Because the traditional measurement of TFP ignores energy input and does not consider the negative externalities caused by environmental pollution, it is easy to bring about a measurement bias and it cannot truly reflect the quality of economic development [6]. Green total factor productivity (hereafter, GTFP), namely, the total factor productivity when considering environmental protection and economic efficiency, has attracted widespread concerns at home and abroad [7,8]. Therefore, the improvement of green total factor productivity and the promotion of a green economic transformation have become research hotspots in recent years [9–11].

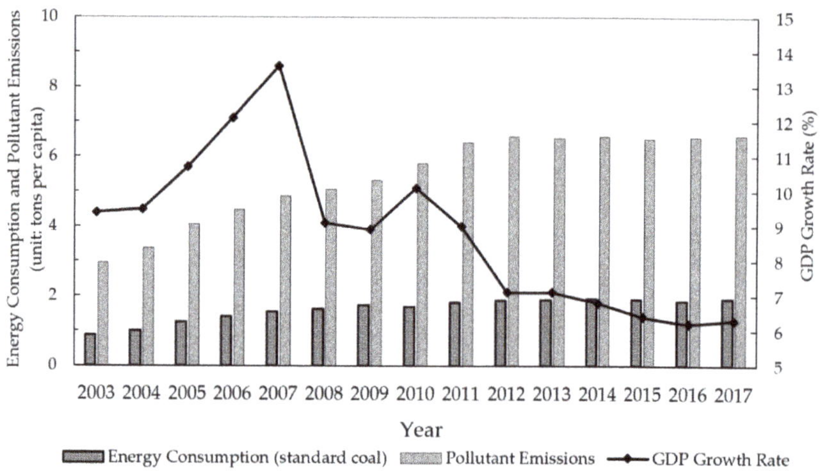

Figure 1. Trends of China's energy consumption, pollutant emissions, and GDP growth. Source: author's calculation with data from China Statistical Yearbook (2004–2018).

With the increasingly sharp contradiction between the environmental carrying capacity and green economic development, strengthening environmental regulation has gradually become a global trend, and China is no exception [12–16]. Faced with severe environmental pressures, Chinese policy makers have formulated a series of strict environmental regulatory policies to address pollution problems. Especially after the 18th CCP National Congress, the central government of China began tightening environmental pollution control, with the enforcement of the new Environmental Protection Law in 2015 and the Thirteenth Five-Year Plan for Ecological Environment Protection in 2016. In addition, 31 provinces in mainland China had been all covered by the central environmental protection supervision system by 2017 and the goals of achieving Ecological Civilization and Beautiful China were also clearly put into the Constitution in 2018. Currently, one of the main objectives of environmental regulation in China is to establish a green and low-carbon circular economic system, in which the driving force of economic growth is changed from investment to innovation [17,18]. In this context, the goal is to reverse the negative environmental impact of economic development and explore the realistic path of green transformation. In view of this, by investigating the effect of environmental regulation on GTFP and its mechanisms, this paper is expected to provide references for formulating reasonable environmental regulation policies for improving GTFP, as well as having important practical significance on the promotion of the high-quality development of China's economy.

It is undeniable that the rapid development of China's economy stems largely from the reform and innovation of the economic system [7,19]. In the process of more than 40 years of reform and expansion, the Chinese government has always adhered to the guidelines for establishing a modern market economic system. The role of the market mechanisms in resource allocation has gradually increased, realizing its fundamental transformation from the auxiliary position, to the basic position, and then to the decisive role [20]. The 19th CCP National Congress in 2017 further proposed to speed up the establishment and improvement of the socialist market economic system. Therefore, the relationship between the government and the market, namely, the governance changing from administrative governance to economic governance, is constantly adjusted [21]. Obviously, the role of governance transformation in promoting sustainable economic growth cannot also be ignored. However, few scholars have deeply explored the growth effect of governance transformation from the perspective of GTFP [22]. As a big developing country, China continues reforming towards the socialist market economy. The relationship between governance transformation and GTFP, as well as whether governance transformation can accelerate the dividend effect of environmental regulation on GTFP, are theoretical and practical issues worthy of in-depth exploration [23–25].

This paper mainly aims to explore the effect of environmental regulation and governance transformation on GTFP in China. Specifically, based on the theoretical analysis, we use Chinese provincial panel data from 2003 to 2017 to empirically investigate the impact of environmental regulation and governance transformation on GTFP, which is analyzed by constructing a dynamic panel data regression model and using a system generalized moment estimation method. The results showed that environmental regulation inhibited the increase in GTFP in the short term but promoted the growth of GTFP in the long term, and there was a nonlinear U-shaped relationship between environmental regulation and GTFP in China. Meanwhile, the impact of governance transformation on GTFP was significantly positive and, therefore, governance transformation can accelerate the realization of the Porter hypothesis, which reflects the promotional effect of environmental regulation on GTFP. In addition, the results also showed that there was regional heterogeneity in the impact of environmental regulation on GTFP based on the significance of the nonlinear impact in the eastern and western regions. The influence was not obvious in the central region.

The main contributions of this study to the literature are as follows. Firstly, we incorporated environmental regulation, governance transformation, and GTFP into a unified analytical framework in which the internal relationship between the three variables was investigated. Therefore, the research conclusions provide a more comprehensive understanding of the inherent mechanisms of the green growth effects on environment regulation. Secondly, we introduced resource exhaustion, environmental pollution, and economic growth into a productivity evaluation system and estimated the GTFP of China's 30 provinces by using the Global Malmquist-Luenberger (GML) index based on the directional distance function. This enabled us to inherit the advantage of traditional productivity indexes, e.g., the Malmquist-Luenberger index, while alleviating the infeasibility problem and providing a more comprehensive calculation process. Thirdly, the linear term and quadratic term of environmental regulation were both introduced into the econometric model to explore the possible nonlinear relationship between environmental regulation and GTFP. In addition, to provide a sound theoretical basis for formulating differentiated environmental policy systems, we further analyzed the regional heterogeneous effects of environmental regulation on GTFP by dividing the balanced panel into three subsamples, namely, the eastern region, the central region, and the western region. Fourthly, the interaction effect of environmental regulation and governance transformation was also added into the empirical model, testing the moderating effect of governance transformation on the relationship between environmental regulation and GTFP. Finally, we empirically investigated the impact of environmental regulation and governance transformation on China's provincial GTFP by using a dynamic panel model and system-generalized methods of moment (SYS-GMM) to overcome the possible endogenous problem.

The remainder of this paper is organized as follows. Section 2 briefly reviews the relevant literature and proposes three theoretical hypotheses. Section 3 describes the data sources and methods used in the empirical analysis. Section 4 discusses the empirical estimation results. Section 5 concludes the study and highlights several policy implications.

2. Literature Review and Research Hypotheses

2.1. Literature Review

When it comes to environmental regulation, governance transformation, and GTFP, previous studies have focused on the relationship between environmental regulation and GTFP, the relationship between governance transformation and GTFP, and the realization of the conditions of the Porter hypothesis. Therefore, in this section, we also review the related literature from these three aspects.

2.1.1. The Relationship between Environmental Regulation and GTFP

With the increasing attention to the quality of the ecological environment, many scholars have adopted various methods to explore the impact of environmental regulation on GTFP [9,26–29]. However, the existing literature has not yet reached a consensus on the relationship between environmental regulation and GTFP [13]. Some studies hold the view that the essence of environmental regulation is to internalize the negative externalities of pollution, for it will inevitably bring additional costs to enterprises. Therefore, environmental regulation will inhibit the improvement of productivity [30,31]. Hancevic [12] claimed that environmental regulation will restrain the improvement of productivity owing to increases in pollution control costs. Zhang and Jiang [32] investigated the effect of the environmental policy on a firm's green productivity by using Chinese coal-fired power plant data from 2005 to 2010 and found that stringent environmental regulation will damage green productivity growth. Cai and Ye [33] discussed the impact of the enforcement of China's new environmental protection law on enterprises' TFP by using DID model and proved that environmental regulation can give rise to a decline in enterprises' TFP due to financial constraints. This conclusion is also supported by Du et al. [15] who indicated that environmental regulation would restrain green technology innovation. Conversely, some scholars believe that strict and well-designed environmental regulation can stimulate corporate innovation activities aimed at reducing compliance costs, enhance enterprises' competitiveness, and promoting their productivity [34]. Lanoie et al. [35], using survey data from seven OECD countries in 2003, examined the effect of environmental regulation on productivity. They confirmed the weak Porter hypothesis and concluded that environmental regulation could promote TFP growth. Wang and Shen [36] focused on the effect of environmental regulation on the environmental productivity of China's industries over the period from 2000 to 2012 and found that environmental regulation and environmental productivity were positively correlated, which, to a certain extent, validates the Porter hypothesis. Based on the panel data of the OECD countries' industrial sectors between 2004 and 2009, Wang et al. [13] discussed the effect of environmental policy stringency on green productivity growth and confirmed that environmental regulation had a positive impact on green productivity growth. Zhang [14] adopted the dynamic panel model to explore the impact of environmental regulation on the green productivity of Chinese manufacturing firms and found that environmental regulation facilitated GTFP, especially in state-owned enterprises. In addition, some people have claimed that the impact of environmental regulation on GTFP is uncertain, for the compliance cost effects and the innovation compensation effects exist simultaneously. Based on the panel data of China's carbon-intensive industries from 2000 to 2014, Zhao et al. [37] found that there was an inverted U-shaped relationship between environmental regulation and GTFP, demonstrating the inexistence of the Porter hypothesis in the long term. Qiu et al. [38] employed the FGLS model and the dynamic GMM model to analyze the effect of environmental regulation on the GTFP of China's industrial sectors and verified a nonlinear U-shaped curve relationship between environmental regulation and GTFP. This result is consistent with that of Shen et al. [39] who found that the effect of environmental regulation on GTFP exhibited a significant U-shaped relationship from a provincial perspective. However, none of the above literature has examined the impact of environmental regulation on China's provincial GTFP, which is of great significance for formulating differentiated environmental regulation policies to promote GTFP growth.

2.1.2. The Relationship between Governance Transformation and GTFP

Regarding the relationship between governance transformation and GTFP, most firm-level evidence showed that market-oriented governance transformation, as an important institutional arrangement, can significantly facilitate GTFP. From the perspective of the influence mechanisms, three research hypotheses have been formed. The first hypothesis is the transaction cost effects. A well-developed marketization mechanism can effectively reduce the transaction costs and the investment risk of enterprises, which contributes to the enhancement of the profitability and production efficiency [21,40,41]. Zhang and Liu [20] argued that enterprises located in more developed market systems were highly related to more bank loans and other financial intermediaries, because efficient financing channels can fully meet the amount of capital investment required by enterprises to achieve the targeted GTFP. Therefore, market-oriented reforms raise the enterprises' return on capital and investment, as well as improving GTFP [19,22]. The second hypothesis is the resource allocation effects. It is widely accepted that market mechanisms can directly enhance the operational flexibility of enterprises through the rebound effect, which can help to decrease the originally expected inputs, as well as increasing outputs [42]. Moreover, high-level market systems can improve the allocation efficiency of resources among and within enterprises and can boost the productivity of enterprises [24]. Bin et al. [23] analyzed the effect of the within-industry allocation efficiency on firm productivities and argued that the improvement of the resource allocation efficiency had a strongly positive influence on TFP growth. This conclusion has been confirmed by Lin and Chen [10] who found that factor market distortion inhibited China's GTFP growth. The third hypothesis is technological innovation effects. Some previous studies found that GTFP growth was significantly positively correlated with innovation and that well-developed market systems stimulated the innovative activities of enterprises aimed at obtaining high profits, which contributed to the promotion of the enhancement of production efficiency [13,43,44]. Audretsch and Belitski [45] adopted firm-level unbalanced panel data to examine the effect of R&D on productivity and verified that the effort of innovation had a positive effect on green productivity by promoting technology transfer in a well-developed marketization environment. Zhang and Vigne [46] found that innovation efficiencies had a positive and significant impact on GTFP because of the benefits of market-oriented reforms. However, few scholars have empirically tested the impact of governance transformation on China's GTFP from the provincial level perspective, especially the impact of regional heterogeneity on the relationship between governance transformation and GTFP, implying that geographic location is an important factor affecting the growth effect of governance transformation.

2.1.3. The Realization Conditions of the Porter Hypothesis

The Porter hypothesis posits that well-designed environmental regulation can stimulate enterprises to carry out technological innovation and engender innovation compensation effects which help to improve the competitiveness of enterprises and their productivity [34,47]. Therefore, taking advantage of the innovation effects of environmental regulation is the key to achieve a win-win situation between environmental protection and economic development [48]. Accordingly, the existing literature mainly discusses the realization of the conditions of the Porter hypothesis from the following two aspects. On the one hand, some scholars discussed the impact of the fiscal policy, foreign direct investment, financial development, industrial structures, and factor endowment on the Porter hypothesis from the macro-level perspective. For example, Song et al. [49] analyzed the compound effects of fiscal decentralization and environmental regulation on GTFP in the Yangtze River economic belt and found that appropriate fiscal decentralization can contribute to the realization of the Porter hypothesis. Qiu et al. [38] explored the relationship between environmental regulation, FDI, and industrial GTFP, based on Chinese provincial panel data, and confirmed that FDI can accelerate the realization of the Porter hypothesis through the channel of the technology spillover effect. Lv et al. [50] examined the impact of financial development on green innovation under environmental regulation and confirmed that the financial structure was conducive to the realization of the Porter hypothesis, while the financial scale and financial efficiency had a negative effect on green development. Wang and Shen [36] investigated the relationship between industry structure changes and environmental productivity by using the Lema index and verified that industrial agglomeration had a significant positive effect on the innovation effects of environmental regulation. Xie et al. [51] employed a panel threshold model to examine the relationship among environmental regulation, human capital, and GTFP, and confirmed that the improvement of human capital structure significantly promoted the realization of the Porter hypothesis. On the other hand, some people discussed the impact of the enterprise ownership structure, the enterprise trade advantage, and enterprise resource misallocation on the Porter hypothesis from the microeconomic perspective. Peng et al. [25] confirmed that state-owned enterprises had lower productivity, on average, than non-state-owned enterprises, based on a large panel of data on Chinese industrial enterprises from 1998 to 2007, indicating that the impact of the ownership structure on the Porter hypothesis was very significant. Tang et al. [52] used a difference-in-difference framework to estimate the impact of export on productivity under environmental regulation and verified that an export advantage contributed to the realization of the Porter hypothesis. Based on the panel data of Chinese listed companies, Cai and Ye [33] confirmed that bank credit misallocation inhibited the realization of the Porter hypothesis. The conclusion is consistent with Lin and Chen [10] who found that factor market distortion had a negative influence on China's GTFP growth. Most notably, the reform of the economic system was an important factor affecting the realization of the Porter hypothesis. To date, few scholars have investigated whether an increase in the environmental regulation intensity will affect China's GTFP growth through the moderating effect of governance transformation.

2.2. Research Hypotheses

Based on the existing research and the reality of China's industrial economic development, in this section we analyze the influence mechanisms of environmental regulation and governance transformation on GTFP systematically, and we put forward three research hypotheses to be tested.

2.2.1. The Theoretical Mechanism of Environmental Regulation on GTFP

From the previous literature, it should be noted that the impact of environmental regulation on GTFP mainly depends on the comprehensive effects of an innovation decline and a value promotion [13]. To be specific, the decline in innovation is due to the decrease in innovation resources, which are mainly encroached by environmental regulation costs. The improvement of value is due to the contribution of the green process innovation, which can be spawned by environmental regulation. On the whole, the previous studies have greatly deepened our understanding of the effect of environmental regulation on GTFP; however, what we need to highlight is that the great majority of these studies ignored the dynamic effects of environmental regulation when analyzing its role. Specifically, when environmental supervision is less strict, the implementation of environmental regulation not only increases the pollution control costs but also stimulates extensive production and restrains green economic efficiency, which are referred to as the "cost effect" and the "crowding-out effect", respectively [34]. However, with the improvement of environmental regulation stringencies, enterprises must continue to increase their environmental investment to carry out green technology innovations. This gradually compensates for the compliance costs and contributes to green productivity in the long run, which is called the "innovation compensation effect" [38,53]. Thus, environmental regulation will weaken the enterprises' competitiveness in the early stages, but it can stimulate innovation and promote productivity over the long term. Hence, the following hypothesis is proposed:

Hypothesis 1 (H1). *Environmental regulation may inhibit GTFP in the short term and can promote GTFP in the long term and there is a U-shaped relationship between environmental regulation and GTFP.*

2.2.2. The Theoretical Mechanism of Governance Transformation on GTFP

Theoretically, governance transformation reflects the persistent improvement of the degree of marketization in a country or a region. The socialist governance transformation can be categorized into two models: the Soviet model, which strongly argues for shock therapy, and the Chinese model, which advocates for a gradual reform. Compared with the Soviet model, the Chinese model can better cultivate a unified and open market economy and can create a fair and orderly institutional environment for private enterprises. In addition, it can improve the innovation incentive mechanisms, optimize resource allocation efficiencies, and promote enterprise productivity. From the previous literature, in order to clarify how market-oriented governance transformation affects GTFP, the key is to find out the way towards the improvement of GTFP. From the perspective of enterprises, the sources of GTFP growth are determined by two fundamental forces [23,54]. The first is the improvement of the corporate internal production efficiency caused by technological progress, which stems from R&D investment, technology introduction, a deepening of division of labor, the enhancement of the management level, and the optimal allocation of internal resources [10]. The second is the improvement of resource allocation efficiencies among enterprises, specifically where production factors flow from low productivity enterprises to high productivity enterprises, including the creative destruction process, in which low productivity enterprises continue to withdraw from the market and high productivity enterprises continue to enter the market [21]. Hence, by relying on the specialized division of labor and the adoption of advanced green technologies, market-oriented governance transformation can not only promote the enhancement of the internal production efficiency of enterprises, but it can also effectively raise the efficiency of resource allocations among enterprises, which can improve the overall green productivity of the whole society. Therefore, the following hypothesis is formulated:

Hypothesis 2 (H2). *Governance transformation can promote GTFP improvement.*

2.2.3. The Theoretical Mechanism of Governance Transformation on the Porter Hypothesis

The previous research showed that the market-oriented governance transformation was helpful for improving the market competition and promoting corporate technological innovation [20]. Whether the governance transformation has a compound effect on the Porter hypothesis depends largely on the nature of the innovation effect of the governance transformation. Ettlie et al. [55] demonstrated that technological innovation can be divided into incremental innovation and radical innovation. Radical innovation refers to a kind of innovation that can produce a significant impact on market rules, the competition situation, and industrial layout, and may even lead to an industrial reshuffle [56,57]. Therefore, strengthening radical innovations and promoting the transformation of corporate technological innovations from incremental innovations to radical innovations are not only an important way for enterprises to break through technological bottlenecks and achieve an innovation catch-up, but they are also the key to the compound effect of governance transformation on the Porter hypothesis [45,58].

From the perspective of corporate governance, state-owned enterprises still contain more administrative governance factors because the reform is not in place, while private enterprises have more economic governance factors. Therefore, the innovation characteristics of enterprises with different ownerships will show differences due to different governance mechanisms. That is, state-owned enterprises prefer incremental innovations, while private enterprises hope to obtain radical innovations for subverting the existing market structure. Specifically, in the early stages of environmental regulation, radical innovation is not easy to realize. State-owned enterprises can achieve incremental innovations because they can obtain many subsidies from the government. Thus, the green competitiveness of state-owned enterprises is stronger than that of private enterprises. In the later stages of environmental regulation, the radical innovations of private enterprises are gradually realized, while the radical innovations of state-owned enterprises are slow due to the difficulty of governance transformation. At this time, the green competitiveness of private enterprises will exceed that of state-owned enterprises. Therefore, the governance transformation can accelerate the realization of radical innovations and can promote the improvement of GTFP. Based on this, the following hypothesis is proposed:

Hypothesis 3 (H3). *Governance transformation can accelerate the realization of the Porter hypothesis; namely, governance transformation contributes to the achievement of the improvement of environmental regulation on GTFP.*

In summary, the theoretical mechanisms of the hypotheses constructed in this paper can be summarized in Figure 2. As can be seen in Figure 2, environmental regulation will affect GTFP through three channels: the innovation compensation effect, the compliance cost effect, and the crowding out effect. Thus, the research Hypothesis 1 (H1) is obtained. Meanwhile, governance transformation can not only improve the internal production efficiency of enterprises, but it can also enhance the allocation efficiency among enterprises, which can promote GTFP. Therefore, the research Hypothesis 2 (H2) is formed. In addition, the innovation characteristics of enterprises with different ownerships will exhibit significant differences due to different governance mechanisms; namely, state-owned enterprises prefer incremental innovation, while private enterprises hope to obtain radical innovation for subverting the existing market structure. Accordingly, we can put forward the research Hypothesis 3 (H3).

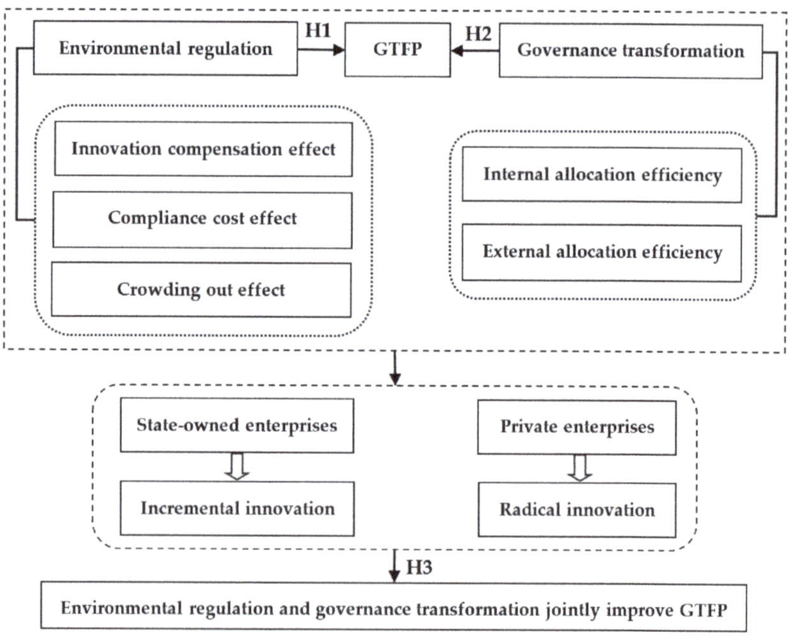

Figure 2. The theoretical mechanism diagrams of hypotheses.

3. Econometric Methodology and Data

3.1. Econometric Model Specification

Under the new growth theory, economic growth is mainly promoted by capital, labor, and technological progress. In addition, previous studies have shown that environmental regulation, the optimization of resource allocation, and R&D investment can give rise to technological progress. Similarly, FDI and export, can bring about technology spillovers under the condition of an open economy [8,59]. Accordingly, the production function can be described as follows:

$$Y(y_{desire}, y_{undesire}) = A(er, gt, rd, fdi, ex, t) \cdot F(K, L) \tag{1}$$

In Equation (1), Y represents the total output, consisting of the desired output and the undesired output; A stands for the green total factor productivity (GTFP) considering undesired output; *er* denotes environmental regulation; and *gt*, *rd*, *fdi*, and *ex* represent governance transformation, R&D investment, foreign direct investment, and export, respectively. K and L indicate capital and labor, respectively. In addition, A indicates the Hicks neutral technology progress function. For simplicity, in reference to the study by Zhang [22], we assume that A in Equation (1) includes a variety of components, as follows:

$$A(er, gt, rd, fdi, ex, t) = A_{i0} e^{\lambda_i t} er_{it}^{\alpha_i} gt_{it}^{\beta_i} rd_{it}^{\gamma_i} fdi_{it}^{\delta_i} ex_{it}^{\tau_i} \tag{2}$$

By substituting Equation (2) into Equation (1), we get the following equation:

$$Y_{it}(y_{desire_{it}}, y_{undesire_{it}}) = A_{i0} e^{\lambda_i t} er_{it}^{\alpha_i} gt_{it}^{\beta_i} rd_{it}^{\gamma_i} fdi_{it}^{\delta_i} ex_{it}^{\tau_i} \cdot F(K_{it}, L_{it}) \tag{3}$$

where i and t denote the region and time, respectively; A_{i0} represents the initial productivity level; $\lambda_i t$ reflects exogenous productivity changes; and α_i, β_i, γ_i, δ_i, and τ_i represent the parameters of environmental regulation, governance transformation, R&D investment, foreign direct investment, and export trade on GTFP, respectively.

In terms of the definition of GTFP, we divide the two sides of Equation (3) by using $F(K_{it},L_{it})$ to obtain the following formula:

$$GTFP_{it} = \frac{Y_{it}(y_{desire_{it}}, y_{undesire_{it}})}{F(K_{it}, L_{it})} = A_{i0} e^{\lambda_i t} er_{it}^{\alpha_i} gt_{it}^{\beta_i} rd_{it}^{\gamma_i} fdi_{it}^{\delta_i} ex_{it}^{\tau_i} \tag{4}$$

By taking the natural logarithm of both sides of Formula (4), we obtain the theoretical framework describing the impact factors of GTFP, as follows:

$$\ln GTFP_{it} = \ln A_{i0} + \lambda_i t + \alpha_i \ln er_{it} + \beta_i \ln gt_{it} + \gamma_i \ln rd_{it} + \delta_i \ln fd_{it} + \tau_i \ln ex_{it} \tag{5}$$

To correctly explore the effect of environmental regulation, governance transformation, and their interaction terms on GTFP, based on the above analysis framework, the linear term and the quadratic term of environmental regulation are both introduced into the econometric model to investigate the possible nonlinear relationship between environmental regulation and GTFP. Since the current productivity growth may be affected by past productivity, the first-order lag term of GTFP is also included in the model as an explanatory variable to examine the dynamic cumulative effect of GTFP growth. Meanwhile, the estimation method, the system generalized method of moments (GMM), is used in this paper mainly because the system GMM can effectively overcome the endogenous problem by introducing instrumental variables. Based on the above considerations, the dynamic panel regression model constructed in this study is as follows:

$$\ln GTFP_{it} = \alpha_0 + \alpha_1 \ln GTFP_{it-1} + \alpha_2 \ln ER_{it} + \alpha_3 (\ln ER_{it})^2 + \alpha_4 \ln GT_{it} + \beta X_{it} + V_i + \varepsilon_{it} \tag{6}$$

where i and t represent the province and year, respectively (i = 1, 2, 3, . . . , 30, t = 2003, 2004, . . . , 2017); V_i indicates the provincial fixed effect; ε_{it} is the random error term; and

$GTFP_{it}$ denotes the green total factor productivity for each province; α_1 is a hysteresis multiplier, indicating the effect of the last period of GTFP on the current GTFP; ER_{it} denotes environmental regulation; GT_{it} represents governance transformation; and X_{it} is the control variables vector, including R&D investment, export trade, foreign direct investment, and the factor endowment structure, respectively. To be specific, the coefficient of the quadratic term of ER illustrates the nonlinear effect of environmental regulation on GTFP. When the estimated value of parameter α_3 is significantly more than 0, Hypothesis 1 is confirmed. Simultaneously, when the result of the parameter α_4 is significantly greater than 0, Hypothesis 2 is confirmed. In addition, the interaction term of *ER* and *GT* is included in the model to verify Hypothesis 3. The dynamic panel regression model with the cross-term is established as follows:

$$\begin{aligned}\ln GTFP_{it} = \alpha_0 + \alpha_1 \ln GTFP_{it-1} + \alpha_2 \ln ER_{it} + \alpha_3 (\ln ER_{it})^2 + \alpha_4 \ln GT_{it} \\ + \alpha_5 \ln ER_{it} \times \ln GT_{it} + \beta X_{it} + V_i + \varepsilon_{it}\end{aligned} \tag{7}$$

In Equation (7), $\ln ER_{it} \times \ln GT_{it}$ indicates the cross-term of environmental regulation and governance transformation. When the estimated result of the coefficient of the interaction term is significantly greater than 0, Hypothesis 3 is confirmed.

3.2. Variable Selection and Description

3.2.1. Dependent Variable

The dependent variable used here is green total factor productivity (GTFP). In general, productivity indexes used in prior studies focused on measuring marketable outputs relative to the paid factors of production. However, the generation of by-products, such as environmental pollutants, was not taken into consideration. In view of this, Chung et al. [60] proposed the Malmquist-Luenberger index, based on the directional distance function, which extends the original Malmquist index to account for undesired outputs, such as industrial sulfur dioxide, industrial smoke and dust, and industrial sewage. Therefore, to overcome the drawback of lacking environmental factors in the traditional productivity index, and to inherit the advantages of the Malmquist-Luenberger index following Chung et al. [60] and Oh [61], this paper uses the global Malmquist-Luenberger index (GML), based on the directional distance function, to measure the GTFP growth for each province in China. The GML index used in this study is defined as follows:

$$GML^{t,t+1}(x^t, y^t, b^t, x^{t+1}, y^{t+1}, b^{t+1}) = \frac{1 + D^G(x^t, y^t, b^t)}{1 + D^G(x^{t+1}, y^{t+1}, b^{t+1})} \tag{8}$$

In Equation (8), $D^G(\bullet)$ represents the directional distance function; x^t represents the input vector constructed by N kind of input factors; y^t represents the desirable output vector constructed by M kind of desired outputs; and b^t represents the undesirable output vector constructed by I kind of undesired outputs. Specifically, the input factors include: (1) capital input, where the capital stock of each province is calculated by employing the perpetual inventory method [9]; (2) labor input, measured by the annual average number of people employed for each province; and (3) energy consumption, expressed by the provincial primary energy consumption, which is converted to standard coal. In addition, the output factors include: (1) the desirable output, denoted by gross industrial output; and (2) the undesirable output, measured by a variety of environmental pollutants, including industrial sewage emissions, industrial sulfur dioxide, and carbon dioxide emissions.

3.2.2. Core Independent Variables

- Environmental regulation (ER). According to the Porter hypothesis, reasonable environmental regulation can effectively stimulate enterprise enthusiasm for green innovation, promote pollution emissions reduction, and improve green productivity. In previous studies, there were no clear and unified criteria to represent environmental regulation, which can mainly be measured by pollutant emission reductions, environmental pollution control investments, pollution reduction expenditures, regulatory enforcement stringencies, and pollution sewage charges [4,39,62,63]. For the consideration of data integrity and availability, this paper selects the ratio of the total investment of provincial industrial pollution control to the gross industrial output as a proxy variable for the provincial environmental regulation level. Usually, the higher the proportion of the investment, the greater the environmental regulation intensity, and the better the effect of regional green development. In addition, we also select the ratio of the total investment of industrial pollution control to the operating cost of industrial enterprises, as a substitute variable for the robustness analysis.

- Governance transformation (GT). China's corporate governance, which is deeply rooted in the transitional economy, is gradually transforming from administrative governance to economic governance. In essence, governance transformation reflects the persistent improvement of the degree of marketization for a region. Generally speaking, private enterprises have better economic governance, while state-owned enterprises have stronger administrative governance in China. Therefore, the governance transformation, which is measured by the ratio of the main business income of private industrial enterprises to the sum of the main business income of state-owned and private-owned industrial enterprises for each region, is selected here. The larger the ratio of governance transformation, the higher the degree of marketization, and the better the resource allocation and productivity of enterprises.

3.2.3. Control Variables

To alleviate the endogenous problem caused by the omitted variables, and to improve the estimation accuracy, a series of control variables are selected in the model by referring to the previous literature. The variables included are as follows:

- R&D investment (RD). Technological innovation is the important driving force for the improvement of regional green total factor productivity, which is conducive to the optimized resource allocation of enterprises, the enhancement of the product quality, and the reduction of pollution emissions [27,48,64]. In this paper, R&D investment is measured by the ratio of R&D internal expenditure to regional industrial GDP.
- Export trade dependence (EX). Previous studies indicate that export is highly correlated with regional green development [9]. China has grown into the world's largest exporter over the past ten years. Export not only helps to expand foreign demand, to finance R&D, and to stimulate green innovation, but it may also increase local pollution emissions. To investigate the effect of export expansions on regional green development, we choose the ratio of the total export volume to the provincial GDP as agent indicators for the analysis [49,65].
- Foreign direct investment (FDI). As a main channel for international industrial linkages and technology spillovers, FDI can not only change domestic capital markets, but it can also promote the improvement of GTFP [38]. Thus, foreign direct investment, which is represented by the proportion of annual foreign investment actually utilized in GDP, is regarded as a control variable in this study.
- Factor endowment structure (K/L). China's industry is gradually transforming from an extensive model to an intensive model. Compared to labor-intensive industries, capital-intensive industries usually use relatively advanced technology and equipment, which is beneficial to the improvement of resource efficiency and the green transformation of industry [5,66]. Therefore, the ratio of capital to labor is used to represent the factor endowment structure for each region.

3.3. Data Sources and Variable Descriptive Statistics

Considering the data availability and the actual needs of the research, this paper selected the Chinese provincial panel data between 2003 and 2017 to empirically investigate the impact of environmental regulation on green total factor productivity. To be specific, our sample covers 30 provinces, municipalities, and autonomous regions in mainland China from 2003 to 2017. Due to a shortage of the portion of required data, Hong Kong, Macao, Taiwan, and Tibet are excluded here. The sample dataset used in the study was mainly derived from the China Statistical Yearbook, the China Energy Statistical Yearbook, the China Environment Statistical Yearbook, the China Industrial Statistical Yearbook, the China Industrial Economic Statistical Yearbook, the China Science and Technology Statistical Yearbook, and each province's Provincial Statistical Yearbook for each sample year. The methods of moving the averages and interpolations were applied to supplement the missing data in some years and regions. In total, a balanced sample set of 450 observations was created for each region during this 15-year period. Furthermore, all variable values in the study were transformed into logarithmic forms to reduce heteroscedasticity. In order to eliminate the price effect, we deflated all the nominal variables in this study into real variables, by a GDP deflator, into the 2003 constant price. The descriptive statistics of all aforementioned variables are summarized in Table 1 below.

Table 1. Descriptive statistics of the variables from 2003 to 2017.

Variable	Definition	Obs	Mean	Min	Max	Std. Dev.
lnGTFP	Green total factor productivity	450	0.134	−0.115	0.690	0.168
lnER	Environmental regulation	450	2.259	−0.451	4.472	0.866
lnGT	Governance transformation	450	9.234	6.613	11.259	1.043
lnRD	R&D investment	450	4.00	1.104	5.054	0.494
lnEX	Export trade dependence	450	6.819	4.285	9.122	1.002
lnFDI	Foreign direct investment	450	5.112	1.351	6.958	1.301
ln(K/L)	Factor endowment structure	450	2.979	1.798	4.773	0.608

4. Empirical Results Analysis

4.1. Unit Root Test and Multicollinearity

In order to eliminate the spurious regression problem and to ensure that the estimation results are accurate and reliable, the stationarity test of all variables was implemented before the regression analysis. The test methods consisted of LLC, IPS, Fisher-ADF, and Fisher-PP tests. As shown in Table 2, the test results showed that almost all of the variables can pass more than three significance tests simultaneously, indicating that the raw data sequence of each variable was stationary. In addition, the variance inflation factor (VIF) was used to test the multicollinearity problem. The results of the VIF test indicated that the VIF values were all less than 10 and ranged from 1.24 to 2.22, showing that there was no multicollinearity among the variables. Therefore, the regression analysis was performed.

Table 2. Unit root and VIF test results.

Variable	LLC	IPS	Fisher-ADF	Fisher-PP	VIF
lnGTFP	−1.0309	−3.0823 **	97.7870 **	65.2958	—
lnER	−2.2471 *	−5.7744 ***	142.7996 ***	66.8284	1.60
lnGT	−7.3828 ***	−6.5908 ***	92.2760 **	94.7653 ***	2.22
lnRD	−5.4882 ***	−1.2160	181.8429 ***	114.186 ***	1.24
lnEX	−1.9065 *	−6.5586 ***	137.0833 ***	150.429 ***	1.79
lnFDI	−2.3105 **	−4.4187 ***	162.0403 ***	62.5083	1.84
ln(K/L)	−3.4148	−5.5994 ***	64.1777	128.726 ***	1.31

Note: ***, **, and * represent mean significance at the 1%, 5%, and 10% levels, respectively.

4.2. The Spatial-Temporal Dynamic Evolution of Regional GTFP in China

Based on the panel data of 30 provinces in China over the period from 2003 to 2017, this study adopted a directional distance function and the GML index to measure the regional GTFP growth, as shown in Figures 3 and 4.

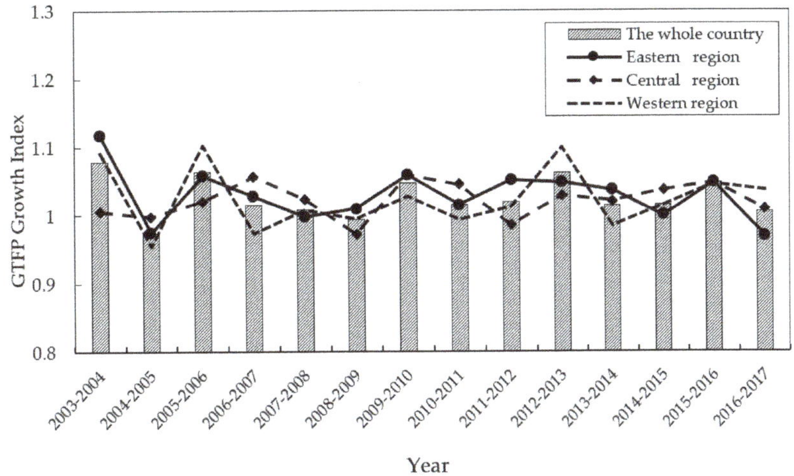

Figure 3. Trends of regional average GTFP growth index in China from 2003 to 2017.

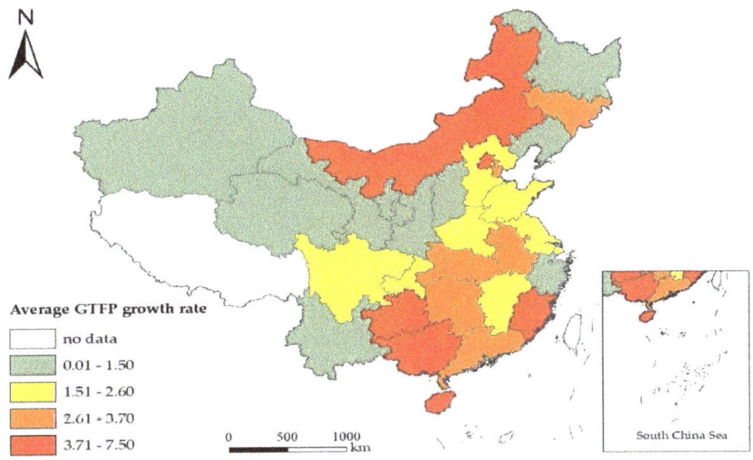

Figure 4. Spatial distribution of regional average GTFP growth rate in China from 2003 to 2017.

Figure 3 shows the overall trend of China's GTFP from 2003 to 2017. The average annual growth rate of GTFP dropped from 7.8375 in 2003 to 0.4687 in 2017, indicating that the GTFP presented an overall downward trend during these 15 years. To be specific, the GTFP declined from 2003 to 2007, followed by a slight rise from 2008 to 2010 and further fluctuates until 2013, although these variation features are not very obvious. During the 11th and 12th Five-Year Plans, the government enhanced the governance of energy conservation and the emission reduction of enterprises, gradually strengthening the responsibility of local governments to control their environmental pollution. Due to the long-term dependence on the extensive economic development model and the occurrence of the financial crisis in 2008, China has implemented a series of stimulus programs to promote infrastructure investment and heavy industries. As a result, the extensive production conditions caused by resource consumption and environmental pollution have not substantially improved. In 2013, the average growth rate of China's GTFP rose to 6.1834, illustrating that environmental supervision has brought about some positive effects. However, since 2013, when China's economy entered a new normal period, the pressure of the growth slowdown caused a decline in GTFP, which decreased to 0.4687 in 2017.

In terms of changes in different regions, the levels of economic development in the eastern, central, and western regions were different, and the changes in GTFP varied accordingly (see Figures 3 and 4). Specifically, between 2008 and 2014, the eastern region experienced rapid economic growth and the contribution of GTFP increased from 0.9425 in 2008 to 3.662 in 2014, after which it began to decline rapidly. From 2006 to 2012, the GTFP growth in the western region fluctuated little. Since 2013, the GTFP growth rate in the western region has shown a downward trend, declining from 9.9725 in 2013 to 3.7044 in 2017. From 2005 to 2015, the GTFP growth in the central region fluctuated little, showing the steady contribution of GTFP to economic development. However, the GTFP growth rate rose to 4.7981 in 2016 and then began to decline rapidly, falling to 0.8975 in 2017.

Since the reform and expansion, the central region has given priority to the development of heavy industry to achieve rapid economic growth. Due to the lack of physical capital, human capital, and advanced technology, the effect of the industrial policy on economic growth was restricted to a great extent. Therefore, the local government relaxed the punishment for resource damage and environmental pollution, trying to sacrifice the environment in exchange for the rapid economic growth. However, this extensive development model is doomed to be unsustainable. Although environmental governance was strengthened in 2015, the region is still unable to get out of the development pattern characterized by high pollution and high energy consumption.

The western region is rich in natural resources and energy and has a strong economic development potential. With the implementation of the Western Development Strategy and the latecomer advantage, some developed areas have witnessed rapid economic growth, which will inevitably accelerate energy consumption and environmental pollutants emission, resulting in a poorer performance of GTFP long-term.

4.3. The Analysis of Baseline Empirical Results

The purpose of this paper is mainly to test whether the nonlinear U-shaped relationship between environmental regulation and GTFP exists or not. Furthermore, considering the background of the Chinese market-oriented reform, governance transformation is also introduced into the model to investigate its impact on GTFP. Specifically, we first used the feasible generalized least squares (FGLS) method, the fixed effect (FE) method, and the random effect (RE) method to explore the effects of environmental regulation and governance transformation on GTFP, respectively. The estimation results are presented in columns 1–6 of Table 3. As we expected above, the coefficients of the quadratic term of environmental regulation were positive, and so were the coefficients of governance transformation. However, the fitting degrees of these six models were all less than 0.4, indicating that these three estimation methods were not able to explain causality effectively. In addition, if the explanatory variables are endogenous, the FGLS method, the FE method, and the RE method may lead to inconsistencies in parameter estimations. Therefore, in order to effectively overcome the endogeneity problem, we used the system generalized method of moments (SYS-GMM) to estimate the models by introducing instrumental variables. The difference generalized method of moments (DIFF-GMM) was also used to ensure that the regression results were robust. The estimation results of the DIFF-GMM method and SYS-GMM method are shown in columns 7 and 8 and columns 9 and 10 of Table 3, respectively. It should be noted that the AR tests, which are used to test the autocorrelation of the residual term, showed that there was a first-order autocorrelation but there was no evidence of a second-order autocorrelation. Meanwhile, the Hansen over-identification tests, which are usually adopted to examine the validity of the instrumental variables, indicated that the null hypothesis cannot be rejected; namely, the instrumental variables were jointly effective. Therefore, the specifications of the dynamic panel data models in this study are reasonable.

Table 3. The regression results of impact of environmental regulation on GTFP for full samples.

Variable	FGLS		FE		RE		DIFF-GMM		SYS-GMM	
	(1)	(2)	(3)	(4)	(5)	(6)	(7)	(8)	(9)	(10)
lnER	−0.0386 *** (0.0146)	−0.0377 *** (0.0141)	−0.0782 ** (0.0393)	−0.0708 * (0.0389)	−0.0765 * (0.0400)	−0.0685 * (0.0395)	−0.0556 *** (0.0217)	−0.0578 ** (0.0275)	−0.0749 ** (0.0354)	−0.0950 ** (0.0424)
$(\text{lnER})^2$	0.0038 (0.0037)	0.0045 (0.0037)	0.0076 (0.0091)	0.0068 (0.0089)	0.0063 (0.0092)	0.0066 (0.0089)	0.0097 * (0.0057)	0.0116 * (0.0070)	0.0100 * (0.0072)	0.0155 * (0.0094)
lnGT		0.0930 *** (0.0142)		0.0504 * (0.0316)		0.0512 ** (0.0222)		0.1277 *** (0.0432)		0.0269 * (0.0146)
lnRD	0.0691 *** (0.0132)	0.0726 *** (0.0144)	0.1025 *** (0.0296)	0.1114 *** (0.0270)	0.1077 *** (0.0256)	0.1051 *** (0.0239)	0.0831 *** (0.0306)	0.1232 *** (0.0389)	0.0924 *** (0.0290)	0.0742 *** (0.0265)
lnFDI	−0.0028 (0.0120)	−0.0043 (0.0108)	0.0117 (0.0203)	0.0084 (0.0202)	0.0142 (0.0183)	0.0082 (0.0192)	0.0232 (0.0177)	0.0153 (0.0191)	0.0188 (0.0149)	0.0120 (0.0133)
lnEX	−0.0019 (0.0144)	−0.0160 (0.0164)	0.0173 (0.0304)	0.0105 (0.0290)	0.0152 (0.0234)	0.0025 (0.0221)	0.0049 (0.0161)	0.0299 (0.0267)	−0.0224 * (0.0142)	−0.0367 * (0.0194)
ln(K/L)	0.0557 *** (0.0178)	−0.0046 (0.0179)	−0.0763 ** (0.0280)	0.0365 (0.0463)	−0.0661 ** (0.0262)	0.0358 (0.0326)	0.0422 * (0.0240)	−0.0278 (0.0425)	−0.0458 *** (0.0170)	−0.0550 *** (0.0166)
L.lnGTFP							0.3794 *** (0.1147)	0.2735 *** (0.1030)	0.6613 *** (0.0980)	0.6381 *** (0.1041)
Inflection point	5.0789	4.1889	5.1447	5.2058	6.0714	5.1894	2.866	2.491	3.745	3.065
R^2	0.0955	0.0956	0.3799	0.3952	0.3790	0.3747				
AR (1)							0.0340	0.0469	0.0332	0.0299
AR (2)							0.4499	0.6814	0.4249	0.4253
Hansen							0.1062	0.1726	0.1811	0.1579
Observations	450	450	450	450	450	450	450	450	450	450

Note: standard errors in parentheses. ***, **, and * represent mean significance at the 1%, 5%, and 10% levels, respectively.

Firstly, the coefficients of the first-order lag term of GTFP were all significantly positive at the 1% level in Models (7)–(10), showing that the growth of GTFP is a dynamic accumulation process with significantly positive feedback and path dependency. The SYS-GMM estimation results of the environmental regulation showed that the coefficients of the linear term of environmental regulation were all significantly negative, while the coefficients of the quadratic term were significantly positive, indicating that there is a nonlinear U-shaped relationship between environmental regulation and GTFP. As a comparison, the DIFF-GMM estimation results showed that the regression results were robust. Therefore, Hypothesis 1 (H1) is verified. The feasible explanation for this nonlinear relationship is that when environmental supervision is less strict, the pollution control costs and the extensive production are higher, and the green economic efficiency is lower. However, with the improvement of environmental regulation stringencies, enterprises must continue to increase environmental investment to carry out green technology innovation, which will gradually compensate for the compliance costs and contribute to green productivity in the long term. Furthermore, taking Model (10) as an example, the inflection point value of environmental regulation is 3.065, which is greater than the mean level of 2.259, shown in Table 1, indicating that the intensity of environmental regulation in China is still located on the left side of the U-shaped curve, meaning that the promotional effect of environmental regulation on GTFP has not been achieved fully.

Secondly, the coefficients of governance transformation were all positive and significant in Model (8) and Model (10), showing that governance transformation can promote the improvement of GTFP. Hypothesis 2 (H2) is, thus, verified. The possible explanation for this is that with the establishment and improvement of the socialist market economic system, the market-oriented governance transformation plays an increasingly important role in the efficiency of the resource allocation among enterprises. Therefore, resources will flow into high efficiency enterprises over time, which contributes to the enhancement of the internal production efficiency of enterprises by the specialized division of labor and the adoption of advanced green technology. This will then improve the overall green productivity of the whole society in the long term.

Finally, among the control variables, the coefficients of R&D investment were significantly positive, showing that R&D investment can promote the growth of GTFP. The credible explanation for the result is that the increase in R&D investment is beneficial to the enhancement of the innovation capacity of enterprises through the promotion of technological progress, thus improving production efficiency. The coefficients of FDI were always positive but not significant, indicating that FDI cannot significantly improve GTFP. This is due to the fact that local governments pay more attention to the quantity of FDI but ignore the quality of FDI. As a result, the introduction of foreign-invested enterprises with a high production efficiency and green technology is insufficient, which affects the improvement of regional productivity. However, export trade dependence and the factor endowment structure have a negative impact on GTFP. The conceivable explanation is that the low-level export product quality and the unreasonable resource allocation models hinder the transformation of the extensive economic development characterized by high input, high emissions, and low efficiency and, thus, inhibit the growth of GTFP.

4.4. The Analysis of Regional Heterogeneity Results

Although the regression results of the full sample show a nonlinear U-shaped relationship between environmental regulation and GTFP, governance transformation can improve GTFP. Due to China's vast territories and the differences in the level of economic development among regions, whether the benchmark regression results are still tenable in different regions is, therefore, unknown. In order to solve this problem, the study divided the full sample into three sub-samples according to geographical locations and economic characteristics, which are the eastern region, the central region, and the western region. Then, we used the SYS-GMM method to estimate three sub-samples. The results are presented in Table 4.

The regression results of Models (1)–(6) in Table 4 show that the effects of environmental regulation on GTFP have regional differences. Specifically, the U-shaped relationship between environmental regulation and GTFP was significant in the eastern and western regions, but it was uncertain in the central region. The reasons can be summarized into three aspects. Firstly, cities in the eastern region have established third-party pollution control mechanisms and have obtained remarkable achievements. Compared to the other regions, industrial enterprises in the eastern region are more adaptable to stricter environmental standards. Secondly, following the findings by Song et al. [49], government subsidies will impair the positive effect of environmental regulation on technological innovation. In the central region, the R&D activities of environmental control are heavily dependent on government investments, so that the enterprise benefits from technological innovation investment are not enough to compensate for the additional production costs caused by environmental regulation. In addition, in order to stimulate economic development, local governments compete to set lower environmental regulatory standards to attract investment projects. For this reason, environmental regulation policies become a mere formality. Thirdly, in the western region, owing to the relatively backward economic development level, many enterprises are able to receive more favorable policies under the national implementation of the Western Development Strategy. With the strengthening of environmental regulation, more green funds provided by local governments are used to support enterprises to carry out green technology innovations, which improves the green production efficiency in the long term.

Table 4. Regression results of different regions with SYS-GMM.

Variable	Eastern Region		Central Region		Western Region	
	(1)	(2)	(3)	(4)	(5)	(6)
lnER	−0.0309 *	−0.0304 *	−0.0250	−0.0410	−0.1949 ***	−0.2207 ***
	(0.0168)	(0.0199)	(0.0360)	(0.0419)	(0.0640)	(0.0571)
$(\text{lnER})^2$	0.0057	0.0089 *	−0.0099	0.0104	0.0289 **	0.0336 ***
	(0.0051)	(0.0051)	(0.0106)	(0.0103)	(0.0131)	(0.0131)
lnGT		0.0202 **		0.0621 ***		0.0215 *
		(0.0092)		(0.0176)		(0.0141)
lnRD	0.0772 **	0.0380 **	0.0303 **	0.0285	0.0829 **	0.0849 *
	(0.0352)	(0.0170)	(0.0137)	(0.0286)	(0.0364)	(0.0522)
lnFDI	0.0566 **	0.0387 ***	0.0008	−0.0074	0.0059	0.0104
	(0.0266)	(0.0113)	(0.0107)	(0.0150)	(0.0100)	(0.0117)
lnEX	−0.0501 *	−0.0510	−0.0089	0.0484 ***	0.0110	-0.0074
	(0.0261)	*** (0.0187)	(0.0089)	(0.0169)	(0.0111)	(0.0148)
ln(K/L)	−0.0557 *	−0.0389 **	−0.0117	0.0104	−0.0200 *	−0.0377 **
	(0.0335)	(0.0188)	(0.0187)	(0.0137)	(0.0110)	(0.0189)
L.lnGTFP	0.8112 ***	0.8520 ***	0.8335 ***	0.7040 ***	0.2630 **	0.2151 **
	(0.0837)	(0.0609)	(0.0913)	(0.0807)	(0.1369)	(0.1164)
Inflection point	2.7105	1.7079	—	—	3.3720	3.2842
AR(1)	0.0133	0.0129	0.0430	0.0411	0.0820	0.0985
AR(2)	0.7593	0.7951	0.2102	0.2336	0.3001	0.3265
Hansen	0.1015	0.1258	0.2136	0.1300	0.5730	0.4749
Observations	165	165	120	120	165	165

Note: Standard errors in parentheses. ***, **, and * represent mean significance at the 1%, 5%, and 10% levels, respectively. The eastern region consists of Liaoning, Hebei, Tianjin, Beijing, Shandong, Jiangsu, Shanghai, Zhejiang, Fujian, Guangdong, and Hainan. The central region consists of Heilongjiang, Jilin, Shanxi, Anhui, Jiangxi, Henan, Hubei, and Hunan. The western region consists of Shanxi, Gansu, Ningxia, Qinghai, Xinjiang, Sichuan, Yunnan, Guangxi, Guizhou, Chongqing, and Inner Mongolia.

Meanwhile, the regression coefficients of governance transformation in the eastern region, central region, and western region were 0.0202, 0.0621, and 0.0215, respectively, indicating that the promotional effect of governance transformation on GTFP in the central region is greater than that in the eastern region and western region. Because of the implementation of the Central Rise Policy, the state and the local governments have issued a series of policies to promote economic development, which stimulates the development of private enterprises in the central region. Under such circumstances, market-oriented governance transformation can effectively strengthen the efficiency of resource allocation among enterprises, which inspires the vitality of private enterprises with a high efficiency and promotes the realization of radical innovation, as well as improving the production efficiency in this region [44,46].

In addition, the influence of other control variables on GTFP also present regional differences. For example, the regression coefficients of export trade dependence in the eastern region were significantly negative, while those in the central and western regions were not significant. The regression coefficients of the factor endowment structure were significantly negative in the eastern and western regions, while those in the central region were not significant. The regression coefficients of FDI were significantly positive in the eastern region, while those in the central and western regions were not significant, mainly because the quality of FDI introduced in the eastern region is improved constantly and GTFP is also promoted. Moreover, the impact of R&D investment on GTFP in all regions was significantly positive, indicating that R&D investment contributes to the enhancement of enterprise innovation capacities, as well as improved production efficiency over time.

4.5. The Analysis of the Robustness Test Results

In order to ensure the reliability and validity of the baseline regression results, this paper used four ways to perform robustness tests. First, we used the dynamic panel threshold model to estimate the full sample. To be specific, according to the threshold variable, namely, the level of environmental regulation, the full sample was classified into a high group and a low group. The SYS-GMM method was then used to estimate the two groups simultaneously. Second, we adjusted the measurement pattern of environmental regulation. Specifically, the ratio of the total investment of industrial pollution control to the operating costs of industrial enterprises was selected as a substitute variable for environmental regulation. Then, the regression analysis was based on the adjusted full sample data. Third, the two-step SYS-GMM method was used to estimate the full sample. Compared with the one-step SYS-GMM, the two-step SYS-GMM can improve the estimation efficiency, as the weight matrix of the instrumental variables can be modified by the residual matrix of the one-step SYS-GMM. Fourth, we adjusted the sample interval for estimation. Specifically, the samples in 2003 and 2017 were excluded to eliminate the impact of the sample time selection on the estimation results. Thus, the provincial panel data from 2004 to 2016 were used for the re-estimation. The robustness test results are shown in Table 5.

Table 5. Robustness test results of impact of environmental regulation on GTFP.

Variable	Panel Threshold Model		Replacing ER Variable		Two-step SYS-GMM		Adjusting Sample Interval	
	(1)Low Group	(2) High Group	(3)	(4)	(5)	(6)	(7)	(8)
lnER	−0.0564 **	0.1727 *	−0.0768 **	−0.1023 **	−0.1811 **	−0.1487 **	−0.0818 **	−0.1404 **
	(0.0274)	(0.1003)	(0.0354)	(0.0540)	(0.0874)	(0.0715)	(0.0356)	(0.0666)
$(\ln ER)^2$			0.0096 *	0.0159 *	0.0322 *	0.0269 **	0.0133 *	0.0262 *
			(0.0066)	(0.0085)	(0.0181)	(0.0141)	(0.0080)	(0.0147)
lnGT	0.1450 ***	0.1107 **		0.0265*		0.0513 **		0.0103
	(0.0473)	(0.0547)		(0.0149)		(0.0247)		(0.0144)
lnRD	0.1682 ***	0.1093 **	0.0923 ***	0.0751 **	0.1030 **	0.0864 *	0.0866 **	0.0901 **
	(0.0462)	(0.0504)	(0.0297)	(0.0277)	(0.0436)	(0.0470)	(0.0389)	(0.0470)
lnFDI	0.0209	0.0107	0.0206	0.0144	0.0092	0.0019	0.0388	0.0346
	(0.0326)	(0.0367)	(0.0151)	(0.0135)	(0.0171)	(0.0146)	(0.0367)	(0.0281)
lnEX	−0.1595 ***	−0.1899 ***	−0.0224	−0.0367 *	−0.0116	−0.0351	−0.0414	−0.0429 **
	(0.0579)	(0.0567)	(0.0149)	(0.0197)	(0.0111)	(0.0275)	(0.0275)	(0.0184)
ln(K/L)	−0.1937 ***	−0.2215 **	−0.0443 **	−0.0525 ***	−0.0313	−0.0339 *	−0.0350 **	−0.0418 ***
	(0.0589)	(0.0891)	(0.0179)	(0.0166)	(0.0295)	(0.0207)	(0.0176)	(0.0142)
L.lnGTFP	0.3303 **	0.6457 ***	0.5854 ***	0.6369 ***	0.5716 ***	0.5569 ***	0.7413 ***	0.7233 ***
	(0.1586)	(0.1174)	(0.1405)	(0.1046)	(0.1152)	(0.1286)	(0.1275)	(0.1485)
Inflection point	3.150 (threshold value)		4.000	3.217	2.812	2.764	3.0752	2.6794
AR (1)	0.0078		0.0317	0.0280	0.0259	0.0194	0.0588	0.0454
AR (2)	0.1964		0.4294	0.4192	0.4346	0.3971	0.3303	0.3166
Hansen	0.6852		0.1922	0.3304	0.2441	0.2910	0.1224	0.4002
Observations	450		450	450	450	450	390	390

Note: Standard errors in parentheses. ***, **, and * represents mean significance at the 1%, 5%, and 10% levels, respectively.

Columns 1 and 2 in Table 5 report the results of the panel threshold regression model, indicating that there is a nonlinear U-shaped relationship between environmental regulation and GTFP. Specifically, when the level of environmental supervision is lower than the threshold value (3.15), environmental regulation inhibits the growth of GTFP. If the level of environmental supervision is greater than 3.15, environmental regulation can facilitate the improvement of GTFP. Furthermore, the coefficients of governance transformation were both significantly positive in the low and high groups. Columns 3 and 4 in Table 5 show the regression results when the measurement of environmental regulation is replaced, demonstrating that the coefficients of the quadratic term of environmental regulation were positive and significant, confirming the nonlinear U-shaped relationship between environmental regulation and GTFP. The coefficients of governance transformation were significantly positive. Columns 5 and 6 in Table 5 show the estimation results of the two-step SYS-GMM, illustrating that the relationship between environmental regulation and GTFP is nonlinear and U-shaped. The coefficients of governance transformation were also significantly positive. Columns 7 and 8 in Table 5 report the regression results of adjusting the sample interval, indicating that the nonlinear U-shaped relationship between environmental regulation and GTFP exists. The coefficients of governance transformation were positive. In addition, the regression results of the four robustness tests showed that the signs and significance of the coefficients of other control variables were consistent with the baseline empirical results. In conclusion, the robustness tests verified the existence of the nonlinear U-shaped relationship between environmental regulation and GTFP and that governance transformation can promote the growth of GTFP. Thereby, the baseline regression results of this study are robust and reliable.

4.6. Further Discussion

With the deepening of the socialist market economic reform, the role of the market mechanism in resource allocation has been increasingly strengthened. In essence, governance transformation reflects a market-oriented resource allocation reform, indicating that the governance model is changing from an administrative governance to an economic governance. Regarding the increasingly serious environmental problems, it is unknown if the market-oriented governance transformation can improve the effect of environmental regulation on GTFP and if the governance transformation can facilitate the realization of the Porter hypothesis and its influencing mechanisms. In order to solve these problems, the interaction term between governance transformation and environmental regulation was added into the model to investigate the influence of governance transformation on the Porter hypothesis. The regression results are shown in Table 6.

Table 6. The regression results of impact of governance transformation on the Porter hypothesis.

Variable	SYS-GMM						DIFF-GMM	
	(1)	(2)	(3)	(4)	(5)	(6)	(7)	(8)
lnER	−0.2481 *** (0.0654)	−0.2732 *** (0.0730)	−0.3034 *** (0.0872)	−0.2756 *** (0.0777)	−0.2258 *** (0.0670)	−0.2498 *** (0.0649)	−0.2408 (0.1884)	−0.5657 *** (0.2176)
$(\ln ER)^2$	0.0155 * (0.0092)	0.0148 * (0.0085)	0.0153 * (0.0085)	0.0151 ** (0.0077)	0.0135 ** (0.0072)	0.0142 * (0.0080)	0.0189 * (0.0101)	0.0325 ** (0.0148)
lnGT	0.0178 *** (0.0052)	0.0078 (0.0053)	0.0273 ** (0.0137)	0.0329 ** (0.0127)	0.0089 (0.0180)		0.0982 ** (0.0500)	
lnER*lnGT	0.0182 *** (0.0060)	0.0212 *** (0.0063)	0.0236 *** (0.0074)	0.0226 *** (0.0065)	0.0165 *** (0.0057)	0.0187 *** (0.0048)	0.0295* (0.0165)	0.0444** (0.0180)
lnRD		0.0615 *** (0.0191)	0.0785 *** (0.0244)	0.0809 *** (0.0218)	0.0828 *** (0.0250)	0.0879 *** (0.0285)	0.1319 *** (0.0441)	0.1316 *** (0.0494)
lnFDI			0.0250 * (0.0138)	0.0203 (0.0158)	0.0016 (0.0143)	0.0027 (0.0140)	0.0149 (0.0175)	0.0179 (0.0179)
lnEX				0.0102 (0.0156)	−0.0183 (0.0229)	−0.0109 (0.0158)	0.0385 (0.0255)	0.0364 (0.0240)
ln(K/L)					−0.0428 ** (0.0209)	−0.0392 ** (0.0176)	−0.0178 (0.0464)	−0.0075 (0.0485)
L.lnGTFP	0.6306 *** (0.0928)	0.5937 *** (0.0999)	0.5738 *** (0.0948)	0.5801 *** (0.0867)	0.5852 *** (0.0910)	0.5831 *** (0.0894)	0.1862 * (0.1106)	0.2348 * (0.1233)
AR (1)	0.0434	0.0363	0.0296	0.0354	0.0389	0.0373	0.0221	0.0129
AR (2)	0.4082	0.4200	0.4027	0.4238	0.4369	0.4363	0.8091	0.5174
Hansen	0.3387	0.5999	0.5471	0.5183	0.3637	0.4029	0.1211	0.1461
Observations	450	450	450	450	450	450	450	450

Note: Standard errors in parentheses. ***, **, and * represent mean significance at the 1%, 5%, and 10% levels, respectively.

The estimation results reported in columns 1–8 show that the coefficients of the interaction term between governance transformation and environmental regulation are significantly positive, indicating that, with the improvement of the environmental regulation intensity, governance transformation plays an increasingly important role in promoting the growth of GTFP. In other words, governance transformation can accelerate the realization of the improvement effects of environmental regulation on GTFP. Hypothesis 3 (H3) is, thus, verified. The reason for the result is probably that as market plays an increasingly important role in resource allocation, the efficiency of resource allocation among enterprises can be improved, which contributes to the inspiration of the innovative enthusiasm of private enterprises in the face of stricter environmental regulations. Radical innovation can, therefore, be realized quickly, and this will promote productivity over the long term. In addition, the signs and significance of the coefficients of environmental regulation, governance transformation, and the other control variables are also consistent with the baseline regression results.

5. Conclusions

How to protect the ecological environment and promote high-quality economic development has gradually become a research hotspot in recent years. Under such circumstances, this paper uses the GML method to measure the GTFP of 30 provinces in China from 2003 to 2017 and investigates the impact and mechanisms of environmental regulation on GTFP by using a dynamic panel model and the SYS-GMM method. The main conclusions are drawn as follows. First, under the dual pressures of severe resource constraints and environmental protection, GTFP is an accurate and meaningful indicator of the measurement of the level of economic development. Second, there is a nonlinear U-shaped relationship between environmental regulation and GTFP, indicating that the Porter hypothesis is verified in China. Most notably, the intensity of environmental regulation is still located on the left side of the U-shaped curve, which means that the promotional effect of environmental regulation on GTFP has not yet been realized fully. Meanwhile, the nonlinear U-shaped relationship shows significant regional differences. It is the western region that presents the highest level of significance, followed by the eastern region, but it is insignificant in the central region. Third, governance transformation can significantly improve GTFP by promoting enterprise technological innovation. Fourth, governance transformation can accelerate the realization of the Porter hypothesis by inspiring the innovation enthusiasm of private enterprises. In other words, governance transformation contributes to the achievement of the realization of the improvement effects of environmental regulation on GTFP. Moreover, R&D investment can significantly improve GTFP, while the impacts of export trade dependence and the factor endowment structure on GTFP are negative and significant. The influence of FDI on GTFP is insignificant.

In order to uphold the guidance of green development and to promote high-quality economic development by preserving the ecological environment, based on the above conclusions, we propose the following policy recommendations.

Firstly, China should firmly hold the conviction that lucid waters and lush mountains are invaluable assets and should always adhere to an ecological priority and green development. Specifically, the Chinese government should closely monitor energy conservation, emission reductions, and ecological environment protection, as well as optimizing the ecological environment of factor allocation and enhancing the value creativity of factor resources, such as labor, capital, and energy. Meanwhile, the state and local governments should formulate a diversified green government performance appraisal system, especially for the official promotion evaluation mechanism, in which the weight of environmental indicators should be considered. Moreover, local governments should strengthen exchanges and cooperation in environmental governance and should establish inter-jurisdiction joint preventions and control coordination mechanisms to improve the ecological environment.

Secondly, the Chinese government should establish a long-term, institutionalized, and standardized environmental regulation policy system that is coordinated with regional economic development as soon as possible. To be specific, the central government should further strengthen the overall planning of environmental regulation across regions and establish a coordinated and unified environmental supervision system, such as setting up an inter-regional transfer payment system characterized by an ecological compensation mechanism. At the same time, the government should vigorously expand environmental regulation tools and comprehensively use legal, economic, technical, and administrative means to establish a fair and diverse environmental regulation tool system. In addition, the state and local governments should enhance the coordination between regional environmental policies and regional economic development policies, as well as implementing flexible and differentiated environmental regulation policies to improve the effectiveness of environmental regulation over time.

Thirdly, China should strive to create a fair and trustworthy market environment and give full play to the decisive role of the market in resource allocation. Specifically, the government should accelerate the market-oriented reform of the factor price in the capital market, labor market, and land market, as well as improving the transparency of market transactions to eliminate the factor price distortion. Meanwhile, the government should strengthen anti-monopoly policies, reduce entry constraints to monopoly industries, and promote the reform of the profit distribution systems of state-owned enterprises. In addition, the government should avoid excessive intervention in the economy, eliminating the differential treatment in credit supplies, interest rates, and market access, as well as improving the official administrative efficiency and public service levels.

Finally, in order to realize the green development of China's economy, we should use the coordination effect of technological innovation, FDI, trade openness, and factor endowment. Specifically, (1) the state and local governments should increase their investment in R&D and should provide financial support for green technology innovation by setting up green development funds. In particular, the government should improve the incentive mechanisms for the commercialization of technological innovation achievements. (2) In order to fully exploit the spillover effect and pollution halo effects of FDI, the local governments should transform the FDI attraction mode from quantity to quality to attract high-quality technological FDI and green FDI based on local economic development circumstances. (3) China should continue to expand and optimize the foreign trade structure. It is important to accelerate the transition of the export trade from quantity to quality, such as reducing the proportion of export volume in low value-added and high pollution industries. Meanwhile, the import volume of new technologies, especially the green technologies, should be enlarged. (4) China should improve the factor market allocation and promote the free flow of capital, labor, and other factors. For example, the government should strengthen financial marketization reforms to effectively reduce the capital cost for enterprises and to deepen the Hukou (household registration) system reform to optimize labor allocations between urban and rural areas.

Limitations and Outlook

This paper mainly explores the impact of environmental regulation on China's regional green development from the governance transformation perspective. Although this study provides valuable insights, it still has certain limitations, which could also be directions for future research. First, owing to the difficulty in collecting relevant data, the sample period of this paper spanned from 2003 to 2017. Specifically, when calculating the GTFP growth of China's 30 provinces, the data of these variables, such as gross industrial output, industrial sulfur dioxide, and industrial sewage emissions, were only updated to 2017. The index of environmental regulation, namely, the amount of industrial pollution control investment, lacks the data for 2018 in all provinces. If additional data had been available, the conclusions would be richer and more reliable. Future research can make progress on data expansion. Second, while this study investigates the nonlinear relationship between environmental regulation and GTFP in an empirical analysis, its driving mechanism and dynamic evolutionary paths have not been clearly explored, which is limited by sample data acquisition. Therefore, the follow-up studies can attempt to establish theoretical models (e.g., the dynamic stochastic general equilibrium model), which could be used to describe the dynamic transmission mechanisms of environmental regulation and governance transformation on GTFP, as well as providing a sound theoretical basis for the empirical results of this paper. Third, the dynamic panel GMM model used in this paper ignores the spatial effects of environmental regulation. However, due to the externality of environmental pollution, there are obvious imitation behaviors and strategic games in inter-regional environmental regulation, which inevitably engenders spatial spillover effects. In the future, we plan to divide environmental regulation into administrative environmental regulation and market-based environmental regulation. This will enable the construction of a dynamic spatial panel GMM model to investigate the direct and indirect effects of different types of environmental regulation on GTFP. Finally, this study uses provincial-level data, and its availability is limited. To be specific, due to the remarkable differences in economic development levels across different cities within a province, it is meaningful and reasonable to explore the relationship among environmental regulation, governance transformation, and the GTFP for different regions when city-level data are available in the future. Specifically, the use of city-level data can not only control the potential heterogeneity across cities within a province, but it can also enhance the credibility due to the significant expansion of the sample size.

Author Contributions: Article research framework design, X.X.; empirical model construction, X.X., X.L. and L.Z.; raw data collection and data processing, X.L. and L.Z.; writing and translating, X.X. and L.Z. All authors have read and agreed to the published version of the manuscript.

Funding: This research is sponsored by the National Social Science Foundation of China (No. 19BRK036), the Humanities and Social Science Youth Foundation of the Ministry of Education in China (No. 18YJC840047), and the Social Science Foundation of Hunan Province (No. 17YBQ104).

Institutional Review Board Statement: This study did not involve humans. No statement from the institutional review board is required.

Informed Consent Statement: Not applicable.

Data Availability Statement: The datasets and computer programs used in this study are available from the corresponding author upon reasonable requests.

Acknowledgments: We are sincerely grateful to the editor and anonymous referees for their insightful remarks and suggestions. They make some pertinent comments on the previous version of this paper, and also give us some suggestions and hints. We also would like to thank Junqi He, Yan Qu, Jia Song and Cui Yuan for their research assistance. Nevertheless, any errors that remain in this paper are solely our responsibility.

Conflicts of Interest: The authors declare no conflict of interest.

References

1. Banerjee, A.; Duflo, E.; Qian, N. On the road: Access to transportation infrastructure and economic growth in China. *J. Dev. Econ.* **2020**, *145*, 102442. [CrossRef]
2. Zhou, J.; Raza, A.; Sui, H.G. Infrastructure investment and economic growth quality: Empirical analysis of China's regional development. *Appl. Econ.* **2021**, *53*, 2615–2630. [CrossRef]
3. Liu, K.; Shi, D.; Xiang, W.; Zhang, W. How has the efficiency of China's green development evolved? An improved non-radial directional distance function measurement. *Sci. Total Environ.* **2022**, *815*, 152337. [CrossRef] [PubMed]
4. Du, J.; Zhang, J.; Li, X. What is the mechanism of resource dependence and high-quality economic development? An empirical test from China. *Sustainability* **2020**, *12*, 8144. [CrossRef]
5. Li, X.; Du, J.; Long, H. Understanding the green development behavior and performance of industrial enterprises (GDBP-IE): Scale development and validation. *Int. J. Environ. Res. Public Health* **2020**, *17*, 1716. [CrossRef]
6. Oh, D.; Heshmati, A. A sequential Malmquist-Luenberger productivity index: Environmentally sensitive productivity growth considering the progressive nature of technology. *Energy Econ.* **2010**, *32*, 1345–1355. [CrossRef]
7. Curtis, C.C. Economic reforms and the evolution of China's total factor productivity. *Rev. Econ. Dyn.* **2016**, *21*, 225–245. [CrossRef]
8. Song, X.; Zhou, Y.; Jia, W. How do economic openness and R&D investment affect green economic growth? Evidence from China. *Resour. Conserv. Recycl.* **2019**, *146*, 405–415.
9. Zhang, Y.; Jin, P.; Feng, D. Does civil environmental protection force the growth of China's industrial green productivity? Evidence from the perspective of rent-seeking. *Ecol. Indic.* **2015**, *51*, 215–227. [CrossRef]
10. Lin, B.; Chen, Z. Does factor market distortion inhibit the green total factor productivity in China? *J. Clean Prod.* **2018**, *197*, 25–33. [CrossRef]
11. Li, J.; Tang, D.; Tenkorang, A.P.; Shi, Z. Research on environmental regulation and green total factor productivity in Yangtze River Delta: From the perspective of financial development. *Int. J. Environ. Res. Public Health* **2021**, *18*, 12453. [CrossRef] [PubMed]

12. Hancevic, P.I. Environmental regulation and productivity: The case of electricity generation under the CAAA-1990. *Energy Econ.* **2016**, *60*, 131–143. [CrossRef]
13. Wang, Y.; Sun, X.; Guo, X. Environmental regulation and green productivity growth: Empirical evidence on the Porter hypothesis from OECD industrial sectors. *Energy Policy* **2019**, *132*, 611–619. [CrossRef]
14. Zhang, D. Marketization, environmental regulation, and eco-friendly productivity: A Malmquist-Luenberger index for pollution emissions of large Chinese firms. *J. Asian Econ.* **2021**, *76*, 101342. [CrossRef]
15. Du, K.; Cheng, Y.; Yao, X. Environmental regulation, green technology innovation, and industrial structure upgrading: The road to the green transformation of Chinese cities. *Energy Econ.* **2021**, *98*, 105247. [CrossRef]
16. Chen, L.; Zhang, X.; He, F.; Yuan, R. Regional green development level and its spatial relationship under the constraints of haze in China. *J. Clean Prod.* **2019**, *210*, 376–387. [CrossRef]
17. Kesidou, E.; Wu, L. Stringency of environmental regulation and eco-innovation: Evidence from the eleventh Five-Year Plan and green patents. *Econ. Lett.* **2020**, *190*, 109090. [CrossRef]
18. Zou, H.; Zhang, Y. Does environmental regulatory system drive the green development of China's pollution-intensive industries? *J. Clean Prod.* **2022**, *330*, 129832. [CrossRef]
19. Li, R.; Ma, Z.; Chen, X. Historical market genes, marketization and economic growth in China. *Econ. Model.* **2020**, *86*, 327–333. [CrossRef]
20. Zhang, D.; Liu, D. Determinants of the capital structure of Chinese non-listed enterprises: Is TFP efficient? *Econ. Syst.* **2017**, *41*, 179–202. [CrossRef]
21. Han, J.; Miao, J.; Du, G.; Yan, D.; Miao, Z. Can market-oriented reform inhibit carbon dioxide emissions in China? A new perspective from factor market distortion. *Sustain. Prod. Consump.* **2021**, *27*, 1498–1513. [CrossRef]
22. Zhang, D. Can export tax rebate alleviate financial constraint to increase firm productivity? Evidence from China. *Int. Rev. Econ. Financ.* **2019**, *64*, 529–540. [CrossRef]
23. Bin, P.; Chen, X.; Fracasso, A.; Tomasi, C. Resource allocation and productivity across provinces in China. *Int. Rev. Econ. Financ.* **2018**, *57*, 103–113. [CrossRef]
24. Li, J.; Liu, H.; Du, K. Does market-oriented reform increase energy rebound effect? Evidence from China's regional development. *China Econ. Rev.* **2019**, *56*, 101304. [CrossRef]
25. Peng, J.; Xie, R.; Ma, C.; Fu, Y. Market-based environmental regulation and total factor productivity: Evidence from Chinese enterprises. *Econ. Model.* **2021**, *95*, 394–407. [CrossRef]
26. Dong, J.; Xue, G.; Dong, M.; Xu, X. Energy-saving power generation dispatching in China: Regulations, pilot projects and policy recommendations: A review. *Renew. Sustain. Energ. Rev.* **2015**, *43*, 1285–1300. [CrossRef]
27. Liu, Y.; Lei, J.; Zhang, Y. A study on the sustainable relationship among the green finance, environment regulation and green total factor productivity in China. *Sustainability* **2021**, *13*, 11926. [CrossRef]
28. Wu, H.; Li, Y.; Hao, Y.; Ren, S.; Zhang, P. Environmental decentralization, local government competition, and regional green development: Evidence from China. *Sci. Total Environ.* **2020**, *708*, 135085. [CrossRef]
29. Zhou, A.; Li, J. Impact of anti-corruption and environmental regulation on the green development of China's manufacturing industry. *Sustain. Prod. Consump.* **2021**, *27*, 1944–1960. [CrossRef]
30. Rexhäuser, S.; Rammer, C. Environmental innovations and firm profitability: Unmasking the Porter hypothesis. *Environ. Resour. Econ.* **2014**, *57*, 145–167. [CrossRef]
31. Tang, K.; Qiu, Y.; Zhou, D. Does command-and-control regulation promote green innovation performance? Evidence from China's industrial enterprises. *Sci. Total Environ.* **2020**, *712*, 136362. [CrossRef]
32. Zhang, N.; Jiang, X. The effect of environmental policy on Chinese firm's green productivity and shadow price: A metafrontier input distance function approach. *Technol. Forecast. Soc. Chang.* **2019**, *144*, 129–136. [CrossRef]
33. Cai, W.; Ye, P. How does environmental regulation influence enterprises' total factor productivity? A quasi-natural experiment based on China's new environmental protection law. *J. Clean Prod.* **2020**, *276*, 124105. [CrossRef]
34. Porter, M.E.; Linde, C. Toward a new conception of the environment-competitiveness relationship. *J. Econ. Perspect.* **1995**, *9*, 97–118. [CrossRef]
35. Lanoie, P.; Laurent-Lucchetti, J.; Johnstone, N.; Ambec, S. Environmental policy, innovation and performance: New insights on the Porter hypothesis. *J. Econ. Manag. Strategy* **2011**, *20*, 803–842. [CrossRef]
36. Wang, Y.; Shen, N. Environmental regulation and environmental productivity: The case of China. *Renew. Sustain. Energ. Rev.* **2016**, *62*, 758–766. [CrossRef]
37. Zhao, X.; Liu, C.; Yang, M. The effects of environmental regulation on China's total factor productivity: An empirical study of carbon-intensive industries. *J. Clean Prod.* **2018**, *179*, 325–334. [CrossRef]
38. Qiu, S.; Wang, Z.; Geng, S. How do environmental regulation and foreign investment behavior affect green productivity growth in the industrial sector? An empirical test based on Chinese provincial panel data. *J. Environ. Manage.* **2021**, *287*, 112282. [CrossRef] [PubMed]
39. Shen, L.; Fan, R.; Wang, Y.; Yu, Z.; Tang, R. Impacts of environmental regulation on the green transformation and upgrading of manufacturing enterprises. *Int. J. Environ. Res. Public Health* **2020**, *17*, 7680. [CrossRef] [PubMed]
40. Boerner, K.; Hainz, C. The political economy of corruption and the role of economic opportunities. *Econ. Transit.* **2009**, *17*, 213–240. [CrossRef]

41. Chen, M.; Guariglia, A. Internal financial constraints and firm productivity in China: Do liquidity and export behavior make a difference? *J. Comp. Econ.* **2013**, *41*, 1123–1140. [CrossRef]
42. Sorrell, S. Energy substitution, technical change and rebound effects. *Energies* **2014**, *7*, 2850–2873. [CrossRef]
43. Cohen, W.M.; Levinthal, D.A. Innovation and learning: The two faces of R&D. *Econ. J.* **1989**, *99*, 569–596.
44. Chen, K.; Wemy, E. Investment-specific technological changes: The source of long-run TFP fluctuations. *Eur. Econ. Rev.* **2015**, *80*, 230–252. [CrossRef]
45. Audretsch, D.B.; Belitski, M. The role of R&D and knowledge spillovers in innovation and productivity. *Eur. Econ. Rev.* **2020**, *123*, 103391.
46. Zhang, D.; Vigne, S.A. How does innovation efficiency contribute to green productivity? A financial constraint perspective. *J. Clean Prod.* **2021**, *280*, 124000. [CrossRef]
47. Li, X.; Long, H. Research Focus, Frontier and knowledge base of green technology in China: Metrological research based on mapping knowledge domains. *Pol. J. Environ. Stud.* **2020**, *29*, 3003–3011. [CrossRef]
48. Shao, S.; Luan, R.; Yang, Z.; Li, C. Does directed technological change get greener: Empirical evidence from Shanghai's industrial green development transformation. *Ecol. Indic.* **2016**, *69*, 758–770. [CrossRef]
49. Song, M.; Du, J.; Tan, K.H. Impact of fiscal decentralization on green total factor productivity. *Int. J. Prod. Econ.* **2018**, *205*, 359–367. [CrossRef]
50. Lv, C.; Shao, C.; Lee, C. Green technology innovation and financial development: Do environmental regulation and innovation output matter? *Energy Econ.* **2021**, *98*, 105237. [CrossRef]
51. Xie, R.; Yuan, Y.; Huang, J. Different types of environmental regulations and heterogeneous influence on green productivity: Evidence from China. *Ecol. Econ.* **2017**, *132*, 104–112. [CrossRef]
52. Tang, H.; Liu, J.; Wu, J. The impact of command-and-control environmental regulation on enterprise total factor productivity: A quasi-natural experiment based on China's Two Control Zone policy. *J. Clean Prod.* **2020**, *254*, 120011. [CrossRef]
53. Lamine, W.; Mian, S.; Fayolle, A.; Wright, M.; Klofsten, M.; Etzkowitz, H. Technology business incubation mechanisms and sustainable regional development. *J. Technol. Transf.* **2018**, *43*, 1121–1141. [CrossRef]
54. Li, X.; Liu, J.; Huo, X. Impacts of tenure security and market-oriented allocation of farmland on agricultural productivity: Evidence from China's apple growers. *Land Use Pol.* **2021**, *102*, 105233. [CrossRef]
55. Ettlie, J.E.; Bridges, W.P.; O'keefe, R.D. Organization strategy and structural differences for radical versus incremental innovation. *Manag. Sci.* **1984**, *30*, 682–695. [CrossRef]
56. Ritala, P.; Hurmelinna-Laukkanen, P. Incremental and radical innovation in coopetition: The role of absorptive capacity and appropriability. *J. Prod. Innov. Manag.* **2013**, *30*, 154–169. [CrossRef]
57. Wang, Y.; Hu, H.; Dai, W.; Burns, K. Evaluation of industrial green development and industrial green competitiveness: Evidence from Chinese urban agglomerations. *Ecol. Indic.* **2021**, *124*, 107371. [CrossRef]
58. Forés, B.; Camisón, C. Does incremental and radical innovation performance depend on different types of knowledge accumulation capabilities and organizational size? *J. Bus. Res.* **2016**, *69*, 831–848. [CrossRef]
59. Drucker, J.; Feser, E. Regional industrial structure and agglomeration economies: An analysis of productivity in three manufacturing industries. *Reg. Sci. Urban. Econ.* **2012**, *42*, 1–14. [CrossRef]
60. Chung, Y.H.; Färe, R.; Grosskopf, S. Productivity and undesirable outputs: A directional distance function approach. *J. Environ. Manag.* **1997**, *51*, 229–240. [CrossRef]
61. Oh, D. A global Malmquist-Luenberger productivity index. *J. Prod. Anal.* **2010**, *34*, 183–197. [CrossRef]
62. Domazlicky, B.R.; Weber, W.L. Does environmental protection lead to slower productivity growth in the chemical industry? *Environ. Resour. Econ.* **2004**, *28*, 301–324. [CrossRef]
63. Cai, X.; Lu, Y.; Wu, M.; Yu, L. Does environmental regulation drive away inbound foreign direct investment? Evidence from a quasi-natural experiment in China. *J. Dev. Econ.* **2016**, *123*, 73–85. [CrossRef]
64. Dong, Z.; He, Y.; Wang, H.; Wang, L. Is there a ripple effect in environmental regulation in China? Evidence from the local neighborhood green technology innovation perspective. *Ecol. Indic.* **2020**, *118*, 106773. [CrossRef]
65. Guo, R.; Yuan, Y. Different types of environmental regulations and heterogeneous influence on energy efficiency in the industrial sector: Evidence from Chinese provincial data. *Energy Policy* **2020**, *145*, 111747. [CrossRef]
66. Fang, C.; Cheng, J.; Zhu, Y.; Chen, J.; Peng, X. Green total factor productivity of extractive industries in China: An explanation from technology heterogeneity. *Resour. Policy* **2021**, *70*, 101933. [CrossRef]

International Journal of
Environmental Research and Public Health

MDPI

Article

The Impact of Grounding in Running Shoes on Indices of Performance in Elite Competitive Athletes

Borja Muniz-Pardos [1,2,3], Irina Zelenkova [2,3], Alex Gonzalez-Aguero [1,2,3], Melanie Knopp [4], Toni Boitz [4], Martin Graham [4], Daniel Ruiz [4], Jose A. Casajus [2,3,5] and Yannis P. Pitsiladis [3,6,7,8,*]

1 Faculty of Health and Sports Science (FCSD), Department of Physiatry and Nursing, University of Zaragoza, 50009 Zaragoza, Spain; bmuniz@unizar.es (B.M.-P.); alexgonz@unizar.es (A.G.-A.)
2 GENUD (Growth, Exercise, Nutrition and Development) Research Group, Department of Physiatry and Nursing, University of Zaragoza, 50009 Zaragoza, Spain; iz@i1.ru (I.Z.); joseant@unizar.es (J.A.C.)
3 International Federation of Sports Medicine (FIMS), 1007 Lausanne, Switzerland
4 adidas Innovation, adidas AG, 91074 Herzogenaurach, Germany; Melanie.Knopp@adidas.com (M.K.); Toni.Boitz@adidas.com (T.B.); martin.william.graham@adidas.com (M.G.); daniel.ruiz@adidas.com (D.R.)
5 Faculty of Medicine, Department of Physiatry and Nursing, University of Zaragoza, 50009 Zaragoza, Spain
6 School of Sport and Health Sciences, University of Brighton, Eastbourne BN20 7SN, UK
7 Centre for Exercise Sciences and Sports Medicine, FIMS Collaborating Centre of Sports Medicine, University of Rome "Foro Italico", 00135 Rome, Italy
8 European Federation of Sports Medicine Associations (EFSMA), 1007 Lausanne, Switzerland
* Correspondence: y.pitsiladis@brighton.ac.uk

Citation: Muniz-Pardos, B.; Zelenkova, I.; Gonzalez-Aguero, A.; Knopp, M.; Boitz, T.; Graham, M.; Ruiz, D.; Casajus, J.A.; Pitsiladis, Y.P. The Impact of Grounding in Running Shoes on Indices of Performance in Elite Competitive Athletes. *Int. J. Environ. Res. Public Health* **2022**, *19*, 1317. https://doi.org/10.3390/ijerph19031317

Academic Editors: Roberto Alonso González Lezcano, Francesco Nocera and Rosa Giuseppina Caponetto

Received: 24 November 2021
Accepted: 23 January 2022
Published: 25 January 2022

Abstract: The introduction of carbon fiber plate shoes has triggered a plethora of world records in running, which has encouraged shoe industries to produce novel shoe designs to enhance running performance, including shoes containing conductor elements or "grounding shoes" (GS), which could potentially reduce the energy cost of running. The aim of this study was to examine the physiological and perceptual responses of athletes subjected to grounding shoes during running. Ten elite runners were recruited. Firstly, the athletes performed an incremental running test for VO_2max and anaerobic threshold (AT) determination, and were familiarized with the two shoe conditions (traditional training shoe (TTS) and GS, the latter containing a conductor element under the insole). One week apart, athletes performed running economy tests (20 min run at 80% of the AT) on a 400 m dirt track, with shoe conditions randomized. VO_2, heart rate, lactate, and perceived fatigue were registered throughout the experiment. No differences in any of the physiological or perceptual variables were identified between shoe conditions, with an equal running economy in both TTS and GS (51.1 ± 4.2 vs. 50.9 ± 5.1 mL kg^{-1} min^{-1}, respectively). Our results suggest that a grounding stimulus does not improve the energy cost of running, or the physiological/perceptual responses of elite athletes.

Keywords: earthing; environmental physiology; running performance; running economy; shoe technology; grounding

1. Introduction

During the past five years, shoe designs have experienced a great technological revolution, which has been accompanied by a plethora of world records in all long-distance running events (i.e., from 5000 m to marathons, in both male and female athletes). Joyner et al., recently suggested that the factors potentially explaining the recent records in long-distance running are the physiological and training factors, in addition to shoe technology and drafting [1]. However, the abrupt drop in world records across all distances since 2017 suggests that shoe technology has a major contribution when compared to the other factors (i.e., training methods, the physiology of athletes, and drafting are factors that have not substantially changed in the last 5 years) [2].

The most popular shoe technology for road running includes a carbon fiber plate (CFP) within the sole, a light and highly reactive foam, and a stack up to 40 mm in thickness. This technology has been shown to reduce the energy cost of running during a fixed exercise intensity (traditionally between 14 and 18 km h^{-1}) by approximately 4%, when compared to non-CFP shoes [3–5]. This improved running economy (RE) seems to be elicited by an increase in energy return caused by the action of passive elastic recoil, which in turn increases stride length and contact times, reduces step frequencies, and slightly increases the peak forces upon ground contact, when compared to non-CFP shoes [3,6,7].

The great popularity and effectiveness of CFP shoes has encouraged the shoe industry to explore new forms of shoe designs to optimize both health and performance during running. The implementation of "grounding" in humans purports to take advantage of the prolonged contact between an individual and the ground, and the potential transmission of energy between the two. Previous research states that the "direct contact of humans with the earth or using a metal conductor changes the electric potential on the surface of the body, as well as within the entire human organism" [8]. While the etiology of this potential effect is difficult to explain from a biophysiological perspective, previous findings have shown that the direct contact of an individual with the ground may reduce inflammatory processes, mood, pain, and stress at rest [9–11] and during exercise [8,9], with some studies suggesting that grounding technology may have a medical application. For example, previous research has suggested that the implementation of grounding is beneficial for mood, and may be especially beneficial in cases of depression, anxiety, stress, and trauma [11,12].

In relation to the existing research on grounding and exercise, an informative pilot study examined the effects of grounding on muscle physiology in response to exercise-induced muscle damage, and observed faster muscle recovery times under the grounding condition compared to the placebo [13]. The same group performed a more comprehensive follow-up study [14], observing that grounding significantly reduced creatine kinase (CK) levels 24 h post-exercise when compared to the placebo, suggesting that grounding may reduce acute muscular damage post-exercise. Following these early studies on grounding and muscle damage, a further study focused on the impact that this technology may have during aerobic exercise [8]. Sokal et al. claimed that the indirect contact of cyclists with the ground (through a metal conductor) while exercising elicited an increase in the electrical potential of the body when compared to those in the control group (not grounded). This study further reported that the observed increase in electrical potential with was accompanied by a greater decrease in blood urea concentrations during and after a 30 min cycling test at 50% of VO_2max, indicating, according to the authors, a decreased physiological stress [8]. While these previous studies showed a benefit of grounding on the muscle recovery and physiological stress of healthy subjects in response to different modes of exercise (i.e., resistance training and cycling), the impact of this technology while running is unknown.

Given the imminent introduction of grounding technology in running shoes, and the absence of rigorous scientific evidence of its effects, adding conductor elements within the shoe and employing a well-controlled experimental design, would allow for the assessment of any putative effects of this technology (i.e., grounding technology in running shoes) during running. This is especially important given the recent controversy that novel shoe technologies are negatively impacting the integrity and fairness within sport [2,15]. A recent critical review [2] highlighted how novel shoe designs are revolutionizing the world of sport, as numerous National, European, World, and Olympic records have been broken over an extraordinarily short time period (i.e., since the introduction of CFP shoes). In addition to this controversy, there is a lack of well-controlled and rigorous studies in the field that focus on the impact of shoe designs on running performance [2], which makes the true performance benefits of certain shoe technologies difficult to determine.

Considering the reduced physiological stress and muscle damage witnessed in subjects while performing other physical activities (i.e., strength exercises and cycling), it is important to examine the impact of grounding on the physiological and perceptual responses to running, especially considering the interest of shoe companies in incorporating grounding technology into running shoes, and the potential fairness/integrity issues that may result if a performance benefit is demonstrated. Therefore, the main aim of the present study was to compare the RE and physiological stress of well-trained runners while running in either grounding shoes (GS) or traditional training shoes (TTS).

2. Materials and Methods

2.1. Participants

Ten highly-trained male runners (age = 27 ± 7 years; weight = 64.6 ± 6 kg; height = 176.3 ± 5.4 cm) were recruited for the present study. Upon recruitment, all subjects received and signed an informed consent form in order to participate in the study. Subjects were required to meet the following inclusion criteria: (1) to train a minimum of 50 km week^{-1}, (2) to have a personal best under 35:00 min:s in 10 km or 17:30 min:s in 5 km, (3) to be healthy and without any musculoskeletal injury.

2.2. Procedures

The present study design required runners to visit either the laboratory or the track on two occasions, both separated by a period of 7 days to avoid any residual fatigue. Visit 1 included a VO_2max test, ventilatory threshold determination, and shoe familiarization in the laboratory; Visit 2 included 20 min RE tests at 80% of the anaerobic threshold, on a 400 m dirt track, with the order of the two shoe conditions randomized (Figure 1). A dirt track was selected over a traditional synthetic PU rubber track to avoid any material interference between the ground and the athlete. The present study was approved by the Ethics Committee of Aragon (CEICA, num. 17/2021).

2.3. Shoe Conditions

Two shoe conditions were tested: the traditional training shoe (TTS) and the grounding shoe (GS), with these being visually identical as shown in Figure 1. Shoes with grounding potential contained a conductor element around the insole, and aimed to diminish the physiological stress experienced by the athlete during running as they run in closer contact with the ground. The insulation and thermal permeability of the shoes were considered similar, given that the same material was used for both experimental and non-experimental shoes, with the exception of the conductor element. Both uppers consisted of the same knitted textile, produced and supplied at the same time for both types of shoe (Figure 1). The GS upper included a textile webbing containing yarn that encouraged electrical charge to flow through the material. The material was stitched into the collar area, and ran through the midsole to connect with the rubber on the outsole that contacts the ground. The TTS outsole included conventional rubber, while the GS outsole included rubber that encouraged the flow of electrical charge. The manufacturers labelled the shoes with a number in red or blue according to the two shoe conditions, and this setting was used by the research team to keep the study design double-blinded (See Figure 1). Additionally, as each athlete may have become subjectively biased during the familiarization trial, all blue/red labels were obscured with tape in Visit 2. All athletes had their own pair of shoes for each shoe condition.

2.4. Visit 1. Maximal Oxygen Uptake and Ventilatory Threshold Determination

On the first day, athletes were subjected to a skin temperature test and a SARS-CoV-2 antigen test, in order to participate in this study. Upon testing negative, informed consent was signed by all participants, and medical history and pre-participation screening was also completed. The laboratory assessments performed during the first day included:

Anthropometric and body composition assessments. The parameters measured were as follows: weight, height, height from sitting position, foot length, calf circumference and fold, and thigh circumference and fold. Percent body fat, muscle mass, and bone mass were assessed with a DXA scan (Hologic Corp., Bedford, MA, USA). Body fat, body water, and muscle mass were also assessed via bioimpedance (TANITA BC 780-S MA, Tanita Corp., Tokyo, Japan).

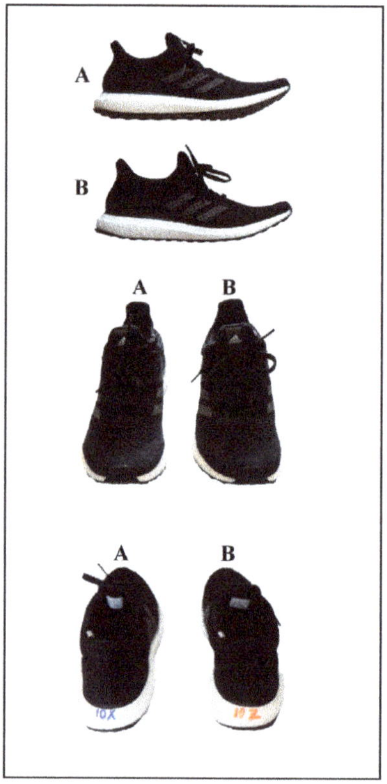

Figure 1. Image of the right grounding shoe (**A**) and traditional training shoe (**B**) for one of the elite athletes.

Maximal aerobic capacity test. All subjects were previously familiarized with VO_2max testing. Prior to the VO_2max test, subjects laid down for 5 min, and resting electrocardiograms and blood pressure tests were performed and assessed by experienced medical doctors to ensure athletes did not have any cardiological issues. Participants breathed through a low dead space mask, with air sampled at 60 mL min^{-1}. Before each test, two-point calibrations of the gas sensors were completed, using a known gas mixture (16% O_2 and 5% CO_2) and ambient air. Ventilatory volume was calibrated using a 3 L (±0.4%) syringe. Firstly, subjects performed a self-paced warm-up, and prior to the commencement of the test, subjects were instrumented with a portable metabolic analyzer (Cosmed K5, Cosmed Srl, Rome, Italy) and a heart rate device (Polar H10, Polar Electro, Kempele, Finland). A short-ramp incremental protocol was used (i.e., 13–16 min) as this has been shown to be the most appropriate assessment for identifying individual physiological events in well-trained runners [16–18]. The protocol consisted of a 3 min run at 10 km h^{-1} and a 1% gradient on a treadmill (h/p/cosmos, Nussdorf—Traunstein, Germany), followed by increases of 1 km h^{-1} min^{-1} until volitional exhaustion. Heart rate was monitored throughout the test, and overall perception of effort (RPE) and specific RPE for the legs were registered immediately after the test. This test enabled the determination of VO_2max (defined as the highest 30 s mean values obtained during the test) and individual anaerobic threshold (IAT), determined through visual assessment conducted by two experienced exercise physiologists. Each individual speed for subsequent shoe trials were determined at the 80% of the IAT velocity. This VO_2max test involved the subjects' preferred shoe, and served to objectively quantify individual running speed for subsequent RE trials (avoiding the impact of the slow component of oxygen uptake given the repeated square-wave design of the RE tests on the second visit). Visit 1 also involved the familiarization of the different running shoes during a light, 5 min run with each pair of shoes, in preparation for Visit 2.

2.5. Visit 2. Running Economy Tests

During the second visit, indices of performance, with particular focus on RE, were assessed for each shoe condition, determined on a 400 m dirt track. Air temperature and humidity were recorded at the beginning and end of the experimental sessions using a portable meteorological station, and all trials were performed either in the early morning or late evening to avoid extreme environmental conditions. Participants breathed through a low dead space mask, with air sampled at 60 mL min^{-1}. Before each subject's first trial, the portable metabolic analyzer was calibrated following the calibration procedures aforementioned. The shoe conditions were randomly assigned, and both runners and assessors were blinded to the shoe condition. Brand new socks were used for each RE trial to avoid excessive humidity within the shoe, as this could impact grounding effect. Body mass was measured before and after each test. Each runner warmed up for 15 min with their preferred training shoes prior to being equipped with the portable metabolic analyzer. Pre-trial blood lactate was measured from a single drop of whole blood from the fingertip using a lactate meter (Lactate Pro 2, Arkray Europe, B.V., Amstelveen, the Netherlands), and pre-trial heart rate and RPE were also collected. Athletes performed two 20 min exercise bouts at 80% of their IAT velocity for each shoe condition, with a 20 min rest in between (Figure 2). The duration of this RE protocol was longer than traditional RE tests (4–6 min) used in previous studies examining shoe designs [3–5]. The reason for this was to allow for a longer contact time between the athlete and the earth, which is crucial for obtaining a dose–response relationship. Lactate, whole-body RPE, and legs-only RPE (1–10 scale) were recorded at min 1, 3, and 15 of recovery following both trials, and heart rate and ventilatory parameters were monitored throughout the test. A researcher (and experienced cyclist) paced all runners at their individual speed using a bicycle. The RE elicited by each shoe condition was determined as the mean VO_2 between min 10 to min 15, as steady state was ensured during this period. To reduce the noise in the ventilatory measurements, a 7-breath averaging method was performed.

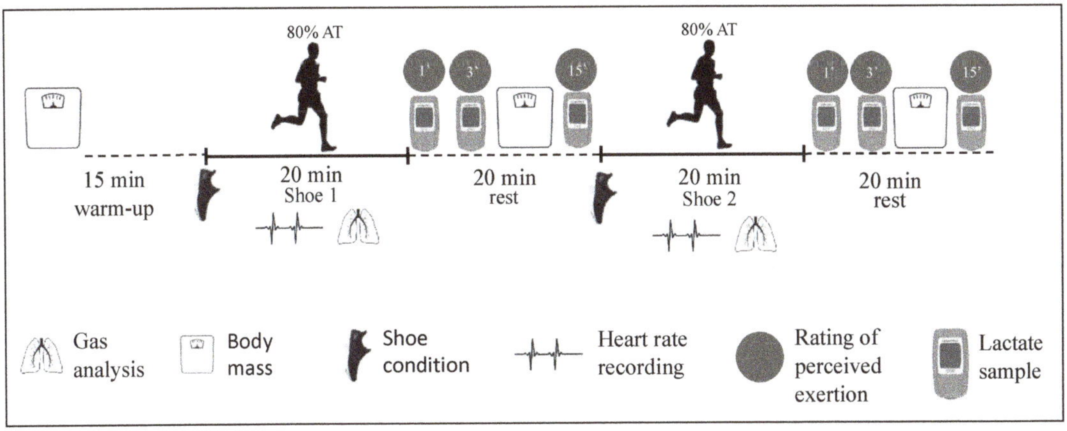

Figure 2. Protocol for the running economy trials at 80% of the anaerobic threshold (AT).

2.6. Statistical Analysis

Means and standard deviations (mean ± SD) were calculated for all variables. An a priori sample size calculation (G*Power software, version 3.1.9.3, Heinrich-Heine-Universität Düsseldorf, Düsseldorf, Germany) was performed using the running economy data reported in a previous study testing different shoe designs in well-trained athletes (Barnes et al., 2018). The VO_2 data for both the control and grounded shoe (53.61 ± 2.20 vs. 51.26 ± 2.23 mL kg^{-1} min^{-1}, respectively) were used to generate a correlation coefficient of 0.45 and a Cohen's d of 1.01. A two-tailed t-test revealed that a total sample size of 10 subjects was required to obtain statistical power of 0.80 and an alpha of 0.05. A Shapiro–Wilk test revealed normal data distributions across all studied variables. Student's t-tests for paired samples were applied between TTS and GS shoe conditions in order to examine the differences between metabolic and RE data (HR, VO_2, RER). Significant values were set at $p \leq 0.05$ and effect sizes (Cohen's d) were also calculated. The Statistical Package for the Social Sciences (SPSS) version 23.0 (SPSS Inc., Chicago, IL, USA) was used to perform the statistical analyses.

3. Results

A final sample of 10 athletes completed the present study, with no drop-outs. These athletes were national to international level runners/triathletes, with two of them having participated in major sporting events (Olympic Games and World Championships). Table 1 presents the mean and individual descriptive characteristics of the sample, showing a fairly homogeneous fitness level across all runners (i.e., mean VO_2max of 78.4 ± 3.8 mL kg^{-1} min^{-1}).

Table 1. Descriptive characteristics of the participants.

ID	Age (years)	Weight (kg)	Height (cm)	BMI ($kg\ m^{-2}$)	Bioimpedance (Fat %)	VO_2max ($mL\ kg^{-1}\ min^{-1}$)
Athlete 1	31.0	78.5	180.3	24.1	12.7	76.0
Athlete 2	25.7	65.7	177.8	20.8	5.5	82.3
Athlete 3	35.0	64	174.3	21.1	10.4	80.3
Athlete 4	20.8	68.9	186.3	19.9	11.8	83.6
Athlete 5	31.1	57.0	171.0	19.5	3.0	78.0
Athlete 6	26.2	59.3	170.2	20.5	11.2	77.8
Athlete 7	38.2	66.0	176.5	21.2	3.8	78.5
Athlete 8	25.0	72.5	177.7	23.0	7.0	77.3
Athlete 9	20.6	64.9	171.2	22.1	8.9	80.5
Athlete 10	18.1	64.0	183.0	19.1	8.5	69.9
Mean ± SD	27.2 ± 6.6	66.1 ± 6.2	176.8 ± 5.4	21.1 ± 1.6	8.3 ± 3.4	78.4 ± 3.8

A Student's t-test for paired samples revealed no significant difference in RE values between TTS and GS conditions (51.1 ± 4.2 vs. 50.9 ± 5.1 mL kg^{-1} min^{-1}, respectively, p = 0.779, Cohen's d = 0.092). Figure 3 shows both mean and individual values for VO_2. Additionally, blood lactate was not different between shoe conditions at min 1 (p = 0.793), min 3 (p = 0.250), and min 15 (p = 0.641) post-exercise (Figure 4). Both whole-body and legs-only RPE values were also not significantly different between TTS and GS at min 1 (p = 1.0 and p = 0.273, respectively), min 3 (p = 0.443 and p = 0.591, respectively), and min 15 (p = 0.168 and p = 0.591, respectively) post-exercise (Figure 4). Finally, HR values were not significantly different between TTS and GS during exercise (150.1 ± 15 vs. 151.0 ± 16 bpm, respectively, p = 0.461, Cohen's d = 0.244; Figure 4).

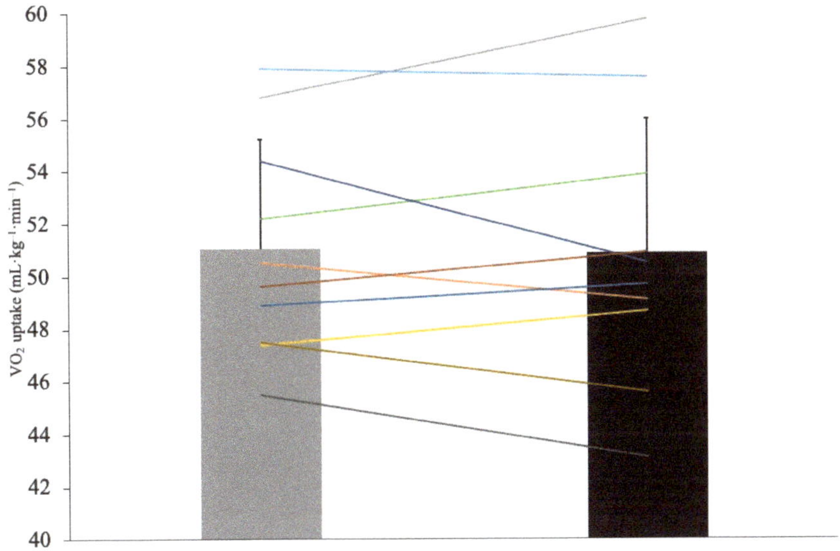

Figure 3. Mean and individual running economy values (mL kg^{-1} min^{-1}) of the 10 athletes running in traditional training shoes (grey column) and in grounding shoes (black column).

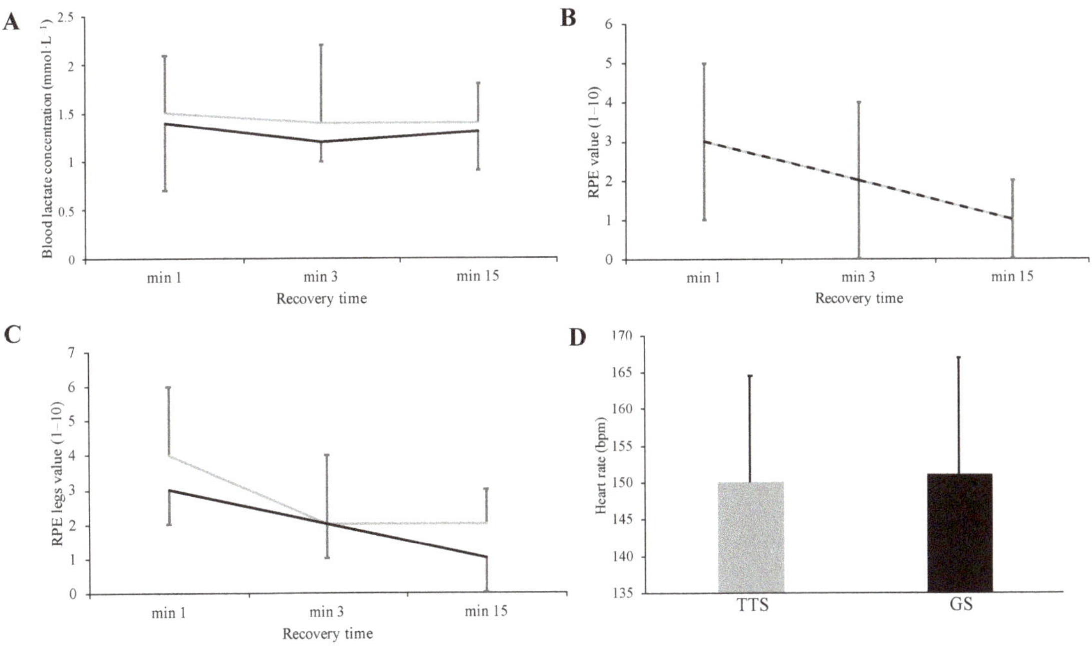

Figure 4. Blood lactate (**A**), whole-body rate of perceived exertion (RPE; **B**), and legs-only RPE (**C**) during the recovery period after running in the traditional training shoe (TTS, gray solid line) or grounding shoe (GS, black solid line). Heart rate during the running economy trial in both TTS and GS trials (**D**). Dashed lines represent overlapping mean values between shoes.

4. Discussion

The main findings of the present study show that grounding technology applied to shoe designs does not provide a physiological/perceptual response over traditional training shoes in well-trained athletes. The RE, blood lactate, heart rate, and perceptual response of these athletes, exercising at 80% of their IAT during 20 min on a 400 m dirt track, were not different between shoes conditions.

Despite previous promising findings suggesting that grounding technology has positive effects on the physiological responses (i.e., reduced acute inflammatory processes) of humans at rest [7,8], very limited research has focused on the implementation of grounding during exercise, with only two studies focusing on the effectiveness of grounding in reducing muscular damage after exercise-induced DOMS. This is the first study to examine the impact of grounding in shoes during running, which makes the comparison with previous studies challenging due to the unique nature of running for the implementation of this technology (i.e., intermittent contact time with the ground). Our findings, however, differ from those of Sokal et al. [8], who claimed that all recreational cyclists within their study experienced physiological attenuation at rest, during a 30 min exercise at 50% of their VO_2max, and during recovery, indicated by decreases in blood urea; however, these authors failed to include any individual data. It is also worth noting that these biochemical parameters were not measured immediately prior to grounding/placebo conditions, and therefore group-by-time interactions could not be determined, which limits the interpretation of these results. Additionally, one would expect both blood urea and creatinine concentrations to remain unchanged following the exercise protocol used by these authors (a single bout of light exercise for 30 min). Blood urea and creatinine levels have been shown to increase after prolonged, strenuous exercise as a result of increased protein catabolism and/or impaired renal function [19], which is unlikely to have occurred during the exercise protocol proposed by Sokal et al. The difference between the groups observed by Sokal et al., interpreted in the context of our present findings, are more likely due to day-to-day inter-individual variability in blood urea, or some potential methodological issues during data collection, rather than due to physiological stress attenuation during exercise. In a subsequent study, Sokal et al. presented additional data from the same aforementioned experiment [20], focusing on the effects of grounding on VO_2 uptake, blood glucose, lactate, and bilirubin concentrations. The 42 subjects included in this study were divided into two subgroups ($n = 21$) according to their VO_2max, therefore, both groups had a comparable cardiorespiratory fitness (Group A = 50.8 vs. Group B = 50.7 mL kg^{-1} min^{-1}). The study design followed a double-blind, crossover protocol between Groups A and B. During the first testing day, Group A was under the placebo condition and Group B was under the grounding stimulus, with these conditions interchanged during the second day of testing. These authors reported a significantly reduced VO_2 uptake (numeric data not shown by the authors) at the end of the exercise with the grounding stimulus only in Group B, when compared to the placebo. The study design employed by Sokal et al. [8,20] has limited reliability, given that their experimental tests were performed on different days, which may have biased the results. Day-to-day variability and the lack of a familiarization trial may have potentiated the learning effects only for Group B (i.e., the group with the grounding stimulus during the second day). These results should, therefore, be interpreted with caution.

To our knowledge, the two aforementioned studies are the only two experiments focusing on the effects of grounding on the biophysiological responses of humans during submaximal exercise. However, the important methodological issues described above, and the use of cycling being the only mode of exercise, limits the interpretation of the current literature and its comparison with the present study. In our experiment, we used a double-blind, randomized, crossover design, with tests for all experimental conditions performed on the same day. We are aware that the conductor element within the shoe was not in permanent contact with the ground (i.e., intermittent contact time during running), and we did not measure muscle activity, nor foot/stride mechanics, during running, which may have provided more information and potentially revealed an effect. However, to ensure a sufficient contact time, we designed a longer than usual RE protocol (i.e., 20 min bouts; Figure 2), so that we could identify a potential dose–response relationship over time. Despite these rigorous experimental procedures, our results show that grounding technology did not have any impact on the measured responses during running when compared to traditional training shoes. Previous research showed a decrease in muscle damage in response to high-intensity strength exercises in subjects under grounding conditions [13,14] when compared to a placebo. These findings would suggest that grounding technology may have a role to play as a muscle recovery method, which in turn could translate into a benefit for runners when performing higher intensity exercise (i.e., above the anaerobic threshold) in which muscle fatigue and acidosis occur to a greater extent. Nonetheless, future research using larger sample sizes and examining foot mechanics (especially contact times) would be required to confirm our findings. Other shoe designs currently available on the market that include a CFP and a high midsole stack height made of compliant, resilient, and lightweight foam, seem the most effective shoe modality to date. This technology has shown to improve RE by increasing the midsole longitudinal bending stiffness, favoring a decrease in the range of motion of the metatarsophalangeal joint [3,21,22].

5. Conclusions

In conclusion, our results suggest that grounding in shoe designs is not an effective alternative for well-trained athletes to improve their running efficiencies, and/or their physiological/perceptual responses during submaximal exercise. However, there are intrinsic limitations that should be considered. Potential grounding effects could have been missed during our study as running does not allow constant contact between the athlete and the ground, which could have potentially biased the results. In relation to this, lower caliber athletes may have benefited from this technology given their ground contact times are greater than faster, elite athletes; an issue that could not be addressed in the current study. Future research may therefore consider additional sports in which athletes remain in constant contact with the ground (e.g., race-walking, cross-country skiing, powerlifting). Despite these limitations, our study followed a high-quality methodological protocol (double-blind, randomized, crossover design) using a homogeneous sample of highly trained athletes (as represented in Table 1), which suggests that our conclusions are reliable for this specific population.

Author Contributions: Conceptualization and methodology: B.M.-P., I.Z., M.K., D.R., J.A.C. and Y.P.P.; formal analysis: A.G.-A., J.A.C., I.Z., B.M.-P.; writing—original draft preparation: B.M.-P., I.Z., A.G.-A.; review and editing: B.M.-P., I.Z., A.G.-A., M.K., T.B., M.G., D.R., J.A.C. and Y.P.P.; supervision: Y.P.P. and J.A.C. All authors have read and agreed to the published version of the manuscript.

Funding: This study was supported by a contract from adidas AG with the University of Zaragoza, Spain (Project: "Testing support for innovation project"; number 2021/0348).

Institutional Review Board Statement: The present study was approved by the Ethics Committee of Aragon, Spain (CEICA, num. 17/2021).

Informed Consent Statement: Informed consent was obtained from all subjects involved in the study.

Data Availability Statement: The datasets used and analyzed within the present manuscript will be available from the corresponding author/first author upon request.

Acknowledgments: We wish to thank the athletes involved in this study for participating.

Conflicts of Interest: M.K., T.B., M.G., D.R. are employees of adidas AG. B.M.P., I.Z., A.G.A., J.A.C., Y.P.P. have no conflicts of interest relevant to the content of this article.

References

1. Joyner, M.J.; Hunter, S.K.; Lucia, A.; Jones, A.M. Physiology and fast marathons. *J. Appl. Physiol.* **2020**, *128*, 1065–1068. [CrossRef] [PubMed]
2. Muniz-Pardos, B.; Sutehall, S.; Angeloudis, K. Recent Improvements in Marathon Run Times Are Likely Technological, Not Physiological. *Sports Med.* **2021**, *51*, 371–378. [CrossRef] [PubMed]

3. Hoogkamer, W.; Kipp, S.; Frank, J.H.; Farina, E.M.; Luo, G.; Kram, R. A comparison of the energetic cost of running in marathon racing shoes. *Sports Med.* **2018**, *48*, 1009–1019. [CrossRef]
4. Barnes, K.R.; Kilding, A.E. A Randomized Crossover Study Investigating the Running Economy of Highly-Trained Male and Female Distance Runners in Marathon Racing Shoes versus Track Spikes. *Sports Med.* **2019**, *49*, 331–342. [CrossRef] [PubMed]
5. Hunter, I.; McLeod, A.; Valentine, D.; Low, T.; Ward, J.; Hager, R. Running economy, mechanics, and marathon racing shoes. *J. Sport Sci.* **2019**, *37*, 2367–2373. [CrossRef] [PubMed]
6. Hoogkamer, W.; Kram, R.; Arellano, C.J. How biomechanical improvements in running economy could break the 2-hour marathon barrier. *Sports Med.* **2017**, *47*, 1739–1750. [CrossRef]
7. Rodrigo-Carranza, V.; González-Mohíno, F.; Santos-Concejero, J.; González-Ravé, J.M. The Effects of Footwear Midsole Longitudinal Bending Stiffness on Running Economy and Ground Contact Biomechanics: A Systematic Review and Meta-analysis. *Eur. J. Sport Sci.* **2021**, *1*, 26. [CrossRef]
8. Sokal, P.; Jastrzębski, Z.; Jaskulska, E.; Sokal, K.; Jastrzębska, M.; Radzimiński, Ł. Differences in blood urea and creatinine concentrations in earthed and unearthed subjects during cycling exercise and recovery. *Evid.-Based Complement Altern Med. Hindawi* **2013**, *2013*, 445. [CrossRef]
9. Menigoz, W.; Latz, T.T.; Ely, R.A.; Kamei, C.; Melvin, G.; Sinatra, D. Integrative and lifestyle medicine strategies should include Earthing (grounding): Review of research evidence and clinical observations. *Explore* **2020**, *11*, 152–160. [CrossRef]
10. Oschman, J.L.; Chevalier, G.; Brown, R. The effects of grounding (earthing) on inflammation, the immune response, wound healing, and prevention and treatment of chronic inflammatory and autoimmune diseases. *J. Inflamm. Res.* **2015**, *8*, 83. [CrossRef]
11. Chevalier, G. The effect of grounding the human body on mood. *Psychol. Reports* **2015**, *116*, 534–542. [CrossRef] [PubMed]
12. de Tord, P.; Bräuninger, I. Grounding: Theoretical application and practice in dance movement therapy. *Arts Psychother.* **2015**, *43*, 16–22. [CrossRef]
13. Brown, D.; Chevalier, G.; Hill, M. Pilot study on the effect of grounding on delayed-onset muscle soreness. *J. Altern. Complementary Med.* **2010**, *16*, 265–273. [CrossRef]
14. Brown, R.; Chevalier, G.; Hill, M. Grounding after moderate eccentric contractions reduces muscle damage. *Open Access J. Sports Med.* **2015**, *6*, 305. [PubMed]
15. Pitsiladis, Y.; Muniz-Pardos, B.; Miller, M.; Verroken, M. Sport integrity opportunities in the time of Coronavirus. *Sports Med.* **2020**, *50*, 1701–1702. [CrossRef]
16. Myers, J.; Bellin, D. Ramp exercise protocols for clinical and cardiopulmonary exercise testing. *Sport Med.* **2000**, *30*, 23–29. [CrossRef]
17. Myers, J.; Buchanan, N.; Walsh, D.; Kraemer, M.; McAuley, P.; Hamilton-Wessler, M. Comparison of the ramp versus standard exercise protocols. *J. Am. Coll. Cardiol.* **1991**, *17*, 1334–1342. [CrossRef]
18. Cerezuela-Espejo, V.; Courel-Ibañez, J.; Moran-Navarro, R.; Martınez-Cava, A.; Pallares, J.G. The relationship between lactate and ventilatory thresholds in runners: Validity and reliability of exercise test performance parameters. *Front. Physiol.* **2018**, *9*, 1320. [CrossRef]
19. Warburton, D.; Welsh, R.; Haykowsky, M.; Taylor, D.; Humen, D. Biochemical changes as a result of prolonged strenuous exercise. *Br. J. Sports Med.* **2002**, *36*, 301. [CrossRef]
20. Sokal, P.; Jastrzębski, Z.; Sokal, K.; Dargiewicz, R.; Jastrzębska, M.; Radzimiński, Ł. Earthing modulates glucose and erythrocytes metabolism in exercise. *Age* **2016**, *21*, 21.
21. Weyand, P.G. Now Afoot: Engineered Running Economy. *J. Appl. Physiol.* **2020**, *128*, 1083.
22. Stefanyshyn, D.J.; Nigg, B.M. Mechanical energy contribution of the metatarsophalangeal joint to running and sprinting. *J. Biomech.* **1997**, *30*, 1081–1085. [CrossRef]

International Journal of
Environmental Research and Public Health

MDPI

Article

Optimization of Ultrasonic-Assisted Extraction of Chlorogenic Acid from Tobacco Waste

Guoming Zeng [1,†], Yujie Ran [1,†], Xin Huang [1], Yan Li [2], Maolan Zhang [1,*], Hui Ding [1], Yonggang Ma [2], Hongshuo Ma [1], Libo Jin [3] and Da Sun [3,*]

1 Chongqing Engineering Laboratory of Nano/Micro Biological Medicine Detection Technology, School of Architecture and Engineering, Chongqing University of Science and Technology, Chongqing 401331, China; 2017015@cqust.edu.cn (G.Z.); glad1232022@163.com (Y.R.); 2019443106@cqust.edu.cn (X.H.); abc05062022@163.com (H.D.); hx17358367180@163.com (H.M.)

2 School of Pharmacy, Taizhou Polytechnic College, Taizhou 225300, China; 20066954@cqu.edu.cn (Y.L.); zml@cqu.edu.cn (Y.M.)

3 Biomedical Collaborative Innovation Center of Zhejiang Province, Institute of Life Sciences, Wenzhou University, Wenzhou 325035, China; 20160121@wzu.edu.cn

* Correspondence: 2019016@cqust.edu.cn (M.Z.); sunday@wzu.edu.cn (D.S.); Tel./Fax: +86-173-6586-6501 (D.S.)

† These two authors contributed equally to this work.

Abstract: Using tobacco waste as raw material, the ultrasonic-assisted extraction of chlorogenic acid was optimized by response surface methodology (RSM). After repeated freezing and thawing of tobacco waste twice, the effect of pH value, ethanol volume fraction, temperature and extraction time on the extraction rate of chlorogenic acid was investigated by a single factor experiment. On the basis of this, the factors affecting the yield of chlorogenic acid were further optimized by using RSM. The optimum extraction conditions for chlorogenic acid were set at pH = 4.1, ethanol volume fraction was 49.57% and extraction time was 2.06 h. Under the above conditions, the extraction rate of chlorogenic acid could reach 0.502%, which was higher than traditional extraction and unpretreated ultrasonic extraction. All these results can be used as a reference for the extraction of effective ingredients in tobacco waste.

Keywords: waste treatment; chlorogenic acid; optimal design; preprocessing; ultrasonic-assisted extraction

Citation: Zeng, G.; Ran, Y.; Huang, X.; Li, Y.; Zhang, M.; Ding, H.; Ma, Y.; Ma, H.; Jin, L.; Sun, D. Optimization of Ultrasonic-Assisted Extraction of Chlorogenic Acid from Tobacco Waste. *Int. J. Environ. Res. Public Health* **2022**, *19*, 1555. https://doi.org/10.3390/ijerph19031555

Academic Editor: Roberto Alonso González-Lezcano

Received: 28 December 2021
Accepted: 27 January 2022
Published: 29 January 2022

1. Introduction

China, as a major tobacco producer, accounts for about half of the world's tobacco production. For tobacco, most of it will be used to produce cigarettes, while about a quarter of the leftover material will be discarded and not reasonably utilized [1]. For this part of tobacco waste, if discarded casually, it may destroy the structure of the soil on the one hand; on the other hand, the harmful components in the tobacco waste will also infiltrate into the groundwater, thus further harming human life [2]. In view of this, if these tobacco wastes can be reasonably used as resources, not only can the above problems be solved, but also a large number of natural chemical raw materials can be obtained, and the income of tobacco farmers can also be increased. In addition to this, it is also in line with China's policy on the resourcefulness of solid waste.

Numerous studies have demonstrated that tobacco leaves contain a number of active substances, such as saccharides, organic acids, alkaloids and proteins [3–7]. However, there are few studies on the contents of these substances in waste materials, such as tobacco stems [8]. Among many bioactive substances, chlorogenic acid has been widely used in the fields of medicine, food and cosmetics because of its good antibacterial, anti-inflammatory, free radical scavenging and anti-cancer properties [9–11]. At present, the extraction of chlorogenic acid in the literature was mainly derived from Chinese herbal medicines, such as honeysuckle, *Eucommia ulmoides* leaves and so on [12–14]. Besides, most of them were extracted directly without any preprocessing. The extraction methods of chlorogenic acid mainly involve water extraction [12], alcohol extraction [14], ultrasonic extraction [15] and microwave extraction [16]. Among these methods, ultrasonic extraction of chlorogenic acid has the advantages of a fast mass transfer process and high extraction efficiency, which has attracted the attention of many researchers [17].

In order to further improve the resource utilization of tobacco waste and provide a reference for the extraction of chlorogenic acid from tobacco stems and other wastes. In the present study, chlorogenic acid was extracted from tobacco stems using double freeze-thaw method ultrasonic technology for the first time. The tobacco waste was first repeated freezing and thawing, and then the effect of ultrasonic time, temperature and ethanol content on the yield of chlorogenic acid was investigated using a single factor method. Finally, the response surface methodology (RSM) was used to find the optimal extraction process parameters.

2. Materials and Methods

2.1. Materials

The tobacco waste samples mainly consisting of tobacco stems were collected from a local cigarette factory in Chongqing, China, in September 2020. Chlorogenic acid standard was purchased from Aladdin Bio-Chem Technology, China. Anhydrous ethanol was purchased from the Chongqing Drug Stock Limited Company (Chongqing, China); the experimental water was double deionized water, and the resistance was 16 MΩ.

2.2. Experimental Methods

2.2.1. Standard Curve of Chlorogenic Acid

Accurately weighed 3.5 mg of chlorogenic acid standard in 25 mL brown volumetric flask, and then added 50% ethanol to the mark to prepare the standard solution. After that, chlorogenic acid solutions of 0.5 mL, 1.0 mL, 1.5 mL, 2.0 mL, 2.5 mL and 3.0 mL were transferred into 25 mL brown volumetric bottles and then the chlorogenic acid solutions of different concentrations were obtained by making volume with 50% ethanol. A 50% ethanol solution was also used as the blank control. The absorbance of chlorogenic acid solution with different concentrations was determined by an uv-vis spectrophotometer at 329 nm. The standard curve of $Y = 0.044X–0.013$, $R^2 = 0.9993$ was drawn with the concentration of chlorogenic acid standard as the X-coordinate and the absorbance as the Y-coordinate. This result indicated a linear relationship between the absorbance values and the concentration of chlorogenic acid in the 2.8 ug/mL to 16.8 ug/mL range.

2.2.2. Pretreatment of Tobacco Waste

Tobacco waste was first cleaned under running water and rinsed in deionized water after removing impurities. After that, it was placed in a 70–75 °C electric constant temperature blast drying oven for drying. The dried tobacco waste was crushed and sifted through a 40-mesh sieve, and then collected in a brown jar for further use. Tobacco waste powder (0.5 g) was weighed and then transferred into a 50 mL centrifuge tube. A certain volume of deionized water was added to make it completely cover the tobacco waste powder, sealed and then the chlorogenic acid was extracted by ultrasonic after two cycles of freezing. The first reaction was performed at 40 °C for 30 min, and then freeze-thawed at −20 °C; the second reaction was performed at 40 °C for 30 min, freeze-thawed at −20 °C, and then cooled at room temperature for use.

2.2.3. Extraction of Chlorogenic Acid from Tobacco Waste

The waste tobacco stem solution was dried after the above pretreatment, and then the anhydrous ethanol solution was added in accordance with the preset proportion to ultrasonic extract, centrifugation and collected the supernatant (the specific preparation process is depicted in Figure 1). The obtained supernatant was then diluted 20 times and the absorbance value at 329 nm was detected by UV spectrophotometer. The concentration of chlorogenic acid was calculated according to the standard curve and then substituted into the following equation to obtain the yield of chlorogenic acid.

$$\text{The yield of Chlorogenic acid} = \frac{C_{(\text{Chlorogenic acid})} \times \text{Dilution ratio} \times V_{(\text{Extraction Solution})}}{W_{(\text{Raw material})}} \times 100\%$$

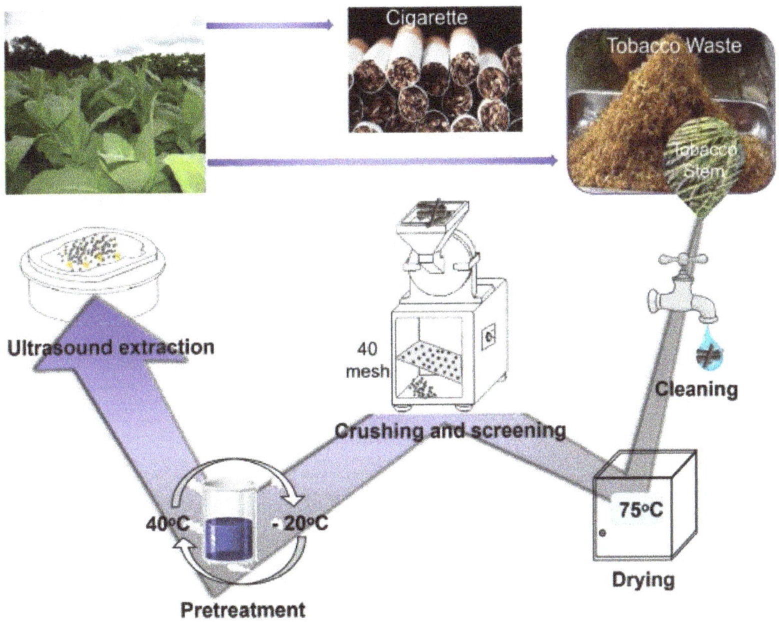

Figure 1. The flow chart of chlorogenic acid extraction from tobacco stem.

2.2.4. HPLC Analysis

Sample preparation and analysis: cut tobacco leaves, dry at 40 °C, pass through a sieve with a 1.0 mm aperture after crushing, and place them in a sample bottle for later use; accurately weigh 40.0 mg of tobacco powder and place it in two 10 mL plugs for quantitative determination. In the test tube, add 45% ethanol solution, ultrasonically extract at a certain temperature, centrifuge, dilute to 10 mL, filter with a 0.22 um filter, and inject and analyze according to the selected chromatographic conditions. Chromatographic conditions: Column: Econosphere C18 column (5 um, 4.6 mm × 250 mm), column temperature: 30, flow rate: 1 mL/min, mobile phase: methanol, water, acetic acid, gradient elution program: 0- Within 20 min, the volume ratio of methanol: water: acetic acid changed from 96:0:4 to 76:20:4; 20–30 min changed to 0:100:0. Detection wavelength: 340 nm, injection volume: 10 uL. Preparation of standard stock solution: Accurately weigh 10.0 mg of chlorogenic acid standard sample into a 10 mL volumetric flask, dissolve it with 45% ethanol solution to volume, use it as a stock solution, and store it at low temperature.

2.2.5. Analytical Method

The results were collated, counted and plotted using Origin 8.0. The data are expressed as the means ± SD (n = 3).

3. Results and Discussion

3.1. HPLC Experiment

Figure 2 is the standard curve of chlorogenic acid.Draw standard stock solution (5, 2, 0.5, and 0.3 mL) and dilute to 10 mL in turn, with concentrations of 5.2, 2.3, 0.8, and 0.04 mg/10 mL, respectively. Dilute the standard stock solution and the above-mentioned 4 concentrations after dilution. The gradient was injected and analyzed according to the selected chromatographic conditions. In the range of 0.04–10.0 mg/10 mL, linear regression was performed with the peak area ratio (Y) and the mass concentration ratio (X), and the linear regression equation Y = 178.15X −10. 12, correlation coefficient: = 0. 9997, based on the signal-to-noise ratio of 3, the minimum detection limit of chlorogenic acid is 0. 41 × 10^{-2} mg/10 mL.

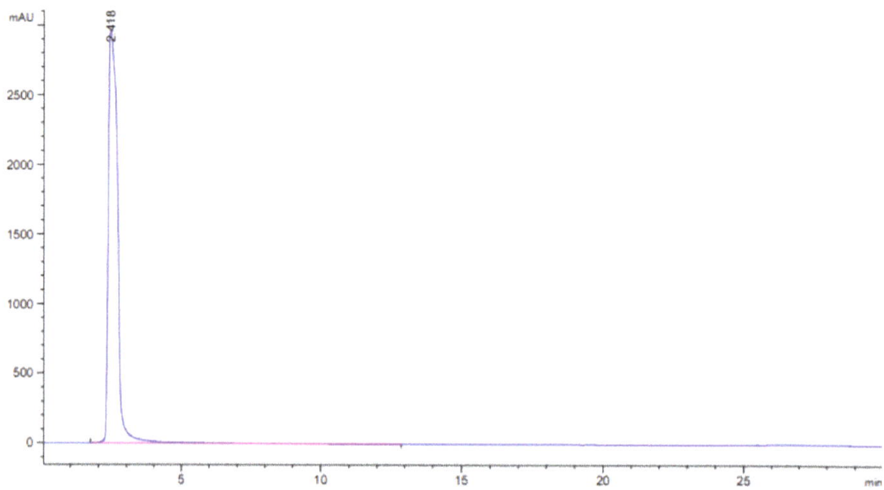

Figure 2. HPLC chromatogram of chlorogenic acid in tobacco.

3.2. Single Factor Experiment

After reviewing the literature on the extraction of chlorogenic acid from biomass by ultrasonic method, four aspects, namely the volume fraction of ethanol, ultrasonic extraction time, temperature and pH value of the extraction solution, were chosen to investigate the effect on the extraction rate of chlorogenic acid from tobacco waste in this experiment. Each group was repeated three times and the average values were taken for the graphs to obtain the optimum ultrasonic extraction conditions for chlorogenic acid in tobacco waste.

3.2.1. Effect of Ethanol Volume Fraction on the Yield of Chlorogenic Acid in Tobacco Waste

The effect of ethanol volume fractions of 40%, 50%, 60% and 70% on the extraction yield of chlorogenic acid was examined. The chlorogenic acid yield first increased and then decreased as the volume fraction of ethanol gradually increased, with a maximum at 50% of the volume fraction of ethanol in Figure 3. This was in accordance with the literature reported [18]. This may be because the molecular structure of chlorogenic acid contained a large number of hydroxyl groups, so an appropriate volume fraction of ethanol could promote the dissolution of chlorogenic acid in tobacco waste. However, when the volume fraction of ethanol was further increased, other fat-soluble substances may also be dissolved, thus interfering with the yield of chlorogenic acid. This may also be caused by the decrease in the diffusion capacity of solute as the volume fraction of ethanol increases [19].

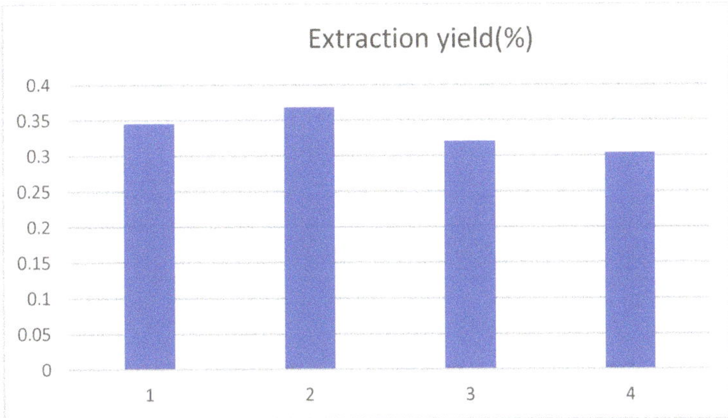

Figure 3. Influence of ethanol volume fraction on the extraction yield of chlorogenic acid, and 1, 2, 3, and 4 represent the ethanol volume fraction of 40%, 50%, 60% and 70%, respectively.

3.2.2. Influence of Ultrasonic Temperature on the Yield of Chlorogenic Acid in Tobacco Waste

The effect of ultrasonic extraction temperature of 50 °C, 60 °C, 70 °C and 80 °C on the extraction yield of chlorogenic acid was investigated, and the results are shown in Figure 4. With the ultrasonic extraction temperature increasing, the extraction yield for chlorogenic acid showed an evident rise first and then decreased, achieving a maximum at 70 °C. This result was slightly higher than the 57 °C reported in the literature [20], which may be caused by the rigorous structure of the tobacco stem compared with the tobacco leaf. The molecular motion speed and dissolution rate of chlorogenic acid will increase with the rising temperature. However, when the ultrasonic temperature was too high, it would cause the destruction of chlorogenic acid, resulting in the reduction of the extraction rate.

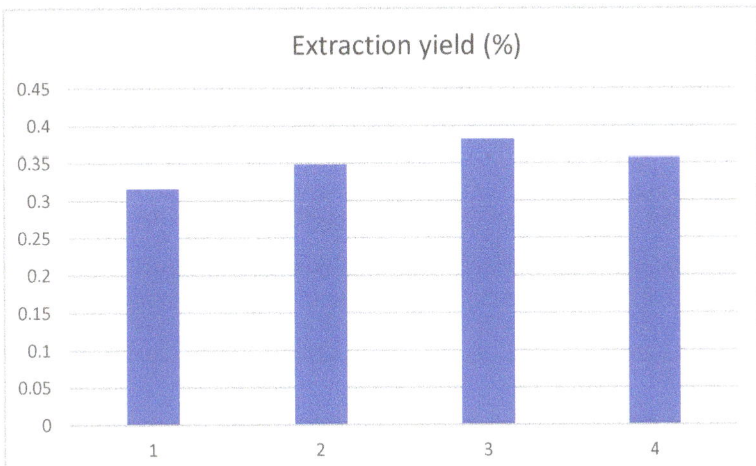

Figure 4. Influence of ultrasonic temperature on the extraction yield of chlorogenic acid, and the 1, 2, 3, and 4 represent the ultrasonic extraction temperature of 50 °C, 60 °C, 70 °C and 80 °C, respectively.

3.2.3. Effect of pH on the Yield of Chlorogenic Acid in Tobacco Waste

The change in chlorogenic acid yield was studied when the pH value of the extract gradually rose from 3 to 6, and the results are shown in Figure 5. The yield of chlorogenic acid in tobacco waste was the highest when the pH of the extract was 4. This may be because the molecular structure of chlorogenic acid contained both carboxyl and hydroxyl groups, which would decompose as the pH of the extract gradually increased, leading to a decline in the extraction rate.

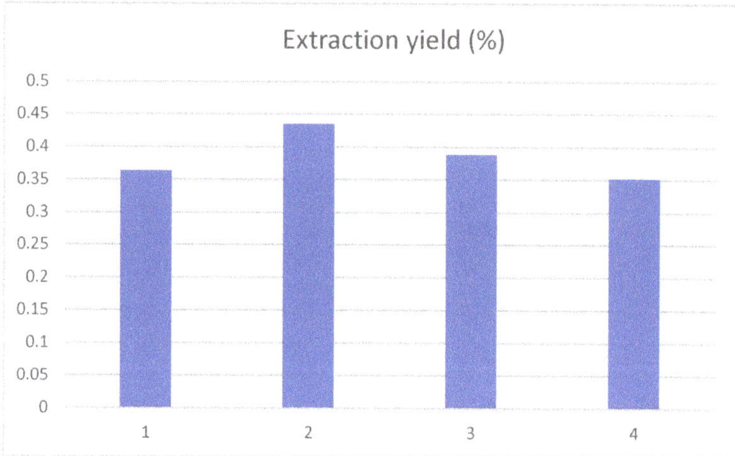

Figure 5. Influence of pH value on the extraction yield of chlorogenic acid, and the 1, 2, 3, and 4 represent the pH value of 3, 4, 5 and 6, respectively.

3.2.4. Influence of Ultrasonic Time on the Yield of Chlorogenic Acid in Tobacco Waste

The ultrasonication extraction times were set at 1.5 h, 2.0 h, 2.5 h and 3.0 h, and the results are shown in Figure 6. The yield of chlorogenic acid increased first and then decreased as ultrasound extraction time went on. When the extraction time increased to 2 h, the yield of chlorogenic acid was the highest. The possible reason was that, with the extension of ultrasonic time, chlorogenic acid was degraded by the thermal effect or photolysis. It was also possible that the prolonged extraction time would lead to the dissolution of other impurities in the tobacco waste, resulting in a decrease in the dissolution rate of chlorogenic acid. In addition, these impurities may also interfere with the experimental measurement.

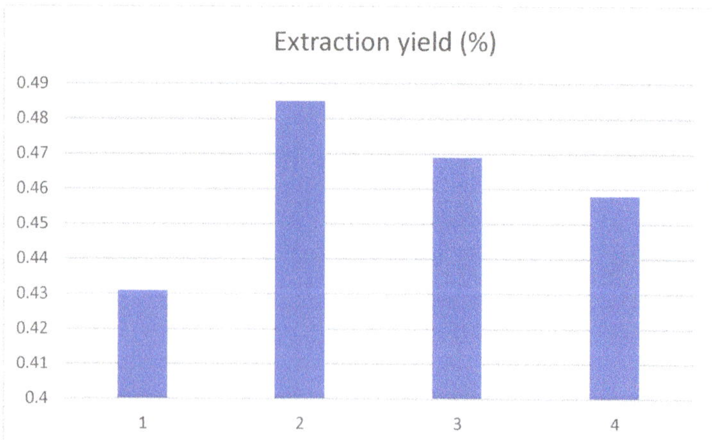

Figure 6. Influence of ultrasound time on the extraction yield of chlorogenic acid, and the 1, 2, 3, and 4 represent the extraction times of 1.5 h, 2.0 h, 2.5 h and 3.0 h, respectively.

3.3. Experimental Methods

3.3.1. Box—Behnken Design

Although the single factor experiment can optimize the experimental conditions to a certain extent, it could not accurately judge the optimal experimental point. Thus, RSM was chosen to obtain the best process parameters in this study. The design was based on the experimental results of the above single-factor experiments, considering the controllability of experimental operation and using chlorogenic acid yield as the index of investigation. The design results are shown in Table 1 by using the Box-Behnken central combination of Design Expert 8.0.6 software. RSM is an optimization method that can intuitively represent the relationship between experimental conditions and dependent variables by using graphical techniques, so it has been applied in many fields [21–24].

Table 1. Response surface analysis and results.

Run	Factors			The Yield of Chlorogenic Acid (%)
	A: Ultrasound Time (h)	B: Ethanol Concentration (%)	C: pH Value of Extraction Solution	
1	2.0	40	3.0	0.336
2	2.0	50	4.0	0.486
3	1.5	60	4.0	0.356
4	2.0	50	4.0	0.527
5	2.0	50	4.0	0.492
6	2.5	50	5.0	0.439
7	2.5	50	3.0	0.349
8	1.5	50	3.0	0.374
9	2.5	60	4.0	0.377
10	2.0	60	3.0	0.360
11	2.0	40	5.0	0.331
12	2.0	50	4.0	0.487
13	2.5	40	4.0	0.426
14	1.5	40	4.0	0.415
15	1.5	50	5.0	0.401
16	2.0	60	5.0	0.360
17	2.0	50	4.0	0.514

3.3.2. Analysis of Variance

Quadratic polynomial regression fitting was performed on Box-Behnken's experimental design and experimental results, and the binary regression equation model was obtained as follows:

$$\text{Chlorogenic acid yield } \% = -2.88 + 0.37A + 0.07B + 0.57C + 5 \times 10^{-4}AB + 0.03AC + 1.25 \times 10^{-4}BC - 0.13A^2 - 7.59 \times 10^{-4}B^2 - 0.08C^2.$$

Significance test was performed on the coefficient of the regression model, and the results were shown in Table 2. It can be seen from the table that the model $p < 0.05$, the difference was significant, indicating that the regression model obtained in this experiment had a good fitting degree for the yield of chlorogenic acid in tobacco waste. The R^2 was 0.9068, indicating that the experimental error was small. According to the value of F, it can be judged that the order of influence of various factors on chlorogenic acid extraction in tobacco waste was as follows: pH of the extraction solution > volume fraction of ethanol > ultrasonic time. The quadratic terms B^2 and C^2 were significant, indicating that they have a great influence on the yield of chlorogenic acid. The missing term $p = 0.0749 > 0.05$, showing no significance, indicates that factors other than the model study had little influence on the response value. Therefore, the regression equation obtained in this study can be used to determine the best ultrasonic-assisted extraction process of chlorogenic acid in tobacco waste.

Table 2. The ANOVA for response surface quadratic model to extraction of chlorogenic acid.

Source	Sum of Squares	DF	Mean Square	F Value	*p* Value Prob > F	Remarks
Model	0.063	9	7.019×10^{-3}	7.57	0.0071	Significant
A-Time	2.531×10^{-4}	1	2.531×10^{-4}	0.27	0.6175	
B-Concentration	3.781×10^{-4}	1	3.781×10^{-4}	0.41	0.5435	
C-pH	1.568×10^{-3}	1	1.568×10^{-3}	1.69	0.2347	
AB	2.500×10^{-5}	1	2.500×10^{-5}	0.027	0.8742	
AC	9.923×10^{-4}	1	9.923×10^{-4}	1.07	0.3354	
BC	6.250×10^{-6}	1	6.250×10^{-6}	6.738×10^{-3}	0.9369	
A^2	4.271×10^{-3}	1	4.271×10^{-3}	4.61	0.0690	
B^2	0.024	1	0.024	26.12	0.0014	
C^2	0.026	1	0.026	28.05	0.0011	
Residual	6.493×10^{-3}	7	9.275×10^{-4}			
Lack of Fit	5.146×10^{-3}	3	1.715×10^{-3}	5.09	0.0749	Not significant
Pure Error	1.347×10^{-3}	4	3.367×10^{-4}			
Cor Total	0.070	16				

3.3.3. Response Surface Map Analysis

The data in Table 2. were fitted by quadratic multiple regression to obtain the corresponding response surface stereogram, as shown in Figure 7.

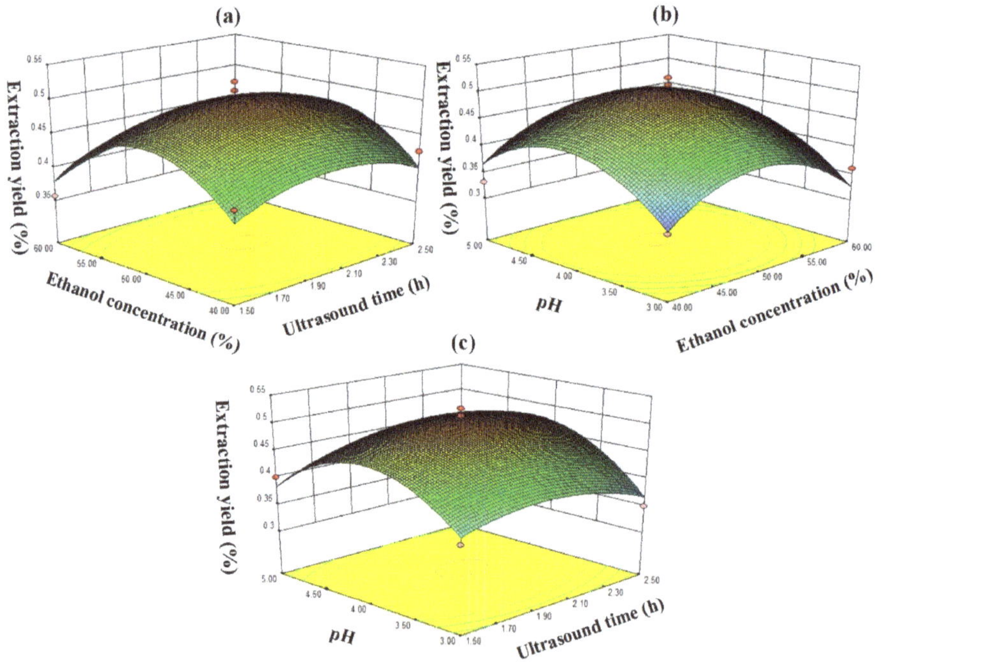

Figure 7. Response surface plots for the effects of (**a**) ethanol concentration vs. extraction time, (**b**) ethanol concentration vs. pH, and (**c**) pH vs. extraction time on the extraction yield of chlorogenic acid.

The contour line indicated that the chlorogenic acid yield in tobacco waste was the same in the same oval area and gradually decreased from the center to the edge [25,26]. Therefore, as shown in Figure 7, the vertex position of the response surface map indicated the highest extraction yield of chlorogenic acid. The opening of the response surface was downward, indicating that the chlorogenic acid yield increased with the increase of the value of each factor in a certain range. Then, after the maximum respective face value was reached, the chlorogenic acid yield decreased as each factor increased further. According to the p value of the significance test of each variable in Table 2, it can be seen that the influence of each factor on the yield of chlorogenic acid is: $C^2 > B^2 > A^2 > C > AC > B > A > AB > BC$, indicating that there is a certain relationship between the factor interactions. The optimal extraction conditions of chlorogenic acid from tobacco waste by RSM were as follows: ultrasonic time of 2.06 h, ethanol volume fraction of 49.57%, pH of 4.1, and the theoretical yield of chlorogenic acid was 0.502%. In order to verify the feasibility of the above method and consider the feasibility of actual operation, the conditions were modified and carried out under the following conditions: ultrasonic extraction time of 2.0 h, ethanol volume fraction of 50% and pH value of 4.1. Finally, the yield of chlorogenic acid extracted from tobacco waste was 0.497% under the above conditions, which was very close to the predicted results.

4. Conclusions

The tobacco waste was first pre-treated by repeated freeze-thawing before ultrasonic extraction of chlorogenic acid. Then, single-factor experiments and RSM were chosen to optimize the extraction process parameters of chlorogenic acid from tobacco waste. The obtained optimal process conditions were as follows: 2.06 h of ultrasonic extraction time, 49.57% of ethanol by volume, and extracting solution pH of 4.1. Under these conditions, the yield of chlorogenic acid could reach 0.502%. This result indicated that the resource utilization of tobacco waste, such as tobacco stems, was an effective way to develop its added value. In addition, the repeated freeze-thawing method adopted in this study has the advantages of being simple, low energy consumption and low cost when compared with other pretreatment methods, such as ionic liquid and steam blasting, so it could provide a reference for the extraction of chlorogenic acid and even other active ingredients in biomass cells.

Author Contributions: Conceptualization, G.Z. and M.Z.; methodology, D.S.; software, Y.R.; validation, X.H., H.D. and H.M.; formal analysis, Y.M.; investigation, L.J.; resources, G.Z.; data curation, Y.L.; writing—original draft preparation, G.Z.; writing—review and editing, M.Z.; visualization, Y.M.; supervision, D.S.; project administration, M.Z.; funding acquisition, D.S. All authors have read and agreed to the published version of the manuscript.

Funding: This research was funded by [National Natural Science Foundation of China] grant number [52103156,51901160]; [Chongqing Science and Technology Commission Project] grant number [cstc2021jcyj-msxmX0663], [Basic scientific research project of Wenzhou] grant number [S2020005]; [Provincial and Ministerial Co-constructive of Collaborative Innovation Center for MSW Comprehensive Utilization] grant number [shljzyh2021-23]; [Taizhou Science and Technology Support (Agriculture) Project] grant number [TN202012, SNY20210008]; [Chongqing Bayu Scholars Young Scholars Project] grant number [YS2021089]; [College Students Innovation Training Program] grant number [2021198,202211551007].

Institutional Review Board Statement: Not applicable.

Informed Consent Statement: Not applicable.

Conflicts of Interest: The authors declare no conflict of interest.

References

1. Yang, J.; Liu, W.; Kong, C.; Dong, H.; Zheng, J. Co-digestion of tobacco waste with different agricultural biomass feedstocks and the inhibition of tobacco viruses by anaerobic digestion. *Bioresour. Technol.* **2015**, *189*, 210–216.
2. Mumba, P.P.; Phiri, R. Environmental Impact Assessment of Tobacco Waste Disposal. *Int. J. Environ. Res.* **2008**, *2*, 225–230.
3. Glaiton, T.; Marcelo, G.; Aline, D.; José, Z.A. Nanofibrillated cellulose from tobacco industry wastes. *Carbohydr. Polym.* **2016**, *148*, 69–77.
4. Ma, X.; Meng, Z.; Qiu, L.; Chen, J.; Guo, Y.; Yi, D.; Ji, T.; Jia, H.; Xue, M. Solanesol extraction from tobacco leaves by Flash chromatographybased on molecularly imprinted polymer. *J. Chromatogr. B* **2016**, *1020*, 1–5. [CrossRef]

5. Li, X.; Liu, F.; Wang, H.; He, F.; Yang, R.; Zhao, M. Gas Chromatography-Mass Spectrometry Method for Simultaneous Detection of Nine Alkaloids in Tobacco and Tobacco Products by QuEChERS Sample Preparation. *Anal. Sci.* **2019**, *35*, 849–854. [CrossRef]
6. Sánchez, L.E.F.; Corigliano, M.G.; Oliferuk, S.; Ramos, D.V.A.; Rivera, M.; Mendoza, M.L.F.; Angel, S.O.; Sander, V.A.; Clemente, M. Oral Immunization with a Plant HSP90-SAG1 Fusion Protein Produced in Tobacco Elicits Strong Immune Responses and Reduces Cyst Number and Clinical Signs of Toxoplasmosis in Mice. *Front. Plant Sci.* **2021**, 726910–726929. [CrossRef]
7. Hu, R.S.; Wang, J.; Li, H.; Ni, H.; Chen, Y.F.; Zhang, Y.W.; Xiang, S.P.; Li, H.H. Simultaneous extraction of nicotine and solanesol from waste tobacco materials by the column chromatographic extraction method and their separation and purification. *Sep. Purif. Technol.* **2015**, *146*, 1–7. [CrossRef]
8. Zhang, M.; Zeng, G.; Pan, Y.; Qi, N. Difference research of pectins extracted from tobacco waste by heat reflux extraction and microwave-assisted extraction. *Biocatal. Agric. Biotechol.* **2018**, *15*, 359–363. [CrossRef]
9. Zhang, X.; Shi, L.; Chen, R.; Zhao, Y.; Ren, D.; Yang, X. Chlorogenic acid inhibits trimethylamine-N-oxide formation and remodels intestinal microbiota to alleviate liver dysfunction in high L-carnitine feeding mice. *Food Funct.* **2021**, *12*, 10500–10512. [CrossRef]
10. Wang, S.; Li, Y.; Huang, D.; Chen, S.; Xia, Y.; Zhu, S. The inhibitory mechanism of chlorogenic acid and its acylated derivatives on α-amylase and α-glucosidase. *Food Chem.* **2022**, *372*, 131334–131343. [CrossRef]
11. Zhang, Z.H.; Pan, T.W. HPLC determination of chlorogenic acid in Verbena officinalis L. extract and its in-vitro antibacterial activity. *Biomed. Res.* **2017**, *28*, 3996–4001.
12. Li, H.; Zhou, Z.; Tang, S. Optimization of Extraction Process of Total Flavonoids and Chlorogenic Acid from Flos Lonicerae by Orthogonal Experiment. *Med. Plant* **2019**, *10*, 5–17.
13. Qin, G.; Ma, J.; Wei, W.; Li, J.; Yue, F. The enrichment of chlorogenic acid from Eucommia ulmoides leaves extract by mesoporous carbons. *J. Chromatogr. B* **2018**, *1087*, 6–13. [CrossRef]
14. Kazem, R.M.; Hejazi, K.S.M.; Sadat, M.P.R. Optimization of chlorogenic acid extraction from Elm tree, Ulmus minor Mill., fruits, using response surface methodology. *Sep. Purif. Technol.* **2021**, *256*, 117773–117784.
15. Saleh, I.A.; Vinatoru, M.; Mason, T.J.; Abdel-Azim, N.S.; Aboutabl, E.A.; Hammouda, F.M. A possible general mechanism for ultrasound-assisted extraction (UAE) suggested from the results of UAE of chlorogenic acid from *Cynara scolymus* L. (artichoke) leaves. *Ultrason Sonochem.* **2016**, *31*, 330–336. [CrossRef]
16. Shao, P.; Zhang, J.F.; Chen, X.X.; Sun, P.L. Microwave-assisted extraction and purification of chlorogenic acid from by-products of Eucommia Ulmoides Oliver and its potential anti-tumor activity. *J. Food Sci. Technol.* **2015**, *52*, 4925–4934. [CrossRef]
17. Kaltsa, O.; Lakka, A.; Grigorakis, S.; Karageorgou, I.; Batra, G.; Bozinou, E.; Lalas, S.; Makris, D.P. A Green Extraction Process for Polyphenols from Elderberry (*Sambucus nigra*) Flowers Using Deep Eutectic Solvent and Ultrasound-Assisted Pretreatment. *Molecules* **2020**, *25*, 921. [CrossRef]
18. Gao, R.; Zhang, Y.; Zhang, H. Optimization of Microwave Extraction of Chlorogenic Acid from Tussilago Farfara by Response Surface Methodology. *Fine Chem.* **2017**, *34*, 1246–1251.
19. Wang, X.; Li, X.; Cai, C.; Dai, J.; Wen, F.; Wang, J. Process optimization of chlorogenic acid extraction from crataegus pinnatifida bge using aqueous ionic liquid. *Trans. CSAE* **2014**, *30*, 270–276.
20. Liu, J.; Mu, T.; Sun, H.; Fauconnier, M.L. Optimization of ultrasonic–microwave synergistic extraction of flavonoids from sweet potato leaves by response surface methodology. *J. Food Process. Preserv.* **2019**, *43*, 13928–13941. [CrossRef]
21. Zhang, Y.; Hou, Z.C. A model updating method based on response surface models of reserved singular values. *Mech. Syst. Signal Pr.* **2018**, *111*, 119–134. [CrossRef]
22. Samae, D.; Debangsu, K.; Bhaskor, J.B.; Pankaj, K.; Vinayak, K. Thermo-economic optimization of a biogas-diesel dual fuel engine as remote power generating unit using response surface methodology. *Therm. Sci. Eng. Prog.* **2021**, *24*, 100935–100943.
23. Omranian, S.R.; Hamzah, M.O.; Valentin, J.; Hasan, M.R.M. Determination of optimal mix from the standpoint of short term aging based on asphalt mixture fracture properties using response surface method. *Constr. Build Mater.* **2018**, *179*, 35–48. [CrossRef]
24. Yin, G.H.; Dang, Y.L. Optimization of extraction technology of the Lycium barbarum polysaccharides by Box-Behnken statistical design. *Carbohyd. Polym.* **2008**, *74*, 603–610. [CrossRef]
25. Tolga, T.; Gürkan, K.; Selin, H.; Zeynep, C.; Selin, S.; Yasser, V. Boron removal from aqueous solutions by chitosan/functionalized-SWCNT-COOH: Development of optimization study using response surface methodology and simulated annealing. *Chemosphere* **2022**, *288*, 132554–132562.
26. Negi, N.; Srihar, S.P.; Wadikar, D.D.; Sharma, G.K.; Semwal, A.D. Optimization of instant foxtail millet based khichdi by using response surface methodology and evaluation of its shelf stability. *J. Food Sci. Technol.* **2021**, *58*, 4478–4485. [CrossRef]

International Journal of
Environmental Research and Public Health

MDPI

Article

Spatial Spillover Effects of Directed Technical Change on Urban Carbon Intensity, Based on 283 Cities in China from 2008 to 2019

Hui Zhang [1] **and Haiqian Ke** [1,2,*]

1 Fanli Business School, Nanyang Institute of Technology, Nanyang 473000, China; zhanghuinylg@163.com
2 Institute of Central China Development, Wuhan University, Wuhan 430072, China
* Correspondence: kehaiqian@whu.edu.cn

Abstract: Technical change essentially drives regional social and economic development, and how technical change influences the regional sustainable development of the ecological environment is also of concern. However, technical change is not always neutral, so how does directed technical change affect urban carbon intensity? Is there a spatial spillover effect between these two? In order to answer these above questions, this article first explores the relationship between directed technical change and carbon intensity through the spatial Durbin model; then, it separately analyses whether the relationship between the two in low-carbon and non-low-carbon cities will differ; finally, we performed a robustness test by replacing weights, replacing the explained variable with a lag of one period, and replacing the explained variable. The conclusions are as follows: (1) There is a positive spatial correlation between the carbon intensity of Chinese cities—that is, there is a positive interaction between the carbon intensity of local cities and of neighboring cities. For every 1% change in the carbon intensity of neighboring cities, the carbon intensity of local cities changes by 0.1027% in the same direction. (2) The directed technical change has a significant inhibitory effect on urban carbon intensity, whether in local cities or neighboring cities. However, it is worth mentioning that the direct negative effect is greater in local cities than in neighboring cities. (3) The directed technical change in low-carbon cities has a stronger inhibitory effect on carbon intensity, with a direct effect coefficient of −0.5346 and an indirect effect coefficient of −0.2616. Due to less green policy support in non-low-carbon cities, the inhibitory effect of directed technical change on carbon intensity is weakened; even if the direct effects and indirect effects are superimposed, it is only −0.0510 rather than −0.7962 for low-carbon cities.

Keywords: directed technical change; spatial durbin model; carbon intensity; urban sustainable development

Citation: Zhang, H.; Ke, H. Spatial Spillover Effects of Directed Technical Change on Urban Carbon Intensity, Based on 283 Cities in China from 2008 to 2019. *Int. J. Environ. Res. Public Health* **2022**, *19*, 1679. https://doi.org/10.3390/ijerph19031679

Academic Editors: Roberto Alonso González Lezcano, Francesco Nocera and Rosa Giuseppina Caponetto

Received: 30 December 2021
Accepted: 31 January 2022
Published: 1 February 2022

1. Introduction

Climate change caused by the greenhouse effect is one of the greatest threats to human life on a global scale, because it endangers the ecological security of the Earth and, thus, the survival and development of human beings [1]. For example, a one meter rise in sea levels caused by the melting of glaciers would directly affect around one billion people, and also approximately one-third of the world's arable land [2]. Hence, the IPCC and the Kyoto Protocol have jointly promoted the process of global cooperation in addressing climate change, and established the goal of preventing the increase in the surface temperature from exceeding 2 degrees Celsius in the future. The core countermeasure is to control and to reduce greenhouse gas emissions globally. In particular, there is an urgent need to control CO_2 emissions and the growth rate of fossil energy consumption [2].

In the past 100 years, developed countries have undergone industrialization successively, consuming a large amount of the Earth's natural resources—especially energy resources. However, some developing countries are currently entering the stage of industrialization, and increased energy consumption is an objective necessity for their economic and social development. Given the speed and scale of China's economic development in recent years, China's total carbon emissions have ranked first in the world since 2005 [3]. Therefore, China should give consideration to how to reduce the total amount of carbon emissions, and make continuous efforts in improving carbon productivity and reducing carbon intensity.

As the most direct and powerful means to reduce regional carbon emissions and the greenhouse effect, energy saving and emissions reduction are the inherent requirements for China to realize its own sustainable development, but also make important contributions to the global mitigation of climate change. The year 2006 was the year that China's energy conservation and emissions reduction policy framework was formed. As China surpassed the US in total energy consumption for the first time in 2009, becoming the world's largest energy consumer [4], China proposed to reduce energy consumption per unit of GDP by ~20% and to reduce the total amount of major pollutants by 10% during the 11th 5-year plan period, consistent with the goals proposed by 2020 to achieve carbon peak by 2030 and carbon neutrality by 2060 [5,6]. From the perspective of international experience, European developed countries have spent 55–60 years on reducing emissions, reaching the peak of carbon dioxide emissions in 1990–1996, and aiming to achieve zero carbon emissions by 2050. China's goal is to achieve carbon peak and carbon neutrality in only 30 years; hence, there is no doubt that China's process of reducing carbon emissions is full of hardships and challenges.

Green policy support and technical change are both important driving forces in reducing carbon emissions. On the one hand, most countries agree that optimizing the energy mix, market regulation, and political regulations are effective measures to reduce greenhouse gas emissions [7]. Additionally, saving non-renewable energy, developing renewable green energy, optimizing the energy structure, and reducing the release of gases harmful to the environment are sufficient and necessary conditions for achieving the targeted reductions in emissions. Additionally, in the process of achieving the above measures, technical change and support are also inseparable—the Porter hypothesis is the most powerful proof of this [8]. On the other hand, the US, Japan, and the European Union have all invested heavily into scientific research and the development of energy-saving and emissions-reducing technologies, and they have also achieved better environmental performance [9]. This confirms that technical change is an important driving force for regional energy conservation and global emissions reduction. However, from the perspective of endogenous economic growth theory, technical change is not always neutral—that is, the effect of technical change on productivity or the accumulation of production factors is not always similar. This may lead to an -unequal increase in the marginal output of factors such as capital and labor [10] which, in turn, can have varying degrees of impact on resource consumption, economic growth, and environmental quality. Simultaneously, as China is in a period of tightening resource and environmental constraints, promoting high-quality economic development, improving the environmental governance system, and committing to achieving green development, it is thus necessary to explore the impact of directed technical change on China's total carbon emissions, as well as how to strengthen or mitigate said impact. Such exploration is thus conducive to an in-depth understanding of how to promote the transformation of China's economic development to a green, low-carbon, and environmentally friendly mode.

2. Literature Review and Theoretical Hypotheses

Through reviewing the relevant literature, reducing carbon emissions mainly depends on the influence of factors such as energy prices, environmental policies, and technical change [11]. First of all, because carbon emissions have certain externalities, they come from unconscious and uncompensated economic activities. Therefore, the government allows a "Pigovian tax" policy to ensure that greenhouse gas emissions are no longer free, forcing enterprises to use greener technologies or fuels, thereby alleviating the decline in environmental quality [12]. The Chinese government has tried to curb the rise in total carbon emissions by controlling the carbon pricing, the related tax price, the number of carbon transactions, and the price of carbon credits [13]. For instance, in 2012 and 2014, China launched a carbon trading pilot in seven provinces and cities to try to internalize the external costs of enterprises' emissions by controlling carbon pricing, and then formed China's largest carbon trading market in 2021 [14]. Therefore, the increasing energy price due to the carbon tax will induce the increasing R&D investment in low-carbon technology, which will benefit the development of greener technologies. Secondly, market-based and command-based policies can impose mandatory emissions reduction targets and standards requiring enterprises to achieve emission reduction targets, respectively. In February 2017, the National Development and Reform Commission announced the third batch of national low-carbon city pilots, for which a total of 45 cities were selected [15], trialing cities with low-carbon economic development, citizens with a low-carbon lifestyle, and a low-carbon society under government management. Therefore, theoretically speaking, the support of low-carbon policies should make cities more successful in reducing carbon emissions. Third, technical change is a key factor in reducing emission reduction costs in the future, because more advanced technologies are often greener. For example, solar energy becomes cheaper faster than coal, so the costs of reducing carbon emissions are lower. The chemical industry, steel industry, construction industry, and other fields have achieved multiple milestones in energy saving, consumption reduction, and pollution reduction due to the embedded energy-saving technology, clean production technology, and the recycling of waste, showing the important role of technical change in China's realization of carbon emission reductions. Specifically, technical change can be used to ease the contradiction between economic growth and the continuously increasing carbon emissions in the following four ways: First, technical changes can effectively reduce the dependence on and overuse of energy, simultaneously expanding green energy use without significantly slowing economic growth [16,17]. For example, the improvement of end-treatment technology and the establishment of a whole-process pollution reduction system can achieve carbon reduction [18]. Second, most scholars generally accept the view that the improvement of energy efficiency means that the same amount of energy input can bring more energy output [19]. Although some scholars have questioned whether higher energy efficiency means more energy consumption [20], it is undeniable that improved energy efficiency can also reduce energy costs. Third, as a terminal solution, carbon capture and storage can decompose the captured and stored carbon dioxide before, during, or after combustion, and transport and store it to a safe place [21], and the realization of all of these effective mitigation measures is inseparable from technical change and support. Fourth, with the advent of the era of big data, cloud technology has enabled the promotion and application of clean technology to be realized on a large scale at a faster speed or lower cost [22]. Therefore, the promotion of green policy support and technical change can help to reduce carbon emissions.

However, technical change is not always neutral. It has been found that technical change may be directed by factors such as factor price changes, R&D activities, trade, and FDI (foreign direct investment) technology spillovers. The idea of directed technical change was first proposed by Hicks (1932) [23], and it has been developed more comprehensively by Kennedy (1964), Samuelson (1965), and Drandakis and Phelps (1966) [24–26]. However, in recent theoretical research, the more commonly accepted theories mainly come from Acemoglu (1998; 2003; 2006; 2007) and Jones (2005) [27–31]. First of all, Acemoglu's (2002) model is driven by the profits of "technology monopolists" rather than being induced by factor prices, so it can effectively distinguish between directed technical change and factor substitution effects [32]. At the same time, on the basis of the CES (constant elasticity of substitution) production function, Acemoglu proposed that technical progress changes the relative marginal productivity of factors in different proportions, so as to have different characteristics of saving or using factors. That is, if technical change increases the marginal productivity of factor i relative to factor j, then technical change is directed towards factor i; if the effect of directed technical change reduces the relative use of factor i, technical change is called "factor i-saving technical change". Later, Jones (2005) argued that the shape of the production function and the direction of technical change were determined by the distribution of innovation [31]. Jones also explored the determinants of directed technical change under the Cobb–Douglas production function [31]. Despite Jones starting from a different perspective, his conclusion was in line with Acemoglu's theory—both of them emphasized the reasonable micro-basis mechanism of directed technical change, and they have made some progress in theoretical models and empirical methods to promote the study area of directed technical change.

More importantly, many papers have confirmed that the energy efficiency of similar activities in different enterprises, fields, and countries is quite different, and the accelerated diffusion of energy technology is helpful in achieving energy conservation and emissions reduction [33–37]. This means that the emissions reduction effects brought by technical change have a certain degree of spatial relevance and spatial difference. In 2010, Sun calculated the average annual energy-saving rate of each province in China from 2006 to 2010, and found that the average annual energy-saving rate of neighboring cities has a certain degree of similarity [38]; this reflects how China's energy-saving rate has a certain geographical correlation. Additionally, the similarity within the four plates and the difference between the four plates in China are also significant reasons for the spatial correlation of regional carbon emissions. Yao and Yu (2011) used the DEA method to reveal that the carbon intensity in the eastern and central provinces was significantly inhibited by technical change, while the carbon intensity in the northeast and western regions was increased by technical change [39]. Based on China's provincial-level data, Wei and Yang (2010) found that there were regional differences in the effects of technology on emissions reduction [40]. In view of this, why does the influence of technical change on carbon emissions have regional agglomeration and differences, and can spatial correlation and difference strengthen or alleviate the influence of directed technical change on carbon emissions? This series of questions are worthy of further in-depth investigation.

Therefore, on the basis of the spatial model, this article will first explore whether there is an urban-directed technical change in China, and attempt to ascertain the effect of directed technical change on urban carbon emissions. In this article, the investment-biased technology change technique (IBTECH) proposed by Fare et al. (1994; 1997) is used to measure the directed technical change of 283 cities in China [41–45]. This method is based on the non-parametric data envelopment analysis (DEA) method, and is further decomposed on the basis of the Malmquist total factor productivity index. The advantage of this method is that it is not restricted by the shape of the production function or factor prices. In addition, carbon intensity is the ratio of the total amount of regional carbon emissions to the total regional GDP; this is mainly because the concept of carbon intensity is more objective than the total amount of carbon emissions itself, because the influence of factors such as population size and area size on the measurement results can be removed. At the same time, carbon intensity reflects the output efficiency of carbon emissions. As per capita GDP continues to increase, carbon intensity is expected to decline. Therefore, carbon intensity can also reflect the balance between economic development and carbon emissions more comprehensively.

Hence, this paper takes 283 prefecture-level cities in China as the research object in order to explore whether there is spatial correlation between urban carbon intensity and directed technical change, and then explores what kind of effect directed technical change will have on urban carbon intensity; the roadmap is reflected in Figure 1. The marginal contributions of this paper are as follows: Firstly, this paper innovatively expands and extends the scope of research on the interaction between directed technical change and urban carbon intensity from a spatial perspective. Secondly, this article examines whether and how official low-carbon policy support will affect the relationship between the two. For example, if directed technical change has a significant inhibitory effect on the local carbon intensity, it may nevertheless have a significant positive effect on the carbon intensity of neighboring cities. This result could be a strong reference for experts who study the spatial relationship between the two. At the same time, when the spatial correlation and mechanism of interaction between the two are more deeply understood, it may also help to explore the different underlying mechanisms of influence on different regions. Finally, this article verifies the relationship between the two from the city level, since cities are specific spatial carriers for achieving peak carbon and carbon neutrality goals, as they are more specific, objective, and realistic than national and provincial levels. Therefore, our findings may be helpful for relevant departments—such as the National Resources Commission of the State Council, the National Development and Reform Commission, the Ministry of Ecology and Environment, city councils, and relevant prefecture-level "carbon neutrality" monitoring and command platforms—helping them to form a better plan in the process of achieving China's peak carbon and carbon neutrality. For example, if the above departments can recognize that the direction of technical change has a certain significant relationship with urban carbon intensity, through guiding or changing the direction of technical change, the inhibitory effect on urban carbon intensity can be enhanced or the enhancement effect on carbon intensity can be weakened.

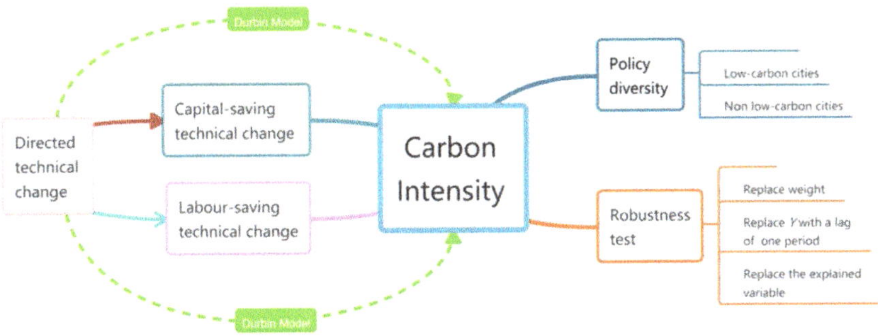

Figure 1. Roadmap of the paper.

3. Data and Models

3.1. Data

3.1.1. Explained Variable: Carbon Intensity

This article adopts the reference method in the greenhouse gas emission inventory guidelines formulated by the IPCC in 2006 [46,47]—that is, to estimate energy consumption, unify the energy units, and then multiply the carbon content coefficient in order to calculate the total carbon emissions, and deduct the amount of carbon used as raw materials as well as the amount of carbon for non-energy use. Finally, the output is corrected with the oxidation coefficient and converted into carbon emissions. Afterwards, we measured China's urban energy consumption from 2008 to 2019 by surveying the regional energy balance, and then calculated the carbon dioxide emissions from each city's energy consumption, divided by the city's gross domestic product, to determine the carbon intensity of one city:

$$E_{co_2} = \frac{\sum_i A_i \cdot c_i}{GDP} \tag{1}$$

where E_{co_2} is the regional total carbon intensity (tons/RMB 10,000), A_i is the consumption of the ith energy (tons), and c_i is the carbon dioxide emission coefficient of this energy.

$$A_i = F_i + T_i + H_i + N_i \tag{2}$$

where F_i is the terminal consumption of the ith energy of the region, T_i is the consumption of the ith energy for power generation of the region, H_i is the ith energy for heating consumption of the region, and N_i is the ith consumption of industrial raw materials of the region.

Due to the scarcity of energy resources, the energy utilization between regions will flow and cross one another. Considering the spillover and diffusion effects of energy-saving technologies, energy consumption is influenced not only by local economic development strategies, technical change, and other factors, but also by these factors in surrounding areas. In addition, the frequent economic cooperation activities, energy-saving scientific and technical exchanges, and the radiation effects of energy-saving policies among Chinese cities have caused carbon emissions to be affected by local regions and adjacent regions; this is also the cause of the spatial concentration and correlation of urban carbon emissions in China. As we can see, this paper uses ArcGIS to draw the spatial distribution map of China's urban carbon intensity from 2008 to 2019 in Figures 2 and 3; we then divided all 283 cities into 7 groups (the urban carbon intensity of China is sorted into seven groups based on one-seventh of 100%. For example, group 1 represents 0–14.29% (1/7), and group 7 represents 85.72–100%). Greener color indicates higher carbon intensity, while yellower color indicates lower carbon intensity; the unit of urban carbon intensity is tons/RMB 10,000. It is natural to expect some correlation between the carbon intensity of Chinese cities. In fact, carbon intensity in 2008–2019 was on a downward trend, especially in the eastern region. However, we can also see that there was little change in carbon intensity in the central and western regions of China.

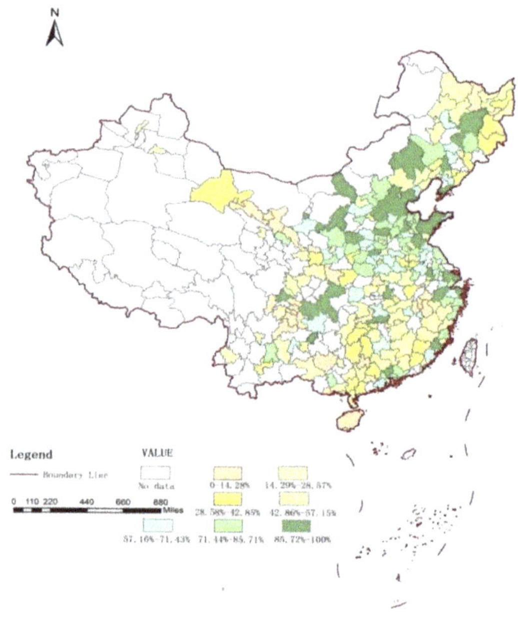

Figure 2. Carbon intensity in China, 2008.

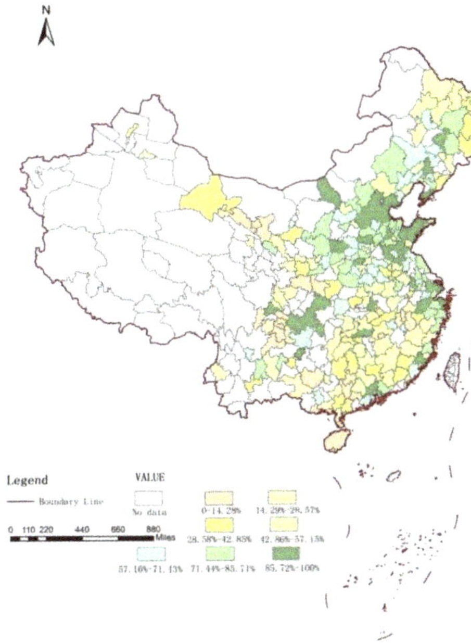

Figure 3. Carbon intensity in China, 2019.

3.1.2. Core Explanatory Variables: Directed Technical Change

Based on the use of DEA/Malmquist index to measure total factor productivity, Fare et al. (1997) decomposed the Malmquist index into the following parts: technical efficiency change index (FFCH) and technology change index (TECH) [41]; they also decomposed the technology change index into the technology scale change (MATECH), the output-biased technology change (OBTECH), and the input-biased technology change (IBTECH) indices. As IBTECH can effectively judge the direction of technical progress after combining the changes in the proportions of element input combinations between two adjacent periods, this article uses the IBTECH index to measure the directed technical progress [46–48], and the calculation method is as follows:

Let $x_t = (x_{1t}, \ldots .., x_{Nt})$ be the vector of factor input in period t, and $yt = (y_{1t}, \ldots .., y_{Nt})$ be the vector of output in period t. The Shephard input distance function in period t can be defined as follows [47]:

$$\mathrm{D}_t{}^i(y,x) = \max\left\{\lambda : \frac{x}{\lambda} \in L^t(y)\right\} \tag{3}$$

$$IBTECH = \sqrt{\frac{D_0^{t+1}(y^{t+1},x^t)}{D_0^t(y^{t+1},x^t)} / \frac{D_0^{t+1}(y^t,x^t)}{D_0^t(y^t,x^t)}} \tag{4}$$

When $x2_{t+1}/x1_{t+1} < x2_t/x1_t$ and $IBTECH$ are both less than 1, the technical change is $x1_{\text{-}saving}$, and the $IBTECH$ becomes smaller the higher the degree of technical change directed towards $x1_{\text{-}saving}$. When $x2_{t+1}/x1_{t+1} > x2_t/x1_t$, the situation is the opposite. When $x2_{t+1}/x1_{t+1} = x2_t/x1_t$, technical change is neutral. In this study, $x1$ is labor input, while $x2$ is capital input. In order to unify the two situations, this article sums up the opposite of the $IBTECH$ value in $x2_{t+1}/x1_{t+1} > x2_t/x1_t$, and $IBTECH$ values under $x2_{t+1}/x1_{t+1} < x2_t/x1_t$ remain unchanged so as to obtain the quantitative index of labor-saving technical change. Therefore, a large value of this index indicates that the directed technical change is more capital-saving [46,47]. This trend is also consistent with the findings of many scholars who investigated directed technical change in China [48]. Additionally, since the calculation process of directed technical change involves multiple indicators, different indicators often have different dimensions and units, which will affect the results of data analysis. To solve the comparability between data indicators, we used data normalization processing to convert the original data into decimals between (0, 1), after which each indicator was in the same order of magnitude, which is suitable for comprehensive comparative evaluation [49,50].

3.1.3. Control Variables

Based on the STIRPAT model (Dietz and Rosa 1994) [51], in addition to directed technical change, population density, and average urban night lights, this paper selects the following five control variables (as shown in Table 1) from the economic, social, and environmental perspectives: the proportion of tertiary industry, foreign direct investment, total road passenger transport, the number of full-time college teachers, and the scale of pollution control investment [11,44,46,47]. Among them, population density, night light data, and total road passenger transport are expected to have the most positive effect on carbon intensity. However, the proportion of tertiary industry, foreign direct investment, the number of full-time college teachers, and the scale of pollution control investment are expected to have a suppressing effect on carbon intensity.

Table 1 provides a description of the explained variables, core explanatory variables, and control variables selected in this article, as well as the unit and the basic data source of each variable. Table 2 is the statistical description of main variables.

Table 1. Data description and source.

Variable	Name	Symbol	Data Source
Explained variables	Carbon intensity	*lncd*	The ratio of urban carbon emissions to GDP; the basic data can be found in *the China Urban Statistical Yearbook* (2009–2020) and *China Urban Environment Yearbook* (2009–2020).
Core explanatory variables	Directed technological change	*lndtc*	The capital stock is estimated by the perpetual inventory method based on the year 2000; total employment and real GDP are derived from the *China Urban Statistical Yearbook* (2009–2020) and *China Science and Technology Yearbook* (2009–2020).
Control variables	Population density (ratio of urban population to urban area)	*lnpop*	Data from the *Statistical Yearbook of Chinese Cities* (2009–2020).
	Average urban night lights	*lnnl*	NPP-VIIRS NTL (2014–2019) and DMSP-OLS RNTL (2009–2013), and using the method of Chen et al. (2021) to calibrate inconsistent data sources around 2013 [52].
	Foreign direct investment	*lnfdi*	Data from the *Statistical Yearbook of Chinese Cities* (2009–2020)
	The proportion of tertiary industry to GDP	*lnthird*	
	Total road passenger transport	*lntrans*	
	The number of full-time college teachers	*lntechs*	
	The ratio of pollution control investment to GDP	*lnpollution*	

Table 2. Statistical description of main variables.

Variable	Symbol	Unit	Observations	Mean	Standard Deviation	Minimum	Maximum
Carbon intensity	*lncd*	Tons/RMB 10,000	3113	0.87	2.3901	0.49	4.23
Directed technological change	*lndtc*	Data have been normalized	3113	0.65	0.7907	0.32	0.98
Population density (ratio of urban population to urban area)	*lnpop*	Number of people/hm^2	3113	2.16	4.0014	1.57	3.05
Average urban night lights	*lnnl*	Candela(cd)	3113	3.70	5.0668	2.11	6.94
Foreign direct investment	*lnfdi*	RMB 10,000	3113	2.60	1.4762	1.70	5.08
The proportion of tertiary industry to GDP	*lnthird*	%	3113	37.8%	0.1825	28.71%	76.30%
Total road passenger transport	*lntrans*	10,000 people	3113	3.59	2.2003	1.04	6.68
The number of full-time college teachers	*lntechs*	10,000 people	3113	1.61	3.2947	2.69	5.74
The ratio of pollution control investment to GDP	*lnpollution*	RMB 10,000	3113	3.98	3.0898	0.91	6.37

3.2. Models

3.2.1. OLS Regression Model

In this study, the STIRPAT model (Dietz and Rosa, 1994) was used as the basic OLS regression model (ordinary least squares, which is the most fundamental form of regression analysis) to study the ecological environmental quality; the equation is expressed as follows [51]:

$$IBTECH = \sqrt{\frac{D_0^{t+1}(y^{t+1},x^t)}{D_0^t(y^{t+1},x^t)} / \frac{D_0^{t+1}(y^t,x^t)}{D_0^t(y^t,x^t)}} \quad (5)$$

where I_{it} represents environmental impact, P_{it} represents population size, A represents per capita wealth, T_{it} refers to technology, and e is the error term. After obtaining the natural logarithms of both sides, more variables were added to the right side of the equation to enhance the richness of the model. Consequently, the benchmark model below was built to examine the relationship between urban carbon intensity and directed technical change:

$$lncd_{it} = \alpha_0 + \alpha_1 lnpop_{it} + \alpha_2 lnnl_{it} + \alpha_3 lndtc_{it} + \alpha_4 X_{it} + \varepsilon_{it} \quad (6)$$

where i is the cross-sectional unit of the 283 Chinese cities investigated (due to the absence of necessary statistical data, 15 western cities among 298 prefecture-level cities were excluded herein), t is the year, population (P_{it}) and technical level (T_{it}) are represented by lnpopit and energy efficiency lndtcit, respectively, urban night light data ($lnnl_{it}$) represent per capita wealth A_{it}, and $lncd_{it}$ represents carbon intensity (the explained variable). X_{it} is a group of control variables, which includes the proportion of tertiary industry, foreign direct investment, total road passenger transport, the number of full-time college teachers, and the scale of pollution control investment; $lndtc_{it}$ is the core explanatory variable, ε is a random disturbance term, and α_0-α_4 are the estimated parameters.

3.2.2. Spatial Regression Model

Because traditional measurement methods do not consider the spatial correlation between observations, there are certain limitations when studying multiple regional related issues. Scholars' tentative research on spatial models mainly comes from SDM, SEM, and SDM, and there are also many academic papers on the impact of technical change on environmental quality [53–55]. However, based on the STIRPAT model, this paper takes the directed technical change as the core explanatory variable and carbon intensity as the explained variable—a method rarely seen in previous studies.

Spatial measurement models are generally divided into three types: spatial lag model (SLM), spatial error model (SEM), and spatial Durbin model (SDM) [56–60]. The SLM adds the spatial lag term of the explained variable to the general panel data model, indicating that the explanatory variable on a certain spatial unit is affected by the explanatory variable of the adjacent spatial unit. The SEM adds spatially related error terms—that is, the error term of a certain spatial unit model is considered to be affected by the adjacent spatial unit model error term. The SDM integrates the characteristics of the spatial lag model and the spatial error model. In all of the above models, the intensity of the influence of adjacent spatial units is represented by a spatial weight matrix. Therefore, this paper tries to propose an SLM model (Formula (7)), an SEM model (Formula (8)), and an SDM model (Formula (9)) to describe in depth the relationship between carbon intensity, population, economic development level, and directed technical change, as follows:

$$lncd_{it} = \delta\sum_{j=1}^{N} W_{ij}lncd_{jt} + \phi + \alpha_1 lnpop_{it} + \alpha_2 lnnl_{it} + \alpha_3 lndtc_{it} + c_i + \alpha_t + \varepsilon_{it} \tag{7}$$

$$\begin{aligned} lncd_{it} &= \phi + \alpha_1 lnpop_{it} + \alpha_2 lnnl_{it} + \alpha_3 lndtc_{it} + c_i + \alpha_t + u_{it} \\ u_{it} &= \rho\sum_{j=1}^{N} W_{ij}u_{jt} + \varepsilon_{it} \end{aligned} \tag{8}$$

$$\begin{aligned} lncd_{it} &= \delta\sum_{j=1}^{N} W_{ij}lncd_{jt} + \phi + \alpha_1 lnpop_{it} + \alpha_2 lnnl_{it} + \alpha_3 lndtc_{it} \\ &+ \sum_{j=1}^{N} W_{ij}(lnpop_{it} + lnnl_{it} + lndtc_{it})\theta + c_i + \alpha_t + \varepsilon_{it} \end{aligned} \tag{9}$$

where δ is the spatial regression coefficient, which represents the influence of the explained variable $lncd_{jt}$ of the adjacent spatial unit on the explained variable $lncd_{it}$ of this spatial unit; if it is significantly positive, this means that the explained variable has obvious positive spatial overflow—that is, the increase in the variable of one spatial unit in the research scope corresponds to the increase in the variables of other spatial units; u_{it} is the spatial autoregressive error term; ρ is the spatial error coefficient, which represents the influence of the adjacent spatial unit error term u_{it} on the spatial unit error term u_{it}; θ is the spatial lag term coefficient of the explanatory variable, which indicates the influence of the adjacent spatial unit explanatory variable $lndtc_{it}$ on the explanatory variable $lncd_{it}$ of this spatial unit; N is the number of spatial units, and $\mathbf{W}$ is the economic geographic spatial weight matrix. First, we used the LM test to determine whether the spatial lag effect and the spatial error effect were significant, and then used the Wald or LR tests to determine whether the spatial Durbin model can be simplified into a spatial lag model or a spatial error model. Assumption 1: $\theta = 0$; Assumption 2: $\theta + \lambda\beta = 0$. If Assumption 1 passes the significance test, the spatial Durbin model can be reduced to a spatial lag model, while if Assumption 2 passes the significance test, the spatial Durbin model can be reduced to a spatial error model [61,62].

3.2.3. Direct and Indirect Effects Regression Model

From the mathematical structure of the SDM, it can be seen that the explanatory variable y_{local} of a certain spatial unit is mainly affected by three aspects: the explained variable y_{neib} of the adjacent space unit, the explanatory variable x_{local} of this space unit, and the explanatory variable x_{neib} of the adjacent space unit. In addition to directly affecting y_{local}, the x_{local} of this space unit can also affect the y_{neib} of adjacent space units, and then transfer it to the space unit y_{local} through the spatial autocorrelation of y_{neib}. This comprehensive effect of x_{local} on y_{local} becomes a direct effect of explanatory variables; the x_{local} of this space unit can directly affect the y_{neib} of the adjacent space unit, or it can affect the y_{local} of this space unit, and then transfer to the y_{neib} of the adjacent space unit through the spatial autocorrelation of y_{local}. This comprehensive effect of x_{local} on y_{neib} becomes an indirect effect, also known as the spatial spillover effect of explanatory variables. Therefore, the spatial Durbin model can be rewritten into the following form [61,62]:

$$Y_{it} = (1 - \lambda W)^{-1}\varphi_N + (1 - \lambda W)^{-1}(X_t\beta + WX_t\theta)^{-1} + (1 - \lambda W)^{-1}v_t^* \quad (10)$$

where φ_N represents the space error term, meaning the error term with time and space effects. Therefore, the partial derivative of the explained variable Y with respect to the kth explanatory variable at a certain moment is:

$$\left[\frac{\partial Y}{\partial X_{1k}} \cdot \frac{\partial Y}{\partial X_{Nk}}\right] = (I - \lambda W)^{-1}\begin{bmatrix} \beta_k & W_{12}\theta_k & \cdots & W_{1N}\theta_k \\ W_{21}\theta_k & \beta_k & \cdots & W_{2N}\theta_k \\ \cdots & \cdots & \cdots & \cdots \\ W_{N1}\theta_k & W_{N2}\theta_k & \cdots & \beta_k \end{bmatrix} \quad (11)$$

where the mean of the diagonal elements on the right is the direct effect, and the mean of the sum of each row (column) of the off-diagonal elements is the indirect effect [63–65].

4. Results Analysis

4.1. OLS Regression Results

The results of Table 3 show the OLS regression results based on Formula (7). The capital-saving technical change suppress the increase in urban carbon intensity in China. One unit of capital-saving technical change could lead to a −0.0162 unit decrease in urban carbon intensity. This may be because highly skilled labor restrains the expansion of production by reducing capital inputs such as plants and machinery, and also reduces carbon intensity to some extent through the accumulation of human capital. Additionally, the population density, foreign direct investment, number of full-time college teachers, and pollution abatement show inhibitory effects on the urban carbon intensity of Chinese cities. However, the average night light data, tertiary industry proportion, and total road passenger transport all increase the urban carbon intensity significantly.

Table 3. OLS regression results.

Explanatory Variable	Coefficient	*t*-Value
lndtc	−0.0162 ***	(−2.83)
lnpop	−0.0024 **	(−2.30)
lnnl	0.0043 ***	(4.37)
lnfdi	−0.0624 ***	(−4.92)
lnthird	0.0003 ***	(5.34)
lntrans	0.0048 ***	(4.98)
lntechs	−0.0055	(−0.84)
lnpollution	−0.2046 *	(−1.86)

Note: the value of t is in parentheses, and ***, **, and * are significant at the levels of 1%, 5%, and 10%, respectively.

4.2. Spatial Regression Results

There are many methods of "spatial correlation or spatial structure test"; Moran's I index is by far the earliest, most used, and most famous test in practice [66], and it is simpler in calculation than Wald and LR tests [67]. However, its disadvantage is that the test was not developed under the framework of the maximum likelihood method, and no alternative hypothesis is proposed [68]. Anselin found that the RS test has an asymptomatic standard when testing the spatial model of cross-sectional data, but the Wald and LR tests do not [69]. For the spatial error autocorrelation cross-sectional model with spatial lag-dependent variables, a robust LM test has further introduced joint, marginal, and conditional tests to verify the spatial model structure [56].

Therefore, as shown in Table 4, we carried out an LM test and a robust LM test for non-spatial interaction models with four forms: time and space are not fixed, space is fixed, time is fixed, and time and space are fixed; the results show that the spatial error effect cannot pass the 1% robustness test, except for the time–space-non-fixed effect, space-fixed effect, and time-fixed effect; the other kinds of spatial lag effect and spatial error effect pass the LM test and robust LM test, and the spatial lag effect is more significant than the spatial error effect, showing that the SDM cannot be reduced to the SLM or the SEM—that is, the SDM is optimal. Therefore, it is necessary to construct the SDM under the fixed form of space and time.

Table 4. LM testing results.

	Time and Space Are Not Fixed	Time and Space Are Fixed	Time Is Fixed	Space Is Fixed
LM test of spatial lag effect (LMlag)	41.47 ***	52.48 ***	51.28 **	47.59 ***
	(0.000)	(0.000)	(0.000)	(0.000)
Robust LM test of spatial lag effect (R-LMlag)	18.93 ***	46.71 ***	30.38 **	25.73 ***
	(0.000)	(0.000)	(0.000)	(0.000)
LM test of spatial error effect (LMerr)	30.65 ***	9.63 ***	38.03 **	17.92 ***
	(0.000)	(0.000)	(0.000)	(0.000)
Robust LM test for spatial error effects (R-LMerr)	1.61	2.30 **	1.91 *	29.37 ***
	(0.107)	(0.021)	(0.057)	(0.000)

Note: the value of t is in parentheses, and ***, **, and * are significant at the levels of 1%, 5%, and 10%, respectively.

Table 5 shows the results based on the SDM. The coefficients and significance levels are overall improved compared to the OLS regression results from Table 3. Firstly, this shows that the spatial regression coefficient δ is significantly positive, indicating that the carbon intensity of Chinese cities is obviously affected by the carbon intensity of neighboring cities in the same direction, and also positively affects the carbon intensity of neighboring cities. This confirms that the carbon intensity of cities has obvious spatial spillovers—that is, for every 1% change in the carbon intensity of neighboring cities, the carbon intensity of the local city will change in the same direction by 0.1027%. Secondly, the significance test of the t-value of the regression coefficient β shows that the carbon intensity of Chinese cities is negatively affected by local capital-saving technical change, population density, foreign direct investment level, and pollution abatement; however, it is positively affected by night light data, the proportion of tertiary industries, and number of road passengers. Once again, the level of urban education shows no significant impact on carbon intensity. Finally, the t-value significance test of the spatial lag coefficient θ shows that the carbon intensity level of 283 cities in China is negatively affected by the capital-saving technical progress of neighboring cities. For neighboring cities, their population density, night light data, foreign direct investment level, proportion of tertiary industries, road passenger traffic, and pollution control investment all contribute to the improvement of the local city's carbon intensity. In summary, the degree of carbon intensity in Chinese cities is affected by the local and neighboring regions' capital-saving technical change, population density, night light data, foreign direct investment level, proportion of tertiary industries, number of road passengers, and pollution control investment. In addition, the capital-saving technical change, night light data, foreign investment level, and proportion of tertiary industries in neighboring cities play more important roles.

Table 5. Results of the SDM.

Variable	Coeffcient	Lag Coefficient
	β	θ
Spatial regression coefficient δ	0.1027 *** (4.91)	–
lndtc	−0.0398 *** (−4.50)	−0.0458 *** (−8.28)
lnpop	−0.0624 *** (−3.66)	0.0620 *** (3.53)
lnnl	0.0426 *** (4.37)	0.3019 *** (6.89)
lnfdi	−0.0109 ** (−2.46)	0.3813 *** (9.37)
ln3rd	0.0167 *** (5.08)	0.0299 ** (2.31)
lntrans	1.5103 *** (5.34)	0.0374 *** (2.46)
lntechs	−0.0070 (−0.79)	−0.0903 (−1.21)
lnpollution	−0.7210 *** (−4.98)	0.4892 *** (−4.50)

Note: the value of *t* is in parentheses, and ***, ** are significant at the levels of 1%, 5%, respectively.

4.3. Results of Direct and Indirect Effects of Variables

Table 6 shows the further calculation of the direct and indirect effects of various influencing factors on urban carbon intensity. The *rho* value was 0.2857 and the significance test was passed at the level of 10%. This shows that urban carbon intensity still has a strong positive spatial correlation. The regression results first show that the direct and indirect effects of capital-saving technical are is significantly negative, and that the direct effect is greater than the indirect effect, indicating that the superposition of the direct effect and the indirect effect significantly inhibits the carbon intensity of the local city and its neighbors—that is, if the level of capital-saving technical change increases by 1 unit, the carbon intensity of the city and neighboring cities will decrease by 0.0472 and 0.0259 units, respectively, which means that the city's overall carbon intensity will decrease by 0.0731 units in total. Secondly, the direct and indirect effects of average night light data, foreign investment level, the proportion of tertiary industries, and road passenger traffic are all in the same direction among local cities and neighboring cities; among them, night light data and road passenger traffic promote the carbon intensity of local cities and neighboring cities, meaning that the economic vitality of the region can drive the economic development of neighboring regions, which will inevitably use and consume more energy and increase the overall carbon intensity level. The increase in the level of local foreign investment is conducive to the imitation and learning of advanced knowledge and technology, and it can also play a demonstrable effect in neighboring areas. Because more advanced technology is often greener and more environmentally friendly, increasing the level of foreign investment can reduce the carbon intensity of local and neighboring cities; although a higher proportion of tertiary industry is accompanied by an increase in consumption, it is lower than the volume of resources consumed by the primary and secondary industries, so the overall increase in carbon emissions is significantly suppressed. The more the road passenger traffic, the wider the scope of social and economic activities between neighboring cities, and the higher the frequency of interaction between cities; therefore, road traffic plays an overall promoting role in carbon intensity. Third, the direct and indirect effects of population density, the number of full-time teachers in colleges and universities, and pollution control investment differ significantly or insignificantly. The increase in population density of local cities has a certain siphoning effect on the total population of neighboring cities. Therefore, the inhibitory effect of population agglomeration on carbon intensity mainly comes from the indirect effect of reducing the carbon intensity level of neighboring cities. The urban education level represented by the number of full-time university teachers does not show a significant correlation with carbon intensity. Meanwhile, a higher scale of pollution control investment has a significant direct inhibitory effect on the local city, and the coefficient is greater than its positive indirect effect. After the combined effect of the two, the overall carbon intensity of the city remains suppressed. In view of this, except for the educational level, all other factors have significant direct and indirect effects; among them, the spatial spillover effects of capital-saving technical change, population density, and the proportion of tertiary industries are the most obvious, significantly reducing the urban carbon intensity.

Table 6. Direct and indirect effects of the SDM.

Variable	Direct Effect	Indirect Effect	Total Effect
lndtc	−0.0472 *** (−4.69)	−0.0259 ** (−2.08)	−0.0731 *** (−3.99)
lnpop	0.4843 (0.56)	−0.5946 * (1.85)	−0.1103 * (1.90)
Lnnl	0.0305 ** (2.11)	0.5858 *** (3.99)	0.6163 *** (5.28)
Lnfdi	−0.1671 * (−1.83)	−0.0053 ** (−2.55)	−0.1724 *** (−6.21)
Ln3rd	−0.0951 *** (−4.93)	−0.0054 ** (−2.38)	−0.1005 *** (−4.91)
lntrans	0.2376 ** (2.11)	0.0374 *** (2.46)	0.2750 *** (3.90)
lntechs	0.0447 (0.16)	0.0013 (0.70)	0.0460 (0.99)
lnpollution	−0.8181 * (−1.83)	0.3024 *** (5.13)	−0.5157 *** (4.02)
rho		0.2857 ** (2.51)	
R^2		0.68	
likelihood ratio		1329.0971	

Note: the value of *t* is in parentheses, and ***, **, and * are significant at the levels of 1%, 5%, and 10%, respectively.

4.4. Robust Test

In order to separate the environmental policy from the regression results, as the former may influence the latter, 45 low-carbon cities and 238 non-low-carbon cities were selected for the regression of the SDM (in February 2017, the National Development and Reform Commission announced the list of the third batch of national low-carbon city pilots, and a total of 45 cities were selected). The results in Table 7 show that *rho* values of 0.1793 and 0.2667 both pass the significance test at the 5% level, indicating that there is still a strong positive spatial correlation of urban carbon intensity with directed technical change in China. Under the SDM, the capital-saving technical change of low-carbon cities has a stronger inhibitory effect on local carbon intensity, with a direct effect coefficient of −0.5346 and an indirect effect coefficient of −0.2616. This shows that the increase in capital-saving technical change can better improve resource utilization, increase the development of new energy technologies, and reduce pollutant emissions in the production process, thereby suppressing the carbon emissions of the local and neighboring areas. For non-low-carbon cities, due to the lack of support for green environmental protection policies, the inhibitory effect of capital-saving technical change on carbon intensity is weakened. Even if the direct effect and the indirect effect are superimposed together, the coefficient is only −0.0510, which is lower than the coefficient of −0.7962 for low-carbon cities. The analysis results of the remaining explanatory variables are generally consistent with the results of Table 3, except for the direct and indirect effects of population density on non-low-carbon cities, which are both shown to significantly promote carbon emissions. Most of the coefficients of the proportion of tertiary industries are significantly positive.

Table 7. Low-carbon cities and non-low-carbon cities.

Variable	Low-Carbon Cities			Non-Low-Carbon Cities		
	Direct Effect	Indirect Effect	Total Effect	Direct Effect	Indirect Effect	Total Effect
lndtc	−0.5346 ***	−0.2616 ***	−0.7962 **	−0.0436 **	−0.0074 **	−0.0510 **
	(−2.72)	(−3.10)	(−2.29)	(−2.29)	(−2.10)	(−1.79)
lnpop	−0.3478 **	−0.1791 *	−0.5269 *	0.0421 **	0.0191 *	0.0612 *
	(−2.13)	(−1.69)	(−1.80)	(2.41)	(1.67)	(1.69)
lnnl	0.1200 ***	0.0132 **	0.1332 **	0.0142 *	0.0124 *	0.0266 **
	(3.62)	(3.30)	(2.06)	(1.74)	(1.81)	(2.40)
lnfdi	−0.1236 **	−0.0981 **	−0.2217 **	−0.0188 ***	−0.0020 ***	−0.0208 ***
	(−2.53)	(−2.07)	(−2.03)	(−5.75)	(−3.96)	(−2.85)
ln3rd	−0.1028 **	0.0145 *	0.0883 *	0.0033 **	0.0174 *	0.0207 **
	(−2.19)	(1.82)	(1.81)	(2.23)	(1.83)	(1.74)
lntrans	0.0337 **	0.0294 *	0.0631 *	0.0013 **	0.0066 *	0.0079 **
	(2.06)	(1.83)	(1.72)	(2.20)	(1.89)	(1.96)
lntechs	0.1394	0.0110	0.1504	0.0411	0.0007	0.0418
	(1.61)	(0.17)	(0.12)	(1.04)	(0.87)	(0.14)
lnpollution	−1.1082 ***	−0.0201 ***	−1.1283 ***	0.1313 **	−0.0507 **	0.0806 **
	(−5.09)	(−2.85)	(−6.20)	(1.96)	(−2.12)	(2.24)
Rho		0.1793 **			0.2667 **	
		(2.23)			(2.50)	
R^2		0.76			0.69	
Likelihood ratio		1319.8709			783.9702	

Note: the value of *t* is in parentheses, and ***, **, and * are significant at the levels of 1%, 5%, and 10%, respectively.

In Table 8, this paper presents three ways to further test the robustness of results: the replacement of geographic weights, the use of the dynamic SDM (the explanatory variable will lag one period), and the replacement of the explanatory variable as the carbon footprint. This shows that the capital-saving technical change still directly or indirectly shows a significant inhibitory effect on the urban carbon intensity in China, proving that the regression results in this article are robust. In addition, by comparing the magnitude of the coefficients, it can be seen that the capital-saving technical change still has a stronger inhibitory effect on the carbon intensity of the local area than that of the neighboring area—that is, the accelerated flow of capital resources in the region and its adjacent areas caused by the capital-saving technical change in the region can not only raise the level of environmental protection technology, but also play a role in reducing the carbon intensity; at the same time, due to the existence of the warning effect, it may also lead to an increasing demand for ecological environment improvement in the surrounding areas; therefore, the governments of the neighboring regions pay more attention to the degree of utilization of technical change, thereby restraining the carbon intensity of the neighboring regions. The performance of the remaining control variables is essentially the same as in Table 3.

Table 8. Robustness test.

Variable	Replacement of Geographic Weights		Dynamic Durbin Model		Replacement of the Explanatory Variable	
	Direct Effect	Indirect Effect	Direct Effect	Indirect Effect	Direct Effect	Indirect Effect
lndtc	−1.0453 ***	−0.0726 **	−0.0203 **	−0.0169 *	−0.0266 ***	−0.0116 **
	(−7.21)	(−2.23)	(−2.14)	(−2.75)	(−2.48)	(−2.48)
lnpop	0.0068 **	0.0205 *	0.0014 *	0.0167 **	0.0031 ***	0.0086 ***
	(2.42)	(1.76)	(1.95)	(2.10)	(2.83)	(4.87)
lnnl	0.0042 ***	0.0076 **	0.1236 **	0.0009 **	0.0051 ***	0.0312 ***
	(2.95)	(2.07)	(2.47)	(2.15)	(3.77)	(3.18)
lnfdi	−0.0136 **	−0.0199 **	−0.0410 ***	−0.0209 ***	−0.5134 **	−0.7758 ***
	(−2.26)	(−2.30)	(−4.39)	(−6.31)	(−2.39)	(5.19)
ln3rd	0.0019 **	0.0025 *	0.0424 **	0.0086 ***	0.0072 **	0.0058 **
	(1.70)	(1.92)	(2.07)	(2.66)	(2.23)	(1.71)
lntrans	0.0414 ***	0.0015 *	0.0009 *	0.0180 **	0.0027 *	−0.0222 **
	(3.04)	(1.95)	(1.78)	(2.05)	(1.73)	(1.88)
lntechs	0.0085	0.0106	0.0007	0.0281	0.0016	0.0459
	(0.94)	(0.38)	(0.96)	(1.06)	(0.55)	(1.35)
lnpollution	−0.0709 ***	0.0172 ***	−0.9781 ***	0.0338 **	−0.0404 **	0.0016 **
	(−4.39)	(2.88)	(−4.22)	(2.12)	(−2.41)	(2.40)
Rho	0.2913 ***		0.1433 ***		0.0136 ***	
	(2.80)		(6.28)		(8.50)	
R^2	0.64		0.49		0.72	
Likelihood ratio	838.7348		1092.5382		1205.9276	

Note: the value of *t* is in parentheses, and ***, **, and * are significant at the levels of 1%, 5%, and 10%, respectively.

5. Conclusions

Based on the SDM, this paper investigates the relationship between directed technical change (capital-saving) and carbon intensity, and then discusses whether the relationship will change in low-carbon cities and non-low-carbon cities. Finally, the robustness of the regression results in the case of replacement of weights, replacement of the *Y* lag period, and replacement of explained variables is explained. The conclusions are as follows: (1) The carbon intensity of Chinese cities is positively and significantly influenced between local cities and the neighboring cities; the carbon intensity of the local city will change by 0.1027% of a unit in the same direction as one unit of a neighboring city—that is, there is a positive spatial correlation between the urban carbon intensity of Chinese cities. (2) The direct effect of capital-saving technical change is greater than the indirect effect, and both the direct and indirect effects are significantly negative—that is, capital-saving technical change has a significant inhibitory effect on local and adjacent carbon intensity. (3) The capital-saving technical change of low-carbon cities has stronger inhibition on local carbon intensity than that of non-low-carbon cities.

Therefore, the policy implications of the results in this paper are as follows: First of all, China is now in a critical period of economic transformation and green development, which requires not only emphasizing and promoting the role of technical change in the coordinated development of urban economy, society, and ecology, but also adjustment of the direction of technical change in a timely manner, in order to contribute to the sustainable development of urban ecological environment in China. Secondly, we should focus on strengthening the interaction and linkage between cities, so that cities with low carbon intensity can play a leading and exemplary role, reducing the growth rate of carbon intensity in adjacent areas. Finally, it should be strongly advocated that the government and relevant departments should appropriately expand the scope of green policies, so that more Chinese cities benefit from the support of green policies and financial investment, and better develop urban energy conservation and emissions reduction activities.

Author Contributions: Conceptualization, H.Z.; methodology, H.K.; software, H.Z.; validation, H.Z.; H.K.; project administration, H.K. All authors have read and agreed to the published version of the manuscript.

Funding: This research received no external funding.

Institutional Review Board Statement: Not applicable.

Informed Consent Statement: Not applicable.

Data Availability Statement: Due to the confidentiality and privacy of the data, they will only be provided upon reasonable request.

Conflicts of Interest: The authors declare no conflict of interest.

References

1. Zemp, M.; Huss, M.; Thibert, E.; Eckert, N.; McNabb, R.W.; Huber, J.; Barandun, M.; Machguth, H.; Nussbaumer, S.U.; Gärtner-Roer, I.; et al. Global glacier mass changes and their contributions to sea-level rise from 1961 to 2016. *Nature* **2019**, *568*, 382–386. [CrossRef] [PubMed]
2. Stainforth, D.A.; Calel, R. New priorities for climate science and climate economics in the 2020s. *Nat. Commun.* **2020**, *11*, 3864. [CrossRef] [PubMed]
3. Li, Z.-Z.; Li, R.Y.M.; Malik, M.Y.; Murshed, M.; Khan, Z.; Umar, M. Determinants of carbon emission in China: How good is green investment? *Sustain. Prod. Consum.* **2021**, *27*, 392–401. [CrossRef]
4. Wang, Y.; Gong, X. Does financial development have a non-linear impact on energy consumption? Evidence from 30 provinces in China. *Energy Econ.* **2020**, *90*, 104845. [CrossRef]
5. He, Y.; Xu, Y.; Pang, Y.; Tian, H.; Wu, R. A regulatory policy to promote renewable energy consumption in China: Review and future evolutionary path. *Renew. Energy* **2016**, *89*, 695–705. [CrossRef]
6. Yu, J.; Shi, X.; Guo, D.; Yang, L. Economic policy uncertainty (EPU) and firm carbon emissions: Evidence using a China provincial EPU index. *Energy Econ.* **2021**, *94*, 105071. [CrossRef]
7. Chinowsky, P.; Hayles, C.; Schweikert, A.; Strzepek, N.; Strzepek, K.; Schlosser, C.A. Climate change: Comparative impact on developing and developed countries. *Eng. Proj. Organ. J.* **2011**, *1*, 67–80. [CrossRef]
8. Porter, M.E. *Competitive Advantage of Nations? The Competitive Advantage of Nations*; The Free Press: New York, NY, USA, 1990; pp. 73–93.
9. Sisco, M.R.; Pianta, S.; Weber, E.U.; Bosetti, V. Global climate marches sharply raise attention to climate change: Analysis of climate search behavior in 46 countries. *J. Environ. Psychol.* **2021**, *75*, 101596. [CrossRef]
10. Antonelli, C.; Feder, C. The new direction of technological change in the global economy. *Struct. Chang. Econ. Dyn.* **2020**, *52*, 1–12. [CrossRef]
11. Nguyen, T.T.; Pham, T.A.T.; Tram, H.T.X. Role of information and communication technologies and innovation in driving carbon emissions and economic growth in selected G-20 countries. *J. Environ. Manag.* **2020**, *261*, 110162. [CrossRef]
12. Sajid, M.J.; Niu, H.; Liang, Z.; Xie, J.; Rahman, M.H.U. Final consumer embedded carbon emissions and externalities: A case of Chinese consumers. *Environ. Dev.* **2021**, *39*, 100642. [CrossRef]
13. Wang, C.; Zhang, L.; Zhou, P.; Chang, Y.; Zhou, D.; Pang, M.; Yin, H. Assessing the environmental externalities for biomass- and coal-fired electricity generation in China: A supply chain perspective. *J. Environ. Manag.* **2019**, *246*, 758–767. [CrossRef] [PubMed]
14. Ke, H.; Dai, S.; Yu, H. Spatial effect of innovation efficiency on ecological footprint: City-level empirical evidence from China. *Environ. Technol. Innov.* **2021**, *22*, 101536. [CrossRef]
15. Khanna, N.; Fridley, D.; Hong, L.X. China's pilot low-carbon city initiative: A comparative assessment of national goals and local plans. *Sustain. Cities Soc.* **2014**, *12*, 110–121. [CrossRef]
16. Mimura, T.; Simayoshi, H.; Suda, T.; Iijima, M.; Mituoka, S. Development of energy saving technology for flue gas carbon dioxide recovery in power plant by chemical absorption method and steam system. *Energy Convers. Manag.* **1997**, *38*, S57–S62. [CrossRef]
17. Adhvaryu, A.; Kala, N.; Nyshadham, A. The light and the heat: Productivity co-benefits of energy-saving technology. *Rev. Econ. Stat.* **2020**, *102*, 779–792. [CrossRef]
18. Almeida, S.T.D.; Borsato, M. Assessing the efficiency of End of Life technology in waste treatment—A bibliometric literature review. *Res. Conserv. Recycl.* **2019**, *140*, 189–208. [CrossRef]
19. Iris, Ç.; Lam, J.S.L. A review of energy efficiency in ports: Operational strategies, technologies and energy management systems. *Renew. Sustain. Energy Rev.* **2019**, *112*, 170–182. [CrossRef]
20. Shove, E. What is wrong with energy efficiency? *Build. Res. Inf.* **2018**, *46*, 779–789. [CrossRef]
21. Raza, A.; Gholami, R.; Rezaee, R.; Rasouli, V.; Rabiei, M. Significant aspects of carbon capture and storage—A review. *Petroleum* **2019**, *5*, 335–340. [CrossRef]
22. Singh, A.; Mishra, N.; Ali, S.I.; Shukla, N.; Shankar, R. Cloud computing technology: Reducing carbon footprint in beef supply chain. *Int. J. Prod. Econ.* **2015**, *164*, 462–471. [CrossRef]
23. Hicks, J.R.S. *The Theory of Wages*; Macmillan: London, UK, 1932.

24. Kennedy, C. Induced bias in innovation and the theory of distribution. *Econ. J.* **1964**, *74*, 541–547. [CrossRef]
25. Samuelson, P.A. Proof that properly anticipated prices fluctuate randomly. *Ind. Manag. Rev.* **1965**, *6*, 41–49.
26. Drandakis, E.M.; Phelps, E.S. A model of induced invention, growth and distribution. *Econ. J.* **1966**, *76*, 823–840. [CrossRef]
27. Acemoglu, D. Why do new technologies complement skills? Directed technical change and wage inequality. *Q. J. Econ.* **1998**, *113*, 1055–1089. [CrossRef]
28. Acemoglu, D. Labor and capital: Augmenting technical change. *J. Eur. Econ. Assoc.* **2003**, *1*, 199–230. [CrossRef]
29. Acemoglu, D.; Aghion, P.; Zilibotti, F. Distance to frontier, selection, and economic growth. *J. Eur. Econ. Assoc.* **2006**, *4*, 37–74. [CrossRef]
30. Acemoglu, D. Equilibrium bias of technology. *Econometrica* **2007**, *75*, 1371–1409. [CrossRef]
31. Jones, C.I. The shape of production function and the direction of technical change. *Q. J. Econ.* **2005**, *120*, 517–549.
32. Acemoglu, D. Directed technical change. *Rev. Econ. Stud.* **2002**, *69*, 781–809. [CrossRef]
33. Chen, Y.H.; Emer, J.; Sze, V. Eyeriss: A spatial architecture for energy-efficient dataflow for convolutional neural networks. *IEEE Micro.* **2016**, *44*, 367–379. [CrossRef]
34. Huang, J.; Xiang, S.; Wu, P.; Chen, X. How to control China's energy consumption through technological progress: A spatial heterogeneous investigation. *Energy* **2022**, *238*, 121965. [CrossRef]
35. Yang, Y.; Liang, S.; Yang, Y.; Xie, G.H.; Zhao, W. Spatial disparity of life-cycle greenhouse gas emissions from corn straw-based bioenergy production in China. *Appl. Energy* **2021**, *305*, 117854. [CrossRef]
36. Vega, S.H.; van Leeuwen, E.; van Twillert, N. Uptake of residential energy efficiency measures and renewable energy: Do spatial factors matter? *Energy Policy* **2021**, *160*, 112659. [CrossRef]
37. Yang, L.; Wang, K.-L.; Geng, J.-C. China's regional ecological energy efficiency and energy saving and pollution abatement potentials: An empirical analysis using epsilon-based measure model. *J. Clean. Prod.* **2018**, *194*, 300–308. [CrossRef]
38. Sun, X. Research on fluctuations and convergency of efficiency in energy conservation and emission reduction in China. *Stat. Inf. Forum* **2010**, *25*, 101–107. [CrossRef]
39. Yao, X.L.; Yu, B. Technical progress, structure change, and carbon dioxide emissions of industry. *Sci. Res. Manag.* **2012**, *33*, 35–40. [CrossRef]
40. Wei, W.X.; Yang, F. Impact of technology advance on carbon dioxide emission in China. *Stat. Res.* **2010**, *27*, 36–44.
41. Färe, R.; Grosskopf, S.; Lovell, C.A.K.; Grifell-Tatjé, E. Biased technical change and the malmquist productivity index. *Scand. J. Econ.* **1997**, *99*, 119–127. [CrossRef]
42. Domazlicky, W. Total factor productivity growth in manufacturing: A regional approach using linear programming. *Reg. Sci. Urban Econ.* **1999**, *29*, 105–122. [CrossRef]
43. Pastor, J.T.; Lovell, C.K.; Aparicio, J. Defining a new graph inefficiency measure for the proportional directional distance function and introducing a new Malmquist productivity index. *Eur. J. Oper. Res.* **2019**, *281*, 222–230. [CrossRef]
44. Kone, A.C.; Buke, T. Factor analysis of projected carbon dioxide emissions according to the ipcc based sustainable emission scenario in turkey. *Renew. Energy* **2019**, *133*, 914–918. [CrossRef]
45. Mulligan, C.; Sala-I-Martin, X. *A Labor-Income-Based Measure of the Value of Human Capital: An Application to the States of the United States*; NBER Working Papers: Cambridge, MA, USA, 1995. [CrossRef]
46. Lu, F.; Liu, M.H.; Sun, Y.Y. Agglomeration, TFP and industrial growth. *Stud. Sci. Sci.* **2018**, *36*, 1575–1584.
47. Wang, B.B.; Qi, S.Z. Biased technological progress, factor substitution and China's industrial energy intensity. *Econ. Res. J.* **2014**, *49*, 115–127.
48. Tu, Z.G.; Chen, L. The direction of technological progress and high-quality economic development: Based on the perspective of TFP and industrial structure upgrading. *J. China Univ. Geosci.* **2019**, *19*, 119–135.
49. Liang, T.; Wang, S.; Lu, C.; Jiang, N.; Long, W.; Zhang, M.; Zhang, R. Environmental impact evaluation of an iron and steel plant in China: Normalized data and direct/indirect contribution. *J. Clean. Prod.* **2020**, *264*, 121697. [CrossRef]
50. Silva, R.; Lbo, R.; Faro, L.E.; Santos, G.; Peixoto, M. Genetic parameters for somatic cell count (scc) and milk production traits of guzerá cows using data normalized by different procedures. *Trop. Anim. Health Prod.* **2020**, *52*, 2513–2522. [CrossRef]
51. Dietz, T.; Rosa, E.A. Rethinking the environmental impacts of population, affluence and technology. *Hum. Ecol. Rev.* **1994**, *1*, 277–300.
52. Chen, J.D.; Wang, B.; Huang, S.; Song, M. The influence of increased population density in China on air pollution. *Sci. Total Environ.* **2020**, *735*, 139456. [CrossRef]
53. Acemoglu, D.; Aghion, P.; Bursztyn, L.; Hemous, D. The environment and directed technical change. *Am. Econ. Rev.* **2012**, *102*, 131–166. [CrossRef]
54. Stengos, T.; Fatouros, N. *Nuclear Energy, Economic Growth and the Environment: Optimal Policies in a Model with Endogenous Technical Change and Environmental Constraints*; University of Guelph: Guelph, ON, Canada, 2020.
55. Wang, X.; Wang, Y.; Lan, Y. Measuring the bias of technical change of industrial energy and environment productivity in China: A global DEA-Malmquist productivity approach. *Environ. Sci. Pollut. Res.* **2021**, *28*, 41896–41911. [CrossRef] [PubMed]
56. Bao, C.; Chen, X.J.; Liang, G.L. Analysis on the influencing factors of water use efficiency in Henan province based on spatial econometric models. *J. Nat. Resour.* **2016**, *31*, 1138–1147.
57. Anselin, L.; Le, G.J.; Jayet, H. Spatial panel econometrics. In *The Econometrics of Panel Data, Fundamentals and Recent Developments in Theory and Practice*, 3rd ed.; Matyas, L., Sevestre, P., Eds.; Kluwer: Dordrecht, The Netherlands, 2006.

58. Druska, V.; Horrace, W.C. Generalized moments estimation for spatial panel data: Indonesian rice farming. *Am. J. Agric. Econ.* **2004**, *86*, 185–198. [CrossRef]
59. Baltagi, B.; Song, S.H.; Koh, W. Testing panel data regression models with spatial error correlation. *J. Econ.* **2003**, *117*, 123–150. [CrossRef]
60. Anselin, L.; Hudak, S. Spatial econometrics in practice: A review of software options. *Reg. Sci. Urban Econ.* **1992**, *22*, 509–536. [CrossRef]
61. Yang, Y.; Zhao, T.; Wang, Y.; Shi, Z. Research on impacts of population-related factors on carbon emissions in Beijing from 1984 to 2012. *Environ. Impact Assess. Rev.* **2015**, *55*, 45–53. [CrossRef]
62. Bai, C.Q.; Zhou, L.; Xia, M.L.; Feng, C. Analysis of the spatial association network structure of China's transportation carbon emissions and its driving factors. *J. Environ. Manag.* **2020**, *253*, 109765. [CrossRef]
63. Elhorst, J.P. Matlab software for spatial panels. *Int. Reg. Sci. Rev.* **2014**, *37*, 389–405. [CrossRef]
64. Lesage, J.P.; Pace, R.K. *Introduction to Spatial Econometrics*; CRC Press: Boca Raton, FL, USA, 2009.
65. Gómez-Rubio, V.; Bivand, R.S.; Rue, H. Estimating spatial econometrics models with integrated nested laplace approximation. *Mathematics* **2021**, *9*, 2044. [CrossRef]
66. Anselin, L.; Bera, A.K.; Florax, R.; Yoon, M.J. Simple diagnostic tests for spatial dependence. *Reg. Sci. Urban Econ.* **1996**, *26*, 77–104. [CrossRef]
67. Baltagi, B.H.; Li, Q. Testing AR(1) against MA(1) disturbances in an error component model. *J. Econ.* **1995**, *68*, 133–151. [CrossRef]
68. Anselin, L. *Spatial Econometrics: Methods and Models*; Kluwer Academic Publishers: Boston, MA, USA, 1988.
69. Zhang, J.F.; Fang, Y. A robust test for spatial errors models. *J. Quant. Tech. Econ.* **2011**, *28*, 152–160. [CrossRef]

International Journal of
Environmental Research and Public Health

MDPI

Article

Study on Regional Differences and Convergence of Green Development Efficiency of the Chemical Industry in the Yangtze River Economic Belt Based on Grey Water Footprint

Yunbo Xiang [1], Wen Shao [1], Shengyun Wang [2,*], Yong Zhang [1] and Yaxin Zhang [2]

[1] School of Architecture and Art Design, Hunan University of Science and Technology, Xiangtan 411201, China; yunb.xiang@hnust.edu.cn (Y.X.); shaowen0921@163.com (W.S.); hnkdzhyong@sina.com (Y.Z.)
[2] Research Center for Economic and Social Development in Central China of Nanchang University, Nanchang University, Nanchang 330031, China; zhangyaxin0926@163.com
* Correspondence: wangshengyun@163.com

Abstract: Grey water footprint is included in the green development efficiency evaluation index system of the chemical industry. From 2002 to 2016, the super efficiency Slack Based Measure (SBM) model was used to measure the green development efficiency of the chemical industry in the Yangtze River Economic Belt. Dagum Gini coefficient and its decomposition method were used to decompose the regional differences of green development efficiency of the chemical industry in the Economic Belt, and the coefficient of variation method and panel data regression model were used to test the convergence characteristics. The following results were obtained. (1) The total grey water footprint of the chemical industry in the Yangtze River Economic Belt showed a fluctuating downward trend from 2002 to 2016. (2) The green development efficiency of the chemical industry in the Yangtze River Economic Belt was significantly improved, and the spatial differentiation law of gradient decline in the upper, middle, and lower reaches of the Economic Belt was shown. (3) The regional difference of green development efficiency of the chemical industry in the Yangtze River Economic Belt initially showed an expanding trend and then a narrowing trend. Regional differences in the upper reaches of the Yangtze River increased while those in the middle reaches first increased and then decreased, whereas those in the lower reaches decreased significantly. The variance in green development efficiency of the chemical industry is the main cause of regional differences. (4) From 2012 to 2016, the Yangtze River Economic Belt had obvious convergence in its whole region, middle reaches, and lower reaches and an inconspicuous convergence in the upstream area. Regional difference of green development efficiency of the chemical industry in the Economic Belt was the combined effect of the results of environmental regulation, industrial structure, foreign investment intensity, and scientific and technological advancements. Our results have high theoretical reference values and practical guiding significance for implementing the green efficiency promotion strategy of the chemical industry in Yangtze River Economic Belt by region and classification.

Keywords: chemical industry; green development efficiency; grey water footprint; regional differences; convergence; Yangtze River Economic Belt

Citation: Xiang, Y.; Shao, W.; Wang, S.; Zhang, Y.; Zhang, Y. Study on Regional Differences and Convergence of Green Development Efficiency of the Chemical Industry in the Yangtze River Economic Belt Based on Grey Water Footprint. *Int. J. Environ. Res. Public Health* **2022**, *19*, 1703. https://doi.org/10.3390/ijerph19031703

Academic Editors: Roberto Alonso González Lezcano, Francesco Nocera and Rosa Giuseppina Caponetto

Received: 2 December 2021
Accepted: 28 January 2022
Published: 2 February 2022

1. Introduction

The Yangtze River Economic Belt is one of the most critical contradiction areas between economic development and environmental protection in China [1]. A total 40% of available freshwater resources and more than 20% of its wetland resources in China are concentrated in the Yangtze River Basin, which covers 204 national aquatic germplasm resources protection zones. The River Basin is one of the important ecological security barriers and economic centers in China [2]. The chemical industry is a basic and pillar industry of the national economy, with high dependence on water and energy as well as high safety and environmental risks [3]. China is the largest chemical producer in the world. In 2018, its chemical turnover was 119.8 million EUR, accounting for 35.8% of the global chemical sales for the year [4]. The production value of chemical products in the Yangtze River Economic Belt accounts for more than 40% of the country's total. At present, "chemical industry encircling the river" poses challenges to the Yangtze River Economic Belt. There are more than 400,000 chemical enterprises, 5 steel bases, 7 oil refineries, and many large petrochemical bases along the Yangtze River, leading to a greater risk of environmental pollution [5]. In the "joint efforts to protect" and under the general requirements of "no large-scale development", the green transformation and development of the chemical industry in the Yangtze River Economic Belt is particularly urgent.

The Chinese economy has entered a high-quality development stage from the high-speed growth stage now. The traditional industrial development mode of high energy consumption, high pollution, and high emission has gradually changed to the intensive, efficient, and sustainable green development mode. The Chinese government has attached great importance to the green development of the chemical industry in the Yangtze River Economic Belt. On 14 November 2020, General Secretary Xi Jinping presided over a forum that aimed to promote the comprehensive development of the Yangtze River Economic Belt, stressing the need to make it the main battlefield of Chinese ecological priority and green development. Relevant departments of the state have also issued a series of policies and regulations, such as guiding opinions on strengthening the green development of industries in the Economic Belt, the ecological environment protection plan for the area, the Law of the People's Republic of China on the Protection of the Yangtze River, and so forth. All of these endeavors actively promote the green transformation and upgrading of the chemical industry in the Yangtze River Economic Belt. In the past five years, more than 8000 chemical enterprises along the Economic Belt have been reformed, relocated, transformed, or closed. Remarkable achievements have been made in the green transformation and development of the chemical industry. The ecological environment has been significantly improved. The proportion of excellent water quality sections in the Yangtze River basin increased from 82.3% in 2016 to 91.7% in 2019 and further increased to 96.3% from January to November 2020. The elimination of poor V water bodies achieved for the first time in 2020. It can be seen that comprehensively promoting the green development of the chemical industry and improving its green development efficiency [6] are key to solving the dilemma of the "chemical industry surrounding the river", which ensures environmental and industrial development safety and realizes the sustainable development of the chemical industry. The Yangtze River Economic Belt includes 9 provinces, 2 cities, and 11 provincial administrative units and covers an area of approximately 2.05 million km^2 [7]. Due to the differences in resource conditions, economic development levels, innovation abilities, and chemical industry development histories, the spatial distribution and green development level of the chemical industry show spatial heterogeneity, which increases the challenge for the Economic Belt to promote the industrial green development. In order to measure the gray water footprint and green development efficiency of the chemical industry in the Yangtze River Economic Belt, to reveal the spatial differences and their convergence in the green development efficiency of the chemical industry in 11 provinces and cities, and to provide policy support for the green development of the chemical industry in the Yangtze River Economic Belt, this research systematically studied the regional differences and convergence of green development efficiency of the chemical industry in the Yangtze River Economic Belt. The results are expected to be valuable in theoretical reference and practical significance for implementing green development promotion strategy of the chemical industry in different regions and categories.

2. Literature Review

The concept of "green development" was first proposed by the United Nations Development Programme in 2002. The essence of green development is to regard resources and the environment as endogenous factors of growth and provide a balance between economic growth and ecological environment protection by changing the dynamic mechanism of economic development to form a new sustainable development model [8,9]. From the perspective of input and output, green development efficiency refers to the proportional relationship between green development output and input. Green development efficiency is an important indicator to analyze the degree of green development of industries and is often used to reflect the completion degree, achievements, and effectiveness of green development. Since data envelopment analysis (DEA) can consider a variety of input and output and does not need to set specific function forms, it has become the mainstream method to measure green development efficiency [10]. Pittman (1983) first included "undesirable" output into the productivity analysis process [11]. Chung et al. (1997) proposed directional distance function and the Malmquist–Luenberger Index (MLI), which carries out productivity evaluation after the "undesirable" output is considered reasonable [12]. Tone (2001, 2002) proposed a SBM model that considers relaxation measures to effectively overcome radial and angular defects [13,14]. A DEA analysis method based on the measurement of slack variables, which puts the input and output slack directly into the objective function so that it can directly measure the inefficiency caused by slack compared to the optimal production frontier, thus solving the problem of input and output slack in the traditional DEA model, removing the inefficiency caused by slack, and also solving the problem of productivity evaluation in the presence of non-expected outputs. Many scholars used the DEA model to discuss the green development efficiency of the chemical industry. Tanzil and Beloff (2006) summarized the sustainability indicators and indicators of the chemical industry, focusing on ecological efficiency and company-specific indicators [15]. Alessandro et al. (2017) measured the environmental economic efficiency of Italian and German chemical enterprises [16]. Yeh Jiahuey et al. (2019) calculated the total factor green energy efficiency of China's chemical industry [17]. Yijun Zhang et al. (2020) used the three-stage SBM–DEA model and MLI to measure the green total factor productivity (GTFP) of China's chemical industry [6]. Sun Honghai (2017) used super-efficiency DEA to calculate the ecological efficiency of 25 petrochemical enterprises in China [18]. Yuan Yaqiong (2018) used DEA and value-driven analysis to evaluate the ecological efficiency of heavy chemical enterprises in Beijing, Tianjin, and Hebei region from 2012 to 2016 [19]. Lu Qiuqin et al. (2020) used the improved three-stage DEA model to evaluate the transformation and upgrading efficiency of China's coal chemical enterprises [20].

When using DEA, researchers usually take labor, capital, and energy as inputs, the output value of the chemical industry as the expected output, and environmental pollutants as the unexpected output to build an evaluation model of green development efficiency of the chemical industry. These indicators do not consider the characteristics of the chemical industry, which has a great impact on water environment. Tony Allan proposed "Virtual Water"; Hoekstra et al. proposed the concept of "Water Footprint". Grey water footprint refers to the volume of freshwater required to dilute certain pollutants on the basis of existing water quality standards and natural background concentration [21]. Given that water footprint and grey water footprint can better represent the water consumption and water pollution accounting of industries [22], they have been gradually incorporated into the evaluation framework of the green development efficiency of regional industries [23,24].

The spatial distribution and environmental risk of the chemical industry in the Yangtze River Economic Belt have always been hot areas of academic concern. For a long time, the spatial layout of the chemical industry in the Economic Belt has reflected two major factors: the proximity to raw materials and market. The chemical industry along the Yangtze River is mainly distributed in the areas of Shanghai and Jiangsu [25]. In recent years, the petrochemical industry had a trend of expansion along the river to the upstream. The environmental pollution load gradient also shifted to the middle and upper reaches, and the environmental risk increased [26,27]. Xiang et al. (2021) found that the spatial differentiation characteristics of green development efficiency of the chemical industry in the Yangtze River Economic Belt were obvious. Economic level, scientific and technological innovation, industrial structure, and industrial agglomeration are the main factors affecting the spatial differentiation of green development efficiency of the chemical industry in the

Economic Belt. The impact of foreign investment intensity and environmental regulation is relatively weak [28]. Therefore, it is necessary to guide the chemical industry of the Yangtze River Economic Belt to gather in large coastal bases and raw material producing or consumption areas, improve the rate of chemical enterprises entering the park, and optimize the spatial layout of the chemical industry [29]. Some scholars also studied the negative effects of the development of the chemical industry on the ecological environment. Zhu Deming et al. (2006) showed that the development of the chemical industry along the Yangtze River in Jiangsu threatened the drinking water source and water supply safety [30]. Intensive chemical enterprises and unreasonable industrial layout along the Yangtze River Economic Belt have brought some potential environmental risks to the environmental protection of the Yangtze River Basin [31,32]. Dong et al. (2020) found that the division level of heavy chemical industry in the middle and upper reaches of the Yangtze River Economic Belt decreased, which promoted the decline of the regional pollution level [33].

The contribution of this research is mainly reflected in the following aspects. Firstly, it makes up for the industry characteristics that little considered the impact of the chemical industry on the water environment in previous studies. In this study, water footprint and grey water footprint are included in the green development efficiency measurement index system of the chemical industry, and the green development efficiency of the chemical industry is established by using DEA, which was calculated from 2002 to 2016 in the Yangtze River Economic Belt. Secondly, Dagum Gini coefficient and its decomposition method are used to decompose the regional differences of green development efficiency of the chemical industry in the Economic Belt. Lastly, the convergence characteristics of green development efficiency of the chemical industry in the Economic Belt and its upstream, middle, and lower reaches are tested with the coefficient of variation method and panel data regression model from three aspects, i.e., convergence, absolute convergence, and conditional absolute convergence.

3. Materials and Methods

3.1. Regional Overview

The Yangtze River Economic Belt consists of the 11 provincial administrative units of Shanghai, Jiangsu, Zhejiang, Anhui, Jiangxi, Hubei, Hunan, Guizhou, Chongqing, Sichuan, and Yunnan (Figure 1) and covers an area of about 2.05 million km^2, accounting for 21% of the country and more than 40% of the total population and economy [7]. It is one of the Chinese chemical industry agglomeration areas. In 2016, 11 provinces and cities in the Yangtze River Economic Belt achieved a total sales value of 8253.40 billion RMB, accounting for 43.46% of the total sales value in China. The sales output values of the chemical industry in downstream areas, middle reaches, and upstream area were 530.18 billion RMB, 1816.96 billion RMB, and 1134.663 billion RMB, accounting, respectively, for 27.91%, 9.57%, and 5.97% of that in China. The sales value of the chemical industry in Jiangsu province was the highest at 2954.89 billion RMB, about 15.56% of the whole country, while that in Yunnan province was the lowest at 139.00 billion RMB, accounting for 0.73% of that in the whole country [28].

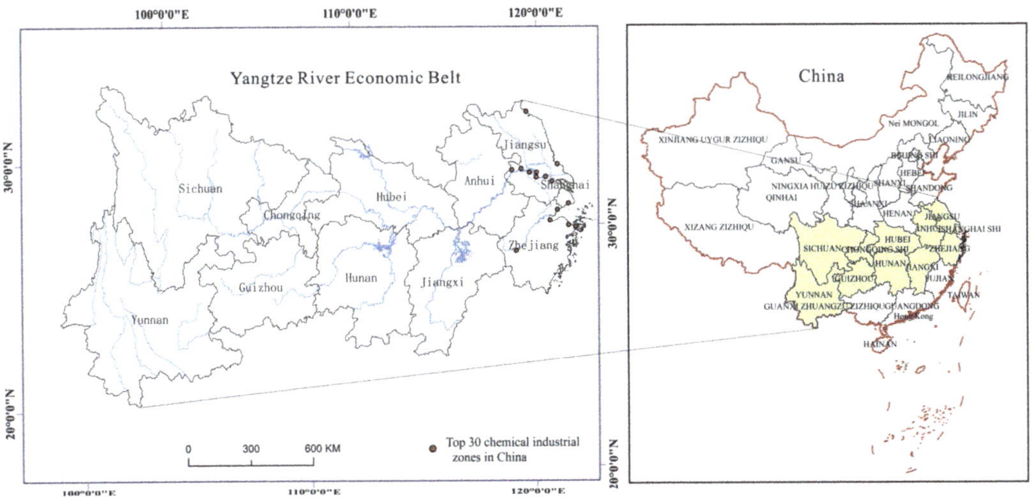

Figure 1. Map of the Yangtze Economic Belt.

3.2. Methods

3.2.1. Calculation of Grey Water Footprint of the Chemical Industry

Industrial wastewater is directly discharged into surface water. The main pollutants in industrial wastewater can be measured directly, such as chemical oxygen demand (COD) and ammonia nitrogen (NH_4^+-N) in chemical industry wastewater. Therefore, COD and NH_4^+-N are used as the main indicators to measure the grey water footprint of the chemical industry. The calculation formula is as follows [23]:

$$GWF_{ind} = \max(GWF_{ind(COD)}, GWF_{ind(NH_4^+-N)})$$

$$GWF_{ind(i)} = \frac{L_{ind(i)}}{C_{\max} - C_{nat}} - W_{ed}$$

$$GWF_{reg} = \sum_{i=1}^{n} GWF_{ind(i)}$$

where GWF_{ind} (billion m^3) is the grey water footprint of the chemical industry, $GWF_{ind(i)}$ (billion m^3) is the grey water footprint of the chemical industry with the standard of category i pollutants, W_{ed} (billion m^3) is the discharge amount of chemical industry wastewater, and GWF_{reg} (billion m^3) is the grey water footprint of the regional chemical industry. China's Standard Limits for Basic Items of Surface Water Environmental Quality Standard (GB 3838-2002) is used as the standard. In the standard, the water quality is required to meet the class III water quality index, and the concentration limits of COD and ammonia nitrogen (NH_4^+-N) in class III water are taken as the environmental concentration standards of COD and ammonia nitrogen (NH_4^+-N) in water.

3.2.2. Measurement Model of Green Development Efficiency of the Chemical Industry

The SBM–undesirable model was proposed to measure the green development efficiency of the chemical industry. It is calculated as [34]: Supposing there are n individual *DMUs*, including input vector, expected output, and unexpected output, respectively, that are recorded as x, $x \in R_m$, $y^g \in R_{s1}$, and $y^b \in R_{s2}$. The matrix is defined as

$$X = [x_1, x_2, \ldots, x_n] \in R_{m\times n},\ Y^g = [y_1^g, y_2^g, \ldots, y_n^g] \in R_{s1\times n},\ Y^b = [y_1^b, y_2^b, \ldots, y_n^b] \in R_{s2\times n}$$

According to the actual input and output, supposing $x_i > 0, y_i^g > 0, y_i^b > 0$, productive collection P, that is, N element input X. All combinations of expected and undesired outputs can be defined as

$$P = \left\{ (x, y^g, y^b) \middle| x \geq X\lambda, y^g \geq Y^b\lambda, y^b \geq Y^b\lambda(\lambda \geq 0) \right\}$$

Therefore, the SBM–undesirable model can be expressed as

$$p* = \min \frac{1 - \frac{1}{m}\sum\limits_{i=1}^{i} \frac{S_i^-}{X_{i0}}}{1 + \frac{1}{S_1+S_2}\left(\sum\limits_{r=1}^{S_1} \frac{S_r^g}{y_{r0}^g} + \sum\limits_{r=1}^{S_2} \frac{S_r^b}{y_{r0}^b} \right)}, \ s.t. \begin{cases} X_0 = X\lambda + S^- \\ y_0^g = Y^g\lambda + S^g \\ y_0^b = Y^b\lambda + S^b \\ S^- \geq 0, S^g \geq 0, S^b \geq 0, \lambda \geq 0 \end{cases}$$

Type: S_i^-, S_r^g, and S_r^b, respectively, represent the first i_0 input redundancy, expected output deficiency, and expected output superscalar of each decision-making unit; S_i^-, S_r^g, and S_r^b, respectively, denote their corresponding vectors; and λ is the weight vector. The optimal solution of the above formula is (λ^*, S^{-*}, S^{g*}, S^{b*}). $P^* = 1$ only when the bad output exists, that is, $S^{-*} = 0$, $S^{g*} = 0$, $S^{b*} = 0$ when DMU_0 is efficient.

3.2.3. Dagum Gini Coefficient and Decomposition Method

By using the Dagum Gini coefficient method, this study analyzes the spatial differences and sources of green development efficiency of the chemical industry in the upper, middle, and lower reaches of the Yangtze River Economic Belt. According to the Gini coefficient and its subgroup decomposition method proposed by Dagum (1997), the definition of Gini coefficient G is as shown in Equation (1) [35]:

$$G = \frac{\sum_{j=1}^{k}\sum_{h=1}^{k}\sum_{i=1}^{n_j}\sum_{r=1}^{n_h}|y_{ji} - y_{hr}|}{2n^2\overline{y}} \tag{1}$$

where j and h are subscripts for different regions; i and r are the indexes of provinces and cities, respectively; n is the total number of provinces and cities; k is the total number of regions; and $n_j(n_h)$ and $j(h)$ are the number of provinces and cities within a region. $y_{ji}(y_{hr})$ is the green development efficiency of the chemical industry in $j(h)$ regional provinces and cities $i(r)$, and $\overline{y}$ is the average value of green development efficiency of the chemical industry in all provinces and cities. On the overall Gini coefficient G by region, according to the average value of green development efficiency of the chemical industry in each region k, the region is sorted and then the Gini coefficient G is divided into three parts: intraregion (intra-group) difference pairs G contribution of G_w, interregional (inter-group) difference pairs G contribution of G_{nb}, and interregional (inter-group) ultra-variable density pairs G contribution of G_t. When the three meet, $G = G_w + G_{nb} + G_t$, in which the area j has a Gini coefficient of G_{jj} and intraregional differences G_w. The calculation formulas are Formulas (2) and (3), respectively; zones j and h have a Gini coefficient between G_{jh} and the regional net difference G_{nb}. The calculation formulas are Formulas (4) and (5), respectively. The calculation formula for the interregional super-variable density G_t is shown in Formula (6).

$$G_{jj} = \frac{\frac{1}{2\overline{y}_j}\sum_{i=1}^{n_j}\sum_{r=1}^{n_j}|y_{ji} - y_{jr}|}{n_j^2} \tag{2}$$

$$G_w = \sum_{j=1}^{k} G_{jj}P_jS_j \tag{3}$$

$$G_{jh} = \sum_{i=1}^{n_j}\sum_{r=1}^{n_h}\frac{|y_{ji} - y_{hr}|}{n_jn_h(\overline{y}_j + \overline{y}_h)} \tag{4}$$

$$G_{nb} = \sum_{j-2}^{k} \sum_{h-1}^{j-1} G_{jh}(p_j s_h + p_h s_j) D_{jh} \tag{5}$$

$$G_t = \sum_{j=2}^{k} \sum_{h=1}^{j-1} G_{jh}(p_j s_h + p_h s_j)(1 - D_{jh}) \tag{6}$$

In Equation (5), $p_j = n_j/n$, $s_j = n_j\overline{y}_j/n\overline{y}$, and $j = 1, 2, 3$. In Equation (7), D_{jh} denotes region j and h. See Formula (7) for the relative influence of green development efficiency of the chemical industry. d_{jh} is the difference of the green development efficiency of the chemical industry between regions (see Equation (8)). j, h all $y_{ji} - y_{hr} > 0$ is the mathematical expectation of the sample summation; p_{jh} is the super-variable first-order moment, representing the region. j, h all $y_{hr} - y_{ji} > 0$ is the mathematical expectation of the sample summation.

$$D_{jh} = \frac{d_{jh} - p_{jh}}{d_{jh} + p_{jh}} \tag{7}$$

$$d_{jh} = \int_0^{\infty} dF_j(y) \int_0^{y} (y - x) dF_h(x) \tag{8}$$

$$p_{jh} = \int_0^{\infty} dF_h(y) \int_0^{y} (y - x) dF_j(x) \tag{9}$$

where $F_j(F_h)$ represents the area $j(h)C$, which is the cumulative distribution function of green development efficiency of the chemical industry.

3.2.4. Convergence Model

To investigate the evolution trend of green development efficiency of the chemical industry in the whole Yangtze River Economic Belt and the upper, middle, and lower reaches, the convergence analysis is carried out, including σ Convergence and β Convergence.

σ Convergence refers to the trend where the deviation of green development efficiency of the chemical industry in different regions is decreasing over time. σ Convergence is measured by the coefficient of variation and can be calculated as [36]:

$$\sigma = \frac{\sqrt{\sum_{i}^{N_j} (F_{ij} - \overline{F}_{ij})^2 / N_j}}{\overline{F}_{ij}}$$

where j indicates the number of areas (j = 1, 2, 3 ...), i indicates the number of provinces and cities in the region (i = 1, 2, 3 ...), N_j is the number of provinces and cities in each region, and F_{ij} denotes that the region j exists t with an average value of green development efficiency of the chemical industry in the period.

The β convergence model is [36]:

$$\ln\left(\frac{F_{i,t+1}}{F_{i,t}}\right) = \alpha + \beta F_{i,t} + \mu_i + \nu_t + \varepsilon_{it}$$

The left side of the model is the growth rate of green development efficiency of the chemical industry calculated by logarithmic difference, where μ_i is a fixed effect, v_t is a time-fixed effect, and ε_{it} is a random error term.

In condition β, the convergence model is absolute β. A series of control variables is added to the convergence model. This study adds environmental regulation, industrial structure, technical level, and foreign investment intensity as control variables. The convergence model for condition β is

$$\ln\left(\frac{F_{i,t+1}}{F_{i,t}}\right) = \alpha + \beta F_{i,t} + \delta X + \mu_i + \nu_t + \varepsilon_{it}$$

In the regression process, each variable is logarithmic. In this paper, a two-way fixed effect model is adopted to improve the coefficient. In the β accuracy of estimation, the robust error standard of clustering is adopted to the provincial and municipal levels. If $\beta < 0$ and is significant, the green development efficiency of the chemical industry in the Yangtze River Economic Belt converges, or it diverges. The rate of convergence $b = -\ln(1+\beta)/T$.

3.3. Index Selection and Data Processing

3.3.1. Measurement Index of Green Development Efficiency of the Chemical Industry

According to existing research results, combined with the classification and characteristics of the chemical industry, the evaluation index system of green development efficiency of the chemical industry is constructed from input and output. Manpower, capital, energy, and water for the chemical industry are selected as investment indexes. The sales output value of the chemical industry is selected as the expected output index and the grey water footprint of the chemical industry as the unexpected output index (Table 1).

Table 1. Evaluation index system of green development efficiency of the chemical industry.

Index		Variable	Variable Declaration
Input index		Human input	Average annual number of employees in chemical industry (10,000)
		Capital input	Net fixed assets of chemical industry (100 million CNY)
		Energy input	Total energy consumption of chemical industry (ten thousand tec)
		Water input	Chemical industry water consumption (100 million m^3)
Output index	Expected output	Chemical industry output value	Sales output value of chemical industry (100 million CNY)
	Unexpected output	Water pollution	Chemical industry grey water footprint (billion m^3)

Considering the availability of data of the chemical industry, the scope of the chemical industry is defined as five subsectors in the manufacturing industry by the *China Industrial Statistics Yearbook*: petroleum processing, coking and nuclear fuel processing; chemical raw materials and chemical products manufacturing; pharmaceutical manufacturing; chemical fiber manufacturing; and rubber and plastic products manufacturing. Relevant data come from the *China Industrial Statistics Yearbook*, *China Environmental Statistics Yearbook*, *China Statistical Yearbook*, and statistical yearbooks of various provinces and cities from 2003 to 2017. *China Industrial Statistical Yearbook*, *China Environmental Statistical Yearbook*, and *China Statistical Yearbook* are the most authoritative and important sources of data for conducting research on China's socioeconomic development, available in both paper and electronic versions, published annually by the National Bureau of Statistics of China, and can be accessed through a variety of official channels for direct access to relevant data. The details are as follows. The missing data are estimated by intermediate interpolation method. There are no direct statistical data of total industrial water consumption and wastewater discharge in the statistical yearbook, so we apply the data of industrial wastewater and pollutant discharge in wastewater for each subsector in China to estimate the data of pollutant discharge in industrial wastewater for each subsector in each province [37]. Energy data of the chemical industry are estimated by reference [38]. For the net fixed capital and industrial sales output value of the chemical industry, the fixed assets investment price index of corresponding provinces and cities and the ex-factory price index of industrial producers are used for price reduction, which is reduced to the level of 2000.

3.3.2. Variables Affecting the Efficiency of Green Development of the Chemical Industry

Using environmental regulations, industrial structure, foreign investment intensity and technological progress as control variables, this paper studied their influence on the green development efficiency of the chemical industry in the Yangtze River Economic Belt. Among them, the total amount of environmental governance for environmental regulation represents the proportion of GDP. Science and technology investment is represented by the proportion of science and technology expenditure in fiscal expenditure, which is representative of the investment amount of foreign-funded enterprises at the end of the year. The proportion of the secondary industry in GDP represents the industrial structure.

4. Results

4.1. Evolution Characteristics of Grey Water Footprint of the Chemical Industry in the Yangtze River Economic Belt

The grey water footprint of the chemical industry in the Yangtze River Economic Belt declined from 2002 to 2016 with a trend of fluctuation. It decreased from 16.03 billion m^3 in 2002 to 12.03 billion m^3 in 2008 and then increased to 14.43 billion m^3 in 2016. In 2008, due to the impact of the financial crisis, the operation of chemical enterprises was impacted, the production capacity decreased, and the total grey water footprint was at its lowest point. After the financial crisis, thanks to the support of relevant national policies, chemical enterprises gradually eliminated the crisis, the output of the chemical industry gradually recovered, and the discharge of wastewater in the chemical industry increased, leading to an increase in the total grey water footprint of the chemical industry.

The grey water footprint of the chemical industry in Jiangsu, Zhejiang, Hubei, Hunan, Sichuan, and Yunnan provinces is relatively high. These provinces are the main concentration provinces of the chemical industry in the Economic Belt, with large-scale enterprises that have high amounts of wastewater discharge. The chemical industry in Shanghai has the lowest wastewater footprint. On the one hand, Shanghai has accelerated the adjustment of its industrial structure, the proportion of the chemical industry in the national economy has decreased, and the overall scale of the chemical industry has shrunk. In 2016, the sales value of its chemical industry only accounted for 2.67% of that in China. On the other hand, the chemical industry in Shanghai is gradually transforming and upgrading to the direction of a high-end, green, and low-carbon chemical industry. Shanghai has carried out the construction of a "Green Industrial zone" earlier in China, and its environmental and economic indicators of 10,000 CNY of output value led the national level of the same industry. The grey water footprint of the chemical industry in Guizhou is relatively low, mainly because of the small scale of the chemical industry. In 2016, the sales value of the chemical industry in Guizhou only accounted for 0.83% of the national total (Figure 2).

4.2. Spatial and Temporal Evolution of Green Development Efficiency of the Chemical Industry in Yangtze River Economic Belt

From 2002 to 2016, the green development efficiency of the chemical industry in the Yangtze River Economic Belt showed an overall development and evolution trend of first decreasing and then increasing, with an average of 0.5163, only reaching the optimal level of 51.63% (Table 2). This trend showed that the overall level of green development efficiency of the chemical industry is not high and still has great growth potential. Note that the green development efficiency of the chemical industry showed a downward trend from 2002 to 2005, which may be due to the reversal of China's economic model in the later stage of its 11th Five-Year Plan. Moreover, the chemical industry turned back to the development model of high consumption, high pollution emission, and low efficiency. The average green development efficiency of the chemical industry in the Yangtze River Economic Belt increased significantly during 2012 and 2016, which is the reason that provinces and cities in the Economic Belt accelerated the green development, transformation, and upgrading of the chemical industry and achieved remarkable results after the 18th National Congress.

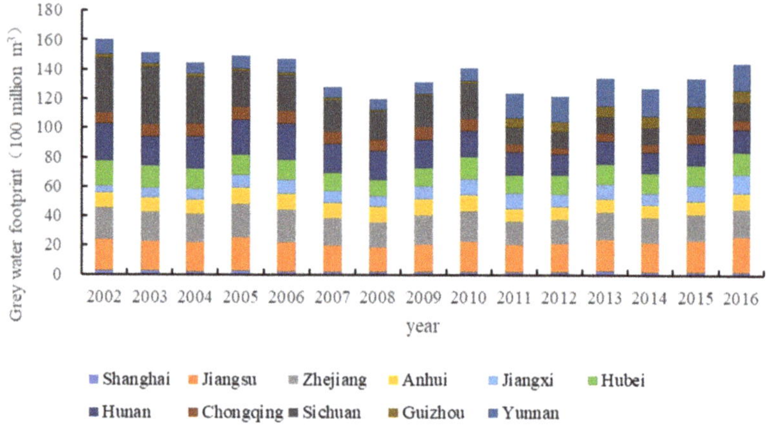

Figure 2. Grey water footprint of the chemical industry in Yangtze River Economic Belt.

Table 2. Green development efficiency of the chemical industry in the Yangtze River Economic Belt from 2002 to 2016.

	2002	2004	2006	2008	2010	2012	2014	2016 Year	Average
Guizhou	0.2809	0.2351	0.2131	0.2176	0.1984	0.1916	0.1973	0.2612	0.2271
Sichuan	0.2390	0.2538	0.2836	0.3366	0.3461	0.3634	0.4109	0.4922	0.3387
Yunnan	0.2243	0.2401	0.2581	0.3114	0.2640	0.2395	0.2422	0.2916	0.2569
Chongqing	0.2508	0.2370	0.2204	0.2526	0.2517	0.2742	0.3041	0.3918	0.2728
Hubei	0.3794	0.3117	0.3173	0.3687	0.3447	0.4368	0.4817	0.5043	0.3883
Hunan	0.2938	0.2609	0.2718	0.3177	0.3363	1.0000	1.0000	1.0000	0.5312
Jiangxi	0.3132	0.2679	0.2746	0.2770	0.3506	0.3521	0.4005	0.4052	0.3273
Anhui	0.3129	0.3177	0.3099	0.3357	0.3410	0.3593	0.4124	0.4346	0.3512
Jiangsu	1.0000	1.0000	1.0000	1.0000	1.0000	1.0000	1.0000	1.0000	0.9860
Shanghai	1.0000	1.0000	1.0000	1.0000	1.0000	1.0000	1.0000	1.0000	1.0000
Zhejiang	1.0000	1.0000	1.0000	1.0000	1.0000	1.0000	1.0000	1.0000	1.0000
Upstream area	0.2488	0.2415	0.2438	0.2795	0.2650	0.2672	0.2886	0.3592	0.2739
Midstream area	0.3288	0.2802	0.2879	0.3211	0.3438	0.5963	0.6274	0.6365	0.4156
Downstream area	0.8282	0.8294	0.8275	0.8339	0.8352	0.8398	0.8531	0.8586	0.8343
Whole area	0.4813	0.4658	0.4681	0.4925	0.4939	0.5652	0.5863	0.6164	0.5163

From the upstream, midstream, and downstream areas, the average green development efficiency from 2002 to 2016 of the chemical industry in the downstream area was 0.8343, which was in a high-level development state with a small overall change range. The average green efficiencies of the chemical industry in the midstream and upstream areas were 0.4156 and 0.2739, respectively, which are relatively low and generally show an evolutionary trend of first declining and then rising (Table 2).

In terms of provinces and cities, the green development efficiency of the chemical industry in Shanghai, Zhejiang, and Jiangsu has been maintained at the optimal state of 1.00 (except when it was at 0.79 in 2005), while that in Hunan province also reached the optimal state of 1.00 from 2012 to 2016. The green development efficiency of the chemical industry in Anhui, Hubei, Chongqing, Sichuan, Guizhou, and Yunnan provinces increased to varying degrees, showing a development trend of first decreasing and then increasing. However, there is still a large gap in the green development efficiency of the chemical industry between these provinces and the Shanghai, Zhejiang, and Jiangsu provinces (Figure 3).

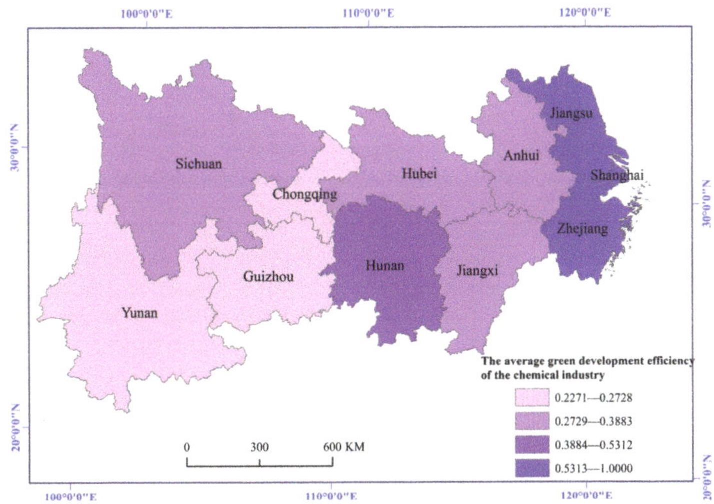

Figure 3. The average green development efficiency of the chemical industry from 2002 to 2016.

4.3. Regional Difference Analysis of Green Development Efficiency of the Chemical Industry in the Yangtze River Economic Belt

To further reveal the regional differences and sources of green development efficiency of the chemical industry in the Yangtze River Economic Belt, Dagum Gini coefficient and its decomposition method were used to calculate and decompose its relative level.

4.3.1. Overall Regional Differences

From 2002 to 2016, the average regional difference of green development efficiency of the chemical industry in the Yangtze River Economic Belt was 0.3080, showing a development trend of first expanding and then narrowing. The maximum and minimum regional differences of green development efficiency of the chemical industry appeared in 2007 and 2016 at 0.3347 and 0.2577, respectively. From 2007 to 2010, the green development efficiency of the chemical industry fluctuated greatly, due mainly to the impact of the financial crisis and the inconsistent degree of recovery of such efficiency in various provinces and cities. From 2012 to 2016, the regional differences in green development efficiency of the chemical industry narrowed, mainly because since the 18th National Congress of the Communist Party of China, the middle and upper reaches with low green development efficiency of the chemical industry have strengthened the treatment of the chemical industry, improved its resource and energy utilization efficiency, reduced waste water discharge, and improved the green development efficiency, thereby reducing the regional differences in green development efficiency of the chemical industry.

4.3.2. Intraregional Differences

On the whole, the regional difference of green development efficiency of the chemical industry in downstream areas is the largest, with an average of 0.1472. The second is the middle reaches, with an average of 0.1043. The upstream area is the smallest, with an average of 0.0873. From the evolution trend, from 2002 to 2012, the regional difference of green development efficiency of the chemical industry in the middle and lower reaches showed an upward trend in fluctuation. From 2012 to 2016, it showed a downward trend. From 2002 to 2016, the green development efficiency of the chemical industry in the upstream region showed an upward trend in fluctuation, indicating that the regional differences are expanding. Note that, although the regional differences of green development efficiency of the chemical industry in the upstream region is the smallest, they are expanding. Hence, it is necessary to strengthen the regulation of regional difference of green development efficiency of the chemical industry in the upstream region. Although there are great regional differences in the green development efficiency of the chemical industry in the middle reaches and downstream areas, these have narrowed significantly since 2012.

4.3.3. Differences between Regions

From the mean value of green development efficiency of the chemical industry among the three regions, the regional difference between the downstream and upstream areas is the largest at 0.5081, between the lower and middle reaches is 0.3805, and between the middle reaches and the upper reaches is the smallest at 0.1872. From the changing trend, the regional difference between the middle and upper reaches tends to expand, whereas those between downstream and upstream and between downstream and midstream tend to narrow (Figure 4).

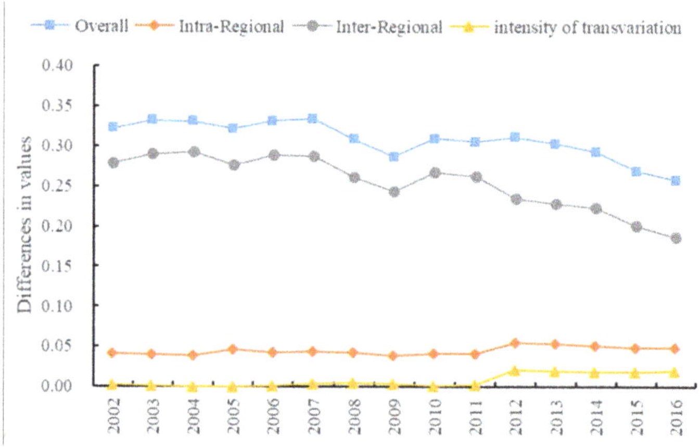

Figure 4. Regional differences in green development performance of the chemical industry in the Yangtze River Economic Belt.

4.3.4. Source of Difference

From the perspective of difference sources, the contribution of inter-group differences is the largest with an average value of 0.2545, which is higher than that of regional differences with an average value of 0.0453, and the contribution of over variable density with an average value of 0.0082. The evolution trend of inter-group differences is similar to that of overall regional differences, and the contribution rate of the average value of inter-group differences is as high as 78.94%. This percentage showed that the difference between groups is the main factor affecting the overall regional difference of green development efficiency of the chemical industry in the Yangtze River Economic Belt. The contribution rates of intra-group difference and hypervariable density were 14.05% and 2.54%, respectively, which have relatively small contributions to the overall regional difference (Table 3).

4.4. Regional Convergence Analysis of Green Development Efficiency of the Chemical Industry in the Yangtze River Economic Belt

4.4.1. σ-Convergence Test

The σ-convergence test method is used to calculate the σ-convergence coefficient of the whole Yangtze River Economic Belt and the upper, middle, and lower reaches, as shown in Figure 5. From 2002 to 2004, the global σ-convergence coefficient of the Economic Belt increased and showed a divergent state. From 2006 to 2016, the global σ-convergence coefficient generally showed a downward trend, indicating that the global σ-convergence occurred. This means that the regional differences in the green development efficiency of the chemical industry in the Yangtze River Economic Belt are shrinking.

Table 3. Regional differences in green development efficiency of the chemical industry in the Yangtze River Economic Belt.

Year	Overall G	Inter Group	Between Groups	Hypervariable Density	Upstream	Midstream	Downstream	Midstream–Upstream	Downstream–Upstream	Downstream–Midstream
2002	0.3224	0.0415	0.2786	0.0023	0.0456	0.0579	0.1556	0.1386	0.5380	0.4413
2003	0.3327	0.0408	0.2900	0.0019	0.0151	0.0597	0.1588	0.1264	0.5540	0.4677
2004	0.3312	0.0392	0.2921	0.0000	0.0153	0.0403	0.1542	0.0741	0.5490	0.4950
2005	0.3220	0.0463	0.2753	0.0003	0.0350	0.0419	0.1829	0.0831	0.5239	0.4621
2006	0.3321	0.0426	0.2885	0.0010	0.0638	0.0351	0.1564	0.0894	0.5448	0.4849
2007	0.3347	0.0446	0.2867	0.0034	0.0832	0.0679	0.1531	0.1058	0.5411	0.4848
2008	0.3089	0.0435	0.2605	0.0049	0.0930	0.0634	0.1494	0.1006	0.4980	0.4487
2009	0.2869	0.0389	0.2438	0.0042	0.0610	0.0405	0.1484	0.1051	0.4767	0.4070
2010	0.3093	0.0412	0.2672	0.0010	0.1074	0.0092	0.1479	0.1325	0.5188	0.4187
2011	0.3054	0.0414	0.2615	0.0025	0.1148	0.0381	0.1394	0.1211	0.5045	0.4253
2012	0.3110	0.0551	0.2345	0.0215	0.1287	0.2414	0.1430	0.3834	0.5178	0.2529
2013	0.3029	0.0541	0.2280	0.0208	0.1227	0.2369	0.1420	0.3654	0.5024	0.2503
2014	0.2933	0.0517	0.2228	0.0188	0.1522	0.2123	0.1291	0.3717	0.4944	0.2264
2015	0.2691	0.0494	0.2003	0.0194	0.1332	0.2122	0.1241	0.3174	0.4421	0.2233
2016	0.2577	0.0493	0.1875	0.0209	0.1380	0.2077	0.1235	0.2931	0.4160	0.2194

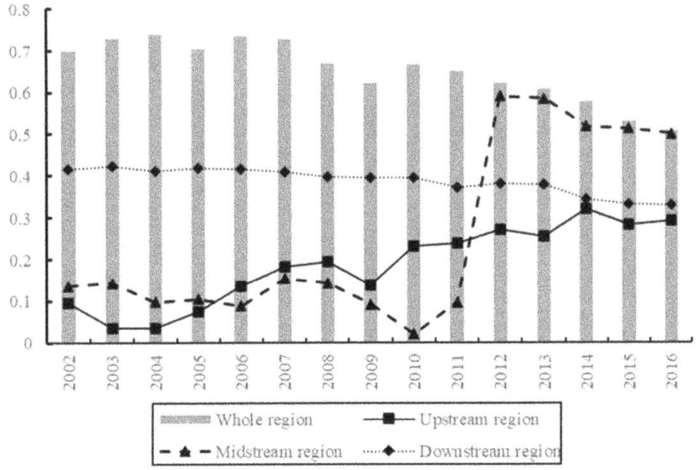

Figure 5. Absolute convergence graph.

From different regions, the σ-convergence coefficient of downstream areas showed a downward trend from 2002 to 2016 and σ-convergence, indicating that the regional difference in green development efficiency of the chemical industry in downstream areas had narrowed. From 2002 to 2012, the σ-convergence coefficient in the middle reaches increased and then decreased, and after 2012, it continued to decline, showing σ-convergence. After 2012, the regional difference of green development efficiency of the chemical industry in the middle reaches was reduced. From 2002 to 2016, the σ-convergence coefficient in the upstream region basically showed an upward trend and no σ-convergence, indicating that the difference in green development efficiency of the chemical industry in the upstream region was expanding.

Overall, the green development efficiency of the chemical industry in the whole region and the downstream areas of the Economic Belt has σ-convergence. After 2012 in the middle reaches, the green development efficiency of the chemical industry also had σ-convergence. There is no σ-convergence in the upstream region, and the regional imbalance of green development efficiency of the chemical industry intensified, which is basically consistent with the analysis results of Gini coefficient.

4.4.2. Absolute Convergence of β

The Hausman test shows that the panel data model with time and individual double fixed effects is more appropriate, and so the β absolute convergence mechanism was tested. The results show that the β absolute convergence coefficients in the whole region and the upper, middle, and lower reaches of the Yangtze River Economic Belt are negative, indicating that the green development efficiency of its chemical industry exists in β absolute convergence. Among them, the significance of the whole region, the upstream region, and the middle reaches region passed the significance test of 1%, 5%, and 5%, respectively. These results showed that the growth rate of green development efficiency of the chemical industry in the whole region, the upstream region, and the middle reaches region of the Yangtze River Economic Belt converged, while the significance of the downstream region did not pass the test. In terms of convergence speed, the upstream region is the fastest, followed by the midstream region (Table 4).

Table 4. β Absolute convergence table.

Variable	Whole Region	Upstream Region	Midstream Region	Downstream Region
β	−0.1734 *** (−4.43)	−0.2545 ** (−3.86)	−0.1806 ** (−7.13)	−0.2691 (−0.92)
Constant term	−0.1996 *** (−5.31)	−0.4009 ** (−4.46)	−0.2761 ** (−9.73)	−0.0877 (−1.31)
R^2	0.0736	0.3676	0.4548	0.1027
Convergence rate	0.0127%	0.0196%	0.0132%	-

Note: ** and ***, respectively, represent significance at the confidence levels of 5% and 1%, and T statistics are in brackets. "-" means empty.

Conditional β convergence does not require different regions to have the same basic characteristics, i.e., different regions can be at different growth paths and steady-state levels. If conditional β convergence exists, they eventually converge to their respective steady states by virtue of their own characteristics. In this paper, the green development efficiency of chemical industry in the Yangtze River Economic Belt is examined in four aspects, namely environmental regulation, industrial structure, foreign investment intensity, and scientific and technological progress, to investigate which factors contribute to the green development efficiency of chemical industry in Yangtze River Economic Belt to reach the conditional convergence. After controlling the control variables, such as environmental regulation, industrial structure, foreign capital intensity, and scientific and technological progress, the β absolute convergence coefficient in the whole region and the upper, middle, and lower reaches of the Yangtze River Economic Belt was still negative. In addition, the significance of the whole region and the middle reaches passed the significance test at 1% and 5%, respectively. This shows that the green development efficiency of the abovementioned regional chemical industry follows the trend of β absolute convergence, which is under the consideration of environmental regulation, industrial structure, foreign capital intensity, and scientific and technological progress. In terms of convergence rate, the convergence rate in the middle reaches is faster.

In the panel data regression model of the whole region and the upper, middle, and lower reaches of the Yangtze River Economic Belt, the regression coefficients of the control variable environmental regulation are negative, and the whole region and the upper reaches pass the 5% and 10% significance tests, respectively. This finding showed that the environmental regulation of the whole region and the upper reaches restricts the reduction in regional difference in the green development efficiency of the chemical industry. The regression coefficients of industrial structure in the whole region, the middle reaches, and the downstream regions are positive, while those of the upstream regions are negative, but they all fail to pass the significance test. The regression coefficient of foreign capital intensity in the whole region, the upstream region, and the downstream region is positive, while that of the middle reach region is negative, but only the upstream region passes the significance test. The results showed that the foreign capital intensity helps reduce the regional difference of green development efficiency of the chemical industry in the upstream region. The regression coefficients of scientific and technological progress in the whole region, upstream, midstream, and downstream regions are positive, but only the whole region passes the significance test. The outcome means that the improvement of scientific and technological level helps reduces the difference in green development efficiency of the chemical industry in these regions but is not the main reason (Table 5).

Table 5. β Conditional convergence table.

Variable	Whole Region	Upstream Region	Midstream Region	Downstream Region
β	−0.1564 ***	−0.2476	−0.1920 **	−0.3976
	(−3.61)	(−1.25)	(−8.18)	(−1.41)
Environmental regulation	−37.6551 **	−11.4104 *	−51.8642	−30.9161
	(−3.04)	(−2.43)	(−1.00)	(−1.01)
Industrial structure	0.3754	−0.4512	1.5735	0.3231
	(1.53)	(−1.93)	(1.02)	(2.01)
Foreign capital intensity	0.8206	7.6279 **	−5.4985	0.9576
	(1.26)	(4.49)	(−0.65)	(2.04)
Science and technology	1.7491 **	6.4771	2.5444	1.8611
	(2.89)	(1.08)	(0.99)	(1.30)
Constant term	−0.3230 ***	−0.3667	−0.6851	−0.3956
	(−3.72)	(−1.79)	(−1.44)	(−2.28)
R^2	0.0250	0.0854	0.1260	0.0748
Convergence rate	0.0113%	-	0.0142%	-

Note: *, **, and ***, respectively, represent significance at the confidence levels of 10%, 5%, and 1%, and T statistics are in brackets. "-" means empty.

5. Discussion

First, the problem of water ecological environment in the Yangtze River Economic Belt has attracted increasing research attention. Grey water footprint has been widely recognized as an indicator of pollution intensity [39,40]. The industrial grey water footprint index can better reflect the water pollution of industrial production activities than the wastewater pollutant discharge index can [23]. In this study, grey water footprint is incorporated into the evaluation framework of green development efficiency of the chemical industry. It can better reflect the impact of chemical industry production activities on the water environment and provide new research ideas for the calculation of green development efficiency of the chemical industry. In recent years, the green development, transformation, and upgrading of the chemical industry in the Economic Belt has achieved remarkable results. Nonetheless, in the future, we should still focus on the dynamic change trend of pollutant discharge in chemical industry wastewater, further strengthen the water pollution control of the chemical industry, optimize the industrial scale, reduce the grey water footprint of the chemical industry, and improve the efficiency of grey water footprint of the chemical industry. On the basis of this calculation model, provinces and cities can also build a measurement model of green development efficiency of the chemical industry based on grey water footprint, monitor the green development of the chemical industry, and put forward governance strategies. However, the water consumption and grey water footprint data of the chemical industry used in this paper were estimated using the provincial and industrial data in the *Yearbook of China Economic Census* (2008) and reference [38], and there is a certain error with the actual value. In future research, it is still necessary to improve the accuracy of data estimation or expand the channels for obtaining water environment data of the chemical industry.

Second, this study showed that the green development efficiency of the chemical industry in the Yangtze River Economic Belt increased significantly from 2002 to 2016 and showed a development and evolution trend of first declining and then rising. Yijun Zhang (2020) found that the overall green development performance of China's chemical industry showed a significant improvement trend from 2007 to 2017 [6]. Yeh Jiahuey (2019) studied the green development performance of China's chemical industry from 1980 to 2013 and found that it showed an evolution law of first declining and then rising from 2002 to 2013 [17]. These results are basically consistent with the results of the present research. In recent years, the Chinese government has strengthened the construction of ecological civilization and actively promoted the green transformation and upgrading of the chemical industry with remarkable results. In particular, the 18th Congress of the Communist Party of China in 2012 proposed to give prominence to the construction of ecological civilization and build a "Beautiful China." According to the data of the China Development and Reform Commission from 2016 to 2020, there were more than 8000 chemical enterprises along the Yangtze River. Furthermore, the proportion of excellent water environment sections in the Yangtze River Basin increased from 82.3% in 2016 to 91.7% in 2019 and further increased to 96.3% from January to November in 2020, and the proportion of inferior class V water quality in the Yangtze River Basin decreased from 3.5% to 0.6% during 2016 and 2019. The elimination of inferior class V water bodies would be realized for the first time in 2020, which showed that the green development of the chemical industry in the Economic Belt has achieved remarkable results, thus supporting the conclusions of this paper from the practical level.

Third, the regional heterogeneity of green development efficiency of the chemical industry in the Yangtze River Economic Belt is very obvious. Affected by the natural geographical environment and socioeconomic conditions, there are obvious gaps in the socioeconomic development level, industrialization level, and scientific and technological innovation ability in the upper, middle, and lower reaches of the Yangtze River Economic Belt. The zonality of industrial ecological efficiency [41] and green development level [42] is significant. This study found that the green development efficiency of the chemical industry in the Yangtze River Economic Belt was the highest in the lower reaches from 2002 to 2016, followed by the middle reaches, and the lowest in the upper reaches. The overall regional difference and interregional difference tended to narrow, and the intraregional difference expanded. Our result is similar to the research conclusions of Yunbo Xiang (2021) on the spatial differences of green development efficiency of the chemical industry in the Yangtze River Economic Belt [28], but there are some differences in specific values, which may be caused by different measurement indicators and used models. According to the above research results, in the future, the focus of the chemical industry governance in the Yangtze River Economic Belt would still be to accelerate the green development, transformation, and upgrading of the chemical industry in the middle and upper reaches, improve the green development efficiency of the chemical industry, and reduce regional differences. At the same time, we should pay attention to controlling regional differences and preventing their expansion. The middle and upper reaches should improve the green development efficiency of the chemical industry by means of technological innovation, optimizing the industrial scale, adjusting industrial structure, and strengthening environmental regulation. At the same time, we should promote the diffusion of technology, capital, and talents in the lower reaches to the middle and upper reaches. We should promote the green and coordinated development of the chemical industry in the Yangtze River Economic Belt.

6. Conclusions

This research studied the regional differences, influencing factors, and convergence of green development efficiency of the chemical industry in the Yangtze River Economic Belt by using the super efficiency SBM model, Dagum Gini coefficient, coefficient of variation method, and panel data regression model. The green development efficiency measurement model of the chemical industry constructed in this paper can more objectively and comprehensively reflect the impact of the chemical industry on the water environment than in previous studies and is very consistent with the industrial characteristics of the chemical industry and the regional water environment problems of the Economic Belt. Accurately measuring the green development efficiency of the chemical industry in the Economic Belt can provide theoretical support for chemical water treatment and green development in the area. Analyzing the difference, influence, and convergence of green development efficiency of the chemical industry in the Yangtze River Economic Belt can provide reference for formulating strategies to improve the green development efficiency of the chemical industry by region and classification.

The main conclusions of this paper are as follows.

First, from 2002 to 2016, the total grey water footprint of the chemical industry in the Yangtze River Economic Belt showed a downward trend, while the green development efficiency of the chemical industry showed an upward trend as a whole. This finding means that remarkable achievements have been made in environmental governance and green development of the chemical industry in the Yangtze River Economic Belt in recent years.

Second, there are significant regional differences in the green development efficiency of the chemical industry in the Yangtze River Economic Belt. From the perspective of space, the green development efficiency of the chemical industry in the lower reaches is high, while that in the middle and upper reaches is low. In terms of time, the overall regional differences and interregional differences tend to narrow, and the intraregional differences expand. From the source of difference, regional difference is the main source of regional difference in green development efficiency of the chemical industry in the Yangtze River Economic Belt.

Third, there is σ-convergence in the green development efficiency of the chemical industry in the whole region, the middle reaches, and the lower reaches of the Yangtze River Economic Belt, while there is no σ-convergence in the upper reaches. There are β absolute convergence and β conditional convergence in the green development efficiency of the chemical industry in the whole region and the upper, middle, and lower reaches of the Yangtze River Economic Belt.

Fourth, there is spatial heterogeneity in the impact of environmental regulation, industrial structure, foreign capital intensity, and scientific and technological progress on the green development efficiency of the chemical industry in the Yangtze River Economic Belt. This spatial heterogeneity suggests that in the governance of the chemical industry in the Yangtze River Economic Belt, common but differentiated policy measures should be formulated and precisely applied according to the characteristics of the region, by region and by industry. The middle and upper reaches should strengthen environmental regulation, adjust the structure of chemical industry, strengthen supervision and management of foreign investment, and improve environmental access standards. The lower reaches should focus on scientific and technological innovation, promote the upgrading of chemical industry value chain, and enhance the resilience of chemical industry.

It should be noted that, due to the limitation of statistical data, the paper uses the proportion of COD and ammonia nitrogen (NH_4^+-N) emissions in industrial wastewater of the chemical industry by industry nationwide to estimate the COD and ammonia nitrogen (NH_4^+-N) emissions in wastewater of the chemical industry by industry in each province when calculating the gray water footprint, without distinguishing the proportion of COD and ammonia nitrogen (NH_4^+-N) emissions in wastewater between provinces and regions differences. To some extent, this underestimates the differences in gray water footprints of chemical industries in the Yangtze River Economic Belt among provinces and cities. Meanwhile, the study of the differences in the overall green development efficiency of the chemical industry in the Yangtze River Economic Belt and its convergence can help to grasp the green development efficiency of the chemical industry in provinces and cities in general, but in-depth studies on the gray water footprint and green development efficiency of five subsectors are needed in the future to reveal the differences between industries and to develop more refined governance strategies for the chemical industry.

Author Contributions: Conceptualization, Y.X. and S.W.; methodology, Y.X., S.W., and Y.Z. (Yaxin Zhang); data curation, W.S. and Y.Z. (Yong Zhang); writing, Y.X., S.W., and W.S.; super-vision S.W.; funding Acquisition, Y.X. and S.W. All authors have read and agreed to the published version of the manuscript.

Funding: This research was supported by regional funds of the National Natural Science Foundation of China (42061026), projects of Jiangxi Social Science Foundation in 2021 (21JL01) and the Humanities and Social Sciences Research Project of the Ministry of Education (20 YJA 790071).

Institutional Review Board Statement: Not applicable.

Informed Consent Statement: Not applicable.

Data Availability Statement: The data presented in this study are available on request from the corresponding author.

Conflicts of Interest: The authors declare no conflict of interest.

References

1. Li, J.; Liang, M.; Zhong, Y. Spatiotemporal pattern and problem area identification of coordinated economic and environmental development in the Yangtze River Economic Belt. *Resour. Environ. Yangtze River Basin* **2020**, *29*, 2584–2596.
2. Liu, L.; Huang, G.; Wang, Z.; Chu, Z.; Li, H. Main problems, situation and Countermeasures of water ecological environment security in the Yangtze River Basin. *Environ. Sci. Res.* **2020**, *33*, 1081–1090.
3. Raza, M.Y.; Lin, B.; Liu, Y. Cleaner production of Pakistan's chemical industry: Perspectives of energy conservation and emissions reduction. *J. Clean. Prod.* **2021**, *278*, 123888. [CrossRef]
4. Cefic Facts and Figures. Facts And Figures of The European Chemical Industry. Available online: http://www.cefic.org (accessed on 30 January 2020).
5. Houming, Z.; Hailin, Q. Study on "Heavy chemical industry encircling the river" in the Yangtze River Economic Belt. *Chinas Natl. Cond. Strength* **2017**, *4*, 38–40.
6. Zhang, Y.; Song, Y.; Zou, H. Transformation of pollution control and green development: Evidence from China's chemical industry. *J. Environ. Manag.* **2020**, *275*, 111246. [CrossRef] [PubMed]
7. Peiyang, C.; Xigang, Z. China's regional economic differences based on different scales. *J. Geogr.* **2012**, *67*, 1085–1097.
8. Lyytimaki, J.; Antikainen, R.; Hokkanen, J.; Koskela, S.; Kurppa, S.; Känkänen, R.; Seppälä, Y. Developing Key Indicators of Green Growth. *Sustain. Dev.* **2018**, *26*, 51–64. [CrossRef]
9. Liu, Y.; Yuan, H.; Hu, K. Green development in China: Characteristics, laws, framework methods and evaluation applications. *J. Jishou Univ. Soc. Sci. Ed.* **2019**, *40*, 16–28.
10. Gao, Y. Research on green development performance and its influencing factors of China's eight comprehensive economic zones *Res. Quant. Econ. Technol. Econ.* **2019**, *36*, 3–23.
11. Pittman, R.W. Multilateral Productivity Comparisons with Undesirable outputs. *Econ. J.* **1983**, *93*, 883–891. [CrossRef]
12. Chung, Y.H.; Färe, R.; Grosskopf, S. Productivity and undesirable Outputs: A Directional Distance Function Approach. *J. Environ. Manag.* **1997**, *51*, 229–240. [CrossRef]
13. Tone, K. A slacks-based Measure of efficiency in Data Envelopment Analysis. *Eur. J. Oper. Res.* **2001**, *130*, 498–509. [CrossRef]
14. Tone, K. A slacks-based Measure of Super-Efficiency in Data Envelopment Analysis. *Eur. J. Oper. Res.* **2002**, *143*, 32–41. [CrossRef]
15. Tanzil, D.; Beloff, B.R. Assessing impacts: Overview on sustainability indicators and metrics. *Environ. Qual. Manag.* **2006**, *15*, 41–56. [CrossRef]
16. Manello, A. Productivity growth, environmental regulation and win–win opportunities: The case of chemical industry in Italy and Germany. *Eur. J. Oper. Res.* **2017**, *262*, 733–743. [CrossRef]
17. Jiahuey, Y.; Liu, Y.; Yu, Y. Measuring green growth performance of China's chemical industry, Resources. *Conserv. Recycl.* **2019**, *149*, 160–167. [CrossRef]
18. Honghai, S.; Yanling, X.; Yanqiu, W. Evaluation of relative ecological efficiency of petrochemical industry. *Ecol. Econ.* **2017**, *33*, 42–45.
19. Yaqiong, Y. *Research on Enterprise Ecological Efficiency Driven by Value*; Beijing University of Chemical Technology: Beijing, China, 2018.
20. Qiuqin, L.; Meng, Y.; Guangqiu, H. Research on efficiency evaluation of transformation and upgrading of coal chemical enterprises excluding environmental factors. *Math. Pract. Underst.* **2020**, *50*, 116–126.
21. Hoekstra, A.Y.; Chapagain, A.K.; Aldaya, M.M.; Mekonnen, M.M. *The Water Footprint Assessment Manual: Setting the Global Standard*; Routledge: London, UK, 2011.
22. Hoekstra, A.Y.; Mekonnen, M.M. The water footprint of humanity. *Proc. Natl. Acad. Sci. USA* **2011**, *109*, 3232–3237. [CrossRef]
23. Caizhi, S.; Xiaodong, Y. Measurement and transfer analysis of grey water footprint of Chinese provinces and industries based on a multi-regional input-output model. *Prog. Geogr.* **2020**, *39*, 207–218.
24. Shengyun, W.; Yajie, H.; Huimin, R.; Jing, L. Performance evaluation and driving effect decomposition of Provincial Ecological Welfare in China. *Resour. Sci.* **2020**, *42*, 840–855.
25. Hui, Z.; Xuejun, D. Spatial pattern evolution and influencing factors of chemical industry along the Yangtze River. *Geogr. Res.* **2019**, *38*, 884–897.
26. Fengqi, Z.; Ning, C. Suggestions on optimizing the layout of chemical industry in the Yangtze River Economic Belt. *Environ. Prot.* **2016**, *44*, 25–30.
27. Qingjun, C.; Xiaofeng, W. Layout analysis and optimization suggestions of chemical industry in the Yangtze River Economic Belt. *Chem. Ind.* **2018**, *36*, 5–9.
28. Yunbo, X.; Shengyun, W.; Chuxiong, D. Spatial differentiation and driving factors of green development efficiency of chemical industry in the Yangtze River Economic Belt. *Econ. Geogr.* **2021**, *41*, 108–117.

29. Xuepeng, J.; Yaya, S.; Yanwei, S.; Danyang, W.; Hao, M.; Shengfeng, L.; Xianjin, H. Temporal and spatial pattern evolution and influencing factors of chemical industry in the Yangtze River Delta from the perspective of admission rate. *Geogr. Res.* **2020**, *39*, 1116–1127.
30. Deming, Z.; Haixia, Z.; Futian, Q. Impact of chemical industry development along the river in Jiangsu on water environment and countermeasures. *Reg. Res. Dev.* **2006**, *1*, 54–57.
31. Yuting, Z.; Yafei, L.; Linyan, D.; Yihan, Y.; Xiaomin, L.; Qihong, S. Environmental risks and Countermeasures of heavy chemical industry in typical basins of the Yangtze River Economic Belt. *Environ. Sci. Res.* **2020**, *33*, 1247–1253.
32. Chuanqing, W.; Yunling, Y. "Hubei sample" and "Jiangsu sample" to solve the problem of "Chemical industry encircling the river". *West Forum.* **2020**, *30*, 71–83.
33. Xinling, D.; Yueyou, Z. Industrial division, environmental pollution and regional economic development—An Empirical Study Based on the heavy chemical industry in the Yangtze River Economic Belt. *Econ. Longit. Latit.* **2020**, *37*, 20–28.
34. Yang, L.; Jianliang, Y.; Yuan, L. Efficiency evaluation and equilibrium characteristics of green development of China's urban agglomeration. *Econ. Geogr.* **2019**, *39*, 110–117.
35. Chuanming, L.; Huitong, W.; Xiaomin, W. Research on regional difference decomposition and convergence of Internet financial development in China's eight urban agglomerations. *Quant. Econ. Tech. Econ. Res.* **2017**, *34*, 3–20.
36. Shuai, L. Regional differences and stochastic convergence of China's economic growth quality. *Res. Quant. Econ. Tech. Econ.* **2019**, *36*, 24–41.
37. Yuanyi, H. *Study on Distribution Characteristics and Driving Factors of Heavy Metal Gray Water Footprint in Industrial Wastewater in China*; Beijing University of Science and Technology: Beijing, China, 2020.
38. Xiang, C.; Xu, X. Study on the dynamic evolution and influencing factors of regional differences in circular economy efficiency of China's industrial industry—An Empirical Study from papermaking and paper products industry. *China Soft Sci.* **2015**, *1*, 160–171.
39. Min, S.; Kaijie, S.; Yanxia, M.; Ang, L. Calculation and analysis of grey water footprint of industries in the Yangtze River Economic Belt Based on input-output table. *Resour. Ind.* **2021**, *23*, 13–22. [CrossRef]
40. Tianbo, F.; Changxin, X.; Lihua, Y.; Siyu, H.; Qing, X. Measurement and driving factors of grey water footprint efficiency in Yangtze River Basin. *Sci. Total Environ.* **2022**, *802*, 149587.
41. Chen, J.; Wang, J.; Fan, Y. Study on temporal and spatial differences and influencing factors of industrial ecological efficiency in the Yangtze River Economic Belt. *J. Henan Univ. Sci. Technol. Soc. Sci. Ed.* **2021**, *39*, 39–46.
42. Shaohong, C.; Gucheng, Z.Z. Measurement of green development level and temporal and spatial evolution characteristics of the Yangtze River Economic Belt. *Econ. Manag. East China* **2021**, *35*, 25–34. [CrossRef]

buildings MDPI

Article

A New Approach to Assessing the Energy Efficiency of Industrial Facilities

Natalia Verstina, Natalia Solopova, Natalia Taskaeva, Tatiana Meshcheryakova * and Natalia Shchepkina

Department of Management and Innovation, Moscow State University of Civil Engineering (National Research University), Yaroslavskoe Shosse 26, 129337 Moscow, Russia; verstinang@mgsu.ru (N.V.); solopovana@mgsu.ru (N.S.); taskayevann@mgsu.ru (N.T.); schepkinann@mgsu.ru (N.S.)
* Correspondence: meshcheryakovats@mgsu.ru

Abstract: The modern climate policy of different countries, decarbonization, the principles of ESG and sustainable development determine the main trends in the world economy, the result of which is a new vision of the energy-saving problem. The authors' research is based on the key idea that in the modern world, systematic measures are needed to improve the energy efficiency of enterprises in the industrial sector of the economy. The article analyzes the systems used for assessing the energy efficiency of objects for various purposes, and on this basis, their advantages and limitations in application are revealed, which were taken by the authors as a basis for developing a new approach to assessing the energy efficiency of industrial facilities. The study gives preference to the point-rating assessment. The authors have developed a system of indicators structured by groups: building energy efficiency, technological process energy efficiency, energy efficiency and environmental friendliness management. The system of indicators of energy efficiency of an industrial facility proposed by the authors has been replaced as a basis for ranking industrial facilities by energy efficiency classes.

Keywords: energy efficiency; energy saving; sustainable development; ESG principles; industrial facility; energy efficiency indicators

Citation: Verstina, N.; Solopova, N.; Taskaeva, N.; Meshcheryakova, T.; Shchepkina, N. A New Approach to Assessing the Energy Efficiency of Industrial Facilities. *Buildings* **2022**, *12*, 191. https://doi.org/10.3390/buildings12020191

Academic Editors: Roberto Alonso González Lezcano, Francesco Nocera and Rosa Giuseppina Caponetto

Received: 8 January 2022
Accepted: 4 February 2022
Published: 8 February 2022

1. Introduction

The modern climate policy of states and decarbonization is currently supported by a number of steps that are being implemented both in individual countries and at the intergovernmental level. Climatic degradation caused by anthropogenic greenhouse gas (GHG) emissions is noted in the paradigms of not only ecological but also energy and economic development of industrialized countries. This encourages states to constantly work to improve international and national so-called "green" standards for various sectors of the economy, including for its industrial sector.

In December 2019, the EU declared a "green course", the goal of which is to achieve climate neutrality by 2050. Scientists and experts consider carbon neutrality as a set of actions aimed at reducing the carbon footprint at all stages of the product life cycle, "intermediate" targets for the way to which will be the reduction in 2030 of CO_2 emissions by 55% to the level of 1990 and an increase in the share of renewable energy sources in the energy balance of countries to 38–40% (in electricity–up to 65%). At the same time, after 10 years, the EU expects, primarily at the expense of the industrial sector of the economy, to reduce the consumption of coal by 70% and oil and gas by 30% and 25% compared to 2015, respectively. In parallel with the EU, similar practical steps are being taken in Asia and North America. Therefore, in September 2020, China announced carbon neutrality by 2060, and from 1 February 2021, the country introduced a national emissions trading system. In October 2020, Japan and South Korea made statements of achieving carbon neutrality by 2050. The United States plans to sign the Paris Agreement and continue the environmental course of development of the industrial and energy sectors of the economy [1–3].

In the above context, the principles of ESG (environmental—ecology, social—social development, governance—corporate governance), which are also called the principles of responsible investment, are becoming more widespread. Both industrialized countries and companies in the industrial sector of the economy are evaluated according to the ESG (World Energy Trilemma Index) index. According to the British audit and consulting company Ernst & Young Global Limited, 97% of investors today are guided by the ESG index, making a decision when choosing an investment object, the provision of high values of which is relevant for all enterprises in the industrial sector of the economy, the problematic part of the activity, in this case, is the improvement of environmental indicators directly related to the energy efficiency of their activities [4,5]. The catalyst for compliance with ESG principles, including environmental friendliness, is the organization of an effective system for monitoring energy consumption and managing energy costs of enterprises in the industrial sector of the economy, focused on reducing them and increasing the energy efficiency of industrial facilities. In view of this, the system for assessing the energy efficiency of industrial facilities is of particular importance, the importance of which in the considered context is increasing.

Let us note another important condition for ensuring energy efficiency of all enterprises in the industrial sector of the economy: the need to revise approaches to assessing their energy efficiency is caused by the instability of the world economy in the context of a pandemic. COVID-19 in 2020 affected the change in the volume of energy consumption in the world, which decreased by 4%. Moreover, in the period from 2000 to 2018. This average annual rate was 2%, and in 2019 fell to 0.8% [6]. In 2020, energy consumption decreased in most countries due to the introduced lockdowns, which affected the activities of enterprises in the industrial sector of the economy in almost all sectors of the economy.

It is obvious that the restoration by enterprises of the industrial sector of the production economy to the "pre-pandemic" level and its further increase after the localization of the pandemic will lead to an increase in energy consumption. It will affect the consumption of fossil fuels, which are currently the main sources of energy for enterprises in the industrial sector of the economy. Such data are based on the dominance in the global energy balance of fossil fuels according to world expert forecasts, despite the most positive forecasts for the development of renewable energy sources. A logical consequence will be an increase in the volume of emissions of pollutants and greenhouse gases, which should be taken under special control at the level of each enterprise in the industrial sector of the economy, first of all, by managing its energy consumption.

In this regard, in the study, the authors focused their attention on enterprises in the industrial sector of the economy as the largest end consumers of energy resources [6]. In the course of the research, the problem of defining a previously not specified concept of the category of "industrial object" was identified, the study of the definitions of which showed the presence of discrepancies and blurred formulations, which became a system-forming task of the study.

The subject of the study is the assessment of the energy efficiency of an industrial facility that characterizes the problem area of the study. The aim of the study is to form a new approach to assess the energy efficiency of industrial facilities, which makes it possible to significantly unify the monitoring of energy consumption at enterprises of the industrial sector of the economy, and on this basis, to ensure the possibility of accelerating their transition to ESG principles and focusing them on the need to form new management tools to improve environmental performance directly related to the energy efficiency of their activities. For the set goal, the corresponding tasks were constructed and solved, the achievements of the consistent solution of which are associated with new scientific results:

- to specify the category "industrial facility" as an object of energy efficiency assessment;
- to determine the factors for assessing the energy efficiency of an industrial facility;
- form a system of indicators for assessing the energy efficiency of industrial facilities;
- develop a formula for calculating energy efficiency indicators of an industrial facility.

The solution to the tasks was carried out in three consecutive stages, which are presented in Table 1.

The first stage, research of information systems, is aimed at systematizing and analyzing the current regulatory and legislative framework, using terms and approaches to assess the energy efficiency of objects for various purposes, relevant for the development of a new approach to assessing the energy efficiency of industrial facilities.

Table 1. Problem-solving logic.

	Stage 1	Stage 2	Stage 3
Tasks	**Research of Public Information Sources**	**Organization of an Expert Survey on the Assessment of the Energy Efficiency of an Industrial Facility**	**Formation of a System of Indicators for Assessing the Energy Efficiency of an Industrial Facility**
1. Specify "industrial facility" as an object of energy efficiency assessment	Systematization: – regulatory and legislative framework for assessing the energy efficiency of objects for various purposes; – terms in the field of energy efficiency; – approaches to the definition of an energy efficiency object; – existing national and international systems for assessing the energy efficiency of various facilities. Definition: – object of energy efficiency assessment; – indicators of consumption of energy resources when assessing the energy efficiency of the facility.	Conducting an expert survey on the topic of the study, taking into account the issue of clarifying the concept of "industrial facility". Consolidation of survey data, processing and interpretation of expert survey results. Clarification of the concept of "industrial facility".	
2. Formulate factors for assessing the energy efficiency of an industrial facility	Systematization of factors affecting the energy efficiency of buildings. Systematization of factors affecting the energy efficiency of technological processes.	Systematization of expert opinions on the importance of factors affecting the energy efficiency of an industrial facility. Identification of factors affecting the energy efficiency of an industrial facility.	Consideration of factors.

Table 1. *Cont.*

Tasks	Stage 1 Research of Public Information Sources	Stage 2 Organization of an Expert Survey on the Assessment of the Energy Efficiency of an Industrial Facility	Stage 3 Formation of a System of Indicators for Assessing the Energy Efficiency of an Industrial Facility
3. Form a system of indicators for assessing the energy efficiency of industrial facilities	Systematization of indicators influencing the assessment of energy efficiency. Systematization of approaches to the formation of indicators for assessing the energy efficiency of facilities. Determination of the principles for the formation of indicators for assessing the energy efficiency of industrial facilities. Systematization of indicators influencing the assessment of energy efficiency.	Systematization of the principles for assessing the energy efficiency of industrial facilities. Systematization of expert opinions on the significance of indicators in assessing the energy efficiency of an industrial facility. Determination of significant indicators for assessing the energy efficiency of an industrial facility. Systematization of the principles for assessing the energy efficiency of industrial facilities.	Substantiation of the systematization of indicators of energy efficiency of an industrial facility. Systematized presentation of energy efficiency indicators of an industrial facility. Allocation of groups of indicators according to the nature of consumption of energy resources. Substantiation of the systematization of indicators of energy efficiency of an industrial facility.
4. Provide a formalized description of the process for assessing the final indicator of the energy efficiency of an industrial facility	Systematization of the applied formulas for calculating the energy efficiency indicators of buildings and technological processes or those proposed in scientific research. Definition of formulas for calculating the energy efficiency indicators of buildings.		Representation of formulas for calculating the integral indicator of an industrial facility.

The second stage is the organization of an expert survey and analysis of the results obtained, aimed at identifying the opinions of experts in the field of the efficiency of an industrial facility as an object for assessing energy efficiency and energy efficiency factors of industrial enterprises that are significant in developing an approach to assessing the energy efficiency of industrial facilities.

The third stage is the formation of a system of indicators for assessing the energy efficiency of an industrial facility, the results of the first two stages on the example of a new approach to assessing the energy efficiency of industrial facilities, based on the updated concept of the object of assessment, a new system of indicators for assessing energy efficiency and methods for determining indicators.

2. Materials and Methods

A study by the authors of the legislative and regulatory framework of various countries of the world, which is significant for assessing energy efficiency, showed that active work towards assessing the energy efficiency of facilities began already in the second half of the 20th century. In economically developed countries (USA, EU countries, Japan, Republic of Korea, etc.) and dynamically developing countries (China, Russia, etc.), by now, basic Laws (Directives) have been developed that define the national energy policy, regulate the consumption of energy by various objects and management of energy efficiency processes [7–17]. In most of these countries, to ensure energy efficiency, an integrated approach to energy conservation is being implemented in practice, while there are programs: in the USA—on the development of energy standards for buildings (Building Energy Codes Program, BECP) [18], on the justification of energy labeling of household appliances and electronic devices (Energy Star [19] and State Energy Program, SEP [20]), to support households in terms of insulation of buildings (Weatherization Assistance Program, WAP) [21]; in the countries of the European Union—on the labeling of energy-consuming equipment (Energy Star Program [19]) and the European Green Deal (action plan to turn Europe into a climate-neutral continent by 2050); in Japan—for equipping industrial facilities with energy-efficient technical means (Building Energy Management Systems Program), for equipping the residential sector with energy-efficient technical means and a smart home system (Home Energy Management Systems Program), for stimulating the development of household electrical appliances and office devices with very low energy consumption (Program "Creation of the best energy efficient products"), on product labeling and implementation of innovations without increasing their cost (Program "Top-Runner-Programs"), on the formation of energy-efficient information technology for the industrial sector and the development of new technologies (Project "Green IT Project") [22,23]. The variety of the considered programs speaks of great opportunities in improving energy efficiency in the modern world, and naturally determines the formulation of the question regarding the standards, which consolidate the already achieved results and principles that are universal in nature for certain objects in relation to which energy efficiency is considered. In the study, the authors examined objects related to industrial real estate and the processes carried out in it related to the consumption of energy.

To date, most countries have energy efficiency standards for residential and commercial buildings, which include design and regulatory indicators for assessing energy consumption and thermal protection of buildings, conducting energy audits and creating an energy management system [24–26]. For certification of buildings, taking into account energy consumption, as a rule, a point-rating system is adopted when assessing indicators (LEED, BREEAM, DGNB, WELL) [27–30]. In the European Union, the standard ISO 52000 of the EPB series (standards in the field of energy efficiency of buildings), which has been in force since 2017 and includes an assessment of energy consumption by a building and its life support systems, is the fundamental standard [31]. The most progressive design standards are considered to be highly efficient green buildings [32] and the international green construction code [33]. The analysis of the materials presented above showed that there is a high degree of elaboration of the issues of assessing the energy efficiency of buildings, including the definition of indicators for assessing energy consumption, their measurement and calculation, which became possible to systematize in this study.

The systematization of the assessment of the energy efficiency of real estate in European countries [34–38] showed that new and existing buildings are considered as the object of assessment: houses (residential and non-residential, multi-apartment and single-family, standard and individual, stone, brick, panel), public (administrative and commercial), industrial and others. Industrial buildings, as objects of energy efficiency assessment, are mentioned in the analytical materials of Italy. Similar objects of assessment are considered in the USA [16,34,35]. Considering the high degree of consumption of energy resources by industrial enterprises, significant energy losses during their operation due to the possible imperfection of building structures and their wear and tear, technological processes in the production of products [39,40], the authors identified the relevance of developing a new approach to assessing the energy efficiency of enterprises in the industrial sector of the economy, and at the same time it was revealed the need to concretize the concept of "industrial facility".

The systematization of materials representing various approaches to the definition of an industrial facility has shown the following options for its identification:

– production facilities—buildings used for production and assembly work, warehouse buildings [41];

- factory, plant—an industrial enterprise that includes one or more interconnected production, administrative and auxiliary buildings [42];
- industrial facility—a stationary technological unit, where one or more types of activities are carried out, stationary equipment and/or structures used in connection with any technological process for industrial production, an enterprise, its workshops, sections or sites for the production of products [43];
- industrial complex—real estate objects used for activities in the field of industry [44];
- production facility—enterprises of various industrial sectors [45];
- industrial enterprise—a complex of buildings and structures for the production of industrial products [45].

To solve the problem of determining the category of "industrial facility" for assessing energy efficiency, the method of analysis and classification of information was used, which made it possible to collect in a single system the available information on assessing the energy efficiency of objects for various purposes, to streamline a significant information resource, to identify the problems of determining the category of "industrial facility". The use of the method of expert assessments determined the significant features of the enterprise in the industrial sector of the economy, which require consideration when assessing their energy efficiency. The application of these methods provided an understanding of the need to concretize the definition of an industrial facility for the purpose of assessing its energy efficiency, which makes it possible to switch to a systematic representation of the assessment of the energy efficiency of industrial facilities, which is invariant to industry affiliation.

The study of the materials collected by the authors showed the need for their analysis in accordance with the tasks set. It is important to note that the interpretation of the concept of an "industrial facility" in the studied sources is generally similar in content, and the specificity of its formulation is due to the difference in tasks solved in the development of documents (programs and standards). In this regard, it became necessary to obtain a qualitatively different material in the study—actual views of leading experts in this field from a number of countries, whom the authors attracted to form a consolidated position on clarifying the concept that is essential for solving the issues of assessing the energy efficiency of enterprises in the industrial sector of the economy—"industrial facility" and related to its specific principles of conducting the assessment. The sample of Russian and foreign experts was formed on the basis of the developed criteria for assessing the competencies of experts corresponding to the objectives of the study.

A questionnaire consisting of two blocks was used as a survey tool. The first block included general questions to collect data on experts, characterizing their professional interests and experience in the field under study. In this block, brief information about the expert was recorded: the name and surname of the expert, their position, E-mail, the country they represent, the region, the name and type of activity of the company in which they work, as well as interest in receiving information about the results of the survey. The questions in this block were mostly open-ended. The second block directly contained questions on the research topic. All the questions in this block were mandatory, which made it possible to get answers from the respondents to all the questions posed in it. Due to the fact that in modern conditions, an online survey is one of the most convenient methods for conducting a survey, the questionnaire was compiled in the simplest application for administering surveys—Google Forms.

As a way of agreeing on the expert opinions, the "majority rule" was used, according to which the interpretation was chosen, which was adhered to by the majority of experts. At the final stage of the study, a report was generated containing a description of the survey results and recommendations for their further application were given. The experts unanimously confirmed the expediency of separating the assessment of the energy efficiency of enterprises in the industrial sector of the economy into an independent research area and the need to clarify the definition of the concept of an "industrial facility". At the same time, they noted the complexity of the object of assessment, which entails considering it as an integral complex, described by a system of energy efficiency indicators, requiring quantitative measurement and formalization of the assessment process. On the basis of the materials obtained, the first of the tasks of the study was solved—the author's definition of the concept of an "industrial facility" as an industrial building (structure) or a complex of adjacent buildings (structures) was proposed, including its entire property complex, which has a single engineering infrastructure that ensures production activities as a business entity.

The transition to the next research task, related to the indicators for assessing the energy efficiency of objects, determined the need to obtain materials regarding the modern practice of its assessment in different countries of the world to determine the essential aspects of the assessment and the results achieved. The solution to the problem of identifying the conditions for assessing the energy efficiency of an industrial facility is based on the use of comparative analysis and the method of expert assessments. The use of these methods made it possible to identify the most disputable areas of research and determine the authors' position on the systemic representation of the object of assessment and the principles of forming a system of indicators when developing a new approach to assessing the energy efficiency of industrial facilities, to make a decision on the choice of factors affecting energy efficiency indicators, to determine the composition of assessment indicators and to determine their significance, which ensured the representativeness of the results.

In general terms, the level of energy efficiency of the object of assessment is determined based on the characteristics of consumption or the consumption of energy resources. Comparative characteristics of materials related to the consumption of energy resources in different countries showed certain differences. These include the following: of total building energy consumption, 89% of the countries in the sample surveyed include heating, 84% of countries include hot water, 79% of countries include cooling, 74% include lighting, and minimum countries account for auxiliary equipment; 21%, household electrical appliances; 16% and air humidification; 11% (Figure 1). It can be concluded that these directions of consumption of energy resources should be reflected in the system of indicators for assessing the energy efficiency of an industrial facility [35].

According to the Comparative Review of Energy Efficiency Standards and Technologies in Buildings in the UNECE Region, the most significant conditions related to energy efficiency in buildings are: availability of heating and hot water supply (40 of the analyzed countries); thermal characteristics and geometry of the building (enclosing structures, floors, etc.) (38 countries); air conditioning (37 countries); forced (mechanical) and natural ventilation (37 countries); location and orientation of buildings (36 countries); passive solar systems and solar protection (36 countries). Conditions such as passive cooling (8 countries), heat recovery (7 countries) and dehumidification (2 countries) [35] (Figure 2) are considered limitedly.

The investigated materials showed a difference in approaches to assessing energy efficiency even at the stage of determining the conditions that affect it. In particular, in the United States, the following are considered as conditions for the energy efficiency of buildings: climatic parameters at the site of an object, parameters of the internal microclimate, dimensions of a building, heat-shielding properties of a building, parameters of engineering systems and the number of people (living in a building) [35]. In the Russian Federation, when assessing energy efficiency, conditions are considered related to architectural and engineering solutions, the characteristics of individual structural elements of a building that are included in projects during construction, overhaul or reconstruction and on the basis of which the specific indicators of energy resource consumption are estimated [14].

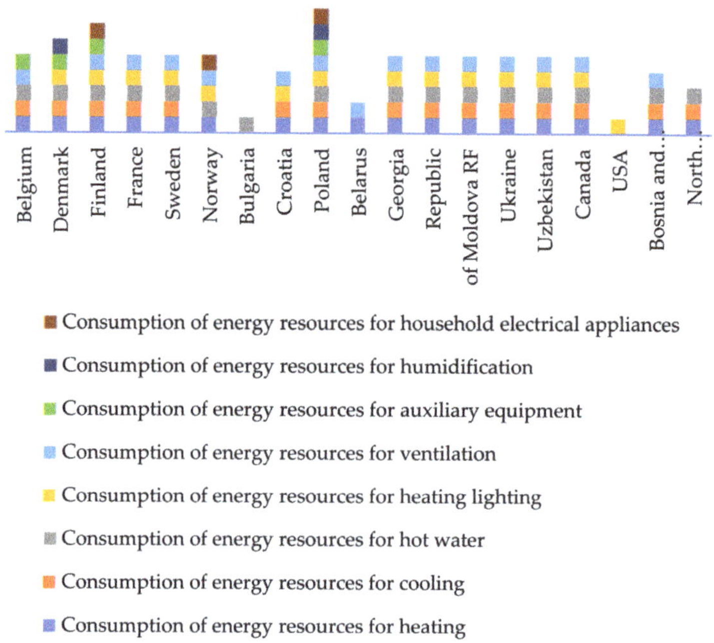

Figure 1. Accounting for the consumption of energy resources in terms of energy efficiency of buildings (built by the authors based on the "Comparative review of existing technologies to improve the energy efficiency of buildings in the UNECE region in 2019" [35]).

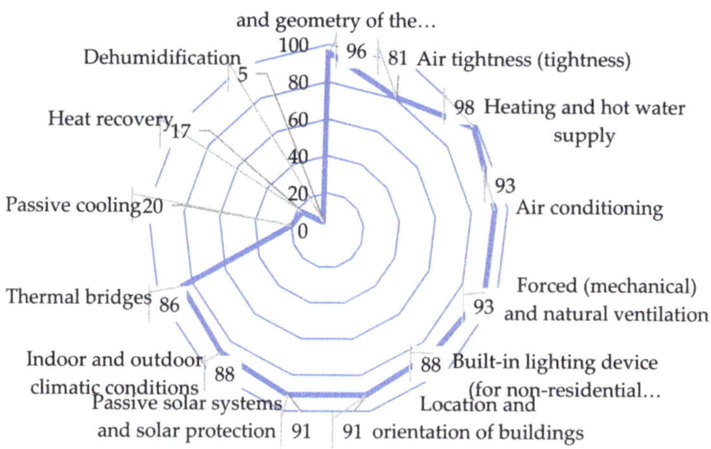

Figure 2. Consideration of energy efficiency conditions when assessing the energy efficiency of buildings (constructed by the authors based on the "Comparative Review of Energy Efficiency Standards and Technologies for Buildings in the UNECE Region for 2018" [35]).

In this regard, the authors summarized the opinions of experts obtained as a result of an expert survey conducted by them, aimed, among other things, at identifying the conditions for ensuring energy efficiency in determining the energy efficiency of an industrial facility (Figure 3).

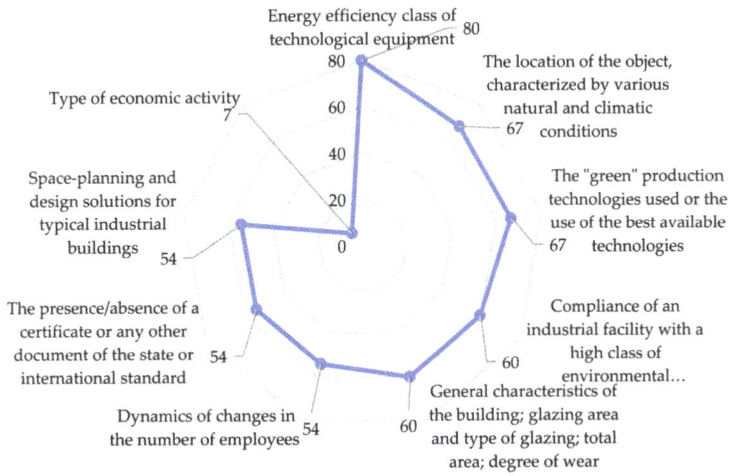

Figure 3. Distribution of expert opinions on the importance of conditions for ensuring energy efficiency of an industrial facility, % of respondents.

According to experts, the most significant conditions include: the location of the assessment object to take into account the natural and climatic features of the territory (67% of experts); general characteristics of the building (year of construction, number of stories), glazing area and type of glazing, area, degree of wear (60% of experts); space-planning and design solutions for typical industrial buildings (54% of experts). Taking into account the specifics of an industrial facility as an object for the production of industrial products, the experts noted the need to take into account the energy efficiency class of technological equipment (80% of experts) and the used "green" production technologies or the use of the best available technologies (67% of experts). Focusing on modern environmental trends, they recommended taking into account the compliance of an industrial facility with an environmental class, confirmed by the presence of a "green" certificate in one or several international systems LEED, BREEAM, DGNB and others (60% of experts) and the presence/absence of a certificate or any other document state or international standard, certifying the existence of an energy policy, strategy or energy management system at the enterprise of the industrial sector of the economy that meets the requirements of ISO 50001 (54% of experts). This emphasizes the importance of accounting in determining the energy efficiency of industrial facilities of technological processes for the production of industrial products, as well as energy efficiency and environmental friendliness management.

The transition in the study to the development of principles and indicators for assessing the energy efficiency of industrial facilities required the use of traditional methods of scientific knowledge related to the studied subject area. In the course of work, at certain stages, the authors widely used research methods included in the group of analytical methods, the system method and mathematical methods (analysis and synthesis, scaling and classification, comparative analysis, induction and deduction, statistical methods, the method of expert assessments, the establishment of quantitative relationships between the studied phenomena, etc.), which made it possible to provide an integrated solution regarding the proposed system of indicators for assessing the energy efficiency of industrial facilities. In particular, based on the methods of analysis and synthesis of previously used approaches to assessing energy efficiency, a new approach has been formed to ensure a meaningful relationship between the definition of an industrial facility and the proposed system of energy efficiency indicators within the selected context. The use of methods for analyzing and classifying information made it possible to collect, in a single system, the available information for assessing the energy efficiency of objects for various purposes, to streamline a significant information resource and to determine the conceptual apparatus for the formation of each of the proposed indicators. This provided not only the specification of the definition of an industrial facility for the purpose of assessing its energy efficiency, presented in the article above but also the development on this basis of an integrated approach to assessment, taking into account the indicators already used in practice for assessing the energy efficiency of non-industrial facilities (residential, public facilities) when creating a new approach for assessing the energy efficiency of industrial facilities.

Comparative analysis was used to analyze the correspondence of energy consumption indicators and their indicative values (set, for example, at the state level), as well as to formulate proposals for discussion on the ranking of the values of energy efficiency indicators of industrial facilities. The systematic method used in the research made it possible to form a general vision of the problem and, in relation to the object of research, to carry out a comprehensive analysis of the current conditions of energy consumption by an industrial facility both during the operation of buildings and in the production of finished products, which are also considered from the standpoint of organizing the management of these processes. In addition, the system method made it possible to take into account the hierarchy of the representation of the object under study, which makes it possible to determine the priority of the processes of energy consumption by an industrial object relative to the control processes. This made it possible to present an assessment of the energy efficiency of an industrial facility in the form of decomposition of interrelated groups of indicators and to structure in the study the processes of energy consumption by an industrial facility. The proposed structuring is presented in the form of three subsystems of indicators characterizing the energy efficiency of the building, the energy efficiency of technological processes and the provision of energy efficiency combined with environmental friendliness in terms of organizing effective management on the principles of ESG. The use of the method of comparative analysis in combination with the systemic method provided the basis for the formation of a new system of indicators for assessing the energy efficiency of industrial facilities, as well as providing formulas for calculating indicators for assessing the energy efficiency of an industrial facility.

The use of the method of expert assessments, which was modified by the authors in relation to the studied subject area, made it possible to concretize the conditions for assessing an industrial facility and give it meaningful characteristics, make a decision on the choice of factors affecting the level of energy efficiency indicators, determine the system of assessment indicators and rank them according to their degree of significance, which ensured the representativeness of the results. When using the method of expert assessments, in addition to questionnaires, interviews were conducted with leading experts, which made it possible to identify the most controversial areas of research and make a reasonable choice of methods that best suit the tasks being solved. The logic of determining the energy efficiency indicators of industrial facilities is described using the mathematical apparatus of formalizing the consumption of energy resources and modeling individual processes for managing energy efficiency and environmental friendliness of an industrial facility, taking into account the principle of multiple options for the types of resources, estimated and standard values of the level of their consumption, which allows a flexible approach to the formation of a system of energy efficiency indicators.

3. Results

In the process of researching the collected material using the considered methods, the author's position was formed regarding the system of energy efficiency indicators of an industrial facility and to solve the assigned tasks.

To solve the problem of determining factors for assessing the energy efficiency of an industrial facility, the consolidated information of the analysis of the regulatory and legal framework in the field of energy efficiency and the results of a comparative analysis of the conditions for ensuring energy efficiency of industrial enterprises, presented in the practice of various countries of the world, was used. Comparative characteristics showed a wide variety of approaches to energy efficiency management in buildings and production processes.

The identified conditions for energy efficiency, taking into account the current focus on compliance with the principles of sustainable development and ESG, were supplemented by new conditions in the management of energy efficiency and environmental friendliness of an industrial enterprise that operates on the basis of the industrial facility being assessed. The question of assessing the significance of energy efficiency conditions in the industry was included in an expert survey conducted by the authors, on the basis of which the factor space for ensuring the energy efficiency of an industrial facility was determined.

The classification of factors for assessing the energy efficiency of an industrial facility is based on signs that reflect conditions essential for ensuring the energy efficiency of an industrial facility. The classification of factors for assessing the energy efficiency of an industrial facility proposed by the authors includes general and specific factors. A sign of distinguishing into the group of general factors for assessing the energy efficiency of an industrial facility is the use of traditional resources necessary for the maintenance of buildings and the implementation of the technological process. This group includes the factors of energy consumption and the need for them. Energy consumption factors are controllable, focus on compliance with standards and take into account technical characteristics of the building and equipment, energy consumption depending on their type (fuel, heat energy, electricity), water consumption for building maintenance and production activities, features of technological processes, specifics activities of industrial facilities, etc. Factors of demand for energy resources are determined by the environment in which the efficient use of energy resources is carried out.

An indication of the selection of specific factors for assessing the energy efficiency of an industrial facility into the group is the use of special resources that are applicable for the maintenance of buildings and the implementation of technological processes. This group includes the factors of using non-traditional and interchangeable types of energy resources, the availability of automation of building engineering systems and technological processes, the environmental characteristics of the building and technological processes. The group of specific factors of energy efficiency of an industrial facility includes the factors of energy efficiency and environmental friendliness, which are determined by the efficiency and timing of those carried out by the enterprise, which operates on the basis of the industrial facility being assessed, investments in energy-saving measures, the presence of a certified energy management system at the enterprise in accordance with the requirements of the international standard ISO 50001 and the monitoring of energy consumption, using technologies from the list of the best available technologies (BAT) in the production process.

The features of the object of assessment and a significant number of specific factors of influence on the characteristics of the consumption of energy resources during the functioning of industrial production during the operation of the building and the creation of products, the importance of which is constantly increasing in modern conditions, determined the need to form a new system of indicators for assessing the energy efficiency of an industrial facility. It was based on the following principles for solving this problem:

- consistency, representing the integrity and interconnectedness of the elements of an industrial facility (buildings, structures, machines, equipment and technological processes) and their consumption of all types of energy resources;
- complexity, taking into account all aspects of energy consumption of an industrial facility, types and quantities of consumed types of energy resources in accordance with technological processes, as well as regulatory and technical documentation, standards and other regulations;
- the sequence that determines the processes for assessing the energy efficiency of industrial facilities and the regulation of the consumption of energy resources by an industrial facility in the context of focusing on the principles of ESG and sustainable development;
- comparability, providing a unified format for presenting energy efficiency indicators of an industrial facility and uniformity of measurements of indicators of consumption of energy resources;

- rationality, which determines the assessment of the energy efficiency of an industrial facility on the basis of determining the necessary and sufficient level of consumption of energy resources for products at an industrial facility of the required quality and quantity;
- functional interconnection, ensuring the need to assess energy efficiency, taking into account the requirements of resource consumption and resource-saving in technological processes of an industrial facility, energy consumption and energy-saving standards, control of energy resources consumption;
- the continuity of processes, which implies the possibility of ensuring the continuity of the processes of strategic, tactical and operational planning of energy-saving and energy-efficiency indicators of industrial facilities, as well as their monitoring at all stages of the life cycle of an industrial facility;
- orientation towards the market situation, which implies the correlation of the assessed indicators of energy saving and energy efficiency in conjunction with the position of an industrial enterprise in specialized markets;
- the unity of the approach, providing an identical presentation of the logic of formation, definition, accounting, analysis, adjustment of indicators of consumption of energy resources, as well as the indicator of energy efficiency of the evaluated industrial facility;
- the obligation to take into account the requirements of the current legislation of the countries and the mandatory standards for the consumption of all types of energy and fuel consumption in the production process;
- environmental friendliness, which determines the need to provide an opportunity to characterize the impact of the results of the activity of an industrial enterprise on the components of the environment when determining the indicators of energy saving and energy efficiency of industrial facilities.

The systematization of the proposed indicators for assessing the energy efficiency of industrial facilities was carried out from the point of view of participation in the final result of the consumption of energy resources. The first group of indicators is associated with the building as a place where the production process is carried out, the second, directly with the technological process of manufacturing products, and the third, with the management process aimed at ensuring energy efficiency and environmental friendliness of the building and the technological process.

The new system of indicators for assessing the energy efficiency of an industrial facility within the framework of the three identified groups takes into account the indicators recommended by experts for use in assessing the energy efficiency of industrial facilities and analyzed by the authors taking into account the above principles (Figure 4).

In the new system of indicators for assessing the energy efficiency of an industrial facility, the authors used the values and characteristics of the conditions for their formation to systematize indicators, which have a decisive influence on the estimated energy efficiency of an industrial facility. Let us briefly characterize the substantive characteristics of the main ones that play a system-forming role. The investigated and selected indicators, first of all, include such indicators as: total power of electrical receiving devices; energy intensity of production per unit of production (consumption of all energy resources referred to the total volume of production in monetary terms); total consumption of energy resources; coefficients of performance (COP) and fuel use (FU) of production equipment used for the main production and auxiliary processes; the share of payments for energy resources in the value of manufactured products; main product range.

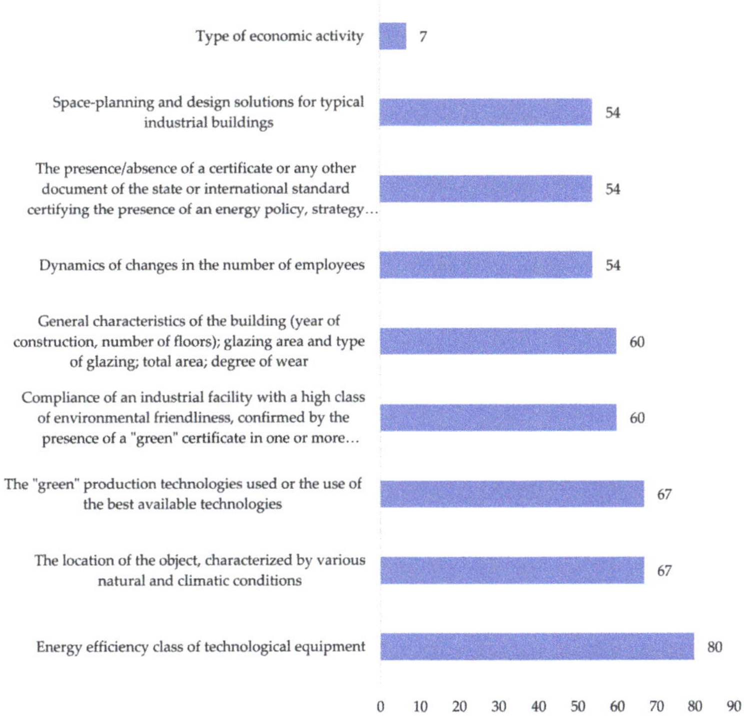

Figure 4. Distribution of expert opinion on the significance of indicators for assessing the energy efficiency of industrial facilities.

The natural indicator of the total power of electrical receiving devices is important, which characterizes the amount of energy consumption depending on the type of electrical equipment and a specific consumer, seasonal load, characteristics of technological processes, installed capacity and efficiency, etc. The natural indicators also include the consumption of energy resources. It reflects the total amount of energy resources consumed by an industrial facility in a comparable form for a certain period of time. Taking these indicators into account in the system of energy efficiency indicators of an industrial facility will make it possible to determine not only the amount of energy resources required for the operation of power equipment and an industrial facility as a whole in the time period but also to ensure control over the processes of their consumption. The specific indicator of the energy intensity per unit of production characterizes the energy efficiency of the production process in terms of the amount of all energy resources in value terms per unit of the value of the production of an industrial enterprise. Relative indicators of efficiency and FU characterize the amount of useful energy resources and fuel to their total amount. In the system of energy efficiency indicators of an industrial facility, their place is ensured not only by a direct influence on the general level of energy efficiency of an industrial facility but also by the information content of its dynamics when organizing energy efficiency management of an industrial facility. The share of payments for energy resources in the value of manufactured products characterizes the energy efficiency of the technological process and, as an integral part, determines the level of energy efficiency of an industrial facility as a whole and how a controlled value ensures its dynamics.

The system of indicators for assessing the energy efficiency of an industrial facility formed by the authors is presented in Table 2.

Table 2. The system of indicators for assessing the energy efficiency of an industry.

Source of Expense	Energy Type	Monitoring Indicator
First group of indicators—Energy efficiency of buildings		
1.1. Resource efficiency in buildings		
Energy consumption	Fuel (boiler-furnace, motor)	Fuel consumption for heating and ventilation of the building, hot water supply
		Fuel consumption system status
	Thermal energy	Heat consumption for heating and ventilation of the building, hot water supply
		Condition of external structures of the building
		Heat consumption system status
	Electricity	Electricity consumption for lighting, utility systems and air conditioning systems
		Power system status
Water consumption		Water consumption for engineering systems
		Condition of the water supply system of the building
1.2. Consumption of non-traditional and other types of energy resources in buildings		
		Renewable energy consumption
		Secondary energy consumption
1.3. Automation of building engineering systems		
		The presence of a centralized dispatching system with the possibility of individual (zonal) regulation
		Availability of local automation systems for engineering support systems
1.4. Environmental characteristics of the building		
		Environmental friendliness of building materials and structures
		Sustainability of the building
		Environmental characteristics of the air environment (microclimate)
Second group of indicators—Energy efficiency of technological processes		
2.1. Efficiency of resource consumption in production		
Energy consumption	Fuel (boiler-furnace, motor)	Fuel consumption for production
		Technical condition of equipment
	Thermal energy	Heat consumption for production
		Technical condition of equipment
	Electricity	Electricity consumption for production
		Technical condition of equipment
2.2. Consumption of non-traditional and other types of energy resources in the production process		
		Renewable energy consumption
		Secondary energy consumption
2.3. Automation of technological processes		
		Availability of modern automation systems for technological processes

Table 2. *Cont.*

Source of Expense	Energy Type	Monitoring Indicator
2.4. Environmental characteristics of technological processes		
		Environmental performance of equipment
		Sustainability of raw materials used in the production process
2.5. Energy efficiency of production		
		Energy intensity of production, thousand tons/thousand rubles.
		The share of payments for energy resources in the value of manufactured products (works, services)
		Efficiency of technological equipment
		The level of electricity losses in the electrical networks of the industrial complex
		The level of heat losses in heating networks
		Application of energy-saving equipment
		Renewable energy consumption
		Secondary energy consumption
2.6. Automation of technological processes		
		Availability of modern automation systems for technological processes
2.7. Environmental characteristics of technological processes		
		Environmental performance of equipment
		Sustainability of raw materials used in the production process
2.8. Energy efficiency of production		
		Energy intensity of production, thousand tons/thousand rubles.
		The share of payments for energy resources in the value of manufactured products (works, services)
		Efficiency of technological equipment
		The level of electricity losses in the electrical networks of the industrial complex
		The level of heat losses in heating networks
		Application of energy-saving equipment
Third group of indicators—Ensuring energy efficiency and environmental friendliness of an industrial facility		
3.1. Energy efficiency management of an industrial facility		
		Efficiency of investments in energy-saving measures
		Energy management system ISO 50001
		Energy monitoring
		Use of technologies from the list of the best available technologies (BAT)
		Payback of energy-saving measures
3.2. Environmental management of an industrial facility		
		The quality of sanitary protection
		Environmental management system ISO 14000
		The quality of waste collection and disposal

The proposed system of indicators for assessing the energy efficiency of an industrial facility includes quantitative and qualitative indicators. It is assumed that quantitative indicators are determined by calculation, and qualitative ones are based on expert opinion. To ensure the comparability of all indicators in the system, quantitative and qualitative indicators should be converted into a single measurement system, for example, into points.

The first group of indicators, "Energy efficiency of the building", includes four subgroups. The subgroup of indicators of resource consumption in a building provides information on the consumption of all types of fuel (boiler, stove, motor), heat energy, electricity and water consumption used to ensure the functioning of the building. These quantitative indicators are supplemented by qualitative indicators reflecting the condition of the building, its structural elements and systems and the possibility of changing the indicators of energy consumption and the structural elements and systems themselves to improve the energy efficiency of an industrial facility. The allocation of quantitative indicators for the consumption of non-traditional and other types of energy resources in buildings into an independent subgroup is due to the focus on ensuring the requirements for environmental friendliness of the building and reducing costs when implementing measures to improve the energy efficiency of an industrial facility. In the subgroup "automation of building engineering systems", qualitative indicators are presented that reflect the presence or absence of dispatching systems and automation of the process of energy consumption during building operation, as well as the ability to manage their implementation in the building operation process when solving the issue of improving the energy efficiency of an industrial facility. The subgroup of quality indicators reflecting the environmental characteristics of the building itself and used in the construction of environmental materials, including taking into account the characteristics of the air environment, is directly related to modern trends in ensuring ESG principles.

The second group of indicators, "Energy efficiency of technological processes", includes five subgroups. The first four subgroups of indicators coincide in content with similar subgroups in the group of indicators "Energy efficiency of the building", but the quantitative and qualitative indicators presented in them are related to the technological processes of production at an industrial facility. At the same time, the indicators of consumption of energy resources and water are supplemented with qualitative indicators of the state of equipment (for example, the degree of wear, innovation), which makes it possible to manage indicators of the consumption of energy resources and water through the management of quality characteristics in order to increase the energy efficiency of an industrial facility. Additionally, this subgroup includes quantitative and qualitative indicators of energy efficiency of production to determine the degree of compliance of the technological process of production with environmental friendliness and ESG principles and obtain information for making management decisions to improve the energy efficiency of an industrial facility in this context.

The third group of indicators, "Ensuring energy efficiency and environmental friendliness of an industrial facility", includes two subgroups of quantitative and qualitative indicators related to the management of energy efficiency of an industrial facility (efficiency of investments in energy-saving measures, the presence of an ISO 50001 energy management system, monitoring of energy consumption, the use of BAT technologies and the return on investment of energy-saving measures) and management of the environmental friendliness of an industrial facility (the quality of sanitary protection, the presence of an ISO 14000 environmental management system and the quality of waste collection and disposal), in accordance with the principles of environmental friendliness and ESG, guaranteeing a focus on improving the energy efficiency of an industrial facility and ensuring its development in line with modern energy-saving trends.

For the values of qualitative and quantitative indicators of energy efficiency of an industrial facility, the task of developing formulas for calculating them using a point assessment was solved.

The energy efficiency of a building in terms of the consumption of energy and non-traditional resources in points is determined by the formula:

$$Sbld\_l = \sum_{i=1}^{m} Sbld_i, \tag{1}$$

where *Sbld_l* is the sum of points assigned to the building in accordance with the consumption of all energy and non-traditional resources, and $Sbld_i$ is the number of points assigned to the building in accordance with the consumption of an energy or non-traditional resource of the i-th type ($i = 1, \ldots m$).

The level of consumption of energy and non-traditional resources of the i-th type in points is determined by the formula:

$$Sbld_i = \sum_{j=1}^{n} di_j, \tag{2}$$

where $Sbld_i$ is the sum of points assigned to the building in accordance with the consumption of the energy and non-traditional resource of the i-th type for each j-th direction of expenditure ($j = 1, \ldots, n$) and di_j is the number of points assigned to the building in accordance with the percentage of deviation of the actual values of the consumption of the energy and non-traditional resource of the i-th type in the j-th direction of expenditure.

When calculating the percentage of deviation in points, the following designations are used: *aij* is the actual value of the energy and non-traditional resource of the i-th type, spent on the building in the j direction, *Nij* is the normative value of the energy and non-traditional resource of the i-th type, spent on the building in the j direction and *Pij* is the percentage value of the indicator of the actual consumption of the energy and non-traditional resource of the i-th type in the j-th direction of consumption, referred to the building, in comparison with the standard indicator.

To calculate the indicator, the formula is used:

$$SPij = aij \times Nij, \tag{3}$$

$$dij = Pij - 100\%. \tag{4}$$

The number of points for a specific percentage of deviation is assigned based on an expert survey.

When assessing the qualitative indicators of the energy efficiency of an industrial facility, the points are assigned based on expert analysis. In this case, the assessment of the quality characteristics of the energy efficiency of the building is determined by the formula:

$$Sbld\_q = \sum_{z=1}^{Z} Sbld\_q_z, \tag{5}$$

where *Sbld_q* is the sum of points, taking into account the quality characteristics of the energy efficiency of the building, and $Sbld\_q_z$ is the sum of points that determines the qualitative characteristics of the energy efficiency of the building based on the opinion of experts on the criterion z (z = 1, ... , Z).

The energy efficiency of buildings in points is determined by the formula:

$$Sbld = Sbld\_l + Sbld\_q, \tag{6}$$

where *Sbld* is the sum of points assigned to the building in accordance with the consumption of all energy and non-traditional resources, and points for the quality characteristics of the building, and *Sbld_l* is the sum of points assigned to the building in accordance with the consumption of all energy and non-traditional resources.

The calculations of the energy efficiency indicator for technological processes are carried out in the same way as the calculation of the energy efficiency indicators of a building.

To determine the qualitative characteristics of the energy efficiency of technological processes, the following formula is used:

$$Stp\_q = \sum_{z=1}^{Z} Stp\_q_z, \tag{7}$$

where *Stp_q* is the sum of points, taking into account the qualitative characteristics of the energy efficiency of technological processes, and Stp_q_z is the number of points assigned to the quality of energy efficiency of technological processes by the opinion of experts to the criterion z ($z = 1, \ldots, Z$).

The energy efficiency of technological processes in points is determined by the formula:

$$Stp = Stp\_l + Stp\_q, \tag{8}$$

where *Stp* is the sum of points assigned to technological processes in accordance with the consumption of all energy and non-traditional resources, and points for the quality characteristics of the building, and *Stp_l*, is the sum of points attributed to technological processes in accordance with the consumption of all energy and non-traditional resources.

The quality characteristics of ensuring energy efficiency and environmental friendliness are determined by the formula:

$$Sem = \sum_{z=1}^{Z} Sem\_q_z, \tag{9}$$

where *Sem* is the sum of points, taking into account the qualitative characteristics of environmental and energy management at the enterprise, and Sem_q_z is the number of points assigned to the quality of environmental and energy management according to experts, with the criterion z ($z = 1, \ldots, Z$).

The final indicator of the energy efficiency of an industrial facility in points:

$$Seff = Sbld + Stp + Sem. \tag{10}$$

The final value of the energy efficiency indicator of an industrial facility is the basis for classifying an industrial facility as a certain energy efficiency class.

4. Discussion

In the course of the analysis of open data and the results of an expert survey, the absence in the world practice of national and international systems for assessing the energy efficiency of industrial facilities was revealed. This fact allows us to assume that the system of indicators for assessing the energy efficiency of industrial facilities proposed by the authors can not only be integrated into the national rating systems but also become the basis for international rating systems for assessing the energy efficiency of industrial facilities. This proposal reflects the possibility and necessity of using the results obtained at different levels of energy efficiency management, at the level of micro, meso and macroeconomic systems, which correspond to the organization of energy efficiency management of industrial facilities at the level of an individual enterprise, region, state as a whole and internationally. At the same time, it is the scale of the possible use of the system for assessing the level of energy efficiency of industrial facilities that determines the need for discussions in solving the problem of ensuring the uniformity of measurements.

Considering the issue of the uniformity of energy efficiency measurements, it should be noted that the expert opinion of the survey participants, combined with the analysis of the researchers' materials, allowed the authors to take into account the most significant factors in ensuring energy efficiency and proposing the corresponding estimated indicators, which are presented above. At the same time, it is provided that the energy efficiency of a building and technological processes is assessed based on the results of an energy survey of an industrial facility, but the assessment of quantitative values, for example, at the levels of "high energy efficiency" and "low energy efficiency" are completely uncertain. The assessment situation is further complicated by the fact that there are no standards for the level of specific energy consumption (energy intensity) of production for all types of industrial activity in the considered reference group of countries. There are standards for building structures (for example, restrictions on heat loss) and, in part, for equipment for some types of industrial production. At the same time, in the new approach to assessing the energy efficiency of industrial facilities proposed by the authors, the issues of ensuring energy efficiency and environmental friendliness are predetermined for the first two groups of indicators, to a greater extent reflecting the realization of the energy-saving potential at an enterprise that operates on the basis of the industrial facility being assessed.

When analyzing acceptable assessment methods, two options were considered, used in combination with each other: an assessment based on the calculation of the specific indicator of energy consumption and its comparison with standard (reference) indicators; a rating score based on the scoring model. In this regard, such a combination of them was used, which excludes contradictions while ensuring the uniformity of energy efficiency measurements, and allows an unambiguous interpretation of the obtained quantitative values according to the proposed formulas. However, as the studies have shown, the use of scoring and the implementation of rating of industrial facilities on this basis, due to the differences in the organization of this activity in different countries of the world, requires the correct choice of the main positions for rating, which are proposed for discussion in this section.

Let us take a look at the context of this discussion. Recently, rating systems for evaluating various objects have become most widespread. This fact is connected not so much with the simplicity of the assessment procedures but with the possibility of providing greater coverage of the factors taken into account in the assessment, the convenience of comparing the results obtained for the assessment objects by a set of heterogeneous indicators, as well as the visibility of the presented results in dynamics, taking into account the assurance of the uniformity of measurements. Moreover, important advantages of the rating assessment are the possibility of comparisons in the presence of not only quantitatively measurable but also qualitatively assessed parameters/characteristics of the object. For example, in the proposed approach to assessing the energy efficiency of industrial facilities, due to the integration of two assessment methods in determining indicators, it became possible to take into account indicators that were previously rarely used, for example, the use of RES and BAT.

It is possible to take into account the presence of the enterprise, which operates on the basis of the assessed industrial facility, a policy of sustainable energy efficient and environmental development, confirmed by the corresponding certificates ISO-50001 and ISO-14001, as part of the third group of indicators proposed by the authors for assessing the processes of ensuring energy efficiency and environmental friendliness. This opportunity is of particular importance in modern conditions due to the trend of transition of the economies of many countries to low-carbon energy on a global scale and the policy measures introduced in a number of countries in this direction, including mandatory "carbon reporting". Therefore, the proposed system includes a group of indicators, which is associated with the organization of processes for achieving sustainable development by ensuring energy efficiency and environmental friendliness of industrial facilities, including through effective enterprise management.

At the same time, there are also known difficulties in the construction of point-rating assessments, which the authors, introducing into discussion issues for discussion, want to avoid. The most common disadvantages include: redundancy of criteria (especially in the case when there is a partial duplication of criteria), which increases the complexity of work with the evaluation system and the subjective nature of the scoring of indicators, which depends on the level of competence of experts. Let us single out several positions for discussion related to the implementation of a point-rating assessment in assessing the energy efficiency of industrial facilities. These include:

- determination of criteria and scales (ranks) for evaluating indicators;
- determination of intervals (standardization) of permissible values;
- interpretation of the data obtained to make a decision regarding the evaluated object.

The simplest and most common method of constructing a rating scale, used in all areas of knowledge, is the method of paired comparisons—the assessment and choice of solutions, widely used in expert assessments when it is necessary to prioritize in the process of any activity or ranking of various objects [46]. To rank according to the importance of indicators for assessing the energy-efficiency of industrial facilities in each group, it is advisable to use the analysis of hierarchies by Thomas Saaty, which includes the following stages:

1. Isolation of the problem and determination of the purpose of the assessment.
2. Determination of the main criteria and alternatives for the assessment.
3. Building a hierarchy: a tree from a goal through criteria to alternatives.
4. Construction of a matrix of "pairwise comparisons" of criteria by purpose and alternatives by criteria.
5. Analysis of the resulting matrices.
6. Determination of the weights of alternatives according to the hierarchy system [46].

When compiling on a scale, you can use the existing practice, which involves the determination of the minimum allowable (threshold value) number of points for each indicator, group of indicators and the total amount of points. The threshold value of the final score can be adjusted according to the results of a survey of experts. The step of the interval value corresponding to a certain level of the energy efficiency class is proposed to be made equivalent. This practice is used when ranking objects of assessment in the systems of international "green" standards for real estate, which at the level of national rating systems in the field of energy efficient and green construction is coordinated by the International Committee on the so-called "green" buildings (Green Building Council) [47]. Therefore, the discussed issues of justifying the approach to rating the set of energy efficiency indicators of industrial facilities in order to ensure the uniformity of its measurements and interpretation of the data obtained are considered by the authors on the basis of a comparison of rating systems for assessing buildings according to international "green" standards. This makes it possible to form a judgment regarding the first two groups of indicators in the system of indicators of energy efficiency of industrial facilities proposed by the authors, which are associated with buildings and the production technologies implemented in them. Table 3 shows the structure of rating systems for assessing "green" standards in construction, for each section of which a set of indicators is used to determine the integral values obtained using the point-rating assessment.

Each section of the assessment includes several assessment indicators, normalized by quantitative values and qualitative characteristics, which are assessed on a scale in credits (points). After summing up the points received for each section, they are compared with the corresponding scaling system (Table 4). According to experts, this scaling system is characterized by the subjectivity of the distribution of final points between the assessment levels. It is also obvious that the set of sections, indicators and assessment criteria is determined in accordance with the individual priorities of expert organizations and national interests [48].

As you can see from Table 3, there is a scatter in the levels (ranks) of the scale in the compared standards. In practice, this leads to the fact that in the case of the "shortage" of several points to the threshold level, for example, in the LEED system, the company can apply for a certificate in the BREEAM system, which has more levels and a more flexible assessment system. For an enterprise, such an opportunity may be positive, but for a national or international monitoring system for data on the assessed objects, it is an obvious distortion of statistics.

Table 3. Sections of the assessment of buildings according to international "green" standards.

BREEAM [28]	LEED [27]	DGNB [29]	WELL [30]
Energy	Location and transport accessibility	Environmental quality	Water
Health and wellness	Sustainable objects	Economical quality	Air
Innovation	Water use efficiency	Sociocultural and functional quality	Nutrition
Land use	Energy and atmosphere	Technical quality (only for new objects)	Lighting
Materials (edit)	Water use efficiency	Process quality (only for new objects)	Physical activity
Management	Indoor environmental quality	Location quality (new properties only)	Thermal comfort
Pollution	Integrative process		Noise control
Transport	Innovations		Materials (edit)
Waste	Regional priorities		Mental health
Water			Community
			Innovations

Table 4. Scales of assessments in the systems of international "green" standards.

	BREEAM	LEED	DGNB	WELL
Ranking levels (scores)	Pass (30–44) Good (45–54) Very good (55–69) Excellent (70–84) Outstanding (≥85)	Certified (40–49) Silver (50–59) Gold (60–79) Platinum (≥80)	Bronze (<35 *) Silver (35–49) Gold (50–64) Platinum (≥65)	Silver (50–59) Gold (60–79) Platinum (≥80)

* For operated buildings.

Regarding the third group of indicators proposed based on the results of studies of the system for assessing the energy efficiency of an industrial facility, which is associated with the organization of processes for achieving sustainable development through measures to ensure energy efficiency and environmental friendliness, the authors used another material for comparison, which focuses on the activities of the enterprise management. Two methodological approaches were chosen for discussion in a similar area of assessment—the determination of an integral point assessment of the sustainable economic condition of an enterprise and a comprehensive rating assessment of enterprises.

In the first of the considered methodological approaches, the integral point assessment of the sustainable economic state of the enterprise, the choice and justification of the criteria for this assessment and the establishment of restrictions on their change are presented in detail [49]. For this, for each indicator included in the corresponding classification group of assessment, either the upper and lower criteria boundaries of the level of the analyzed indicators are determined, or their optimal values, and for some indicators (for example, in terms of performance indicators), the trend of their change is taken as a criterion. Depending on the deviation of the achieved level of the indicator from the selected criterion, a point estimate is established according to the existing scale, which allows the company to be attributed to one of six classes of solvency. Thus, it can be noted that there is a principle of differentiation for choosing a scale (ranks) for assessing indicators, which takes into account their specific features.

In the second of the considered methodological approaches, the complex rating of enterprises is based on their comparison for each indicator of economic condition with a conditional reference enterprise that has the best results for all compared indicators, which is determined by actual data [50]. Thus, the basis for obtaining the rating of an enterprise is not the subjective assumptions of experts but the highest results of enterprises from the entire set of compared objects that have developed in real market competition. The benchmark for comparison is the most successful competitor, which has the best indicators. When implementing rating within the framework of this methodological approach, the main problem is finding a "reference" object.

Returning to the discussion of the point-rating assessment when making a decision regarding the assessed object when assessing the energy efficiency of an industrial facility, we can consider the following scale as a proposal: all assessment levels can be conditionally divided into "very high", "high", "medium", "low" and "critically low" energy efficiency. This can be used, for example, to develop various measures along the entire "vertical" energy efficiency management, from the state level to the enterprise level. In the case of establishing a high level of energy efficiency of the assessed object, the state can stimulate an enterprise that operates on the basis of the assessed industrial facility with tax incentives (for example, exemption from property tax) and other economic preferences. The most significant result for the enterprise itself is the identification of the potential for its even more successful development and the attraction of investments through "green" and "white" certificates. If a "low" and "critically low" level is identified, the enterprise needs to take urgent measures to bring the facility to a higher level of energy efficiency.

The considered disputable aspects in the study make it possible to determine its prospects associated with the development of the proposed new approach to assessing the energy efficiency of industrial facilities, namely, the need for:

- development of criteria and scales for assessing the energy efficiency of industrial facilities while ranking the indicators according to the degree of significance. Taking into account the analyzed experience, it is necessary to use the method of paired comparison of energy efficiency indicators with the involvement of experts;
- to define intervals (standardization) of permissible values of indicators. Studies have shown that it is advisable to determine the minimum threshold value for the sum of points, determined by the minimum permissible (according to regulatory documents and expert opinion) values for individual indicators and corresponding groups;
- to form recommendations for the interpretation of the data obtained when making decisions regarding the evaluated object. Based on the estimates obtained, the management of the enterprise will be able to make decisions on the choice of priority areas for increasing the level of energy efficiency of an industrial facility, create long-term and current plans containing organizational, methodological, technological and incentive measures to carry out the necessary energy-saving measures.

Thus, at the next stage of the study, it is planned, taking into account the debatable issues (the calculation basis for determining the indicators while using the possibilities of using data arrays of domestic and international standards), to rank the obtained values based on the pairwise comparison, and also to form a scale of energy efficiency levels of industrial facilities.

5. Conclusions

In the process of analyzing the subject area of the research, scientific and practical problems were identified and solved, which ensured the formation of a new approach to the system for assessing the energy efficiency of industrial facilities. The results obtained have been achieved through the use of a set of research methods, primarily based on materials from authoritative publications, the information provided on the official websites of state authorities in various countries, as well as a survey of the expert community.

The primary issue resolved in the study was the clarification of the category of "industrial facility", which is the object of the study. A common problem was identified—the lack of a unified approach to its definition in many countries, which was confirmed during a survey of representatives of the authoritative expert community. The proposed definition made it possible to concretize an industrial facility, generalizing the existing formulations, taking into account expert opinion, which made it possible to implement subsequent tasks. For an objective description of the factor space of the evaluated object of research, which determines the characteristics of its energy efficiency, specially formulated questions on this problem area were included in the expert survey conducted by the authors. The results of the survey made it possible to determine a set of factors affecting the energy efficiency of an industrial facility, as well as their distribution according to the degree of importance.

The most important result of the study was the formed system of indicators of energy efficiency of industrial facilities, formed into three groups: energy efficiency of a building, energy efficiency of technological processes, ensuring energy efficiency and environmental friendliness. The proposed system of indicators takes into account the accumulated practical experience in ensuring energy efficiency in many countries and the actual theoretical developments presented in scientific works, which made it possible to form a new approach to assessing the energy efficiency of an industrial facility and to develop methodological provisions for determining the assessment indicators. On the basis of these provisions, it is possible to conduct a point-rating assessment of the energy efficiency of an industrial facility using formalized procedures lined up by the authors in a certain sequence.

It is assumed that the developed system of indicators can be integrated into the national standards of countries and used in international rating systems for assessing the energy efficiency of industrial facilities. In the context of the transition of the world energy sector to the principles of sustainable development and low-carbon energy, the restrictions imposed by many countries on the volume of greenhouse emissions, a new approach to assessing the energy efficiency of industrial facilities will provide not only an effective tool for large-scale monitoring of the efficiency of energy-saving measures at industrial facilities of countries but also the implementation of the principles of sustainable development and ESG at the enterprises of the industrial sector of the economy.

The questions proposed by the authors for discussion determine the need for further research in the direction of developing a methodology for assessing energy efficiency indicators of industrial facilities. The expert assessment of energy saving and energy efficiency of industrial facilities proposed after discussions by the authors on the basis of a "reference" indicator for each group of types of economic activities of industrial facilities will provide an opportunity to classify industrial facilities by the level of energy efficiency and will allow unambiguous determination of the position of the facility in solving state-important problems, including in the field of subsidizing and lending measures to reduce energy intensity and optimize energy costs, to develop and implement alternative technologies with low energy intensity and will also create an important component of financial planning at the macro, meso and micro levels.

The applied significance of the results lies in solving the most important state tasks to ensure the implementation of energy conservation and energy efficiency policies by systematizing information on the energy characteristics of the key end consumers of energy resources, industrial facilities, and forming an objective idea of the potential for reducing the energy intensity of industrial products across the country.

Author Contributions: Conceptualization, N.V., T.M., N.T. and N.S. (Natalia Shchepkina); methodology, T.M., N.T. and N.S. (Natalia Shchepkina); validation N.V. and T.M.; formal analysis, N.T. and N.S. (Natalia Shchepkina); investigation, T.M., N.T. and N.S. (Natalia Shchepkina); writing—review and editing, N.V., N.S. (Natalia Solopova), N.T., N.S. (Natalia Shchepkina) and T.M.; visualization, N.T., N.S. (Natalia Shchepkina) and T.M.; supervision, N.V.; project administration, N.V. All authors have read and agreed to the published version of the manuscript.

Funding: This research was funded by RFBR, grant number 20-010-00754.

Data Availability Statement: Not applicable.

Conflicts of Interest: The authors declare no conflict of interest.

References

1. Leonard, M.; Pisani-Ferry, J.; Shapiro, J.; Tagliapietra, S.; Wolff, G. The Geopolitics of the European Green Deal. Policy Contribution 04/2021, Bruegel. 2021. Available online: https://www.bruegel.org/wp-content/uploads/2021/02/PC-04-GrenDeal-2021-1.pdf (accessed on 1 December 2021).
2. Mitronova, T. The Fourth Energy Transition: Risks and Challenges for RussiaVedomosti. 2021. Available online: https://www.vedomosti.ru/opinion/articles/2021/01/31/856101-chetvertii-energoperehod (accessed on 1 December 2021).
3. Corporate Strategies for Carbon Neutrality. An Overview of the Climate Commitments of Global Companies. Available online: https://www.economy.gov.ru/material/file/f55d57f8dcbb8ec195b1575e857610dc/03062021.pdf (accessed on 1 December 2021).
4. How Will ESG Performance Shape Your Future? Available online: https://www.ey.com/en_gl/assurance/how-will-esg-performance-shape-your-future (accessed on 1 December 2021).
5. ESG Investment. Available online: https://www.bwfa.com/esg-investing/ (accessed on 1 December 2021).
6. Statistical World Energy Yearbook 2021. Available online: https://yearbook.enerdata.net/total-energy/world-consumption-statistics.html (accessed on 1 December 2021).
7. Directive 2012/27/EU of the European Parliament and of the Council of 25 October 2012 on Energy Efficiency, Amending Directives 2009/125/EC and 2010/30/EU and Repealing Directives 2004/8/EC and 2006/32/EC. Available online: https://eur-lex.europa.eu/legal-content/EN/TXT/?qid=1399375464230&uri=CELEX:32012L0027 (accessed on 1 December 2021).
8. Directive (EU) 2018/844 of the European Parliament and of the Council of 30 May 2018 Amending Directive 2010/31/EU on the Energy Performance of Buildings and Directive 2012/27/EU on Energy Efficiency. Available online: https://eur-lex.europa.eu/legal-content/EN/TXT/?uri=uriserv%3AOJ.L_.2018.156.01.0075.01.ENG (accessed on 1 December 2021).
9. Proposal for a Directive of the European Parliament and Council on Energy Efficiency (Revised). Available online: https://eur-lex.europa.eu/legal-content/EN/TXT/?uri=CELEX:52021PC0558 (accessed on 1 December 2021).
10. Energy Efficiency Law. Available online: https://www.meti.go.jp/english/information/data/laws.html#anre (accessed on 1 December 2021).
11. Gebäudeenergiegesetz (GEG). Available online: https://www.bgbl.de/xaver/bgbl/start.xav?startbk=Bundesanzeiger_BGBl&bk=Bundesanzeiger_BGBl&start=//*[@attr_id=%27bgbl107s1519.pdf%27]#__bgbl__%2F%2F*%5B%40attr_id%3D%27bgbl120s1728.pdf%27%5D__1611934877837 (accessed on 1 December 2021).
12. Law of the People's Republic of China "On Energy Saving". Available online: http://www.nea.gov.cn/2017-11/03/c_136725225.htm (accessed on 1 December 2021).
13. Foreign Electric Power Industry. Available online: https://www.np-sr.ru/ru/market/cominfo/foreign/index.htm#11 (accessed on 1 December 2021).
14. Law on Energy Saving and Energy Efficiency Improvement and on Amendments to Certain Legislative Acts of the Russian Federation: Federal Law No. 261-FZ от 23.11.2009 г. Available online: https://docs.cntd.ru/document/9017693 (accessed on 1 December 2021).
15. CIS Electric Power Council. Anniversary Publication of the Summary Report on Key Issues of Ecology, Energy Efficiency and RES in the Electric Power Industry of the CIS Participants. Available online: http://energo-cis.ru/wyswyg/file/57-Moscow%202020/After%20SUP/17.11.2020%20%D0%AE%D0%A1%D0%9E%D1%81%20%D1%83%D1%87%D0%B5%D1%82%D0%BE%D0%BC%20%D0%BF%D1%80-%D0%BA%20%D0%9F%D0%9D%D0%90_%D0%9F%D0%B5%D1%82%D1%80%D0%BE%D0%B2%D0%B0.pdf (accessed on 1 December 2021).
16. Energy Policy Act (EPAct). The Energy Policy Act (EPAct) of 2005 (P.L. 109–58). 2005. Available online: https://www.ferc.gov/enforcement/enforce-res/EPAct2005.pdf (accessed on 1 December 2021).
17. Electricity Regulation in South Korea. Available online: https://www.lexology.com/library/detail.aspx?g=4a7f6594-b6b4-4249-a928-a0e02ed683e5 (accessed on 1 December 2021).
18. The Official Website of the Building Energy Codes Program (BECP). Available online: https://www.energycodes.gov/ (accessed on 1 December 2021).
19. The Official Website of the Energy Star Program. Available online: https://www.energystar.gov/about/origins_mission/energy_star_numbers (accessed on 1 December 2021).
20. The Official Website of the State Energy Program (SEP). Available online: https://www.energy.gov/eere/wipo/state-energy-program (accessed on 1 December 2021).
21. The Official Website of the Weatherization Assistance Program. Available online: https://nascsp.org/wap/ (accessed on 1 December 2021).
22. Japanese Programs. Energy Policy of Japan Magyar Tudományos Journal № 40. 2020. Available online: https://cyberleninka.ru/article/n/energeticheskaya-politika-yaponii/viewer (accessed on 1 December 2021).
23. Japanese Programs. Podoba Energy Strategy and Green Energy Transition in Japan. Available online: https://cyberleninka.ru/article/n/energeticheskaya-strategiya-i-perehod-k-zelyonoy-energetike-v-yaponii/viewer (accessed on 1 December 2021).
24. PD CEN ISO/TR 52000-2: 2017 Energy Performance of Buildings—Indicators, Requirements, Ratings and Certifications—Part 2: Explanation and Rationale for ISO 52003-1. Available online: https://www.iso.org/obp/ui/#iso:std:iso:tr:52000:-2:ed-1:v1:en (accessed on 1 December 2021).
25. ISO 50001:2018 Energy Management Standard. Available online: https://www.iso.org/standard/69426.html (accessed on 1 December 2021).

26. Standard ANSI/ASHRAE/IES 90.1-2019—Energy Standard for Buildings, Excluding Low-Rise Residential Buildings. Available online: https://www.ashrae.org/technical-resources/bookstore/standard-90-1 (accessed on 1 December 2021).
27. LEED. Available online: http://leed.usgbc.org/leed.html (accessed on 1 December 2021).
28. BREEAM. Available online: https://www.breeam.com/ (accessed on 1 December 2021).
29. DGNB. Available online: https://www.dgnb-system.de/en/system/ (accessed on 1 December 2021).
30. WELL. Available online: https://www.wellcertified.com/ (accessed on 1 December 2021).
31. ISO 52000-1:2017 Energy Performance of Buildings—EPB Overall Assessment—Part 1: General Framework and Procedures. Available online: https://www.iso.org/standard/65601.html (accessed on 1 December 2021).
32. Standard for the Design of High-Performance Green Buildings Except Low-Rise Residential Buildings. Available online: https://www.ashrae.org/file%20library/technical%20resources/standards%20and%20guidelines/standards%20addenda/189_1_2020_ax_20210126.pdf (accessed on 1 December 2021).
33. International Green Construction Code (IGCC). Available online: https://www.ashrae.org/file%20library/technical%20resources/bookstore/2018-igcc_preview_1102.pdf (accessed on 1 December 2021).
34. Existing Energy Certification Systems for Buildings Around the World. UNDP/GEF Project "Improving Energy Efficiency in the Housing Construction Sector of Turkmenistan" Ashhadab. 2016. Available online: https://docviewer.yandex.ru/view/0/?*=TSwcSs3CZ%2B5%2B6LLNw2GdSw1vwjR7InVybCI6Imh0dHBzOi8vd3d3LnVuZHAub3JnL2NvbnRlbnQvZGFtL3R1cmttZW5pc3Rhbi9kb2NzL2xhdGVzdC1yZXBvcnRzL1dFQl9zeXN0ZW1zJTIwb2YlMjBlbmVyZ3klMjBjZXJ0aWZpY2F0ZXMlMjBvZiUyMGJ1aW (accessed on 1 December 2021).
35. Comparative Overview of Energy Efficiency Standards and Technologies in Buildings in the United Nations Economic Commission for Europe Region. Geneva. 2018. Available online: https://unece.org/fileadmin/DAM/hlm/Meetings/2018/09_05-07_St._Petersburg/EE_Standards_in_Buildings_full_version.ENG.pdf (accessed on 1 December 2021).
36. ISO 52003-1:2017 Energy Performance of Buildings—Indicators, Requirements, Ratings and Certificates—Part 1: General Aspects and Application to the Overall Energy Performance. Available online: https://www.iso.org/standard/65662.html (accessed on 1 December 2021).
37. ISO/TR 52003-2:2017 Energy Performance of Buildings—Indicators, Requirements, Ratings and Certificates—Part 2: Explanation and Justification of ISO 52003-1. Available online: https://www.iso.org/standard/65661.html (accessed on 1 December 2021).
38. Methodology for Determining (Calculating) the Energy Efficiency Classes of Apartment Buildings. Available online: https://sro150.ru/metodiki/1034-opredelenie-raschet-klassov-energeticheskoj-effektivnosti-mnogokvartirnykh-domov (accessed on 1 December 2021).
39. Tusnin, V.M. *Architecture of Civil and Industrial Buildings: Textbook*; ASV Publishing House: Moscow, Russia, 2016; 328p.
40. Fisenko, A.A.; Basse, M.E. Architecture and Modern Information Technologies. -№ 1 (19). 2012. Available online: http://marhi.ru/AMIT/2013/2kvart13/basse/abstract.php (accessed on 1 December 2021).
41. Order of the Ministry of Regional Development of Russia Dated 5 July 2011 No. 320 "On the Approval of the Set of Rules" Ensuring Anti-Terrorist Security of Buildings and Structures; General Design Requirements "(together with SP 132.13330.2011. Set of Rules; Ensuring Anti-Terrorist Protection of Buildings and Structures; General Design Requirements)". Available online: https://www.economy.gov.ru/material/dokumenty/prikaz_minekonomrazvitiya_rossii_ot_29_iyulya_2019_g_468.html (accessed on 1 December 2021).
42. Order of the Federal Agency for Technical Regulation and Metrology Dated 19 December 2017 No. 2031-st "On Approval of the National Standard of the Russian Federation GOST R 58033-2017" Buildings and Structures. Dictionary, Part 1. General Terms. Available online: https://docs.cntd.ru/document/556324271 (accessed on 1 December 2021).
43. Order of the Federal Agency for Technical Regulation and Metrology Dated 26 October 2016 No. 1519-st "On Approval of the National Standard of the Russian Federation GOST R 56828.15-2016" Best Available Technologies. Terms and Definitions. Available online: https://docs.cntd.ru/document/456028927?marker (accessed on 1 December 2021).
44. Law "On the Industrial Policy of the City of Moscow" No. 55 Dated 7 October 2015. Available online: https://docs.cntd.ru/document/537981669 (accessed on 1 December 2021).
45. Order of the Ministry of Construction, Housing and Communal Services of the Russian Federation of 17 September 2019 No. 544/pr "On approval of SP 18.13330.2019" Production Facilities. Planning Organization of the Land Plot "(SNiP II-89-80" General Plans of Industrial Enterprises)". Available online: https://docs.cntd.ru/document/564407614?marker=7D20K3 (accessed on 1 December 2021).
46. Thomas, L.S. Decision Making with the Analytic Hierarchy Process. *Int. J. Serv. Sci.* **2008**, *1*, 83–98. Available online: https://web.archive.org/web/20170918192816/http://www.colorado.edu/geography/leyk/geog_5113/readings/saaty_2008.pdf (accessed on 1 December 2021).
47. World Green Building Council (WorldGBC). Available online: https://www.worldgbc.org/ (accessed on 1 December 2021).
48. Tabunshchikov, Y.A.; Granev, V.V.; Naumov, A.L. Rating System for Assessing the Quality of Buildings. AVOK No. 6'2010/Indoor Microclimate. Available online: https://www.abok.ru/for_spec/articles.php?nid=4690 (accessed on 1 December 2021).

49. Nikiforova, N.A.; Dontsova, L.V.; Dontsov, E.V. Data Mining in Modeling the Financial Condition of Enterprises. Available online: https://www.nifi.ru/images/FILES/Journal/Archive/2011/2/statii/2011_02_01_.pdf (accessed on 1 December 2021).
50. Pchelintsev, A.D.; Pchelintsev, V.A. Methods for Determining Comparative Rating Economic State of Industrial Enterprises. *Bull. Nizhny Novgorod Univ.* **2010**, *3*, 583–593. Available online: http://www.unn.ru/pages/e-library/vestnik/99999999_West_2010_3(2)/37.pdf (accessed on 1 December 2021).

energies

MDPI

Article

Spatial Network Structure of China's Provincial-Scale Tourism Eco-Efficiency: A Social Network Analysis

Qingfang Liu [1], Jinping Song [1,*], Teqi Dai [1], Jianhui Xu [2,3], Jianmei Li [2] and Enru Wang [4]

1 Faculty of Geographical Science, Beijing Normal University, Beijing 100875, China; m13155029850@163.com (Q.L.); daiteqi@bnu.edu.cn (T.D.)
2 School of Geographic Information and Tourism, Chuzhou University, Chuzhou 239099, China; xjhgx@chzu.edu.cn (J.X.); lijianmei@126.com (J.L.)
3 Finnish Meteorological Institute, FI-00101 Helsinki, Finland
4 Department of Geography & Geographic Information Science, University of North Dakota, Grand Forks, ND 58202, USA; enru.wang@email.und.edu
* Correspondence: jinpingsong@163.com

Abstract: While tourism eco-efficiency has been analyzed actively within tourism research, there is an extant dearth of research on the spatial network structure of provincial-scale tourism eco-efficiency. The Super-SBM was used to evaluate the tourism eco-efficiency of 30 provinces (excluding Tibet, Hong Kong, Macao and Taiwan). Then, social network analysis was employed to examine the evolution characteristics regarding the spatial network structure of tourism eco-efficiency. The main results are shown as follows. Firstly, tourism eco-efficiency of more than two thirds' provinces witnessed an increasing trend. Secondly, the spatial network structure of tourism eco-efficiency was still loose and unstable during the sample period. Thirdly, there existed the multidimensional nested and fused spatial factions and condensed subsets in the spatial network structure of tourism eco-efficiency. However, there was still a lack of low-carbon tourism cooperation among second or third sub-groups. These conclusions can provide references for policymakers who expect to reduce carbon emissions from the tourism industry and to achieve sustainable tourism development.

Keywords: low-carbon tourism; tourism eco-efficiency; spatial network correlation; Super-SBM; social network analysis

Citation: Liu, Q.; Song, J.; Dai, T.; Xu, J.; Li, J.; Wang, E. Spatial Network Structure of China's Provincial-Scale Tourism Eco-Efficiency: A Social Network Analysis. *Energies* **2022**, *15*, 1324. https://doi.org/10.3390/en15041324

Academic Editors: Roberto Alonso González Lezcano, Francesco Nocera and Rosa Giuseppina Caponetto

Received: 18 January 2022
Accepted: 8 February 2022
Published: 11 February 2022

1. Introduction

Tourism has solidified its role as the strategic-pillar industry in China [1], accounting for 6.69% of the total gross domestic product (GDP) in 2019. For a long time, tourism has been regarded as an industry with low-carbon and environmental protections [2]. Therefore, adequate attention is not paid to the pollution brought by tourism industry in China. With the expansion and improvement of the tourism economy, the negative environment impacts of the tourism industry have gradually been exposed [3]. The Fourteenth Five Year Plan, issued by the central government in March 2021, emphasized the high-quality development is the main direction of the tourism industry in the next five years. Tourism eco-efficiency is defined as creating more economic value in tourism products and service, while eliminating negative environmental effects and reducing resource consumption [4–6]. The improvement of tourism eco-efficiency cannot only be in accordance with the goal of carbon emission peaking and carbon neutrality (Two Carbon) but also promote the high-quality development of tourism industry [7].

With the exposure of the negative impacts of tourism development on ecological environment, quite a few scholars have gradually begun to concentrate how to achieve low-carbon development in tourist destinations. Moreover, the Sustainable Tourism Development Action Strategy (STDAS) put forward the concept of sustainable tourism, and pointed out that both ecological environment and economic benefit should be taken into consideration [7]. Based on the core principles of sustainable tourism, Gössling, Peeters, Ceron, Dubois, Patterson and Richardson [6], calculating the carbon emissions from the tourism industry, put forward the concept of tourism eco-efficiency. Since then, it has triggered a huge wave in academic tourism circle. Extant assessment methods are divided into two types, namely, the single indicator method, and the model method [4]. With regard to the single indicator method, tourism eco-efficiency can be expressed by the ratio of tourism economic benefit to the environmental effect [8]. During the application of the single indicator method, the tourism receipt and the carbon dioxide emission from tourism industry were defined as the tourism input and the environmental effects, respectively, by Perch-Nielsen, et al. [9] Additionally, some scholars regarded tourism-related carbon footprint as the environmental effect of tourism [10–12]. However, the superior rational is not obtained by the single indicator method; meanwhile, this method is suitable for a single object or item. Thus, the single indicator method may not provide more targeted implications for tourist destination management (TDM) [2]. In terms of the model method, constructing the index system of input-output is a prerequisite for evaluating tourism eco-efficiency; the choice of evaluation models can reduce error, and make the results more scientific [4]. The index system of input–output mainly contains capital, labor, energy consumption, tourism receipt and the environmental effects [4,13]. Moreover, the non-convex metafrontier DEA-based model, Super-DEA model, and Super-EBM model are used to take into consideration the undesired output, such as carbon emissions from the tourism industry, tourism solid waste discharge, and tourism wastewater discharge [2,13,14]. In addition, some scholars have also investigated the factors driving the evolution of tourism eco-efficiency. The main factors include the level of tourism economy [7], technological innovation [15], industrial structure of tourism [16] and environmental regulation [17].

With the improvement of market mechanism and regional integration, the production factors such as talent, technology, and capital of the low-carbon tourism development flow among various areas, resulting in tourism eco-efficiency in different areas, has grown more connected [18]. Due to the implementation of eco-environmental policies, there is more communication and cooperation regarding tourism sustainable development. Therefore, technologies relevant to low-carbon tourism and the experience of managers are exchanged among various regions, resulting in the formation of a spatial network structure of tourism eco-efficiency [2]. What's more, exploring the spatial network structure of tourism eco-efficiency can provide reference for the cooperation and communication of sustainable tourism development. Some scholars have explored the spatiotemporal evolution characteristics regarding tourism eco-efficiency by adopting exploratory spatial data analysis (ESDA) based on the attribute data [15–17,19,20]. However, scholars failed to devote to enough attentions to the spatial network structure of tourism eco-efficiency based on the relational data. In particular, the roles that various provinces play in the spatial network structure of tourism eco-efficiency have seldom been studied.

In order to fill this gap, taking 30 provinces in China as the case studies, this study explored the evolution characteristics regarding spatial network structure of tourism eco-efficiency. To our best knowledge, this study is among the first to explore the spatial network structure of provincial-scale tourism eco-efficiency. Our research makes three contributions to the extant literature on tourism eco-efficiency. First, this study casts new light on our understanding of the spatial connection and spatial spillover of tourism eco-efficiency from the relational data rather than attribute data. Secondly, the previous literature mainly concentrated on the evaluation of tourism eco-efficiency, whereas this study enriched and broadened research topics such as spatial characteristics. Thirdly, our research sought to advance original methodological and empirical contributions. To be more specific, this study established a comprehensive research framework regarding the spatial network structure of tourism eco-efficiency. Although the example is limited to China, this research framework is, to a certain extent, universalizable.

The rest of this study is structured as follows. Section 2 introduced the main research method, the index system and the data source. The empirical results were presented in

Section 3, in which this study evaluated the tourism eco-efficiency and explored the evolution characteristics regarding the spatial network structure of tourism eco-efficiency. The discussion and conclusions were presented in Section 4, in which this study discussed the empirical results, summarized the literature contributions, and provided recommendations for tourist destination management.

2. Materials and Methodology

2.1. Method

2.1.1. Super-SBM

Data envelopment analysis (DEA) is a model that evaluates multiple decision units with similar inputs and outputs [21]. However, there are two main shortcomings in the traditional DEA morel. First, the slack variables may affect the accuracy of the evaluation results. Second, there solely exists expected output, and the undesirable output is not fully taken into account. In order to make up the for above-mentioned deficiencies, Tone [22] proposed the slack-based model (SBM) based on the undesirable output, which not only takes into consideration the issue of slack, but also includes undesirable output. There is no doubt that the modifications of the model can make the evaluation more accurate. Nevertheless, when the SBM is employed to assess the efficiency of several decision-making units (DMUs), it is easy to generate the phenomenon wherein the efficiency values of DMUs all reach the optimal frontier production surface [23]. In other words, the efficiency values of multiple DMUs are 1, which makes the comparison of DMUs' efficiency impossible. Considering this issue, Tone [24] put forward the Super-SBM model based on the traditional SBM. The formula of Super-SBM is as follows.

$$\begin{cases} Min = \dfrac{\frac{1}{m}\sum\limits_{i=1}^{m}(\overline{x}/x_{ik})}{\frac{1}{r1+r2}\left(\sum\limits_{s=1}^{r1}\overline{y^d}/y^d_{sk}+\sum\limits_{q=1}^{r2}\overline{y^u}/y^u_{qk}\right)} \\ \overline{x} \geq \sum\limits_{j=1,\neq k}^{n} x_{ij}\lambda_j;\ \overline{y^d} \leq \sum\limits_{j=1,\neq k}^{n} y^d_{sj}\lambda_j;\ \overline{y^d} \geq \sum\limits_{j=1,\neq k}^{n} y^d_{qj}\lambda_j \\ \overline{x} \geq x_k;\ \overline{y^d} \leq y^d_k;\ \overline{y^u} \geq y^u_k;\ \lambda_j \geq 0, i = 1,2,\ldots,m \\ j = 1,2,\ldots,n;\ j = 1,2,\ldots,n;\ q = 1,2,\ldots,r_2 \end{cases} \tag{1}$$

where, ρ is the tourism eco-efficiency; x, y^d and y^u are input, expected output and undesirable output, respectively. m, r_1, and r_2 are the quantities of inputs, expected outputs and undesirable outputs, respectively. A value of tourism eco-efficiency greater than or equal to 1 indicates that the tourism eco-efficiency is in an effective state; otherwise, it is in an invalid state.

2.1.2. Modified Gravity Model

A province is a point in the spatial network structure of tourism eco-efficiency, and the spatial connection of tourism eco-efficiency among provinces is the line [25]. At present, the vecto autoregressive (VAR) model, and the modified gravity model are universally used to establish the spatial correlation matrix of tourism eco-efficiency. Given that the sensibility regarding the choice of lag order may reduce the accuracy of examining the network structure characteristics [26], the modified gravity model has been universally applied to construct the spatial correlation matrix. More importantly, this model can take consideration into the "quality" and "distance", and reflect the evolution characteristics regarding the spatial network structure [27]. Based on the above-mentioned advantages, this study applied the modified gravity model. The formula is as follows.

$$F_{ij} = K_{ij}\frac{E_i \cdot E_j}{{D_{ij}}^2}, K_{ij} = \frac{E_i}{E_i + E_j} \tag{2}$$

where F_{ij} denotes the gravity between province i and province j. E_i and E_j represent the tourism eco-efficiency in province i and province j, respectively. D_{ij} represents the distance between province i and province j, which is represented by the shortest straight-line distance among two provincial capitals [25]. K_{ij} is the correction coefficient. Generally speaking, provinces with high tourism eco-efficiency possess a stronger radiation effect on provinces than that of provinces with low tourism eco-efficiency, through radiation of tourism low-carbon technology and spillovers of tourism low-carbon information [2]. In this study, K_{ij} is calculated by the proportion of tourism eco-efficiency of province i in the sum of tourism eco-efficiency of province i and province j.

2.1.3. Social Network Analysis

Social network analysis (SNA), an interdisciplinary research method, aims to describe the relationship among members in a network and the influence of different relationship patterns on the characteristics regarding network structure based on graph theory and algebra [1,28]. Due to the advantages of intuitive graphics and accurate characterization, the application of SNA has been gradually expanded from sociology to economics, management, psychology, geography and other disciplines [27,29,30]. This study mainly adopted the SNA to explore the overall and individual characteristics regarding spatial network structure of tourism eco-efficiency in China and to reveal the actual or potential relationship between provinces. The relevant formulas can be seen in Table 1.

Table 1. Formulas of indicators regarding social network analysis.

Index	Formula	Number	Explanation of Formula
Network density	$D = \frac{L}{N \times (N-1)}$	(3)	Where D is the network density, L is the actual relationship number, and N is the number of research areas.
Network hierarchy	$H = 1 - \frac{K}{\max(K)}$	(4)	Where H is the network hierarchy, K is the symmetric reachable points, and max(K) is the maximum possible point logarithm.
Network efficiency	$E = 1 - \frac{M}{\max(M)}$	(5)	Where E is the network efficiency, M is the number of redundant lines, and max(M) is the maximum number of possible redundant lines.
Clustering coefficient	$C_i = \frac{2e_i}{k_i(k_i-1)}$	(6)	Where C_i is the clustering coefficient, e_i represents the number of edges between k neighbors of province I, k_i is the number of edges of node i.
Average path length	$L = \frac{1}{1/2N(N-1)} \sum_{i \geq j} d_{ij}$	(7)	Where N is the total of network nodes, d_{ij} is distance between province i and province j.
Degree centrality	$De = \frac{n}{N-1}$	(8)	Where De is the point centrality, n is the number of nodes connected with the province, and N is the maximum number of nodes connected with the province.
Betweenness centrality	$Cb_i = \frac{2\sum_{i}^{n}\sum_{j}^{n} b_{ij}(l)}{N^2-3N+2}, i \neq j \neq l, i < j$	(9)	Where Cb_i is betweenness centrality; b_{ij} is the number of the shortcuts between city i and city j; and $b_{ij}(l)$ represents the number of shortcuts between province i and province j.
Closeness centrality	$C_{APi}^{-1} = \sum_{i=1}^{n} d_{ij}$	(10)	Where C_{APi}^{-1} is closeness centrality; and d_{ij} is the shortest distance between province i and province j.

(1) The overall network structure characteristics. The overall network structure characteristics are mainly reflected by six indexes, namely, network density, network connectedness, network hierarchy, network efficiency, clustering coefficient and average path length. Network density and network connectedness mainly reflect the density degree of spatial network structure. The higher the network density is, the more connectedness there is, and the closer the spatial network structure is. The network hierarchy mainly assess the asymmetric accessibility of network individual. The higher the network hierarchy, the

more rigid the network structure, and more provinces play the role of edge in the spatial network structure. Network efficiency mainly reflects the connection efficiency among nodes in the spatial network structure. If the network efficiency is lower, there will be more spillover channels among various provinces, and the more stable the network structure is. The clustering coefficient and the average path length are used to mirror the characteristics of "small-world" regarding the spatial network structure [31], among which, the clustering coefficient mainly represents the cohesion of the spatial network structure. The higher the clustering coefficient is, the more frequent the network connections are. The average path length can indicate the distance between nodes.

(2) The individual network structure characteristics. The individual network structure characteristics are mainly reflected by three indexes, namely degree centrality, betweenness centrality and closeness centrality. Specifically, the point centrality reflects the central position of the node in the network structure. The greater power in the network structure, and the more prominent the central position of the node in the network structure. Betweenness centrality mirrors the degree to which nodes control the connections among other nodes. The higher the betweenness centrality, the greater the priority and control of the node. Closeness centrality reflects the ability a node to be controlled by other nodes. The greater closeness centrality, the more direct spatial associations among nodes, and the easier it is for the node to play the role of the center.

(3) Network cohesive sub-groups analysis. Cohesive sub-groups can explain the substructure within a group, which is a broad concept of sub-group [28]. Nodes in a sub-group possess relatively strong, relatively close and relatively direct relationships, whose fundamental purpose is to reveal the actual or potential relationship between nodes [32].

2.2. Index System Selection

This study regards capital, labor and energy as the tourism input indicators. Land is one of the most basis production factors in economic activities, but it is not a decisive factor affecting the intensive or extensive management of tourism industry in the process of tourism economic development [33]. More seriously, there is a dearth of the dataset on the number of tourism land-use [1]. Therefore, the land is not seen as the basis input in this study. Capital input has a significant influence on the development pathway to a certain extent, thus, playing an indispensable role in the low-carbon tourism development. In this study, the total of fixed asset investment regarding tourist attractions, travel agencies and star-hotels is used to represent the level of tourism capital investment [28]. Additionally, tourism industry is regarded as a labor-intensive industry with significant employment attributes. In this study, the number of tourism employees is used to represent the labor input of tourism [34]. Tourism energy input is of great importance in evaluating tourism eco-efficiency; this study selects tourism energy consumption to represent tourism energy input [13].

With respect to the expected output index, the total tourism revenue is the direct embodiment of economic benefits from tourism. Moreover, the total number of tourists can better reflect the spillover effect of the tourism industry [35]. In terms of undesired output, this study adopts carbon emissions from the tourism industry to reflect the negative impact of tourism-related economic development on the ecological environment [7,13].

2.3. Data Source

In this study, 30 provinces (excluding Tibet, Hong Kong, Macao and Taiwan) were taken as the case studies. The data on inbound tourism revenue, inbound tourist arrival, and fixed asset investment in the tourism industry were mainly received from the China Statistical Yearbook (2001~2018) and China Tourism Statistical Yearbook (2001~2018). Domestic tourism revenue and domestic tourist arrival were mainly taken from the statistical yearbooks of 11 provinces during the period of 2001~2018. Quite a few data were supplemented and improved by the statistical bulletins of national economic and social development of each province. With regard to carbon emissions and energy consumption, this study adopted the "bottom-up" method, including decomposition and summation based on determining the key areas, overall tourism energy consumption and carbon emissions [36,37]. The specific calculation process was played in Appendix A. The data involved in the calculation of energy consumption and carbon emissions from the tourism industry were mainly received from the China Transport Statistical Yearbook (2001~2018) and the China Energy Statistical Yearbook (2001~2018). A part of the data is collected from the Tourism Sample Survey Data (2001~2018) and the Statistical Bulletin of National Economic and Social Development. Additionally, in order to avoid the interference of price factors on the empirical results, the data of income nature is adjusted, with year 2000 as the baseline period.

3. Results

3.1. Measurement of Tourism Eco-Efficiency

China's tourism eco-efficiency, shown in Table 2, witnessed a fluctuating growth trend during the study period, which increased from 0.441 in 2000 to 0.525 in 2017, with an average annual growth rate of 1.1%. This indicated that tourism-related economic development in China still relied on resources and harmed the environment; thus, there is tremendous room for progress in low-carbon tourism development. According to the partition criterion, formulated by the *National Bureau of Statistics* in 2011, 30 provinces were divided into four areas, namely Eastern area, Central area, Western area, and Northeastern area. From the perspective of the sub-area, the tourism eco-efficiency in the Eastern, Central, Western and Northeastern areas all showed a fluctuating growth trend, with the largest growth rate (32.70%), and the smallest growth rate (14.31%), respectively (Figure 1). The order of the spatial heterogeneity distribution pattern regarding the mean of tourism eco-efficiency by area was Eastern (0.740), Northeastern (0.440), Central (0.429) and Western (0.217) during the period of 2000~2017. At the provincial level, except for Beijing, Tianjin, Liaoning, Henan, Hunan, Chongqing, Sichuan, Qinghai and Ningxia, tourism eco-efficiency of the remaining 21 provinces experienced varying degrees of increase during the study period; the largest increase was in Jilin Province (197.18%); the largest decrease was in Qinghai Province (43.33%), indicating that, due to the differences in the input of the material elements of the tourism economy, there was great spatial heterogeneity in the tourism eco-efficiency among these provincial areas in China.

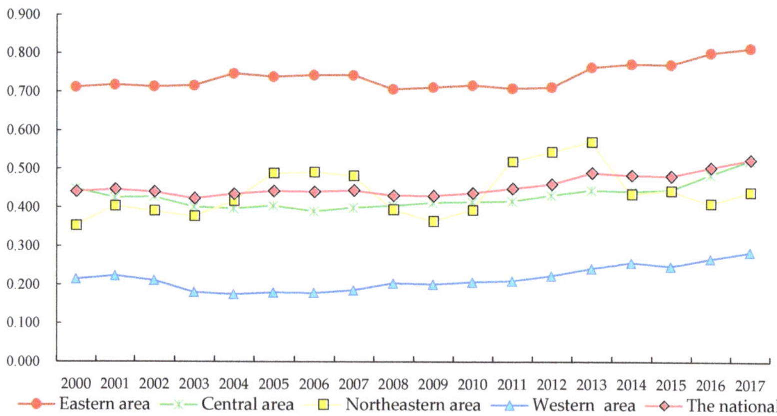

Figure 1. The evolution trend of tourism eco-efficiency in China and four sub-regions from 2000 to 2017. Eastern area includes Beijing, Tianjin, Hebei, Shanghai, Jiangsu, Zhejiang, Fujian, Shandong, Guangdong, and Hainan. Central area consists of Shanxi, Jiangxi, Anhui, Henan, Hubei, Hunan. Western area includes Inner Monglia, Guangxi, Chongqing, Sichuang, Guizhou, Yunan, Shannxi, Gansu, Qinghai, Ningxia, and Xinjiang. Northeastern area includes Liaoning, Jilin, and Heilongjiang.

Table 2. Tourism eco-efficiency of 30 provinces from 2000 to 2017.

Province	2000	2003	2006	2009	2012	2015	2017	Mean
Beijing	0.440	0.523	0.577	0.504	0.419	0.397	0.421	0.469
Tianjin	1.670	1.749	1.763	1.517	1.460	1.461	1.548	1.595
Hebei	0.380	0.297	0.296	0.328	0.380	0.423	0.502	0.362
Shanxi	0.221	0.184	0.175	0.242	0.326	0.400	0.551	0.277
Inner Monglia	0.295	0.287	0.296	0.344	0.434	0.591	0.621	0.399
Liaoning	0.628	0.732	1.016	0.583	1.031	0.631	0.608	0.783
Jilin	0.140	0.156	0.200	0.233	0.299	0.415	0.415	0.256
Heilongjiang	0.291	0.244	0.257	0.278	0.304	0.286	0.298	0.282
Shanghai	1.164	1.139	1.139	1.189	1.131	1.214	1.156	1.174
Jiangsu	1.052	1.069	1.095	1.112	1.119	1.137	1.139	1.105
Zhejiang	0.486	0.493	0.609	0.564	0.662	1.031	1.160	0.707
Anhui	0.215	0.204	0.198	0.224	0.217	0.245	0.320	0.229
Fujian	0.262	0.243	0.277	0.315	0.283	0.298	0.315	0.284
Jiangxi	0.304	0.262	0.253	0.293	0.338	0.326	0.433	0.308
Shandong	0.390	0.356	0.384	0.343	0.369	0.449	0.579	0.407
Henan	1.394	1.355	1.322	1.267	1.218	1.217	1.219	1.283
Hubei	0.269	0.198	0.222	0.260	0.286	0.293	0.370	0.267
Hunan	0.289	0.209	0.173	0.188	0.204	0.192	0.245	0.209
Guangdong	1.122	1.151	1.149	1.113	1.132	1.129	1.132	1.134
Guangxi	0.130	0.121	0.138	0.171	0.219	0.292	0.369	0.205
Hainan	0.153	0.143	0.144	0.134	0.170	0.176	0.189	0.158
Chongqing	0.368	0.282	0.294	0.283	0.268	0.276	0.316	0.298
Sichuan	0.198	0.142	0.143	0.160	0.177	0.167	0.170	0.166
Guizhou	0.271	0.268	0.255	0.336	0.366	0.383	0.406	0.328
Yunnan	0.249	0.179	0.162	0.215	0.255	0.253	0.327	0.227
Shaanxi	0.286	0.244	0.229	0.258	0.272	0.258	0.336	0.264
Gansu	0.194	0.151	0.153	0.141	0.157	0.177	0.221	0.166
Qinghai	0.139	0.102	0.097	0.101	0.092	0.083	0.079	0.100
Ningxia	0.079	0.071	0.066	0.058	0.054	0.055	0.053	0.062
Xinjiang	0.161	0.146	0.140	0.150	0.170	0.200	0.245	0.171
Mean	0.441	0.423	0.441	0.430	0.460	0.482	0.525	0.456

Notes: Due to the length limitation, the results of 2000, 2003, 2006, 2009, 2012, 2015, and 2017 are only represented in Table 2.

3.2. The Spatial Network Structures

3.2.1. Overall Network Characteristics

In this study, ArcGIS10.3 software was used to draw the network structure of China's provincial-scale tourism eco-efficiency, which can reflect the overall network structure characteristics of tourism eco-efficiency in China. Figure 2 showed that with the implementation of the ecological civilization strategy and the high-quality development strategy, the cooperation among different provinces in promoting the transformation of the tourism development mode has been deepening. Therefore, the spatial network structure of tourism eco-efficiency was complex and dense. The overall network structure of China's tourism eco-efficiency, shown in Figure 2, was relatively loose during the study period. The average number of network relationships in each province was 107; the average network density was 0.123; the average clustering coefficient was 0.417, and the average path length was 2.98. Low network agglomeration, connectivity, and closeness were not only conducive to the diffusion and spillovers of tourism low-carbon production factors, such as technologies, talents and capital among provinces, but also affected the stability of the spatial network structure of tourism eco-efficiency.

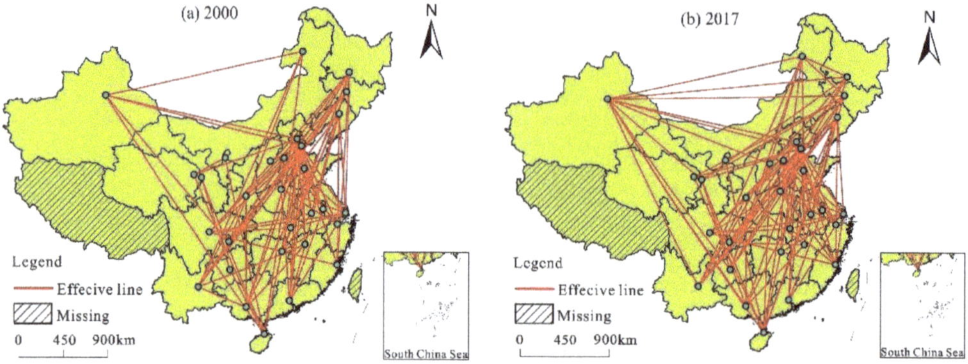

Figure 2. Spatial network structure of tourism eco-efficiency in year 2000 (**a**), and 2017 (**b**), China.

In terms of the evolution trend, the network density, and the number of network relationships, were both increasing slowly in the fluctuation; however, the increase degree was still small, which indicated that the scale, level and standard of low-carbon tourism cooperation among these provinces were still low (Figure 3). It was noteworthy that the clustering coefficient witnessed a slight downward trend, while the average path length experienced a slight upward trend, revealing that the connectivity of the tourism eco-efficiency transmission and the cohesion of the overall network structure among provinces have decreased. Additionally, this highlights that the low-carbon technology between provinces used to promote low-carbon tourism development still faces obstacles and constraints, such as administrative boundaries.

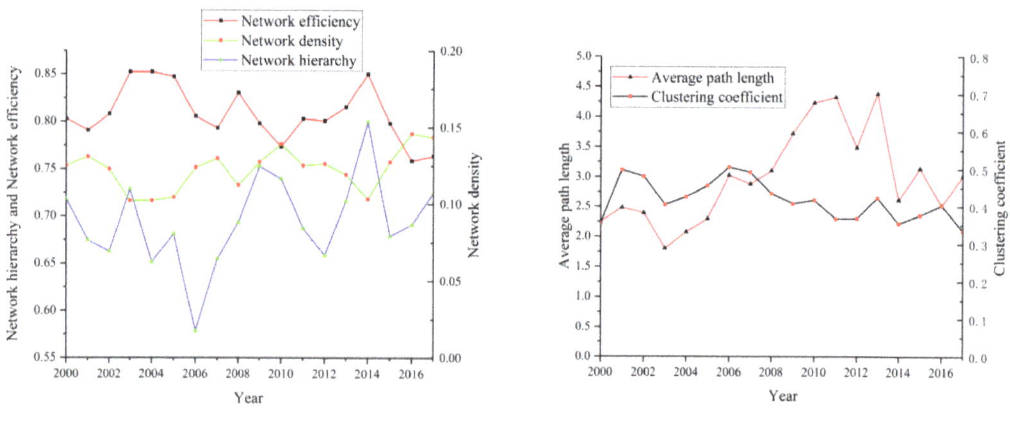

Figure 3. Overall spatial network structure of tourism eco-efficiency.

Figure 3 revealed that the network hierarchy regarding spatial network structure of China's provincial-scale tourism eco-efficiency increased from 0.718 in 2000 to 0.725 in 2017; the network hierarchy always remained above the value of 0.57, indicating that there was a hierarchical network structure in the spillover effect of tourism eco-efficiency among provinces and that this hierarchical structure was becoming increasingly intense. Additionally, the spatial equilibrium of tourism eco-efficiency in each province was relatively poor; the internal environment in which the spill occurred was as terrible as the radiation.

On the contrary, while the network efficiency experienced a downward trend in the fluctuation, decreasing from 0.803 in 2000 to 0.764 in 2017, which revealed that the connectivity of network structure of tourism eco-efficiency has increased, the routes of tourism ecological resource elements spillovers among provinces has been raised, and the stability of spatial correlation has been improved. However, there was also a risk that with the increase of redundant cables, the transmission efficiency of the network structure would be reduced. Therefore, maintaining reasonable network efficiency can optimize the allocation of network resources.

3.2.2. Individual Network Characteristics

In this study, three indexes, i.e., degree centrality, betweenness centrality and closeness centrality, were used to analyze the characteristics regarding individual network structure of tourism eco-efficiency. Furthermore, the spatio-temporal evolution characteristics of the above-mentioned three indicators, adopting the ArcGIS10.2 software, were visually played by the inverse distance weight (IDW) method (Figure 4).

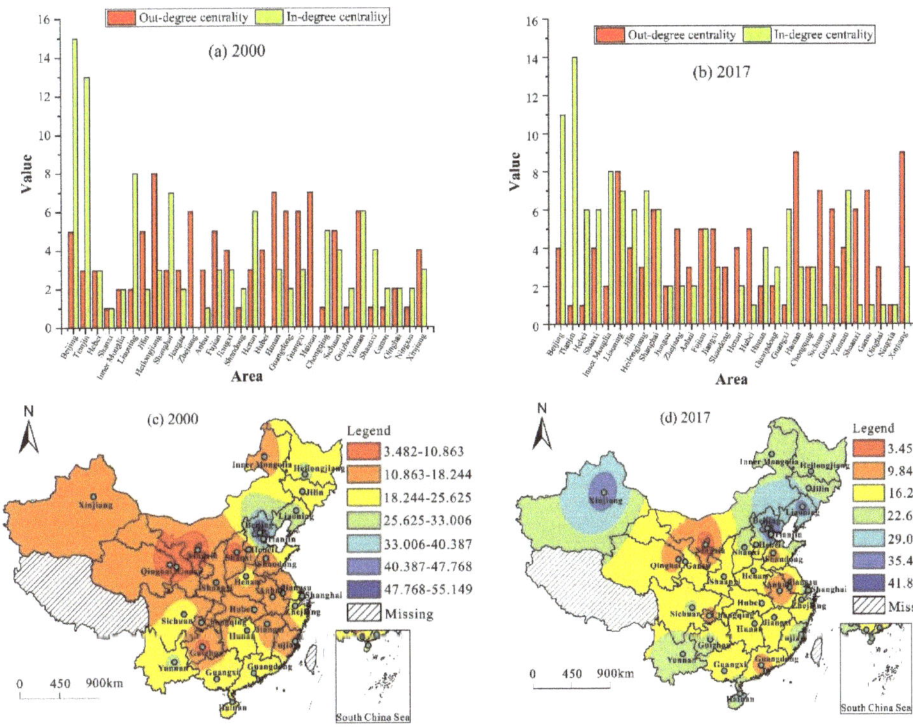

Figure 4. The spatial distribution of point degree in year 2000 (**a**,**c**) and 2017 (**b**,**d**).

(1) Point Degree

Out-degree centrality and in-degree centrality can reflect the interaction relationships among provinces in the spatial network structure of tourism eco-efficiency. Specifically, the out-degree centrality and the in-degree centrality represents the spillover effect and agglomeration effect from tourism eco-efficiency, respectively. The average values of in-degree centrality and out-degree centrality, shown in Figure 4a,b, experienced an overall growth trend during the sample period, which indicated that the inflow and outflow of tourism eco-efficiency among provinces were strengthening constantly, and that the mutual connection of tourism eco-efficiency between provinces was strengthening. To be more specific, in 2000, there were 14 provinces with higher out-degree centrality than mean value, in which Heilongjiang, Hunan, Hainan, Guangxi, Guangdong, Zhejiang and Yunnan ranked TOP 7, while Ningxia, Gansu, Guizhou and other regions exhibited less spillover effect for other provinces. Moreover, there were nine provinces with above-average in-degree centrality, with Beijing, Tianjin, Liaoning and Henan in the top tier, and Hubei, Hainan and Shanxi in the lowest tier. In contrast, the number of provinces that exhibited an above-average out-degree centrality dropped by two in 2017, with Hainan, Fujian, Jiangxi and Sichuan still remaining in the top ranks, whereas the number of provinces with above-average in-degree centrality increased to 12, showing that China's provincial-scale tourism eco-efficiency network was more closely structured; the number of provinces that can receive other radiation effects is increasing, and the cooperation and exchanges among different provinces in low-carbon tourism technologies were also continuously strengthening.

In 2000 and 2017, the interval of point centrality was [3.482, 55.149] and [3.455, 48.202], respectively. The interval range of point centrality saw a narrow trend, indicating that the spatial differences of point centrality among various provinces witnessed a trend of constant balance. The spatial network structure of tourism eco-efficiency tended to be balanced; provinces increasingly played a core role. As can be seen from Figure 4c,d, the spatial distribution pattern of point centrality has been expanded from a high value area in 2000 (with Beijing and Tianjin as the core) to two high value areas in 2017 (with Beijing as the core of the Northern area around Bohai Sea and Urumqi as the core of the northern Xinjiang region). While the coverage of the low-value areas of point centrality has been shrinking, its spatial distribution pattern has been reduced from a continuous low-value area in 2000 (the continuous low-value area with the core of Urban Agglomeration along the Yellow River in Ningxia and the Lanzhou-Xining Urban Agglomeration) and three scattered-point areas with low-value (Shanxi, Shandong and Guizhou) to one low-value area in 2017 (the low-value area with the core of Urban Agglomeration along the Yellow River in Ningxia). Some of the provinces with high point centrality, such as Tianjin, were able to share modern low-carbon tourism technology and management experience with other provinces, and, thus, improve their point centrality by increasing out-degree centrality. Other provinces, such as Xinjiang, become the province with high point centrality in 2017, which was mainly due to the deep implementation of the Aid-Xinjiang program. Xinjiang can absorb the management experience of developing low-carbon tourism products, designing low-carbon tourism routes, establishing low-carbon tourism enterprise, and so on, which improved the point centrality by strengthening in-degree centrality.

(2) Closeness Centrality

In 2000 and 2017, the ranges of closeness centrality were (32.957, 64.430) and (33.727, 64.390), respectively. On the one hand, the overall provincial closeness centrality tended to increase. On the other hand, the regional differences of closeness centrality among provinces gradually contracted. This indicated that more provinces can make full use of the transmission effect of the spatial network structure, quickly generate spatial connections with other provinces, and play the role of "central actors" in the spatial network structure of tourism eco-efficiency. As shown in Figure 5, similar to the geographical distribution pattern of point centrality, the areas covered with high closeness centrality were mainly distributed around the northern part of the Bohai Sea with Beijing and Tianjin as the core; the low-value areas were mainly distributed along the urban agglomeration along the Yellow River in Ningxia. With the spatial association of the tourism eco-efficiency among the provinces increasing, the spatial scope of the high closeness centrality saw an expanding trend to a certain extent, while the coverage of the low closeness centrality was reduced to a certain extent. On the one hand, the low-value areas with the core of the urban agglomeration along the Yellow River in Ningxia were difficult to spill over into the surrounding provinces due to the behindhand low-carbon tourism technology. On the other hand, due to their unfavorable transport accessibility, it was difficult to connect with the provinces located in the Central area or the Eastern area. Therefore, it played the role of marginal actor in the spatial network structure of tourism eco-efficiency.

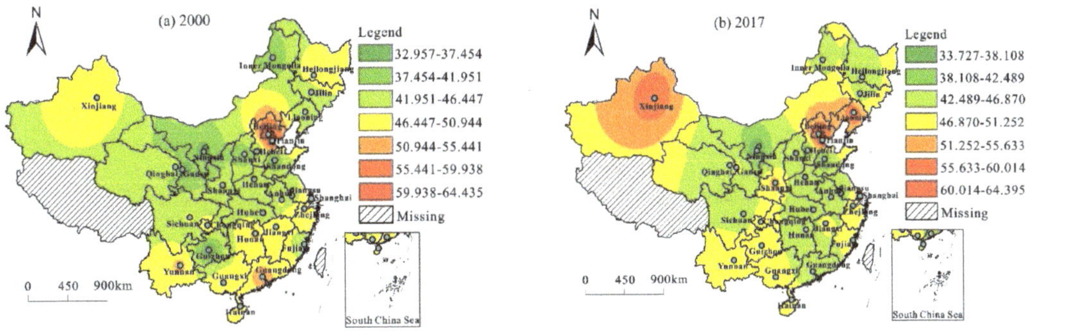

Figure 5. The spatial distribution of closeness centrality in year 2000 (**a**) and 2017 (**b**).

(3) Betweenness Centrality

The ranges of the provincial betweenness centrality were (0, 33.334) and (0.001, 25.612) in 2000 and 2017, respectively. The betweenness centrality saw a decreasing trend during the sample period, indicating that the spatial equilibrium of the betweenness centrality tended to be intensive, and the spatial network structure of tourism eco-efficiency gradually transformed from simple to complex (Figure 6). In 2000, the high-value areas of betweenness centrality were mainly located in Beijing, Tianjin, Guangdong, Hainan and Yunnan, which controlled at least two communication channels for tourism eco-efficiency, showing that the above-mentioned provinces played a role of bridge and intermediary in the transmission of low-carbon tourism technologies, and were the key nodes of the tourism eco-efficiency network structure. Significantly, some of the above provinces are provinces with a developed tourism economy in China, such as Beijing and Guangdong, which possess favorable low-carbon tourism technologies and management. Moreover, the other provinces were pilot low-carbon tourism provinces in China, such as Hainan and Yunnan, with a relatively perfect regulation of the tourism-related ecological environment; they can take on the role of intermediary to other provinces' tourism ecological protection resource elements.

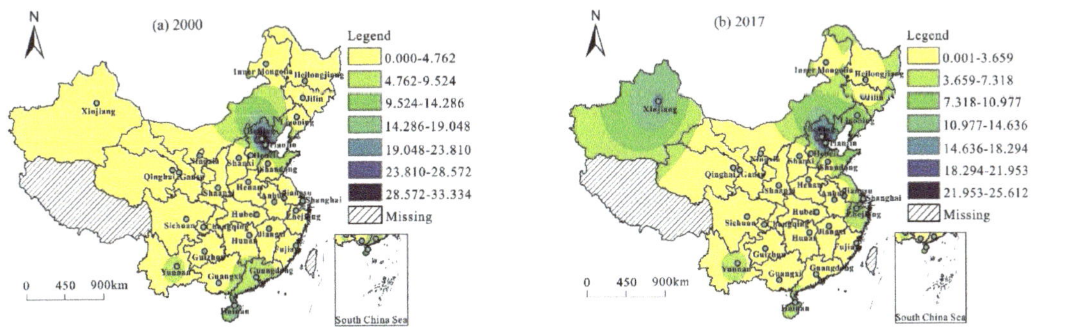

Figure 6. The spatial distribution of Betweenness centrality in year 2000 (**a**) and 2017 (**b**).

3.3. Cohesive Sub-Group

The convergent correlation (CONCOR) model in UCINET (University of California at Irvine Network) software was used for the cluster analysis. Figure 7 shows that the spatial network structure of tourism eco-efficiency in 2000 and 2017 was divided into four secondary sub-groups and eight tertiary sub-groups, forming multidimensional nested and fused spatial cliques and condensed subsets. The boundary of each sub-group faced with several obstacles due to the large number of sub-groups; the spatial connection and overflow of tourism eco-efficiency among provinces were not close. From the perspective of time evolution, the constituent provinces of each subgroup were constantly changing on the whole; however, the individual provinces under most sub-groups remained unchanged, such as Beijing and Hebei in the first sub-group, Hainan and Xinjiang in the seventh sub-group, and Qinghai, Ningxia and Gansu among the eighth sub-group, which fully demonstrated that the sub-groups of the spatial network structure of tourism eco-efficiency had gradually become stable, and the functions and roles of some provinces had not changed a lot, especially the eighth sub-group, except that Guizhou moved to other sub-groups. Qinghai, Ningxia and Gansu provinces were always located in the eighth sub-group. These three provinces were mainly restricted by geographical location and held weak connections with other provinces; they were situated at the edge of the tourism eco-efficiency network.

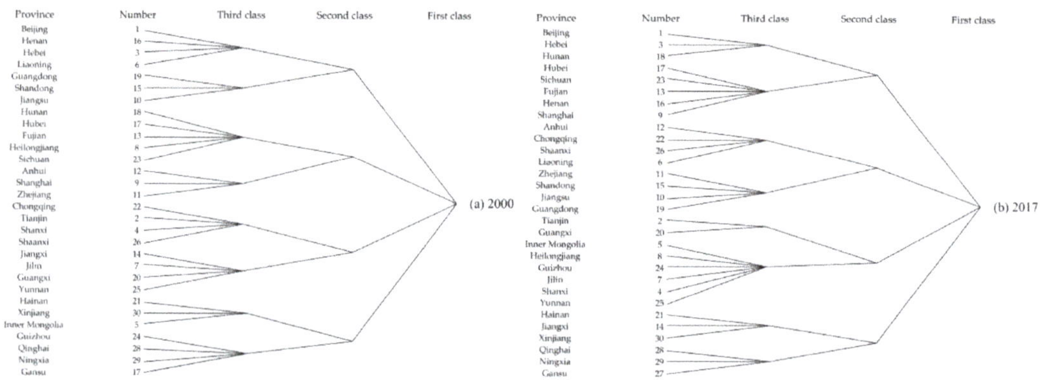

Figure 7. Subgroup of the tourism eco-efficiency network in China in year 2000 (**a**) and 2017 (**b**).

4. Discussion and Conclusions

4.1. General Discussion

Tourism eco-efficiency is an important indicator to assesses the degree of low-carbon development in the tourism industry. Additionally, the low-carbon development of the tourism industry is one of the most important goals of the high-quality development of tourism. Against the background of high-quality development, it is imperative that tourism eco-efficiency should be explored. Although increasing attention has been paid to tourism eco-efficiency, there is scant work on the spatial network structure of tourism eco-efficiency in China. Therefore, the practical background and theoretical gap have driven us to concentrate on this topic. This study adopted Super-SBM, considering undesired output and social network analysis to explore the evolution characteristics of spatial network structure of tourism eco-efficiency.

There was been a slight rise of tourism eco-efficiency in China; the order of spatial distribution characteristics by areas were Eastern, Northeastern, Central, and Western. From the perspective of a single province, tourism eco-efficiency of more than two thirds of the provinces presented an increasing trend, indicating that provinces have increasingly begun to pay more attention to the quality improvement of the tourism industry rather than solely to quantity growth [5]. More specifically, improving tourism eco-efficiency has been a crucial strategy that coordinates tourism-related economic development and eco-environmental protection in tourists' destinations in China [7,38].

There are significant spatial connections of tourism eco-efficiency among various provinces, which is in accordance with the findings of Wang, Xia, Dong, Li, Li, Ba and Zhang [15]. In terms of overall network, although spatial connection of tourism eco-efficiency among various provinces has heightened during the sample period to a certain extent, the spatial network structure of tourism eco-efficiency was still loose and unstable.

Moreover, there existed rigid stratification in the spillover relationship of tourism eco-efficiency among different provinces. More seriously, the above-mentioned phenomenon has not been profoundly changed. From the perspective of the small-world characteristic, there was a lack of cohesive force and connection convenience in spatial network structures of tourism eco-efficiency, demonstrating that it is imperative that the central government establish tourism eco-environmental protection and supervision mechanisms across provinces, which is in line with the conclusion of Sun, Hou, Huang and Zhong [7].

With regard to an individual network, the spatial network structure of tourism eco-efficiency has become more compact, complicated, and balanced, which demonstrates that, increasingly, provinces can rapidly generate connections between other provinces and play the role of intermediary in the spatial network structure of tourism eco-efficiency. Generally, due to the limitation of geographical location, provinces located in the Western area play a marginal role in the network structure, which results from the fact that there is a lack of modern low-carbon tourism technology, and not enough investment in environmental protection in the Western area [17]. With respect to the results of the cohesive group, there existed the multidimensional nested and fused spatial factions and condensed subsets in the spatial network structure of tourism eco-efficiency; however, there was a dearth of effective connection among second or third sub-groups, which further confirmed that the spatial network structure of tourism eco-efficiency was incompact.

4.2. Theoretical Contributions

Our study makes three contributions to the new body of knowledge. To our knowledge, our research may be among the first study efforts to explore the evolution characteristics of the spatial network structure of provincial-level tourism eco-efficiency. Firstly, the extant literature mainly concentrates on a single tourism sector, such as scenic spots and hotels; this study can enrich and broaden the literature about the tourism efficiency of all tourist destinations. Secondly, this study grasps the spatial relationship of tourism eco-efficiency among different tourist destinations based on the relational data, providing new research perspectives for other scholars who expect to investigate spatiotemporal characteristics of tourism eco-efficiency. Thirdly, our research constructs the spatial connection matrix of tourism eco-efficiency by using the modify gravity model. Although the empirical investigation takes 30 provinces of China as a case study, this model is universal and applicable across other countries.

4.3. Practical Implications

This conclusion of our research is of great significance to the sustainable development of the tourism industry in China. Based on these conclusions, this study put forward recommendations for destination management organizations (DMOs). First, the spatial differences of tourism eco-efficiency across four areas must be taken into account by the central government. More capital investment and policy support should be brought into the Central and Western areas by the implementation of the Western Development Strategy and Central Risen Strategy, thus, achieving the coordinated improvement of tourism eco-efficiency. Second, the spatial network structure of tourism eco-efficiency was still loose and unstable. Therefore, the spatial connection of tourism eco-efficiency must be strengthened by accelerating the flow of information and technology among different provinces. For example, Anhui Province can gain the spillover of technology and the radiation of management from the other provinces in Yangtze River Delta Urban Agglomeration. Third, the barrier of administrative division needs to be broken by combining macroeconomic regulation and market disposition, which aims to generate more channels of the communication regarding low-carbon development. Given that there was a dearth of connections of tourism eco-efficiency among the second or third sub-groups, the cooperation and connection of sustainable tourism development should also be optimized by the construction of a low-carbon tourism market and the decrease of connection cost.

4.4. Limitations and Future Research

This study is not without limitations, which should not be overlooked; however, it also paves the potential road for future study. Firstly, with tourism-related economic development, the coefficients or the calculation method of carbon emissions from the tourism industry need to be adjusted in future research. Secondly, the data on the use of tourism land cannot be included in an input–output index system due to the size of the dataset. Therefore, the index system must be improved in future research. Thirdly, future scholars should explore the factors driving the spatial network structure of tourism eco-efficiency.

Author Contributions: Conceptualization, Q.L. and J.S.; methodology, T.D. and J.X.; formal analysis, Q.L. writing—original draft preparation, E.W. and J.L.; writing—review and editing, Q.L. and J.S. All authors have read and agreed to the published version of the manuscript.

Funding: This research was funded by The National Natural Science Foundation of China, grant number 42171170, 41801154, and 41901193. Meanwhile, The Chuzhou Science and Technology Plan Project, grant number 2021ZD007, and The Key University Science Research Project of Anhui Province, grant number KJ2021A1078 also provided supports for this study.

Institutional Review Board Statement: Not applicable.

Informed Consent Statement: Not applicable.

Data Availability Statement: Data available from the authors upon request.

Acknowledgments: We acknowledge the precious advice of the referees and editors. Meanwhile, we thank An Shi for his contribution that he modified all pictures.

Conflicts of Interest: The authors declare no conflict of interest.

Appendix A

Evaluation on Carbon Dioxide Emission and Energy Consumption from the Tourism Industry

Based on the existing results at home and abroad, this study chose to use the "bottom-up" method to calculate energy consumption and carbon dioxide emissions from the tourism industry. This study calculated the energy consumption/carbon dioxide emissions in three key tourism sectors, namely tourism transportation, tourism accommodation and tourism activities, and then summarized the total energy consumption/carbon dioxide emissions. The calculation formula is as follows:

$$C^t = \sum_{j=1}^{3} C_j^t = C_1^t + C_2^t + C_3^t \quad \text{(A1)}$$

where, C^t represents the total energy consumption/carbon dioxide emissions of tourism industry in year t; C_j^t represents the energy consumption/carbon dioxide emissions of department j in year t; C_1^t represents energy consumption/carbon dioxide emissions of tourism and transportation sectors in year t; C_2^t represents energy consumption/carbon dioxide emissions of tourism and accommodation sector in year t; C_3^t represents energy consumption/carbon dioxide emissions from tourism activities in year t.

$$C_1^t = \sum_{i=1}^{30} C_{i1}^t = \sum_{i=1}^{30} \sum_{x=1}^{4} Q_{ix}^t \cdot f_x \cdot \alpha_x \quad \text{(A2)}$$

where, C_{i1}^t represents the energy consumption/carbon dioxide emissions of tourism and transportation sectors in region i in year t; Q_{ix}^t represents the passenger turnover of category x mode of transportation in region i in year t; f_x represents the proportion of tourists in the passenger traffic volume of class x mode. The values of highway, civil aviation, railway and water transportation can be determined as 13.8%, 64.7%, 31.6%, and 10.6%, respectively, by referring to the existing research results. α_x represents the energy consumption/carbon dioxide emissions coefficient of class x transportation mode, where the α value of highway is 133 g CO_2/pkm, the value of civil aviation is 137 g CO_2/pkm, and the railway and water transport are 27 g CO_2/pkm and 106 g CO_2/pkm.

$$C_2^t = \sum_{i=1}^{30} C_{i2}^t = \sum_{i=1}^{30} N_i^t \cdot l_i^t \cdot \beta \tag{A3}$$

where, C_{i2}^t represents the energy consumption/carbon dioxide emissions of the tourism and accommodation sector in region i in year t; N_i^t is the number of beds in tourist hotels in region i in year t; l_i^t represents the average room occupancy rate in region i in year t; β is the energy consumption/carbon dioxide emissions coefficient (g/p visitor-night) per bed per night, and the value is 2.458 g/p visitor-night.

$$C_3^t = \sum_{i=1}^{30} C_{i3}^t = \sum_{i=1}^{30} \sum_{s=1}^{5} P_{is}^t \cdot \gamma_s \tag{A4}$$

where, C_{i3}^t represents the energy consumption/carbon dioxide emissions of regional tourism activities in year t; P_{iS}^t denotes the number of tourists participating in category s tourism activities in region i in year t; γ_S is the energy consumption/carbon dioxide emissions coefficient of class s tourism activities, and the energy consumption/carbon dioxide emissions coefficient of tourism, vacation tourism, business trip, visiting friends and relatives and other tourism activities are, respectively, 417 g/p visitor, 1670 g/p visitor, 786 g/p visitor, 591 g/p visitor and 172 g/p visitor.

References

1. Wang, Z.; Liu, Q.; Xu, J.; Fujiki, Y. Evolution characteristics of the spatial network structure of tourism efficiency in China: A province-level analysis. *J. Destin. Mark. Manag.* **2020**, *18*, 100509. [CrossRef]
2. Sun, Y.; Hou, G. Analysis on the Spatial-Temporal Evolution Characteristics and Spatial Network Structure of Tourism Eco-Efficiency in the Yangtze River Delta Urban Agglomeration. *Int. J. Environ. Res. Public Health* **2021**, *18*, 2577. [CrossRef] [PubMed]
3. Scott, D.; Peeters, P.; Gössling, S. Can tourism deliver its "aspirational" greenhouse gas emission reduction targets? *J. Sustain. Tour.* **2010**, *18*, 393–408. [CrossRef]
4. Peng, H.; Zhang, J.; Lu, L.; Tang, G.; Yan, B.; Xiao, X.; Han, Y. Eco-efficiency and its determinants at a tourism destination: A case study of Huangshan National Park, China. *Tour. Manag.* **2017**, *60*, 201–211. [CrossRef]
5. Liu, J.; Zhang, J.; Fu, Z. Tourism eco-efficiency of Chinese coastal cities—Analysis based on the DEA-Tobit model. *Ocean. Coast. Manag.* **2017**, *148*, 164–170. [CrossRef]
6. Gössling, S.; Peeters, P.; Ceron, J.-P.; Dubois, G.; Patterson, T.; Richardson, R.B. The eco-efficiency of tourism. *Ecol. Econ.* **2005**, *54*, 417–434. [CrossRef]
7. Sun, Y.; Hou, G.; Huang, Z.; Zhong, Y. Spatial-Temporal Differences and Influencing Factors of Tourism Eco-Efficiency in China's Three Major Urban Agglomerations Based on the Super-EBM Model. *Sustainability* **2020**, *12*, 4156. [CrossRef]
8. Gössling, S.; Broderick, J.; Upham, P.; Ceron, J.-P.; Dubois, G.; Peeters, P.; Strasdas, W. Voluntary Carbon Offsetting Schemes for Aviation: Efficiency, Credibility and Sustainable Tourism. *J. Sustain. Tour.* **2007**, *15*, 223–248. [CrossRef]
9. Perch-Nielsen, S.; Sesartic, A.; Stucki, M. The greenhouse gas intensity of the tourism sector: The case of Switzerland. *Environ. Sci. Policy* **2010**, *13*, 131–140. [CrossRef]
10. Yu, L.; Bai, Y.; Liu, J. The dynamics of tourism's carbon footprint in Beijing, China. *J. Sustain. Tour.* **2019**, *27*, 1553–1571. [CrossRef]
11. Lin, L. Research on the spatio-temporal evolution of tourism eco-efficiency by using the ecological footprint model. *Fresenius Environ. Bull.* **2021**, *30*, 10665–10674.
12. Yang, G.; Li, P.; Zheng, B.; Zhang, Y. GHG Emission-Based Eco-Efficiency Study on Tourism Itinerary Products in Shangri-La, Yunnan Province, China. *Curr. Issues Tour.* **2008**, *11*, 604–622. [CrossRef]
13. Zha, J.; Yuan, W.; Dai, J.; Tan, T.; He, L. Eco-efficiency, eco-productivity and tourism growth in China: A non-convex metafrontier DEA-based decomposition model. *J. Sustain. Tour.* **2020**, *28*, 663–685. [CrossRef]
14. Zha, J.; He, L.; Liu, Y.; Shao, Y. Evaluation on development efficiency of low-carbon tourism economy: A case study of Hubei Province, China. *Socio-Econ. Plan. Sci.* **2019**, *66*, 47–57. [CrossRef]
15. Wang, R.; Xia, B.; Dong, S.; Li, Y.; Li, Z.; Ba, D.; Zhang, W. Research on the Spatial Differentiation and Driving Forces of Eco-Efficiency of Regional Tourism in China. *Sustainability* **2020**, *13*, 280. [CrossRef]

16. Lu, F.; Qin, W.; Wang, Y.-X.; Gupta, P. Research on Spatial Pattern Dynamic Evolution Algorithm and Optimization Model Construction and Driving Mechanism of Provincial Tourism Eco-Efficiency in China under the Background of Cloud Computing. *Sci. Program.* **2021**, *2021*, 1951264. [CrossRef]
17. Qiu, X.; Fang, Y.; Yang, X.; Zhu, F. Tourism Eco-Efficiency Measurement, Characteristics, and Its Influence Factors in China. *Sustainability* **2017**, *9*, 1634. [CrossRef]
18. Pan, F.; Hall, S.; Zhang, H. The spatial dynamics of financial activities in Beijing: Agglomeration economies and urban planning. *Urban Geogr.* **2020**, *41*, 849–864. [CrossRef]
19. Li, B.; Ma, X.; Chen, K. Eco-efficiency measurement and spatial-temporal evolution of forest tourism. *Arab. J. Geosci.* **2021**, *14*, 568. [CrossRef]
20. Su, L.; Ji, X. Spatial-temporal differences and evolution of eco-efficiency in China's forest park. *Urban For. Urban Green.* **2021**, *57*, 126894. [CrossRef]
21. Nurmatov, R.; Fernandez Lopez, X.L.; Coto Millan, P.P. Tourism, hospitality, and DEA: Where do we come from and where do we go? *Int. J. Hosp. Manag.* **2021**, *95*, 102883. [CrossRef]
22. Tone, K. A slacks-based measure of efficiency in data envelopment analysis. *Eur. J. Oper. Res.* **2001**, *130*, 498–509. [CrossRef]
23. Zhang, J.; Su, Y.; Wu, J.; Liang, H. GIS based land suitability assessment for tobacco production using AHP and fuzzy set in Shandong province of China. *Comput. Electron. Agric.* **2015**, *114*, 202–211. [CrossRef]
24. Tone, K. Dealing with Undesirable Outputs in DEA: A Slacks-based Measure (SBM) Approach. *GRIPS Res. Rep. Ser.* **2003**, *2003*, 44–45.
25. Bai, C.; Zhou, L.; Xia, M.; Feng, C. Analysis of the spatial association network structure of China's transportation carbon emissions and its driving factors. *J. Environ. Manag.* **2020**, *253*, 109765. [CrossRef] [PubMed]
26. He, Y.-Y.; Wei, Z.-X.; Liu, G.-Q.; Zhou, P. Spatial network analysis of carbon emissions from the electricity sector in China. *J. Clean. Prod.* **2020**, *262*, 121193. [CrossRef]
27. Shen, W.; Liang, H.; Dong, L.; Ren, J.; Wang, G. Synergistic CO_2 reduction effects in Chinese urban agglomerations: Perspectives from social network analysis. *Sci. Total Environ.* **2021**, *798*, 149352. [CrossRef]
28. Gan, C.; Voda, M.; Wang, K.; Chen, L.; Ye, J. Spatial network structure of the tourism economy in urban agglomeration: A social network analysis. *J. Hosp. Tour. Manag.* **2021**, *47*, 124–133. [CrossRef]
29. Pierce, P.P.; Kabo, F.; Killian, J.; Stucky, C.; Huffman, S.; Migliore, L.; Braun, L. Social network analysis: Exploring connections to advance military nursing science. *Nurs. Outlook* **2021**, *69*, 311–321. [CrossRef]
30. Yao, Q.; Li, R.Y.M.; Song, L.; Crabbe, M.J.C. Construction safety knowledge sharing on Twitter: A social network analysis. *Saf. Sci.* **2021**, *143*, 105411. [CrossRef]
31. Dai, L.; Derudder, B.; Liu, X. The evolving structure of the Southeast Asian air transport network through the lens of complex networks, 1979-2012. *J. Transp. Geogr.* **2018**, *68*, 67–77. [CrossRef] [PubMed]
32. Zhang, P.; Zhao, Y.; Zhu, X.; Cai, Z.; Xu, J.; Shi, S. Spatial structure of urban agglomeration under the impact of high-speed railway construction: Based on the social network analysis. *Sustain. Cities Soc.* **2020**, *62*, 102404. [CrossRef]
33. Song, M.; Li, H. Estimating the efficiency of a sustainable Chinese tourism industry using bootstrap technology rectification. *Technol. Forecast. Soc. Chang.* **2019**, *143*, 45–54. [CrossRef]
34. Chaabouni, S. China's regional tourism efficiency: A two-stage double bootstrap data envelopment analysis. *J. Destin. Mark. Manag.* **2019**, *11*, 183–191. [CrossRef]
35. Castilho, D.; Fuinhas, J.A.; Marques, A.C. The impacts of the tourism sector on the eco-efficiency of the Latin American and Caribbean countries. *Socio-Econ. Plan. Sci.* **2021**, *78*, 101089. [CrossRef]
36. Wu, P.; Shi, P.H. An estimation of energy consumption and CO_2 emissions in tourism sector of China. *J. Geogr. Sci.* **2011**, *21*, 733–745. [CrossRef]
37. Wu, P.; Han, Y.; Tian, M. The measurement and comparative study of carbon dioxide emissions from tourism in typical provinces in China. *Acta Ecol. Sin.* **2015**, *35*, 184–190. [CrossRef]
38. He, L.; Zha, J.; Loo, H.A. How to improve tourism energy efficiency to achieve sustainable tourism: Evidence from China. *Curr. Issues Tour.* **2019**, *23*, 1–16. [CrossRef]

International Journal of
Environmental Research and Public Health

MDPI

Article

Can Artificial Intelligence Improve the Energy Efficiency of Manufacturing Companies? Evidence from China

Jun Liu [1,2,*], Yu Qian [1], Yuanjun Yang [1] and Zhidan Yang [1]

1 School of Management Science and Engineering, Nanjing University of Information Science & Technology, Nanjing 210044, China; qianyu7098@gmail.com (Y.Q.); yyjwork1995@163.com (Y.Y.); hannahyeung1226@gmail.com (Z.Y.)
2 Institute of Free Trade Zone, Nanjing University of Information Science & Technology, Nanjing 210044, China
* Correspondence: liujun@nuist.edu.cn; Tel.: +86-13776572972

Abstract: Improving energy efficiency is an important way to achieve low-carbon economic development, a common goal of most nations. Based on the comprehensive survey data of enterprises above a designated size in Guangdong Province, this paper studies the impact of artificial intelligence on the energy efficiency of manufacturing enterprises. The results show that: (1) artificial intelligence, as measured by the use of industrial robots, has significantly improved the energy efficiency of manufacturing enterprises. This conclusion is still robust after introducing data on industrial robots in the United States over the same time period as the instrumental variable for the endogeneity test. (2) The mechanism test shows that artificial intelligence mainly promotes the improvement in energy efficiency by promoting technological progress; the impact of artificial intelligence on the technological efficiency of enterprises is not significant. (3) Heterogeneity analysis shows that the age of the manufacturing enterprises inhibits a promoting effect of artificial intelligence on energy efficiency; manufacturing enterprises' performance can enhance the promoting effect of artificial intelligence on energy efficiency, but this promoting effect can only be shown when the enterprise performance is positive. The paper clarifies both the impact of artificial intelligence on the energy efficiency of manufacturing enterprises and its mechanism of action; this will help provide a reference for future decision-making designed to improve manufacturing enterprises' energy efficiency.

Keywords: artificial intelligence; manufacturing enterprises; energy efficiency; heterogeneity

Citation: Liu, J.; Qian, Y.; Yang, Y.; Yang, Z. Can Artificial Intelligence Improve the Energy Efficiency of Manufacturing Companies? Evidence from China. *Int. J. Environ. Res. Public Health* **2022**, *19*, 2091. https://doi.org/10.3390/ijerph19042091

Academic Editor: Nir Krakauer

Received: 12 December 2021
Accepted: 11 February 2022
Published: 13 February 2022

1. Introduction

For some time, the global energy issue has been a major concern, hindering the development of human society [1,2]. The 2019 BP World Energy Statistical Yearbook shows that, in 2018, global primary energy demand increased 2.9% and carbon emissions increased 2.0%. This was the fastest growth year since 2010. In 2019, affected by the new coronavirus epidemic, the growth rate of global primary energy consumption slowed to 1.3% as compared to 2018, but carbon emissions caused by energy consumption increased significantly, by 2.0% [3]. China accounts for more than three-quarters of the net increase in global energy consumption and has become its largest driving force. For the sustainable development of both the economy and society, the Chinese government has put energy conservation and emissions reduction front and center [4]. At the 2021 China Energy Work Conference, there was a call for the strict implementation of a "dual control" system involving both total energy consumption and intensity, with total energy consumption to be limited to within five billion tons of standard coal at an average annual growth rate of less than 3%.

The industrial sector is the largest consumer of energy. According to data from the United Nations Industrial Development Organization, in developing countries and countries with economies in transition, the growth rate of industrial energy use will be 1.8–3.1% per year, with 50% of energy to be supplied to industrial systems. At the same time, the contradiction between economic development and limited energy supply has become increasingly prominent. Therefore, how to manage the energy demand of Chinese manufacturing enterprises and improve their energy efficiency is very important for achieving regional and global reductions in greenhouse gas emissions and reducing corporate energy intensity [5]. Studies to date have pointed out that technology can indeed improve energy efficiency and reduce energy consumption [6,7], but current industrial energy efficiency is far below the best technically feasible levels.

With the rise of a new global scientific and technological revolution, AI has developed rapidly around the world and has now become an important developmental trend in global manufacturing. The use of industrial robots is an important manifestation of the application of AI in the manufacturing sector [8,9]. From the perspective of the application of industrial robots in China (see Figure 1), although the number of industrial robots put into use is increasing year by year, its growth rate is far lower than that for the number of industrial robots purchased in China. That is, companies have purchased artificial intelligence (AI) equipment, but the proportion of production applications is not high. There is a practical problem: the operation of artificial intelligence requires a lot of energy. After it is put into production, can artificial intelligence improve manufacturing enterprises' energy efficiency? Manufacturing enterprises may have more stringent technical conditions for using AI and may face higher investment costs, resulting in the number of purchases of AI being greater than the number of applications for their use. Will this lead to a waste of resources for the company, thereby inhibiting energy efficiency? The questions to be studied in this paper are as follows:

- What impact does artificial intelligence have on the energy efficiency of Chinese manufacturing enterprises? How specific is the impact?
- In what ways does artificial intelligence affect the energy efficiency of manufacturing enterprises?
- What kind of heterogeneity is there in the impact of artificial intelligence on the energy efficiency of manufacturing enterprises?

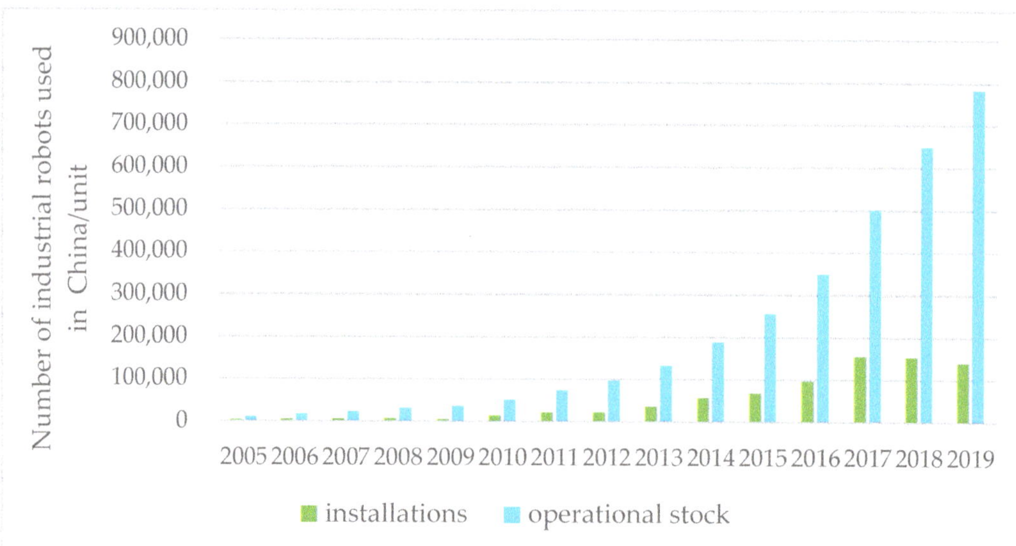

Figure 1. Installation and use of industrial robots in China.

To answer the above questions, it is necessary to conduct empirical research on the basis of looking at related theories and combining them with real world data in China.

Most of the existing research on artificial intelligence and industrial robots has focused on the labor market, economic growth, carbon emissions, etc. [10–12]. However, empirical research between AI and energy efficiency is relatively rare. We aim to supplement this research herein. The purpose of this paper is to analyze the impact mechanism of artificial intelligence on the energy efficiency of manufacturing enterprises and to answer the question of how artificial intelligence affects energy efficiency. This paper uses the data of manufacturing enterprises to construct a DEA-Malmquist model and multiple fixed effect model for empirical testing. We further analyze the role of firm age and firm performance in moderating the impact of AI on energy efficiency. This paper provides micro-evidence for the impact of artificial intelligence on energy efficiency, and expands the research on artificial intelligence and enterprise energy efficiency.

The structure of this article is as follows: This first part reviews the related research on the factors affecting energy efficiency. Through the method of literature review, it analyzes how artificial intelligence has an impact on energy efficiency and proposes research hypotheses. The second part is the literature review and research hypothesis. The third part is model design, and mainly deals with model design, variable selection and descriptive statistics of data. The main goal is to build an econometric model that empirically tests the impact of AI on energy efficiency. A data envelopment model is established to measure the energy efficiency of manufacturing enterprises. Finally, select the relevant control variables and describe the data. The fourth part is the empirical test. This part mainly analyzes the empirical results and uses the instrumental variable method (IV) to alleviate the endogeneity problem of the model and to discuss the heterogeneity of enterprises. The fifth part is discussion. This part will use the literature comparison method to compare the conclusions of this paper with the published literature, answer the research questions of this paper and summarize its contributions. The last part is the conclusion and policy recommendations.

2. Literature Review and Research Hypothesis

With the increasingly prominent energy problem, discovering the factors that affect energy efficiency has become the focus of scholars' research, including urbanization level [13], energy cost [14], environmental regulation [15,16], and resource endowment [17], etc.

Relevant research on the impact of technological progress on corporate energy efficiency can be divided into two categories. One view is that technological advancement can improve corporate energy efficiency and thereby reduce energy consumption [18–20] Popp [21] used patent data to estimate the impact of technological progress on energy consumption. The results of the study proved that technological advancement can save enterprises more energy in the long run. Welsch and Ochsen [22] demonstrated, through an empirical study in the Federal Republic of Germany, that technological progress can improve corporate energy efficiency, while factor substitution and biased technological progress are important factors for fluctuations in energy intensity. Technological progress can effectively narrow the energy efficiency gap between European companies. In the future, the EU should support European manufacturing companies in introducing and using both sustainable processes and product innovation to narrow the energy efficiency gap [23]. Wang and Wang [24], using the number of patents granted to measure technological innovation, found that technological innovation in China has significantly improved urban energy efficiency. Sun et al. [25], based on their research on 24 innovative countries, found that there is a significant positive relationship between technological innovation and energy efficiency.

Other scholars believe that innovations in artificial intelligence, information and communication technology have led to a decrease in the unit cost of energy. This will stimulate enterprises to expand production, bring on a "rebound effect" to energy consumption and thus lead to a more complex kind of energy efficiency for manufacturing enterprises [26,27].

Currently, academia has widely accepted the existence of the rebound effect [28–30], although it is still controversial as to whether the rebound effect will completely offset increases in energy efficiency brought about by technological progress (that is, the rebound effect is greater than 100%). A study by Jin [31], based on the electricity consumption data of 3500 households in South Korea, gave empirical calculations showing that the energy rebound effect was about 30%. Vélez-Henao et al. [32] believed that every 1% drop in energy prices in Colombia would increase the rebound effect by 38.56%. Adha et al. [33] found that the short-term and long-term rebound effects in Indonesia were 87.2% and −45.5%, respectively, indicating that technological improvements can improve energy efficiency in the long-term. Therefore, technological progress has become an important factor affecting energy efficiency.

Artificial intelligence is considered to be a general technology that can support other innovations [34]. While enterprises use AI to achieve technological progress, the use of AI further promotes new technological innovations, thus forming a new virtuous circle [35]. Therefore, considering that related research on the impact of AI on corporate energy efficiency is still relatively rare, we look first at research showing how technological progress impacts corporate energy efficiency. This will significantly affect energy efficiency [34].

First, artificial intelligence can accelerate knowledge spillover and creation and promote technological progress of enterprises in energy saving and cleaner production, and thereby improve energy efficiency [25]. The stronger the ability of an enterprise to learn and absorb, the higher its ability to innovate [36]. Through deep learning and computer vision technology, artificial intelligence can screen out a large amount of effective information and create new knowledge and new computing solutions more efficiently than ever before, thereby accelerating the process of knowledge reorganization [37]. The acceleration of knowledge reorganization can promote the re-creation of knowledge and information [38]. At the same time, artificial intelligence breaks the boundaries of knowledge dissemination within and between enterprises and can accelerate knowledge spillover and information sharing, thereby promoting technological innovation [39]. With the improvement in the level of artificial intelligence, this information contribution ability has been further strengthened. The learning and absorptive capacity of the employees of the enterprise is also continuously improved, thereby promoting the absorption and creation of knowledge within the enterprise [34]. In turn, this promotes technological innovation of enterprises, results in more optimized equipment and energy use decisions, and improves energy efficiency [35].

Second, artificial intelligence promotes technological progress and improves energy efficiency by increasing investment in R&D and talent. The development of artificial intelligence will bring more intelligent devices such as industrial robots, thereby producing a labor substitution effect [40]. The shortage of high-skilled labor caused by this complementary substitution of labor will further force manufacturing enterprises to increase investment in talents and R&D [41]. Talent and R&D investment can further promote technological progress [42]. At the same time, with the increasing global trend of using industrial robots, companies are actively improving their production processes and manufacturing skills. Among them, the use of artificial intelligence technology to improve product processes has become an important way to gain competitive advantage [43]. In turn, through technological progress, the production process is optimized, thereby improving energy efficiency [44]. In the waste management sector, the application of neural networks and machine learning can predict the amount of waste generated, promote waste reuse and improve energy efficiency [45].

In addition, artificial intelligence can improve energy efficiency by increasing technological efficiency. That is, AI can also shorten the gap between businesses and optimal energy efficiency by improving technological efficiency. On the one hand, artificial intelligence can improve production efficiency. Manufacturing companies can use industrial robots to replace low-skilled production workers [46]. Using intelligent technology for production can effectively improve product quality and reduce energy consumption caused by repeated production due to substandard products [47]. With the help of artificial intelligence technology, such as machine learning, deep learning, etc., enterprises can complete the design, production and sales of products faster [48,49]. On the other hand, artificial intelligence can improve the efficiency of resource allocation. Enterprises use advanced intelligent equipment to make equipment self-perceive, self-analyze, and self-decide. This results in real-time feedback and optimization of production information, reduces equipment response time, reduces energy waste and significantly improves resource allocation efficiency and energy efficiency [50,51].

Artificial intelligence has been widely used in various sectors to improve energy efficiency [52,53]. For example, in the construction sector, the combination of artificial intelligence and big data can improve the energy efficiency of buildings and the comfort of houses [54]. In the energy supply sector, the application of smart meter data can help to accurately predict the consumption of electricity and natural gas so as to better plan and operate the energy supply system [55,56]. Huang and Koroteev [45] believe that AI technologies such as neural networks and machine learning are more successful in energy and waste management, which can then be used to improve the efficiency of electricity, heat and gas in the future. Chen et al. [57] believe that artificial intelligence can optimize equipment scheduling and operation, and their proposed AIEM model can effectively improve energy efficiency and promote the use of renewable energy.

Based on the above analysis, we propose the following hypothesis:

Hypothesis 1: *AI can improve the energy efficiency of manufacturing companies.*

Hypothesis 2: *AI can improve corporate energy efficiency by promoting technological progress and technical efficiency.*

3. Model Design

3.1. The Model

Referring to the research of Bloom et al. [58], we take total factor productivity (TFP) as the explained variable and establish the following regression equation:

$$TFP_{ijct} = \alpha + \beta AI_{ijct} + \gamma X'_{ijct} + \varphi_{ind} + \phi_{year} + \theta_{city} + \delta_{ijct} \quad (1)$$

where TFP_{ijct} represents the total factor productivity of manufacturing enterprises in industry j in city i in year t, AI_{ijct} represents the intelligence level of manufacturing enterprises and X'_{ijct} represents other control variables in the model that affect the total factor energy efficiency of manufacturing enterprises. φ_{ind}, ϕ_{year} and θ_{city} represent industry fixed effects, time fixed effects and city fixed effects, respectively. δ_{ijct} is the random error term. β is the most concerned coefficient of this article. If β is statistically significantly positive, it means that the application of artificial intelligence has improved energy efficiency.

3.2. The Variables

(1) Dependent variable: total factor energy efficiency (TFP).

This paper refers to the research of Wang et al. [59] and calculates the total factor productivity of manufacturing enterprises based on the DEA-Malmquist index method. In recent years, Data Envelopment Analysis (DEA) has been often used by scholars to measure total factor productivity. The DEA method uses linear optimization to estimate the boundary production function and distance function, without making assumptions about the form and distribution of the production function, and so avoids strong theoretical constraints [60,61]. At the same time, the DEA-Malmquist index method is now one of the mainstream DEA measurement methods. It can decompose changes in total factor productivity into technological progress and changes in technical efficiency, thereby facilitating in-depth analysis of the causes of changes in total factor productivity. It has been widely used by scholars in energy efficiency research [62]. In this light and, referring to the research of Wang et al. [59], we assume that the form of the production function of the firm is in the form of the Cobb–Douglas production function, and its natural logarithm can be converted to a linear form:

$$\ln(Y_{jt}) = A + a\, ln(K_{jt}) + b \ln(L_{jt}) + c\, ln(E_{jt}) + \varepsilon_{jt} \tag{2}$$

where j and t represent the manufacturing enterprises and year, respectively, and Y_{jt} represents the output, which is measured by the company's operating income. K_{jt}, L_{jt} and E_{jt} represent the three production input factors of capital, labor and energy, respectively, which are measured by the total assets of the enterprise, the number of employees and the electricity consumption. A is a constant term, ε_{jt} is a residual term and a, b and c are the coefficients of the elements. Therefore, by constructing the DEA- Malmquist model, we can calculate the total factor productivity (TFP) of manufacturing enterprises. According to the research of Fare et al., under the conditions of fixed returns to scale (c) and strong disposal of factors, the minimum technical efficiency (CRS) can be decomposed into:

$$F_j^t(y^t, x^t \big| c, s = s_j^t(y^t, x^t \big| s) \cdot CN_j^t(y^t, x^t \big| v) \cdot F_j^t(y^t, x^t \big| v, w) \tag{3}$$

where $F_j^t(y^t, x^t \big| c, s$ is the technical efficiency, $s_j^t(y^t, x^t \vee s)$ is the scale efficiency, $CN_j^t(y^t, x^t \vee v)$ is the degree of strong disposal of the measuring element and $F_j^t(y^t, x^t \vee v, w)$ is the pure technical efficiency. The input distance function is the reciprocal of technical efficiency, namely:

$$D_j^t(y^t, x^t) = \frac{1}{F_j^t(y^t,\ x^t | c, s)} \tag{4}$$

In Equation (4), the input distance function can be regarded as the distance moved from a certain production point (y^t, x^t) to the ideal input point, $D_j^t(y^t, x^t) \geq 1$, when $D_j^t(y^t, x^t) = 1$, (y^t, x^t) is on the best front and the technology is valid; if $D_j^t(y^t, x^t) > 1$, then (y^t, x^t) is outside the best front and the technology is invalid.

Therefore, the Malmquist indices based on periods t and $t+1$ are:

$$M_j^t = \frac{D_j^t(x^{t+1}, y^{t+1})}{D_j^t(x^t, y^t)}$$

$$M_j^{t+1} = \frac{D_j^{t+1}(x^{t+1}, y^{t+1})}{D_j^{t+1}(x^t, y^t)} \tag{5}$$

The above indexes are symmetrical in economic meaning. Referring to the method of Fare et al. (1994) [63], their geometric average is defined as a composite index, that is, total factor productivity TFP:

$$TFP_{jt} = M_j\left(x^t, y^t, x^{t+1}, y^{t+1}\right) = \left(M_j^t \cdot M_j^{t+1}\right)^{\frac{1}{2}} = \left[\frac{D_j^t(x^{t+1}, y^{t+1})}{D_j^t(x^t, y^t)} \cdot \frac{D_j^{t+1}(x^{t+1}, y^{t+1})}{D_j^{t+1}(x^t, y^t)}\right]^{\frac{1}{2}} \tag{6}$$

We further decompose the Malmquist index into:

$$TFP_{jt} = M_j(x^t, y^t, x^{t+1}, y^{t+1}) = \frac{D_j^{t+1}(x^{t+1}, y^{t+1})}{D_j^{t+1}(x^t, y^t)} \times \left[\frac{D_j^t(x^t, y^t)}{D_j^{t+1}(x^t, y^t)} \cdot \frac{D_j^t(x^{t+1}, y^{t+1})}{D_j^{t+1}(x^{t+1}, y^{t+1})}\right]^{\frac{1}{2}} \times \left[\frac{D_j^t(x^{t+1}, y^{t+1})/D_j^t(x^{t+1}, y^{t+1})}{D_j^t(x^t, y^t)/D_j^t(x^t, y^t)} \cdot \frac{D_j^{t+1}(x^{t+1}, y^{t+1})/D_j^{t+1}(x^{t+1}, y^{t+1})}{D_j^{t+1}(x^t, y^t)/D_j^{t+1}(x^t, y^t)}\right]^{\frac{1}{2}} = pech \times techch \times sech \tag{7}$$

where *pech* is pure technical efficiency change, which is the change in technical efficiency under the assumption of variable returns to scale. *sech* is the change in scale efficiency, indicating the influence of scale economy on total factor energy efficiency. $pech \times sech$ is the change in technical efficiency (eff), which measures the degree of catching up to the best practice of each observation object from t to $t+1$. Greater than 1 means that the technical efficiency is improved, less than 1 means that the technical efficiency is reduced and equal to 1 means that there is no change in the technical efficiency.

Techch is the change in technological progress and reflects the contribution of the movement of the production front to the change in total factor productivity. It measures the movement of the technological boundary from t to the $t+1$ period. Greater than 1 means technological progress, less than 1 means technological regression and equal to 1 means no change in technological level.

(2) Independent variable: Enterprise intelligence level (AI).

This article refers to the research of Acemoglu and Restrepo [40] and uses the number of industrial robots to measure the level of artificial intelligence of manufacturing enterprises. With reference to the research of Yang and Hou [64], we calculate the use of industrial robots in manufacturing enterprises based on the ratio of the output value of the enterprise to the total output value of the industry to measure the level of enterprise intelligence.

(3) Control variables: The debt-to-asset ratio (Lcv).

The debt-to-asset ratio measures the ability of manufacturing enterprises to use creditors to provide funds for operating activities. Companies with high levels of debt lack sufficient capital to use advanced technology and optimize production processes; it is difficult to improve their energy efficiency. This article uses the ratio of the total amount of corporate liabilities to total assets to measure debt-to-asset ratio.

Corporate age (Firmage). Generally speaking, the rigidity of the corporate structure, caused by the age of manufacturing enterprises, will affect the company's energy structure adjustment, thereby affecting the energy efficiency of manufacturing enterprises. We take the company's incorporation date as the benchmark and add the company's age variable to the model.

Ownership of enterprises (Ownership). Generally speaking, private enterprises are more likely to take measures to reduce the cost of production and operation, which will affect the total factor energy efficiency of manufacturing enterprises. If the company is a private company, it is 1, and for the rest it is 0.

Corporate performance (Ros). Corporate performance often has positive and negative effects on total factor energy efficiency. When the company's performance is good, the company may choose to expand the scale of production and invest in more factor resources. The positive effect lies in the scale economy effect and output growth brought about by the expansion of production scale, which leads to the growth of the company's total factor energy efficiency. The negative effect is when the marginal increase in output is smaller than the increase in input energy, which leads to a reduction in total factor energy efficiency. Referring to the study of Boubakri et al. [65], we use the ratio of corporate net profit to operating income to measure *ros*.

Enterprise energy consumption level (Energy). Differences in enterprise energy consumption levels will lead to changes in total factor energy efficiency. Manufacturing enterprises with higher levels of energy consumption may have greater marginal room for growth in their total factor energy efficiency. At the same time, energy dependence may also lead to smaller changes in their total factor energy efficiency. According to the "2010 National Economic and Social Development Statistical Report", companies in the six highest energy consumption industries specified by the state are assigned a value of 1, and the rest are assigned a value of 0.

3.3. Data Sources

The data of industrial robots in this article come from the International Federation of Robotics (IFR), which counts the global number of industrial robots by industry. The enterprise-level data come from a comprehensive survey conducted by the Guangdong Provincial Economic and Information Technology Commission on the situation of enterprises above a designated size in the province. The data span from 2013 to 2015. As the database counts more than 110,000 manufacturing enterprises in Guangdong Province, the data are considered comprehensive and can be used to scientifically measure the energy utilization of micro-enterprises.

On this basis, this article processes the data as follows: (1) The World Robot Association data are first sorted according to the "Classification of National Economic Industries" (2019). (2) Non-manufacturing industry data and samples of manufacturing enterprises with less than ten employees are excluded, following which abnormal values of various variables are processed. (3) In order to further alleviate the problem of heteroscedasticity caused by variable measurement, this paper performs winsorized processing for both dependent variables and independent variables below the 1% quantile and above the 99% quantile. The explanation and data sources of variables are listed in Table 1. The descriptive statistics of the processed variables are shown in Table 2.

Table 1. Description of variables.

Variables	Symbol	Definition Measuring Method	Unit	Data Sources
Industrial robots	AI	Installation amount of industrial robots	1 unit	International Federation of Robotics (IFR)
Total factor energy efficiency	TFP	DEA-Malmquist model	/	The comprehensive survey conducted by the Guangdong Provincial Economic and Information Technology Commission on the situation of enterprises above a designated size in the province
Debt-to-asset ratio	Lcv	The ratio of the total amount of corporate liabilities to total assets	/	
Enterprise age	Firmage	The current date minus the enterprises' registered date	year	
Ownership of enterprises	Owner-ship	If the enterprise is a private company, it is 1, and for the rest it is 0	/	
Enterprise performance	Ros	The ratio of net profit to operating revenue	/	
Enterprise energy consumption level	Energy	If enterprise is in the six high energy consumption industries, it is 1, and for the rest it is 0	/	

Table 2. Descriptive statistics of variables.

Variable	Obs	Std.Dev.	Mean	Min	Max
AI	40,053	0.3052	0.7087	0.0000	7.6321
Lcv	40,053	0.5480	0.3756	0.0000	2.9998
Firmage	40,053	8.1580	5.4697	0.0000	26.0000
Ros	40,053	0.0588	0.1409	−0.6713	0.7897
Ownership	40,053	0.9959	0.0641	0.0000	1.0000
Energy	40,053	0.1638	0.3701	0.0000	1.0000
TFP	40,053	1.1728	0.9552	0.0902	11.5830

4. Empirical Test

4.1. Benchmark Regression

In order to exclude the influence of individual manufacturing enterprises' characteristics on the robustness of the model, we use a two-way fixed effects model for empirical testing. Compared with the general static panel model that only fixes individual corporate effects that does not change with time, the two-way fixed effects model fixes the individual corporate effects and time effects, respectively; this makes the empirical results more credible. The benchmark regression results are shown in Table 3.

Table 3. Benchmark regression.

Variable	(1)	(2)	(3)	(4)
	M1	M2	M3	M4
AI	0.0469 ***	0.1450 ***	0.0458 ***	0.1449 ***
	(5.99)	(8.70)	(5.79)	(8.74)
Control	NO	NO	YES	YES
Industry_FE	NO	YES	NO	YES
City_FE	NO	YES	NO	YES
Year_FE	NO	YES	NO	YES
cons	1.1585 ***	0.9974 ***	1.1898 ***	0.9708 ***
	(228.53)	(178.77)	(22.26)	(6.03)
N	40,053	40,053	40,053	40,053
Adj_R^2	0.0012	0.0234	0.0027	0.0246

Note a: (1) The values in parentheses are standard errors. (2) *** indicate that the variable coefficients have passed the 1% significance tests, respectively. Note b: N represents the number of sample observations.

Model (1) only adds independent variables. The results show that the coefficient of the Ai variable is 0.0469 and that it passes the 1% significance test. Model (2) controls the fixed effects of industry, region and time on the basis of Model (1). The results also show that artificial intelligence is positively correlated with energy efficiency of manufacturing enterprises. The coefficient of artificial intelligence is 0.1450 and passes the 1% significance test. In Model (3), we add control variables; the results show that the coefficient of artificial intelligence is 0.0458, and that it passes the 1% significance test. Model (4) controls the fixed effects of industry, region and time on the basis of Model (3). The results show that the artificial intelligence coefficient is 0.1449, and that it passes the 1% significance test, further proving that artificial intelligence has a significant positive correlation with manufacturing companies. From this, we deduce that artificial intelligence has a significant positive impact on the energy efficiency of manufacturing enterprises, which is consistent with Hypothesis 1. Artificial intelligence can improve energy efficiency by improving both the production efficiency and the management efficiency of manufacturing enterprises.

4.2. Endogenous Test

There may be an endogenous problem in Equation (1) in this paper. First, there is the problem of missing unobservable variables, such as production and operation problems that may affect both the artificial intelligence level and the energy efficiency of manufacturing enterprises at the same time. The second is that manufacturing enterprises with higher energy efficiency in production may often be manufacturing enterprises with higher levels of artificial intelligence, so there are synergy biases. Therefore, this article alleviates the endogenous problem by looking for an instrumental variable method. The Acemoglu and Restrepo [40] study pointed out that, due to the obvious international competition among several major manufacturing countries in the world, countries have shown a high degree of convergence in the scale of new technologies and equipment applications. Therefore, it is reasonable to use the number of industrial robots in the same industry in other major manufacturing countries as an instrumental variable.

Considering the specific situation of China's manufacturing industry, the competition between China's manufacturing industry and the United States has become increasingly fierce in recent years, with the manufacturing industries of the two countries having a strong competitive relationship. At the same time, data from the International Federation of Robotics (IFR) show that the number of industrial robots used in China and the United States is also increasing sharply, with a strong positive correlation. Therefore, this article draws on the ideas of Acemoglu and Restrepo [40] and uses the number of industrial robots in the same industry in the United States during the same period as the instrumental variable *iv*, which conforms to the correlation assumption of instrumental variables. On the other hand, the use of artificial intelligence in the United States has a relatively small impact on the energy efficiency of manufacturing enterprises in Guangdong Province, China, which conforms to the exogenous hypothesis of instrumental variables. The test results are shown in Table 4.

Table 4. Endogenous test.

Variable	(5) First	(6) 2SLS
AI		0.8875 **
		(2.07)
IV	0.0185 ***	
	(7.92)	
Control	YES	YES
Industry_FE	YES	YES
City_FE	YES	YES
Year_FE	YES	YES
N	39854	39,854
Underidentificationtest		
Kleibergen–PaaprkLMstatistic	60.52 ***	
Weakidentificationtest		
Cragg–DonaldWaldFstatistic	14.48 ***	
Kleiberge–PaapWaldrkFstatistic	62.68 ***	
	(16.38)	
Weakinstrumentrobustinference		
Anderson–RubinWaldtest	4.54 **	

Note a: (1) The values in parentheses are standard errors. (2) ***, ** indicate that the variable coefficients have passed the 1% and 5% significance tests, respectively. Note b: The blanks indicate that the relevant variables are not included in the model.

This paper uses the two-stage least squares method to estimate Equation (1). The one-stage regression results in the Model (5) in Table 3 show that the instrumental variables selected in this paper are significantly positively correlated with the endogenous variables. The correlation coefficient is 0.0185, which passes the 1% significance test and satisfies the correlation hypothesis. The two-stage regression result in Model (6) shows that the sign of the coefficient of artificial intelligence is positive, the coefficient is 0.8875 and that it is significant at the 5% level, which is consistent with the benchmark regression result and further proves Hypothesis 1. At the same time, this article further tests the rationality of the instrumental variables and rejects the null hypothesis, which proves that the instrumental variables used in this article are appropriate.

4.3. Robustness Test

In order to further prove the robustness of the model, we conducted a robustness test as shown in Table 5.

The first step is to replace the explanatory variables. In Model (7), we take the industrial robot inventory ($Ai2$) of manufacturing enterprises as a substitute independent variable to measure the level of artificial intelligence. The estimation results show that the inventory coefficient of industrial robots is 0.0511 and that it passes the 1% significance test, indicating that there is a significant positive correlation between industrial robot inventory and energy efficiency of manufacturing enterprises. This result is consistent with the benchmark regression results and proves that artificial intelligence has a significant positive impact on the energy efficiency of manufacturing enterprises.

The second is to replace the explained variable. In Model (8), referring to the study of Bloom et al. [58], energy intensity (*ee*) is used as a substitute dependent variable. Energy intensity reflects the energy consumption of a company's unit output value and can measure the energy efficiency of a company to a certain extent. The results show that the coefficient of influence of artificial intelligence on the energy intensity variables of manufacturing enterprises is −0.0053, which passes the 1% significance test. It shows that artificial intelligence has significantly reduced the energy intensity of manufacturing enterprises and that manufacturing enterprises have enjoyed improved economic energy benefits. This proves that artificial intelligence can improve the energy efficiency of manufacturing enterprises.

Table 5. Robustness test.

Variable	(7)	(8)	(9)	(10)
	Replace Explanatory Variables	**Replace Dependent Variable**	**Tobit**	**Sys-GMM**
AI		−0.0053 ***	0.0143 ***	0.2991 ***
		(−3.80)	(4.30)	(7.84)
AI2	0.0511 ***			
	(8.00)			
L.tfee				−0.1094 ***
				(−6.83)
Control	YES	YES	YES	YES
Industry_FE	YES	YES	YES	YES
City_FE	YES	YES	YES	YES
Year_FE	YES	YES	YES	YES
_cons	0.9656 ***	0.0616 ***	3.4522	1.5660 ***
	(5.97)	(3.53)	(0.14)	(5.91)
N	40,053	40,053	40053	24,729
Adj_R^2	0.0243	0.0053		

Note a: (1) The values in parentheses are standard errors. (2) *** indicate that the variable coefficients have passed the 1% significance tests, respectively. Note b: The blanks indicate that the relevant variables are not included in the model.

The third step is to replace the regression model. In Model (9), taking into account the possible censorship features in the dependent variable, we use the Tobit model for regression. Under the Tobit regression model, the coefficient of influence of artificial intelligence on enterprise energy efficiency variables is 0.2991 and passes the 1% significance test. It shows that there is still a significant positive correlation between artificial intelligence and enterprise energy efficiency variables. The conclusions obtained are consistent with the OLS regression results, which proves that artificial intelligence can significantly promote the energy efficiency of manufacturing enterprises. In addition, we use the Sys-GMM method for regression in Model (10). The Sys-GMM method can further alleviate the endogenous problems that may exist in the model to a certain extent [66]. Under the Sys-GMM model, the impact of artificial intelligence on energy efficiency variables is still significantly positive.

4.4. Heterogeneity Test

Considering that the level of artificial intelligence of manufacturing enterprises will be affected by the characteristics of individual enterprises, we expand Equation (1) to increase the interaction term between the individual heterogeneity characteristic variable ($char_{ijct}$) of manufacturing enterprises and artificial intelligence (AI). To test the effect of artificial intelligence on the energy efficiency of manufacturing enterprises under conditions of differing individual enterprise heterogeneity, the expanded equation is as follows:

$$TFP_{ijpt} = \alpha + \beta AI_{ijpt} + \gamma X'_{ijpt} + \tau rob_{ijpt} * char_{ijct} + \varphi_{ind} + \phi_{year} + \theta_{city} + \delta_{ijpt} \quad (8)$$

For the characteristics of individual heterogeneity variables, this paper examines the two dimensions of firm age ($firmage$) and firm performance (ros), and the measurement method is the same as that of Equation (1). Regression results are shown in Table 6.

Table 6. Heterogeneity test.

Variable	(11) Firmage	(12) Ros
AI	0.2473 ***	0.1172 ***
	(6.77)	(6.54) *
AI ∗ Firmage	−0.0107 ***	
	(−3.60)	
AI ∗ Ros		0.6229 ***
		(2.88)
Control	YES	YES
Industry_FE	YES	YES
City_FE	YES	YES
Year_FE	YES	YES
cons	0.9462 ***	0.9688 ***
	(5.87)	(6.00)
N	40053	40053
Adj_R^2	0.0252	0.0260

Note a: (1) The values in parentheses are standard errors. (2) ***, * indicate that the variable coefficients have passed the 1% and 10% significance tests, respectively. Note b: The blanks indicate that the relevant variables are not included in the model.

According to Model (11) in Table 6, the artificial intelligence coefficient is 0.2473 and passes the 1% significance test, indicating that artificial intelligence indeed has a significant positive impact on energy efficiency. The coefficient of the interaction term between enterprise age and artificial intelligence is significantly negative, showing that the age of the company will weaken the role of artificial intelligence in promoting energy efficiency in manufacturing enterprises. That is, the longer the enterprise has been established, the smaller the effect of artificial intelligence on its energy efficiency. According to the analysis of the inter-effect on the left side of Figure 2a, when the firm age does not exceed 18 years, the marginal effect of artificial intelligence on the energy efficiency of manufacturing enterprises gradually decreases and is statistically significant. When the age of manufacturing enterprise ($firmage$) exceeds 18 years, the marginal effect of artificial intelligence on energy efficiency gradually decreases and is not statistically significant. At the same time, according to Model (12) in Table 6, the artificial intelligence coefficient is 0.1172 and passes the 1% significance test. This also supports the results of the benchmark regression. The coefficient of the interaction term ($AI \times ros$) between corporate performance and artificial intelligence is significantly positive, indicating that the performance of manufacturing enterprises can strengthen the role of artificial intelligence in promoting energy efficiency. That is, the higher the performance of manufacturing enterprises, the greater the effect of artificial intelligence in improving its energy efficiency. According to the analysis on the right side of Figure 2b, the marginal effect of artificial intelligence on the energy efficiency of manufacturing enterprises is negative and statistically significant when the enterprise performance term (ros) does not exceed −0.57. When the performance of manufacturing enterprise (ros) does not exceed −0.17, the marginal effect of artificial intelligence on the energy efficiency of manufacturing companies turns from negative to positive, but it is not statistically significant. When the company's age exceeds −0.07, the marginal effect of artificial intelligence on the energy efficiency of manufacturing companies gradually increases and is statistically significant.

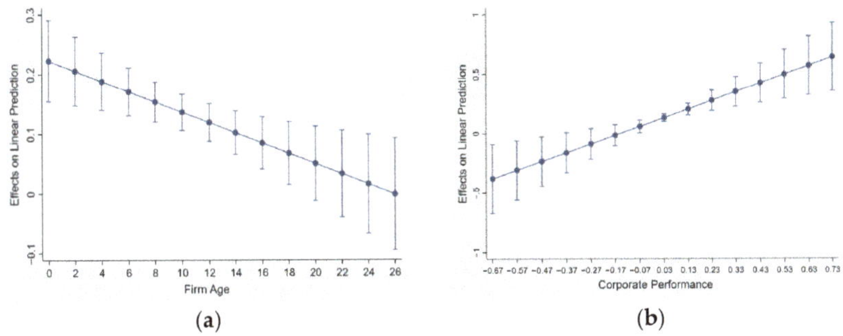

Figure 2. The average marginal effect of enterprise individual characteristic variables.

4.5. Influence Mechanism Test

Impact mechanism analysis shows that artificial intelligence can promote the improvement of energy efficiency by promoting technological progress and improving technical efficiency. Therefore, based on the Malmquist theory, we take the two decomposition indexes of technological progress (*techch*) and technical efficiency (eff) as dependent variables, and observe the different effects of intelligence on the two. The results are shown in Table 7, where Model (13) represents technological progress and Model (14) represents technical efficiency. According to the results, the influence coefficient of artificial intelligence on the technological progress variable is 0.1419, and it has passed the 1% significance test. This is consistent with Hypothesis 2. It shows that artificial intelligence can significantly promote the technological progress of manufacturing enterprises. However, the relationship between AI and technological efficiency failed the significance test. It shows that the impact of artificial intelligence on the technical efficiency of manufacturing enterprises is not obvious, which is different from Hypothesis 2.

Table 7. Heterogeneity test.

Variable	(13) Techch	(14) Eff
AI	0.1419 ***	−0.0061
	(9.31)	(−1.53)
Control	YES	YES
$\text{Industry}_{\text{FE}}$	YES	YES
City_{FE}	YES	YES
Year_{FE}	YES	YES
cons	0.9644 ***	1.0276 ***
	(6.38)	(23.43)
N	39785	38905
Adj^2_{R}	0.0128	0.0887

Note a: (1) The values in parentheses are standard errors. (2) *** indicate that the variable coefficients have passed the 1% significance tests, respectively. Note b: The blanks indicate that the relevant variables are not included in the model.

5. Discussion

The application of AI technologies has had a significant impact on the energy sector [67]. The empirical evidence in this paper shows that artificial intelligence can significantly improve the energy efficiency of manufacturing enterprises. This conclusion is similar to that of Chen et al. (2021). Chen et al. (2021) proposed a new algorithm based on artificial intelligence technology and an evaluation model using AIEM for energy efficiency and conservation prediction. It is concluded that the use of artificial intelligence technology can improve energy efficiency and renewable energy use [57]. Furthermore, based on algorithms, Lee et al. (2022) concluded that artificial intelligence can achieve energy savings in different fields [68]. In contrast, we are not an algorithm or forecasting study, but based on econometrics, using micro-data of manufacturing companies, we have proved the impact of AI on energy efficiency. To the best of our knowledge, the paper is one of the few to provide evidence of the impact of AI on energy efficiency through econometric methods.

We believe that the promotion of artificial intelligence in energy efficiency mainly comes from two aspects. First, as a general-purpose technology, artificial intelligence can accelerate knowledge learning and creation, increase the R&D and talent investment of manufacturing enterprises and promote technological progress of manufacturing enterprises, thereby improving energy efficiency. This was also verified in the mechanism inspection. This conclusion is similar to the research conclusion of Fisher-Vanden et al. [69]. Technological progress has a significant effect on the improvement of energy efficiency in Chinese manufacturing enterprises. Artificial intelligence can significantly improve the progress of enterprise energy utilization technology by accelerating both enterprise knowledge learning and creation and increasing enterprise R&D and talent investment.

Second, artificial intelligence promotes energy efficiency by improving technical efficiency. However, this has not been verified in the mechanism test. We believe that, on the one hand, this may be due to the existence of the productivity paradox. Generally speaking, technological progress can effectively promote improvements in technical efficiency, but when it comes to computer-related technology, this experience is often proved to be wrong. The excessive automation brought about by artificial intelligence may restrict the growth of technical efficiency [40]. Excessive intelligence will not only directly lead to the reduction of technical efficiency, but may also cause an energy "rebound effect" through wastage of resources and labor mismatch and, in this way, indirectly inhibit the growth of energy efficiency. Judging from the current status of corporate energy efficiency, the impact of artificial intelligence on corporate energy efficiency is more from technological progress. The level of technical efficiency in various industries is still relatively average, and the growth rate is relatively slow. As predicted by Li and Zhou [70], as the market gradually improves, technological progress will continue to play a greater role in the energy efficiency growth of manufacturing companies, while the contribution of technical efficiency will be relatively reduced.

The test results of the heterogeneity of individual characteristics of manufacturing enterprises show that: On the one hand, the role of artificial intelligence in promoting energy efficiency will decrease as companies age. The reason may be that the older the enterprise, the higher the cost of coordinating various business units. Disadvantages such as high transformation costs and rigid corporate structure brought about by the age of manufacturing enterprises often inhibit the improvement of energy efficiency in manufacturing enterprises. On the other hand, the role of artificial intelligence in promoting energy efficiency will increase with the growth of corporate performance. This shows that an improvement in corporate performance is conducive to the rational operation of artificial intelligence companies. The application of artificial intelligence requires continuous capital investment by manufacturing enterprises. The better the performance of the enterprise, the more sufficient funds the manufacturing enterprises have to play the role of intelligent transformation. The study by Huang et al. (2022) also came to a similar conclusion. It is believed that the use of industrial robots will improve corporate performance, expand production scale and then improve energy efficiency through scale effects [71]. The previous literature, although analyzing the industry heterogeneity of the impact of industrial robots on energy intensity, believed that industrial robots mainly affect the energy intensity of labor-intensive industries. However, it is not specific to the level of firm heterogeneity [72].

Based on the above analysis and comparison with existing literature, the marginal contribution of this paper is as follows: (1) From the perspective of AI promoting technological progress and improving technical efficiency, this paper analyzes the impact mechanism of AI on the energy efficiency of manufacturing enterprises. (2) It constructs a DEA-Malmquist model to measure the total factor energy efficiency of micro-enterprises and empirically tests the impact of AI on the total factor energy efficiency of manufacturing enterprises and its heterogeneity. (3) To alleviate the endogenous problems in the model as much as possible, the number of industrial robots in the same industry in the United States during the same period is taken as an instrumental variable for the use of AI in Chinese manufacturing enterprises. (4) Using the data of manufacturing enterprises, this paper provides the first microscopic evidence that AI can improve the energy efficiency of manufacturing enterprises. It thus expands current research on the relationship between AI and manufacturing enterprises' energy efficiency.

6. Conclusions

This paper studies the impact of artificial intelligence on the energy efficiency of manufacturing enterprises and its mechanism of action from both theoretical and empirical aspects. Research shows that: Artificial intelligence significantly improves the energy efficiency of manufacturing companies. After introducing the US industrial robot data as an instrumental variable for endogeneity testing, the results are still stable.

In addition, we found that the impact of artificial intelligence on the energy efficiency of manufacturing enterprises is mainly achieved by accelerating knowledge learning and creation, increasing the R&D and talent investment of manufacturing enterprises and promoting the technological progress of manufacturing enterprises. This paper further analyzes the heterogeneity of manufacturing enterprises. The results show that the age of manufacturing firms inhibits the promotion of artificial intelligence on energy efficiency. Manufacturing firm performance enhances AI's boost to energy efficiency, but this boost can only be seen when firm performance is positive.

Based on the above conclusions, the following policy recommendations are put forward:

(1) Increase the application scope of artificial intelligence in manufacturing enterprises and give full play to the positive impact of technological progress on enterprise energy efficiency. Encourage manufacturing enterprises to continuously increase investment in research and development of intelligent technology. Shift technological innovation from production efficiency-oriented to energy saving-oriented innovation.

(2) Improve the contribution of artificial intelligence to the technical efficiency of energy utilization. Through intelligent decision-making, intelligent control and intelligent management, manufacturing enterprises can allocate resources more reasonably in the process of production and operation, save energy costs, reduce energy waste and improve energy utilization efficiency.

(3) With artificial intelligence applications, focus on enterprise heterogeneity. Encourage high-tech manufacturing enterprises to vigorously develop artificial intelligence, give full play to the knowledge and technology spillovers brought by artificial intelligence, promote enterprise energy technology innovation and improve energy efficiency.

Due to data limitations, the data used in this article are the data of manufacturing enterprises from 2013 to 2015; the time span is relatively short. The conclusions drawn can only represent the short-term impact of artificial intelligence on the energy efficiency of manufacturing enterprises. The research conclusions in this paper are based on samples from Guangdong Province, China and may not be suitable for other countries. In addition, although this paper uses enterprise micro-survey data, there is still a lack of data to directly measure the level of artificial intelligence in enterprises. In the future, based on the global data, the long-term effects of artificial intelligence for manufacturing enterprises can be studied further.

Author Contributions: Conceptualization, J.L. and Y.Q.; methodology, Y.Q.; software, Y.Q. and Y.Y.; formal analysis, Y.Q.; investigation, J.L.; resources, J.L.; data curation, Y.Y.; writing—original draft preparation, Y.Q. and Y.Y.; writing—review and editing, Z.Y.; visualization, Z.Y.; supervision, J.L.; project administration, J.L. and Y.Q.; funding acquisition, J.L. and Y.Q. All authors have read and agreed to the published version of the manuscript.

Funding: This study was collectively funded by the National Natural Science Foundation of China [No. 71973068], Social Science Foundation Major Project of Jiangsu, China [No.18ZD003], Humanities and Social Sciences Research Planning Foundation of China's Ministry of Education [No. 19YJA790055], and Postgraduate Research and Innovation Project of Jiangsu Province [No. KYCX21_1022].

Institutional Review Board Statement: Not applicable.

Informed Consent Statement: Not applicable.

Data Availability Statement: The data of industrial robots in this article comes from the International Federation of Robotics (IFR). This data can be found here: https://ifr.org/worldrobotics/ (accessed on 12 December 2021). The enterprise-level data comes from a comprehensive survey conducted by the Guangdong Provincial Economic and Information Technology Commission on the situation of enterprises above a designated size in the province. The data are survey data and have not been made public.

Conflicts of Interest: The authors declared no potential conflict of interest with respect to the research, authorship and/or publication of this article.

References

1. Macharia, K.K.; Gathiaka, J.K.; Ngui, D. Energy efficiency in the Kenyan manufacturing sector. *Energy Policy* **2022**, *161*, 112715. [CrossRef]
2. Su, B.; Goh, T.; Ang, B.W.; Ng, T.S. Energy consumption and energy efficiency trends in Singapore: The case of a meticulously planned city. *Energy Policy* **2022**, *161*, 112732. [CrossRef]
3. BP. *BP Statistical Review of World Energy*; BP Statistical Review: London, UK, 2020. Available online: https://www.bp.com/en/global/corporate/energy-economics/statistical-review-of-world-energy.html (accessed on 1 December 2021).
4. Zhu, J.; Lin, B. Economic growth pressure and energy efficiency improvement: Empirical evidence from Chinese cities. *Appl. Energy* **2022**, *307*, 118275. [CrossRef]
5. Rai, V.; Henry, A.D. Agent-based modelling of consumer energy choices. *Nat. Clim. Chang.* **2016**, *6*, 556–562. [CrossRef]
6. He, Y.; Fu, F.; Liao, N. Exploring the path of carbon emissions reduction in China's industrial sector through energy efficiency enhancement induced by R&D investment. *Energy* **2021**, *225*, 120208.
7. Shan, S.; Genç, S.Y.; Kamran, H.W.; Dinca, G. Role of green technology innovation and renewable energy in carbon neutrality: A sustainable investigation from Turkey. *J. Environ. Manag.* **2021**, *294*, 113004. [CrossRef]
8. Jung, J.H.; Lim, D. Industrial robots, employment growth, and labor cost: A simultaneous equation analysis. *Technol. Forecast. Soc.* **2020**, *159*, 120202. [CrossRef]
9. Lambrecht, J.; Kästner, L.; Guhl, J.; Krüger, J. Towards commissioning, resilience and added value of Augmented Reality in robotics: Overcoming technical obstacles to industrial applicability. *Robot Comput.-Int. Manuf.* **2021**, *71*, 102178. [CrossRef]
10. Ni, B.; Obashi, A. Robotics technology and firm-level employment adjustment in Japan. *Jpn. World Econ.* **2021**, *57*, 101054. [CrossRef]
11. Aghion, P.; Jones, B.F.; Jones, C.I. *Artificial Intelligence and Economic Growth*; University of Chicago Press: Chicago, IL, USA, 2019; pp. 237–282.
12. Liu, J.; Liu, L.; Qian, Y.; Song, S. The effect of artificial intelligence on carbon intensity: Evidence from China's industrial sector. *Socio-Econ. Plan Sci.* **2021**, 101002. [CrossRef]
13. Liu, W.; Zhan, J.; Zhao, F.; Wei, X.; Zhang, F. Exploring the coupling relationship between urbanization and energy eco-efficiency: A case study of 281 prefecture-level cities in China. *Sustain. Cities Soc.* **2021**, *64*, 102563. [CrossRef]
14. Liu, H.; Zhang, Z.; Zhang, T.; Wang, L. Revisiting China's provincial energy efficiency and its influencing factors. *Energy* **2020**, *208*, 118361. [CrossRef] [PubMed]
15. Wang, Y.; Deng, X.; Zhang, H.; Liu, Y.; Yue, T.; Liu, G. Energy endowment, environmental regulation, and energy efficiency: Evidence from China. *Technol. Forecast. Soc.* **2022**, *177*, 121528. [CrossRef]
16. Curtis, E.M.; Lee, J.M. When do environmental regulations backfire? Onsite industrial electricity generation, energy efficiency and policy instruments. *J. Environ. Econ. Manag.* **2019**, *96*, 174–194. [CrossRef]
17. Sun, P.; Liu, L.; Qayyum, M. Energy efficiency comparison amongst service industry in Chinese provinces from the perspective of heterogeneous resource endowment: Analysis using undesirable super efficiency SBM-ML model. *J. Clean. Prod.* **2021**, *328*, 129535. [CrossRef]
18. Lin, B.; Moubarak, M. Renewable energy consumption–economic growth nexus for China. *Renew. Sustain. Energy Rev.* **2014**, *40*, 111–117. [CrossRef]
19. Wurlod, J.; Noailly, J. The impact of green innovation on energy intensity: An empirical analysis for 14 industrial sectors in OECD countries. *Energy Econ.* **2018**, *71*, 47–61. [CrossRef]
20. Sun, H.; Edziah, B.K.; Sun, C.; Kporsu, A.K. Institutional quality, green innovation and energy efficiency. *Energy Policy* **2019**, *135*, 111002. [CrossRef]

21. Popp, D.C. The effect of new technology on energy consumption. *Resour. Energy Econ.* **2001**, *23*, 215–239. [CrossRef]
22. Welsch, H.; Ochsen, C. The determinants of aggregate energy use in West Germany: Factor substitution, technological change, and trade. *Energy Econ.* **2005**, *27*, 93–111. [CrossRef]
23. Gerstlberger, W.; Knudsen, M.P.; Dachs, B.; Schröter, M. Closing the energy-efficiency technology gap in European firms? Innovation and adoption of energy efficiency technologies. *J. Eng. Technol. Manag.* **2016**, *40*, 87–100. [CrossRef]
24. Wang, H.; Wang, M. Effects of technological innovation on energy efficiency in China: Evidence from dynamic panel of 284 cities. *Sci. Total Environ.* **2020**, *709*, 136172. [CrossRef] [PubMed]
25. Sun, H.; Edziah, B.K.; Kporsu, A.K.; Sarkodie, S.A.; Taghizadeh-Hesary, F. Energy efficiency: The role of technological innovation and knowledge spillover. *Technol. Forecast. Soc.* **2021**, *167*, 120659. [CrossRef]
26. Saunders, H.D. Fuel conserving (and using) production functions. *Energy Econ.* **2008**, *30*, 2184–2235. [CrossRef]
27. Lange, S.; Pohl, J.; Santarius, T. Digitalization and energy consumption. Does ICT reduce energy demand? *Ecol. Econ.* **2020**, *176*, 106760. [CrossRef]
28. González, J.F. Empirical evidence of direct rebound effect in Catalonia. *Energy Policy* **2010**, *38*, 2309–2314. [CrossRef]
29. Lemoine, D. General equilibrium rebound from energy efficiency innovation. *Eur. Econ. Rev.* **2020**, *125*, 103431. [CrossRef]
30. Gillingham, K.; Rapson, D.; Wagner, G. The rebound effect and energy efficiency policy. *Rev. Env. Econ. Policy* **2020**, *10*, 1. [CrossRef]
31. Jin, S. The effectiveness of energy efficiency improvement in a developing country: Rebound effect of residential electricity use in South Korea. *Energy Policy* **2007**, *35*, 5622–5629. [CrossRef]
32. Vélez-Henao, J.; García-Mazo, C.; Freire-González, J.; Vivanco, D.F. Environmental rebound effect of energy efficiency improvements in Colombian households. *Energy Policy* **2020**, *145*, 111697. [CrossRef]
33. Adha, R.; Hong, C.; Firmansyah, M.; Paranata, A. Rebound effect with energy efficiency determinants: A two-stage analysis of residential electricity consumption in Indonesia. *Sustain. Prod. Consum.* **2021**, *28*, 556–565. [CrossRef]
34. Liu, J.; Chang, H.; Forrest, J.Y.; Yang, B. Influence of artificial intelligence on technological innovation: Evidence from the panel data of china's manufacturing sectors. *Technol. Forecast. Soc.* **2020**, *158*, 120142. [CrossRef]
35. Vocke, C.; Constantinescu, C.; Popescu, D. Application potentials of artificial intelligence for the design of innovation processes. *Procedia CIRP* **2019**, *84*, 810–813. [CrossRef]
36. Vlačić, E.; Dabić, M.; Daim, T.; Vlajčić, D. Exploring the impact of the level of absorptive capacity in technology development firms. *Technol. Forecast. Soc.* **2019**, *138*, 166–177. [CrossRef]
37. Catania, L.J. 3-The science and technologies of artificial intelligence (AI). In *Foundations of Artificial Intelligence in Healthcare and Bioscience*; Catania, L.J., Ed.; Academic Press: Cambridge, MA, USA, 2021; pp. 29–72.
38. O'Leary, D.E. Artificial intelligence and big data. *IEEE Intell. Syst.* **2013**, *28*, 96–99. [CrossRef]
39. Goldfarb, A.; Trefler, D. *AI and International Trade*; National Bureau of Economic Research: Cambridge, MA, USA, 2018.
40. Acemoglu, D.; Restrepo, P. The race between man and machine: Implications of technology for growth, factor shares, and employment. *Am. Econ. Rev.* **2018**, *108*, 1488–1542. [CrossRef]
41. Ma, H.; Gao, Q.; Li, X.; Zhang, Y. AI development and employment skill structure: A case study of China. *Econ. Anal. Policy* **2022**, *73*, 242–254. [CrossRef]
42. Jiang, X.; Fu, W.; Li, G. Can the improvement of living environment stimulate urban Innovation?—Analysis of high-quality innovative talents and foreign direct investment spillover effect mechanism. *J. Clean. Prod.* **2020**, *255*, 120212. [CrossRef]
43. Du, C.J.; Hu, J.; Chen, W.X. Development model and countermeasures of china's new generation of artificial intelligence industry. *Econ. Rev. J.* **2018**, *4*, 41–47.
44. Ahmad, T.; Zhang, D. Using the internet of things in smart energy systems and networks. *Sustain. Cities Soc.* **2021**, *68*, 102783. [CrossRef]
45. Huang, J.; Koroteev, D.D. Artificial intelligence for planning of energy and waste management. *Sustain. Energy Technol. Assess.* **2021**, *47*, 101426. [CrossRef]
46. Edler, D.; Ribakova, T. The impact of industrial robots on the level and structure of employment in Germany—A simulation study for the period 1980–2000. *Technol. Forecast. Soc.* **1994**, *45*, 255–274. [CrossRef]
47. Deng, Z. Promoting the deep integration of artificial intelligence and manufacturing industry: Difficulties and policy suggestions. *Econ. Rev. J.* **2018**, *11*, 13–20.
48. Jarrahi, M.H. Artificial intelligence and the future of work: Human-AI symbiosis in organizational decision making. *Bus. Horiz.* **2018**, *61*, 577–586. [CrossRef]
49. Sowa, K.; Przegalinska, A.; Ciechanowski, L. Cobots in knowledge work: Human–AI collaboration in managerial professions. *J. Bus. Res.* **2021**, *125*, 135–142. [CrossRef]
50. Kusiak, A. Smart manufacturing. *Int. J. Prod. Res.* **2018**, *56*, 508–517. [CrossRef]
51. Gallaher, M.P.; Oliver, Z.T.; Rieth, K.T.; O'Connor, A.C. *Economic Analysis of Technology Infrastructure Needs for Advanced Manufacturing: Smart Manufacturing*; National Institute of Standards and Technology: Gaithersburg, MD, USA, 2016. [CrossRef]
52. Supekar, S.D.; Graziano, D.J.; Riddle, M.E.; Nimbalkar, S.U.; Das, S.; Shehabi, A.; Cresko, J. A framework for quantifying energy and productivity benefits of smart manufacturing technologies. *Procedia CIRP* **2019**, *80*, 699–704. [CrossRef]
53. Sarkar, M.; Sarkar, B. How does an industry reduce waste and consumed energy within a multi-stage smart sustainable biofuel production system? *J. Clean. Prod.* **2020**, *262*, 121200. [CrossRef]

54. Mehmood, M.U.; Chun, D.; Zeeshan; Han, H.; Jeon, G.; Chen, K. A review of the applications of artificial intelligence and big data to buildings for energy-efficiency and a comfortable indoor living environment. *Energy Build.* **2019**, *202*, 109383. [CrossRef]
55. Smajla, I.; Sedlar, D.K.; Vulin, D.; Jukić, L. Influence of smart meters on the accuracy of methods for forecasting natural gas consumption. *Energy Rep.* **2021**, *7*, 8287–8297. [CrossRef]
56. Tang, W.; Wang, H.; Lee, X.; Yang, H. Machine learning approach to uncovering residential energy consumption patterns based on socioeconomic and smart meter data. *Energy* **2022**, *240*, 122500. [CrossRef]
57. Chen, C.; Hu, Y.; Karuppiah, M.; Kumar, P.M. Artificial intelligence on economic evaluation of energy efficiency and renewable energy technologies. *Sustain. Energy Technol. Assess.* **2021**, *47*, 101358. [CrossRef]
58. Bloom, N.; Genakos, C.; Martin, R.; Sadun, R. Modern management: Good for the environment or just hot air? *Econ. J.* **2010**, *120*, 551–572. [CrossRef]
59. Wang, Q.; Zhao, Z.; Zhou, P.; Zhou, D. Energy efficiency and production technology heterogeneity in China: A meta-frontier DEA approach. *Econ. Model* **2013**, *35*, 283–289. [CrossRef]
60. Battese, G.E.; Rao, D.P.; O'Donnell, C.J. A metafrontier production function for estimation of technical efficiencies and technology gaps for firms operating under different technologies. *J. Prod. Anal.* **2004**, *21*, 91–103. [CrossRef]
61. Gökgöz, F.; Güvercin, M.T. Energy security and renewable energy efficiency in EU. *Renew. Sustain. Energy Rev.* **2018**, *96*, 226–239. [CrossRef]
62. Tang, L.; He, G. How to improve total factor energy efficiency? An empirical analysis of the Yangtze River economic belt of China. *Energy* **2021**, *235*, 121375. [CrossRef]
63. Färe, R.; Grosskopf, S.; Norris, M.; Zhang, Z. Productivity growth, technical progress, and efficiency change in industrialized countries. *Am. Econ. Rev.* **1994**, *84*, 66–83.
64. Yang, G.; Hou, Y. The use of industrial robots, technological upgrading and economic growth. *China Ind. Econ.* **2020**, *10*, 140–158.
65. Boubakri, N.; Cosset, J.; Saffar, W. The role of state and foreign owners in corporate risk-taking: Evidence from privatization. *J. Financ. Econ.* **2013**, *108*, 641–658. [CrossRef]
66. Harris, M.N.; Mátyás, L. A comparative analysis of different IV and GMM estimators of dynamic panel data models. *Int. Stat. Rev.* **2004**, *72*, 397–408. [CrossRef]
67. Lyu, W.; Liu, J. Artificial Intelligence and emerging digital technologies in the energy sector. *Appl. Energy* **2021**, *303*, 117615. [CrossRef]
68. Lee, D.; Chen, Y.; Chao, S. Universal workflow of artificial intelligence for energy saving. *Energy Rep.* **2022**, *8*, 1602–1633. [CrossRef]
69. Fisher-Vanden, K.; Jefferson, G.H.; Jingkui, M.; Jianyi, X. Technology development and energy productivity in China. *Energy Econ.* **2006**, *28*, 690–705. [CrossRef]
70. Li, L.S.; Zhou, Y. Can technological progress improve energy efficiency: Based on the empirical study on Chinese industrial sectors. *Manag. World* **2006**, *10*, 82–89.
71. Huang, G.; He, L.; Lin, X. Robot adoption and energy performance: Evidence from Chinese industrial firms. *Energy Econ.* **2022**, *107*, 105837. [CrossRef]
72. Wang, E.; Lee, C.; Li, Y. Assessing the impact of industrial robots on manufacturing energy intensity in 38 countries. *Energy Econ.* **2022**, *105*, 105748. [CrossRef]

International Journal of
Environmental Research and Public Health

MDPI

Article

Carbon-Emission Characteristics and Influencing Factors in Growing and Shrinking Cities: Evidence from 280 Chinese Cities

Xinhua Tong [1], Shurui Guo [1], Haiyan Duan [2,*], Zhiyuan Duan [2,*], Chang Gao [1] and Wu Chen [3]

1 Northeast Asian Studies College, Jilin University, Changchun 130012, China; tongxinhua@jlu.edu.cn (X.T.); guosr20@mails.jlu.edu.cn (S.G.); changgao20@mails.jlu.edu.cn (C.G.)
2 College of New Energy and Environment, Jilin University, Changchun 130012, China
3 Auditing Office of Jinniu, Chengdu 610036, China; chenwu19@mails.jlu.edu.cn
* Correspondence: duanhy1980@jlu.edu.cn (H.D.); duanzy18@mails.jlu.edu.cn (Z.D.)

Abstract: The CO_2 emission-mitigation policies adopted in different Chinese cities are important for achieving national emission-mitigation targets. China faces enormous inequalities in terms of regional economic development and urbanization, with some cities growing rapidly, while others are shrinking. This study selects 280 cities in China and divides them into two groups of growing cities and two groups of shrinking cities. This is achieved using an index called "urban development degree," which is calculated based on economic, demographic, social, and land-use indicators. Then, the 280 cities' CO_2 emission characteristics are examined, and extended STIRPAT (stochastic impacts by regression on population, affluence, and technology) is used to verify the influencing factors. We find that rapidly growing cities (RGCs) present a trend of fluctuating growth in CO_2 emissions, rapidly shrinking cities (RSCs) show an inverted U-shaped trend, and slightly growing (SGCs) and slightly shrinking cities (SSCs) show a trend of rising first, followed by steady development. Moreover, for growing cities, the population, economy, and proportion of tertiary industry have positive effects on carbon emissions, while technology has negative effects. For shrinking cities, the population and economy have significant positive effects on carbon emissions, while technology and the proportion of tertiary industry have negative effects.

Keywords: CO_2 emissions; growing cities; shrinking cities; STIRPAT; comprehensive index; China

Citation: Tong, X.; Guo, S.; Duan, H.; Duan, Z.; Gao, C.; Chen, W. Carbon-Emission Characteristics and Influencing Factors in Growing and Shrinking Cities: Evidence from 280 Chinese Cities. *Int. J. Environ. Res. Public Health* **2022**, *19*, 2120. https://doi.org/10.3390/ijerph19042120

Academic Editors: Roberto Alonso González Lezcano, Francesco Nocera and Rosa Giuseppina Caponetto

Received: 18 January 2022
Accepted: 8 February 2022
Published: 14 February 2022

1. Introduction

China has become one of the world's major consumers of energy and emitters of carbon dioxide. The Chinese government has therefore set a goal to reach peak carbon emissions by 2030 and carbon neutrality by 2060 [1,2]. Cities, as highly concentrated places of population and industry, typically produce about 80% of total carbon emissions; in Chinese cities, the proportion is as high as 85% [3]. Therefore, controlling urban carbon emissions is crucial for achieving emission-reduction targets [4,5]. In China, with rapid urbanization and enormous imbalances in regional development, some cities are growing, while others are shrinking [6,7]. The populations and economies of growing and shrinking cities are varied, resulting in divergent effects on carbon emissions. Accordingly, CO_2 emission-mitigation policies need to be adjusted according to the characteristics of different cities [5]. It is necessary, therefore, to explore the characteristics and driving factors of carbon emissions in growing and shrinking cities to more effectively achieve emission targets.

2. Literature Review

Urban carbon emission trends, peak forecasting, and the related influencing factors have attracted considerable research attention. Regarding carbon-emission trends, the research clearly indicates that emissions are on the rise in China. Zhou et al. [8], for example, found that carbon emissions increased continuously from 1992 to 2013 in all Chinese cities, growing faster in eastern China than in central and western China. Zhu et al. [9] found that carbon emissions doubled from 1997 to 2012 in Tianjin. However, while total carbon emissions have shown an overall growth trend, emissions are decreasing in certain sectors. For instance, using multiscale input–output analysis, Hung et al. [10] found that carbon emissions in Hong Kong's construction industry decreased from 2004 to 2011. Meanwhile, with China's stated aim to reach carbon peak by 2030, many studies have assessed its feasibility, arriving at two opposing views: "can achieve" and "cannot achieve." For example, using data for 50 Chinese cities, Wang et al. [11] predicted that emissions in those cities would peak between 2021 and 2025. Huang et al. [12] similarly found that under existing policies, Guangzhou would reach peak carbon in 2023. However, Lin et al. [13] found that the limited use of clean energy and ongoing rapid economic growth in Xiamen would cause it to reach carbon peak later than the 2030 target. Likewise, Zhang et al. [14] conducted three simulations on the timing of peak carbon in Baoding, and two of the scenarios indicated that peak carbon would not be achieved until 2040.

The factors affecting carbon emissions are another important area investigated in the research. Many studies have shown that socioeconomic factors, such as economic development, population growth, technology, industrial structure, and energy structure, have important effects on urban carbon emissions [8,15–17]. Generally speaking, economic development and population growth increase the demand for energy, resulting in an increase in carbon emissions. Ou et al. [18], for example, studied the socioeconomic factors affecting carbon emissions in cities with different developmental levels in China and found that economic and population growth increased emissions in cities at all levels. Taking 128 countries as samples, Dong et al. [19] found that countries with larger populations consumed more energy and thus generated more carbon emissions. Economic growth, however, does not always increase emissions. When economic development reaches a certain level, carbon emissions will decline; that is, the economy has an inverted U-shaped effect on carbon emissions. Studying 276 large cities around the world, Fujii et al. [20], for example, found that emissions first rose and then decreased with economic growth. Technological progress and industrial structure optimization typically improve energy efficiency and reduce emissions. Wang et al. [21], for instance, found that technology was negatively correlated with carbon emissions. Meanwhile, Li et al. [22] suggested that reducing the proportion of secondary industry and prioritizing the development of tertiary industry could be beneficial for reducing emissions in Chinese cities. Optimizing the energy mix means increasing the use of clean energy, which directly leads to a decrease in carbon emissions. Boluk et al. [23], for example, found that electricity generation using renewable energy helped to improve environmental conditions in Turkey. Similarly, Xu et al. [24] suggested that if China slows down its energy consumption and shifts toward low-carbon fuels, its emission targets could be feasible. Although the abovementioned socioeconomic factors affect carbon emissions, the effects are different. Economic development and population growth tend to increase emissions, while technological progress and industrial and energy structure optimization can decrease emissions.

The existing research tends to study all cities together without distinguishing between them. In fact, with ongoing economic development and population mobility, cities currently face two different development states: growth and shrinkage [25,26]. Different cities have different characteristics in terms of economies and population, and their effects on the environment are also different [27–29]. Studies have confirmed that growing and shrinking cities exhibit different energy-efficiency and carbon-emission characteristics. For example, after classifying growing and shrinking cities based on a population index, Xiao et al. [30] found that emissions in rapidly shrinking cities presented a continuously increasing trend, while growing cities reached their emission peaks during 2011–2013. Liu et al. [31] also used a population index to study emissions in growing and shrinking cities and found that urban shrinkage increased emissions and that the energy efficiency of shrinking cities was lower than that of growing ones.

Our review of the literature reveals limitations in the existing research. First, although many studies have focused on the characteristics of and factors affecting urban carbon emissions, they tend to ignore the potential differences between different types of cities. Second, although some studies have comparatively investigated the emissions of shrinking and growing cities, the classifications of those cities are mostly based on a single population index, lacking comprehensive classification. In truth, in addition to population changes, urban growth and shrinkage also involve economic, social, and land-use factors [32]. In light of the above, this study constructs an index, called "urban development degree," using economic, demographic, social, and land-use indicators. Then, cities are divided into growing and shrinking cities, and their carbon-emission characteristics and related influencing factors are investigated. The findings can provide a reference for emission-mitigation policies.

There are three contributions of this paper. First of all, we focus our research on the city level rather than the national or provincial level, which is a further complement to the micro-level research on carbon emissions. Secondly, we divide different types of urban development patterns by using a comprehensive indicator calculated from socioeconomic indicators, rather than researching all cities under a unified framework. Thirdly, we conduct an in-depth analysis of the influencing factors of carbon emissions in different types of cities, and analyze the reasons for the differences in carbon emissions, so as to provide a targeted reference for the formulation of carbon emission reduction policies and low-carbon development paths for cities with similar characteristics.

3. Method

3.1. Research Framework

Figure 1 presents a schematic framework of this study's methodological approach. The framework consists of three parts. The first divides the growing and shrinking city groups and calculates their carbon emissions. The second part compares the social development and carbon-emission characteristics of four groups of cities and uses extended STIRPAT (stochastic impacts by regression on population, affluence, and technology) to test the factors affecting carbon emission. Finally, the third part involves discussing the results and presenting the conclusions.

3.2. Categorization of Shrinking and Growing Cities

There are two ways to classify growing and shrinking cities. One is to consider the change in population over a certain period, where an increase in population is identified as urban growth, and a decrease is identified as urban shrinkage [6,28,33]. The other way is to consider the change in nighttime light over a certain period; when nighttime light brightens, the city is growing, and when it dims, the city is shrinking [34–36]. However, population division can only reflect changes in the urban population, and while nighttime light can reflect the economy and population, the data are not continuous in time and are characterized by uncertainty, which will affect the results. Therefore, some scholars try to use a comprehensive index to identify growing and shrinking cities. For example, Lin et al. [37] believe that urban growth and shrinkage are characterized by the changes in economy, population, land use and finances. Then, they construct a comprehensive index called urban development degree by using total population, economic growth, employment and unemployment and built-up area data to evaluate growing and shrinking cities in China. Zhang et al. [38] determine that the growth and shrinkage of cities are characterized by the changes in population, economy and social consumption, and shrinking cities often face economic downturns, shrinking population and declining spending power. Referring to Lin et al. [37] and Zhang et al. [38], this study, therefore, constructs an index of urban development degree (UDD) to divide growing and shrinking cities.

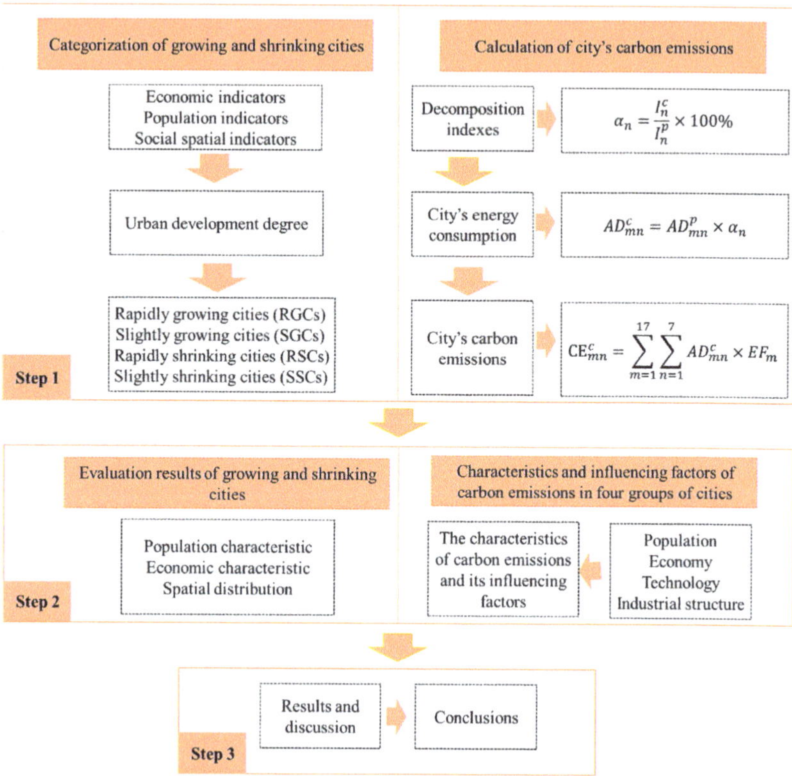

Figure 1. Research framework.

Calculating UDD requires the following demographic, economic, and social indicators: (1) Population includes three indicators, natural population growth rate, total population, and population density. Natural population growth rate refers to the difference between birth rate and death rate, which represents the change in natural population growth. Total population refers to the registered urban population, representing the change in the total population. Population density refers to the number of people per unit of land, representing the change in population density. (2) The economy includes per capita GDP (gross domestic product), per capita fiscal revenue, and GDP growth rate. Per capita GDP is the output level of unit population, and per capita fiscal income is the fiscal income of unit population, representing the level of urban economic development. GDP growth rate is the percentage increase in urban output, representing the speed of economic development. (3) The social and land-use dimensions include three indicators: total retail sales of consumer goods, per capita fiscal expenditure, and built-up area. Total retail sales of consumer goods represent a city's consumption capacity. Per capita fiscal expenditure is the level of fiscal expenditure per unit of population, representing the government's service capacity. Built-up area refers to the actual developed area in a city, representing the spatial change in urban land use. See Table 1 for details.

Table 1. Urban development degree indicators selection.

Dimensions	Indicators	Unit
Population	Natural population growth rate	‰
	Total population	10^4 Person
	Population density	Person/km^2
Economic	Per capita GDP	Yuan
	Per capita fiscal revenue	Person/yuan
	GDP growth rate	%
Social and Land use	Total retail sales of consumer goods	10^4 yuan
	Per capita fiscal expenditure	Person/yuan
	Built-up area	Km^2

Equations (1)–(8) show the calculation process for UDD.

When X_{ij} is positive,

$$X'_{ij} = \frac{X_{ij} - \min X_j}{\max X_j - \min X_j}, \tag{1}$$

When X_{ij} is negative,

$$X'_{ij} = \frac{\max X_j - X_{ij}}{\max X_j - \min X_j}, \tag{2}$$

$$Y_{ij} = X'_{ij} / \sum_{i=1}^{m} X'_{ij}, \tag{3}$$

$$e_j = -k \sum_{i=1}^{m} (Y_{ij} \times \ln Y_{ij}),\ k = \frac{1}{\ln(m)}, \tag{4}$$

$$d_j = 1 - e_j, \tag{5}$$

$$W_j = d_j / \sum_{j=1}^{n} d_j, \tag{6}$$

$$\text{index}_{it} = \sum_{j=1}^{n} (W_j \times X'_{ij}), \tag{7}$$

$$\text{UDD}_{(it_0, it_1)} = \text{index}_{it_1} - \text{index}_{it_0}, \tag{8}$$

where i represents the city, j represents the indicator, t represents the year, n represents the number of indicators, and m represents the number of cities. Equations (1) and (2) are the process for standardizing the original data. X_{ij} and X'_{ij} represent the original data and standardized data of the j index of city I, respectively. Equations (3)–(6) show the process for calculating the index weight; W_j is the index weight. Equations (7) and (8) show the process for calculating UDD. index_{it} represents the urban development index, and $\text{UDD}_{(it_0, it_1)}$ represents UDD from t_0 to t_1.

Following the literature on growing and shrinking cities [6,28], we identify a city whose $\text{UDD}_{(it_0, it_1)} < 0$ as a shrinking city and a city whose $\text{UDD}_{(it_0, it_1)} \geq 0$ as a growing city. In addition, based on research on group divisions and the development characteristics of urban populations and economies [29], we divide the cities into the following four groups: (1) rapidly growing cities (RGCs), UDD ≥ 0.05, which have rapid population, economic, and consumption development; (2) slightly growing cities (SGCs), $0 \leq$ UDD < 0.05, in which the population increases and the economy and consumption develop steadily; (3) rapidly shrinking cities (RSCs), UDD < -0.02, which show sharp declines in population, economy, and consumption; and (4) slightly shrinking cities (SSCs), $-0.02 \leq$ UDD < 0, which are characterized by population decreases and slow growth in consumption and the economy.

3.3. CO_2 Emission Accounting

Since carbon emissions from fossil fuel consumption account for more than 90% of total carbon emissions, this study only calculates carbon emissions from urban fossil-energy consumption. In addition, in the absence of an urban energy balance table in China, following Shan et al. [39,40], we scale down the provincial energy balance table to the city level based on GDP, demographic data, and industrial output. The calculation of CO_2 follows the Intergovernmental Panel on Climate Change (IPCC). The calculation formula for carbon emissions is as follows:

$$CE^{c}_{mn} = \sum_{m=1}^{17} \sum_{n=1}^{7} AD^{c}_{mn} \times EF_{m}, \quad (9)$$

where CE^{c}_{mn} represents CO_2 emissions from 17 fuel types, m is the energy type, n represents the main industry sector, AD^{c}_{mn} is the consumption of m fuel in sector n, and EF_m is the emission factor. The default IPCC emission factors are used in this study.

3.4. STIRPAT Model

STIRPAT is widely used to examine the factors affecting CO_2 emissions. It is based on Ehrich and Holdren's (1971) IPAT (impact of population, affluence, and technology) model and has been widely used to examine the effects of human activity on environmental change. The STIRPAT formula is as follows:

$$I = aP^{b}A^{c}T^{d}\varepsilon, \quad (10)$$

where I is environmental impact, P is population, A is affluence, and T is technology level. a is the dominant factor; b, c, and d are the parameters to be estimated; and ε denotes the random error. Taking the logarithm form to both sides, the STIRPAT model can be expressed as below:

$$\ln I = \ln a + b\ln P + c\ln A + d\ln T + \ln \varepsilon, \quad (11)$$

where ln () is the natural logarithm, and b, c, and d are equivalent to elasticity coefficients in economics, which can be regarded as the percentage change in the environment caused by a 1% change in one influencing factor under the condition that other factors remain unchanged.

The STIRPAT model allows additional explanatory factors to be added. In this study, referring to Cai et al. [16] and Wang et al. [41], we augment STIRPAT by adding industrial structure. The augmented model is given as

$$\ln I = \ln a + \beta_1 \ln P_{it} + \beta_2 \ln A_{it} + \beta_3 \ln T_{it} + \beta_4 \ln Q_{it} + \ln \varepsilon, \quad (12)$$

where I represents CO_2 emissions, a is the intercept term, P is the total population, and T is the technological level, which is represented by the reciprocal of energy intensity and is obtained by the ratio of GDP to energy consumption. Q is the industrial structure, represented by the proportion of output value of tertiary industry; β_1, β_2, β_3, and β_4 are the elastic coefficients of population, economy, technology, and industry structure, respectively.

In this study, the panel data method based on extended STIRPAT model was used to empirically investigate the relationship between influencing factors and CO_2 emissions. The panel data analysis is a statistical method to analyze two-dimensional observations collected from multiple entities over multiple times. Compared with conventional models using only time-series or cross-sectional data, this method has the advantages of providing more degrees of freedom and reducing the effects of multi-collinearity [18]. Three models are commonly used in panel data analysis: mixed-effects model, fixed-effects model and random-effects model. F-test and Hausman test are required to determine which model to use for regression. We conduct regressions on the four groups of cities to test whether there are differences in the factors affecting carbon emissions in different groups. After using the F-test and Hausman test on the four groups, a panel fixed-effect model was selected for regression (see Section 4.3 for the empirical results).

3.5. Research Objects and Data Sources

Research objects: The research object of this paper involves cities at the prefecture level and above. Due to the lack of data in some cities, 280 cities were finally identified and their economy and population accounted for more than 80% of China's. At the same time, they cover all provinces in China and are widely distributed.

Data sources: The data used to construct UDD (i.e., registered population, population density, natural population growth rate, per capita GDP, per capita fiscal expenditure, GDP growth rate, built-up area, population fiscal expenditure, and total retail sales of consumer goods) are from The Statistical Yearbook of Chinese Cities, covering the two years of 2010 and 2019. The GDP of each industry and population used for scaling are derived from cities and their corresponding provincial statistical yearbooks from 2010 to 2019. The province energy balance tables are from the China Energy Statistical Yearbook for 2010–2019. Missing population density data for 2018 were calculated from the ratio of the registered population to land area, which was obtained from the China Urban Statistical Yearbook. Some missing data are supplemented with data for adjacent years.

4. Results and Discussion

4.1. Results for Growing and Shrinking Cities

Based on the value of UDD and the categorization rules, 145 cities shrank during 2009–2018, accounting for 51.79%, mostly distributed in northeastern, central, and western China. A total of 135 cities grew, accounting for 48.21%, mostly distributed in the eastern coastal areas (Figure 2). Among the growing cities, 126 had slight growth, and 9 had rapid growth, accounting for 45% and 3.21%, respectively. Among the shrinking cities, 33 were rapidly shrinking, and 112 were slightly shrinking, accounting for 11.79% and 40%, respectively. Cities with slight growth account for the highest proportion, while those with rapid growth account for the lowest proportion. Most cities in China are SGCs or SSCs, while only a few are RGCs or RSCs.

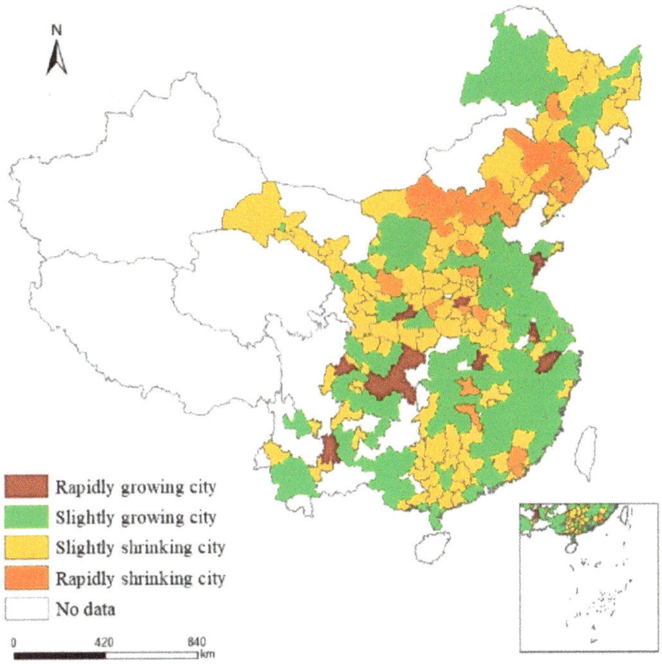

Figure 2. Spatial distribution of shrinking and growing cities in China, 2009–2018.

4.1.1. Characteristics of Growing Cities

The UDD of RGCs exceeds 0.05; these include Nanjing, Hangzhou, Zhengzhou, Wuhan, Xi'an, Chongqing, Chengdu, Kunming, and Qingdao. Most of these cities are provincial capitals with convenient transportation, good medical conditions, and high levels of education. Their economic development is at the highest level, with per capita GDPs of 50,000–110,000 yuan, and their economies are rapidly expanding. All of these RGCs have populations close to 10 million and are growing rapidly. Moreover, these cities have completed their industrial transformation and upgrading. In 2018, tertiary industry accounted for more than 55% of all industry in these cities (Figure 3a).

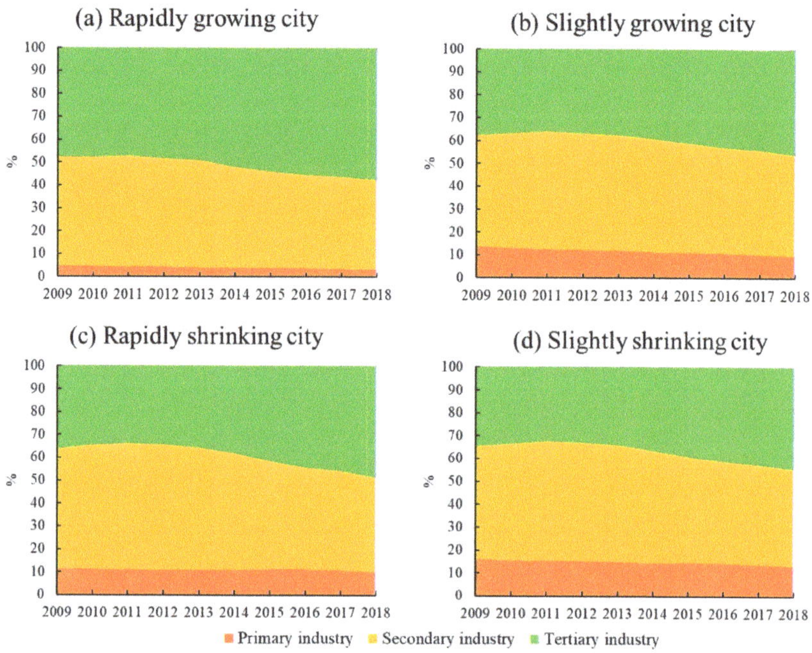

Figure 3. Industrial structure of growing and shrinking cities.

The UDD of SGCs ranges from 0 to 0.05; examples include Jinan, Suzhou, Ningbo, Jiaxing, Xiamen, and Fuzhou, mostly distributed in Shandong, Jiangsu, Zhejiang, and Fujian Provinces. Most of these cities are economically developed provincial capitals, with per capita GDPs of 40,000–80,000 yuan. Their economic development levels are lower than those of RGCs, but their economic growth is steady. Furthermore, the SGCs have established a leading position in tertiary industry by optimizing their industrial structures, with the proportion of tertiary industry accounting for more than 45% of the total (Figure 3b). This means that the service industry is constantly improving in these cities. Finally, their total populations show a trend of steady growth.

4.1.2. Characteristics of Shrinking Cities

The UDD of RSCs is below −0.02. Examples include Anshan, Fushun, Zhangjiakou, Tangshan, Baotou, and Daqing, which are mostly distributed in Liaoning, Hebei, and Inner Mongolia. Most of these cities are resource based, mainly relying on mineral resources during their early stage of development, with secondary industry accounting for more than 50% of the total (Figure 3c). Adjustments to the industrial structure started late in these cities. Their economic development is below the middle level, with per capita GDPs mostly between 30,000 and 60,000 yuan. RSCs are experiencing economic decline and population loss.

The UDD of SSCs is between −0.02 and 0. This includes Yichun, Liaoyuan, Datong, Kaifeng, Zigong, and other cities, mostly distributed in Heilongjiang, Jilin, Shanxi, Henan, Gansu, and Sichuan Provinces. Compared with RSCs, SSCs are mostly resource-based cities, taking secondary industry as the leading industry. After industrial restructuring, however, secondary industry accounted for less than 50%, while the service industry accounted for nearly 45% (Figure 3d). In addition, these cities are far away from economically developed cities, have poor geographical location conditions and transportation accessibility, and have relatively low levels of economic development. Their per capita GDP is 20,000–50,000 yuan. Their economies are growing but their populations are diminishing.

4.2. Emission Characteristics of Growing and Shrinking Cities

The carbon emissions of RGCs show a trend of fluctuating growth, RSCs present an inverted U-shaped trend, and SGCs and SSCs rise first and then develop steadily (Figure 4). The carbon-emission trends of the four groups are different, and their driving factors may be different as well. Here, we analyze the possible effects of economies, industrial structure, and technology on the carbon-emission characteristics of the four city groups.

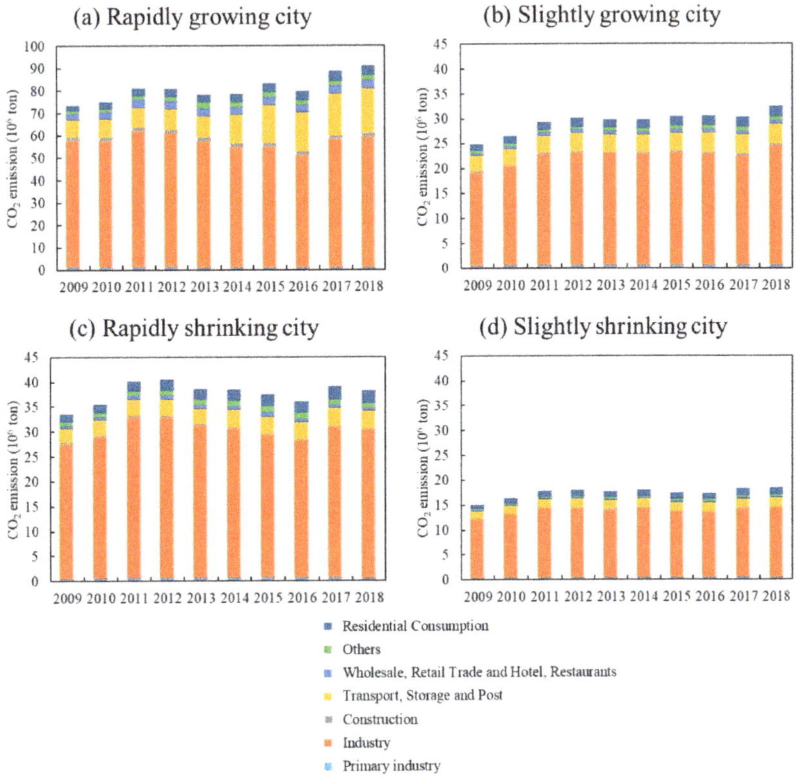

Figure 4. CO_2 emission characteristics of growing and shrinking cities.

4.2.1. Rapidly Growing Cities (RGCs)

The carbon emissions of RGCs are the highest among the four groups, with a trend of fluctuating growth (Figure 4a). From 2009 to 2012, carbon emissions grew at an annual rate of 3.3%. They fluctuated from 2013 to 2016 and continued to grow at an average annual rate of 2.4% in 2017 and 2018. In terms of economic growth, the GDP of RGCs shows an increase of 298.9%, with primary, secondary, and tertiary industries increasing by 202.9%, 247.6%, and 361.7%, respectively. This indicates rapid economic expansion, which contributes to increases in emissions. Between 2013 and 2016, however, the growth rate of GDP slowed down (annual GDP growth during this period was around 10%, lower than in other periods) (Figure 5a), which slowed the growth of carbon emissions over the period. In terms of industrial structure, the proportion of primary and secondary industry continues to decline, while the proportion of tertiary industry continues to rise. The service industry in RGCs is relatively mature and has occupied a dominant position for a long time, making increasing contributions to the economy. Therefore, the development of services may contribute to the increase in carbon emissions. In terms of energy structure, the proportion of coal in RGCs generally shows a downward trend, especially during 2012–2015. The proportion of coal shows a rapid decline (Figure 6), which may help to reduce carbon emissions. In terms of technology, energy intensity drops from 0.74 to less than 0.26 (tec/10^4 yuan), an annual decrease of about 11%, showing a rapid downward trend (Figure 7). This means that technology was greatly improved during the study period. We can see that the energy structure and technology of RGCs have been optimized and improved, which helps reduce carbon emissions. However, the carbon-increasing effect of rapid economic expansion and expanded tertiary industry is greater than the carbon-reducing effect of energy structure optimization and technological progress. Therefore, overall urban carbon emissions show an increasing trend.

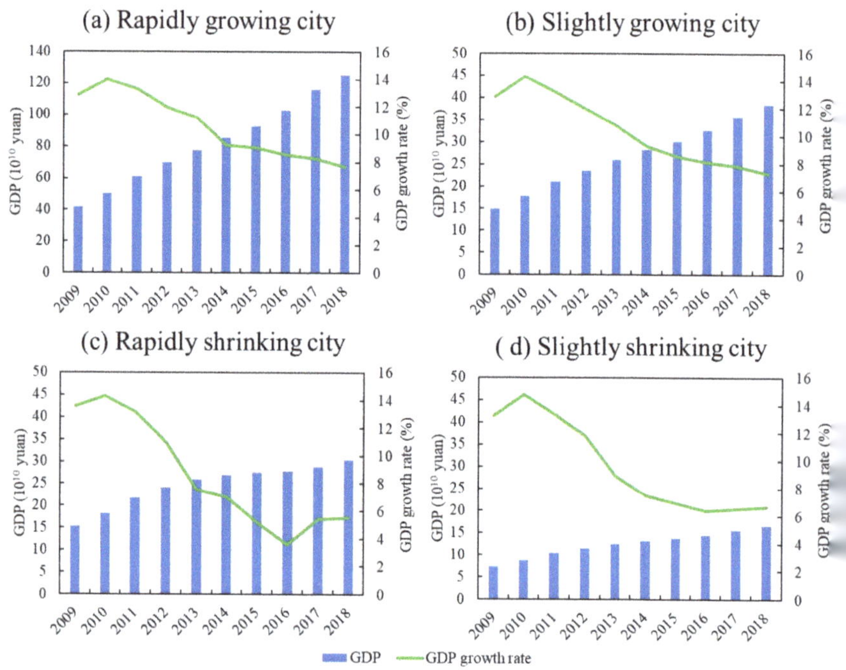

Figure 5. GDP and GDP growth rate of the four city groups.

4.2.2. Slightly Growing Cities (SGCs)

The carbon emissions of SGCs are low among the four city groups, showing a trend of first rising and then changing only slightly (Figure 4b). Specifically, from 2009 to 2012, the carbon emissions of SGCs increased from 24.83 million tons to 30.18 million tons, with an annual growth rate of 5%. Between 2013 and 2018, emissions were around 30 million tons, a small change. In economic terms, the economies of SGCs show an increase of 258.2% However, GDP growth generally shows a downward trend after 2012 (Figure 5b). Although economic expansion may increase carbon emissions, a decline in economic growth might also slow down the growth of emissions, accounting for the slowed growth of emissions after 2012. In terms of industrial structure, the proportion of primary and secondary industry continues to decline, while that of tertiary industry keeps rising. Especially after 2012, the proportion of secondary industry dropped rapidly (annual decline of 2%). This means that the cities reduced their dependence on energy-intensive industries, which helps reduce carbon emissions. In terms of energy structure, the proportion of coal in SGCs is 62%–66%, and there is a small decline (Figure 6). The urban energy structure has been optimized, and the decline in the proportion of coal is conducive to reducing carbon emissions. In terms of technology, the energy intensity of SGCs decreases year by year, from 0.7 in 2009 to 0.34 (tec/10^4 yuan) in 2018, an annual decrease of 7.6% (Figure 7). This could be another reason for the slowed growth of carbon emissions. In general, economic expansion in the SGCs increased carbon emissions. After 2012, however, with slowed economic growth, accelerated changes in industrial structure, energy structure optimization, and technological progress, the growth of carbon emissions was restrained, stabilizing changes in emissions.

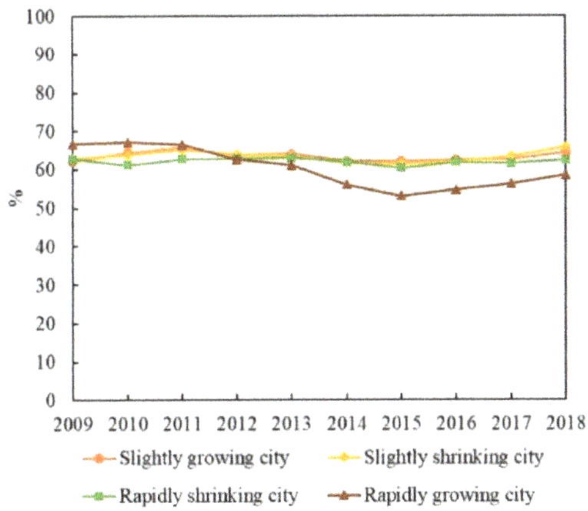

Figure 6. Coal share of growing and shrinking cities.

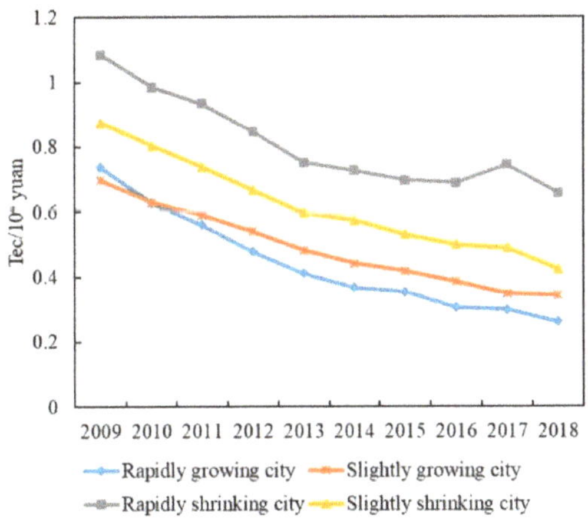

Figure 7. Energy intensity of growing and shrinking cities.

4.2.3. Rapidly Shrinking Cities (RSCs)

Among the four city groups, RSCs' carbon emissions are high, presenting an inverted U-shaped trend; 2013 is a turning-point year (Figure 4c). Regarding the economy, despite RSC economies showing growth, their GDP growth rate first rises and then declines rapidly, indicating that their economies declined after a period of growth (Figure 5c). This is consistent with the change characteristics of carbon emissions. We can infer, therefore, that economic changes triggered the changes in emissions. In terms of industrial structure, the proportion of secondary industry increases first and then decreases, while tertiary industry shows the opposite trend. This means that the cities gradually reduced their dependence on secondary industry and developed tertiary industry, which could curb carbon emission growth. In terms of energy structure, the overall change in coal consumption is relatively small (Figure 6), which differs greatly from the change in carbon emissions. Therefore, energy structure might not have an effect on carbon emissions. Meanwhile, the energy intensity of RSCs decreases from 0.88 to 0.42 (tec/10^4 yuan) (Figure 7); technology was improved, which is conducive to reducing carbon emissions. This analysis reveals that economic and industrial structure (secondary industry) and carbon emissions show the same change characteristics; thus, they may be the main reasons for changes in emissions. Although technological progress can restrain carbon emissions, emissions still show an increasing trend in the early stage. Therefore, technological progress had a weak effect on reducing emissions in the early part of the study period but might account for the reduced emissions in the latter part.

4.2.4. Slightly Shrinking Cities (SSCs)

SSCs have the lowest total carbon emissions among the four city groups. Their carbon-emission trend is similar to that of SGCs, showing a trend of first rising and then changing only a little (Figure 4d). Specifically, carbon emissions rose from 15.14 million tons to 18.09 million tons from 2009 to 2012 and then remained around 18 million tons. In terms of economic development, the GDP of SSCs expanded overall, but the GDP growth rate declined year by year, especially after 2012 (Figure 5d). In terms of industrial structure, the change characteristics for SSCs are similar to those of RSCs, with the proportion of secondary industry first rising and then falling and that of tertiary industry first falling and then rising. Specifically, the proportion of secondary industry rose from 49.3% in 2009 to 51.16% in 2013, and then dropped to 42.18% in 2018. The proportion of tertiary industry fell from 34.5% to 32.8% and then rose to 44.6%. The expansion of economic scale increased carbon emissions, but the slowdown of economic growth and the adjustment of industrial structure after 2012 helped to curb emissions, making them relatively stable. In terms of energy structure, the proportion of coal in SSCs increased from 62.9% in 2009 to 65.8% in 2018 (Figure 6); this means that the energy structure did not improve. Therefore, the energy structure might not be the reason for reduced carbon-emission growth. The energy intensity of SSCs declined annually by 5.4% (Figure 7). The development of low-carbon technologies might be the reason for the reduced growth of emissions.

4.3. *Regression Results*

According to the F-test and Hausman test results, for SGCs, RSCs and SSCs, the fixed-effects model should be used for regression, while the mixed-effects model should be used for RGCs, as shown in Table 2. However, by comparing the mixed-effects regression results with the fixed-effects regression results, the significance of the coefficients of influencing factors has not changed a lot. Therefore, in order to be comparable with the regression results for the other three groups of cities, a fixed-effects model was used for RGCs.

Table 2. F-test and Hausman test for four city groups.

City Groups	F-Test		Hausman Test	
	F-Value	**Prob**	**Shi-Sq. Statistic**	**Prob**
RGCs	F = 1.07	0.3960	5.29	0.2587
SGCs	F = 54.78	0.0000	193.76	0.0000
RSCs	F = 14.74	0.0000	109.76	0.0000
SSCs	F = 13.77	0.0000	300.80	0.0000

Table 3 shows the estimation results of the fixed-effects model for four city groups. It can be found that the regression results of the models in SGCs, RSCs and SSCs perform better, showing that the R-squared values are more significant. The regression result for RGCs is relatively insignificant, mainly due to the small samples, which makes its explanatory power limited. However, the regression result for RGCs is similar to SGCs, mainly because they belong to growing cities, so the results are reasonable to a certain extent.

Table 3. Regression results.

Explanatory Variables	RGCs	SGCs	RSCs	SSCs
lnA	0.351	0.743 ***	0.68 ***	0.74 ***
lnP	0.449	0.943 ***	0.722 ***	0.605 ***
lnT	−0.424	−0.709 ***	−0.518 ***	−0.547 ***
lnQ	1.337 *	0.042	−0.111 ***	−0.097 ***
C	−6.7864	−12.129	−7.824	−12.55
R-squared	0.2025	0.8912	0.9286	0.9486
F	1.91	972.17	146.13	655.53
Number of obs	90	1260	330	1120

Note: *** $p < 0.01$, * $p < 0.1$.

Based on the regression results, population and economic growth have a positive effect on carbon emissions, while technological progress has a negative effect on carbon emissions. The proportion of tertiary industry has a positive impact on growing cities, but has a negative impact on shrinking cities. For RGCs, the proportion of tertiary industry has the largest and most significant impact on emissions, which means that the proportion of tertiary industry is the primary influencing factor for carbon emissions in RGCs. An increase of 1% in the proportion of tertiary industry increases carbon emissions by 1.337%. For SGCs and RSCs, population is the most important factor affecting carbon emissions, showing that carbon emissions increase by 0.943% and 0.722% for every 1% increase in population. The technological progress has the greatest negative impact on SGCs, RSCs and SSCs. For every 1% increase in technological level, carbon emissions decrease by 0.709%, 0.518% and 0.547%. For SSCs, the economic growth has the largest positive impact, as every 1% increase in the economy increases carbon emissions by 0.74%.

In order to further verify the robustness of the regression results, we run a Stochastic Frontier Analysis (SFA) model on the extended STIRPAT, and the SFA results are in high agreement with the regression results, indicating our result is robust. Moreover, referring to Wang et al. [21], we compare the fitting data of CO_2 emission ($lnCO_{2'}$) calculated by the regressions coefficients in Table 3 with the actual CO_2 emissions ($lnCO_2$). The margin of error is within 10%, and most are less than 5%, as shown in Table 4, indicating that the regression model is available.

Table 4. Error statistics of actual CO_2 emissions and estimated values.

Year	RGCs			SGCs			RSCs			SSCs		
	$lnCO_{2'}$	$lnCO_2$	Error (%)	$lnCO_{2'}$	$lnCO_2$	Error (%)	$lnCO_{2'}$	$lnCO_2$	Error (%)	$lnCO_{2'}$	$lnCO_2$	Error (%)
2009	8.51	8.86	4.01	7.46	7.43	0.41	8.07	7.78	3.72	6.99	7.00	0.03
2010	8.56	8.89	3.64	7.54	7.52	0.29	8.15	7.86	3.67	7.10	7.09	0.02
2011	8.60	8.96	4.00	7.62	7.62	0.01	8.25	7.99	3.21	7.19	7.19	0.06
2012	8.62	8.96	3.88	7.64	7.65	0.11	8.26	8.00	3.27	7.23	7.22	0.05
2013	8.68	8.94	2.90	7.65	7.66	0.04	8.24	7.96	3.59	7.19	7.21	0.33
2014	8.60	9.26	7.11	7.66	7.66	0.07	8.24	7.93	3.83	7.23	7.21	0.22
2015	8.61	9.00	4.26	7.67	7.68	0.13	8.20	7.89	3.97	7.21	7.20	0.21
2016	8.61	8.95	3.88	7.67	7.67	0.03	8.19	7.84	4.45	7.21	7.18	0.41
2017	8.68	9.06	4.20	7.67	7.67	0.01	8.21	7.88	4.14	7.24	7.22	0.20
2018	8.66	9.10	4.77	7.69	7.71	0.31	8.14	7.90	3.06	7.16	7.22	0.82

4.4. Discussion

In China, slightly growing and slightly shrinking cities account for the majority, while rapidly growing and rapidly shrinking ones account for a small proportion. Growing cities are mostly distributed in the eastern region and shrinking cities in the northeastern, central, and western regions. This is consistent with Yang et al. [36]. After China's "reform and opening up," the eastern region attracted an inflow of FDI (foreign direct investment) by virtue of geographical advantage. This created many jobs, and many laborers came there in search of work, prompting rapid urban expansion. The northeast, as the old industrial base of China, has long relied on mineral resources for development. In recent years, with the exhaustion of resources and the emergence of excess capacity, cities have been forced to adjust their industrial structures. However, such adjustment has been sluggish, and new economic growth points have not been fostered. As a result, many people lost their jobs and left the region, resulting in the emergence of shrinking cities. The central and western regions are relatively closed geographically and backward in their economic development. A large number of laborers thus migrated out to seek employment opportunities, and urban populations gradually shrunk.

Growing and shrinking cities have different carbon-emission characteristics. The emissions of RGCs show a trend of fluctuating growth, while RSCs present an inverted U-shaped trend. SGCs and SSCs show a trend of first rising and then developing steadily. This differs from Xiao et al. [30] but supports Qiang et al. [42], namely, that air pollution is reduced in shrinking cities. RGCs have developed economies and high urbanization levels, which all contribute to increases in carbon emissions. At the same time, the rapid development of transportation and tertiary industry also increase emissions. As for RSCs, most depend on heavy industry. With the exhaustion of resources and the emergence of overcapacity, cities have been forced to reduce the scale of secondary industry, causing urban economies to decline rapidly, which correspondingly reduces emissions. The economic growth of SGCs and SSCs is relatively flat, and technology is improving, causing emissions to tend to be stable.

The results indicate that economic development and population growth positively affect emissions in the four city groups, while technological progress has a negative effect. The proportion of tertiary industry positively affects emissions in growing cities and negatively affects them in shrinking cities. Supporting Zheng et al. [43], economic development and population growth both increase energy consumption and therefore play obvious roles in increasing emissions. Technological advancement can produce more output using less energy, which reduces carbon emissions. The reason the industrial structure of different groups has different effects on emissions might be related to tertiary industry development. If tertiary industry is fully developed, services such as urban transport will require more energy, contributing to higher emissions. However, if urban tertiary industry development is immature, tertiary industry will consume less energy than secondary industry, which will reduce emissions.

5. Conclusions and Policy Implications

Aiming to support emission-reduction policy making, this study investigates the characteristics of and factors affecting carbon emissions in growing and shrinking Chinese cities. Taking 280 cities as samples, a UDD index developed by the authors was used to divide the cities into four groups: RGCs, SGCs, RSCs, and SSCs. Emission characteristics are discussed in terms of economics, population, energy intensity, and industry structure. The main findings are summarized below.

For RGCs, their economies and populations grow rapidly, their industrial transformation takes place early, and their tertiary industry development is sufficient. Correspondingly, carbon emissions show a fluctuating growth trend. The regression results show that the proportion of tertiary industry has a significant positive effect on carbon emissions while other factors have no significant effects. For RSCs, economic growth is declining, population loss occurs with the decline of secondary industry, and industrial structure adjustment is belated. Their carbon emissions show an inverted U shape. The regression results show that economics and population have significant positive effects on emissions while technology and the proportion of tertiary industry have significant negative effects. For SGCs, their economies and populations have both grown steadily, and tertiary industry has developed continuously with the optimization of industrial structure. Their carbon emissions first rise and then develop steadily. The regression results show that economics and population have significant positive effects on emissions, while technology has a significant negative effect. For SSCs, the level of economic development is low but continues to grow, and the population tends to decrease. Their carbon emissions are similar to those of SGCs, first rising and then developing steadily. The regression results show that economics and population have a significant positive effect on emissions, while technology and the proportion of tertiary industry have a significant negative effect.

The policy implications are as follows. For growing cities with sufficient human capital, they can vigorously develop industries with high-added value and low-carbon emissions. Meanwhile, the government should devote more financial funds to improving the level of low-carbon technology. For shrinking cities, future policies should continue to optimize the industrial structure and encourage the development of the tertiary industry. In addition, the government should increase subsidies for high-quality talents to provide sufficient human capital for technological upgrading.

This study has some limitations. First, in the accounting of urban carbon emissions, only energy-related carbon emissions are accounted, and the carbon emissions generated in cement production processes are not accounted. The accounting scopes will be further expanded to improve data quality in future work. Second, in terms of the influencing factors of carbon emissions, this study focuses on social factors, such as population, economy, and technology. In fact, urban growth and shrinkage, as a comprehensive reflection of population, economic, and social changes, have also been proven to have an impact on carbon emissions and environmental conditions [31,42]. In the future, we will further explore the impact of urban growth and shrinkage on carbon emissions.

Author Contributions: Conceptualization, methodology, formal analysis, writing—original draft preparation, S.G.; writing—review and editing, supervision, X.T. and H.D.; data curation, Z.D., C.G. and W.C. All authors have read and agreed to the published version of the manuscript.

Funding: This research was funded by National Natural Science Foundation of China (Grant Numbers: 71773034 and 71704157).

Institutional Review Board Statement: Not applicable.

Informed Consent Statement: Not applicable.

Data Availability Statement: The data presented in this study are available on request from the corresponding author.

Conflicts of Interest: The authors declare no conflict of interest.

References

1. Yuan, J.H.; Xu, Y.; Hu, Z.; Zhao, C.H.; Xiong, M.P.; Guo, J.S. Peak energy consumption and CO_2 emissions in China. *Energy Policy* **2014**, *68*, 508–523. [CrossRef]
2. den Elzen, M.; Fekete, H.; Hohne, N.; Admiraal, A.; Forsell, N.; Hof, A.F.; Olivier, J.G.J.; Roelfsema, M.; van Soest, H. Greenhouse gas emissions from current and enhanced policies of China until 2030: Can emissions peak before 2030? *Energy Policy* **2016**, *89*, 224–236. [CrossRef]
3. Dhakal, S. Urban energy use and carbon emissions from cities in China and policy implications. *Energy Policy* **2009**, *37*, 4208–4219. [CrossRef]
4. Dhakal, S. GHG emissions from urbanization and opportunities for urban carbon mitigation. *Curr. Opin. Environ. Sustain.* **2010**, *2*, 277–283. [CrossRef]
5. Shan, Y.L.; Guan, D.B.; Hubacek, K.; Zheng, B.; Davis, S.J.; Jia, L.C.; Liu, J.H.; Liu, Z.; Fromer, N.; Mi, Z.F.; et al. City-level climate change mitigation in China. *Sci. Adv.* **2018**, *4*, eaaq0390. [CrossRef]
6. Long, Y.; Wu, K. Shrinking cities in a rapidly urbanizing China. *Environ. Plan. A* **2016**, *48*, 220–222. [CrossRef]
7. He, S.Y.; Lee, J.; Zhou, T.; Wu, D. Shrinking cities and resource-based economy: The economic restructuring in China's mining cities. *Cities* **2017**, *60*, 75–83. [CrossRef]
8. Zhou, C.S.; Wang, S.J. Examining the determinants and the spatial nexus of city-level CO_2 emissions in China: A dynamic spatial panel analysis of China's cities. *J. Clean. Prod.* **2018**, *171*, 917–926. [CrossRef]

9. Zhu, Z.Q.; Liu, Y.; Tian, X.; Wang, Y.F.; Zhang, Y. CO_2 emissions from the industrialization and urbanization processes in the manufacturing center Tianjin in China. *J. Clean. Prod.* **2017**, *168*, 867–875. [CrossRef]
10. Hung, C.C.W.; Hsu, S.C.; Cheng, K.L. Quantifying city-scale carbon emissions of the construction sector based on multi-regional input-output analysis. *Resour. Conserv. Recycl.* **2019**, *149*, 75–85. [CrossRef]
11. Wang, H.K.; Lu, X.; Deng, Y.; Sun, Y.G.; Nielsens, C.P.; Li, Y.F.; Zhu, G.; Bu, M.L.; Bi, J.; McElroy, M.B. China's CO_2 peak before 2030 implied from characteristics and growth of cities. *Nat. Sustain.* **2019**, *2*, 748–754. [CrossRef]
12. Huang, Y.; Liao, C.P.; Zhang, J.J.; Guo, H.X.; Zhou, N.; Zhao, D.Q. Exploring potential pathways towards urban greenhouse gas peaks: A case study of Guangzhou, China. *Appl. Energ.* **2019**, *251*, 113369. [CrossRef]
13. Lin, J.Y.; Kang, J.F.; Khanna, N.; Shi, L.Y.; Zhao, X.F.; Liao, J.F. Scenario analysis of urban GHG peak and mitigation co-benefits: A case study of Xiamen City, China. *J. Clean. Prod.* **2018**, *171*, 972–983. [CrossRef]
14. Zhang, Y.Q.; Liu, C.G.; Chen, L.; Wang, X.F.; Song, X.Q.; Li, K. Energy-related CO_2 emission peaking target and pathways for China's city: A case study of Baoding City. *J. Clean. Prod.* **2019**, *226*, 471–481. [CrossRef]
15. Sun, L.; Liu, W.J.; Li, Z.L.; Cai, B.F.; Fujii, M.; Luo, X.; Chen, W.; Geng, Y.; Fujita, T.; Le, Y.P. Spatial and structural characteristics of CO_2 emissions in East Asian megacities and its indication for low-carbon city development. *Appl. Energ.* **2021**, *284*, 116400. [CrossRef]
16. Cai, B.F.; Guo, H.X.; Cao, L.B.; Guan, D.B.; Bai, H.T. Local strategies for China's carbon mitigation: An investigation of Chinese city-level CO_2 emissions. *J. Clean. Prod.* **2018**, *178*, 890–902. [CrossRef]
17. Meng, Z.S.; Wang, H.; Wang, B.N. Empirical Analysis of Carbon Emission Accounting and Influencing Factors of Energy Consumption in China. *Int. J. Environ. Res. Public Health* **2018**, *15*, 2467. [CrossRef]
18. Ou, J.P.; Liu, X.P.; Wang, S.J.; Xie, R.; Li, X. Investigating the differentiated impacts of socioeconomic factors and urban forms on CO_2 emissions: Empirical evidence from Chinese cities of different developmental levels. *J. Clean. Prod.* **2019**, *226*, 601–614. [CrossRef]
19. Dong, K.Y.; Hochman, G.; Zhang, Y.Q.; Sun, R.J.; Li, H.; Liao, H. CO_2 emissions, economic and population growth, and renewable energy: Empirical evidence across regions. *Energ. Econ.* **2018**, *75*, 180–192. [CrossRef]
20. Fujii, H.; Iwata, K.; Chapman, A.; Kagawa, S.; Managi, S. An analysis of urban environmental Kuznets curve of CO_2 emissions: Empirical analysis of 276 global metropolitan areas. *Appl. Energ.* **2018**, *228*, 1561–1568. [CrossRef]
21. Wang, S.J.; Wang, J.Y.; Li, S.J.; Fang, C.L.; Feng, K.S. Socioeconomic driving forces and scenario simulation of CO_2 emissions for a fast-developing region in China. *J. Clean. Prod.* **2019**, *216*, 217–229. [CrossRef]
22. Li, L.; Lei, Y.L.; Wu, S.M.; He, C.Y.; Chen, J.B.; Yan, D. Impacts of city size change and industrial structure change on CO_2 emissions in Chinese cities. *J. Clean. Prod.* **2018**, *195*, 831–838. [CrossRef]
23. Boluk, G.; Mert, M. The renewable energy, growth and environmental Kuznets curve in Turkey: An ARDL approach. *Renew. Sustain. Energy Rev.* **2015**, *52*, 587–595. [CrossRef]
24. Xu, G.Y.; Schwarz, P.; Yang, H.L. Adjusting energy consumption structure to achieve China's CO_2 emissions peak. *Renew. Sustain. Energy Rev.* **2020**, *122*, 109737. [CrossRef]
25. Turok, I.; Mykhnenko, V. The trajectories of European cities, 1960–2005. *Cities* **2007**, *24*, 165–182. [CrossRef]
26. Blanco, H.; Alberti, M.; Olshansky, R.; Chang, S.; Wheeler, S.M.; Randolph, J.; London, J.B.; Hollander, J.B.; Pallagst, K.M.; Schwarz, T.; et al. Shaken, shrinking, hot, impoverished and informal: Emerging research agendas in planning. *Prog. Plan.* **2009**, *72*, 195–250. [CrossRef]
27. Schetke, S.; Haase, D. Multi-criteria assessment of socio-environmental aspects in shrinking cities. Experiences from eastern Germany. *Environ. Impact Asses.* **2008**, *28*, 483–503. [CrossRef]
28. Martinez-Fernandez, C.; Weyman, T.; Fol, S.; Audirac, I.; Cunningham-Sabot, E.; Wiechmann, T.; Yahagi, H. Shrinking cities in Australia, Japan, Europe and the USA: From a global process to local policy responses. *Prog. Plan.* **2016**, *105*, 1–48. [CrossRef]
29. Wiechmann, T.; Pallagst, K.M. Urban shrinkage in Germany and the USA: A Comparison of Transformation Patterns and Local Strategies. *Int. J. Urban Reg. Res.* **2012**, *36*, 261–280. [CrossRef]
30. Xiao, H.J.; Duan, Z.Y.; Zhou, Y.; Zhang, N.; Shan, Y.L.; Lin, X.Y.; Liu, G.S. CO_2 emission patterns in shrinking and growing cities: A case study of Northeast China and the Yangtze River Delta. *Appl. Energ.* **2019**, *251*, 113384. [CrossRef]
31. Liu, X.J.; Wang, M.S.; Qiang, W.; Wu, K.; Wang, X.M. Urban form, shrinking cities, and residential carbon emissions: Evidence from Chinese city-regions. *Appl. Energ.* **2020**, *261*, 114409. [CrossRef]
32. Martinez-Fernandez, C.; Audirac, I.; Fol, S.; Cunningham-Sabot, E. Shrinking Cities: Urban Challenges of Globalization. *Int. J. Urban Reg. Res.* **2012**, *36*, 213–225. [CrossRef]
33. Yang, Z.; Dunford, M. City shrinkage in China: Scalar processes of urban and hukou population losses. *Reg. Sustain.* **2018**, *52*, 1111–1121. [CrossRef]
34. Dong, B.Y.; Ye, Y.; You, S.X.; Zheng, Q.M.; Huang, L.Y.; Zhu, C.M.; Tong, C.; Li, S.N.; Li, Y.J.; Wang, K. Identifying and Classifying Shrinking Cities Using Long-Term Continuous Night-Time Light Time Series. *Remote Sens.* **2021**, *13*, 3142. [CrossRef]
35. Zhou, Y.; Li, C.G.; Zheng, W.S.; Rong, Y.F.; Liu, W. Identification of urban shrinkage using NPP-VIIRS nighttime light data at the county level in China. *Cities* **2021**, *118*, 103373. [CrossRef]
36. Yang, Y.; Wu, J.G.; Wang, Y.; Huang, Q.X.; He, C.Y. Quantifying spatiotemporal patterns of shrinking cities in urbanizing China: A novel approach based on time-series nighttime light data. *Cities* **2021**, *118*, 103346. [CrossRef]

37. Lin, X.B.; Yang, C.W.; Zhang, X.C.; Cao, H. The measurement and influenceing factors analysis of urban shrinkage in China: Based on the perspective of demographic and economic changes. *Hum. Geogr.* **2017**, *32*, 82–89. (In Chinese)
38. Zhang, S.; Wang, C.X.; Wang, J.; Yao, S.M.; Zhang, F.; Yin, G.W.; Xu, X.Y. A comprehensive measure of urban shrinkage in China and its spatial and temporal differences. *Popul. Resour. Environ.* **2020**, *30*, 72–82. (In Chinese)
39. Shan, Y.L.; Guan, D.B.; Liu, J.H.; Mi, Z.F.; Liu, Z.; Liu, J.R.; Schroeder, H.; Cai, B.F.; Chen, Y.; Shao, S.; et al. Methodology and applications of city level CO_2 emission accounts in China. *J. Clean. Prod.* **2017**, *161*, 1215–1225. [CrossRef]
40. Shan, Y.L.; Guan, D.B.; Zheng, H.R.; Ou, J.M.; Li, Y.; Meng, J.; Mi, Z.F.; Liu, Z.; Zhang, Q. Data Descriptor: China CO_2 emission accounts 1997–2015. *Sci. Data* **2018**, *5*, 170201. [CrossRef]
41. Wang, S.J.; Liu, X.P. China's city-level energy-related CO_2 emissions: Spatiotemporal patterns and driving forces. *Appl. Energ.* **2017**, *200*, 204–214. [CrossRef]
42. Qiang, W.; Lin, Z.W.; Zhu, P.Y.; Wu, K.; Lee, H.F. Shrinking cities, urban expansion, and air pollution in China: A spatial econometric analysis. *J. Clean. Prod.* **2021**, *324*, 129308. [CrossRef]
43. Zheng, J.L.; Mi, Z.F.; Coffman, D.; Milcheva, S.; Shan, Y.L.; Guan, D.B.; Wang, S.Y. Regional development and carbon emissions in China. *Energ. Econc.* **2019**, *81*, 25–36. [CrossRef]

MDPI
St. Alban-Anlage 66
4052 Basel
Switzerland
Tel. +41 61 683 77 34
Fax +41 61 302 89 18
www.mdpi.com

MDPI Books Editorial Office
E-mail: books@mdpi.com
www.mdpi.com/books

www.ingramcontent.com/pod-product-compliance
Lightning Source LLC
Chambersburg PA
CBHW061448220926
51850CB00004B/42
* 9 7 8 3 0 3 6 5 8 2 2 2 1 *